MW00844108

Anesthesia and Analgesia in Laboratory Animals

American College of Laboratory Animal Medicine Series

Steven H. Weisbroth, Ronald E. Flatt, and Alan L. Kraus, eds.:
The Biology of the Laboratory Rabbit, 1974

Joseph E. Wagner and Patrick J. Manning, eds.:
The Biology of the Guinea Pig, 1976

Edwin J. Andrews, Billy C. Ward, and Norman H. Altman, eds.:
Spontaneous Animal Models of Human Disease, Volume 1, 1979; Volume II, 1979

Henry J. Baker, J. Russell Lindsey, and Steven H. Weisbroth, eds.:
The Laboratory Rat, Volume I: Biology and Diseases, 1979; Volume II: Research Applications, 1980

Henry L. Foster, J. David Small, and James G. Fox, eds.:
The Mouse in Biomedical Research, Volume I: History, Genetics, and Wild Mice, 1981; Volume II: Diseases, 1982; Volume Ill: Normative Biology, Immunology, and Husbandry, 1983; Volume IV: Experimental Biology and Oncology, 1982

James G. Fox, Bennett J. Cohen, and Franklin M. Loew, eds.:
Laboratory Animal Medicine, 1984

G. L. Van Hoosier, Jr., and Charles W McPherson, eds.:
Laboratory Hamsters, 1987

Patrick J. Manning, Daniel H. Ringler, and Christian E. Newcomer, eds.:
The Biology of the Laboratory Rabbit, 2nd Edition, 1994

B. Taylor Bennett, Christian R. Abee, and Roy Henrickson, eds.:
Nonhuman Primates in Biomedical Research, Volume I: Biology and Management, 1995; Volume II: Diseases, 1998

Dennis F. Kohn, Sally K. Wixson, William J. White, and G. John Benson, eds.:
Anesthesia and Analgesia in Laboratory Animals, 1997

James G. Fox, Lynn C. Anderson, Franklin M. Loew and Fred W. Quimby, eds.:
Laboratory Animal Medicine, 2nd Edition, 2002

Mark A. Suckow, Steven H. Weisbroth and Craig L. Franklin, eds.:
The Laboratory Rat, 2nd Edition, 2006

James G. Fox, Muriel T. Davisson, Fred W. Quimby, Stephen W. Barthold, Christian E. Newcomer and Abigail L. Smith, eds.:
The Mouse in Biomedical Research, 2nd Edition, Volume I: History, Wild Mice, and Genetics, 2007; Volume II: Diseases, 2007; Volume III: Normative Biology, Husbandry, and Models, 2007; Volume IV: Immunology, 2007

David Backer, ed:
Flynn's Parasites of Laboratory Animals, 2007 (Wiley)

Richard E. Fish, Marilyn J. Brown, Peggy J. Danneman and Alicia Z. Karas, eds.:
Anesthesia and Analgesia in Laboratory Animals, 2nd Edition, 2008

Jack R. Hessler and Noel D.M. Lehner, eds.:
Planning and Designing Animal Research Facilities, 2009

Mark A. Suckow, Karla A. Stevens, and Ronald P. Wilson, eds.:
The Laboratory Rabbit, Guinea Pig, Hamster and other Rodents, 2011

J. Harkness, P Turner, S VandeWoude, C Wheler, eds:
Biology and Medicine of Rabbits and Rodents, 5th Ed, 2012 (Wiley)

Christian R. Abee, Keith Mansfield, Suzette Tardif and Timothy Morris, eds.:
Nonhuman Primates in Biomedical Research, 2nd Edition, Volume I: Biology and Management, 2012; Volume II: Diseases, 2012

Kathryn Bayne and Patricia V. Turner, eds.:
Laboratory Animal Welfare, 2013

James G. Fox and Robert P. Marini eds.:
Biology and Diseases of the Ferret, 2E, 2014 (Wiley)

M. Michael Swindle, ed.:
Swine in the Laboratory: Surgery, Anesthesia, Imaging and Experimental Techniques, 3E, 2015 (Taylor & Francis)

James Fox, (Editor-in-Chief), Lynn Anderson, Glen Otto, Kathleen Pritchett-Corning, and Mark Whary, eds.:
Laboratory Animal Medicine, 3rd edition, 2015

Trenton Schoeb and Kathryn Eaton, eds.:
Gnotobiotics, 2017

Robert Marini, Lynn Wachtman, Suzette Tardif, Keith Mansfield and James Fox, eds.:
The Common Marmoset in Captivity and Biomedical Research, 2018

Mark A. Suckow, F. Claire Hankenson, Ronald P. Wilson, and Patricia L. Foley, eds.:
The Laboratory Rat, 3E, 2019

Samuel C. Cartner, Judith S. Eisen, Susan C. Farmer, Karen J. Guillemin, Michael L. Kent, George E. Sanders
The Zebrafish in Biomedical Research: Biology, Husbandry, Diseases, and Research Applications, 2019

Anesthesia and Analgesia in Laboratory Animals

Third Edition

Edited by

Melissa C. Dyson
Unit for Laboratory Animal Medicine, University of Michigan, Ann Arbor, MI, United States

Paulin Jirkof
Office for Animal Welfare and 3Rs, University of Zurich, Zurich, Switzerland

Jennie Lofgren
Animal Welfare Compliance, Novartis Institutes for Biomedical Research, Cambridge, MA, United States

Elizabeth A. Nunamaker
Charles River Laboratories, Global Animal Welfare and Training, Wilmington, MA, United States

Daniel Pang
Faculty of Veterinary Medicine, University of Calgary, Calgary, AB, Canada

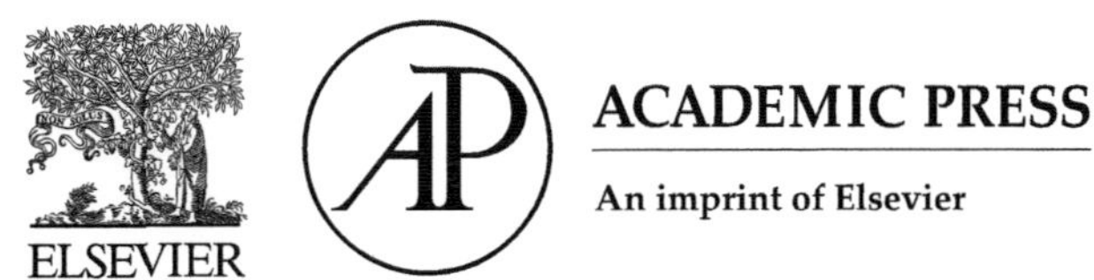

Academic Press is an imprint of Elsevier
125 London Wall, London EC2Y 5AS, United Kingdom
525 B Street, Suite 1650, San Diego, CA 92101, United States
50 Hampshire Street, 5th Floor, Cambridge, MA 02139, United States
The Boulevard, Langford Lane, Kidlington, Oxford OX5 1GB, United Kingdom

ISBN: 978-0-12-822215-7

For information on all Academic Press publications visit our website at https://www.elsevier.com/books-and-journals

Publisher: Stacy Masucci
Acquisitions Editor: Andre G. Wolff
Editorial Project Manager: Barbara Makinster
Production Project Manager: Punithavathy Govindaradjane
Cover Designer: Matthew Limbert

Typeset by TNQ Technologies

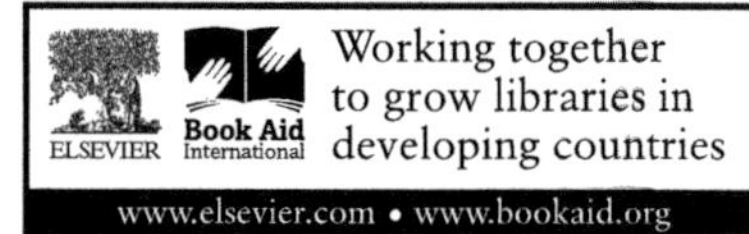

Contents

Section II
Principles of anesthesia and analgesia

4. Injectable anesthetics

Bridget V. Willeford, Steven E. Davison and Robert E. Meyer

5. Tranquilizers, sedatives, local anaesthetics and antimuscarinic agents

Chiara Adami, Alessandra Bergadano and Daniela Casoni

6. Inhalant anesthetics and safety

Cholawat Pacharinsak, Patrick Sharp and C. Tyler Long

7. Pharmacology of Analgesics

Lon V. Kendall, Vanessa L. Oliver and Trinka W. Adamson

Section IV
Periprocedural care

11. General care: periprocedural management considerations for research animals

F. Claire Hankenson, K. Andrew Claude and Vengai Mavangira

12. Pain assessment in laboratory species

Alexandra L. Whittaker and Chalette Brown

13. Basic considerations for pain management in laboratory animals

James O. Marx and Mark A. Suckow

Section V
Practical considerations by species

14. Anesthesia and analgesia in laboratory rodents

Paulin Jirkof and Jennie Lofgren

Section VI
Special topics

27. Management of chronic pain

Klas Abelson and Carsten Grøndahl

28. Anesthesia and analgesia in the fetus and neonate

Gerry Hish

29. Anesthesia for in vivo imaging studies: practical considerations for experimental outcomes and animal welfare

Jordi L. Tremoleda and Christoph W. Blau

Contributors

Klas Abelson, Department of Experimental Medicine, University of Copenhagen, Copenhagen, Denmark

Chiara Adami, Department of Veterinary Medicine, University of Cambridge, Cambridge, United Kingdom

Trinka W. Adamson, Animal Resources Department, Salk Institute for Biological Studies, La Jolla, CA, United States

David B. Anderson, Pentlands Management Systems, Edinburgh, Scotland, United Kingdom

Nick Andrews, Behavior Testing Core, Salk Institute for Biological Studies, La Jolla, CA, United States

Luis Antunes, School of Agrarian and Veterinary Sciences (ECAV), Department of Veterinary Sciences; Centre for the Research and Technology of Agro-Environmental and Biological Sciences (CITAB) UTAD, Vila Real, Portugal

Alessandra Bergadano, Experimental Animal Center (EAC), University of Bern, Bern, Switzerland

Mads F. Bertelsen, Center for Zoo and Wild Animal Health, Copenhagen Zoo, Copenhagen, Denmark

Christoph W. Blau, Charles River Laboratories Edinburgh Ltd., Tranent, Scotland, United Kingdom

Chalette Brown, Cerberus Sciences, Adelaide, SA, Australia

Monika A. Burns, Animal Welfare Compliance, Novartis Institutes for BioMedical Research, Cambridge, MA, United States

Larry Carbone, San Francisco, CA, United States

Daniela Casoni, Experimental Surgical Facility, Experimental Animal Center (EAC), University of Bern, Bern, Switzerland

Carol Clarke, Animal and Plant Health Inspection Service, U.S. Department of Agriculture, Riverdale, MD, United States

K. Andrew Claude, Department of Clinical Science, Carlson College of Veterinary Medicine, Oregon State University, Corvallis, OR, United States

R. Eddie Clutton, Large Animal Research and Imaging Facility, The Roslin Institute, The University of Edinburgh, Roslin, United Kingdom

Chereen Collymore, Laboratory Animal Medicine and Surgery, Charles River Laboratories, Senneville, QC, Canada

Jennifer Davis, School of Veterinary Medicine, Murdoch University, Murdoch, WA, Australia; Animalius Vet, Bayswater, WA, Australia

Steven E. Davison, School of Medicine, University of Louisville, Louisville, KY, United States

Cathy Dwyer, Animal and Veterinary Sciences, Animal Welfare, Safe & Improved Food Challenge Centre, Scotland's Rural College, Edinburgh, United Kingdom

Karin Finger-Baier, Max Planck Institute of Neurobiology (Now: Max Planck Institute for Biological Intelligence, Martinsried), Planegg, Germany

Thea Fleischmann, Center of Surgical Research, University Hospital Zurich, University of Zurich, Zurich, Switzerland

Manuel Martin Flores, Department of Clinical Sciences, College of Veterinary Medicine, Cornell University, Ithaca, NY, United States

Anna E. Goodroe, Southwest National Primate Research Center at Texas Biomedical Research Institute, San Antonio, TX, United States

Carsten Grøndahl, Veterinarian Department, Copenhagen Zoo, Copenhagen, Denmark

Kathryn A. Guerriero, National Institutes of Health, Bethesda, MD, United States

Henning Andreas Haga, Anaesthesia Unit, Faculty of Veterinary Medicine, Norwegian University of Life Sciences, Ås, Norway

F. Claire Hankenson, Laboratory Animal Medicine, School of Veterinary Medicine, University of Pennsylvania, Philadelphia, PA, United States

Craig A. Harms, College of Veterinary Medicine and Center for Marine Sciences and Technology, North Carolina State University, Morehead City, NC, United States

Debra L. Hickman, Department of Comparative Pathobiology, Purdue University, West Lafayette, IN, United States

Gerry Hish, Unit for Laboratory Animal Medicine, University of Michigan, Ann Arbor, MI, United States

Jenelle Izer, Department of Comparative Medicine, College of Medicine, The Pennsylvania State University, Hershey, PA, United States

Paulin Jirkof, Office for Animal Welfare and 3Rs, University of Zurich, Zurich, Switzerland

Cathy Johnson-Delaney, Washington Ferret Rescue & Shelter, Everett, WA, United States

Lon V. Kendall, Laboratory Animal Resources, Colorado State University, Fort Collins, CO, United States

Lucy Kennedy, Unit for Laboratory Animal Medicine, University of Michigan, Ann Arbor, MI, United States

Almut Köhler, Safety and Environment, Karlsruhe Institute of Technology (KIT), Eggenstein-Leopoldshafen, Germany

Angela Lennox, Avian & Exotic Animal Clinic of Indianapolis, Indianapolis, IN, United States

Patrick A. Lester, Unit for Laboratory Animal Medicine, University of Michigan, Ann Arbor, MI, United States; Conrad Jobst Vascular Research Laboratories, University of Michigan, Ann Arbor, MI, United States

Gregory A. Lewbart, College of Veterinary Medicine, North Carolina State University, Raleigh, NC, United States

Jennie Lofgren, Animal Welfare Compliance, Novartis Institutes for Biomedical Research, Cambridge, MA, United States

Judy MacArthur Clark, JMC Welfare International, Sandwich, Kent, United Kingdom

Carolyn M. Malinowski, The University of Texas MD Anderson Cancer Center, Bastrop, TX, United States

Tara L. Martin, Unit for Laboratory Animal Medicine, University of Michigan, Ann Arbor, MI, United States

James O. Marx, Department of Pathobiology, School of Veterinary Medicine, University of Pennsylvania, Philadelphia, PA, United States

Vengai Mavangira, Department of Veterinary Diagnostic and Production Animal Medicine, College of Veterinary Medicine, Iowa State University, Ames, IA, United States

Robert E. Meyer, Clinical Sciences College of Veterinary Medicine, Mississippi State, MS, United States

Jeffrey S. Mogil, Departments of Psychology and Anesthesia, Alan Edwards Centre for Research on Pain, McGill University, Montreal, QC, Canada

Gabrielle C. Musk, School of Veterinary Medicine, Murdoch University, Murdoch, WA, Australia; Animal Care Services, University of Western Australia, Crawley, WA, Australia

Daniel D. Myers, Unit for Laboratory Animal Medicine, University of Michigan, Ann Arbor, MI, United States; Conrad Jobst Vascular Research Laboratories, University of Michigan, Ann Arbor, MI, United States

Elizabeth A. Nunamaker, Charles River Laboratories, Global Animal Welfare and Training, Wilmington, MA, United States

Vanessa L. Oliver, Department of Comparative Biology and Experimental Medicine, Faculty of Veterinary Medicine, University of Calgary, Calgary, AB, Canada; Animal Health Unit, University of Calgary, Calgary, AB, Canada

Cholawat Pacharinsak, Department of Comparative Medicine, Stanford University, Stanford, CA, United States

Heidrun Potschka, Institute of Pharmacology, Toxicology, and Pharmacy, Ludwig-Maximilians-University Munich, Munich, Germany

Catharine E. Pritchard, Office of Laboratory Animal Welfare, National Institutes of Health, Bethesda, MD, United States

Kathleen R. Pritchett-Corning, Office of Animal Resources, Harvard University Faculty of Arts and Sciences, Cambridge, MA, United States; Department of Comparative Medicine, University of Washington, Seattle, WA, United States

Petra Seebeck, Zurich Integrative Rodent Physiology (ZIRP), University of Zurich, Zurich, ZH, Switzerland

Patrick Sharp, Office of Research and Economic Development, Merced, CA, United States

Adam Shriver, Harkin Institute for Public Policy and Citizen Engagement, Drake University, Des Moines, IA, United States

Bhupinder Singh, Comparative Medicine Resources, Rutgers University, Piscataway, NJ, United States

Mark A. Suckow, Department of Biomedical Engineering, University of Kentucky, Lexington, KY, United States

Douglas K. Taylor, Division of Laboratory Animal Services, Augusta University, Augusta, GA, United States

Jordi L. Tremoleda, Queen Mary University of London, London, England, United Kingdom

C. Tyler Long, BD Technology Innovation (BDTI), Durham, NC, United States

Hugo van Oostrom, IVC/Evidensia, Utrecht, the Netherlands

Sarah J. Wahltinez, College of Veterinary Medicine, University of Florida, Gainesville, FL, United States

Miriam Weisskopf, Center of Surgical Research, University Hospital Zurich, University of Zurich, Zurich, Switzerland

Alexandra L. Whittaker, School of Animal and Veterinary Sciences, The University of Adelaide, Adelaide, SA, Australia

Bridget V. Willeford, Laboratory Animal Resources, Mississippi State University, Mississippi State, MS, United States

Catherine J.A. Williams, Zoophysiology, Department of Biology, Aarhus University, Aarhus, Denmark; Department of Biomedical Sciences, Ontario Veterinary College, University of Guelph, Guelph, ON, Canada

Ronald P. Wilson, Department of Comparative Medicine, College of Medicine, The Pennsylvania State University, Hershey, PA, United States

Jeff Wyatt, School of Medicine & Dentistry, University of Rochester, Rochester, NY, United States

Stephan Zeiter, AO Research Institute Davos (ARI), Davos, GR, Switzerland

Preface

Similar to the first and second editions, this book presents a comprehensive review of anesthesia and analgesia as applied to animals needed for research and education. It differs in approach from other veterinary anesthesia texts in that it takes into account the demands of the research environment and reflects the very wide range of species currently encountered in research. It will be useful to those engaged in biomedical research, including veterinarians, investigators, technical staff, and institutional animal care and use committees.

In the biomedical research setting, it is important not only to choose anesthetic and analgesic agents and methods that ensure the well-being of the research animal. It is also critically important to select agents that allow or even enhance scientifically valid and reproducible measurements to be obtained. Wherever possible, background information and appropriate references have been provided to alert the reader to important effects and interactions of various drugs on physiology and metabolism.

The third edition has been updated, expanded, and partially reorganized. We have added additional materials about the ethical, regulatory, and scientific considerations of the use of anesthetics and analgesics, the study of pain, and management of chronic pain. This edition is arranged into six sections including several chapters, each with a lengthy bibliography where readers can find additional information in the primary literature on individuals topics.

Section I provides the reader with detailed overviews of our current ethical, regulatory, and scientific considerations for the use of anesthetics and analgesics in laboratory animals.

Sections II and III contain chapters that provide reviews of the principles of anesthesia and analgesia, as well as how to effectively deliver anesthetic and analgesic agents. These chapters provide the reader with detailed reviews of the anatomy and physiology of pain and the pharmacology of the agents used to relieve pain. Those who have limited experience in administering anesthetics and analgesics to laboratory animals should consult these chapters for the background information required to understand the nature of these agents, including their mechanisms of action.

Section III contains chapters that provide thorough discussions of the practical aspects of providing and monitoring anesthesia. Although later species-specific chapters address some of these issues as they apply to individual species, this section provides useful discussions of essential topics that would be useful for all readers.

Section IV provides information about periprocedural care of animals that are being sedated or anesthetized. This includes recognizing and assessing pain in research animals and providing supportive care in the postprocedural period.

Section V includes chapters that are oriented toward species-specific aspects of anesthesia and analgesia in traditional and nontraditional species. They provide the reader with a comprehensive discussion of agents, methods, and procedures, with an emphasis on peer-reviewed literature. Because the published data on many agents and species are quite limited, unpublished observations are included to give the reader a useful starting point in some instances. These observations are identified as such. To further aid those who have limited experience in anesthetizing a particular species, the authors' preferences for agents and dosages are noted. Each chapter contains tables of useful doses of anesthetics and analgesics for the given species. The reader is encouraged to consult the extensive reference lists for more detail on specific agents and their use in specific research settings.

Section VI, the final section, contains three chapters that summarize the literature about several special topics of interest. These include management of chronic pain, anesthesia and analgesia in the fetus and neonate, anesthetic considerations for imaging studies, and the study of pain itself.

This volume is one of a series of texts that the American College of Laboratory Animal Medicine has sponsored since 1974 as a means to nurture continuing education for its Diplomates, trainees, and their colleagues who have responsibilities for the care and use of laboratory animals. We are indebted to the chapter authors for their dedication and effort during the development of this book and to the authors and editors of the first and second editions, whose work in many cases provided the foundation for the current effort. Finally, this book could not have been completed without the support and resources of the authors' and editors' parent institutions. Royalties from the ACLAM-sponsored texts are used to help support future continuing education programs.

Melissa C. Dyson
Paulin Jirkof
Jennie Lofgren
Elizabeth A. Nunamaker
Daniel Pang

Abbreviations

2-PE	2-phenoxyethanol
3Rs	replacement, reduction, refinement
5-HT	5-hydroxy-tryptamine (serotonin)
6-MAM	6-monoacetylmorphine
18F-FDG	2-deoxy-2-[18F]fluoro-D-glucose
AAALAC	Association for the Assessment and Accreditation of Laboratory Animal Care—International
AALAS	American Association for Laboratory Animal Science
AANA	American Association of Nurse Anesthetists
ABGs	arterial blood gases
AC	Animal Care (APHIS)
ACGIH	American Conference of Governmental Industrial Hygienists
ACH	acetylcholinesterase
ACLAM	American College of Laboratory Animal Medicine
ACTH	adrenocorticotrophic hormone
ACVA	American College of Veterinary Anesthesiologists
AD	atopic dermatitis
ADH	antidiuretic hormone
AEP	auditory evoked potential
AI	apneic index
ALT	alanine aminotransferase
AMPA	α-amino-3-hydroxyl-5-methyl-4-isoxazolepropionic acid
AP	action potential
APHIS	Animal and Plant Health Inspection Service
APL	adjustable pressure limiting valve
APV	Association of Primate Veterinarians
AQUI-S	AQUI-S (2-methoxy-4 propenyl phenol)
ASA	American Society of Anesthesiologists
ASICs	acid-sensing ion channels
AST	aspartate aminotransferase
atm	atmospheres of pressure
ATP	adenosine triphosphate
AtrE	atropinesterase
AV	attending veterinarian
AVMA	American Veterinary Medical Association
AWA	Animal Welfare Act
AWAR	Animal Welfare Act Regulations
AWIC	Animal Welfare Information Center
AWR	Animal Welfare Act Regulations
BDNF	brain-derived neurotrophic factor
BG	blood glucose
BIS	bispectral Index
BP	blood pressure
BSC	biosafety cabinet
BUN	blood urea nitrogen
CBC	complete blood count
CBF	cerebral blood flow
CCAC	Canadian Council on Animal Care
CCD	charge-coupled device
CCI	chronic constriction injury
CFA	compete Freund's adjuvant
CFD	Computational fluid dynamics
CFR	Code of Federal Regulations
CGRP	calcitonin gene–related product
CI	cardiac index
CIP	chronic inflammatory pain
CK	creatine kinase
Cl	chloride
cm	centimeter
cm H_2O	centimeter of water
CMS	composite measurement scale
CNS	central nervous system
CO_2	carbon dioxide
COX 1, 2, and 3	three different forms of cyclooxygenase
CPB	cardiopulmonary bypass
CREB	CAMP responsive element–binding protein
CRF	corticotropin-releasing factor
CRH	corticotrophin-releasing hormone
CRIs	constant rate infusions
CRT	capillary refill time
CS	central sensitization
CSA	Controlled Substances Act
CVP	central venous pressure
CYP2D6	cytochrome P2D6
D5W	dextrose 5% in Water
DEA	Drug Enforcement Agency
DEXA	dual-energy X-ray absorptiometry
DH	dorsal horn
DHPNs	dorsal horn projection neurons

DISS	diameter index safety system
DMSO	dimethyl sulfoxide
DP	prostaglandin receptor
DPPC	dipalmitoyl phosphatidyl choline
DRG	dorsal root ganglion
EAAs	excitatory amino acids
ECG	electrocardiogram, electrocardiography
ED_{50}	effective dose when 50% of subjects are affected
ED_{95}	effective dose when 95% of subjects are affected
EEG	electroencephalogram, electroencephalography
EMS	electrical muscle stimulation
EP	prostaglandin receptor
EP-1	prostaglandin receptor
EPSP	excitatory postsynaptic potential
ERK-CREB	extracellular signal-regulated kinase-CREB
ET	embryo transfer
$ETCO_2$	end-tidal carbon dioxide partial pressure
ET tube	endotracheal tube
Fa	arterial gas
FASEB	The Federation of American Societies for Experimental Biology
FDA	Food and Drug Administration
F_ECO_2	expired CO_2 concentration
FHCs	fluorinated hydrocarbons (sevoflurane and desflurane)
Fi	inspired gas
fMRI	functional magnetic resonance imaging
FP	prostaglandin receptor
GABA	gamma-amino-butyric acid gm gram
GABAA	gamma aminobutyric acid type A receptors
GRAS	generally regarded as safe
GTE	given to effect
Guide	guide for the care and use of laboratory animals
H–CFCs	halogenated chlorofluorocarbons (halothane, enflurane, isoflurane)
HIV	human immunodeficiency virus
HPA	hypothalamic–pituitary–adrenal axis
HR	heart rate
HRV	heart rate variability
HCFCs	halogenated chlorofluorocarbons
HVAC	heating, ventilation, and air-conditioning
I:E ratio	inspiratory-expiratory phase time
IACUC	Institutional Animal Care and Use Committee
IASP	International Association for the Study of Pain
ICP	intracranial pressure
ICS	intercostal space
ID	inner diameter
IINs	inhibitory interneurons
IL-1	interleukin-1
ILAR	Institute for Laboratory Animal Research
IM	intramuscular, intramuscularly
IO	institutional official
IP	intraperitoneal, intraperitoneally
IP	prostaglandin receptor
IPCs	intrapulmonary chemoreceptors
IPPV	intermittent positive pressure ventilation
IRAC	Interagency Research Animal Committee
IT	intrathecal
IV	intravenous, intravenously
IVBP	invasive blood pressure
IVRA	intravenous regional anesthesia
kg	kilogram
KLH	keyhole limpet hemocyanin
kPa	kilopascal
L	liter
LA	left arm
LAWA	Laboratory Animal Welfare Act of 1966
LDH	lactate dehydrogenase
LDI	laser Doppler imaging
LED	light emitting diode
LL	left leg
LMA	laryngeal mask airway
LOX	lipoxygenase
lpm	liters per minute
LPS	lipopolysaccharide
LRS	Lactated Ringer's solution
LTP	long-term potentiation
M1	1st metabolite
MAC	minimal alveolar concentration
MAP	mean arterial pressure
MAPK	mitogen-activated protein kinase
MD	medical doctor
mg	milligrams
MgCl2	magnesium chloride
mGlu5	metabotropic glutamate receptor 5
MH	malignant hyperthermia
MHz	megahertz
ml	milliliter
mm	millimeter
mmHg	millimeters of mercury
MOF	methoxyflurane
MRI	magnetic resonance imaging
MRI/S	magnetic resonance imaging or spectroscopy
mRNA	messenger RNA (ribonucleic acid)
MS-222	tricaine methanesulfonate
N–NOC	non–nociceptive-specific neurons

N_2	nitrogen
N_2O	nitrous oxide
NASA	National Aeronautics and Space Administration
NaV	voltage-gated sodium ion channels
NE	norepinephrine
NHPs	nonhuman primates
NIBP	noninvasive blood pressure
NIH	National Institutes of Health
NIOSH	National Institute for Occupational Safety and Health
NK	natural killer (cell)
NK-1	neurokinin-1
NMB	neuromuscular blocker
NMBD	neuromuscular blocking agent drug
NMDA	*N*-methyl-D-aspartic acid
NMES	neuromuscular electrical stimulation
NO	nitric oxide
NP	neuropathic pain
NRC	National Research Council
NRS	numeric rating scale
NS	nociceptive specific neurons
NSAID	nonsteroidal antiinflammatory drug
NWP	new world primate
O_2	oxygen
OR	operating room
OD	outer diameter
OLAW	Office of Laboratory Animal Welfare
OSHA	Occupational Safety and Health Administration
OSHE	occupational health safety and environment
P.L.	Public Law
PA	primary afferent
PA	pulmonary artery
$PaCO_2$	arterial partial pressure of carbon dioxide
PACU	post-anesthesia care unit
PAG	periaqueductal grey
PaO_2	arterial partial pressure of oxygen
PC	phosphatidyl choline
PCO_2	partial pressure of carbon dioxide
PCV	packed cell volume
P_ECO_2	carbon dioxide in end-parabronchial gas
PEEP	positive end-expiratory pressure
PELs	permissible exposure limits
P_EO_2	oxygen in end-parabronchial gas
PET	positron-emission tomography
PG	prostaglandin
PGD2, PGE2, PGG2, PGF2a, PGH2, PGI2	different prostaglandins
PHS	Public Health Service
PIMs	pulmonary intravascular macrophages
PISS	Pin Index Safety System
PPM	parts per million
PSI	pounds per square inch (pressure)
PSIG	pounds per square inch gauge
PSL	partial sciatic nerve ligation
PT	prothrombin time
PTT	partial thromboplastin time
PVC	polyvinyl chloride
PVG	periventricular grey
q30 min, q20–30 min	refers to "every etc 30 minutes," or "every 20–30 min"
RA	right arm
RBC	red blood cell
RELs	Recommended exposure levels
REM	rapid eye movement
RVM	rostroventral medulla
SC	subcutaneous
SDS	simple descriptive scale
SD	standard deviation
SHF	simian hemorrhagic fever
SHR	spontaneously hypertensive rat
SHT	spinohypothalamic tract
SIV	simian immunodeficiency virus
SMT	spinomesencephalic tract
SNI	spared nerve injury
SNL	spinal nerve ligation
SNR	signal-to-noise ratio
SNS	sympathetic nervous system
SP	substance P
SPECT	single-photon emission computed tomography
SPF	specific pathogen free
SQ	subcutaneous
SRT	spinoreticular tract
STT	spinothalamic tract
TBE	tribromoethanol
TENS	transcutaneous electrical nerve stimulation
TIVA	total intravenous anesthesia
TLV-TWA	Threshold limit value-time-weighted average
TNF	tumor necrosis factor
TP	thromboxane receptor
TV	tidal volume
trkB	tyrosine kinase B
TRPs	transient receptor potential ion channels
TRPV1	transient receptor potential, family V, member 1
TTX	tetrodotoxin
TWA	time-weighted average
TxA2	thromboxane A2
U.S. Government	"U.S. Government Principles for the Principles Utilization and Care of Vertebrate Animals Used in Testing, Research, and Training"
UK	United Kingdom
UN	United Nations
UOP	urinary output

US	United States
USDA	United States Department of Agriculture
V/Q	ventilation/perfusion
VAP	vascular access port
VAS	visual analog scale
VBGs	venous blood gases
VLF	ventrolateral funiculus
VPCs	ventricular premature contractions
WAGs	waste anesthetic gases
WDR	wide dynamic range neurons
WHO	World Health Organization
μCT or microCT	microcomputed tomography
μg	microgram
μPET or microPET	micropositron emission tomography

Section I

Ethical, regulatory, and scientific considerations

Chapter 1

Ethics

Larry Carbone[1] and Adam Shriver[2]
[1]San Francisco, CA, United States; [2]Harkin Institute for Public Policy and Citizen Engagement, Drake University, Des Moines, IA, United States

Chapter outline

I. Introduction

Laboratory animals live dual lives. They are the sentient, feeling subjects of their own lives. They are also the objects of biological research projects that very rarely benefit those animals themselves. This volume presents up-to-date information on how anesthetics, analgesics, and tranquilizers affect animals' welfare as subjects and their use as objects. This chapter complements the technical information in this volume by asking, "What ethical obligations do we have to animals in laboratories? How should we use our available knowledge of animal suffering and its amelioration to conduct experiments?" We focus mostly on ethical questions in which the use of—or decisions not to use—anesthetics, analgesics, tranquilizers, or sedatives figure prominently.

Anesthetics, analgesics, and tranquilizers allow scientists to perform experiments that would otherwise be technically impossible with unrestrained and uncooperative animals. More importantly, used correctly these drugs complement humane training and habituation practices to reduce animal pain, anxiety, distress, and suffering (Gouveia and Hurst, 2017; Graham et al., 2012; LaFollette et al., 2017). Their use is integral to the ethical conduct of animal research and is mandated in most legal and regulatory systems for laboratory animal welfare. Unfortunately, powerful drugs can have serious side effects that may diminish animal welfare, as well as effects on the biological functions scientists try to study. This creates an occasional mismatch between what is best for the animals' welfare and what is best for the scientific project, which is a technical challenge for scientists and veterinarians, and an ethical challenge for them and the oversight bodies reviewing their work.

We begin this chapter in the middle of the story. The first and most basic question is whether using nonhuman animals for humans' interests is justifiable, especially when the individual animals may suffer harm (Garrett, 2012; Kahn, 2014; Nobis, 2016). We do not address that primary question here. Instead, we situate this chapter in the current regulatory and societal context, in which society has already decided, for the time being, that it approves and will even fund and demand animal experimentation (Pew Research Center, 2018) (Chapter 2). The approval is not *carte blanche*, allowing scientists to do whatever they want with animals. Rather, in the laboratory, as in agriculture, entertainment, and other areas, animals' interests receive some ethical consideration, though far less than human

Anesthesia and Analgesia in Laboratory Animals. https://doi.org/10.1016/B978-0-12-822215-7.00005-6

interests receive. Respect for animals' interests may slow some projects, or add inconvenience or expense, but rarely do animal welfare concerns stop research once the humans involved have decided it is important.

In this chapter, we ask the ethical question, "How should we use anesthetics and related medications in laboratory animal care and use?" Consistent ethical action will often mean going beyond the minimum standards in regulations and will always require translating the general language of regulation into more specific standards and practices. This requires technical and veterinary expertise as well as ethical discussions that are broader than what technical experts alone can contribute.

We review the obligation to use our best knowledge of animal welfare to minimize the moral costs of animal research. We also discuss the ethical implications of the limits to our scientific knowledge: how should we treat animals when our abilities to recognize and treat pain and suffering are still in the early stages?

We note that some authors writing on this topic distinguish between "morals" and "ethics." The definitions between different authors are not always consistent, but the main distinction typically refers to the idea that ethics describes a code of rules whereas a morals applies to individuals. However, for our purposes, we will use the terms interchangeably to simply refer to the normative commitments being used to evaluate particular decisions.

II. Consequentialist ethics in laboratory animal use

The standard reasoning about the use of animals in biomedical research is roughly as follows: though the research may involve the animals enduring some harm, the moral significance of these harms may be greatly outweighed by the potential benefits that may result from the research. As such, as long as unnecessary and superfluous harms are eliminated from the process, the practice of rigorous, important research is morally unobjectionable (United States Interagency Research Animal Committee, 1985).

This is more or less a consequentialist approach to ethics (Frey, 1997; Singer, 1990; Sprigge, 1985). In consequentialism, the rightness or wrongness of actions rests entirely on the consequences that result from those actions. Actions are right if they have the best, or at least a sufficiently good balance of good consequences and bad consequences. The term 'consequentialism' refers only to a general view about how consequences are related to assessments of right and wrong actions, but particular consequentialist theories have to additionally fill in details about what counts as good consequences, what counts as bad consequences, and how these consequences are aggregated and compared, and for present purposes, whose consequences—human and or nonhuman—matter (John and Sebo, 2020; Sinnott-Armstrong, 2021).

The most familiar of consequentialist theories are utilitarianism, according to which happiness and positive mental states constitute good consequences while pain, distress, suffering, and negative mental states constitute bad consequences. As such, according to utilitarianism, the right actions are those that maximize happiness and minimize suffering. Utilitarian theories of ethics lend themselves well to moral consideration of animals since animals also presumably suffer pain and distress and have pleasures and other positive experiences. Early utilitarians such as Jeremy Bentham discussed extending moral consideration to animals, and the contemporaneous philosopher Peter Singer has spelled out in detail how utilitarianism requires that we include animals in our moral circle (Bentham, 1789; Singer, 1990).

In animal research, utilitarians mostly work to balance the harmful consequences for laboratory animals against the positive consequences for humans, the environment, or other animals. By contrast, bioethical frameworks for research involving humans are decidedly nonconsequentialist. Deontological, or nonconsequentialist, ethical theories (Kantianism is a version of these) hold that our moral evaluation of actions isn't fully determined by consequences. The notion of human rights, for example, implies that actions are wrong if they violate those rights, even if performing the action might result in a positive balance of consequences. And while a risk-benefit ratio is one important criterion in human subjects research, it resides amongst many other criteria that are more deontological in flavor. For example, if a person does not provide informed consent in the course of the research, the research is deemed unethical, regardless of whether it may result in overall positive consequences by contributing to a medical breakthrough.

This discrepancy in approaches to research on human subjects and nonhuman animal objects is what the philosopher Robert Nozick described as "utilitarianism for animals, Kantianism for people." (Nozick, 1974) So while research on humans is required to adhere to a number of deontological rules, such as respect for autonomous persons, informed consent, and nonmaleficence, research on animals is typically thought to be justified so long as expected harms in a utilitarian calculus are outweighed by potential benefits (Beauchamp and Childress, 1994). By contrast, utilitarianism allows invasive and potentially painful research on animals for the sake of large future benefits for others, though only if we eliminate "unnecessary" pains and only if we are confident that there is a good chance of obtaining the requisite benefits. The human-nonhuman divide is so great in current practices that, starting with the Nuremberg Code that followed war crime prosecutions for Nazi studies of human prisoners, a key component of human research ethics is that animal studies must typically precede any plans to do experiments on humans (Eccles, 1971; National Commission for the Protection of Human Subjects of Biomedical and Behavioral Research, 1978; United States Government Printing Office, 1949; World Medical Association, 1997).

III. Minimizing harms and maximizing pleasures for animals in laboratories

Bentham wrote about animals, "[The question is not, Can they *reason*? nor, Can they *talk*? but, Can they *suffer*?]" (Bentham, 1789) Though some utilitarians use the term "pain" to refer to almost all negative mental states, "suffering" is the better term (Crisp, 2006; Shriver, 2006; Weary, 2014). Not all pains are severe or long-lasting enough to cause suffering of moral significance. A vaccine injection, for example, falls below most regulatory thresholds of distressful pain that should be alleviated. And humans and nonhumans alike will voluntarily endure some pain to achieve a desired reward or prize.

On the other hand, many nonpainful states such as hunger, fear, and anxiety can cause morally significant suffering that should be kept to a minimum. Olsson et al. have proposed a definition of severe suffering as the degree of suffering that so overwhelms the animal (or person's) attention that there is little room for anything else, little possibility of distraction, and little ability to carry on everyday procedures (Olsson et al., 2020).

Currently applied ethics focuses on the subjective experiences of conscious, sentient animals, that is, of animals capable of experiencing mental states of pleasure and suffering (DeGrazia, 1996). Anesthetics and analgesics are important tools for minimizing animal pain, while tranquilizers and other adjuncts can manage anxiety and other distress. General anesthesia renders an animal unconscious, or functionally insentient, but care must be taken to monitor the depth of anesthesia, especially if animals are paralyzed with neuromuscular blocking agents, so that they remain fully unconsciousness and pain-free.

Long-term welfare is usually of the lower concern than animals' short-term and immediate experiences, given how relatively few laboratory animals live long lives. Analgesics, tranquilizers, and antidepressants can mitigate chronic pain and nonpain suffering, though their long-term use is not common with laboratory animals other than nonhuman primates.

The basic ethic underlying current laboratory animal welfare policies is that

Harming sentient animals requires justification.

In this chapter, we use the word *harm* to encompassing both the suffering of significant pain and distress (i.e., negative mental states) as well as depriving sentient animals of opportunities for happiness and pleasure (i.e., positive mental states). We understand sentience to be a neurobiological capacity, or more precisely, a suite of such capacities. Like most such capacities, it occurs to varying degrees in various species and among individuals and life stages within a species (Mellor, 2019). It seems clear with current knowledge that mammals and most vertebrates have morally relevant sentience once they reach a certain stage of development (Mellor, 2019; Sneddon, 2015). Some invertebrates such as octopus and other cephalopods appear to as well (Crook, 2021; Godfrey-Smith, 2016; Mason, 2011; Mather, 2019) (Chapter 26).

Other welcome and unwelcome common species in the animal laboratory, such as *Drosophila* fruit flies, fur mites, and pinworms do not have morally relevant sentience, at least based on present animal welfare cognitive science, though there are notable dissenters from this view (Klein and Barron, 2016; Mikhalevich and Powell, 2020). The range of species that possess at least some degree of morally relevant sentience is broader than the range of species covered by laboratory animal welfare laws, especially in the United States, where even highly sentient rats, mice, and birds are excluded from the Animal Welfare Act's protections.

Do ethical obligations stop with reducing or preventing suffering, with no concurrent obligation to maximize positive mental states (Carbone, 2004; Makowska and Weary, 2020; Tannenbaum and Bennett, 2015)? Pleasure and suffering are different neurobiological processes, modulated by distinctive brain regions. Rather than a single linear scale ranging from extreme suffering to extreme pleasure, there seem to be at least two separate scales, both of them modifiable with analgesics and related drugs, and both deserving of ethical consideration (Shriver, 2014). Picture a beagle chasing a tennis ball at the beach, or a monkey making the rounds grooming her troop-mates. Do we harm these animals if we deprive them of these opportunities? What if they have never before experienced them in their lives? Might we have an even higher obligation to find such positive experiences for laboratory animals whose pain or suffering we will cause for our science than we do for companion animals? Behavior-modifying drugs serve to minimize negative experiences for animals, while other approaches are necessary for enhancing positive experiences. The term "environmental enrichment" is unfortunate; it can sound like some special but optional nicety for animals, something offered within the constraints of standard laboratory housing conditions, not fully rising to the level of a "must" norm in the *Guide*, rather than a high-level obligation to expansively maximize pleasures and positive emotional states (Burghardt, 1999; Lahvis, 2017; Watters, 2009).

For the most part, killing laboratory animals is not treated as a harm in current applied and regulatory situations, though it deprives animals of future potential pleasures. Quite the contrary, euthanasia is an obligation in situations where killing an animal can end their suffering (Carbone, 2004; Cigman, 1989; Regan, 1989; United States Interagency Research Animal Committee, 1985). Setting intervention endpoints is an important tool for limiting the severity and duration of animal suffering. Most discussion of laboratory animal euthanasia therefore focuses not on why we kill animals but on how, minimizing pain, fear and other distress to animals at the time of their deaths (AVMA Panel on Euthanasia, 2020).

Chapter 2 describes the regulations for scientists who conduct animal experiments. While details vary, most countries require some sort of in-house oversight committee, an animal ethics committee (AEC), the common term in most countries, or an Institutional Animal Care and Use Committee, the common term in the United States. Both for simplicity, and to emphasize the ethical work these committees must do, we use the term AEC in this chapter (Chapter 2).

Regardless of the merit and importance of the research, scientists, veterinarians, and AECs must work together, using anesthetics and analgesics as needed, to identify, diagnose, prevent, and/or treat significant animal pain and suffering. In many countries, this starts with the AEC's *severity assessment* of the projected work's effect on the animals' welfare (Bleich et al., 2020). In the United States, a common system, though not required by law, is to prospectively assign pain and distress categories based on the procedure. Procedures that cross a threshold of more than minor or momentary pain or distress are in category D if drugs are used to mitigate the animals' suffering, or in category E, if there is a scientific need to avoid treating the animals (Carbone, 2019). Animal use in these categories is reported retrospectively to the United States Department of Agriculture (USDA), though only for the minority of animals covered by the Animal Welfare Act (AWA) (Chapter 2). Either way, identifying potential harms to animals is the first step in brainstorming ways to prevent, minimize, or treat them.

IV. The Three Rs approach to minimizing harms to animals

By far, the most common organizing framework for minimizing harm to animals in laboratories is the "Three Rs" of reduce, replace, and refine. Russell and Burch published their *Principles of Humane Experimental Techniques* outlining what we now also call collectively "Alternatives" (not their term) to minimize animal suffering in laboratories (Russell and Burch, 1959). Their "Three Rs" are endorsed in a wide range of regulations, professional standards, and ethical statements on animal use (Institute for Laboratory Animal Research, 2011; National Center for the Replacement, 2020; Tannenbaum and Bennett, 2015; The North American 3Rs Collaborative (NA3RsC), 2021). Lobbying groups for tighter restrictions on the scientific use of animals and for greater freedoms from restrictions converge on their value (Chapter 2).

The Three Rs as Russell and Burch described them:

- *Replacement means the substitution for conscious living higher animals of insentient material.*
- *Reduction means a reduction in the number of animals used to obtain information of a given amount and precision.*
- *Refinement means any decrease in the incidence or severity of inhumane procedures applied to those animals which still have to be used (p. 64)* (Russell and Burch, 1959) (Table 1.1).

The Three Rs apply to experimental procedures as well as to housing and all aspects of the animals' lives. Harms in Russell and Burch's framework may be direct—as when scientists knowingly cause pain or distress in order to study them—or contingent, in which harm is an undesirable side effect of the housing or the experiment. However, the fact that contingent harms are undesirable does not mean they can always be eliminated.

Refinement is particularly germane to this volume on anesthetics and related drugs. Anesthesia for surgery and analgesia for acute (e.g., postsurgical) pain are obvious applications. Analgesics are also useful for chronic and nonsurgical pain, though their use apart from postsurgical care is less common (Chapter 27). Expanded use of drugs

TABLE 1.1 Russell and Burch's Three Rs of alternatives in laboratory animals use and Beauchamp and DeGrazia's six principles of animal research ethics.

Three Rs
• Replacement
• Reduction
• Refinement
Six principles of animal research ethics
Core value: social benefit
• Principle of no alternative method
• Principle of expected net benefit
• Principle of sufficient value to justify harm
Core value: animal welfare
• Principle of no unnecessary harm
• Principle of basic needs
• Principle of upper limits to harm

to manage nonpain distress is less common, especially in smaller animals, but are used for managing self-injurious behaviors in nonhuman macaques and might be useful for improving the welfare of other species experiencing chronic distress (Committee on Recognition and Alleviation of Distress in Laboratory Animals, 2008; Kummrow and Brune, 2018) (Chapter 18).

As such, tailoring analgesia and anesthesia to minimize suffering in laboratory animals is a central component of the ethical justification of research on animals. The occurrence of pains that are not necessary for research is impermissible in a utilitarian assessment of the project, since as it fails to produce the optimal ratio of positive to negative states. Circumstances, where anesthetics or other drugs to reduce suffering may interfere with the research goals require a careful technical evaluation and ethical deliberation, as we discuss later in this chapter.

That so many people with different perspectives on the permissibility of animal use in science converge on the value of the Three Rs is at once testimony to their utility but also, paradoxically, to their ethical neutrality. Consideration of the Three Rs is necessary for an ethical animal project, as they comprise all of the tools for reducing harm to animals. Everyone can agree that reducing animal suffering increases the ethical acceptability of animal experiments. But the Three Rs framework alone does not answer important questions such as how aggressively a scientist must pursue alternatives or importantly, which projects justify situations where harm to animals cannot be reduced to zero.

V. Justifying harms to animals, beyond the Three Rs

Beauchamp and DeGrazia's *Six Principles of Research Animal Ethics* aims to build on Russell and Burch's Three Rs framework with consideration of the types of research that could justify harming animals (Beauchamp and DeGrazia, 2019). Their six principles expand on two core values they espouse, that of substantial social benefit and that of consideration for animal welfare, that must be weighed in evaluating the ethical justification of any proposed animal experiments. Table 1.1. Their three principles of animal welfare—the principles of no unnecessary harm, basic needs, and upper limits to harm—map onto and supplement the Three Rs, though more explicitly calling, as do Olsson et al., for upper limits to harms to research animals (Olsson et al., 2020). Anesthetics and analgesics are vital to reducing "necessary" harms and, along with euthanasia options, to staying below upper limits to harms.

The core value of social benefit comprises three principles that flesh out what would be required for a sound justification of harming animals in biomedical science. There must be no reasonable alternative to harming sentient animals (principle of no alternative method). The research must be likely to produce a net benefit when one factors in potential costs and risks to humans as well as the likelihood of successfully achieving the goals (principle of expected net benefit). Third, the net benefit must be substantial, especially when greater animal welfare harms are expected (principle of sufficient value to justify harm).

In the 1980s and 1990s, many countries updated their animal welfare laws with widespread requirements for animal ethics committees amid interdisciplinary discussions of justifications for using laboratory animals (Chapter 2). Bateson, an ethologist in the UK, proposed a three-axis system (Bateson's Cube) for evaluating when to experiment on animals (Bateson, 1986; Carbone, 2020b; Pound and Nicol, 2018). Our version of the cube reflects the US system, in which the harm to animals, the importance of the scientific project, and the quality or merit of the proposed studies are evaluated and determined by separate bodies in no set sequence (Fig. 1.1).

The US system differs from most European countries, where committees are required to conduct some sort of harm-benefit analysis (HBA) (Brønstad et al., 2016; The European Parliament, 2010). In the United State, the Animal Welfare Act carries no such requirement, while the National Institutes of Health sees scientific merit review and ethics committee reviews as somewhat overlapping but distinct; the NIH Scientific Review Groups (SRG) that evaluate merit may indeed require changes in proposed animal use, that the scientist must pass on to the AEC, presumably for AEC review and approval (Office of Laboratory Animal Welfare, 2010). This information flow is unidirectional, and the AEC review does not go to the SRG, even should the AEC have concerns about the merit of the project. Not all animal projects undergo NIH SRG reviews, as not all research is NIH-funded, but even for those that do, no one body formally evaluates the merits, benefits, and animal harms of research proposals.

Following Bateson, a project must score high on all three axes to be considered justified, though we propose that justification is quantitative, not the yes-or-no binary that the figure suggests. And just as justification is quantitative, ethics committee approval can be also. Rather than a binary approved/not approved outcome, AECs may grant limited approvals for pilot work or frequent progress reports before the scientist may expand the animal numbers and range of procedures.

For more than a century, scientists have stated that they only use animals in essential research when animal use is absolutely necessary. Of particular relevance to this text, they never subject animals to unnecessary pain. The United States principles for the utilization and care of vertebrate animals used in testing, research, and training of 1985 are a

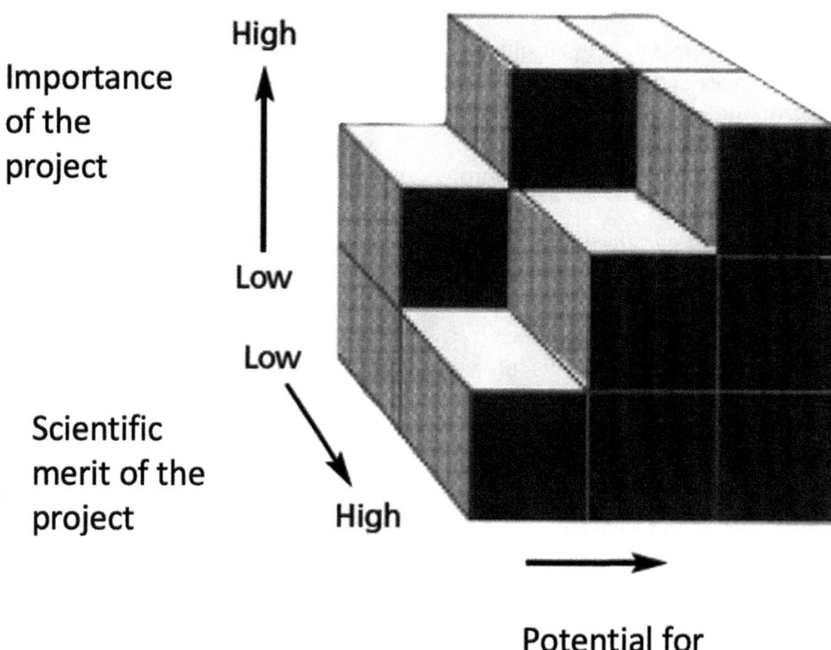

FIGURE 1.1 Modified Bateson's cube. The ethical acceptability of proposed research increases as all three axes move from low toward high.

legal mandate for United States laboratories receiving federal funding:

> *II. Procedures involving animals should be designed and performed with due consideration of their relevance to human or animal health, the advancement of knowledge, or the good of society.*

Moreover, the Principles imply the occasional need to limit treatment of pain if a research project requires such, stating:

> *IV. Proper use of animals, including the avoidance or minimization of discomfort, distress, and pain when consistent with sound scientific practices is imperative.*
>
> United States Interagency Research Animal Committee (1985) (Chapter 2).

But how should scientists operationalize their justification to use animals in ways that may harm them? A limited permission to harm sentient animals in science seems to imply some sort of weighing of the possible harms (or welfare costs) to animals against the potential benefits of the science, i.e., a (HBA). Most European countries now require that an AEC conduct a prospective HBA of animal projects, though only fairly recently (Brønstad et al., 2016; The European Parliament, 2010).

In the United States, the mid-1980s requirement for AECs followed a different path, where the term of choice was "scientific merit" and the question was who, if anyone, should review the merit of a proposed animal project other than the individual scientists themselves (Dresser, 1990; Mann and Prentice, 2004). The Animal Welfare Act does not explicitly call for such a review, while the National Institutes of Health position has been that AECs do not review the scientific merit of a projected use of animals, leaving that to expert reviewers at the funding agencies, while "the IACUC will consider in its review the general scientific relevance of the proposal." (Carbone and Shriver, 2022 - in press; NIH Office of Laboratory Animal Welfare, 2011). This is problematic insofar as even those federally funded institutions under NIH oversight conduct many experiments that are not specifically outlined in grants and may thus elude rigorous merit review from any one body.

> *The* Guide for the Care and Use of Laboratory Animals, *first published in 1963, is the main regulatory document in the United States. Only in its 8th edition in 2011 has it broached something like a call for HBA, stating that "for protocols with the potential for unrelieved pain or distress or other animal welfare concerns … the IACUC is obliged to weigh the objectives of the study against potential animal welfare concern" (Institute for Laboratory Animal Research, 2011). As of 2021, there is no clear guidance from the NIH or the accrediting agency, AAALAC, on just what this means or how to operationalize this.*
>
> AAALAC International (2018), Leland et al. (2019) and NIH Office of Laboratory Animal Welfare (2016).

In reality, as regulatory requirements move toward committee reviews of the harms and benefits of proposed animal projects, we have no established procedure or consensus on what that should entail. Following Bateson's lead, Brønstad et al. and others have proposed approaches for conducting HBA (Animals in Science Committee Harm-Benefit Analysis Subgroup, 2017; Brønstad et al., 2016; Laber et al., 2016; Stafleu et al., 1999).

The challenges for HBA lie not so much in evaluating the scientific quality of the project; peer reviewers at funding agencies or in pharmaceutical companies do that. Russell and Burch launched 60 years of dialogue on how to categorize and evaluate harms. The main objection to HBA is the difficulty of prospectively evaluating the potential benefits of a particular research program when the benefits, or the losses from not performing a project, may not be apparent until years later (Grimm et al., 2017, 2019; Niemi, 2020). In actual practice, human benefits are accorded such a high priority compared to animals' harms that ethics reviews mostly are exercises in harm reduction to the animals, and the quality of the science and importance of the research topic would need to be extremely poor for them to affect the outcome of an HBA (Carbone, 2004; Ferdowsian et al., 2020).

And yet, review bodies do evaluate all three axes of importance, merit and harm, but separately, following no particular sequence, and with minimal cross-talk among reviewers. Only the individual scientist receives and can synthesize the three different bodies' evaluations. To see the significance of this sequencing, consider that human IRB boards are required to *both* ensure that risks to subjects are minimized *and* ensure that risks to subjects are reasonable in light of anticipated benefits (Department of Health and Human Services, 2017). If merely minimizing harm after funding was awarded was sufficient for harm-benefit analysis, the second requirement would be redundant. But they choose to include both, because both clauses have independent contributions to the evaluation of research.

Moreover, merit reviews may cover a large project that contains numerous experiments and assays, not all of which have been spelled out and reviewed in detail by a funding agency's advisory boards. AEC reviews may be more granular. For example, a large-scale grant application to investigate stem cell therapies may not specify the use of a teratoma assay used to verify that the stem cells are truly pluripotent, an assay that Niemi describes as invasive and poorly validated (Niemi, 2020). Should an AEC assume that merit reviewers approved the necessity for this assay, and focus solely on pain management for the surgeries involved? NIH guidance certainly misses this mismatch of granularity of review in its confidence that AECs need not concern themselves with reviewing the quality of science for projects that have received grant funding (NIH Office of Laboratory Animal Welfare, 2011).

Scientists devise their experimental methods to harmonize with the literature in their field, aiming for maximum reproducibility among related experiments. All too often, they publish insufficient methodological detail in their materials and methods sections to allow others to robustly replicate their methods (Landis et al., 2012; Percie du Sert, Ahluwalia, et al., 2020; Percie du Sert, Hurst, et al., 2020). This general challenge to reproducibility has an added moral cost when insufficient detail about welfare-relevant methods such as enrichment, training, anesthesia, and analgesia leads scientists, veterinarians, and AECs to conclude that humane refinements are not consistent with published practices in the field (Carbone and Austin, 2016; Wurbel, 2007).

VI. Veterinarians as anesthesia and analgesia experts and advocates: responsibilities and authority

Veterinarians and others will find this revised edition of *Anesthesia and Analgesia for Laboratory Animals* brimful of updated and useful information. We propose that adequate veterinary care for research animals should go beyond providing technical guidance on pain, anesthesia, and analgesia, with veterinarians not just having the authority to intervene in individual cases, but also an obligation to actively advocate for maximum pain management for research animals' health and welfare (American College of Laboratory Animal Medicine, 2016). The veterinarian's role "includes the *promotion* and monitoring of an animal's well-being [emphasis added]." (American College of Laboratory Medicine, 2016) Researchers may have various reasons of convenience, cost, and most importantly, effects on data, to resist a veterinarian's pain management proposals, and ethics committees with the ultimate decision may favor the investigator's plans over the veterinarian's recommendations (American College of Laboratory Animal Medicine, 2016; Carbone, 2020a). Veterinarians have a unique combination of expert knowledge and institutional authority. The expertise of veterinarians is an essential component of ethical research, and this expertise should play a central role in decisions about research design. We thus propose that there is both a professional obligation and oath to "continual improvement of professional knowledge and competence", but beyond that, a moral obligation for veterinarians to actively advocate for maximum animal welfare (American Veterinary Medical Association, 2021).

VII. Significant unalleviated pain and distress (Category E experiments)

This volume updates readers' knowledge of how to treat laboratory animal pain, greatly advancing animal welfare in science. However, sometimes, scientists see a need to perform experiments that cause pain or distress, and a need to leave the pain untreated out of concern for what drugs might do to the body and to research outcomes. This sort of situation is covered by the USDA's "Category E" in facilities' annual reports (USDA, 2019) (Chapter 2). Every year, some 7%–8% of AWA-covered animals are listed as Category E, with no data on the mice and rats that the Animal Welfare Act excludes (Carbone, 2021; Marx et al., 2021). The ethics committee review of "Category E" requires two types of justification (Carbone, 2014). *Scientific justification* means that the data truly will be diminished if pain medicines are used, and committees vary in how stringent their standards are (Carbone, 2014). Alongside scientific justification is *ethical justification*, in which "necessary" pain that cannot be alleviated without invalidating the data should only be permissible in studies that address important questions with scientific rigor, and without reasonable alternatives that are less painful. Presumably, if the scientific justification is weak, the ethical justification will also be weak, but a strong scientific or technical justification is not sufficient to assure ethical justification.

Animal Ethics Committees make an ethical decision regarding what level of evidence, or scientific justification, they need to conclude that the use of analgesics or other refinements will have a significant deleterious effect on an experiment, and at least in one survey, they varied widely on this (Carbone, 2014). Is it sufficient to state, for example, that nonsteroidal analgesics affect immune function and therefore cannot be used in any study of cancer, sepsis, infection, or other disciplines in which immune function plays a role? Or must a scientist point to specific data that a specific drug has a significant effect on data outcomes in a particular model, and that it is clear the treated animal yields less valid data than the animal with untreated pain? There are times when treating pain and inflammation may yield a somehow truer model than leaving the pain untreated (Carbone, 2019; Committee on Recognition and Alleviation of Pain in Laboratory Animals, 2009; Franchi et al., 2007; Page et al., 2001; Peterson et al., 2017) (Chapter 3) Clearly, animals receive different levels of pain management where AEC standards of evidence differ.

The United States C-D-E system of "pain categories" is actually a system of pain and distress categories. It is not a linear severity scale, and many category D experiments ("with pain, with drugs" in the USDA's language) may be of greater severity than some category E experiments (with Pain, without drugs) (USDA, 2019). For example, the USDA places a hamster undergoing a single 24-hour fast in Category E, while another undergoing multiple major survival surgeries would be in Category D, so long as the investigator does not request approval to withhold analgesics (National Research Council, 2000). In these two cases, the Category D project requires a much higher level of skill to anesthetize the hamster and monitor and manage postoperative care, and a commensurate ethical review.

Scientists have legitimate concerns about the ways in which anesthetics, analgesics, and other refinements to improve animal welfare may affect their data outcomes, or their ability to see their work published if they use analgesics in fields where the common practice is to withhold them. If their field's literature is silent on questions of pain management, humane endpoints, enrichment, training, and other welfare enhancements, they can easily believe, rightly or wrongly, that these moves to improve welfare are unacceptable in their line of research. We see an ethical duty for scientists to publish full information on the use of analgesics and other refinements to establish a robust literature that animal welfare is often consistent with publication in high-caliber journals, and may even improve cross-laboratory reproducibility (Carbone and Austin, 2016; Committee on Guidelines for Scientific Publications Involving Animal Studies, 2011; Percie du Sert, Ahluwalia, et al., 2020; Percie du Sert, Hurst, et al., 2020; Wurbel, 2007). At the risk of yet more regulatory work, we suggest that AECs should pay attention to what their scientists publish, and include training on publication practices as part of their research education mission.

Rabbits in ocular toxicity tests—the Draize test—are at high risk of severe eye pain. As originally developed, rabbits received no analgesic treatment and lived in neck restraints that blocked their freedom to rub their eyes. The test dates back to 1944 and includes standardized methods for restraining rabbits, instilling potentially irritating or caustic chemicals in their eyes, and scoring the damage to their eyes (Draize et al., 1944; Parascandola, 1991). The likely suffering of the rabbits drove a successful public campaign in the 1970s to ban the test for cosmetics and other chemicals and to fund research into replacement alternatives (Singer, 1998; Zurlo et al., 1994). As validated replacements increasingly gain regulatory acceptance, and rabbit numbers are continually reduced, the Draize test is nearly, but not yet complete, a thing of the past (Clippinger et al., 2021).

With reduction and replacement still works in progress, a government panel convened in 2010 to develop refinements that would reduce rabbits' suffering. The refinement of standards for ocular toxicity testing in rabbit eyes is illustrative if cautionary, case study in the application of expert analgesia knowledge.

Historically, the standardized Draize test did not include the use of topical or systemic analgesics, leaving concerned scientists unclear on whether refinement with pain medicines would lead regulators to reject their toxicity tests. In 1990, the United States Interagency Coordinating Committee on the Validation of Alternative Methods published recommendations that the use of topical analgesics with subcutaneous buprenorphine and meloxicam could be acceptable welfare improvements that would not interfere with the test (Interagency Coordinating Committee on the Validation of Alternative Methods, 2010). However, there are no empirical studies of the efficacy or side effects of systemic analgesics in rabbits undergoing Draize testing. A challenge here is that later work has found those subcutaneous analgesic doses largely ineffective in rabbits in other models, and still no assessment of their utility for ocular pain (Askar et al., 2020). It is an open question whether regulators would accept more effective pain management regimens for rabbit Draize tests without demonstration that more aggressive medication, including topical medication, will not confound the ocular irritation scores (Chapter 15).

We urge caution in believing Draize tests using the 2010 ICCVAM guidelines truly refine the procedure as the rabbits experience it and meet ethical norms to eliminate pain. If this tests use must continue, updated guidance for pain management—keeping the ICCVAM's recommendations for euthanasia of severely affected animals—is warranted. Until then, ethics committees reviewing ocular toxicity testing protocols, or any other surgical or painful rabbit experiments should not be lulled into believing that current analgesic protocols will significantly abolish rabbit pain, a crucial caveat for any harm-benefit analysis.

VIII. Ethics of uncertainty

All of the foregoing discussion requires that veterinarians, scientists, and Animal Ethics Committees work with solid information on a range of questions:

- How much suffering will this experiment cause for the animals?
- How much will anesthetic, analgesic, or related drugs improve the animals' welfare?
- How and in what time frame will suffering occur?
- How will these drugs affect data outcomes?
- How well will the animal data predict, or translate into, human outcomes?
- How well will the sample size yield statistically sound findings without animal overuse?

Sprigge writes that in animal experimentation, the harm to animals is certain while the benefits of research are potential, unknowns that may or may not be realized. He argues that in any sort of comparative harm-benefit analysis different weighting should accompany different levels of certainty (Sprigge, 1985). But what if the animal harms are not so certain, obscured by challenges of accurately diagnosing pain or scoring welfare for the millions of animals in laboratories? What is the ethical response, for example, to learning that there validated cage-side pain assays for laboratory rodents or other species are few, and require specialized training (Carbone, 2019; Leung et al., 2016; Mogil et al., 2020; Zhang et al., 2019) (Chapter 12)?

Consider two veterinarians advising a scientist and AEC on a novel model of pancreatic inflammation in mice. The scientist proposes some pilot work, with frequent pain evaluations and analgesic interventions if warranted. One veterinarian believes they can train the scientist to do accurate real-time mouse pain evaluations via observation of the mice in the cage, and endorse approval of the pilot work with "analgesia as needed." The other veterinarian believes this approach leaves mice at high risk of undiagnosed (and untreated) pain, and requests either proactive analgesic treatment with doses and durations from peer-reviewed studies, or a rigorous pilot study with multi-modal pain assessment from experienced pain biologists, trained to assess real-time and image/video-based markers of pain, such as twitching and facial grimaces (Mogil et al., 2020; Roughan and Flecknell, 2004; Zhang et al., 2019). This simple difference in interpreting the facts about animal pain diagnosis can put the different cohorts of mice at very different risk of suffering. Veterinarians, scientists, and AECs would modify their HBA and their approved use of animals if they factored in the uncertainties in pain diagnosis documented throughout this volume, taking a more precautionary approach in approving invasive procedures.

IX. Critical anthropomorphism

As the scientists writing in this volume demonstrate, we still have much to learn about pain recognition in research animals, and much to learn about the safe and effective anesthetic and analgesic regimens for various species and model systems. Recognizing the uncertainty in animal pain recognition, the United States Interagency Research Animal Committee elaborated its Principle IV, that "Unless the contrary is established, investigators should consider that procedures that cause pain or distress in human beings may cause pain or distress in other animals." (United States Interagency Research Animal Committee, 1985). This judicious application of human experience to try to fill in gaps of experimentally derived knowledge of nonhuman animals' subjective experience is called *critical anthropomorphism* and is used correctly, can improve the ethical review of animal experiments (Karlsson, 2011; Nuffield Council on Bioethics, 2005).

Scientists use animals as objects of study hoping that their data will translate to human biology, with no illusion that absolutely everything we learn from animals applies equally in kind and degree to people. Critical anthropomorphism is essentially a reverse translation from human to animal. The advances described throughout this volume reveal how much we still do not know; critical anthropomorphism partially fills those knowledge gaps. Clinical data from humans may be particularly illuminating for chronic conditions accompanied by intermittent or intractable pain in some percentage of the human patient population, such as multiple sclerosis, diabetes, metastatic bone or lung disease, or postoperative craniotomy pain (Ceruti, 2018; Flexman et al., 2010; Hebert et al., 2017; Luger et al., 2005). One of us (Carbone) has read many animal-use protocols in which the investigator has assured the AEC that these are rarely painful conditions in their human patients, thus requiring minimal pain management in their animals. Those claims need a fact-check, for example, by reviewing patient information handouts for various diseases and procedures, as well as via rigorous peer-reviewed published severity assessments in nonhuman animals. Clinicians strive to do their best for the conditions that their patients spontaneously develop. Intentionally creating illness and injury in one's research animals calls for at least that high a standard of care.

A corollary of Principle IV is that human pain treatment may inform nonhuman pain treatment, but again, with caution. If a condition's pain is frequently refractory to treatment in human patients, we cannot assume, without rigorous animal studies, that some short-term buprenorphine or meloxicam will be sufficient for animals with a comparable condition. Clinician-investigators may state that they send their human patients home after a procedure without prescribing pain medications, and so will not plan on analgesics for their animals. But if they allow patients to self-medicate with ibuprofen in their medicine cabinets, an option research animals do not have, is it ethical to withhold analgesics for the animals or to treat "as needed" if no one will be able to rigorously monitor for pain throughout the night?

X. Conclusion

Scientists have an ethical responsibility to consider animal welfare as they plan their research, including the appropriate use of the anesthetics, analgesics, and related drugs that are the subject of this volume. The prevailing applied ethic is a utilitarian approach that considers the consequences of actions and calls at a minimum for efforts to reduce harm to animals in laboratories by decreasing negative states of pain and distress and maximizing positive states and pleasures. The Three Rs—reduce, replace, and refine—are an organizing framework for reducing harm, but increasingly, regulators and scholars are pointing out that they do not address the justifications for causing harm. European policies for prospective harm-benefit analyses, the *Guide*'s recommendation to weigh the objectives of studies against animal welfare concerns, Beauchamp and DeGrazia's six principles, and other efforts seek ways to evaluate the potential benefits (primarily to humans) that might justify the harms to animals. Departing from utilitarian calculations, various experts are calling on scientists and their regulators to set upper limits on harm to animals, no matter the claims to human benefits in studies that entail severe suffering (Beauchamp and DeGrazia, 2019; Beauchamp and Morton, 2015; Olsson et al., 2020).

We have stressed the importance of clear information in terms of whether animals are suffering, whether analgesics and other refinements are helping, and whether scientists can provide good evidence that a project addresses important questions with a high-merit research plan. Often, animal ethics committees lack the information necessary for these determinations and must make ethical choices, in the face of uncertainty, of where to give the benefit of the doubt, requiring, perhaps, that an investigator may feel the AEC's requirements are unnecessary or even disruptive.

Veterinarians and those charged with providing pain relief occupy a central role in efforts to make animal research as ethical as possible. Though there are numerous perspectives on the ethics of animal research, all involved in the debate are agreed that pain and suffering that are unnecessary for research should be eliminated, and these can only be eliminated if veterinarians use their expertise to properly ensure maximal pain relief within the scope of the experimental parameters and if this expertise is given a central role in experimental design. Veterinarians are uniquely situated to influence the ethical dimensions of research, and they have a duty to ensure that pain and suffering in laboratory research are kept to a minimum. Anything less is hollow platitudes that do not benefit the research or the animals.

References

AAALAC International, 2018. Harm-Benefit Analysis. Retrieved December 13 from. https://www.aaalac.org/accreditation/faq_landing.cfm.

Amercan College of Laboratory Medicine, November 2016. ACLAM position statement on adequate veterinary care. J. Am. Assoc. Lab. Anim. Sci. 55 (6), 826–828. https://www.ncbi.nlm.nih.gov/pubmed/27931327.

American College of Laboratory Animal Medicine, November 2016. ACLAM position statement on pain and distress in research animals. J. Am. Assoc. Lab. Anim. Sci. 55 (6), 821. https://www.ncbi.nlm.nih.gov/pubmed/27931324.

American Veterinary Medical Association, 2021. Veterinarian's Oath. Retrieved July 19 from. https://www.avma.org/resources-tools/avma-policies/veterinarians-oath.

Animals in Science Committee Harm-Benefit Analysis Sub-Group, 2017. Review of Harm-Benefit Analysis in the Use of Animals in Research: Report of the Animals in Science Committee Harm-Benefit Analysis Sub-Group Chaired by Professor Gail Davies. https://ore.exeter.ac.uk/repository/bitstream/handle/10871/31153/Review%20of%20harm%20benefit%20analysis%20in%20use%20of%20animals.pdf?sequence=4&isAllowed=y.

Askar, R., Fredriksson, E., Manell, E., Hedeland, M., Bondesson, U., Bate, S., Olsen, L., Hedenqvist, P., November 11, 2020. Bioavailability of subcutaneous and intramuscular administrated buprenorphine in New Zealand White rabbits. BMC Vet. Res. 16 (1), 436. https://doi.org/10.1186/s12917-020-02618-7.

AVMA Panel on Euthanasia, 2020. AVMA Guidelines for the Euthanasia of Animals: 2020 Edition. American Veterinary Medical Association. www.avma.org/KB/Policies/Documents/euthanasia.pdf.

Bateson, P., February 20, 1986. When to experiment on animals. New Sci. 30–32. https://www.umces.edu/sites/default/files/BatesonPaper_0.pdf.

Beauchamp, T., DeGrazia, D., 2019. Principles of Animal Research Ethics. Oxford University Press.

Beauchamp, T.L., Childress, J.F., 1994. Principles of Biomedical Ethics, forth ed. Oxford University Press.

Beauchamp, T.L., Morton, D.B., October 2015. The upper limits of pain and suffering in animal research. Camb. Q. Healthc. Ethics 24 (4), 431–447. https://doi.org/10.1017/S0963180115000092.

Bentham, J., 1789. Excerpt from chapter XVII, section 1. In: The Principles of Morals and Legislation.

Bleich, A., Bankstahl, M., Jirkof, P., Prins, J.B., Tolba, R.H., February 2020. Severity assessment in animal based research. Lab. Anim. 54 (1), 16. https://doi.org/10.1177/0023677219898105.

Brønstad, A., Newcomer, C.E., Decelle, T., Everitt, J.I., Guillen, J., Laber, K., June 2016. Current concepts of harm-benefit analysis of animal experiments—report from the AALAS-FELASA working group on harm-benefit analysis—part 1. Lab. Anim. 50 (1 Suppl. l), 1–*20*. https://doi.org/10.1177/0023677216642398.

Burghardt, G.M., 1999. Deprivation and enrichment in laboratory animal environments. J. Appl. Anim. Welfare Sci. 2 (4), 263–266. https://doi.org/10.1207/s15327604jaws0204_1.

Carbone, L., 2004. What Animals Want: Expertise and Advocacy in Laboratory Animal Welfare Policy. Oxford.

Carbone, L., 2014. Justification for the use of animals. In: Silverman, J., Suckow, M.A., Murthy, S. (Eds.), The IACUC Handbook, third ed. CRC Press, pp. 211–251.

Carbone, L., December 1, 2019. Ethical and IACUC considerations regarding analgesia and pain management in laboratory rodents. Comp. Med. 69 (6), 443–450. https://doi.org/10.30802/AALAS-CM-18-000149.

Carbone, L., January 2020a. Less than full analgesia can leave significant pain under-treated. Lab. Anim. (NY) 49 (1), 5. https://doi.org/10.1038/s41684-019-0442-3.

Carbone, L., 2020b. The potential and impacts of practical application of Beauchamp and DeGrazia's six principles. In: Beauchamp, T., DeGrazia, D. (Eds.), Principles of Animal Research Ethics. Oxford University Press.

Carbone, L., 2021. Estimating mouse and rat use in American laboratories by extrapolation from Animal Welfare Act-regulated species. Sci. Rep. 11 (493). https://doi.org/10.1038/s41598-020-79961-0.

Carbone, L., Austin, J., 2016. Pain and laboratory animals: publication practices for better data reproducibility and better animal welfare. PLoS ONE 11 (5), e0155001. https://doi.org/10.1371/journal.pone.0155001.

Carbone, L., Shriver, A., 2022 - in press. Ethical considerations in anesthesia and analgesia in laboratory animals. In: Pang D., Jirkof P., Lofgren J., Flecknell P. (Eds.), Anesthesia and Analgesia in Laboratory Animals, third ed. Academic Press, Elsevier, pp. 561–568.

Ceruti, S., January 2018. What role does multiple sclerosis play in the development of untreatable painful conditions? Pain Manag. 8 (1), 37–44. https://doi.org/10.2217/pmt-2017-0038.

Cigman, R., 1989. Why death does not harm animals. In: Regan, T., Singer, P. (Eds.), Animal Rights and Human Obligations, Second ed. Prentice Hall, pp. 150–152.

Clippinger, A.J., Raabe, H.A., Allen, D.G., Choksi, N.Y., van der Zalm, A.J., Kleinstreuer, N.C., Barroso, J., Lowit, A.B., June 2021. Human-relevant approaches to assess eye corrosion/irritation potential of agrochemical formulations. Cutan. Ocul. Toxicol. 40 (2), 145–167. https://doi.org/10.1080/15569527.2021.1910291.

Committee on Guidelines for Scientific Publications Involving Animal Studies, 2011. Guidance for the Description of Animal Research in Scientific Publications. National Academy of Sciences. http://www.ncbi.nlm.nih.gov/books/NBK84205/.

Committee on Recognition and Alleviation of Distress in Laboratory Animals, I. f. L. A. R, National Research Council, 2008. Recognition and Alleviation of Distress in Laboratory Animals. The National Academies Press.

Committee on Recognition and Alleviation of Pain in Laboratory Animals, N. R. C, 2009. Recognition and Alleviation of Pain in Laboratory Animals. The National Academies Press.

Crisp, R., 2006. Hedonism reconsidered. Philos. Phenomenol. Res. 73 (3), 619–645. https://doi.org/10.1111/j.1933-1592.2006.tb00551.x.

Crook, R.J., 2021. Behavioral and neurophysiological evidence suggests affective pain experience in octopus. iScience 24 (3), 102229. https://doi.org/10.1016/j.isci.2021.102229.

DeGrazia, D., 1996. Taking Animals Seriously. Cambridge University Press.

Department of Health and Human Services, 2017. Federal policy for the protection of human subjects. Fed. Regist. 82 (12), 7149–7274.

Draize, J.H., Woodard, G., Clavery, H.O., 1944. Methods for the study of irritation and toxicity of substances applied topically to the skin and mucous membranes. J. Pharmacol. Exp. Therapeut. 82, 377–390.

Dresser, R., 1990. Review standards for animal research: a closer look. ILAR News (Inst. Lab. Anim. Resour.) 32 (4), 2–7.

Eccles, J.C., 1971. Animal experimentation versus human experimentation (t. i. t. c. p. f. t. I. I. S. o. t. I. C. o. L. A. Actually, held in DC, April 8–11, 1969, Trans.). In: Defining the Laboratory Animal. National Academy Press, pp. 285–293.

Ferdowsian, H., Johnson, L.S.M., Johnson, J., Fenton, A., Shriver, A., Gluck, J., January 2020. A Belmont report for animals? Camb. Q. Healthc. Ethics 29 (1), 19–37. https://doi.org/10.1017/S0963180119000732.

Flexman, A.M., Ng, J.L., Gelb, A.W., October 2010. Acute and chronic pain following craniotomy. Curr. Opin. Anaesthesiol. 23 (5), 551–557. https://doi.org/10.1097/ACO.0b013e32833e15b9.

Franchi, S., Panerai, A.E., Sacerdote, P., August 2007. Buprenorphine ameliorates the effect of surgery on hypothalamus-pituitary-adrenal axis, natural killer cell activity and metastatic colonization in rats in comparison with morphine or fentanyl treatment [Comparative Study Research Support, Non-U.S. Gov't]. Brain Behav. Immun. 21 (6), 767–774. https://doi.org/10.1016/j.bbi.2007.01.001.

Frey, R.G., 1997. Moral community and animal research in medicine. Ethics Behav. 7 (2), 123–136. https://doi.org/10.1207/s15327019eb0702_4.

Garrett, J.R., 2012. The Ethics of Animal Research: Exploring the Controversy. MIT Press.

Godfrey-Smith, P., 2016. Other Minds: The Octopus, the Sea, and the Deep Origins of Consciousness, first ed. Farrar, Straus and Giroux.

Gouveia, K., Hurst, J.L., March 21, 2017. Optimising reliability of mouse performance in behavioural testing: the major role of non-aversive handling. Sci. Rep. 7, 44999. https://doi.org/10.1038/srep44999.

Graham, M.L., Rieke, E.F., Mutch, L.A., Zolondek, E.K., Faig, A.W., Dufour, T.A., Munson, J.W., Kittredge, J.A., Schuurman, H.J., April 2012. Successful implementation of cooperative handling eliminates the need for restraint in a complex non-human primate disease model. J. Med. Primatol. 41 (2), 89–106. https://doi.org/10.1111/j.1600-0684.2011.00525.x.

Grimm, H., Eggel, M., Deplazes-Zemp, A., Biller-Andorno, N., September 11, 2017. The road to hell is paved with good intentions: why harm-benefit analysis and its emphasis on practical benefit jeopardizes the credibility of research. Animals (Basel) 7 (9). https://doi.org/10.3390/ani7090070.

Grimm, H., Olsson, I.A.S., Sandoe, P., February 2019. Harm-benefit analysis—what is the added value? A review of alternative strategies for weighing harms and benefits as part of the assessment of animal research. Lab. Anim. 53 (1), 17–27. https://doi.org/10.1177/0023677218783004.

Hebert, H.L., Veluchamy, A., Torrance, N., Smith, B.H., April 2017. Risk factors for neuropathic pain in diabetes mellitus. Pain 158 (4), 560–568. https://doi.org/10.1097/j.pain.0000000000000785.

Institute for Laboratory Animal Research, N. R. C, 2011. Guide for the Care and Use of Laboratory Animals, eighth ed. National Academies Press (Record #5712 is using a reference type undefined in this output style.).

Interagency Coordinating Committee on the Validation of Alternative Methods, 2010. ICCVAM Test Method Evaluation Report: Recommendations for Routine Use of Topical Anesthetics, Systemic Analgesics, and Humane Endpoints to Avoid or Minimize Pain and Distress in Ocular Safety Testing. Published by National Toxicology Program, Research Triangle Park, NC.

John, T.M., Sebo, J., 2020. Consequentialism and nonhuman animals. In: Portmore, D.W. (Ed.), The Oxford Handbook of Consequentialism. Oxford University Press, pp. 564–591. https://doi.org/10.1093/oxfordhb/9780190905323.013.32.

Kahn, J., 2014. Lessons learned: challenges in applying current constraints on research on chimpanzees to other animals. Theor. Med. Bioeth. 35 (2), 97–104. https://doi.org/10.1007/s11017-014-9284-6.

Karlsson, F., 2011. Critical anthropomorphism and animal ethics. J. Agric. Environ. Ethics 25, 707–720. https://link.springer.com/article/10.1007/s10806-011-9349-8.

Klein, C., Barron, A.B., 2016. Insects have the capacity for subjective experience. Anim. Sentience 1 (9). https://doi.org/10.51291/2377-7478.1113.

Kummrow, M.S., Brune, M., June 2018. Review: psychopathologies in captive nonhuman primates and approaches to diagnosis and treatment. J. Zoo Wildl. Med. 49 (2), 259–271. https://doi.org/10.1638/2017-0137.1.

Laber, K., Newcomer, C.E., Decelle, T., Everitt, J.I., Guillen, J., Bronstad, A., June 2016. Recommendations for addressing harm-benefit analysis and implementation in ethical evaluation—report from the AALAS-FELASA working group on harm-benefit analysis—part 2. Lab. Anim. 50 (1 Suppl. 1), 21–42. https://doi.org/10.1177/0023677216642397.

LaFollette, M.R., O'Haire, M.E., Cloutier, S., Blankenberger, W.B., Gaskill, B.N., 2017. Rat tickling: a systematic review of applications, outcomes, and moderators. PLoS ONE 12 (4), e0175320. https://doi.org/10.1371/journal.pone.0175320.

Lahvis, G.P., June 29, 2017. Unbridle biomedical research from the laboratory cage. Elife 6. https://doi.org/10.7554/eLife.27438.

Landis, S.C., Amara, S.G., Asadullah, K., Austin, C.P., Blumenstein, R., Bradley, E.W., Crystal, R.G., Darnell, R.B., Ferrante, R.J., Fillit, H., Finkelstein, R., Fisher, M., Gendelman, H.E., Golub, R.M., Goudreau, J.L., Gross, R.A., Gubitz, A.K., Hesterlee, S.E., Howells, D.W., Huguenard, J., Kelner, K., Koroshetz, W., Krainc, D., Lazic, S.E., Levine, M.S., Macleod, M.R., McCall, J.M., Moxley 3rd, R.T., Narasimhan, K., Noble, L.J., Perrin, S., Porter, J.D., Steward, O., Unger, E., Utz, U., Silberberg, S.D., October 11, 2012. A call for transparent reporting to optimize the predictive value of preclinical research. Nature 490 (7419), 187–191. https://doi.org/10.1038/nature11556.

Leland, S.E., Straeter, P.A., Gnadt, B.J., December 31, 2019. The role of the IACUC in the absence of regulatory guidance. ILAR J. 60 (1), 95–104. https://doi.org/10.1093/ilar/ilz003.

Leung, V., Zhang, E., Pang, D.S., August 17, 2016. Real-time application of the Rat Grimace Scale as a welfare refinement in laboratory rats. Sci. Rep. 6, 31667. https://doi.org/10.1038/srep31667.

Luger, N.M., Mach, D.B., Sevcik, M.A., Mantyh, P.W., May 2005. Bone cancer pain: from model to mechanism to therapy. J. Pain Symptom Manag. 29 (5 Suppl. 1), S32–S46. http://www.ncbi.nlm.nih.gov/entrez/query.fcgi?cmd=Retrieve&db=PubMed&dopt=Citation&list_uids=15907645.

Makowska, I.J., Weary, D.M., 2020. A good life for laboratory rodents? ILAR J. https://pubmed.ncbi.nlm.nih.gov/11657070/.

Mann, M.D., Prentice, E.D., 2004. Should IACUCs review scientific merit of animal research projects? Lab. Anim. 33 (1), 26–31. http://www.unmc.edu/iacuc/documents/scientific_merit.pdf.

Marx, J.O., Jacobsen, K.O., Petervary, N.A., Casebolt, D.B., March 1, 2021. A survey of laboratory animal veterinarians regarding mouse welfare in biomedical research. J. Am. Assoc. Lab. Anim. Sci. 60 (2), 139–145. https://doi.org/10.30802/AALAS-JAALAS-20-000063.

Mason, G., 2011. Invertebrate welfare: where is the real evidence for conscious affective states? Trends Ecol. Evol. 5, 212–213.

Mather, J., 2019. What is in an octopus's mind? Anim. Sentience 26 (1). https://doi.org/10.51291/2377-7478.1370.

Mellor, D.J., July 13, 2019. Welfare-aligned sentience: enhanced capacities to experience, interact, anticipate, choose and survive. Animals (Basel) 9 (7). https://doi.org/10.3390/ani9070440.

Mikhalevich, I., Powell, R., 2020. Minds without spines: evolutionarily inclusive animal ethics. Anim. Sentience 5 (29). https://doi.org/10.51291/2377-7478.1527.

Mogil, J.S., Pang, D.S.J., Silva Dutra, G.G., Chambers, C.T., September 2020. The development and use of facial grimace scales for pain measurement in animals. Neurosci. Biobehav. Rev. 116, 480–493. https://doi.org/10.1016/j.neubiorev.2020.07.013.

National Centre for the Replacement, R.a.R.o.A.i.R.N. R., 2020. The NC3Rs: Pioneering Better Science. Retrieved December 22 from. https://www.nc3rs.org.uk.

National Commission for the Protection of Human Subjects of Biomedical and Behavioral Research, 1978. The Belmont Report (DHEW Publication OS 78-0012 ed.). Department of Health, Education, and Welfare.

National Research Council, 2000. Definition of Pain and Distress and Reporting Requirements for Laboratory Animals: Proceedings of the

Workshop Held June 22, 2000. The National Academies Press. https://doi.org/10.17226/10035.

Niemi, S.M., August 12, 2020. Harm-benefit analyses can be harmful. ILAR J. https://doi.org/10.1093/ilar/ilaa016.

NIH Office of Laboratory Animal Welfare, 2011. Frequently Asked Questions: PHS Policy on Humane Care and Use of Laboratory Animals. Retrieved September 15 from. http://grants.nih.gov/grants/olaw/faqs.htm.

NIH Office of Laboratory Animal Welfare, 2016. Balancing Public Interests, Benefits, and Risks in Animal Research. Retrieved September 20 from. https://olaw.nih.gov/sites/default/files/160609_seminar_transcript.pdf (Record #5698 is using a reference type undefined in this output style.).

Nobis, N., 2016. Animals & ethics 101: thinking critically about animal rights. Open Philosophy Press.

Nozick, R., 1974. Anarchy, State, and Utopia. Basic Books.

Nuffield Council on Bioethics, 2005. The Ethics of Research Involving Animals. Nuffield Council on Bioethics.

Office of Laboratory Animal Welfare, N.I.o.H., 2010. Clarification on the Roles of NIH Scientific Review Groups (SRG) and Institutional Animal Care and Use Committees (IACUC) in Review of Vertebrate Animal Research. Retrieved April 7 from. http://grants.nih.gov/grants/guide/notice-files/not-od-10-128.html.

Olsson, I.A.S., C, J.N., Niemi, S.M., Sandoe, P., January 30, 2020. From unpleasant to unbearable-why and how to implement an upper limit to pain and other forms of suffering in research with animals. ILAR J. https://doi.org/10.1093/ilar/ilz018.

Page, G.G., Blakely, W.P., Ben-Eliyahu, S., February 1, 2001. Evidence that postoperative pain is a mediator of the tumor-promoting effects of surgery in rats. Pain 90 (1–2), 191–199. http://www.ncbi.nlm.nih.gov/entrez/query.fcgi?cmd=Retrieve&db=PubMed&dopt=Citation&list_uids=11166986.

Parascandola, J., 1991. The development of the Draize test for eye toxicity. Pharm. Hist. 33 (3), 111–117.

Percie du Sert, N., Ahluwalia, A., Alam, S., Avey, M.T., Baker, M., Browne, W.J., Clark, A., Cuthill, I.C., Dirnagl, U., Emerson, M., Garner, P., Holgate, S.T., Howells, D.W., Hurst, V., Karp, N.A., Lazic, S.E., Lidster, K., MacCallum, C.J., Macleod, M., Pearl, E.J., Petersen, O.H., Rawle, F., Reynolds, P., Rooney, K., Sena, E.S., Silberberg, S.D., Steckler, T., Wurbel, H., July 2020. Reporting animal research: explanation and elaboration for the ARRIVE guidelines 2.0. PLoS Biol. 18 (7), e3000411. https://doi.org/10.1371/journal.pbio.3000411.

Percie du Sert, N., Hurst, V., Ahluwalia, A., Alam, S., Avey, M.T., Baker, M., Browne, W.J., Clark, A., Cuthill, I.C., Dirnagl, U., Emerson, M., Garner, P., Holgate, S.T., Howells, D.W., Karp, N.A., Lazic, S.E., Lidster, K., MacCallum, C.J., Macleod, M., Pearl, E.J., Petersen, O.H., Rawle, F., Reynolds, P., Rooney, K., Sena, E.S., Silberberg, S.D., Steckler, T., Wurbel, H., July 2020. The ARRIVE guidelines 2.0: updated guidelines for reporting animal research. PLoS Biol. 18 (7), e3000410. https://doi.org/10.1371/journal.pbio.3000410.

Peterson, N.C., Nunamaker, E.A., Turner, P.V., December 1, 2017. To treat or not to treat: the effects of pain on experimental parameters. Comp. Med. 67 (6), 469–482. https://www.ncbi.nlm.nih.gov/pubmed/29212578.

Pew Research Center, 2018. Americans are Divided Over the Use of Animals in Scientific Research. Retrieved January 28 from. https://www.pewresearch.org/fact-tank/2018/08/16/americans-are-divided-over-the-use-of-animals-in-scientific-research/.

Pound, P., Nicol, C.J., 2018. Retrospective harm benefit analysis of pre-clinical animal research for six treatment interventions. PLoS ONE 13 (3), e0193758. https://doi.org/10.1371/journal.pone.0193758.

Regan, T., 1989. Why death does harm animals. In: Regan, T., Singer, P. (Eds.), Animal Rights and Human Obligations, second ed. Prentice Hall, pp. 153–157.

Roughan, J.V., Flecknell, P.A., November 2004. Behaviour-based assessment of the duration of laparotomy-induced abdominal pain and the analgesic effects of carprofen and buprenorphine in rats. Behav. Pharmacol. 15 (7), 461–472. https://www.ncbi.nlm.nih.gov/pubmed/15472568.

Russell, W.M.S., Burch, R.L., 1959. The Principles of Humane Experimental Technique. Methuen & Co. Ltd.

Shriver, A., 2006. Minding mammals. Phil. Psychol. 19 (4), 433–442. https://doi.org/10.1080/09515080600726385.

Shriver, A.J., April 2014. The asymmetrical contributions of pleasure and pain to animal welfare. Camb. Q. Healthc. Ethics 23 (2), 152–162. https://doi.org/10.1017/S0963180113000686.

Singer, P., 1990. Animal Liberation, second ed. Avon Books.

Singer, P., 1998. Ethics into Action: Henry Spira and the Animal Rights Movement. Rowman and Littlefield Publishers, Inc.

Sinnott-Armstrong, W., 2021. Consequentialism. In: Zalta, E.N. (Ed.), Stanford Encyclopedia of Philosophy. https://plato.stanford.edu/archives/fall2021/entries/consequentialism/.

Sneddon, L.U., April 2015. Pain in aquatic animals. J. Exp. Biol. 218 (Pt 7), 967–976. https://doi.org/10.1242/jeb.088823.

Sprigge, T.L.S., 1985. Philosophers and antivivisectionism. ATLA 13, 99–106.

Stafleu, F.R., Tramper, R., Vorstenbosch, J., Joles, J.A., July 1999. The ethical acceptability of animal experiments: a proposal for a system to support decision-making. Lab. Anim. 33 (3), 295–303. https://doi.org/10.1258/002367799780578255.

Tannenbaum, J., Bennett, B.T., 2015. Russell and burch's 3Rs then and now: the need for clarity in definition and purpose. J. Am. Assoc. Lab. Anim. Sci. 54 (2), 120–132. http://www.ncbi.nlm.nih.gov/pubmed/25836957.

The European Parliament, 2010. Directive 2010/63/EU of the European Parliament and of the Council of 22 September 2010 on the Protection of Animals Used for Scientific Purposes. https://eur-lex.europa.eu/legal-content/EN/TXT/?uri=celex%3A32010L0063.

The North American 3Rs Collaborative (NA3RsC), 2021. Advancing Science, Innovation and Research Animal Welfare. Retrieved January 22 from. https://www.na3rsc.org.

United States Department of Agriculture, A.a.P.H. I.S., 2019. Annual Report Animal Usage by Fiscal Year. Fiscal Year: 2018. Retrieved January 22 from. https://www.aphis.usda.gov/animal_welfare/annual-reports/Annual-Report-Summaries-State-Pain-FY18.pdf.

United States Government Printing Office, 1949. The Nuremberg code. In: Trials of War Criminals before the Nuremberg Military Tribunals under Control Council Law No. 10, vol 2.

United States Interagency Research Animal Committee, May 20, 1985. Principles for the utilization and care of vertebrate animals used in testing, research, and training [US government policy statement]. Fed. Regist. 50 (97), 20864–20865. http://www.ncbi.nlm.nih.gov/pubmed/11655791.

Watters, J.V., November 2009. Toward a predictive theory for environmental enrichment. Zoo Biol. 28 (6), 609–622. https://doi.org/10.1002/zoo.20284.

Weary, D.M., 2014. What is suffering in animals. In: Appleby, M.C., Weary, D.M., Sandøe, P. (Eds.), Dilemmas in Animal Welfare. CABI. https://www.cabi.org/cabebooks/ebook/20143138804.

World Medical Association, 1997. Declaration of Helsinki. J. Am. Med. Assoc. 277 (11), 925–926.

Wurbel, H., March 15, 2007,. Publications should include an animal-welfare section. Nature 446 (7133), 257. https://doi.org/10.1038/446257a.

Zhang, E.Q., Leung, V.S., Pang, D.S., March 1, 2019. Influence of rater training on inter- and intrarater reliability when using the rat grimace scale. J. Am. Assoc. Lab. Anim. Sci. 58 (2), 178–183. https://doi.org/10.30802/AALAS-JAALAS-18-000044.

Zurlo, J., Rudacille, D., Goldberg, A.M., 1994. Animals and Alternatives in Testing: History, Science, and Ethics. Mary Ann Liebert, Inc.

Chapter 2

Regulatory issues

David B. Anderson[1], Judy MacArthur Clark[2], Carol Clarke[3], Chereen Collymore[4] and Catharine E. Pritchard[5]

[1]*Pentlands Management Systems, Edinburgh, Scotland, United Kingdom;* [2]*JMC Welfare International, Sandwich, Kent, United Kingdom;* [3]*Animal and Plant Health Inspection Service, U.S. Department of Agriculture, Riverdale, MD, United States;* [4]*Laboratory Animal Medicine and Surgery, Charles River Laboratories, Senneville, QC, Canada;* [5]*Office of Laboratory Animal Welfare, National Institutes of Health, Bethesda, MD, United States*

Chapter outline

I. Introduction

This chapter provides a review of the regulations, policies, and standards governing the proper use of anesthesia, analgesia, tranquilizers, and other agents used to prevent or minimize pain and distress in animals used in research, teaching, and testing. It covers the Animal Welfare Act (AWA) and regulations, the Public Health Service (PHS) Policy on Humane Care and Use of Laboratory Animals (Policy), and the *Guide for the Care and Use of Laboratory Animals* (*Guide*). Information regarding the responsibilities of veterinarians, Institutional Animal Care and Use Committees (IACUCs), and research scientists for eliminating or controlling animal pain and distress are summarized. A brief overview of the U.S. federal regulations for the management and use of controlled substances, as well as occupational health and safety concerns associated with anesthetic and analgesic drug use, are also included along with a brief description of related international regulations and policies.

Anesthesia and Analgesia in Laboratory Animals. https://doi.org/10.1016/B978-0-12-822215-7.00014-7

II. Regulations, standards, and policies on humane animal care in the United States

A. Animal Welfare Act and Animal Welfare Regulations and Standards

The AWA was signed into law in August 1966. The original intent of the AWA was to protect pets, such as dogs and cats, from being stolen for use in research. Amendments to the AWA significantly expanded the scope of coverage. The AWA regulations and standards (AWA regulations) provide details on how to comply with the law. The amendments to AWA resulted in regulations that established minimum standards for the care and use of animals in research, teaching, and testing and added institutional responsibilities for oversight of animal care and use. The amendments also resulted in regulations for the sale, exhibition, and commercial transport of covered species. The AWA and regulations are enforced by the United States Department of Agriculture-Animal and Plant Health Inspection Service (USDA-APHIS). Compliance with the regulatory requirements under the AWA and AWA regulations is monitored through the inspection process conducted by APHIS-Animal Care. The inspections are unannounced, and the reports are available online to the public.

The AWA regulations provide minimum requirements for the humane handling, care, and treatment of dogs, cats, guinea pigs, hamsters, rabbits, nonhuman primates, and other warm-blooded species used in research, teaching, and testing. The AWA regulatory definition of "animal," however, specifically excludes from coverage rats of the genus *Rattus*, mice of the genus *Mus*, birds bred for research, and horses not used for research. It also excludes livestock/poultry used for food, fiber; or used or intended for use for improving animal nutrition, breeding management, or production efficiency; or for improving the quality of food or fiber. The AWA regulations require the provision of adequate veterinary care and outline the responsibilities for the attending veterinarian, the principal investigator (PI), and the research facility to minimize animal pain and distress.

To help assure the humane use of experimental animals, the 1985 amendment to the AWA required every animal research facility to establish a committee, designated under the AWA regulations as an IACUC, to assess the research facility's program of animal care, animal housing areas, procedures, and facilities. The members are appointed by the chief executive officer of the institution. At a minimum, the IACUC must be comprised of three members: a chairman; a veterinarian with training or experience in laboratory animal science and medicine, who has direct or delegated program responsibility for animal activities; and a nonaffiliated member who is not personally affiliated or has an immediate family member affiliated in any way with the facility. If the IACUC is comprised of more than three members, not more than three members are to be from the same administrative unit [9 C.F.R. Chapter 1 Subchapter A Section 2.31(b)].

Some of the functions of the IACUC are to review and approve or require modifications to secure approval of all proposed animal research activities or significant changes in those activities; investigate complaints, and suspend animal activities where warranted. Prior to approving the proposed research activity, the IACUC shall ensure that all aspects of the research will be conducted in accordance with the AWA and regulations, medical care is provided by a qualified veterinarian, and that animal pain and distress will be avoided or minimized [9 C.F.R. Chapter 1 Subchapter A Section 2.31(d)]. The IACUC also reviews the animal care and use program and conducts inspections of animal facilities and animal study areas. Animal study areas containing free-living wild animals in their natural habitat need not be inspected. A semiannual report is generated and submitted to the Institutional Official; the person authorized to legally commit on behalf of the facility that the AWA regulatory requirements will be met [9 C.F.R. Chapter 1 Subchapter A Section 2.31(c)].

The attending veterinarian for each research institution has the authority to ensure the provision of adequate veterinary care. Adequate veterinary care must include the availability of appropriate facilities, personnel, equipment, and services within the research institution; along with appropriate methods to prevent, control, diagnose, and treat diseases and injuries. Adequate veterinary care includes the availability of emergency, weekend, and holiday care. In addition, daily observations must occur to assess animal health and well-being. The attending veterinarian also provides guidance to the PI and other personnel associated with animal care and use on handling, immobilization, anesthesia, analgesia, tranquilization, and euthanasia. For surgical procedures, all pre and postprocedural care must be performed in accordance with currently established veterinary medical and nursing procedures (9 C.F.R. Chapter 1 Subchapter A Section 2.33).

If a procedure causes or may cause more than momentary or slight pain or distress, the PI is required to consider alternatives and involve a veterinarian in their planning to ensure appropriate sedatives, analgesics, or anesthetics are provided. The IACUC reviews proposed animal activities to ensure the procedure will be performed with appropriate use of pain-relieving agents. If these agents are withheld, withholding will only occur for a necessary period of time, and there must be a written scientific justification. No animal is to undergo more than one major operative procedure unless scientifically justified and approved by the IACUC, or in the case of a Special

Circumstance, approved by the IACUC and USDA-APHIS. In addition, the IACUC reviews proposed activities to determine whether the PI considered alternatives to procedures that cause more than momentary or slight pain. A written narrative is to be provided of the methods and sources used to determine that no alternatives were available. Animal activities are also reviewed to ensure paralytics are not used without anesthesia, appropriate pre and postoperative care for surgical procedures is provided in accordance with established nursing and veterinary practices, and euthanasia is addressed where appropriate. The method of euthanasia is to be in accordance with the definition as set forth in the AWA regulations unless a deviation is justified for scientific reasons by the PI in writing. Animals that would otherwise experience severe or chronic pain or distress that cannot be relieved must be painlessly euthanized during or at the end of the procedure [9 C.F.R. Chapter 1 Subchapter A Section 2.31(d)].

Facilities that use animals for research, teaching, testing, and experimentation are required under the AWA regulations to submit an annual report to USDA-APHIS that includes the numbers of animals used by species and the level of pain/distress experienced during the reporting period. The report is due December 1st, and encompasses the prior federal fiscal year, which is October 1st to September 30th of the following year. The pain/distress categories in summary are: procedures that involve no pain/distress or do not require pain-relieving drugs; procedures with accompanying pain/distress where appropriate anesthetics, analgesics, or tranquilizers were used; and procedures with accompanying pain/distress where appropriate anesthetics, analgesics, or tranquilizers were withheld because they would adversely affect procedures, results, or interpretation of results. An explanation of the procedures producing pain/distress along with the reason for withholding the appropriate pain-relieving drugs is to be included in the annual report [9 C.F.R. Chapter 1 Subchapter A Section 2.36]. Annual Reports are available online to the public.

In addition to the submission of the annual report, the research facility is responsible for ensuring all scientists, research technicians, animal technicians, and other personnel involved in animal care, treatment, and use, are qualified to perform their duties. Training and instruction must be made available, and qualifications reviewed with sufficient frequency to fulfill the facility's responsibility. Instruction must include guidance on (1) the humane methods of animal maintenance and experimentation; (2) the concept, availability, and use of research or testing methods that limit the use of animals or minimize animal distress; (3) the proper use of anesthetics, analgesics, and tranquilizers for animal species used by the facility, and (4) the utilization of services such as the National Agricultural Library (NAL) and the National Library of Medicine [9 C.F.R. Chapter 1 Subchapter A Section 2.32].

Regarding NAL services, it is a resource for information on the intent and requirements of the AWA, appropriate methods of animal care and use, and alternatives to the use of live animals in painful procedures during research, teaching, and testing. The use of these services could also provide information that would prevent unintended/unnecessary duplication of research involving animals. The Animal Welfare Information Center (AWIC) was established in 1986, as part of NAL. It is an information service to fulfill these functions. It offers free classroom and virtual instruction on performing literature searches for alternatives to live animal use in teaching, testing, and experimentation within the context of the Three Rs (reduction, replacement, and refinement). Its website serves as a resource for information that includes techniques on finding alternatives in the literature, provides information on technologies and approaches that highlight any of the Three Rs, and provides information on the reduction of pain/distress using anesthetics and analgesics. In addition, AWIC also serves as a resource for the history of the AWA and AWA regulations.

B. Public Health Service Policy on Humane Care and Use of Laboratory Animals

The Health Research Extension Act of 1985 (PL 99−158; HREA), Animals in Research, Section 495, mandates the Secretary of Health and Human Services to establish guidelines for the proper care and treatment of animals used in biomedical and behavioral research funded by the PHS. The Act specifically requires the appropriate use of tranquilizers, analgesics, anesthetics, paralytics, and euthanasia. It also outlines the organization and operation of animal care committees. The HREA provides the legislative mandate for the PHS Policy on Humane Care and Use of Laboratory Animals (Policy; olaw.nih.gov/policies-laws/phs-policy.htm), which was last updated in 2015. The National Institutes of Health (NIH) Office of Laboratory Animal Welfare (OLAW) provides guidance and interpretation on the PHS Policy, supports educational programs, and monitors compliance with the PHS Policy to ensure the humane care and use of laboratory animals.

The PHS Policy applies to research conducted or supported by several U.S. federal agencies, including PHS agencies (the National Institutes of Health, the Biomedical Advanced Research and Development Authority, the Centers for Disease Control and Prevention, and the Food and Drug Administration). Through memoranda of understanding with OLAW, the PHS Policy also applies to animal activities supported or conducted by the National Aeronautics and Space Administration, the National Science Foundation, and the Department of Veterans Affairs.

Minimum standards for humane animal care and use referenced in the PHS Policy require institutions to:

- Comply, as applicable, with the AWA and other federal statutes and regulations relating to animals.
- Endorse the United States Government Principles for the Utilization and Care of Vertebrate Animals used in testing, research, and training (United States Government Principles).
- Use the *Guide for the Care and Use of Laboratory Animals* (*Guide*) as a basis for developing and implementing an institutional program for activities involving animals.
- Use methods of euthanasia that are consistent with the recommendations of the most current edition of the American Veterinary Medical Association (AVMA) Guidelines for the Euthanasia of Animals unless a deviation is justified for scientific reasons in writing by the investigator and reviewed and approved by an IACUC.

The United States Government Principles were promulgated in 1985 and provide an ethical framework for conducting research in accordance with the PHS Policy. Three of the nine principles specifically address pain and distress in animals. United States Government Principle IV states that the "proper use of animals," including the avoidance or minimization of discomfort, distress, and pain when consistent with sound scientific practices, is imperative. "Unless the contrary is established, investigators should consider that procedures that cause pain or distress in human beings may cause pain or distress in other animals." Principle V further goes on to state that "Procedures with animals that may cause more than momentary or slight pain or distress should be performed with appropriate sedation, analgesia, or anesthesia." It further emphasizes that "Surgical or other painful procedures should not be performed on unanesthetized animals paralyzed by chemical agents." Principle VI states that "Animals that would otherwise suffer severe or chronic pain or distress that cannot be relieved should be painlessly killed at the end of the procedure or, if appropriate, during the procedure."

The PHS Policy III.B. defines an animal as "any live, vertebrate animal used or intended for use in research, research training, experimentation, biological testing, or for related purposes." The PHS Policy addresses the entire institutional program of animal care and use for these animals, not just the humane use of animals. The program must include, among other things, an Institutional Official (IO), an Institutional Animal Care and Use Committee (IACUC), a veterinarian with the authority and responsibility for the animals, provisions for adequate veterinary care, formal training for animal care and use personnel, an occupational health and safety program, and maintenance of animal facilities. The HREA and PHS Policy require research institutions to provide training for scientists, animal technicians, and others involved in animal care, treatment, or use. This training must include information on humane animal care and use, and research or training methods that would minimize the number of animals required to obtain valid results and minimize animal distress.

No activity involving animals may be conducted or supported by the agencies under OLAW's oversight authority, as listed above, until the institution conducting the activity has provided a written Assurance in compliance with the PHS Policy IV.A. to OLAW. For recipient organizations within the United States, the Assurance is a document describing the institution's proposed program for the care and use of animals and commits the institution to comply with the PHS Policy and standards listed above. It must also include a synopsis of the training that is offered to all animal users, including the humane practice of animal care and use, and research or testing methods that minimize animal pain and distress. Foreign institutions, with direct or indirect funding, must comply with the PHS Policy or provide evidence that acceptable standards for the humane care and use of animals will be met, including all laws, regulations, and policies in their jurisdiction. They must also follow the International Guiding Principles for Biomedical Research Involving Animals developed by the Council for International Organizations of Medical Sciences. These principles align closely with the United States Government Principles as they pertain to the minimization of pain and distress. In addition, OLAW conducts site visits to Assured institutions to assess the adequacy and accuracy of an institution's compliance with the PHS Policy. Site visits may be announced or random and unannounced, and may, on occasion, result from a risk assessment based on reports of noncompliance or review of Assurance documents and Annual Reports to OLAW. Site visits may be conducted in collaboration with the USDA and may be conducted with, or by request of other government agencies or funding components.

The intent of the PHS Policy is to have a diversity of perspectives in IACUC membership, and the members are appointed by the Chief Executive Officer of the institution. The IACUC must consist of no fewer than five members (PHS Policy IV.A.3.) and include: at least one Doctor of Veterinary Medicine with training or experience in laboratory animal science and medicine; one practicing scientist experienced in research involving animals; one member whose primary concerns are in a nonscientific area (e.g., ethicist, lawyer), and one individual who is not affiliated with the institution in any other way than as an IACUC member.

The responsibilities of the IACUC are described in PHS Policy IV.B. and include conducting program reviews and facility inspections and submitting the resulting reports to the IO at least once every 6 months, using the *Guide* as a basis for the evaluation. The IACUC is also responsible for making recommendations to the IO on any aspect of the animal program, facilities, or personnel training. Additionally, it reviews concerns involving the care and use of animals and can authorize the suspension of an animal activity, including for animal welfare concerns.

Another critical function of the IACUC is to review and approve, require modification to secure approval, or withhold approval for animal research activities. PHS Policy IV.C. requires the IACUC to review each proposed animal research project or proposed significant change in an ongoing research project to ensure it is conducted in accordance with the AWA, is consistent with the *Guide*, and conforms with the institution's Assurance. As part of the review, the IACUC must determine that procedures with animals will avoid or minimize discomfort, distress, and pain to the animals, consistent with sound research design. If procedures cause more than momentary or slight pain or distress, they must also be performed with appropriate sedation, analgesia, or anesthesia, unless justified for scientific reasons in writing by the investigator. Whether the procedure is classified as major or minor, the IACUC must ensure that the appropriate analgesia, sterile technique, and perioperative monitoring are employed.

If animals would experience severe or chronic pain or distress that cannot be relieved, they should be euthanized at the end of the procedure, or, if appropriate, during the procedure. The living conditions for research animals also need to be appropriate for their species and contribute to their health and comfort.

The housing, feeding, and nonmedical care of the animals must be directed by a veterinarian or other scientist trained and experienced in the proper care, handling, and use of the species being maintained or studied. Medical care for animals must also be available and provided as necessary by a qualified veterinarian, and personnel conducting animal procedures need to be appropriately qualified and trained in those procedures. Veterinary consultation must occur when pain or distress is beyond the level anticipated in the protocol description or when interventional control is not possible (*Guide*, p. 5). Because of wide individual variation in response to analgesics, regardless of the initial plan for pain relief, animals should be closely monitored during and after painful procedures and should receive additional drugs, as needed, to ensure appropriate analgesic management (*Guide*, p. 122). Lastly, the methods of euthanasia must be consistent with the recommendations of the AVMA Guidelines for the Euthanasia of Animals, unless a deviation is scientifically justified.

Applications and proposals for awards submitted to the agencies listed above that involve the care and use of animals must include the species and approximate number of animals to be used, the rationale for involving animals, and the appropriateness of the species and numbers used. It is incumbent that investigators include a complete description of the proposed animal use with special consideration of procedures designed to assure that discomfort and injury to animals will be limited to that which is unavoidable and that analgesic, anesthetic, and tranquilizing drugs will be used where indicated and appropriate to minimize discomfort and pain to animals. Prior to award, PHS Policies IV.D.2. and V.B., require recipient institutions to verify to the funding agency that the IACUC has reviewed and approved the components of applications and proposals related to the care and use of animals.

Importantly, the PHS Policy is based on the concept of enforced self-regulation. Institutions are required to report to OLAW, through the IO:

1. Reports of any serious or continuing noncompliance with the PHS Policy,
2. Serious deviations from the *Guide*, or
3. Suspension of an activity by the IACUC.

If the institution fails to self-regulate, the Assurance may be restricted or withdrawn by OLAW. Noncompliance with 1-3 above, regardless of whether it involves pain or distress, is reportable to OLAW.

C. Guide for the Care and Use of Laboratory Animals

The *Guide for the Care and Use of Laboratory Animals* (the *Guide*), last published in 2011, is a document written and published by the Institute for Laboratory Animal Research (ILAR), National Research Council, that establishes the minimum ethical, practical, and care standards for researchers and their institution to promote the humane care and use of laboratory animals (*Guide*, p. 1). It provides information to enhance animal well-being, the quality of research, and the advancement of scientific knowledge that is relevant to both humans and animals, and establishes performance standards for the care and use of all vertebrate animals (*Guide*, p. 2). The *Guide* asserts that all who care for, use, or produce animals for research, testing, or teaching must assume responsibility for their well-being (*Guide*, p. 1). The *Guide* was developed by scientists and veterinarians for scientists and veterinarians to uphold the scientific rigor and integrity of biomedical research with laboratory animals as expected by their colleagues and society at large (*Guide*, p. 1).

The *Guide* considers regulatory requirements relevant to many United States-based activities, including the Animal Welfare Regulations (AWR), the PHS Policy on Humane Care and Use of Laboratory Animals (Policy), and the United States Government Principles for the Utilization and Care of Vertebrate Animals Used in Testing, Research, and Training. The use of the *Guide* by non-United States entities also presumes adherence to all regulations relevant to the humane care and use of laboratory animals applicable in those locations (*Guide*, p. 12). The *Guide* recommendations are based on published data, scientific principles, and expert opinions. It is recognized by both the PHS and Association for Assessment and Accreditation of Laboratory Animal Care International (AAALAC International) as a primary reference on which to build and evaluate programs of laboratory animal care and use. In the *Guide*, laboratory animals (also referred to as 'animals') are generally defined as any vertebrate animal (i.e., traditional laboratory animals, agricultural animals, wildlife, and aquatic species) produced for or used in research, testing, or teaching. Animal use is defined as the proper care, use, and humane treatment of laboratory animals produced for or used in research, testing, or teaching (*Guide*, p. 2).

The *Guide* is a comprehensive document that requires an animal care and use program that comprises all activities conducted at an institution with direct impact on animal well-being and personnel safety. This includes key concepts (e.g., ethical considerations), animal and veterinary care, policies and procedures, personnel and program management and oversight, occupational health and safety, IACUC functions, and animal facility design and management (*Guide*, p. 11). Similar to the AWR and the PHS Policy, the *Guide* holds the research institution responsible for ensuring that all personnel involved with the care and use of animals, including investigators, technical personnel, trainees, and visiting investigators are qualified through education, training, and/or experience to accomplish their tasks in a humane and scientifically justifiable manner. Each institution should provide and document formal or on-the-job training to implement an effective and humane program of animal care and use. This may include but not be limited to husbandry, surgical procedures, species-specific behaviors (e.g., signs of pain or distress), and humane endpoints.

Although the role of the IACUC described in the *Guide* remains congruent with its responsibilities as described in the AWRs and the PHS Policy, the *Guide* contrasts with the AWRs and the PHS Policy in that it does not specify a minimum number of members but suggests that the size of the institution, nature, and extent of the program will determine the number of committee members (*Guide*, p. 25). According to the *Guide*, the IACUC includes a doctor of veterinary medicine, at least one practicing scientist experienced in research involving animals, at least one member from a nonscientific background either affiliated or not affiliated with the institution, and at least one public member to represent general community interests (*Guide*, p. 24).

The *Guide* reinforces that veterinary care is an essential part of an animal care and use program and specifies the responsibility of the veterinarian. The primary focus of the veterinarian is to oversee the well-being and clinical care of animals used in research, testing, teaching, and production. This responsibility extends to monitoring and promoting animal well-being during all phases of the animal's life (*Guide*, p. 11). Well-being is determined by considering physical, physiologic, and behavioral indicators, which vary by species. Institutions must provide a veterinarian with the authority, resources, and access to all animals to manage the program effectively (*Guide*, p. 14). An effective veterinary medical program assesses animal welfare and effective management of surgery and perioperative care, pain and distress, anesthesia and analgesia, and euthanasia. It also assesses and manages clinical or protocol related disease or disability, and surgery and perioperative care (*Guide*, pp. 105–106).

The *Guide* acknowledges, "pain is a stressor and, if not relieved, can lead to unacceptable levels of stress and distress in animals" (*Guide*, p. 120). It also emphasizes United States Government Principle IV, that unless the contrary is known or established, if a procedure would cause pain in humans, it may cause pain in animals. The *Guide* goes on to state that unrelieved pain may lead to allodynia, and for these reasons, providing proper use of anesthetics and analgesics is an ethical and scientific imperative (*Guide*, p. 120).

Investigators preparing animal use protocols and IACUC members reviewing such protocols must consider the impact of the proposed procedures on the animals' well-being, the conduct of surgical procedures, and must consider alternative, less-invasive procedures to avoid pain or distress. The IACUC must also ensure the adequacy of training and experience of personnel performing the procedure. In addition, the IACUC must confirm that the protocol: (1) includes the use of appropriate sedation, analgesia, and anesthesia; (2) provides proper pre and postprocedural care; (3) articulates the criteria and process for timely intervention to minimize pain and distress, if necessary; and (4) describes the endpoints for removal of animals from a study. Lastly, euthanasia should be conducted if unrelieved painful or stressful outcomes are anticipated (*Guide*, pp. 25–26).

Minimization of pain, stress, and distress may be accomplished, in part, by providing proper guidance on appropriate animal handling, immobilization, and euthanasia to all research and husbandry personnel involved in animal care and use. Veterinary medical guidance or oversight of surgery programs and pre and postsurgical care is essential to prevent or minimize pain. Providing preoperative or intraoperative analgesia is encouraged as it may improve patient pain relief and well-being after surgery. Guidelines for the selection and proper use of analgesic and anesthetic drugs should be developed and periodically reviewed and updated as standards and techniques are refined (*Guide*, p. 122). Agents that provide anesthesia and analgesia must be used before their expiration dates and should be acquired, stored, their use recorded, and disposed of legally and safely (*Guide*, p. 122). Some classes of drugs such as sedatives, anxiolytics, and neuromuscular blocking agents may not provide analgesia but may be useful when used in combination with appropriate analgesics and anesthetics to provide balanced anesthesia and to minimize stress associated with perioperative procedures (*Guide*, p. 122–123). It is imperative to ensure that a variety of vital signs are closely monitored to ensure complete absence of painful responses. Nonpharmacological control of pain is also emphasized as an element of post or perioperative care. Such care may include providing a quiet, darkened recovery area, a warm and soft resting place, rehydration with fluids, and highly palatable foods or treats (*Guide*, p. 122).

The *Guide* also has expectations regarding the use of nonpharmaceutical-grade substances (*Guide*, p. 31). A pharmaceutical-grade substance is any active or inactive drug, biologic, reagent, etc., manufactured under Good Manufacturing Practices (GMP) which is approved, conditionally approved, or indexed by the Food and Drug Administration (FDA) or for which a chemical purity standard has been written or established by a recognized compendium (e.g., United States Pharmacopeia-National Formulary, British Pharmacopeia). A listing of pharmaceutical-grade drugs and biologics is available through an FDA database (https://www.fda.gov/drugs/development-approval-process-drugs/drug-approvals-and-databases). Pharmaceutical-grade substances, when available, should be used to avoid toxicity or side effects that may threaten the health and welfare of vertebrate animals and/or interfere with the interpretation of research results. However, it may be necessary to use nonpharmaceutical-grade substances such as investigational substances, veterinarian- or pharmacy-compounded substances, and/or Schedule I controlled substances to meet scientific and research goals. Veterinary compounding is the customized manipulation of an approved drug by a veterinarian, or by a pharmacist upon the prescription of a veterinarian, to meet the needs of a research study. The use of nonpharmaceutical-grade chemicals or substances should be described and justified in the animal use protocol and be approved by the IACUC (Wolff et al., 2003). The IACUC is responsible for evaluating the potential adverse consequences of nonpharmaceutical-grade substances when used for research. The evaluation may consider factors including grade, purity, sterility, acid-base balance, pyrogenicity, osmolality, stability, site and route of administration, compatibility of components, side effects and adverse reactions, storage, and pharmacokinetics, as well as animal welfare and scientific issues relating to its use (NIH, 2008).

D. AAALAC International

AAALAC International is a private, nonprofit organization that promotes the humane treatment of animals in science. The AAALAC accreditation program started in 1965 as an activity of the American Association for the Accreditation of Laboratory Animal Care, which accredited institutional animal care and use programs throughout the United States. In 1996, the name was changed to underscore that AAALAC International accredits institutional animal care and use programs around the world. This voluntary accreditation and assessment program is based primarily on the principles outlined in Three Primary Standards: the *Guide for the Care and Use of Laboratory Animals*, the *Guide for the Care and Use of Agricultural Animals in Research and Teaching*, and the European Convention for the Protection of Vertebrate Animals Used for Experimental and Other Scientific Purposes, Council of Europe (ETS 123).

Other references listed on the AAALAC International website (https://www.aaalac.org) may also be used as the basis for assessing animal care and use programs and include species-specific resources such as cephalopod, nonhuman primate, and wild animal guidelines. AAALAC International publishes position statements that can be used as supplemental guidance related to the use of farm animals in research, occupational health and safety, and adequate veterinary care.

AAALAC International recognizes that veterinary care is an essential part of an animal care program and supports the regulations and policies that require the veterinarian to either be board certified by the American College of Laboratory Animal Medicine or have training or experience in laboratory animal science and medicine in the species being housed and used. The veterinarian should also contribute to the establishment of appropriate policies and procedures for ancillary aspects of veterinary care. The veterinarian must provide guidance to all personnel involved in the care and use of animals to ensure appropriate animal handling, immobilization, sedation, analgesia, anesthesia, and euthanasia, as well as provide oversight of animal surgery, and pre and postsurgical care.

By attaining AAALAC International accreditation, a research institution demonstrates that it has established practices that meet or exceed existing regulations and standards to achieve excellence in animal care and use. Institutions that apply for AAALAC accreditation must provide a written program description covering: (1) institutional policies and responsibilities; (2) animal environment, housing, and management; (3) veterinary medical care; and (4) physical plant. Under the section on veterinary medical care, surgical activities, assessment of animal pain and distress, use of analgesia and anesthesia, euthanasia methods, and drug storage and control are described in detail.

A pharmaceutical-grade compound is defined as any active or inactive drug, biologic, or reagent for which a chemical purity standard has been established by a recognized national or regional pharmacopeia (e.g., the United States Pharmacopeia [USP], the British Pharmacopeia [BP], the National Formulary [NF], the European Pharmacopoeia [EP], the Japanese Pharmacopeia [JP], etc.). These standards are used by manufacturers to help ensure that products are of the appropriate chemical purity and quality, in the appropriate solution or compound, to ensure stability, safety, and efficacy.

AAALAC International acknowledges that in an animal care and use program nonpharmaceutical-grade compounds may be necessary for scientific research. AAALAC expects that the IACUC or comparable oversight body has established acceptable criteria for use of such compounds within the institution and for review and approval of their use.

AAALAC International also acknowledges that it is a common veterinary practice to mix and/or dilute pharmaceutical-grade drugs. Once a drug has been adulterated by dilution, addition, or undergone change in formulation outside of the product insert instructions, it is classified as nonpharmaceutical grade (NPG) because the altered product no longer falls into one of the major pharmacopeias. AAALAC expects the institution to establish criteria for review and approval of this drug product use, and develop referenced guidelines on drug labeling and storage. In addition, an appropriate use-by-date should be established, with consideration given to the formulation's sterility, compatibility, and efficacy (see AAALAC FAQ on nonpharmaceutical-grade compounds).

E. Institutional policies

Each research institution should develop, communicate, and implement policies that support the humane care and use of animals within their institution. These policies should help to assure compliance with applicable laws, regulations, and policies, and address the specific requirements of the institution. The scope and complexity of institutional policies will depend on the nature of the research and species of animals used and may exceed the minimal regulatory requirements. For example, an institution may appoint more than the minimal number of members required to serve on the IACUC. Institutional policies may also address the specific provisions for preventing pain or distress and the use of pain-relieving agents. Another example would be a policy outlining the institution-specific process for IACUC review of concerns involving the care and use of animals. As described in the AWA regulations, these concerns may result from public complaints received and from reports of noncompliance received by research facility personnel or employees. This may include investigating inappropriate use of anesthetics or analgesics or withholding the use of pain-relieving agents when it is warranted.

III. Drug enforcement regulations and policies

Many of the agents used to prevent or minimize pain in laboratory animals are subject to laws and regulations that govern their manufacture, importation, possession, and distribution. In general, these agents are referred to as "controlled substances." There are three tiers of law that provide the structure governing the medical use and diversion of controlled substances: international conventions, federal laws and regulations, and state laws and regulations. These laws are supplemented by policy statements on the responsible use of controlled substances by various veterinary and medical practitioner organizations and state and federal governmental departments.

A. International conventions

There are three main international drug control conventions that govern the international manufacture, use, and distribution of controlled substances: the 1961 Single Convention on Narcotic Drugs, the 1971 Convention on Psychotropic Substances (also known as the Vienna Convention), and the United Nations Convention Against Illicit Traffic in Narcotic Drugs and Psychotropic Substances of 1988. The United Nations Commission on Narcotic Drugs is responsible for maintaining and updating the controlled drug schedules in these conventions.

B. Federal laws and regulations

The Drug Enforcement Administration (DEA) within the Department of Justice was established in 1973 as the primary federal agency responsible for the enforcement of federal drug laws in the United States. It is responsible for enforcing the Controlled Substances Act of 1970 (CSA; Title 21 United States Code [USC]), which places all substances which were in some manner regulated under existing federal law into one of five schedules. This placement is based upon various factors related to the substance's medical use, the potential for abuse, and safety or dependence liability (21 USC §811(c)). The Pharmacist's Manual (Revised, 2020; https://www.deadiversion.usdoj.gov/pubs/index.html), published by the DEA, Diversion Control Division, is a comprehensive document intended to summarize and explain the basic requirements for prescribing, administering, and dispensing controlled substances. Individuals establishing controlled substance record-keeping and acquisition systems for a laboratory animal facility should consult this document.

1. *Controlled Substances Act, Title 21 CFR*

The Controlled Substances Act (CSA) sets forth the federal laws regarding both legitimate and illicit use of controlled substances. The CSA establishes five categories of controlled substances, referred to as Schedules I through V. The schedule on which a controlled substance is placed determines the level of restriction imposed on its production, distribution, and possession, as well as the penalties applicable to any improper handling of the substance. A lower schedule number corresponds to greater restrictions, so controlled substances in Schedule I are subject to the most stringent controls, while substances in Schedule V are subject to the least stringent. An alphabetical listing of controlled substances can be found here: https://www.dea.gov/drug-information/drug-scheduling.

2. *Food, Drug, and Cosmetic Act*

Drugs classified as controlled substances subject to the CSA are also subject to other legal regimes. For example, all drugs, including those subject to the CSA, are subject to the Federal Food, Drug, and Cosmetic Act (FD&C Act). The United States Food and Drug Administration (FDA) is the agency primarily responsible for enforcing the FD&C Act.

The key aims of the FD&C Act are related to but distinct from those of the CSA. The CSA establishes distribution controls to prevent the misuse of substances deemed to pose a potential danger to the public welfare. The FD&C Act, by contrast, is a consumer protection statute that seeks to protect consumers from obtaining unsafe or ineffective drugs (and other public health products) through commercial channels. Any person or organization that produces, distributes, or otherwise works with prescription drugs that are also controlled substances must comply with the requirements of both the CSA and the FD&C Act.

FDA-approved animal drugs are reviewed for safety—including safety to the animal, safety of food products derived from the animal, safety to persons administering the drug or otherwise associated with the animal, and safety to the environment. They are also reviewed for effectiveness, meaning that the FDA evaluates evidence that the product will consistently and uniformly do what the labeling claims it will do (https://www.fda.gov/animal-veterinary/resources-you/fda-regulation-animal-drugs). Most FDA-approved animal drugs are included in a searchable publicly available list. This list is known as the Green Book, and FDA updates it in its entirety every month (https://animaldrugsatfda.fda.gov/adafda/views/#/search). It contains information about patents and exclusivity periods, and it is divided into sections that list approved animal drugs alphabetically by trade name, numerically by application number, and alphabetically by active ingredient.

The Animal Medicinal Drug Use Clarification Act of 1994 (AMDUCA) permits veterinarians to prescribe extra-label uses of certain approved new animal drugs and approved human drugs for animals under certain conditions. Extra-label use refers to the use of an approved drug in a manner that is not in accordance with the approved label directions. Under AMDUCA and its implementing regulations published at Title 21, Code of Federal Regulations, Part 530 (21 CFR 530), any extra-label use of an approved new animal or human drug must be by or on the lawful order of a veterinarian within the context of a valid veterinarian-client-patient relationship. Extra-label use must also comply with other provisions of 21 CFR 530. A list of drugs specifically prohibited from extra-label use appears in 21 CFR 530.41 (https://www.fda.gov/animal-veterinary/guidance-regulations/animal-medicinal-drug-use-clarification-act-1994-amduca). Information on marketed animal and human drugs, including their labeling, is available on a site hosted by the NIH, DailyMed, https://dailymed.nlm.nih.gov/dailymed/index.cfm.

Conditional approval allows certain new animal drugs to become available before the sponsor collects all effectiveness data necessary for approval of a new animal drug application (NADA), but after proving the drug is safe in accordance with the full FDA approval standard and showing that there is a reasonable expectation of effectiveness. Conditional approval is available for drugs for minor uses or minor species. A minor use is the intended use of a drug in a major species for an indication that occurs infrequently only in a small number of animals, annually, or in limited geographical areas and in only a small number of animals, annually (Section 201(pp) of the FD&C Act (21 U.S.C. § 321(pp))). Minor species are animals other than humans that are not major species (Section 201 (oo) of the FD&C Act). Major species are dogs, cats, horses, pigs, cattle, turkeys, and chickens (Section 201 (nn) of the FD&C Act). FDA may permit the drug sponsor to keep the conditionally approved new animal drug on the market for up to 5 years, through annual renewals, while collecting the remaining required effectiveness data. Guidance for Industry 261, Eligibility Criteria for Expanded Conditional Approval of New Animal Drugs, also introduced expanded conditional approval. For these drugs, eligibility for conditional approval was expanded beyond minor uses in major species and use in minor species to include certain major uses in major species to incentivize the development of new animal drugs for serious or life-threatening conditions or unmet animal or human health needs where demonstration of effectiveness would require a complex or particularly difficult study or studies.

The index of legally marketed unapproved new animal drugs for minor species (the Index) is a list of new animal drugs that have had their safety and effectiveness affirmed through an alternative FDA review process that includes a report from an outside panel of experts. The Index is available only for new animal drugs intended for use in nonfood-producing minor species. In many cases, drug products intended for use in these species cannot reasonably go through the standard drug approval process. These species may be too rare or varied to be used in traditional safety and effectiveness studies. The Index is especially helpful to individuals treating animals or classes of animals representing markets too small to support the costs of the drug approval process, even with the incentives of the minor use and minor Species (MUMS) Animal Health Act of 2004. Examples include exotic pets, zoo animals, and laboratory rodents.

The extra-label use of medicated feeds conditionally approved and indexed animal drugs is not legal.

Drug compounding is the process of combining, mixing, or altering ingredients to create a medication tailored to the needs of an individual animal or a small group of animals. These drug formulations can play a critical role in veterinary medicine. Compounded animal drugs are typically made by pharmacists or veterinarians. Under the FD&C Act, compounding of animal drugs is legal only when the source of the active ingredient is a finished FDA-approved drug, because such compounding is considered an extra-label use of an approved drug.

While there are cases in which FDA-approved animal or human drugs can be used to treat an animal under the extra-label use provisions of the FD&C Act and related regulations, FDA recognizes that there are circumstances in which no FDA-approved, conditionally approved, or indexed drug (including the extra-label use of an FDA-approved animal or human drug) can be used to treat an animal with a particular condition. In those limited circumstances, an animal drug compounded from bulk drug substances may be a medically appropriate treatment. The FDA regulations define a bulk drug substance and an active pharmaceutical ingredient as "any substance that is intended for incorporation into a finished drug product and is intended to furnish pharmacological activity or other direct effects in the diagnosis, cure, mitigation, treatment, or prevention of disease, or to affect the structure or any function of the body." The terms do not include intermediates used in the synthesis of the substance (21 CFR 207.1).

Because of the safety benefits and protections of the premarket review process and postmarket monitoring of FDA-approved, conditionally approved, and indexed drugs, veterinarians should only use drugs compounded from bulk drug substances if FDA-approved, conditionally approved, or indexed drugs cannot be used to treat the animal. Animal drugs compounded from bulk drug substances have not been reviewed by the FDA for evidence that they are safe, effective, properly manufactured, and accurately labeled. Further, when the compounded drug is for a food-producing animal, the FDA has not reviewed the evidence supporting the conditions of use to protect against harmful drug residues in edible products from that animal. Finally, unlike sponsors of approved, conditionally approved, or indexed animal drugs, compounders are not required to report to the FDA adverse events and product defects regarding animal drugs compounded from bulk drug substances.

Under the FD&C Act, compounding from bulk substances results in a violative product. However, the FDA has generally refrained from taking enforcement action against animal drugs compounded from bulk drug substances under certain circumstances when no other medically appropriate treatment options exist.

In November 2019, FDA issued Draft Guidance for Industry (GFI) #256, Compounding Animal Drugs From Bulk Drug Substances. When finalized, the guidance will describe the types of drugs compounded from bulk drugs substances that the FDA has determined present the greatest risk to human and animal health and intends to prioritize for enforcement action. The draft guidance identifies these as drugs that:

- Present particular human or animal safety concerns
- Are intended for use in food-producing animals
- Are copies of marketed FDA-approved, conditionally approved, or indexed drugs, or
- Are compounded without a patient-specific prescription (i.e., office stock).

The GFI, when finalized, will also describe the circumstances under which the FDA does not generally intend to take enforcement action against drugs compounded from bulk drug substances for violations of the FD&C Act's approval requirements and certain other requirements. As drafted, the GFI separately describes these circumstances for drugs compounded:

- To fill patient-specific prescriptions for nonfood-producing animals
- As office stock to be kept on hand by a veterinarian to treat nonfood-producing animals, and
- Antidotes for food-producing animals.

The draft guidance can be found at https://www.fda.gov/animal-veterinary/animal-drug-compounding/qa-draft-gfi-256-compounding-animal-drugs-bulk-drug-substances. As of this writing, the FDA is reviewing the public comments and revising the guidance to issue it in its final form, at which time it will be implemented.

C. State regulations

There is not a complete overlap between drugs subject to federal and state control for several reasons. First, states may elect to impose controls on substances that are not subject to the CSA. Second, states may wish to adopt federal scheduling decisions at the state level but lag behind federal regulators due to the need for a separate state scheduling process. Third, states may decide not to impose state controls on substances subject to the CSA, or they may choose to impose modified versions of federal controls at the state level.

Crucially, however, the states cannot alter federal law, and when state and federal law conflict, the federal law controls. Thus, when states "legalize" or "decriminalize" a federally controlled substance (as many have done recently with respect to marijuana), the sole result is that the substance is no longer controlled *under state law*. Any federal controls remain in effect and potentially enforceable in those states.

The National Association of State Controlled Substances Authorities (NASCSA; nascsa.org) consists of agencies that oversee the controlled substances in nearly all 50 states. Their website includes state-controlled substance contacts, and state profiles, including state statutes, rules, and DEA exceptions. State agencies should be contacted directly, also, to ensure the most current statutes and rules are adhered to.

D. Institutional policies

Institutions may develop specific policies to enforce the relevant laws regarding controlled substances. For example, the institution may establish policies that identify specific requirements for employees who are responsible for the receipt, storage, and record-keeping of controlled substances, according to the regulations. They may also determine specifically which employees are permitted to administer controlled substances under the institution's DEA license.

IV. Occupational health and safety considerations

An important component of any animal care and use program is the consideration of occupational health and safety. Each activity should be undertaken only after accurately identifying and taking appropriate steps to prevent accidents and injuries.

A. Anesthetic safety issues

The United States Occupational Safety and Health Administration (OSHA) works to ensure safe and healthful working conditions for workers by setting and enforcing standards and by providing training, outreach, education, and assistance. OSHA establishes many hazard-specific safety and health standards. Although OSHA standards do not specifically address waste anesthetic gases, which may expose personnel to health hazards during research procedures, they do address chemicals relevant to anesthetics, such as nitrous oxide, chloroform, enflurane, halothane, and isoflurane (osha.gov/waste-anesthetic-gases/hazards). Chemical-specific details for sampling and exposure limits may be found in the OSHA Occupational Chemical Database. OSHA recognizes that many of its permissible exposure limits (PELs) are outdated and inadequate for ensuring the protection of worker health. Therefore, although OSHA's mandatory PELs remain in effect, the agency recommends that employers consider using the following alternative occupational exposure limits: California Division of Occupational Safety and Health (Cal/OSHA) PELs, National Institute for Occupational Safety and Health recommended exposure limits, and ACGIH threshold limit values and biological exposure indices. These alternative exposure limits are presented side-by-side in OSHA's annotated PELs tables, known as Z-Tables (osha.gov/annotated-pels). There are also 28 OSHA-approved State Plans which may address waste anesthetic gases. State Plans are required to have standards and enforcement programs that are at least as effective as OSHA's and may have different or more stringent requirements (https://www.osha.gov/waste-anesthetic-gases/standards).

An effective waste anesthetic gas management program should be designed and implemented where gas anesthesia is utilized in a research facility. This program should not only provide for environmental mechanisms for adequate WAG scavenging to minimize employee exposure but also include a written hazard communication program. Additionally, monitoring of the environment should be performed either continuously or periodically.

OSHA also maintains standards for the storage and use of compressed gases in any number of work scenarios. These industry standards from 29 CFR 1910 should be utilized in determining the proper storage conditions of compressed gas cylinders as well as the procedures to secure cylinders in use. Many states have additional standards and policies regarding the storage and use of compressed gas cylinders, some of which are OSHA-approved and similar to those standards set forth by federal OSHA guidelines. Refer to each individual state's statutes for applicable guidelines for your state, available at osha.gov/compressed-gas-equipment.

B. Needle and syringe safety issues

In 1991, OSHA issued the Bloodborne Pathogens Standard (29 CFR 1910.1030). In response to the Needlestick Safety and Prevention Act (PL 106–430, 2000), the Bloodborne Pathogens Standard was revised in 2001 to provide standards for using safer needle devices and requiring logs of sharps-related injuries (osha.gov/needlesticks/needlefaq.html).

C. Drug abuse regulations and issues

Opioid misuse and related overdoses led the United States Department of Health and Human Services to declare a public health emergency to address the national opioid crisis in 2017 (https://www.hhs.gov/opioids/about-the-epidemic/index.html). Because of their access and ability to prescribe opioids, physicians, pharmacists, and veterinarians may be affected by the epidemic of opioid abuse. They also have an important role to play in preventing the diversion of opioids for misuse (Mason et al., 2018). The FDA suggests the following to veterinarians to protect themselves, their staff, and their clients: (1) follow all state regulations on prescribing opioids; (2) follow all federal regulations on prescribing opioids; (3) use alternatives to opioids; (4) educate pet owners on safe storage and disposal of opioids; (5) know what to do if a dog overdoses on fentanyl or other opioids; and (6) have a safety plan and know the signs of opioid abuse (https://www.fda.gov/animal-veterinary/resources-you/opioid-epidemic-what-veterinarians-need-know).

The United States Department of Health and Human Services, Substance Abuse and Mental Health Services Administration, provides a drug-free workplace toolkit, which provides step-by-step guidance for starting and maintaining drug-free workplace policies and programs (samhsa.gov/workplace).

V. International considerations

International collaborations in research are increasing, and there is thus a need to be familiar with standards of oversight in different countries. There is no single concise global summary of laws, guidelines, and policies, but there is a steady evolution towards enhanced oversight with a focus on ethical review and implementing the principles of the Three Rs. This is reinforced by the World Organization for Animal Health (OIE), whose 182 member countries, in 2018, signed up to Chapter 7.8 of the Terrestrial Animal Health Code outlining the principles for the use of animals in research and education. For a comprehensive overview of global legislation, regulations, and policies, please see Bayne et al., (2021).

A. Canada

Canada does not have federal legislation on the use of animals in science, as animal welfare is a provincial responsibility (Cloutier, 2018). The Canadian Council on Animal Care (CCAC) is a national nonprofit organization responsible for establishing, maintaining, and overseeing the implementation of standards for animal care and the use of programs that work with animals for research, teaching, and testing (CCAC, 2015). While CCAC certification is not mandatory on a federal level, institutions receiving funds from federal granting agencies (the Canadian Institutes of Health Research, the Natural Sciences and Engineering Research Council of Canada, and the Social Sciences and Humanities Research Council of Canada) and conducting animal-based research must be CCAC certified. Further, the Canadian Food Inspection Agency imposes conformance with CCAC standards as part of the agency's requirements for the importation of nonhuman primates and other species into Canada and veterinary biologics guidelines. Currently, eight provinces make specific references to CCAC standards in their provincial regulations (CCAC, 2006, 2016a). A more detailed review of CCAC creation and function is available in the *Management of Animal Care and Use in Research, Education, and Testing* (Cloutier, 2018).

The CCAC establishes guidelines and policies categorized as General Guidelines (e.g., antibody production, endpoints, euthanasia, husbandry, etc.) and Types of Animals (e.g., amphibians, cats, dogs, various rodents, nonhuman primates, etc.; see https://www.ccac.ca/en/standards/guidelines/). These standards are developed with input from subcommittees of experts and undergo extensive peer and public review. The Three Rs are embedded and are at the heart of all CCAC standards (Cloutier, 2018). In addition to the development of its own guidelines and standards, the CCAC also references these additional documents:

- Canadian Association for Laboratory Animal Medicine (CALAM) Standards of Veterinary Care (CALAM, 2020).
- The National Farm Animal Care COA Codes of Practice for the Care and Handling of Farm Animals.
- The Public Health Agency and Canadian Food Inspection Agency Canadian Biosafety Standards and Guidelines.
- The Canadian Food Inspection Agency Containment Standards for Facilities Handling Aquatic Animal Pathogens.

CCAC standards place the responsibility for institutional program oversight with the Animal Care Committee (ACC). The ACC must be minimally composed of a veterinarian, community representative, scientist/instructor, institutional nonanimal user, a facility manager, a technical staff representative, and the ACC coordinator. The ACC must ensure that no work involving animals occurs prior to the approval of the protocol, scientific merit is obtained, protocols respect all applicable guidelines and policies, appropriate veterinary care is available, and institutional SOPs and policies are developed and reviewed every 3 years.

Regarding anesthesia and analgesia, the CCAC has various overlapping guidelines, including on Categories of Welfare Impact (under review), Scientific Humane Intervention Points and Cumulative Endpoints (under review),

Animal Welfare Assessment, and Experimental Procedures (Part B—Analgesia, Anesthesia, and Surgery). All of these guidelines consider that all vertebrate animals have the capacity to feel pain and that society has a scientific, ethical, and moral imperative to relieve that pain whenever possible. Overall guidance is provided on ways to assess pain in animals, as well as the collaborative process required to select appropriate anesthetics and analgesics for scientific work involving animals. The species-specific guidelines provide some additional information for ACCs to use when evaluating the appropriateness of the regimens selected for specific species and the procedure they will undergo.

The CCAC also has an assessment and certification program whereby panels of experts conduct on-site reviews on a 6-year basis, and interim visits are conducted mid-cycle (at 3 years) by a smaller review panel. Assessments of animal care and use programs are based on the CCAC guidelines, policies, and other reference documents. Based on the assessment, institutions in compliance with CCAC guidelines and policies may receive a CCAC Certificate of Good Animal Practice (GAP). Sustained noncompliance with CCAC standards can ultimately result in withdrawal of all federal animal-based research funding to the institution and/or limit the importation of some species by the institution.

Combinations of federal, provincial, and municipal laws are also in place for the use of controlled substances as well as occupational health and safety programs. Each certified institution is responsible for ensuring compliance with these regulations.

B. Europe

1. European Union

In 1986, the Council of Ministries of the European Economic Communities (EEC) adopted Directive 86/609/EEC for the Protection of Vertebrates Used for Experimental and Other Scientific Purposes. Although the main intention was to harmonize practices throughout the European Union (EU), various differing practices remained. As new technologies (e.g., genetic modification) and increasing considerations on the ethical use and understanding of the welfare needs of animals emerged, the Directive was replaced in 2010 by EU 2010/63.

As with the previous directive, all nonhuman vertebrate animals are protected, but this was further extended to include fetal forms of mammals in the last third of development and, for the first time, a group of invertebrates, all cephalopods. In addition, new specific requirements were introduced to ensure the implementation of the Three Rs (replacement, reduction, and refinement).

Expectations on the implementation of the Three Rs are embedded throughout the Directive, at the national level and at local establishments (through animal welfare bodies), and in all applications for the use of animals in scientific procedures. The application of the Three Rs is a key cornerstone of the directive and is underpinned within the training requirements for scientists and care staff. Directive 2010/63 requires that member states ensure that no animal procedure is performed if another suitable method or testing strategy not entailing the use of a live animal, is recognized under EU legislation. Animal studies must also use the minimum number of animals, use those animals with the lowest capacity to experience pain, suffering, distress, or lasting harm, which cause the least pain, suffering, distress, or lasting harm, and are most likely to provide satisfactory results. Further, death as an endpoint must be avoided as far as possible and replaced by early and humane endpoints.

The application of the Three Rs is subject to continuous review throughout the duration of a project (which can be up to 5 years), such that scientists and establishments are required to introduce new knowledge/developments (e.g., improved anesthesia or analgesic practices) which will further advance the goals of the Three Rs as these become available, having regard for the potential impact on scientific outcomes. The more detailed provisions of the new directive, combined with commonly agreed guidance material, have enabled a more uniform platform for the scientific community and animal welfare provision.

The main requirements of 2010/63/EU are:

- All establishments using, breeding, or supplying animals for use under the directive must be authorized.
- All scientific projects must be authorized. Project applications must contain sufficient information on the scientific objectives and on the harms to the animals to enable a favorable harm/benefit assessment to be made. Applicants also have to provide information on compliance with the Three Rs. In addition, a nontechnical summary of the project is published, and certain projects, for example, those involving nonhuman primates or severe procedures, are subject to retrospective assessment. Each procedure has to be given a prospective severity classification. The classifications are mild, moderate, severe, and nonrecovery (where the animal is maintained entirely under general anesthesia throughout the procedure, and is not allowed to recover consciousness). The assignment of the severity category shall take into account any intervention or manipulation of the animal within a defined procedure, and shall be based on the most severe effects likely to be encountered by an individual animal after applying all refinement techniques (for example, the use of anesthesia and/or analgesia). At the end of the procedure, the actual severity experienced by each animal is reported and published annually. The assessment of actual severity should be undertaken using the observations taken from the

animals during day to day monitoring. It should reflect the highest severity experienced at any stage during the procedure and not based on the severity at the end of the procedure. Nor should the evaluation be considered a simple additive process, e.g., moving from four injections or samplings to five, does not automatically move the categorization from mild to moderate. It should be based on an overall assessment of the animal's experience from the start of the procedure to the end.

- Each establishment has to have a designated veterinarian (DV) to provide advice on welfare and care. The DV contributes to the establishment's Animal Welfare Body, which is responsible for advice on animal acquisition, accommodation, care, and use, advice on the application of the Three Rs, and following and reviewing the outcome of projects. The DV also advises on the reuse of animals and rehoming them where appropriate.
- Standards of accommodation and care are included for all commonly used species.
- Obligations on the use of anesthesia, and restrictions on the use of neuro-muscular blockers.
- Appropriate methods of killing—others may be used where scientifically justified.
- Requirements for training, competence assessment, and continued development for persons involved in care, use, killing, and in the design of projects and procedures.

Guidance on training for the role of DV has been published.

2. United Kingdom

The Animals (Scientific Procedures) Act 1986 (ASPA), the regulation covering the use of laboratory animals in the United Kingdom, was updated in 2013 based on EU Directive 2010/63/EU. Although the United Kingdom formally left the EU in 2020, the relevant regulations have remained essentially unchanged. Responsibility for the administration and enforcement of ASPA in England, Scotland, and Wales rests with the Animals in Science Regulation Unit (ASRU), acting on behalf of the Home Secretary.

ASRU evaluates the scientific merit of all animal-based research, and project licenses are granted after considering the potential benefits and likely adverse effects of the proposed research. In addition to advising on applications for licenses, ASRU also provides the professional inspectorate, members of which visit establishments to assess compliance with licenses, the quality of work being conducted, and the facilities for the housing and care of animals. Northern Ireland follows the same regulatory system, which is administered and enforced by the Department of Health.

The regulations also require an independent committee, the Animals in Science Committee, to advise the Home Secretary on animal use, including the promotion of the Three Rs and the methods used to prevent pain and distress.

The Misuse of Drugs Act 1971 is the main UK law controlling and classifying drugs that are "dangerous or otherwise harmful" when misused. It lists all controlled drugs by classes A, B, and C.

- Class A for the most harmful substances such as ecstasy, LSD, heroin, cocaine, and crack cocaine, magic mushrooms, methadone, and methamphetamine;
- Class B for amphetamines, barbiturates, cannabis, codeine, ketamine, methylphenidate (Ritalin), synthetic cannabinoids, and synthetic cathinones (for example, mephedrone and methoxetamine);
- Class C for anabolic steroids, benzodiazepines (diazepam), gamma-hydroxybutyrate, gamma-butyrolactone, piperazines, and khat.

The Misuse of Drugs Regulations 2001 (extended in 2012) allows for the lawful possession and supply of controlled (illegal) drugs for legitimate purposes. They cover prescribing, administering, safe custody, dispensing, record keeping, destruction, and disposal of controlled drugs to prevent diversion for misuse.

The Inspectorate and Licensing Section of the Home Office Drug Branch is the authority for this Act. A Home Office domestic license is required for the production, supply, or possession of controlled drugs. Security and SOPs compliance must be documented. An annual statement of compliance with the requirements of the Misuse of Drugs legislation is necessary.

C. Central and South America

Mexico: At a federal level, Mexico regulates the production, care, and use of laboratory animals through a 1999 regulation (NOM 062/1999) which covers all the main species, including rodents, dogs, cats, swine, and nonhuman primates. It is based on three documents: the 1996 edition of the ILAR *Guide* (NRC, 1996); the guidelines of the CCAC; and the AVMA Guide on Euthanasia. Each facility must have a veterinarian, an IACUC, and an occupational health program, be registered with the relevant authority, and provide an annual report of activity. In addition, local rules apply generally to implementing the Three Rs by requiring experimental protocols to be designed to minimize or prevent suffering and mandating euthanasia by appropriate means. Efforts to revise and update the 1999 regulation are ongoing but, so far, unproductive.

Argentina: Argentina has no specific national legislation protecting animals used in research, although some standards are included in regulations related to the standards of manufacture of medical products and related testing. A proposal was formulated in 1994 and revised in 2001 which takes into consideration the Three Rs and would require the maintenance of records. This proposal has not been passed, but a national committee is working on the Law Project to develop appropriate regulations. Meanwhile, universities, laboratories, and industries have their own procedures for the care of animals as well as the design and maintenance of animal facilities.

Brazil: Legislation in Brazil in 2008 required the creation of CONCEA, the National Council on the Control of Animal Experiments. The Ministry of Science and Technology (MOST) presides over CONCEA and appoints its coordinator. Each institution must appoint a local ethics committee, which must register with CONCEA. In addition to developing regulations and guidelines regarding animal use, CONCEA also ensures compliance through appropriate monitoring. In 2015, CONCEA wrote the *Brazilian Guide for the Care and Use of Laboratory Animals*, which emphasizes the implementation of the Three Rs. In 2016, four chapters of the *Guide* as well as the Brazilian directive and *Guidelines for Euthanasia* were approved.

Peru: The Animal Welfare Law was published in Peru in 2016 and requires the Ministry of Agriculture to create standards for the protection and welfare of animals used in research. It permits animals to be used in academic and specialized facilities and requires animal welfare ethics committees to guarantee that animals will suffer only if the results cannot be obtained by any other methods. The law also established a National Animal Welfare Ethics Committee and includes an ethical code for the use of animals for experimental, investigation, and teaching purposes based largely on Three Rs principles.

Most other Latin American countries, including Uruguay, have some legislation protecting research animals and implementing the Three Rs, though often this is part of general animal welfare legislation.

D. Asia

The importance of laboratory animal science is becoming more recognized in Asian countries, and this is exemplified by greater professional governance. The Asian Federation of Laboratory Animal Science Associations was established in 2003 and provides a forum for information exchange including legislation. Recent revisions of laws, regulations, and guidelines in Asia emphasize the Three Rs and the need for ethical review of research proposals.

Japan: In Japan, the relevant legislation was most recently revised in 2017. Prior to that revision, the greatest focus was on "refinement" but the principles of "replacement" and "reduction" have now been added to the Act on the Welfare and Management of Animals. Further, guidelines to the standards for the care of laboratory animals, including reducing pain, were also published in 2017 and closely resemble the ILAR *Guide* (NRC, 2011). Veterinary care is included, as well as the role of the laboratory animal veterinary specialist. The establishment of a local ethics committee is suggested in various guidelines but is not a requirement.

Korea: The Animal Protection Act in Korea was most recently amended in 2017 and includes several articles which relate specifically to animals used in research. It is arguably the most stringent animal experimentation law in Asia. By contrast with Japan, Korea mandates the establishment of an ethics committee and the membership is defined by the law. Animal experiments must be conducted in compliance with the Three Rs, ensuring that animals experience the least pain and distress. The law requires the use of sound veterinary practices including, analgesics, sedatives, and anesthetics, and euthanasia must be performed with the least pain and distress.

China: The development of laboratory animal science in China is overseen by the MOST. A regulation was issued by MOST in 2002 which has resulted in almost all of the 31 provinces establishing administrative offices of laboratory animals (AOLAs) which license facilities for animal breeding and use. In 2018, the Chinese government issued a new National Standard pertaining to research animals which has been translated into English (MacArthur Clark and Sun, 2020). This covers all aspects of husbandry, veterinary care, implementation of the Three Rs and ethical review and provides a comprehensive guide to the regulations.

Taiwan: The Animal Protection Law in Taiwan was revised in 2016 and incorporates the principles of the Three Rs as well as requiring the establishment of an ethics committee and a management group including veterinary representation. Guidelines were published in 2018 addressing institutional policy and veterinary care and management. These are largely consistent with the ILAR *Guide* (NRC, 2011).

Thailand: The Animals for Scientific Purposes Act of 2015 was the first to address research animal welfare in Thailand. The Act requires a national committee to establish policies and processes and advise the government. In addition, institutional ethics committees provide local oversight and ensure implementation of the Three Rs, including standards of analgesia and anesthesia.

E. Australasia

Animal research in both Australia and New Zealand is strictly regulated under systems not dissimilar to those in the USA and Europe.

Australia: In Australia, each state (or territory) is responsible for implementing legislation relating to the use of animals in research. At a national level, the National Health and Medical Research Council (NHMRC) requires those receiving funding to comply with the Australian Code for the Care and Use of Animals for Scientific Purposes, last revised in 2013. The Code sets out guiding principles, including the Three Rs, requires animal ethics committees, defines the program of veterinary care, and covers all aspects of the care and use of animals throughout their lifetime. While in theory, the Code covers only NHMRC-funded research, in practice it is applied to all research both in academia and in industry.

New Zealand: In New Zealand, animal use in research is controlled under part six of the AWA of 1999, and overseen by the National Animal Ethics Advisory Committee. Institutions wanting to use animals must work under an approved code of ethical conduct that sets out policies and procedures which must be followed, including the principles of the Three Rs, requirements for veterinary oversight and regular inspection, and institutional reporting which includes the number of animals used as well as the impact of the research, testing, and teaching activities on their welfare. A national report on animal use is published annually by the Ministry for Primary Industries.

Acknowledgments

The authors of this chapter would like to acknowledge the generous contributions of subject matter experts. Neera Gopee, NIH OLAW was incredibly generous with her time and reviewed and edited multiple sections of this chapter relating to animal care and welfare standards in the United States. Patricia Brown, OLAW, reviewed and edited content relating to the PHS Policy. Helen E. Diggs, AAALAC International, developed section content regarding AAALAC International. Representatives from the United States Food and Drug Administration (FDA), Diana Link, Jan Linkenhoker, Amber McCoig, and Margret Oeller reviewed and provided content regarding the FDA. Robert Gibbens and the AWIC from the United States department of agriculture (USDA), reviewed and provided content regarding the USDA. Kathyrn Bayne generously assisted with the international perspective. From the CCAC, we could like to acknowledge Michael Baar and Sylvie Coutier for their efforts in reviewing and editing content relevant to Canadian standards.

References

Animals for Scientific Purposes Act (Thailand), 2015. https://www.aaalac.org/pub/?id=E905D91B-D97F-04BB-41FA-41E9D139B064. (Accessed 27 July 2021).

Bayne, K., Howard, B.R., Kurosawa, T.M., Najera, M.E.A., 2021. Chapter 35: An overview of global legislation, regulations, and policies. In: Handbook of Laboratory Animal Science, fourth ed. CRC Press, pp. 899–921.

Canadian Council on Animal Care (CCAC), 2015. https://ccac.ca/.

Korea Animal Protection Act, 2017. https://elaw.klri.re.kr/eng_mobile/viewer.do?hseq=33572&type=part&key=25. (Accessed 27 July 2021).

MacArthur Clark, J.A., Sun, D., 2020. Guidelines for the Ethical Review of Laboratory Animal Welfare; People's Republic of China National Standard GB/T 35892-2018. https://doi.org/10.1002/ame2.12111.

Mason, D.S., Tenney, L., Hellyer, P.W., Newman, L.S., 2018. Prescription opioid epidemic: do veterinarians have a dog in the fight? Am. J. Publ. Health 108, 1162–1163. https://doi.org/10.2105/AJPH.2018.304603.

National Research Council, 1996. Guide for the Care and Use of Laboratory Animals. National Academy Press, Washington, D.C.

National Research Council, 2011. Guide for the Care and Use of Laboratory Animals. National Academy Press, Washington, D.C.

Wolff, A., Garnett, N., Potkay, S., Wigglesworth, C., Doyle, D., Thornton, D., 2003. Frequently asked questions about the public health service policy on humane care and use of laboratory animals. Lab. Anim. 32 (9), 33–36.

World Organisation for Animal Health (OIE), 2018. Chapter 7.8: Use of Animals in Research and Education. Terrestrial Animal Health Code. http://www.oie.int/index.php?id=169&L=0&htmfile=chapitre_aw_research_education.htm. (Accessed 27 July 2021).

Further reading

Act on Welfare and Management of Animals (Japan), 1973. http://www.japaneselawtranslation.go.jp/law/detail/?id=61&vm=04&re=02. (Accessed 27 July 2021).

Kong, Q., Qin, Q., 2010. Analysis of current laboratory animal science policies and administration in China. ILAR J. 51 (1), E1–E10.

National Institutes of Health, 2021. Guidelines for the use of non-pharmaceutical-grade chemicals/compounds in laboratory animals. Animal Research Advisory Committee Guidelines. https://oacu.oir.nih.gov/animal-research-advisory-committee-guidelines.

Newcomer, C.E., Cloutier, S., 2018. Chapter 9: Assessment and accreditation programs for research animal care and use. In: Weichbrod, R.H., Thompson, G.A.H., Norton, J.N. (Eds.), Management of Animal Care and Use Programs in Research, Education, and Testing, second ed. CRC Press/Taylor & Francis, Boca Raton (FL).

Ogden, B., Pang, W., Agui, T., et al., 2016. Laboratory animal laws, regulations, guidelines and standards in China Mainland, Japan, and Korea. ILAR J. 57 (3), 301–311.

Retnam, L., Chatikavanij, P., Kunjara, P., et al., 2016. Laws, regulations, guidelines and standards for animal care and use for scientific purposes in the countries of Singapore, Thailand, Indonesia, Malaysia, and India. ILAR J. 57 (3), 312–323.

Science Council of Japan, 2006. Guidelines for Proper Conduct of Animal Experiments. http://www.scj.go.jp/ja/info/kohyo/pdf/kohyo-20-k16-2e.pdf. (Accessed 27 July 2021).

Taiwan (Chinese-Taipei): Animal Protection Law, 1998. https://www.animallaw.info/statute/taiwan-cruelty-taiwan-animal-protection-law. (Accessed 27 July 2021).

Chapter 3

Optimizing anesthesia and analgesia for specific research projects

Paulin Jirkof[1], Heidrun Potschka[2] and Douglas K. Taylor[3]

[1]*Office for Animal Welfare and 3Rs, University of Zurich, Zurich, Switzerland;* [2]*Institute of Pharmacology, Toxicology, and Pharmacy, Ludwig-Maximilians-University Munich, Munich, Germany;* [3]*Division of Laboratory Animal Services, Augusta University, Augusta, GA, United States*

Chapter outline

I. General implications of anesthesia and analgesia on study design

A. Introduction

It is of utmost importance to recognize that untreated pain can significantly impact animal welfare as well as the experimental outcomes and model validity in a hard-to-predict manner (e.g., Jirkof, 2017; Peterson et al., 2017). Pain management using anesthesia and analgesia is therefore essential in animal research. Nevertheless, making the optimal choice of an anesthesia and/or analgesia protocol for a specific research question can be challenging. The ideal protocol will effectively relieve pain and lack side effects that might hamper science and animal welfare. In light of the many aspects that must be considered, there is no universally perfect anesthesia or analgesia regimen. Therefore, careful planning with input from experts in veterinary pain management is needed.

B. Choice of agents

Reliable induction of unconsciousness and muscle relaxation, e.g., for surgical procedures, is important for animal welfare and procedural success. In order to provide efficacious pain management, the anticipated level and type of pain need to be considered to avoid therapeutic failure. Visceral, somatic, and nociceptive pain exhibit profound differences in the response to specific analgesic drugs (Orr et al., 2017). More details on anesthesia protocols and analgesia protocols for different pain types, pain severity, and pain duration will be discussed in other chapters of this book.

Beyond animal welfare concerns, the impact of untreated pain, anesthesia, and analgesic protocols on the

Anesthesia and Analgesia in Laboratory Animals. https://doi.org/10.1016/B978-0-12-822215-7.00002-0

experimental design and outcome must also be considered in scientific projects. Protocols should have no negative, or at most a controllable effect on the specific system targeted by the experiment or on experimental procedures. The varying modes of action of pain and different anesthetics and analgesics should be known before protocols are implemented as interference with the model is always possible. We will introduce some typical side effects and interactions later in this chapter. For detailed information on the action of different substances, we refer to the following substance-specific chapters in this book.

Anesthetics and analgesics can impact experimental procedures or may be contraindicated in some animal models. For example, some commonly used analgesics have side effects, such as respiratory depression or increased risk of bleeding, that might complicate anesthetic or surgical procedures. If a partial μ-receptor agonist such as buprenorphine is used in premedication, the effect of a μ-receptor full agonist such as fentanyl is weakened due to the higher receptor affinity of buprenorphine. In animal models, which are associated with a compromised renal or hepatic function, it needs to be considered that the excretion of drugs can be attenuated with delayed excretion, a longer duration of action, and a potential increase of side effects. In the respective cases, it might be necessary to adjust the dosing or the administration intervals or to use alternate drugs. Moreover, any model with compromised bronchial and lung function due to alterations in bronchosecretion, emphysema, or edema should be considered as a relative or absolute contraindication for inhalation anesthesia.

To account for the impact of agents on the model and depending on the research hypothesis and the outcome parameters, drug-exposed control groups (i.e., those that receive the chosen anesthetic and analgesic but do not undergo a painful procedure or surgery) can be crucial for the interpretation of data. Decisions about the necessity for respective control groups require careful consideration focused on the reduction principle of the 3Rs concept.

C. Timing and duration of treatment

For procedures reasonably expected to induce pain, preventive approaches must be considered. Preventive measures are typically initiated before a painful intervention and are extended into the postsurgical phase. With regards to the various mechanisms contributing to peripheral and central sensitization (Ji et al., 2018; McKune et al., 2015; Pogatzki-Zahn et al., 2018), any effort should be made to avoid gaps in pain management as these may result in pain states that are more difficult to control. Efficacious preventive actions should be based on multimodal regimens with a combination of analgesics that limit the development of hypersensitivity (Clutton, 2018; Flecknell, 2018). The potential advantages of multimodal protocols over monotherapy are the maximization of analgesic effects and the minimization of side effects, as reduced amounts of each drug are needed (Wickerts et al., 2011). Nevertheless, combinations of drugs might also have additive side effects; for example, the combination of acetylsalicylic acid and nonsteroidal antiinflammatory drugs (NSAIDs) escalates the effect on the gastrointestinal mucosa (Aronson, 2009). Thus, the pharmacokinetics, the side effects, and the potential interactions with test compounds must be analyzed carefully for all drugs involved when used in animal experimentation.

A possible impact on outcome parameters of a scientific study should not only be considered for the choice of the anesthetic and analgesic regime but also for the timeline of the study. In addition, the choice of an analgesic regimen also needs to consider tolerance development, which in the case of opioids can occur following prolonged administration but also rapidly even during short-term drug exposure (KuKanich and Wiese, 2015). In case of concerns about an influence on parameters of interest in the study, the time course can be very important. Therefore, instead of avoiding a specific anesthetic or analgesic compound, which may serve as a confounding factor, it may also be possible to adjust and extend the time span between surgical intervention and the assessment of the study parameters to allow for a "wash out" period. Thereby, one can avoid the impact of the acute effects of anesthetics and analgesics on the data obtained at a later time point. On the other hand, respective decisions about the plan need to consider the cumulative burden for the animals, which is relevant when the animal model is associated with chronic pain.

D. Administration route

There are multiple routes of administration for analgesic and anesthetic substances. All routes carry with them both desired and undesired effects on well-being, physiology, and behavior. One should weigh the respective advantages and disadvantages, considering factors such as the frequency of handling and restraint necessary and the chemical properties of the compound itself when deciding which route is optimal.

Oral administration of compounds can be generally carried out by gavage, micropipette dosing, or by self-administration. Voluntary oral administration of analgesia avoids the negative effects of handling. Several methods for oral administration have been described, such as mixing analgesics with flavored gelatin (Liles et al., 1998), Nutella (Goldkuhl et al., 2010; Taylor et al., 2016), a regular diet (Molina-Cimadevila et al., 2014), or (sweetened) drinking water (Sauer et al., 2016). These studies, in mice and rats, have shown that several analgesics are efficacious when administered orally and voluntarily. Nevertheless, oral self-administration has been criticized as being less effective than subcutaneous (SQ) treatment (e.g., Cho et al., 2019; Thompson et al., 2006). Reduced bioavailability caused by metabolizing the drug before it reaches systemic circulation is a known obstacle in the oral administration route (Brewster et al., 1981). Moreover, latency to ingestion as well as the total amount ingested by the animals, especially during the resting phase, as well as gastrointestinal motility is difficult to anticipate and clearly variable for each individual. Thus, voluntary ingestion protocols might be applicable only when pain is mild, or in combination with drug injections, at least during the resting phase of rodents (Sauer et al., 2016), or when the methods allow drug intake control (Scarborough et al., 2020).

As an alternative, injectable agents may be administered intraperitoneally, subcutaneously, intramuscularly, or intravenously. For all methods, the frequency of handling and restraint necessary for repeated administration should be considered and weighed against any potential uncertainties in sufficient dosing associated with self-administration (Foley, 2014).

Transdermal administration of some drugs via patches as a minimally intrusive method has also been described for different species, including dogs, cats, and rabbits (Foley, 2014). Drug absorption from transdermal patches, for example, can provide a continuous delivery for days, but can also significantly vary in an interindividual manner with a pronounced influence on the preparation of the administration site, the skin thickness, and the regional temperature (Foley, 2014).

With the exception of the transdermal method, chronic administration via injection or gavage requires repeated handling and restraint of the animal, which can cause additional stress in small laboratory species (Cinelli et al., 2007) and might increase existing pain. This may be a substantial confounder of experimental data and may increase inter- and intra-animal variation (Moberg, 1999). To overcome the negative impact of repeated handling for serial administration and ensure adequate administration of analgesia, depot formulations have been developed for some drugs and species (e.g., Carbone et al., 2012; Foley, 2014; Kendall et al., 2016; Nunamaker et al., 2014; Seymour et al., 2016). These formulations, due to their long-release duration, significantly reduce the necessary frequency of drug administration. Reports suggest that sustained-release formulations can improve the tolerability of buprenorphine in rats (Foley et al., 2011). As with oral administration, a first-pass effect needs to be considered for compounds that are metabolized and inactivated in the liver with intraperitoneal administration. Drugs that can cause gastrointestinal irritation may exert more pronounced adverse effects due to direct exposure of the mucosa to higher concentrations of the compound. Administration via any injection route also needs to consider the local tolerability as the compound and its formulation may cause skin or tissue irritation, which can even result in local necrosis. In this context, all components of a formulation need to be taken into account. Local anesthetic formulations can, for instance, contain vasoconstriction compounds such as epinephrine or vasopressin analogues (Garcia, 2015). These vasoconstrictors result in an earlier onset and longer duration of action and limit the risk of resorptive intoxication. On the other hand, they need to be avoided in the area of terminal capillaries at the extremities. Different administration modes and formulations of drugs also result in different time intervals until therapeutic concentrations are reached at the target site. This needs to be considered when deciding about pretreatment times during study design.

II. Specific implications of anesthesia and analgesia on study design

In the subsequent sections, we discuss the main effects of analgesic drugs routinely used in animal studies, which may exert an impact on possible outcome parameters in experimental studies focusing on three scientific fields using animals: neuroscience, cardiovascular, and cancer studies (e.g., European Commission, 2020). Please note that we can only provide a rough overview with selected specific examples in this chapter and that during study planning it will be of utmost relevance to carefully check the literature for a description of effects that may be relevant for the specific parameters studied. In this context, we would also like to refer the reader to more specific reviews focusing on the selection of analgesics and/or anesthetics in specific research areas (e.g., Hoffmann et al., 2016; Larson et al., 2019).

A. Neuroscience studies

1. Neuroscience models and interventions that require anesthesia and analgesia

Craniotomy is a frequent procedure in neuroscientific research. The types of surgical interventions range from the transient insertion of an injection cannula to permanent implants of recording electrodes and devices, stimulation electrodes, and guide cannulas. Trauma-related to craniotomy procedures can comprise damage to the soft tissue, periosteum, and cranial muscles. The surgical wound area is characterized by an inflammatory pain reaction. Moreover, craniotomy procedures can be associated with post-surgical alterations in intracranial pressure and blood flow, which may cause headaches. In this context, it is of interest that recent reviews critically discussed pain management procedures applied in human patients with craniotomy, which in the past often refrained from the application of multimodal analgesic regimes. Concern has been raised that these approaches may result in insufficient control of postsurgical pain in humans (Dunn et al., 2016; Lutman et al., 2018). Along this line, an efficacious pain management plan with carefully selected analgesic drugs is also of the utmost importance for experimental neurosurgical procedures. Considering evidence for the beneficial effects of local anesthesia in human patients (Dunn et al., 2016; Lutman et al., 2018), it is recommended to always consider infiltration and epiperiostal local anesthesia in addition to the administration of analgesic drugs. When applying parameters suggested for pain assessment (e.g., reviewed by Turner et al., 2019; Tappe-Theodor et al., 2019) in models of neurological disorders, model-specific alterations, including motor dysfunction and behavioral alterations characterizing different models of neurological disorders need to be considered.

Untreated pain may affect many outcome parameters in neuroscience models. Nociceptive signals reach the brain via ascending pathways projecting to different brain regions, which play a key role in the integration and induction of autonomic and endocrine responses (McKune et al., 2015). The sensation of pain is initiated once the nociceptive signal reaches the cerebral cortex. In consideration of the complex signaling mechanisms, and the impact on various brain regions, it is not surprising that uncontrolled nociceptive signaling and pain can have tremendous consequences on multiple molecular and cellular mechanisms. The fact that the perception of pain is associated with an affective component implies an impact on behavioral patterns that can, for instance, reflect an increase in fear or tension (McKune et al., 2015). At the level of the spinal cord and the brain, changes in neurotransmitter signaling among others can involve enhanced glutamatergic signaling (McKune et al., 2015). In addition, excessive inflammatory signaling with microglia activation and elevated levels of proinflammatory mediators can affect the excitability of dorsal horn neurons and other CNS neurons (Chen et al., 2018). In the brain, microglia activation seems to play an important role in the emotional impact of chronic pain states (Inoue and Tsuda, 2018).

Alterations in behavioral patterns are used as parameters for severity and pain assessment in laboratory animals (e.g., Turner et al., 2019; Jirkof, 2014). Thus, in turn, respective changes need to be considered when applying behavioral outcome parameters in neuroscientific research. Alterations in activity and sleep patterns, circadian rhythmicity, social interaction, and exploratory behavior can characterize insufficiently controlled acute and chronic pain states (e.g., Turner et al., 2019; Tappe-Theodor et al., 2019; Jirkof, 2014; Toth, 2019; Jirkof et al., 2019). Reduced burrowing, nest building, and grooming activity has, for instance, been reported in the early postsurgical phase in mice (Arras et al., 2007; Jirkof et al., 2010, 2013; Oliver et al., 2018). The impact of chronic pain on the affective state of laboratory rodents can be reflected by changes in anxiety- and depression-associated behavior (Chen et al., 2022; Hisaoka-Nakashima et al., 2019).

The influence of nociception and pain on neuronal activity can significantly influence electrophysiological recordings, immediate early gene expression, as well as imaging data (Davis et al., 2017; Morton et al., 2016). Structural and molecular alterations occurring in chronic pain states can also affect neuroimaging approaches (Morton et al., 2016) (for further details, see Chapter 29) and postmortem protein or RNA analyses.

2. Impact of analgesia and anesthesia on neuroscience outcome parameters

Some analgesic drugs, including NSAIDs, can influence the functional state of glial cells and inflammatory signaling cascades. Excessive neuroinflammatory signaling has been described in models of encephalitis, multiple sclerosis, traumatic brain injury, cerebral ischemia, Alzheimer's disease, Parkinson's disease, epilepsy, psychiatric disorders, and neuromuscular disorders. An impact of NSAID exposure on clinical symptoms, neuronal damage or loss, glial activation, and blood-brain barrier function needs to be carefully considered in respective models. As evidence exists that cyclooxygenase-2 can also regulate the expression of blood-brain barrier transporters, including P-glycoprotein, the administration of NSAIDs may influence the brain penetration rates of transporter substrates.

An impact on inflammatory signaling in the brain has also been reported for anesthetic drugs, including isoflurane (Bar-Klein et al., 2016). Studies in models of different neurological disorders pointed to the potential neuroprotective effects of isoflurane, propofol, and ketamine (Hoffmann et al., 2016). Indirect neuroprotective effects on neuronal damage can also be related to an influence on the neuronal metabolic rate by different drugs, including inhalation anesthetics, propofol, benzodiazepines, barbiturates, dexmedetomidine, etomidate, and fentanyl (Larson et al., 2019).

In models of ischemic and hemorrhagic stroke, the impact of anesthetics on cerebral blood flow and intracranial pressure can critically influence various outcome parameters (Hoffmann et al., 2016). Interestingly, ketamine can affect cerebral blood flow with opposing effects depending on the brain region. Moreover, it needs to be considered that different drugs, including inhalation anesthetics, propofol, and dexmedetomidine, can exert effects on the cerebral reflex autoregulation of blood flow, which is triggered by ischemic damage (Larson et al., 2019).

While the influence of drugs on neuronal excitability can bias various electrophysiological outcome parameters, drug effects on synaptic activity and plasticity can result in consequences for learning and memory performance. An age-dependent influence on cognitive function and on long-term potentiation has, for instance, been reported following repeated exposure to isoflurane or sevoflurane (Long et al., 2016; Makaryus et al., 2015; Shen et al., 2013; Zhu et al., 2010).

Behavioral parameters are highly sensitive to confounding factors, including drug effects. Thereby, effects largely depend on species, dosing regimens, and drug combinations. Opioid exposure can influence behavioral patterns with changes in activity, stereotypic behavior, and alterations in circadian rhythmicity and sleep patterns (Jirkof et al., 2015; Johnson, 2016; Toth, 2019). Pica behavior (allotriphagia) can be triggered by the uptake of nonnutritious material (Clark et al., 1997; Takeda et al., 1993). A general impact of opioids and other drugs on food intake and body weight development must also be considered for studies analyzing appetite regulation.

Recent research has demonstrated that ketamine can exert significant antidepressant effects (Zanos and Gould, 2018). Thus, the pharmacodynamic effects of ketamine should be considered for experimental studies focused on neuropsychiatric disorders. Moreover, ketamine can trigger hallucinogenic phases.

The fact that inadequately controlled pain and medication may influence scientific outcome parameters should be carefully considered during study planning. In this context, it is emphasized that the choice of an appropriate anesthesia and an effective analgesia regime is a matter of course from an ethical point of view. Thus, potential drug effects should be considered through thoughtful study design with a careful selection of anesthetic and analgesic drugs. In addition, the possible influence of anesthetic and analgesic drugs can also be taken into account by extended time periods following exposure or the inclusion of additional control groups.

B. Cardiovascular studies

1. *Cardiovascular studies: models and interventions that require anesthesia and analgesia*

Cardiovascular diseases (coronary, rheumatic, or congenital heart disease, cerebrovascular or peripheral arterial disease, thrombosis, and embolisms) and the subsequent heart attacks and strokes are a leading cause of death in humans (WHO website, 2021). These conditions are therefore frequently modeled in preclinical animal research. While in most cases no analgesia will be given to an animal with, for example, an induced stroke, procedures to induce, treat or measure physiological outcomes in these conditions might include surgery, and therefore anesthesia and analgesia become important protocol components.

Examples for such surgical interventions are the occlusion of coronary vessels, stenosis of large vessels, coronary artery dilatation, atherosclerosis induction, myocardial infarction, microembolization, heart valve replacement, pericardial surgery, heart transplantation, cardiac catheter, stent implantation, or telemetry transponder implantation. All of these procedures will induce severe pain and require deep anesthesia and multimodal analgesic treatment. Interventions without surgery include the induction of pathological alterations like inflammation or calcification of the heart via the administration of toxic substances. Here, pain levels are variable, and analgesic treatment may not always be needed or possible.

Pain that is not treated or not sufficiently treated can have many effects on the outcome of cardiovascular studies. The mere activation of the nociceptive system can directly cause autonomic nervous system responses. As nerves of the autonomous nervous system innervate almost every organ system, the effects are manifold. Ascending pain impulses lead to hypothalamic activation and increased sympathetic-adrenergic system activity, which affects the body's unconscious actions. This activation results in substantial respiratory and cardiovascular effects, such as changes in blood pressure, heart rate, heart rate variability, stroke volume, cardiac contractility, blood flow, and vasoconstriction. In many species, including laboratory mice (e.g., Arras et al., 2007), the elevation of heart rate and typical changes in heart rate variability can therefore also be a sensitive indicator of pain. The same is true for respiratory rate and body temperature, which like heart rate and heart rate variability, may provide an estimation of the sympathetic and parasympathetic components of autonomic system activity (Conzemius et al., 1997; Gehrmann et al., 2000).

2. *Impact of analgesia and anesthesia on cardiovascular outcome parameters*

The most used inhalation anesthetics have an impact on parameters of interest in cardiovascular studies. Isoflurane causes decreased systemic vascular resistance with hypotension. In a compensatory manner, the heart rate can slightly increase (Evers et al., 2006). While isoflurane acts as a bronchodilator, it can irritate and stimulate tracheal and bronchial reflexes and can trigger laryngospasm. The vasodilatory effect of isoflurane can result in a slightly increased cerebral blood flow with minor risk for increased intracranial pressure (Evers et al., 2006). Sevoflurane exerts hypotensive effects and can decrease cardiac output. In contrast to other inhalation anesthetics, sevoflurane does not cause tachycardia. Thus, it can be preferable in animals with a respective risk. While sevoflurane is not irritating to the airways, exposure results in a reduction of minute ventilation due to a decrease in respiratory volume. The effects on cerebral blood flow and skeletal muscle function are comparable to those of isoflurane (Evers et al., 2006).

Also, the injectable anesthesia agent propofol might lead to vasodilatation and a mild negative ionotropic effect; it therefore can lower blood pressure (Evers et al., 2006; Trapani et al., 2000). Based on peripheral vasoconstriction thiopental can increase blood pressure and the bleeding tendency during a surgical intervention (Berry, 2015). α2-sympathomimetics (e.g., xylazine, medetomidine, dexmedetomidine) are frequently used for surgical procedures in combination with benzodiazepines or the dissociative anesthetic ketamine (Rankin, 2015). Following a short phase with a transient sympathomimetic effect associated with a short increase in arterial blood pressure, α2-sympathomimetics reduce the central sympathetic tone, resulting in hypotension, bradycardia, hypothermia, and respiratory depression (Rankin, 2015). Fast intravenous (IQ) administration of benzodiazepines can exert relevant effects on the regulation of cardiovascular and respiratory function (Ammer et al., 2016).

On the contrary, the side effects of other agents might be minor. Etomidate seems to be without relevant depressant effects on the respiratory and cardiovascular systems and alphaxalone has only minor adverse effects. These include a minor impact on respiration and cardiovascular function with a slight vasodilatation and negative inotropic effect (Berry, 2015).

Like many common anesthesia agents, analgesics of several substance classes can have a distinct impact on cardiovascular outcomes. Opioids and opioid receptors, for example, play a certain role in the cardiovascular system. Of high interest for cardiovascular studies is that endogenously released opioid peptides, as well as exogenously administered opioids, can have cardioprotective effects (Rawal and Patel, 2018; Tanaka et al., 2014). Opioids like fentanyl, for example, limit myocardial damage during ischemia-reperfusion (Headrick et al., 2015; Xu et al., 2015). Other well-known effects of opioids are reduced sympathetic outflows to the heart, bradycardia, increased heart rate, effects on heart contractility, arterial fibrillation, or vasodilation depending on species and substance (Chen and Ashburn, 2015; Gordon, 1990; Ilbäck et al., 2008; Molina, 2006). Morphine causes histamine release, and several species show a pseudo-allergic reaction after administration. Tramadol may lead to serotonin syndrome, including an increase in heart rate and blood pressure as well as cardiac arrhythmia. Cardiac effects of opioids might be accelerated in combination with, for example, benzodiazepine or inhaled anesthetics (Chen and Ashburn, 2015) and may therefore have implications on study design and anesthesia protocols.

Also, NSAIDs have cardiovascular effects. Especially selective cox-2 inhibitors but also nonselective cox-inhibitors may carry cardiovascular risks. They may have effects on vasodilation and may increase the risk of myocardial infarction, arterial fibrillation, bleeding, or worsening of existing heart failure (Schjerning et al., 2020; Tacke et al., 2008). Careful use of NSAIDs in animal experimentation is therefore recommended. Nevertheless, as especially postsurgical treatment is likely short, observed effects are rare (Pawlosky, 2013).

It must be kept in mind that also every kind of restraint, manipulation, or housing-related stress may have a profound impact on physiological outcome parameters that might be of high interest in this field of research. Gentle and refined procedures, e.g., stress-free drug administration and handling, and appropriate housing conditions might be of high importance for the validity of cardiovascular research.

C. Cancer studies

1. Cancer studies: models and interventions that require anesthesia and analgesia

Cancer is a complex disease process defined by unregulated cell growth, categorized into 200 different types identified by tissue of origin and location, and then further classified in the individual patient by stage and grade (Song et al., 2015). The methods used to study cancer are necessarily diverse in order to address the myriad types of cancers that exist. Xenograft models are among the most commonly used, although several carcinogen-induced and genetic-based approaches also exist (Cheon and Orsulic, 2011).

For xenograft models, transplanted cells or tissue could be established and well-characterized immortalized cell lines or uncharacterized clinical specimens obtained directly from human cancer patients—commonly called "patient-derived xenografts". The method of implantation into the recipient is often relatively noninvasive, via IV or SQ injection, thus requiring no anesthesia or analgesia in most cases. In contrast, some models of brain, bone, pancreatic, and liver cancer, for example, where material is placed orthotopically may require a surgical procedure for implantation. Such invasive methods of implantation should be classified as a major survival surgery requiring general anesthesia and postprocedural pain management. Anesthetic and analgesic regimens appropriate in these instances are the same as those used for any surgical manipulation and will not be discussed further here.

In addition to acute surgical pain, chronic pain arising from cancer progression and metastasis in an animal model should be acknowledged and addressed, as it is often significant in humans. The human experience suggests that cancers involving the bones, either as a primary tumor or via metastasis, cause the most significant pain. Rodent models to study bone cancers such as sarcomas have been developed and commonly involve the injection of cancerous cells directly into bone marrow (Pacharinsak and Beitz, 2008), leading to significant pain as tumors increase in size and destroy bone. The same can be said of prostate cancer models with high rates of bone metastasis

(Grabowska et al., 2014). Examples of other models with significant potential to cause pain include the 4T1 cell line breast cancer model due to the high rate of metastasis to the liver and lungs (Yang et al., 2012), and genetically engineered mouse models of aggressive pancreatic ductal adenocarcinoma that cause bile duct obstruction and related pathology (Lee et al., 2016). Pain management plans for all models of cancer, especially those known to be aggressive, are critical to animal welfare and should be thoroughly considered.

2. *Impact of anesthesia and analgesia on cancer studies outcome parameters*

For decades, there has been substantial discussion in human medicine regarding the impact of anesthesia regimens on long-term outcomes in cancer patients. The prevailing thesis has been that some general anesthetic regimens have the potential to increase the risk of distant metastasis subsequent to surgical resection of primary tumors (Byrne et al., 2016). Despite the widespread use of animal models of cancer, studies specifically addressing this question are surprisingly sparse. The few in existence tend to support human clinical data. A review of animal models suggests that volatile anesthetics increase the number of distant metastases (Hooijmans et al., 2016). For example, mice receiving IV injections of melanoma cancer cell lines under halothane or isoflurane show higher rates of metastasis compared to control animals administered only oxygen (Moudgil and Singal, 1997). Despite data showing some untoward effects from anesthetic administration, it remains part and parcel of human cancer management plans where surgical resection of primary tumors is required and necessary to some animal models for reasons of both animal welfare and animal model validity.

In mouse models of breast cancer it has been shown that metastasis increased in animals administered sevoflurane when compared to those receiving propofol (Li et al., 2020). This effect was likely mediated by proinflammatory cytokines. Mice receiving either lidocaine or propofol combined with sevoflurane during tumor cell inoculation exhibited lower rates of metastasis to the liver and lungs compared to those receiving sevoflurane alone (Freeman et al., 2019). Propofol has been shown to possess anticancer properties in vitro (Melamed et al., 2003).

The few published studies of opioid impact on cancer behavior in animal models paint a complex picture; data suggest that this drug class directly enhances tumor growth by reducing natural killer cell function but indirectly inhibit tumor growth by relieving pain. Morphine, for example, reduced tumor cell retention in the lungs of rats following surgery (Page et al., 2001). Fentanyl and bupivacaine combined with morphine show a similar reduction in lung retention (Page et al., 1993). Buprenorphine slightly increased lung metastasis in F344 rats that did not undergo surgery, but significantly reduced lesions in animals concurrently undergoing laparotomy (Franchi et al., 2007). Morphine and fentanyl increased lung metastasis more than saline or buprenorphine.

Morphine led to reduced primary tumor growth and pulmonary metastasis of melanoma cells (Sandler et al., 2003), which was ameliorated by sciatic neurectomy on the effected limb suggesting pain relief played a role. Morphine and fentanyl individually reduced bone cancer lesions (Exadaktylos et al., 2006), but mice treated continuously with morphine showed an increase in bone loss (Khaled and Liu, 2014). Buprenorphine given concurrently with IV inoculation of melanoma cells to mice had no effect on seeding in the lungs compared to saline controls (Liu et al., 2015). A similar study of breast cancer cells implanted subcutaneously in nude mice showed a different result with morphine accelerating tumor growth and increasing vascular density (Gupta et al., 2002). Naloxone abolished this effect.

Studies examining the effect of NSAID administration on mouse models of cancer are abundant with the majority showing that NSAIDs have antitumor properties. NSAIDs appear to exert their effect on tumor growth and metastasis in several ways. Meloxicam, ibuprofen, and celecoxib have been shown to induce apoptosis and reduce cell proliferation using in vitro assays (Dunn et al., 2004; Langley and Rothwell, 2014; Retsky et al., 2012). Decreased VEGF production and a coincident reduction in angiogenesis have been observed in vivo, and the data suggest that these are capable of exerting their effects through mechanisms other than COX inhibition (Patel et al., 2005). Meloxicam is among the most commonly used analgesics in rodents and significantly inhibited pulmonary seeding of melanoma cells (Lofgren et al., 2017). Ibuprofen reportedly slows the growth of ovarian cancer cells (Li et al., 2009). Celecoxib, a COX-2-specific NSAID, has been studied extensively and shown to significantly slow tumor growth. Colon, mammary, and prostate cell lines all show in vivo tumor growth inhibition in mouse and rat models (Kawamori et al., 1998; Leahy et al., 2002; Patel et al., 2005; Rosas et al., 2014).

III. Conclusions

Pain in animal experimentation is a major welfare issue, which must be minimized for ethical and legal reasons. Unrelieved pain also may have substantial and poorly controllable effects on the organism. It may affect complex behavioral traits such as circadian rhythmicity or goal-directed behaviors via motivational changes, may change the sensory capacities of animals via allodynia and hyperalgesia, or affect the physiological and endocrine systems via HPA activation. Thus, untreated pain carries the potential to increase the variability of research data significantly, meaning that anesthesia and pain management has also an important scientific and methodological dimension.

Analgesia and anesthesia are two of the many experimental interventions applied to laboratory animals, and everyone involved with in vivo experiments should be aware of their potential effects. Nevertheless, if analgesia and anesthesia protocols are chosen with care and on a case-by-case basis, effects are controllable. If the information on the effects of new analgesia and anesthesia protocols in specific experiments is missing, the inclusion of an analgesia and/or anesthesia control group might be advisable. The publications based on such applied approaches can provide valuable insights for the scientific community working with laboratory animals.

It should be noted that an important prerequisite for reproducible animal experiments is the proper and complete reporting of every analgesic and anesthetic intervention. Unfortunately, reviews on reporting practices for anesthesia and analgesia protocols after invasive animal procedures reveal that many published studies still do not report, or do not completely report, the anesthetic and analgesic measures involved (e.g., Carbone and Austin, 2016).

Although standardized anesthesia and analgesia protocols are highly appreciated, both need continuous learning and require assessment and adjustment for individual animals, even for animals undergoing similar procedures. Standard, rule-of-thumb protocols are often not appropriate. In addition to promoting animal welfare, providing laboratory animals with optimal analgesia and anesthesia might also improve the clinical relevance of animal models, as customized anesthesia and analgesia protocols are more reflective of the medical treatment of human patients.

It is important to keep in mind that there might be distinct strain, age, and sex differences in regard to pain perception and the effects of analgesia or anesthesia in many species (see for example Smith, 2019).

Any pain management plan must be accompanied by a suitable pain assessment and monitoring plan (see also Chapter 12). Score sheets may help to formalize and standardize the assessment and monitoring of pain, especially for smaller species. Pain assessment should be frequent during expected pain peaks, for example, during the first 12-h to the first days after surgery or during the late stages of painful progressing diseases. The mode of detection of residual pain and the maximum scores that will trigger any following action should be established in advance and be followed up by adequate remedial measures (such as providing additional rescue analgesia or termination of the experiment).

The following chapters will guide the reader through this challenging task.

References

Ammer, H., Potschka, H., Hrsg: Löscher, W., Richter, A., 2016. Lehrbuch der Pharmakologie und Toxikologie für die Veterinärmedizin. In: Chapter 4: Pharmakologie des zentralen Nervensystems (ZNS), pp. 125–180.

Aronson, J.K., 2009. Meyler's Side Effects of Analgesics and Anti-inflammatory Drugs, first ed. Elsevier.

Arras, M., Rettich, A., Cinelli, P., Kasermann, H.P., Burki, K., 2007. Assessment of post-laparotomy pain in laboratory mice by telemetric recording of heart rate and heart rate variability. BMC Vet. Res. 3 (1), 16.

Bar-Klein, G., Klee, R., Brandt, C., Bankstahl, M., Bascuñana, P., Töllner, K., Dalipaj, H., Bankstahl, J.P., Friedman, A., Löscher, W., 2016. Isoflurane prevents acquired epilepsy in rat models of temporal lobe epilepsy. Ann. Neurol. 80 (6), 896–908.

Berry, S.H., 2015. Veterinary anesthesia and analgesia. In: Grimm, K.A., Lamont, L.A., Tranquilli, W.J., Greene, S.A., Robertson, S.A. (Eds.), Chapter 15: Injectable Anesthetics, pp. 277–297.

Brewster, D., Humphrey, M.J., McLeavy, M.A., 1981. The systemic bioavailability of buprenorphine by various routes of administration. J. Pharm. Pharmacol. 33 (8), 500–506. https://doi.org/10.1111/j.2042-7158.1981.tb13848.x.

Byrne, K., Levins, K.J., Buggy, D.J., 2016. Can anesthetic-analgesic technique during primary cancer surgery affect recurrence or metastasis? Can. J. Anesth. 63 (2), 184–192. https://doi.org/10.1007/s12630-015-0523-8.

Carbone, L., Austin, J., 2016. Pain and laboratory animals: publication practices for better data reproducibility and better animal welfare. PLoS One 11 (5), e0155001. https://doi.org/10.1371/journal.pone.0155001.

Carbone, E.T., Lindstrom, K.E., Diep, S., Carbone, L., 2012. Duration of action of sustained-release buprenorphine in 2 strains of mice. J. Am. Assoc. Lab. Anim. Sci. 51 (6), 815–819.

Chen, A., Ashburn, M.A., 2015. Cardiac effects of opioid therapy. Pain Med. 16 (Suppl. 1), S27–S31. https://doi.org/10.1111/pme.12915.

Chen, G., Zhang, Y.Q., Qadri, Y.J., Serhan, C.N., Ji, R.R., 2018. Microglia in pain: detrimental and protective roles in pathogenesis and resolution of pain. Neuron 100 (6), 1292–1311. https://doi.org/10.1016/j.neuron.2018.11.009.

Chen, W.H., Lien, C.C., Chen, C.C., 2022. Neuronal basis for pain-like and anxiety-like behaviors in the central nucleus of the amygdala. Pain 163 (3), e463–e475. https://doi.org/10.1097/j.pain.0000000000002389.

Cheon, D.-J., Orsulic, S., 2011. Mouse models of cancer. Annu. Rev. Pathol. 6 (1), 95–119. https://doi.org/10.1146/annurev.pathol.3.121806.154244.

Cho, C., Michailidis, V., Lecker, I., Collymore, C., Hanwell, D., Loka, M., Danesh, M., Pham, C., Urban, P., Bonin, R.P., Martin, L.J., 2019. Evaluating analgesic efficacy and administration route following craniotomy in mice using the grimace scale. Sci. Rep. 9 (1), 359. https://doi.org/10.1038/s41598-018-36897-w.

Cinelli, P., Rettich, A., Seifert, B., Bürki, K., Arras, M., 2007. Comparative analysis and physiological impact of different tissue biopsy methodologies used for the genotyping of laboratory mice. Lab. Anim. 41 (2), 174–184. https://doi.org/10.1258/002367707780378113.

Clark Jr., J.A., Myers, P.H., Goelz, M.F., Thigpen, J.E., Forsythe, D.B., 1997. Pica behavior associated with buprenorphine administration in the rat. Lab. Anim. Sci. 47 (3), 300–303. https://www.ncbi.nlm.nih.gov/pubmed/9241634.

Clutton, R.E., 2018. A review of factors affecting analgesic selection in large animals undergoing translational research. Vet. J. 236, 12–22. https://doi.org/10.1016/j.tvjl.2018.04.006.

Conzemius, M.G., Hill, C.M., Sammarco, J.L., Perkowski, S.Z., 1997. Correlation between subjective and objective measures used to determine severity of postoperative pain in dogs. J. Am. Vet. Med. Assoc. 210 (11), 1619–1622.

Davis, K.D., Flor, H., Greely, H.T., Iannetti, G.D., Mackey, S., Ploner, M., Pustilnik, A., Tracey, I., Treede, R.D., Wager, T.D., 2017. Brain imaging tests for chronic pain: medical, legal and ethical issues and recommendations. Nat. Rev. Neurol. 13 (10), 624–638. https://doi.org/10.1038/nrneurol.2017.122.

Dunn, G.P., Old, L.J., Schreiber, R.D., 2004. The immunobiology of cancer immunosurveillance and immunoediting. Immunity 21 (2), 137–148. https://doi.org/10.1016/j.immuni.2004.07.017.

Dunn, L.K., Naik, B.I., Nemergut, E.C., Durieux, M.E., 2016. Post-craniotomy pain management: beyond opioids. Curr. Neurol. Neurosci. Rep. 16 (10), 93. https://doi.org/10.1007/s11910-016-0693-y.

European-commission, 2020. REPORT from the COMMISSION to the European Parliament and the Council Report on the Statistics on the Use of Animals for Scientific Purposes in the Member States of the European Union in 2015-2017. https://ec.europa.eu/info/sites/default/files/com-2020-16-f1-en-main-part-1.pdf.

Evers, A., Crowder, A., Balser, J., 2006. Goodman and Gilman's the pharmacological basis of therapeutics. In: Brunton, L., Lazo, J., Parker, K. (Eds.), Chapter 13: General Anesthetics, pp. 341–369.

Exadaktylos, A.K., Buggy, D.J., Moriarty, D.C., Mascha, E., Sessler, D.I., 2006. Can anesthetic technique for primary breast cancer surgery affect recurrence or metastasis? Anesthesiology 105 (4), 660–664. https://doi.org/10.1097/00000542-200610000-00008.

Flecknell, P., 2018. Analgesics in small mammals. Vet. Clin. North Am. Exot. Anim. Pract. 21 (1), 83–103. https://doi.org/10.1016/j.cvex.2017.08.003.

Foley, P.L., 2014. Current options for providing sustained analgesia to laboratory animals. Lab. Anim. 43 (10), 364–371.

Foley, P.L., Liang, H., Crichlow, A.R., 2011. Evaluation of a sustained-release formulation of buprenorphine for analgesia in rats. JAALAS 50 (2), 198–204.

Franchi, S., Panerai, A.E., Sacerdote, P., 2007. Buprenorphine ameliorates the effect of surgery on hypothalamus–pituitary–adrenal axis, natural killer cell activity and metastatic colonization in rats in comparison with morphine or fentanyl treatment. Brain Behav. Immun. 21 (6), 767–774. https://doi.org/10.1016/j.bbi.2007.01.001.

Freeman, J., Crowley, P.D., Foley, A.G., Gallagher, H.C., Iwasaki, M., Ma, D., Buggy, D.J., 2019. Effect of perioperative lidocaine, propofol and steroids on pulmonary metastasis in a murine model of breast cancer surgery. Cancers 11 (5). https://doi.org/10.3390/cancers11050613.

Garcia, E.R., 2015. Veterinary anesthesia and analgesia. In: Grimm, K.A., Lamont, L.A., Tranquilli, W.J., Greene, S.A., Robertson, S.A. (Eds.), Chapter 17: Local Anesthetics, pp. 332–357.

Gehrmann, J., Hammer, P.E., Maguire, C.T., Wakimoto, H., Triedman, J.K., Berul, C.I., 2000. Phenotypic screening for heart rate variability in the mouse. Am. J. Physiol. Heart Circ. Physiol. 279 (2), H733–H740. https://doi.org/10.1152/ajpheart.2000.279.2.H733.

Goldkuhl, R., Jacobsen, K.R., Kalliokoski, O., Hau, J., Abelson, K.S.P., 2010. Plasma concentrations of corticosterone and buprenorphine in rats subjected to jugular vein catheterization. Lab. Anim. 44 (4), 337–343. https://doi.org/10.1258/la.2010.009115.

Gordon, F.J., 1990. Opioids and central baroreflex control: a site of action in the nucleus tractus solitarius. Peptides 11 (2), 305–309. https://doi.org/10.1016/0196-9781(90)90087-L.

Grabowska, M.M., DeGraff, D.J., Yu, X., Jin, R.J., Chen, Z., Borowsky, A.D., Matusik, R.J., 2014. Mouse models of prostate cancer: picking the best model for the question. Cancer Metastasis Rev. 33 (2), 377–397. https://doi.org/10.1007/s10555-013-9487-8.

Gupta, K., Kshirsagar, S., Chang, L., Schwartz, R., Law, P.Y., Yee, D., Hebbel, R.P., 2002. Morphine stimulates angiogenesis by activating proangiogenic and survival-promoting signaling and promotes breast tumor growth. Cancer Res. 62 (15), 4491–4498.

Headrick, J.P., See Hoe, L.E., Du Toit, E.F., Peart, J.N., 2015. Opioid receptors and cardioprotection—'opioidergic conditioning' of the heart. Br. J. Pharmacol. 172 (8), 2026–2050. https://doi.org/10.1111/bph.13042.

Hisaoka-Nakashima, K., Tomimura, Y., Yoshii, T., Ohata, K., Takada, N., Zhang, F.F., Nakamura, Y., Liu, K., Wake, H., Nishibori, M., Nakata, Y., Morioka, N., 2019. High-mobility group box 1-mediated microglial activation induces anxiodepressive-like behaviors in mice with neuropathic pain. Prog. Neuro-Psychopharmacol. Biol. Psychiat. 92, 347–362. https://doi.org/10.1016/j.pnpbp.2019.02.005.

Hoffmann, U., Sheng, H., Ayata, C., Warner, D.S., 2016. Anesthesia in experimental stroke research. Transl Stroke Res 7 (5), 358–367. https://doi.org/10.1007/s12975-016-0491-5.

Hooijmans, C.R., Geessink, F.J., Ritskes-Hoitinga, M., Scheffer, G.J., 2016. A systematic review of the modifying effect of anaesthetic drugs on metastasis in animal models for cancer. PLoS One 11 (5), e0156152. https://doi.org/10.1371/journal.pone.0156152.

Ilbäck, N.G., Siller, M., Stålhandske, T., 2008. Effects of buprenorphine on body temperature, locomotor activity and cardiovascular function when assessed by telemetric monitoring in rats. Lab. Anim. 42 (2), 149–160. https://doi.org/10.1258/la.2007.06002e.

Inoue, K., Tsuda, M., 2018. Microglia in neuropathic pain: cellular and molecular mechanisms and therapeutic potential. Nat. Rev. Neurosci. 19 (3), 138–152. https://doi.org/10.1038/nrn.2018.2.

Ji, R.R., Nackley, A., Huh, Y., Terrando, N., Maixner, W., 2018. Neuroinflammation and central sensitization in chronic and widespread pain. Anesthesiology 129 (2), 343–366. https://doi.org/10.1097/ALN.0000000000002130.

Jirkof, P., 2014. Burrowing and nest building behavior as indicators of well-being in mice. J. Neurosci. Methods 234, 139–146. https://doi.org/10.1016/j.jneumeth.2014.02.001.

Jirkof, P., 2017. Side effects of pain and analgesia in animal experimentation. Lab. Anim. 46 (4), 123–128. https://doi.org/10.1038/laban.1216.

Jirkof, P., Cesarovic, N., Rettich, A., Nicholls, F., Seifert, B., Arras, M., 2010. Burrowing behavior as an indicator of post-laparotomy pain in mice. Front. Behav. Neurosci. 4, 165. https://doi.org/10.3389/fnbeh.2010.00165.

Jirkof, P., Fleischmann, T., Cesarovic, N., Rettich, A., Vogel, J., Arras, M., 2013. Assessment of postsurgical distress and pain in laboratory mice by nest complexity scoring. Lab. Anim. 47 (3), 153–161. https://doi.org/10.1177/0023677213475603.

Jirkof, P., Tourvieille, A., Cinelli, P., Arras, M., 2015. Buprenorphine for pain relief in mice: repeated injections vs sustained-release depot formulation. Lab. Anim. 49 (3), 177–187. https://doi.org/10.1177/0023677214562849.

Jirkof, P., Rudeck, J., Lewejohann, L., 2019. Assessing affective state in laboratory rodents to promote animal welfare-what is the progress in applied refinement research? Anim.: Open Access J. MDPI 9 (12), 1026. https://doi.org/10.3390/ani9121026.

Johnson, R.A., 2016. Voluntary running-wheel activity, arterial blood gases, and thermal antinociception in rats after 3 buprenorphine formulations. J. Am. Assoc. Lab. Anim. Sci. 55 (3), 306–311. https://www.ncbi.nlm.nih.gov/pubmed/27177564.

Kawamori, T., Rao, C.V., Seibert, K., Reddy, B.S., 1998. Chemopreventive activity of celecoxib, a specific cyclooxygenase-2 inhibitor, against colon carcinogenesis. Cancer Res. 58 (3), 409–412.

Kendall, L.V., Wegenast, D.J., Smith, B.J., Dorsey, K.M., Kang, S., Lee, N.Y., Hess, A.M., 2016. Efficacy of sustained-release buprenorphine in an experimental laparotomy model in female mice. J. Am. Assoc. Lab. Anim. Sci. 55 (1), 66–73.

Khaled, W.T., Liu, P., 2014. Cancer mouse models: past, present and future. Semin. Cell Dev. Biol. 27, 54–60. https://doi.org/10.1016/j.semcdb.2014.04.003.

KuKanich, B., Wiese, A.J., 2015. Veterinary anesthesia and analgesia. In: Grimm, K.A., Lamont, L.A., Tranquilli, W.J., Greene, S.A., Robertson, S.A. (Eds.), Chapter 11: Opioids, pp. 207–227.

Langley, R.E., Rothwell, P.M., 2014. Aspirin in gastrointestinal oncology: new data on an old friend. Curr. Opin. Oncol. 26 (4). https://journals.lww.com/co-oncology/Fulltext/2014/07000/Aspirin_in_gastrointestinal_oncology__new_data_on.15.aspx.

Larson, C.M., Wilcox, G.L., Fairbanks, C.A., 2019. Defining and managing pain in stroke and traumatic brain injury research. Comp. Med. 69 (6), 510–519. https://doi.org/10.30802/AALAS-CM-19-000099.

Leahy, K.M., Ornberg, R.L., Wang, Y., Zweifel, B.S., Koki, A.T., Masferrer, J.L., 2002. Cyclooxygenase-2 inhibition by celecoxib reduces proliferation and induces apoptosis in angiogenic endothelial cells in vivo. Cancer Res. 62 (3), 625–631.

Lee, J.W., Komar, C.A., Bengsch, F., Graham, K., Beatty, G.L., 2016. Genetically engineered mouse models of pancreatic cancer: the KPC model (LSL-Kras(G12D/+) ;LSL-Trp53(R172H/+);Pdx-1-Cre), its variants, and their application in immuno-oncology drug discovery. Curr. Protoc. Pharmacol. 73, 14.39.11–14.39.20. https://doi.org/10.1002/cpph.2.

Li, W., Xu, R.-j., Lin, Z.-y., Zhuo, G.-c., Zhang, H.-h., 2009. Effects of a cyclooxygenase-1-selective inhibitor in a mouse model of ovarian cancer, administered alone or in combination with ibuprofen, a nonselective cyclooxygenase inhibitor. Med. Oncol. 26 (2), 170–177. https://doi.org/10.1007/s12032-008-9104-9.

Li, R., Huang, Y., Lin, J., 2020. Distinct effects of general anesthetics on lung metastasis mediated by IL-6/JAK/STAT3 pathway in mouse models. Nat. Commun. 11 (1), 642. https://doi.org/10.1038/s41467-019-14065-6.

Liles, J.H., Flecknell, P.A., Roughan, J., Cruz-Madorran, I., 1998. Influence of oral buprenorphine, oral naltrexone or morphine on the effects of laparotomy in the rat. Lab. Anim. 32 (2), 149–161. https://doi.org/10.1258/002367798780600025.

Liu, B., Qu, L., Yan, S., 2015. Cyclooxygenase-2 promotes tumor growth and suppresses tumor immunity. Cancer Cell Int. 15, 106. https://doi.org/10.1186/s12935-015-0260-7.

Lofgren, J., Miller, A.L., Lee, C.C.S., Bradshaw, C., Flecknell, P., Roughan, J., 2017. Analgesics promote welfare and sustain tumour growth in orthotopic 4T1 and B16 mouse cancer models. Lab. Anim 52 (4), 351–364. https://doi.org/10.1177/0023677217739934.

Long, I., Robert, P., Aroniadou-Anderjaska, V., Prager, E.M., Pidoplichko, V.I., Figueiredo, T.H., Braga, M.F., 2016. Repeated isoflurane exposures impair long-term potentiation and increase basal gabaergic activity in the basolateral amygdala. Neural Plast. 2016.

Lutman, B., Bloom, J., Nussenblatt, B., Romo, V., 2018. A contemporary perspective on the management of post-craniotomy headache and pain. Curr. Pain Headache Rep. 22 (10), 69. https://doi.org/10.1007/s11916-018-0722-4.

Makaryus, R., Lee, H., Feng, T., Park, J.-H., Nedergaard, M., Jacob, Z., Enikolopov, G., Benveniste, H., 2015. Brain maturation in neonatal rodents is impeded by sevoflurane anesthesia. Anesthesiology 123 (3), 557.

McKune, C.M., Murrell, J.C., Nolan, A.M., White, K.L., Wright, B.D., 2015. Veterinary anesthesia and analgesia. In: Grimm, K.A., Lamont, L.A., Tranquilli, W.J., Greene, S.A., Robertson, S.A. (Eds.), Chapter 29: Nociception and Pain, pp. 584–627.

Melamed, R., Bar-Yosef, S., Shakhar, G., Shakhar, K., Ben-Eliyahu, S., 2003. Suppression of natural killer cell activity and promotion of tumor metastasis by ketamine, thiopental, and halothane, but not by propofol: mediating mechanisms and prophylactic measures. Anesth. Analg. 97 (5). https://journals.lww.com/anesthesia-analgesia/Fulltext/2003/11000/Suppression_of_Natural_Killer_Cell_Activity_and.24.aspx.

Moberg, G.P., 1999. When does stress become distress? Lab. Anim.

Molina, P.E., 2006. Opioids and opiates: analgesia with cardiovascular, haemodynamic and immune implications in critical illness. J. Intern. Med. 259 (2), 138–154. https://doi.org/10.1111/j.1365-2796.2005.01569.x.

Molina-Cimadevila, M.J., Segura, S., Merino, C., Ruiz-Reig, N., Andrés, B., de Madaria, E., 2014. Oral self-administration of buprenorphine in the diet for analgesia in mice. Lab. Anim. 48 (3), 216–224. https://doi.org/10.1177/0023677214532454.

Morton, D.L., Sandhu, J.S., Jones, A.K., 2016. Brain imaging of pain: state of the art. J. Pain Res. 9, 613–624. https://doi.org/10.2147/jpr.S60433.

Moudgil, G.C., Singal, D.P., 1997. Halothane and isoflurane enhance melanoma tumour metastasis in mice. Can. J. Anaesth. 44 (1), 90–94. https://doi.org/10.1007/bf03014331.

Nunamaker, E.A., Stolarik, D.F., Ma, J., Wilsey, A.S., Jenkins, G.J., Medina, C.L., 2014. Clinical efficacy of sustained-release buprenorphine with meloxicam for postoperative analgesia in beagle dogs undergoing ovariohysterectomy. J. Am. Assoc. Lab. Anim. Sci. 53 (5), 494–501.

Oliver, V.L., Thurston, S.E., Lofgren, J.L., 2018. Using cageside measures to evaluate analgesic efficacy in mice (*Mus musculus*) after surgery. J. Am. Assoc. Lab. Anim. Sci. 57 (2), 186–201.

Orr, P.M., Shank, B.C., Black, A.C., 2017. The role of pain classification systems in pain management. Crit. Care Nurs. Clin. 29 (4), 407–418. https://doi.org/10.1016/j.cnc.2017.08.002.

Pacharinsak, C., Beitz, A., 2008. Animal models of cancer pain. Comp. Med. 58 (3), 220–233. https://pubmed.ncbi.nlm.nih.gov/18589864.

Page, G.G., Ben-Eliyahu, S., Yirmiya, R., Liebeskind, J.C., 1993. Morphine attenuates surgery-induced enhancement of metastatic colonization in rats. Pain 54 (1). https://journals.lww.com/pain/Fulltext/1993/07000/Morphine_attenuates_surgery_induced_enhancement_of.4.aspx.

Page, G.G., Blakely, W.P., Ben-Eliyahu, S., 2001. Evidence that postoperative pain is a mediator of the tumor-promoting effects of surgery in rats. Pain 90 (1). https://journals.lww.com/pain/Fulltext/2001/02010/Evidence_that_postoperative_pain_is_a_mediator_of.23.aspx.

Patel, M.I., Subbaramaiah, K., Du, B., Chang, M., Yang, P., Newman, R.A., Cordon-Cardo, C., Thaler, H.T., Dannenberg, A.J., 2005. Celecoxib inhibits prostate cancer growth: evidence of a cyclooxygenase-2-independent mechanism. Clin. Cancer Res. 11 (5), 1999–2007. https://doi.org/10.1158/1078-0432.Ccr-04-1877.

Pawlosky, N., 2013. Cardiovascular risk: are all NSAIDs alike? Can. Pharm. J. 146 (2), 80–83. https://doi.org/10.1177/1715163513481569.

Peterson, N.C., Nunamaker, E.A., Turner, P.V., 2017. To treat or not to treat: the effects of pain on experimental parameters. Comp. Med. 67 (6), 469–482. https://pubmed.ncbi.nlm.nih.gov/29212578.

Pogatzki-Zahn, E., Segelcke, D., Zahn, P., 2018. Mechanisms of acute and chronic pain after surgery: update from findings in experimental animal models. Curr. Opin. Anaesthesiol. 31 (5), 575–585. https://doi.org/10.1097/ACO.0000000000000646.

Rankin, D.C., 2015. Veterinary anesthesia and analgesia. In: Grimm, K.A., Lamont, L.A., Tranquilli, W.J., Greene, S.A., Robertson, S.A. (Eds.), Chapter 10: Sedatives and Tranquilizers, pp. 196–207.

Rawal, H., Patel, B.M., 2018. Opioids in cardiovascular disease: therapeutic options. J. Cardiovasc. Pharmacol. Therapeut. 23 (4), 279–291. https://doi.org/10.1177/1074248418757009.

Retsky, M., Rogers, R., Demicheli, R., Hrushesky, W.J.M., Gukas, I., Vaidya, J.S., Baum, M., Forget, P., DeKock, M., Pachmann, K., 2012. NSAID analgesic ketorolac used perioperatively may suppress early breast cancer relapse: particular relevance to triple negative subgroup. Breast Cancer Res. Treat. 134 (2), 881–888. https://doi.org/10.1007/s10549-012-2094-5.

Rosas, C., Sinning, M., Ferreira, A., Fuenzalida, M., Lemus, D., 2014. Celecoxib decreases growth and angiogenesis and promotes apoptosis in a tumor cell line resistant to chemotherapy. Biol. Res. 47 (1), 27. https://doi.org/10.1186/0717-6287-47-27.

Sandler, R.S., Halabi, S., Baron, J.A., Budinger, S., Paskett, E., Keresztes, R., Petrelli, N., Pipas, J.M., Karp, D.D., Loprinzi, C.L., Steinbach, G., Schilsky, R., 2003. A randomized trial of aspirin to prevent colorectal adenomas in patients with previous colorectal cancer. N. Engl. J. Med. 348 (10), 883–890. https://doi.org/10.1056/NEJMoa021633.

Sauer, M., Fleischmann, T., Lipiski, M., Arras, M., Jirkof, P., 2016. Buprenorphine via drinking water and combined oral-injection protocols for pain relief in mice. Appl. Anim. Behav. Sci. 185, 103–112.

Scarborough, J., Mueller, F., Arban, R., Dorner-Ciossek, C., Weber-Stadlbauer, U., Rosenbrock, H., Meyer, U., Richetto, J., 2020. Preclinical validation of the micropipette-guided drug administration (MDA) method in the maternal immune activation model of neurodevelopmental disorders. Brain Behav. Immun. 88, 461–470. https://doi.org/10.1016/j.bbi.2020.04.015.

Schjerning, A.M., McGettigan, P., Gislason, G., 2020. Cardiovascular effects and safety of (non-aspirin) NSAIDs. Nat. Rev. Cardiol. 17 (9), 574–584. https://doi.org/10.1038/s41569-020-0366-z.

Seymour, T.L., Adams, S.C., Felt, S.A., Jampachaisri, K., Yeomans, D.C., Pacharinsak, C., 2016. Postoperative analgesia due to sustained-release buprenorphine, sustained-release meloxicam, and carprofen gel in a model of incisional pain in rats (*Rattus norvegicus*). J. Am. Assoc. Lab. Anim. Sci. 55 (3), 300–305.

Shen, X., Liu, Y., Xu, S., Zhao, Q., Guo, X., Shen, R., Wang, F., 2013. Early life exposure to sevoflurane impairs adulthood spatial memory in the rat. Neurotoxicology 39, 45–56.

Smith, J.C., 2019. A review of strain and sex differences in response to pain and analgesia in mice. Comp. Med. 69 (6), 490–500. https://doi.org/10.30802/aalas-cm-19-000066.

Song, Q., Merajver, S.D., Li, J.Z., 2015. Cancer classification in the genomic era: five contemporary problems. Hum. Genom. 9, 27. https://doi.org/10.1186/s40246-015-0049-8.

Tacke, S., Henke, J., Erhardt, W., 2008. Metamizol (dipyrone) for pain therapy. Tierärztliche Praxis Ausgabe K: Kleintiere/Heimtiere 36 (01), 19–25.

Takeda, N., Hasegawa, S., Morita, M., Matsunaga, T., 1993. Pica in rats is analogous to emesis: an animal model in emesis research. Pharmacol. Biochem. Behav. 45 (4), 817–821. https://doi.org/10.1016/0091-3057(93)90126-e.

Tanaka, K., Kersten, J.R., Riess, M.L., 2014. Opioid-induced cardioprotection. Curr. Pharmaceut. Des. 20 (36), 5696–5705. https://doi.org/10.2174/1381612820666140204120311.

Tappe-Theodor, A., King, T., Morgan, M.M., 2019. Pros and cons of clinically relevant methods to assess pain in rodents. Neurosci. Biobehav. Rev. 100, 335–343. https://doi.org/10.1016/j.neubiorev.2019.03.009.

Taylor, B.F., Ramirez, H.E., Battles, A.H., Andrutis, K.A., Neubert, J.K., 2016. Analgesic activity of tramadol and buprenorphine after voluntary ingestion by rats (*Rattus norvegicus*). J. Am. Assoc. Lab. Anim. Sci. 55 (1), 74–82.

Thompson, A.C., DiPirro, J.M., Sylvester, A.R., Martin, L.B., Kristal, M.B., 2006. Lack of analgesic efficacy in female rats of the commonly recommended oral dose of buprenorphine. J. Am. Assoc. Lab. Anim. Sci. 45 (6), 13–16.

Toth, L.A., 2019. Interacting influences of sleep, pain, and analgesic medications on sleep studies in rodents. Comp. Med. 69 (6), 571–578. https://doi.org/10.30802/AALAS-CM-19-000029.

Trapani, G., Altomare, C., Sanna, E., Biggio, G., Liso, G., 2000. Propofol in anesthesia. Mechanism of action, structure-activity relationships, and drug delivery. Curr. Med. Chem. 7 (2), 249–271.

Turner, P.V., Pang, D.S., Lofgren, J.L., 2019. A review of pain assessment methods in laboratory rodents. Comp. Med. 69 (6), 451–467. https://doi.org/10.30802/AALAS-CM-19-000042.

WHO website. (2021). https://www.who.int/health-topics/cardiovascular-diseases#tab=tab_1.

Wickerts, L., Warrén Stomberg, M., Brattwall, M., Jakobsson, J., 2011. Coxibs: is there a benefit when compared to traditional non-selective NSAIDs in postoperative pain management? Minerva Anestesiol. 77 (11), 1084–1098.

Xu, Y.C., Li, R.P., Xue, F.S., Cui, X.L., Wang, S.Y., Liu, G.P., Yang, G.Z., Sun, C., Liao, X., 2015. κ-Opioid receptors are involved in enhanced cardioprotection by combined fentanyl and limb remote ischemic postconditioning. J. Anesth. 29 (4), 535–543. https://doi.org/10.1007/s00540-015-1998-8.

Yang, S., Zhang, J.J., Huang, X.Y., 2012. Mouse models for tumor metastasis. Methods Mol. Biol. 928, 221–228. https://doi.org/10.1007/978-1-62703-008-3_17.

Zanos, P., Gould, T.D., 2018. Mechanisms of ketamine action as an antidepressant. Mol. Psychiatr. 23 (4), 801–811.

Zhu, C., Gao, J., Karlsson, N., Li, Q., Zhang, Y., Huang, Z., Li, H., Kuhn, H.G., Blomgren, K., 2010. Isoflurane anesthesia induced persistent, progressive memory impairment, caused a loss of neural stem cells, and reduced neurogenesis in young, but not adult, rodents. J. Cerebr. Blood Flow Metabol. 30 (5), 1017–1030.

Section II

Principles of anesthesia and analgesia

Chapter 4

Injectable anesthetics

Bridget V. Willeford[1], Steven E. Davison[2] and Robert E. Meyer[3]

[1]*Laboratory Animal Resources, Mississippi State University, Mississippi State, MS, United States;* [2]*School of Medicine, University of Louisville, Louisville, KY, United States;* [3]*Clinical Sciences College of Veterinary Medicine, Mississippi State, MS, United States*

Chapter outline

Anesthesia and Analgesia in Laboratory Animals. https://doi.org/10.1016/B978-0-12-822215-7.00028-7

I. Introduction

The term "injectable anesthetic," as applied to this chapter, covers a broad range of substances with varied effects. This chapter does not cover sedatives or analgesics, but rather only drugs that produce general anesthesia, with additional information regarding mixtures of these drugs with other agents. Readers are encouraged to consult previous editions of this chapter, which may have more in-depth information for some drugs and mixtures, as well as information about drugs that are no longer commonly used.

The use of injectable anesthetics in laboratory animals is preferred by many for a variety of reasons: ease of administration, a widely available database supporting the use in laboratory animals, fewer specialized equipment needs, avoidance of endotracheal intubation, and fewer potential occupational health concerns for laboratory workers (Fish, 1997). The use of continuous infusion techniques has attracted attention in veterinary and human medicine, not only to account for individual variation but also to improve anesthetic stability by approaching a steady-state blood concentration (Hedenqvist and Hellebrekers, 2003; Ilkiw and Pascoe, 2003; Ting et al., 2004; White, 1989). There has also been interest in developing injectable anesthetic agents that may approach inhalants in the speed of recovery or that have the potential for pharmacologic antagonism (Nunn et al., 1989).

By definition, an injectable anesthetic agent is a compound that by itself produces a state of general anesthesia; this can be further characterized as pharmacologically induced central nervous system (CNS) depression that permits invasive surgical or experimental procedures to be performed. The basic components of general anesthesia include amnesia, unconsciousness, and immobility in response to noxious stimulation.

When evaluating research literature on anesthetic agents, one must consider the importance of defining the parameters of anesthetic duration, and the distinction between depth of anesthesia and antinociceptive potency (Antognini et al., 2005; Whelan and Flecknell, 1992; Wixson et al., 1987a); the shortcomings of control data, such as the absence of nonmedicated animal data and the use of conscious but restrained animals, or animals evaluated shortly after recovery from instrumentation surgery/anesthesia; and failure to maintain normal body temperature and ventilation status. It should also be remembered that, although a pharmacologic effect may be attributed to a particular anesthetic agent, many reported effects are a more generalized feature of the anesthetic state. For example, barbiturate anesthesia has been reported to reduce ionizing radiation effectiveness in killing tumor cells. Although this effect has been attributed to a direct effect on cellular respiration (Aldridge and Parker, 1960), it is instead due to anesthetic-mediated reduction and redistribution of tumor blood flow in anesthetized animals (Meyer et al., 2002).

Injectable anesthetic agents producing adequate anesthesia in one strain or species may be insufficient or may provide different signs of anesthesia at similar doses in other strains or species. There are several possible reasons for this. Anesthetic uptake, distribution, and effect are governed by the pharmacokinetic and pharmacodynamic properties of the anesthetic agent in that strain or species. As is true for other drugs, individual variation plays an important role in biodisposition and pharmacokinetics, as well as in therapeutics. Components of this variation include genotype (breed, stock, or strain), sex, age, body composition, and nutritional and disease status.

Allometric scaling is often applied when extrapolating drug disposition across species. Allometric scaling is based on the empirical observation that certain physiological functions, such as renal glomerular filtration rate, oxygen consumption, cardiac output, and basal metabolic rate, can be scaled across species as a function of body size or surface area according to a power function or its log-transformed linear equivalent:

$$Y =_a W^b$$

where Y is the parameter under study, a is allometric coefficient (intercept) that is constant for a drug, W is the species average body weight, and b is the allometric exponent, generally between 0.67 and 1.0 (Nair et al., 2016). Huang and Riviere (2014) have reviewed the application of allometric scaling principles to predict pharmacokinetic parameters across species.

Abundant, detailed information on the pharmacology of injectable anesthetics is available in both human and veterinary literature. While it is presumed that the cellular mechanisms underlying anesthetic effects are well conserved among species, it is clear that pharmacokinetics (or biodisposition) and clinical effects differ markedly among species. The focus of this chapter, therefore, is on the pharmacologic aspects of injectable agents in experimental animals, with particular emphasis on nondomestic species, and the effects of these agents on the physiology and metabolism of the animal (Tables 4.1 and 4.2).

TABLE 4.1 Considerations when choosing an anesthetic protocol.

• Restraint? Sedation? Invasive procedure?
• Terminal procedure or recovery?
• Procedural duration? Is redosing anticipated? Potential effect?
• Known species, sex, and strain considerations?
• Dose required and appropriate monitoring signs?
• Effect on target tissue perfusion?
• Effect on physiologic and metabolic homeostasis?

II. γ-aminobutyric acid receptor agonists

A. Mechanism of action

The barbiturates, chloral hydrate, alpha-chloralose, tribromoethanol (TBE), propofol, metomidate, etomidate, steroid anesthetics, and the benzodiazepines all exert sedative and hypnotic effects through interactions with the inhibitory γ-aminobutyric acid (GABA) neurotransmitter system (Im et al., 1990; Krasowski and Harrison, 2000; Macdonald and McLean, 1986; Olson et al., 1987; Saunders and Ho, 1990; Stoelting and Hillier, 2006; Suzdak et al., 1986; Turner et al., 1989). Both the GABA and adrenergic neurotransmitter systems act to counterbalance the action of excitatory neurotransmitters. The GABA type A receptor ($GABA_A$) is comprised of five glycoprotein subunits (α′, β, and γ2 subunits). Transmembrane chloride conductance increases when the $GABA_A$ receptor is activated, resulting in postsynaptic cell membrane hyperpolarization and postsynaptic neuron resistance to stimulation by excitatory transmitters. Barbiturates and propofol appear to decrease the rate of dissociation of GABA from its receptor, thus increasing the duration of the GABA-activated opening of chloride channels. Barbiturates also can mimic the action of GABA by activating the chloride channels directly. Etomidate augments GABA-gated chloride currents (indirect modulation) and produces chloride currents in the absence of GABA at higher concentrations (direct modulation). Although propofol, like barbiturates, enhances GABA-activated chloride channel activity, it also has ion-channel-blocking effects in the cerebral cortex and nicotinic acetylcholine receptors and inhibits lysophosphatidate signaling in lipid mediator receptors. Thus, by acting on a single receptor via different mechanisms, quite different anesthetic agents can act synergistically to increase $GABA_A$ receptor-mediated inhibition of the CNS. The use of $GABA_A$-targeted mutant knockout and knockin mice has greatly assisted in determining the role of individual receptor subtypes in anesthetic action (Rudolph and Mohler, 2004; Wafford et al., 2004).

It is important to realize that although $GABA_A$-agonist injectable anesthetics can produce sedation, hypnosis, and, with the exception of the benzodiazepines, general anesthesia, they are generally considered to be poor analgesics and therefore may be insufficient for extensive or highly invasive surgery. However, even large doses of opioids or α2-adrenergic agonists (covered elsewhere in this text) induce an incomplete anesthetic state and usually require the addition of a hypnotic $GABA_A$-agonist (or NMDA-antagonist) to cause unconsciousness (Stoelting and Hillier, 2006).

TABLE 4.2 Anesthetic Considerations when evaluating research literature.

• How are parameters of the duration of effect defined?
• Is a distinction made between depth of anesthesia and antinociceptive potency?
• Is control data missing? (e.g., absence of nonmedicated animal data; use of restrained conscious animals or animals not at rest; insufficient time for full recovery from instrumentation surgery/anesthesia)
• Was normal body temperature and respiration maintained throughout?

B. Barbiturates

1. Pharmacokinetics and metabolism

Most barbiturates are metabolized by oxidation in the liver into inactive, water-soluble compounds and then excreted by renal excretion in the urine (Mihic et al., 2017).

2. Absorption

Barbiturates in general are readily absorbed by most sites, including the gastrointestinal tract; however, the highly alkaline pH of some barbiturate solutions limits their administration via the intravenous (IV) route.

3. Distribution and fate

Generally speaking, barbiturates are widely distributed throughout the body. Highly lipid-soluble, most barbiturates readily cross the blood-brain barrier. Redistribution can then occur to less vascular tissues like muscle and fat, resulting in decreased levels in the brain. Following oral or parenteral administration, barbiturates readily cross the placental barrier and are distributed throughout fetal tissues, with the highest concentrations found in the placenta, fetal liver, and brain. Fetal blood levels approach maternal blood levels following parenteral administration. Barbiturates are excreted in milk and can result in clinical signs in nursing offspring (Branson, 2001).

Species differences in barbiturate response are directly related to pharmacokinetics rather than differences in drug receptor sensitivity (Davis et al., 1973; Dos Santos and Bogan, 1974). For example, pentobarbital half-life is 38, 85, 100, and 200 min in the mouse, rabbit, rat, and dog, respectively (Thurmon, 1985), and thiopental elimination half-life and steady-state volume of distribution in the rabbit are markedly lower than those in the dog or sheep (Ilkiw et al., 1991). Differences in plasma protein binding of barbiturates may contribute to both species and individual differences in drug disposition (Sharma et al., 1970; Thurmon, 1985).

4. Preparation and route of administration

Barbiturates are derived from barbituric acid, which itself is nondepressant, but appropriate side-chain substitutions result in CNS depressant activity that varies in potency and duration with carbon chain length, branching, and saturation. Oxybarbiturates retain an oxygen atom on number 2-carbon atom of the barbituric acid ring. Thiobarbiturates replace this oxygen atom with a sulfur atom, which confers greater lipid solubility. Generally speaking, a substitution such as sulfuration that increases lipid solubility is associated with greater hypnotic potency and a more rapid onset but a shorter duration of action. Addition of a methyl group to the nitrogen atom of the barbituric acid ring, as with oxybarbiturate methohexital, also results in a compound with a short duration of action.

Barbiturate administration is not associated with increased sympathetic activity (Zimpfer et al., 1982). They selectively suppress transmission in sympathetic nervous system ganglia at concentrations that have no detectable effect on nerve conduction. This effect may contribute to decreased systemic blood pressure that is sometimes observed with IV administration of barbiturates or associated with barbiturate overdose. High doses of barbiturates decrease the sensitivity of postsynaptic membranes to acetylcholine at the neuromuscular junction.

5. Side effects

As with other $GABA_A$ agonists, barbiturates are generally considered to be good hypnotic agents, but relatively poor analgesics (Booth, 1988a; Tomemori et al., 1981). Barbiturates at low doses may not provide reliable sedation in the presence of pain without supplemental analgesia, such that the barbiturates may be classified as hypnotic sedatives, reflecting their dose-dependent ability to produce either sedation or a deeper hypnotic state (Heavner, 1986). Instead of sedation, paradoxical excitement can occur, especially at low doses or with slow IV administration, but this is likely due to barbiturate-induced depression of CNS inhibitory centers. Although hyperalgesic properties have been attributed to the barbiturates, spinal cord analgesic effects can be demonstrated (Jewett et al., 1992), as well as peripheral antihyperalgesia effects in a rat intraplantar formalin injection model (da Motta et al., 2004).

a. Immune system effects

The in vitro antiinflammatory effects of anesthetics have been reviewed by Schneemilch et al. (2004). Thiopental directly inhibits cell-mediated immune responses and has a strong antiinflammatory effect. Long-term administration of high doses of thiopental is associated with increased nosocomial infection and mortality, possibly due to the inhibition of nuclear transcription factor kappaB, which is a central regulator of the immune response (Loop et al., 2002). At clinically used concentrations, thiopental has been shown to inhibit the bactericidal functions of leukocytes as well as polarization, chemotaxis, adherence, phagocytosis, the respiratory burst of neutrophils, and the chemotaxis of monocytes, while at high concentrations, thiopental affects neutrophil and monocyte phagocytosis.

Pentobarbital causes injury to lymphocytes and to hepatic Kupffer and endothelial cells in ICR mice within 6 h of administration, as indicated by elevated hepatic aspartate transferase and alanine transaminase levels (Thompson et al., 2002). Lipopolysaccharide (LPS) administration to animals under anesthesia is often used to study proinflammatory cytokine release. Thiopental inhibits endotoxin-induced production of tumor necrosis factor (TNFα), IL-1, and IL-8 and increases IL-10 release in vitro (Taniguchi and Yamamoto, 2005). In adult male HsdBrl:WH Wistar rats, pentobarbital enhances basal expression of IL-1β and IL-6 mRNA in the rat spleen; TNFα mRNA is unaffected (Bette et al., 2004). In C57BL/6 mice anesthetized with 90 mg/kg pentobarbital IP, 40 mg/kg LPS causes endotoxemia and results in hypoglycemia and increased serum alanine aminotransferase, lipase, and creatinine levels, suggesting LPS damage to the liver, exocrine pancreas, and kidney (Kazerani and Furman, 2006). Importantly, lung myeloperoxidase activity, an indicator of neutrophil infiltration, is also increased by LPS, implying that pentobarbital does not protect mice against LPS-mediated damage to the lung and is a suitable anesthetic for studies of endotoxemia (Kazerani and Furman, 2006). In contrast, Yang et al. (2007) report pentobarbital suppression of LPS-induced TNFα mRNA, possibly due to decreased nuclear factor kappaB and activator protein 1 and reduced expression of p38 mitogen-activated protein kinase; these authors conclude pentobarbital protects cells from death directly and indirectly induced by TNFα during the LPS-induced inflammatory response.

b. Other pharmacologic effects

Other reported pharmacologic effects of the barbiturates include the following: progressive decrease in core temperature in rats (Commissaris et al., 1982; Wixson et al., 1987d) and mice (Johnson et al., 1976); decreased renal blood flow and urine output, secondary to lowered blood pressure (Booth, 1988); increased sensitivity to barbiturate anesthesia in uremia, probably due to reduced protein binding (Booth, 1988); reduced renal blood flow and glomerular filtration rate in rats (Gumbleton et al., 1990a; Walker et al., 1986), apparently responsible for decreased elimination rate of aminoglycoside antibiotics (Higashi et al., 1982); decreased packed cell volumes in dogs (Usenik and Cronkite, 1965), miniature swine (Sawyer et al., 1971), and mice (Friedman, 1959); hyperglycemia in hamsters, unrelated to duration of anesthesia or degree of surgical manipulation (Turner and Howards, 1977), not seen in rats (Hinton, 1982); and neuroprotection in gerbils given 50 mg/kg of pentobarbital 30 min before global ischemia (Ishimaru et al., 1995). Barbiturates decrease cerebral blood flow (CBF) and thus decrease intracranial pressure (ICP); cerebral vascular reactivity to carbon dioxide is preserved (Ilkiw, 1992). Although amelioration of neuronal damage through decreased cerebral metabolic rate is provided by barbiturates following a focal ischemic event (Hall and Murdoch, 1990), the ability of barbiturates to improve brain survival after global cerebral ischemia is unlikely, as these drugs are only effective when the EEG remains active and metabolic suppression is possible. For a more extensive review of pharmacologic effects, see the previous edition.

c. Tolerance

Tolerance to barbiturate effects, due to hepatic NADPH-dependent cytochrome P450 enzyme induction, can be demonstrated following previous exposure to the same or different barbiturate drug. For example, rats treated with phenobarbital and later with hexobarbital were anesthetized only 5% as long as untreated rats (Conney et al., 1960), and the pentobarbital plasma half-life following chronic pentobarbital pretreatment was only 12% that of control rats (Commissaris et al., 1982). Chronic exposure to barbiturates, particularly phenobarbital and pentobarbital, has been associated with the induction of cytochrome P450 2B monooxygenase activity and implicated in hepatic tumor carcinogenesis in male F344/NCr rats initiated with *N*-nitrosodiethylamine (Rice et al., 1994). In contrast to tolerance phenomena, drugs that suppress hepatic microsomal enzyme function may prolong the barbiturate effects. The antibiotic chloramphenicol prolongs pentobarbital anesthesia in the rat, mouse, dog, cat, and monkey (Adams, 1970; Adams and Dixit, 1970; Azadegan et al., 1980; Teske and Carter, 1971).

6. *Thiopental, thiamylal, and methohexital*

As thiamylal, thiopental, and methohexital are either no longer commercially available or no longer used, see the previous edition for a description of these anesthetics.

7. *Thiobutabarbital*

Although Inactin, the product name for ethyl-(1-methyl-propyl) malonyl-thiourea (also referred to as thiobutabarbital, or EMTU), is no longer available, it continues to be used for its prolonged and stable anesthetic state in rats for renal studies (Buelke-Sam et al., 1978; Cupples et al., 1982; Rieg et al., 2004; Schiffer et al., 2018; Turner and Howards, 1977) and neuroscience studies (Bu et al., 2020; Jackson et al., 2016). In rats, thiobutabarbital decreases arterial pressure, renal blood flow, and glomerular filtration rate (Walker et al., 1983); renal and single nephron function during thiobutabarbital and thiopental anesthesia were judged to be similar (100 mg/kg intraperitoneal (IP) for each agent) (Haberle et al., 1993). In rabbits, however, thiobutabarbital is ineffective and results in both short periods of anesthesia and death (Hobbs et al., 1991). Reagent-grade thiobutabarbital can be obtained from chemical suppliers such as Sigma–Aldrich. As thiobutabarbital is a nonpharmaceutical-grade compound, its use should be scientifically justified over other pharmaceutical-grade compounds.

8. *Pentobarbital*

The oxybarbiturate pentobarbital continues to be used to produce rodent anesthesia despite its increasing limited availability and expense. The use of pentobarbital stems from a widely available database encompassing decades of use, rapid anesthetic onset, nonirritant nature, and ease of IP injection to rodents of varying ages and body weights (Wixson and Smiler, 1997). Pentobarbital provides inadequate or inconsistent analgesia in mice (Erhardt et al., 1984), rats (Wixson et al., 1987b), and rabbits (Borkowski et al., 1990). IP administration of pentobarbital in rats is associated with mild excitement both on induction and on recovery (Wixson et al., 1987a).

a. Preparation and route of administration

Commercial preparations of pentobarbital are racemic mixtures. The (+) isomer causes a transient period of hyperexcitability before CNS depression, while the (−) isomer produces relatively smooth and progressively deeper hypnosis (Huang and Barker, 1980). At anesthetic doses, pentobarbital suppresses high-frequency neuronal firing by inhibiting voltage-dependent Na^+ channels; higher doses reduce voltage-dependent K^+ conductances (Hardman et al., 1996). Pentobarbital is metabolized primarily by hepatic cytochrome P450 microsomal enzymes and hydroxylation of the 3-carbon methyl butyl side chain (Freudenthal and Carroll, 1973). In sheep, excretion via routes other than urine is negligible (Dos Santos and Bogan, 1974), in contrast to the rat, in which 28% of a dose is excreted in bile within 6 h (Klaassen, 1971). Pentobarbital can be administered either intravenously or intraperitoneally.

b. Cardiovascular effects

Reduced blood pressure, stroke volume, pulse pressure, and central venous pressure are common findings in pentobarbital-anesthetized animals (Parker and Adams, 1978). Although pentobarbital is reported to produce prolonged hypotension in the rat (Svendsen and Carter, 1985; Wixson et al., 1987c), other investigators have reported an increased arterial pressure (Folle and Levesque, 1976). Cardiac output in the rat is reduced (Gumbleton et al., 1990a; Kawaue and Iriuchijima, 1984; Lee et al., 1985; Seyde et al., 1985), and cardiovascular reflex responses are altered (Aisaka et al., 1991; Fluckiger et al., 1985; Wang et al., 1991). Myocardial contractility is impaired following pentobarbital anesthesia in the dog (Vatner et al., 1971), and has been demonstrated in vitro (Parker and Adams, 1978).

The cardiovascular effects of pentobarbital are less pronounced following IP administration. Peak blood concentration is reached more slowly than with IV injection, and the portion of drug absorbed into the portal system is subject to early metabolism in the liver.

Pentobarbital anesthesia in dogs typically increases heart rate (Booth, 1988a; Manders and Vatner, 1976). Heart rate in pentobarbital-anesthetized rats (Wixson et al., 1987c) and rabbits (Borkowski et al., 1990; Flecknell et al., 1983) is not significantly altered, although tachycardia is seen in rabbits with subanesthetic doses (Murthy et al., 1982). The increased heart rate observed with barbiturates is not due to increased sympathetic activity (Zimpfer et al., 1982).

Pharmacologic activation of adenosine triphosphate-regulated K_{ATP} channels mimics ischemic myocardial preconditioning and may decrease infarct size and improve functional recovery of ischemic-reperfused stunned myocardium. Pentobarbital inhibits the ischemic preconditioning-like cardioprotective effect of inhalational anesthetics (Kohro et al., 2001). In a cellular model of simulated myocardial ischemia, diazoxide-induced cell protection of mitochondrial K_{ATP} channel activity was blocked by pentobarbital (Zaugg et al., 2002).

c. Effect on ventilation and blood gases

Pentobarbital can be a potent dose-dependent ventilatory depressant. Respiratory depression is reported in the rat (Folle and Levesque, 1976; Seyde et al., 1985; Svendsen and Carter, 1985; Wixson et al., 1987c), mouse (Erhardt et al., 1984), rabbit (Borkowski et al., 1990; Flecknell et al., 1983), and hamster (Reid et al., 1989). In the dog, pentobarbital decreases the hypercapnic and hypoxic drives of respiration and attenuates carbon dioxide augmentation of the hypoxic response (Hirshman et al., 1975). Wixson et al. (1987c) reported that 40 mg/kg pentobarbital administered IP to male Sprague—Dawley rats decreased pH by 1.2%, or 0.09—0.10 pH units, and increased $PaCO_2$ by 46% (11 mmHg); 30 and 40 mg/kg pentobarbital decreased PaO_2 by 19%—20% (34 mmHg). Even at doses insufficient to produce antinociception, similar ventilatory effects were observed in mice (Erhardt et al., 1984): pentobarbital (50 mg/kg IP) in male adult BALB/c mice decreased arterial pH almost 0.15 units, from 7.285 to 7.137, while arterial PCO_2 increased from 26.5 to 38.8 mmHg and PaO_2 dropped from 111.7 to 93.0 mmHg.

In contrast, Skolleborg et al. (1990) reported arterial blood gas values for pH, PCO_2, and PO_2 within the normal awake range in male Mol: WIST rats following administration of 50 mg/kg IP pentobarbital. Similar findings of minimal respiratory depression have been reported for female Fischer 344 rats anesthetized with 50 mg/kg IP pentobarbital (Dewhirst et al., 1996) and for male Sprague—Dawley rats anesthetized with 40 mg/kg IP pentobarbital (Taie et al., 1999). It has been speculated that these respiratory effects may have been due to the maintenance of body temperature (Collado et al., 1987; Heys et al., 1989).

d. Tolerance and strain differences

Barbiturate sleep time in rats and mice has been used in pharmacologic and toxicologic studies as a noninvasive measure of liver function. Although pentobarbital blood levels also decrease, in part, due to redistribution (Thurmon, 1985), sleep time is inversely proportional to the rate of drug metabolism (Lovell, 1986b). A variety of factors affect sleep time, including age, sex, strain, feed, and nutritional status, bedding material, and temperature (Collins and Lott, 1968; Cunliffe-Beamer et al., 1981; Hall et al., 1976; Jondorff et al., 1958; Lovell, 1986a—c; Quinn et al., 1958; Taber and Irwin, 1969; Vesell, 1968; Westenberg and Bolam, 1981; Westfall et al., 1964). Sleep time can be prolonged by the administration of sulfonamides, salicylates, doxycycline, and phenylbutazone, each of which acts by displacing barbiturates from serum protein-binding sites (Booth, 1988a; Chaplin et al., 1973). At doses of 30—55 mg/kg, female rats take three times longer to recover than males, and mortality is higher in females (Holck et al., 1937).

There are significant differences in pentobarbital dose response among strains of mice, such that underdosage or overdosage frequently occurs. A dose of 50 mg/kg provided adequate sedation, but insufficient analgesia in male adult BALB/c mice (Erhardt et al., 1984); some mortality was noted at doses of 60 mg/kg, indicating a narrow safety margin. Lovell studied the effects of 60 mg/kg pentobarbital administered by IP to 23 strains of inbred mice (Lovell, 1986a–1986c). The variation in sleep time among strains of mice is considerable, ranging from 50 min for female NZW mice to 250 min for male dibromoacetaldehyde mice. Male mice generally sleep longer than female mice. C57BL/6 mice sleep longer than CBA mice, which sleep longer than BALB/c mice. There are also within-strain differences for age, sex, litter size, and fasting prior to anesthesia. Environmental variables affecting sleep time include diet, environmental temperature, and bedding material, with inbred strains showing greater variation than F1 hybrids. At an environmental temperature of 18°C, sleep time in BALB/c mice administered 60 mg/kg pentobarbital IP is 195 min, and raising the environmental temperature to 26°C decreases sleep time to 100 min. However, at an environmental temperature of 18°C, C57BL/10ScSn mice sleep for over 400 min. It is likely that strain and environmental factors have contributed to the confusion surrounding anesthetic effect on tumor physiology and radiotherapy outcome (Meyer et al., 2002).

9. *Barbiturate antagonists*

Although concurrent use of preanesthetic agents can substantially reduce the dosage of barbiturates needed for anesthesia (Booth, 1988a; Muir et al., 1991), there are no clinically useful specific barbiturate antagonists. Bicuculline and picrotoxin, as $GABA_A$-antagonists, are used experimentally for confirmation of GABA-mediated effects (Bloom, 2006). Barbiturate sleep time in rats is decreased by the neurostimulatory neurosteroid pregnenolone sulfate, which is consistent with its antagonist action on the $GABA_A$ receptor (Akwa and Baulieu, 1999). Thyrotropin-releasing hormone (TRH) reduces pentobarbital sleep time in dogs (Hernandez et al., 1987), likely due to pharmacodynamic effects associated with sympathoadrenal activation (Schaefer et al., 1989). Effects of thiopental anesthesia are reduced in dogs and cats following the administration of nonspecific agents such as 4-aminopyridine, amphetamine, or yohimbine (Hatch, 1973; Hatch et al., 1984).

C. Chloral hydrate

1. *Pharmacokinetics and metabolism*

The rate of metabolism of chloral hydrate varies with species but is generally rapid in mammals and occurs predominately in the liver (Daniel et al., 1992). Most of the drug is reduced by hepatic alcohol dehydrogenase to trichloroethanol, an active metabolite that accounts for most of its hypnotic action. Trichloroethanol is metabolized primarily by hepatic conjugation with glucuronic acid to form an inactive metabolite that is excreted in the urine; a small portion of the drug is excreted unchanged (Branson and Booth, 1995; Charney et al., 2006). Although the hypnotic action of chloral hydrate is attributed to trichloroethanol, both chloral hydrate and trichloroethanol enhance the response to submaximal concentrations of GABA on $GABA_A$ receptor subunits expressed in *Xenopus laevis* oocytes (Garrett and Gan, 1998) and human embryonic kidney 239 cells (Krasowski and Harrison, 2000).

Trichloroacetic acid is a quantitatively lesser metabolite of chloral hydrate without a sedative effect. There are species-specific differences in the predominant pathway of its formation, by either oxidation of trichloroethanol or direct oxidation of chloral hydrate. There are significant differences in the rates of metabolism of chloral hydrate, trichloroethanol, and trichloroacetic acid in rats, mice, and humans (Daniel et al., 1992; Lash et al., 2000; Lipscomb et al., 1996).

The metabolism of chloral hydrate has received increased attention because of its place in the metabolism of trichloroethylene, a common metal-degreasing solvent that is a rodent carcinogen (Caldwell and Keshava, 2006; Lash et al., 2000). Hepatocarcinogenicity of trichloroethylene in the mouse is believed to be due primarily to trichloroacetic acid (Bronley-DeLancey et al., 2006), which also may be responsible for the cardiac effects of high doses of chloral hydrate (Laurent et al., 2006).

2. *Absorption*

Chloral hydrate is readily absorbed from the GI tract, but onset of full effect by this route is slow (Green, 1979).

3. *Distribution and fate*

Following IP injection, chloral hydrate is quickly metabolized to form trichloroethanol, which is subsequently eliminated by the kidney (Silverman and Muir, 1993).

4. *Preparation and route of administration*

Chloral hydrate (trichloroacetaldehyde monohydrate) is a Schedule IV (Controlled Substances Act) sedative and hypnotic agent that has been in human clinical use since 1869 and in veterinary use since shortly thereafter (Branson, 2001). Its use has declined steadily over the years as a result of improved drugs and concerns over drug safety.

Current use of chloral hydrate in veterinary practice is limited, and generally not recommended (Hall et al., 2001).

In the research setting, chloral hydrate has been used to achieve medium-duration, light anesthesia with minimal effects on cardiovascular function or reflexes. However, at doses required for surgical anesthesia, the safety margin is reduced significantly, and recovery is prolonged (Flecknell, 1996). There have been few, if any, controlled studies of the anesthetic or analgesic actions of chloral hydrate (Silverman and Muir, 1993).

Chloral hydrate is no longer available as an FDA-approved drug in the United States, so it must be compounded. It has historically been used either intravenously or orally for sedation in horses and cattle. For research purposes, it has been given intraperitoneally to rodents but has also been reported at both IV and subcutaneous doses (Silverman and Muir, 1993). As chloral hydrate is a nonpharmaceutical-grade compound, its use should be scientifically justified over other pharmaceutical-grade compounds.

5. Side effects

In hypnotic doses, the depressant effect of chloral hydrate is limited to the cerebrum, with minimal effects on medullary centers. Motor and sensory nerves are not affected except at high doses, and analgesia is minimal (Branson and Booth, 1995; Flecknell, 1987). Cerebral depression occurs slowly and the use of chloral hydrate for euthanasia of small animals may be preceded by gasping, muscle spasms, and vocalization (Leary et al., 2020). Hypnotic doses of chloral hydrate have minimal effects on cardiorespiratory function (Branson and Booth, 1995), but anesthetic doses may be severely depressive (Field et al., 1993; Rodrigues et al., 2006). In the dog, IV administration results in respiratory depression, lowered blood pressure, and sensitization of the heart to sudden vagal arrest or arrhythmias (Soma, 1983; Strobel and Wollman, 1969).

Chloral hydrate solution is irritating to the stomach mucosa and causes severe inflammation and necrosis with perivascular injection (Booth, 1988a; Ogino et al., 1990). Adynamic ileus, with morbidity and death, has been attributed to the IP administration of high concentrations of chloral hydrate in the rat (Fleischman et al., 1977) and hamster (Dada et al., 1992); lower concentrations will minimize this effect (Vachon et al., 2000). Transient adynamic ileus has also been observed following IP administration in the calf and pig (Silverman and Muir, 1993); this route cannot be recommended for survival procedures. Chloral hydrate in relatively large and repeated doses is carcinogenic in the mouse (Caldwell and Keshava, 2006). Genotoxic effects have been demonstrated in a number of in vivo and in vitro studies (Ikbal et al., 2004).

D. Alpha-chloralose

1. Pharmacokinetics and metabolism

Chloralose is metabolized to glucose and chloral, which, in turn, is metabolized to trichloroethanol. Its metabolism and action, therefore, should resemble those of chloral hydrate (Branson and Booth, 1995). However, the duration of effect following a single dose is much longer with chloralose than with chloral hydrate, and it has been reported in human toxic exposures that alpha-chloralose, but not trichloroethanol, could be detected in blood and urine (Kintz et al., 1996). Furthermore, alpha-chloralose directly enhances the response to submaximal concentrations of GABA on $GABA_A$ receptor subunits expressed in *X. laevis* oocytes (Garrett and Gan, 1998) and human embryonic kidney 239 cells (Krasowski and Harrison, 2000).

2. Distribution and fate

Alpha-chloralose produces hypnosis of long duration (8–10 h), with minimal effect on reflexes. Analgesia generally has been considered poor (Flecknell, 1987; Strobel and Wollman, 1969), although it may be adequate for some procedures (Silverman and Muir, 1993). The effectiveness of alpha-chloralose as an anesthetic appears to vary among species; it is probably not effective in dogs (Holzgrefe et al., 1987). Chloralose use alone in veterinary practice, or experimentally for survival procedures is not recommended due to rough induction, prolonged recovery, and seizure-like activity in some species (Hall et al., 2001; Silverman and Muir, 1993).

Alpha-chloralose is still used in physiological studies to preserve respiratory and cardiac reflexes (Branson and Booth, 1995; Beam et al., 2015), in long-term neuroscience regimens (Storer et al., 1997), and for functional MRI studies in rats (Steward et al., 2005). Surgical manipulations should not be performed with chloralose alone, and physiological experiments typically involve induction with a short-acting anesthetic.

3. Preparation and route of administration

Chloralose is the weakly water-soluble reaction product of glucose with anhydrous chloral (trichloroacetaldehyde); the reaction produces α and β isomers. While hypnotic activity resides almost exclusively with alpha-chloralose, the β isomer is thought to be responsible for convulsions and toxicity (Branson and Booth, 1995). Alpha-chloralose is solubilized for administration by several routes, including oral, by heating to 60°C, or mixing with 25% urethane or other solubilizing agents (Storer et al., 1997). As with other nonpharmaceutical-grade compounds, the use of alpha-chloralose should be scientifically justified over other pharmaceutical-grade compounds.

4. Side effects

Alpha-chloralose is used especially for chemical restraint with minimal cardiac and respiratory depression (Flecknell, 1987), although assisted respiration may be required at the higher doses necessary when the agent is used alone (Holzgrefe et al., 1987). Spinal reflexes may be increased, and strychnine-like convulsions have been reported in dogs and cats. Spontaneous movements are common, and animals may respond to tactile and auditory stimuli (Branson and Booth, 1995; Soma, 1983). Alpha-chloralose is commonly considered to preserve normal autonomic reflex activity, including baroreceptor and chemoreceptor reflexes (see review by Holzgrefe et al., 1987). However, chloralose alters the baroreceptor reflex in lambs (Covert et al., 1988), rats (Fluckiger et al., 1985; Shimokawa et al., 1998; Wang et al., 1991), and rabbits (Ishikawa et al., 1984); the somato-sympathetic-adrenal reflex (Gaumann and Yaksh, 1990) and micturition reflex (Rudy et al., 1991) in cats; and the response to carotid chemoreceptor stimulation in the dog (Zimpfer et al., 1981). Myocardial contractility is impaired (Parker and Adams, 1978). Beam et al. (2015) found that pigs anesthetized with alpha-chloralose lacked an increase in heart rate, which suggested either blunting of the baroreceptor reflex or induction of another method to increase stroke volume. Based on their study, alpha-chloralose appeared to be useful in swine studies of acute pulmonary embolism due to its protection of the sympathetic drive and cardiac output. Steward et al. (2005) has reviewed the effect of several anesthetics, including alpha-chloralose, on neurotransmitter systems in the context of the rat brain blood oxygen level-dependent (BOLD) contrast pharmacological MRI. For a more detailed description of side effects, please see the previous edition.

E. Metomidate and etomidate

1. Pharmacokinetics and metabolism

Etomidate pharmacokinetics were determined in cats after IV administration (3.0 mg/kg); disposition best conformed to a 2- and a 3-compartment open pharmacokinetic model. The first and most rapid distribution half-life was 0.05 h, with a second distribution half-life of 0.35 h. Other data included elimination half-life (2.89 h), apparent volume of distribution (11.87 L/kg), apparent volume of distribution at steady state (4.88 L/kg), apparent volume of the central compartment (1.17 L/kg), and total clearance (2.47 L/kg/h) (Wertz et al., 1990). Hemorrhagic shock in swine produces minimal changes in etomidate pharmacokinetics and no change in pharmacodynamics (Johnson et al., 2003). Increased hypnotic effects attributed to pharmacokinetic changes are observed in hemorrhaged rats (De Paepe et al., 1999).

The pharmacokinetics of IV (3 mg/kg), external bath treatment (9 mg/L), and oral administration of metomidate (7 mg/kg) were described for halibut (*Hippoglossus hippoglossus*) and turbot (*Scophthalmus maximus*) (Hansen et al., 2003). Metomidate had a shorter elimination half-life and higher plasma concentrations in turbot compared with halibut, with both species displaying rapid uptake, distribution, and excretion phases. Following IV administration, the volumes of distribution at steady state were 0.21 L/kg (halibut) and 0.44 L/kg (turbot). Plasma clearance was 0.099 L/h/kg in halibut and 0.26 L/h/kg in turbot, and the elimination half-life was calculated to be 5.8 and 2.2 h in halibut and turbot, respectively. Mean residence time was 2.2 h in halibut and 1.7 h in turbot. Following oral administration, the elimination half-life was 3.5 h in turbot. The maximum plasma concentration was 7.8 mg/L in turbot 1 h after administration. The oral bioavailability was calculated to be 100% in turbot. The maximum plasma concentration following 5 min of external bath treatment was 9.5 and 13.3 mg/L in halibut and turbot, respectively.

2. Absorption

Etomidate is lipophilic (octanol/water partition coefficient: 1000) and a weak base ($pKa = 4.5$; $pH = 8.2$; 99% unionized at physiological pH). It is rapidly distributed following IV administration with peak brain levels reached in less than 1 min and has a biologic half-life of about 40 min in rats.

3. Distribution and fate

Etomidate is rapidly metabolized by ester hydrolysis in the liver (primarily) and plasma to inactive products that are excreted in the urine (Heykants et al., 1975; Lewi et al., 1976). The therapeutic index in rats and mice is wide for loss of the righting reflex (LD50:ED50 = 29:1) (Green et al., 1981).

4. Preparation and route of administration

Etomidate is a hypnotic agent with no analgesic effect and minimal cardiorespiratory effects. Metomidate is a hypnotic agent used in a variety of animal species. It has strong central muscle-relaxant effects, but little to no analgesic properties in larger animals; muscular tremors and involuntary movements may occur. Both metomidate and etomidate generally require addition of an opioid for surgical anesthesia (Flecknell, 1987). (*R*)-metomidate hydrochloride is approved by the FDA and marketed as Aquacalm for use in the aquarium and nonfood fish (Western Chemical, Ferndale, WA). Metomidate was previously available as Hypnodil for use in swine; however, it was banned in the European Union in 1997 (Ungemach et al., 1997). These imidazole agents are potentially useful for long-term, continuous infusion anesthesia due to minimal cumulative effect and good preservation of cardiovascular function.

Despite the lack of analgesic properties in larger mammals, Green et al. (1981) found that short-term, light surgical anesthesia lasting 12–15 min could be produced in the mouse with either metomidate (50 mg/kg) or etomidate (30 mg/kg) given IP; side effects included jerking and twitching movements, but cardiorespiratory depression was minimal. Anesthetic duration and depth were improved by a metomidate–fentanyl combination (60 mg/kg: 0.06 mg/kg) given subcutaneously (Green et al., 1981). Adverse reactions, including marked bradycardia, were observed in chickens using metomidate (Christensen et al., 1987).

Although not approved for use in food fish, metomidate immersion produces dose-dependent sedation and anesthesia in hybrid striped bass (*Morone chrysops* × *M. saxatilis*), channel catfish (*Ictalurus punctatus*), and Chinook salmon (*Oncorhynchus tshawytscha*). In channel catfish, 16 ppm metomidate caused 65% mortality, while 6 ppm was judged the minimum concentration required for sedation and anesthesia (Small, 2003). In Chinook salmon, 6–10 ppm was judged effective, with no change in cardiovascular parameters (Hill and Forster, 2004). Cortisol levels were not increased in both hybrid striped bass or channel catfish, implying that metomidate may be useful in reducing fish stress (Davis and Griffin, 2003; Small, 2003). This conclusion, however, may not hold true considering the inhibiting effect of imidazole drugs on steroidogenesis (see below).

5. Side effects

The neurophysiologic actions of etomidate are similar in many respects to barbiturates and other injectable anesthetic agents such as alfaxalone (Way and Trevor, 1986). Etomidate decreases cerebral metabolic rate and ICP, and has anticonvulsant properties (Batjer, 1993; Milde et al., 1985; Robertson, 1992; Wauquier, 1983). In contrast to other IV anesthetics, the depressive effects of etomidate on myocardial contractility are minimal at concentrations necessary to produce anesthesia. In dogs, anesthetic doses of etomidate have little or no effect on heart rate, blood pressure, myocardial performance, or respiratory function (Muir and Mason, 1989; Pascoe et al., 1992). In artificially ventilated rats, there is minimal effect on heart rate and blood pressure, but the aortic flow is markedly decreased (De Wildt et al., 1983). Imidazole compounds, including etomidate and metomidate, inhibit adrenal steroidogenesis through the inhibition of 11 beta-hydroxylase (Mitterhauser et al., 2003; Preziosi and Vacca, 1988). The role for etomidate has been reduced due to its well-recognized adrenal suppression, especially in septic or critical patients (Forman and Warner, 2011). Adrenal suppression is important, as several researchers have erroneously concluded that medetomidine does not cause stress by assessing the lack of corticosteroid production (Jackson, 2005). Compared with thiopental, a single bolus injection of etomidate (2 mg/kg IV) suppresses adrenocortical function in dogs for 2–6 h (Dodam et al., 1990). Compared with diazepam–ketamine, etomidate (2 mg/kg IV) suppresses adrenocortical function in cats for at least 5 h (Moon, 1997). Additional side effects of etomidate use include pain on injection, nausea, vomiting, and myoclonic movements during induction (Booth, 1988). These effects are reduced following IV administration of diazepam, acepromazine, or morphine immediately prior to etomidate (Muir and Mason, 1989).

Due to its formulation in propylene glycol, hemolysis may occur following IV administration of etomidate (Doenicke et al., 1997; Moon, 1994). An etomidate formulation in aqueous sulfobutyl ether β-cyclodextrin has been developed. Pharmacokinetic and pharmacodynamic parameters were not statistically different for the two formulations in dogs (McIntosh et al., 2004). In vivo hemolysis after IV administration of etomidate in propylene glycol was 10-fold higher than that in the case of sulfobutyl ether β-cyclodextrin enabled formulation. Although etomidate in propylene glycol cannot be given subcutaneously because of the cosolvent in the formulation, a 12 mg/mL aqueous solution of etomidate in 20% (w/v) sulfobutyl ether β-cyclodextrin was well tolerated by this route (McIntosh et al., 2004).

F. Propofol

1. Pharmacokinetics and metabolism

The context-sensitive half-time describes the time required for drug concentration to decrease by 50% after terminating infusion and reflects both distribution and metabolism. In humans, the context-sensitive half-time is less than 40 min for propofol infusions lasting up to 8 h (Hughes et al., 1992). The duration of propofol infusion minimally influences the context-sensitive half-time because rapid metabolic clearance of drug returning from tissue storage sites to the circulation does not slow the decrease in drug plasma concentration.

The clearance of propofol is slower in greyhounds compared with other dog breeds. At a substrate concentration of 20 μM, propofol hydroxylase activity was significantly lower in greyhound microsomes (1.7 nmol/mg/min) compared with beagle dog microsomes (5.1 nmol/mg/min), but was not statistically different compared with mixed-breed dog microsomes (3.1 nmol/mg/min). These results indicate breed-specific differences in propofol hydroxylase activity and that a lower level of hydroxylation of propofol by one or more hepatic cytochrome P450 isoforms may contribute to slow pharmacokinetic clearance of propofol by greyhounds (Court et al., 1999).

Brain sensitivity to propofol is influenced by age and administration rate. In male Sprague–Dawley rats (MOL:SPDR:Han) ranging in age from 23 to 776 days, younger animals require higher induction doses of propofol and have higher serum concentrations than older animals. Older animals, however, have higher brain concentrations of propofol at the EEG endpoint than younger animals

(Larsson and Wahlstrom, 1998). These differences can be explained by pharmacokinetic rather than pharmacodynamic differences.

2. Absorption

The anesthetic properties of propofol are similar in most respects to those of the thiobarbiturates. Recovery from a single dose of propofol is more rapid, however, and there is greater potential as a continuous infusion agent due to the minimal cumulative effect (Glen, 1980; Sebel and Lowdon, 1989). Pulmonary uptake of propofol is significant and can influence its initial availability. Redistribution of propofol is extensive. Propofol clearance from plasma exceeds hepatic blood flow, such that tissue uptake, as well as hepatic oxidative metabolism by cytochrome P450 2B6 and 2C9, is an important factor (Court et al., 2001).

3. Distribution and fate

Hepatic metabolism results in inactive, water-soluble sulfate and glucuronic acid metabolites that are excreted by the kidneys. Propofol also undergoes ring hydroxylation by cytochrome P450 to form 4-hydroxypropofol, which has approximately one-third of the hypnotic activity of propofol; 4-hydroxypropofol is subsequently glucuronidated or sulfated to inactive metabolites. Metabolism is sufficiently rapid that the speed of IV injection can affect both the time to induction and the dose needed (Glen, 1980).

In a sheep model, propofol crosses the placenta and reaches the fetus within 2 min of administration (Andaluz et al., 2003). Maternal levels are three times higher than fetal levels following a single bolus IV dose and six to nine times higher following a 1-h continuous infusion, demonstrating a placental barrier effect. Mean residence times are similar for the mother and fetus following a single IV bolus but increased in the fetus with continuous infusion. Fetal elimination is prolonged following a single bolus or continuous infusion, with half-life times more than twice that observed for the mother. Plasma protein binding is higher in the mother than in the fetus (Gin et al., 1991), which tends to limit placental transfer as only unbound drugs can pass. However, as propofol may bind less to fetal plasma proteins than to maternal plasma proteins, Andaluz et al. (2003) speculate that the free fraction of fetal drug may be higher and is likely to be pharmacologically active. Hence, the use of continuous infusion or multiple bolus injections of propofol is not recommended for cesarean section anesthesia.

4. Preparation and route of administration

Propofol is a substituted isopropylphenol (2,6-diisopropylphenol), chemically distinct from barbiturates, steroids, and imidazoles. Propofol is an oil at room temperature and insoluble in aqueous solution. Unlike the thiobarbiturates, etomidate, and ketamine, propofol is not a chiral drug.

The currently available 1% commercial preparation is an aqueous emulsion of 10% soybean oil, 2.25% glycerol, and 1.2% purified egg phosphatide (Sebel and Lowdon, 1989; Stoelting and Hillier, 2006). Commercially available soybean emulsion preparations differ with respect to pH and the presence of preservatives, either disodium edentate (EDTA) or metabisulfite (Marik, 2004; Stoelting and Hillier, 2006); these formulations, however, are not considered antimicrobially preserved products under USP standards (Sklar, 1997). The soybean emulsion supports bacterial growth such that strict asepsis must be used during handling, administration, and storage; the manufacturer of PropoFlo (Abbott Animal Health, North Chicago, IL) recommends discarding unused products within 6 h of opening. PropoFlo 28 (Zoetis, Kalamazoö, MI) is now available, with the recommendation of discarding unused products within 28 days of opening. This formulation contains 2% benzyl alcohol as a preservative, which has shown to be effective for both induction and short-term maintenance of anesthesia with a 28-day shelf life.

Propofol is degraded in the presence of oxygen and supplied in single-dose vials under nitrogen. Initial clinical formulations of the oil used the solubilizing agent Cremophor EL (polyoxyethylated castor oil); however, Cremophor is known to result in histamine release in the dog and has been associated with pain on injection and anaphylactoid reactions in the rat and pig (Glen and Hunter, 1984). The currently available 1% soybean emulsion is also associated with pain on IV injection, but this can be reduced by selecting a larger vein or prior administration of 1% lidocaine through the same vein. Mixing propofol with other drugs is not recommended, as the coalescence of oil droplets may pose a risk for pulmonary embolism. Hypertriglyceridemia and pancreatitis are uncommon complications with the soybean emulsion preparation. Other alternatives have been investigated, including 1% and 5% nanodroplet microemulsions (Boscan et al., 2006; Morey et al., 2006a, 2006b), the water-soluble propofol prodrug propofol phosphate (Banaszczyk et al., 2002), and an 80% propofol–propylene glycol transdermal preparation (Takahashi et al., 2005).

5. Side effects

As with other $GABA_A$ agonists, propofol is generally considered to be poorly analgesic, but spinal cord analgesic effects can be demonstrated (Frolich et al., 2005; Jewett et al., 1992). The anesthetic properties and hemodynamic effects of propofol are similar for the Cremophor and soybean emulsion formulations, although the soybean formulation has slightly greater potency in mice and male rats (Glen and Hunter, 1984).

Propofol is less effective in rabbit than in other species (Flecknell, 1996). Administration at relatively high doses (≥10 mg/kg IV) results in the sedation of very short duration with little reflex depression or antinociception, while higher doses or longer infusions produce respiratory arrest and death (Aeschbacher and Webb, 1993a, 1993b; Banaszczyk et al., 2002; Blake et al., 1988; Glen, 1980; Ko et al., 1992; Ypsilantis et al., 2006). A starting dose of 10 mg/kg and then incremental increases in dose as needed for relaxation does allow intubation and maintenance of anesthesia by inhalants (Allweiler et al., 2010). In mice, induction time and time to recover coordination are shorter with propofol than with thiopental; the "utilization rate" of propofol, the amount required to maintain prolonged anesthesia, is greatest in mice compared with several other species (Glen, 1980). Apnea commonly occurs in mice, rabbits, cats, and pigs, especially at higher doses; in rhesus monkeys, it is seldom seen. In rabbits, there is a dose-dependent decrease in minute volume (Bellman and Pleuvry, 1981); respiratory arrest may follow the administration of doses high enough to prevent the pain response (Glen, 1980). Apnea occurred in cats at 10 mg/kg propofol, but not in dogs at 6 mg/kg, administered IV on three consecutive days (Matthews et al., 2004).

Propofol decreases cerebral oxygen consumption, reduces ICP, and has anticonvulsive activity (Marik, 2004); it is also a potent antioxidant, has antiinflammatory properties, and is a bronchodilator. Propofol is associated with excitatory motor activity, such as myoclonic jerking and opisthotonos; however, barbiturate-like EEG changes are observed in rats (Glen, 1980). Propofol has anticonvulsive properties in mice and rats (Lee et al., 1998; Lowson et al., 1990), as well as in other species, presumably due to GABA-mediated presynaptic and postsynaptic inhibition of chloride channels. Steward et al. (2005) have reviewed the effects of several anesthetics, including propofol, on brain neurotransmitter systems in the context of rat BOLD contrast pharmacological MRI.

Hypotension associated with propofol administration has raised concerns regarding its use in patients with cardiovascular disease, particularly volume depletion or endotoxemia; changes other than hypotension are more variably reported (Ilkiw et al., 1992). Heart rate is elevated following propofol in rats (Rocchiccioli et al., 1989) and rabbits (Blake et al., 1988). Blood pressure is maintained during light propofol anesthesia in the rabbit (Blake et al., 1988), but decreased at higher doses; cardiac output may be elevated, reduced, or remain unchanged (Aeschbacher and Webb, 1993b; Blake et al., 1988; Glen, 1980; Van Leeuwen et al., 1990). Antinociceptive doses of propofol in the rat result in lowered arterial pressure and heart rate (Tan et al., 1993). Carmichael et al. (1993) confirmed a dose-dependent decrease in blood pressure in rats. There was no effect on cardiac output or coronary or renal blood flows, and splanchnic hemodynamics and liver oxygenation were not adversely affected. Propofol dose-dependently antagonizes β-adrenoceptors in rat myocardial membranes (Zhou et al., 1999). Oxygen utilization is impaired and electron flow is inhibited in the guinea pig cardiomyocyte, and ventricular performance is significantly depressed in the isolated perfused heart (Schenkman and Yan, 2000). In swine, propofol causes a dose-dependent decrease in myocardial contractility (Coetzee et al., 1989; Glen, 1980; Glen and Hunter, 1984). A negative inotropic response has been demonstrated in vitro along with marked attenuation of coronary flow autoregulation (Stowe et al., 1992). Rat atrial and portal vein contractions are inhibited in vitro by propofol addition (Bunting et al., 1989).

The baroreceptor-heart rate reflex is suppressed following propofol administration in rats (Rocchiccioli et al., 1989) and rabbits. The suppression is much less than with alfaxalone/alphadolone (Blake et al., 1988), thiopentone, or ketamine (Blake et al., 1982; Van Leeuwen et al., 1990). In the rabbit and cat, carotid artery infusion of propofol suppresses afferent impulses from single chemoreceptor fibers in response to hypoxia and hypercapnia (Ponte and Sadler, 1989). Pharmacologic activation of adenosine triphosphate-regulated K_{ATP} channels mimics ischemic preconditioning and decreases infarct size or improves functional recovery of ischemic-reperfused stunned myocardium; propofol does not affect cardiac myocyte K_{ATP} channel activity (Zaugg et al., 2002), and may inhibit the ischemic preconditioning-like cardioprotective effect of inhalational anesthetics (Kohro et al., 2001).

In cats, repetitive daily anesthesia with propofol is associated with Heinz body formation; this may be due to propofol being a phenol compound. Heinz bodies developed following three consecutive days of induction with 6 mg/kg IV propofol combined with 30 min of maintenance anesthesia at a constant rate infusion (CRI) of 0.2−0.3 mg/kg/min; generalized malaise, anorexia, and diarrhea were reported after five consecutive days of propofol anesthesia (Andress et al., 1995). On the other hand, clinically insignificant increases in the number of Heinz bodies were reported in cats anesthetized for three consecutive days with 10 mg/kg propofol (Matthews et al., 2004).

Propofol infusion syndrome is a real, albeit rare, entity. It is characterized by metabolic acidosis, acute cardiomyopathy, and skeletal myopathy is often lethal, and is strongly associated with propofol infusions rates of 5 mg/kg/h and greater for more than 48 h. There is evidence that the syndrome is caused by the failure of free fatty acid metabolism due to inhibition of entry into the mitochondria and specific sites in the mitochondrial respiratory chain. The syndrome therefore mimics mitochondrial myopathies (Short and Young, 2003).

Immune system effects

Propofol impairs several monocyte and neutrophil functions of the nonspecific immune system, including polarization, chemotaxis, oxidative burst, and phagocytosis; however, these changes are thought to be due to the soybean emulsion rather than propofol itself (Schneemilch et al., 2004).

On the other hand, propofol has been reported to attenuate proinflammatory cytokine responses, alter the expression of nitric oxide, and decrease neutrophil activation in a rat model of endotoxemia (Marik, 2005; Taniguchi et al., 2000, 2002). The molecular mechanism for these effects is not clear. Unlike thiopental, propofol does not inhibit the activation of nuclear factor kappaB (Loop et al., 2002). Propofol is also a potent antioxidant. The added preservatives may have biological activity: EDTA has antiinflammatory properties, and metabisulfite may cause lipid peroxidation (Marik, 2005). In a swine model of aortic reconstructive surgery, propofol anesthesia was associated with less neutrophil infiltration, lower plasma proinflammatory cytokine levels, lower production of oxygen free radicals, less lipid peroxidation, and reduced inducible nitric oxide synthase activity compared with sevoflurane (Rodriguez-Lopez et al., 2006).

6. Propofol antagonists

Although concurrent use of preanesthetic agents can substantially reduce the dosage of propofol needed for anesthesia (Pablo et al., 1997; Watney and Pablo, 1992), there are no specific propofol antagonists that are clinically useful. Picrotoxin, a noncompetitive $GABA_A$ antagonist, and gabazine, a competitive $GABA_A$ antagonist, both increase propofol ED_{50} in male Sprague–Dawley [Crl:CD(SD)Br] rats by 379% and 362%, respectively (Sonner et al., 2003). TRH reduces propofol sleep time in rats (Larsson et al., 1996), likely due to pharmacodynamic effects associated with sympathoadrenal activation (Schaefer et al., 1989).

G. Tribromoethanol

1. Pharmacokinetics and metabolism

TBE acts at the $GABA_A$ and glycine receptors (Krasowski and Harrison, 2000). The high-affinity states of dopamine D2 and D3 receptors, serotonin 5HT-2A receptors, β2-adrenoceptors, α2-1 and α2-2 adrenoceptors, opiate receptors, and muscarinic receptors are inhibited in vitro by clinical concentrations of ethanol anesthetics (Seeman and Kapur, 2003). The pharmacokinetics of TBE have not been described yet.

2. Absorption

TBE is absorbed quickly when administered IP to rodents, as loss of righting reflex occurs within 5 min of injection.

3. Distribution and fate

TBE is metabolized in the liver by conjugation with glucuronic acid and is excreted in the urine as TBE glucuronate (Green, 1979).

4. Preparation and route of administration

TBE solutions are often referred to as Avertin, which is a misnomer. Avertin was the trade name for Winthrop Laboratories proprietary TBE formulation, which is no longer available. Pharmaceutical-grade TBE was marketed under several proprietary names, including Avertin, Bromethol, Ethobrom, Narcolan, and Narkolan, each as a 66.7% w/w solution of TBE in *t*-amyl alcohol where each milliliter contained 1 g TBE (The Merck Index, 1976; Reynolds, 1982).

As TBE is a nonpharmaceutical-grade compound, and in consideration of the possible side effects and questionable reliability to provide adequate anesthesia, its use is discouraged, and pharmaceutical-grade alternatives are recommended. TBE is light-and heat-sensitive, so preparations should be stored in the dark at cooler temperatures or prepared fresh as needed. When exposed to heat or light, toxic byproducts are produced that can be both nephrotoxic and hepatotoxic. If stored improperly, the risk of peritonitis and intestinal ileus increases.

TBE produces a generalized CNS depression, including both the respiratory and cardiovascular centers. Depression of respiration and circulation, together with its general unpredictability, eventually discouraged clinical use. The duration of TBE anesthesia in mice varies considerably with strain and sex, even among a wide range of dosages (Avila et al., 2001; Buetow et al., 1999; Gardner et al., 1995; Hill et al., 2013; Hogan et al., 1986; Koizumi et al., 2002; Papaioannou and Fox, 1993; Wixson and Smiler, 1997). In female Crl:CD-1(ICR)BR, Icolbm:OF-1, and Hanlbm:NMRI mice, xylazine (16 mg/kg) and ketamine (120 mg/kg), administered IP at a volume of 10 mL/kg, produces embryo transfer success rate similar to that observed with TBE (82% surviving offspring with X/K compared with 85% with TBE) (Zeller et al., 1998). In comparison, Papaioannou and Fox (1993) reported an embryo transfer success rate of 60% with TBE.

5. Side effects

Since TBE produces inflammation and peritonitis, its use should be reserved only for acute terminal studies when administered IP to laboratory animals (Meyer and Fish, 2005).

The concerns regarding the efficacy and safety of TBE, combined with the availability of effective pharmaceutical-grade alternatives, have made the continued routine use of TBE for rodent anesthesia controversial (Silverman, 2003). Acute concentration-dependent abdominal muscle necrosis, peritoneal inflammation, fibrinous splenic serositis, visceral adhesions, and death have been described in CD-1, OF-1, NMRI, ICR, and NCR (nu/nu) mice, as well as in Mongolian gerbils and Sprague–Dawley rats, following a single IP dose of TBE (Buetow et al., 1999; Goelz, 1994; Lieggi et al., 2005a, 2005b; Norris and Turner, 1983; Reid et al., 1999; Zeller et al., 1998). Even with freshly prepared solutions, high mortality has been reported following a second TBE injection (Green, 1979; Norris and Turner, 1983; Papaioannou and Fox, 1993). High death losses in mice after recovery were associated with fluid distension of the stomach and small intestine, suggesting intestinal ileus as the cause of death (Tarin and Sturdee, 1972). Similar results have been reported in Mongolian gerbils; these effects could be reduced, but not eliminated by dilution to 1.25% and by reducing the dosage to 300 mg/kg or less (Norris and Turner, 1983).

Generally speaking, cardiac performance is better in mice during TBE anesthesia than with ketamine combinations, but cardiac performance with TBE is not as repeatable over time as with the inhaled anesthetic isoflurane (Hart et al., 2001; Roth et al., 2002). Hart et al. (2001), using a combination of transthoracic echocardiography and closed chest cardiac catheterization, examined cardiac performance in male Swiss Webster mice administered xylazine/ketamine anesthesia (4.1 mg/kg xylazine and 65 mg/kg ketamine) or TBE (375 mg/kg). TBE produced less bradycardia and had a less effect on cardiac loading and ventricular function than xylazine/ketamine.

H. Alfaxalone

1. Pharmacokinetics and metabolism

The anesthetic effects of steroids have been recognized for more than 70 years (Sutton, 1972). While a number of anesthetic steroids have been investigated, most early clinical work focused on the combination of alfaxalone and alphadolone formulated in 20% polyoxyethylene castor oil (Cremophor-EL; Althesin-human product; Saffan-veterinary product). Most of the reported side effects of alfaxalone/alphadolone were attributed to Cremophor, which induces histamine release and may result in major anaphylactic reactions. The reformulated water-soluble version of alfaxalone (Alfaxan) replaced the Cremophor formulation.

Alfaxalone is a neuroactive steroid molecule with the properties of a general anesthetic. Chemically, it is described as 3-α-hydroxy-5-α-pregnane-11, 20-dione, with a molecular weight of 332.5. The primary mechanism for the anesthetic action of alfaxalone is the modulation of neuronal cell membrane chloride ion transport, induced by binding of alfaxalone to $GABA_A$ cell surface receptors. In dogs administered a single dose of 2 mg/kg alfaxalone IV, the mean volume of distribution at steady state was 2.0 L/kg, the mean terminal plasma elimination half-life was 34 min, and the mean total body clearance was 59.4 mL/kg/min. Similarly, in cats administered a single dose of 5 mg/kg IN, the mean volume of distribution at steady state was 1.3 L/kg, the mean terminal plasma elimination half-life was 43 min, and the mean total body clearance was 24.0 mL/kg/min (Jurox, NADA 141–342 Alfaxan IV injectable anesthetic for use in cats and dogs). Product Insert 2012, USFDA).

In adult female Wistar rats, the mean t1/2elim for 2 and 5 mg/kg i.v. was 16.2 and 17.6 min, respectively, but could not be estimated for IP dosing due to sustained plasma levels for up to 60 min after injection (Lau et al., 2013). Clp for i.v. the injection was calculated at 57.8 ± 23.6 and 54.3 ± 6.8 mL/min/kg, which were 24.5% and 23% of cardiac output, respectively. The observed Cmax was 3.0 mg/L for IP administration, and 2.2 ± 0.9 and 5.2 ± 1.3 mg/L for 2 and 5 mg/kg i.v. administration, respectively. AUC0–60 was 96.2 min mg/L for IP dosing. The relative bioavailability for IP dosing was 26% and 28% compared to i.v. dosing. Differences in the pharmacokinetics of IV alfaxalone between sexes have been identified in rats in plasma clearance, half-life, and mean residence time when administered at a constant rate of infusion (White et al., 2017).

Alfaxalone has nonlinear pharmacokinetics in cats; however, for cats dosed with sequential maintenance doses, there was no clinically relevant pharmacokinetic accumulation (Whittem et al., 2008). In European shorthair cats given 5 mg/kg alfaxalone IM or IV, the mean half-life and mean residence time of alfaxalone were longer after IM (1.28 (SD 0.21) and 2.09 (SD 0.36) hours, respectively) than after IV (0.49 (SD 0.07) and 0.66 (SD 0.16) hours, respectively) administration ($P < .05$) (Rodrigo-Mocholí et al., 2018). Bioavailability after IM injection of alfaxalone was 94.7 (SD 19.8)%. The mean intervals to sternal and lateral recumbency were longer in the IM (3.73 (SD 1.99) and 6.12 (SD 0.90) minutes, respectively) compared to IV (0 min for all animals) treated cats ($P < .01$). Sedation scores indicative of general anesthesia (scores >15) were recorded from 5 to 15 min after IV administration, and deep sedation (scores 11–15) at 20 and 30 min. Deep sedation was observed from 10 to 45 min after IM administration.

One cat from each group showed hyperkinesia during recovery, and the remainder had an uneventful recovery. While IM administration is convenient in cats, it must be noted that the onset of sedation will be slower and a state of general anesthesia will not be achieved.

Dehuisser and coworkers evaluated the pharmacokinetics of a CRI of alfaxalone in intact female Beagle dogs (Dehuisser et al., 2019). Following an IV alfaxalone bolus (3 mg/kg), anesthesia was maintained using an alfaxalone CRI at 0.15 mg/kg/min for 90 (short CRI) or 180 min (long CRI). No significant difference was noted between protocols for any PK parameter. Volume of distribution at steady state (935.74 ± 170.25 vs. 1119.15 ± 190.65 mL/kg), elimination half-life (12 ± 2 vs. 13 ± 3 min), clearance from the central compartment (26.02 ± 4.41 vs. 27.74 ± 5.65 mL/kg/min), and intercompartmental clearance (8.47 ± 4.06 vs. 12.58 ± 7.03 mL/kg/min) were comparable for short CRI and long CRI. Cardiovascular variables remained within physiological limits. Mechanical ventilation was necessary (short CRI: n = 1, long CRI: n = 4). The manufacturer's recommended dose rate resulted in a superficial plane of anesthesia with poor recovery characteristics.

2. *Absorption*

Alfaxalone as the sole agent has variable effects on sleep time and the ability to create a state of surgical anesthesia in laboratory rodents. In female ICR mice, IP, or SC alfaxalone was relatively ineffective at producing an anesthetic state; a combination of medetomidine, midazolam, and alfaxalone at 60 or 80 mg/kg IP did not produce surgical anesthesia at any dose tested, while the same doses given SC produced surgical anesthesia (Higuchi et al., 2016). In adult female Wistar rats, 20 mg/kg IP alfaxalone caused sustained levels of sedation, no apnea, and longer sleep times than IV dosing at 2–5 mg/kg, although immobilization was not induced in 30% of rats given alfaxalone IP (Lau et al., 2013). The duration was dose-dependent, but generally short, and recovery was rapid. Plasma half-life was approximately 7 min and serum protein binding was about 40%. Arenillas and Gomez de Segura (2018) found a combination of IP alfaxalone with dexmedetomidine and fentanyl allowed for more prolonged anesthesia than alfaxalone alone, but a much higher dose was required for males than females. D'Ovidio et al. (2018) found IM alfaxalone 5 mg/kg to be safe for healthy guinea pigs undergoing minor noninvasive procedures lasting 15–20 min, with both respiratory function and body temperature preserved during the time of anesthesia. Doerning and coworkers reported SC alfaxalone 20 mg/kg produced uncomplicated sedation in guinea pigs sufficient for nonpainful procedures not requiring complete immobility; the addition of dexmedetomidine and buprenorphine increased the duration of sedation and immobility but did not result in general anesthesia (Doerning et al., 2018).

In male New Zealand White rabbits, Huynh and coworkers reported that intramuscular administration of alfaxalone at 4, 6, or 8 mg/kg produced dose-dependent sedation with potential respiratory depression in rabbits at the highest dose (Huynh et al., 2015). The time to maximal effect ranged from 8 to 16 min, and the sedation duration varied from 36.9 (95% CI (31.6–42.3)) min to 58.4 (52.8–63.9) min for a dose of 4 and 8 mg/kg, respectively. The authors concluded that a 4 mg dose produces rapid sedation and fast recovery with minimal cardiovascular effects in rabbits, but bradypnea was observed such that oxygen support was recommended. Additional analgesia will be required to perform invasive procedures.

IV alfaxalone has been used to immobilize several species of reptiles, chelonians, and amphibians. In squamate lizards, alfaxalone 9 mg/kg IV via the ventral coccygeal vein produced effective sedation in most species examined with no obvious complications observed; however, loss of righting reflex was not achieved in four (57.1%) blotched bluetongue lizards (*Tiliqua nigrolutea*), two (33.3%) coastal carpet pythons (*Morelia spilota mcdowelli*), and one (50%) red-bellied black snake (*Pseudechis porphyriacus*) (Scheelings et al., 2011). Righting reflex following alfaxalone 5 mg/kg administered intravenously was lost within 12–45 s (17.52 ± 8.80 s) in inland bearded dragons (*Pogona vitticeps*), 15–40 s (24.60 ± 9.61 s) in Rankin's dragons (*Pogona henrylawsoni*), and 12–40 s (21.70 ± 9.53 s) in Chinese water dragons (*Physignathus cocincinus*) (Knotek 2017). Perrin and Bertelsen compared IV 10 mg/kg propofol with 12 mg/kg alfaxalone in the central inland bearded dragon (*Pogona vitticeps*) (Perrin and Bertelsen, 2017). Both protocols resulted in smooth and rapid induction and subsequent intubation. A surgical plane of anesthesia, defined as a loss of reaction to noxious stimuli and absent muscle tone, was achieved in 5/8 (62.5%) alfaxalone animals and 0/8 of the propofol animals. Reflexes and muscle tone were regained from a cranial to caudal direction. There was no effect on heart rate; however, both protocols resulted in respiratory depression, including 5- and 20-min durations of apnea in two of the alfaxalone animals.

In loggerhead turtles (*Caretta caretta*), the median anesthetic induction time following alfaxalone IV at 3 mg/kg, 5 mg/kg, or 10 mg/kg was 2 min. Endotracheal intubation was accomplished in all turtles following induction. Heart rate significantly increased after the 3- and 5-mg/kg doses were administered. The median interval from alfaxalone administration to first spontaneous respiration was 16, 22, and 54 min for the 3-, 5-, and 10-mg/kg doses, respectively, and the median intervals to recovery were 28, 46, and 90 min, respectively. Assisted ventilation was required for one turtle after receiving the 5-mg/kg dose and for five turtles after receiving the 10-mg/kg dose. The 10-mg/kg dose resulted in respiratory acidosis and marked hypoxemia at 30 min.

Alfaxalone has been evaluated as an immersion agent and as an intramuscular agent in fish. Bailey and coworkers evaluated 1 mg/kg, 5 mg/kg, or 10 mg/kg of IM alfaxalone in koi carp (*Cyprinus carpio*) (Bailey et al., 2014). Fish were assessed every 15 min for opercular rate, and a sedation score from 0 to 5 awarded, with 0 indicating no response and 5 indicating as absent righting reflex and anesthesia. Anesthetized koi were subsequently maintained on a recirculating water system. Time to anesthesia/recovery was recorded and heart rate was recorded every 15 min. Anesthesia was achieved in 0/6, 1/6, and 5/6 fish at 1, 5, and 10 mg/kg, respectively. The duration of anesthesia for one fish at 5 mg/kg was 2 h. At 10 mg/kg, median anesthesia duration was 6.5 (3−10) hr. At 10 mg/kg, prolonged apnea (2−3 h) was observed in 3/6 fish, 2/3 died under anesthesia, and 1/3 recovered 10 h postinjection. The median peak sedation scores were 1.5, 2.5, and 5, at 1, 5, and 10 mg/kg, respectively. A dosage of 10 mg/kg alfaxalone resulted in 33% mortality, and the duration of anesthesia and opercular rate were unpredictable at all doses. Due to variation in response as well as risk of mortality, the authors concluded that intramuscular alfaxalone cannot be recommended for anesthesia in koi carp.

Using immersion, Koi carp were immobilized in water containing 10 mg/L alfaxalone and then maintained with alfaxalone at either 1 or 2.5 mg/L via a recirculating water system (Minter et al., 2014). The median anesthesia induction time for all fish was 5.4 min. Median recovery time was 11.8 and 26.4 min in the 1.0 and 2.5 mg/L doses, respectively. Cessation of opercular movement occurred in 0/6 and 4/6 fish exposed to 1.0 and 2.5 mg/L dose, respectively. No difference was observed in the median heart rate over the duration of the anesthetic events. Response to noxious stimulation was 4/6 and 0/6 in the 1.0 and 2.5 mg/L doses, respectively. Oxygenation and ventilation did not change during the experiment, but there was a significant decrease in blood pH noted along with an increase in blood lactate concentration. The authors concluded the maintenance dose of 2.5 mg/L was sufficient to prevent response to noxious stimuli but was associated with a clinically relevant depression in opercular rate.

Immersion anesthesia of oscar fish (*Astronotus ocellatus*) with alfaxalone 5 mg/L was sufficient for the collection of diagnostic samples in all fish (Bugman et al., 2016). Mean ± SD induction time was 11 ± 3.8 min (minimum, 5 min; maximum, 15 min), and the mean recovery time was 37.5 ± 13.7 min (minimum, 20 min; maximum, 55 min). There was a significant difference in opercular movement rate over time, with respiratory rates significantly decreasing between baseline and anesthesia and then significantly increasing between anesthesia and recovery. There was no significant difference in heart rate over time. Median lactate concentrations were significantly increased in all anesthetized fish. Other physiologic or blood gas variables did not change significantly.

Alfaxalone immersion with branchial/cutaneous irrigation has been reported for Mexican axolotls (McMillan and Leece, 2011). Anesthesia was induced by immersion in water containing (5 mg/L) alfaxalone. Anesthesia was maintained through continuous irrigation of the branchial gills and skin with alfaxalone 5 mg/L and additional 30 μL drops of 10 mg/mL alfaxalone applied to the branchial gills and skin as needed. The depth was adjusted by branchial irrigation of alfaxalone solutions and lightened by irrigation using fresh water. Branchial and gular respiratory movements persisted at what was considered an appropriate anesthetic depth. Anesthesia lasted approximately 1 h with recovery in 15 min. Recovery was assisted through branchial and cutaneous irrigation with fresh water.

Zebrafish exposed to either alfaxalone or alfaxalone with preservatives 10 mg/L showed similar times to loss of equilibrium and response to von Frey fibers and subsequent time to recovery, with no deaths and no gross external pathology (Farry et al., 2019).

3. Distribution and fate

This clearance of alfaxalone is suggestive of rapid metabolic clearance of the parent moiety (Whittem et al., 2008). Rapid hepatic metabolic clearance by the liver has been identified in other species as a likely mechanism of recovery from alfaxalone anesthesia (Sear and McGivan, 1981). Renal, pulmonary, and potentially cerebral metabolism are also speculated to be involved in the elimination of this drug. Studies in humans and rats have demonstrated that metabolites of alfaxalone are primarily excreted in the urine, with a small amount likely to be excreted in the bile (Sear, 1996). Although the exact metabolic clearance and excretion mechanisms are unknown in cats, the alfaxalone metabolites produced are similar to those of humans and rats, allowing for the extrapolation that renal elimination is probably also important in this species (Warne et al., 2015).

4. Preparation and route of administration

Alfaxan Multidose IDX (Jurox) is currently available for use in multiple nonfood-producing minor species, including many laboratory animals (https://todaysveterinarypractice.com/alfaxalone-an-old-drug-in-a-new-formulation/accessed May 1, 2022). This formulation uses 2-hydroxypropyl-β cyclodextrin as a solubilizing agent and ethanol, benzethonium chloride, and chlorocresol as preservatives. It may be administered IV, SQ, IM, and IP with variable results (see 2. Absorption). It can also be administered by dilution in water and immersion of fish and amphibians.

5. Side effects

In beagle dogs administered etomidate (3 mg/kg IV) or alfaxalone (4 mg/kg IV), alfaxalone caused significant tachycardia and increased cardiac index, and statistically (but not clinically) decreased arterial pressures and systemic vascular resistance index (Rodríguez et al., 2012). Etomidate caused no significant cardiovascular changes. Quality of recovery was judged as better with alfaxalone. Both agents caused short-lived hypoxia. Ventilatory depression has been observed with alfaxalone given alone to rats (7). Recovery quality is noted to be improved in most species when sedatives and/or analgesics are coadministered.

III. NMDA-antagonists

A. Mechanism of action

The neuropharmacology of the phencyclidine derivatives is complex, with interactions at *N*-methyl D-aspartate (NMDA) and nonNMDA glutamate/nitric oxide/cGMP receptors, as well as nicotinic and muscarinic cholinergic, and monoaminergic and opioid receptors (Kohrs and Durieux, 1998). Although ketamine does weakly bind at GABA receptors, NMDA receptor antagonism accounts for most of its analgesic effects (Kohrs and Durieux, 1998; Pozzi et al., 2006). Glutamate and its analog, NMDA, are excitatory amino acids. Group 1 metabotropic glutamate receptors are reported to regulate NMDA receptor function (Sou et al., 2006). In addition, interactions with voltage-dependent Na^+ and L-type Ca^{++} channels have been described. When glutamate occupies the binding site on the NMDA subtype of the glutamate receptor in the presence of glycine, the ligand-gated (ionotropic) channel opens, allowing Ca^{++}, Na^+, and K^+ to either enter or leave the cell, which leads to postsynaptic neuronal depolarization. Ketamine binds to the phencyclidine receptor in the NMDA channel and prevents further ion flux, thus inhibiting glutamate activation of the channel in a noncompetitive manner. The blockade is time-, concentration-, and stimulation frequency-dependent. The phencyclidine-binding site partly overlaps with a binding site for Mg^{++}. In addition, ketamine can produce a mild local anesthetic effect through neuronal Na^+ channel inhibition, as well as cerebral vasodilation through Ca^{++} channel inhibition.

B. Cyclohexamines

1. Pharmacokinetics and metabolism

The cyclohexamine anesthetics, phencyclidine, and its congeners ketamine and tiletamine, have been categorized as dissociative anesthetics and sympathomimetic anesthetics (Soma, 1983). "Dissociative" refers to the apparent dissociation of the patient from its environment, believed to be caused by interruption of CNS impulses as well as differential depression and activation of various areas of the brain (Muir, 1985; Reich and Silvay, 1989). The anesthetic action of ketamine requires a functioning cerebral cortex (Wright, 1982). There is depression or disorganization of the associative areas of the brain, while subcortical areas may be activated (Haskins, 1992; Oguchi et al., 1982). The subject seems completely unaware of the environment, and suggested mechanisms include electrophysiologic inhibition of the thalamocortical pathways and stimulation of the limbic system. Ocular and pharyngeal reflexes are retained, or attenuated less with ketamine than with other anesthetic agents, which can make traditional monitoring of anesthetic depth using observation of physical signs misleading. The pharmacology of ketamine and tiletamine, as well as their use in veterinary medicine, has been reviewed (Li and Vlisides, 2016; Lin, 1996; Lin et al., 1993).

Ketamine is metabolized by the liver in most species. Upon its administration, it is rapidly metabolized by microsomal enzymes CYP3A4 into a series of compounds of which norketamine and hydroxynorketamine are considered the most important. The most important pathway is *N*-demethylation by cytochrome P450 to norketamine (metabolite I), an active metabolite with one-third to one-fifth of the initial activity. Norketamine is hydroxylated and conjugated to water-soluble products that are excreted by the kidney; reduced renal output can thus result in prolonged ketamine action. The cyclohexanone ring also undergoes oxidative metabolism. The so-called metabolite II is apparently not a naturally occurring in vivo metabolite, but a by-product of the chromatographic process (Reich and Silvay, 1989). Ketamine pretreatment decreases the plasma half-life of intravenously administered ketamine by induction of hepatic microsomal enzyme activity (Marietta, 1977). Tolerance has been demonstrated in rats (Livingston and Waterman, 1978) and nonhuman primates (Pouget et al., 2010).

2. Absorption

Ketamine has high lipid solubility, a pK of 7.5 at physiologic pH, and is associated with rapid induction and return to consciousness following redistribution from the CNS to other body tissues (Thurmon, 1985). The 10% aqueous solution has a pH of 3.5, which may result in pain on injection and muscle necrosis in small animals (Wright, 1982). It has high bioavailability following IV or IM administration (Reich and Silvay, 1989), although IM injection may result in more variable peak plasma concentrations (Löscher et al., 1990). It is not significantly bound to plasma proteins, leaves the blood rapidly following injection, and is initially distributed to highly perfused tissues, such as the brain, where its high lipid solubility ensures rapid transfer across the blood–brain barrier. It is subsequently redistributed away from the brain to other, less well-perfused tissues.

3. Distribution and fate

Peak brain levels of ketamine are reached within 1 min following IV injection in the rat, and brain: plasma ratios remain at 6.5:1 for more than 10 min (Cohen et al., 1973). Over half of an oral, IM, or IP dose of radiolabeled ketamine in the rat is recovered in urine and feces within 24 h. By 72 h, 53%–75% is recovered in urine and 23%–25% in feces. Ketamine is transferred readily across the placenta in dogs, monkeys, and humans (Chang and Glazko, 1974). There are significant species differences in the relative amounts of free ketamine and ketamine metabolites in the urine (Chang and Glazko, 1974), and protein binding in serum (Wright, 1982). Löscher et al. (1990) present a detailed analysis of pharmacokinetic data in swine, compared with the data in other domestic species.

The plasma half-life of tiletamine in cats is 2–4 h; in dogs, monkeys, and rats, it is 1.2 h, 1–1.5 h, and 30–40 min, respectively (Lin, 1996).

4. Preparation and route of administration

The wide veterinary use of ketamine stems from its low cost, wide margin of safety, ease of administration, and initial introduction as a Drug Enforcement Administration noncontrolled anesthetic (presently DEA Class III). Ketamine can be administered intravenously, intramuscularly, or intraperitoneally. There is, however, concern that IM injection of ketamine can cause discomfort and tissue reactions in small rodents, and, therefore, this route should be avoided (Flecknell, 1996; Wixson and Smiler, 1997).

Ketamine is water-soluble and structurally resembles phencyclidine. The presence of an asymmetric carbon atom produces two optical isomers, *R*(−) and *S*(+); these isomers differ in anesthetic potency and effect (Muir and Hubbell, 1988; Reich and Silvay, 1989; Ryder et al., 1978). Commercial racemic mixtures of ketamine consist of equal parts of the *R*(−) and *S*(+) isomers; however, only *S*(+) ketamine is commercially available. *S*(+) ketamine produces more intense analgesia, more rapid metabolism and recovery, less salivation, and a lower incidence of emergence reactions than *R*(−) ketamine. *S*(+) ketamine has analgesic potency approximately twice that of racemic ketamine and four times greater than *R*(−) ketamine. Like cocaine, both ketamine isomers inhibit the postganglionic sympathetic nerve reuptake of catecholamines.

Ketamine is generally considered to be a potent analgesic, blocking the conduction of pain impulses to thalamic and cortical areas. Although analgesia is reportedly more effective for procedures involving the musculoskeletal system than the abdomen (Wright, 1982), NMDA antagonists have been shown to provide visceral analgesia in animals as well as humans (Olivar and Laird, 1999; Strigo et al., 2005). Ketamine has recently reemerged as an important drug for the prevention and management of chronic pain, as spinal cord dorsal horn NMDA receptors are important mediators in the "wind-up" chronic pain phenomenon.

Tiletamine was initially developed in an effort to find an agent with potency and duration intermediate between phencyclidine and ketamine. Its current use in veterinary medicine is primarily in a 1:1 combination with the benzodiazepine zolazepam, marketed as the product Telazol.

5. Side effects

The cardiovascular effects of ketamine are modified by the concurrent administration of other anesthetic agents. Ketamine in vitro causes direct myocardial depression (Schwartz and Horwitz, 1975). Because of its receptor profile, however, ketamine increases myocardial contractility through increased sympathetic nervous system activity, and ketamine administration to dogs and cats typically increases hemodynamic variables (Muir, 1985; Wright, 1982). The sympathetically mediated positive inotropic and chronotropic effects of ketamine can be blocked by inhaled anesthetics, ganglionic blockade, cervical epidural anesthesia, and spinal cord transection (Stanley, 1973; Traber et al., 1970). Baroreceptor reflex response is altered in ketamine-anesthetized rats (Wang et al., 1991) and rabbits (Blake et al., 1982). Ketamine alone results in a short vasodepression followed by a longer-lasting strong pressor response (Altura et al., 1980). Increases in heart rate and mean arterial pressure have been reported following ketamine administration in rats and rabbits (Kumar and Kumar, 1984; Wang et al., 1991). Other studies in rabbits have found an elevated heart rate (Dhasmana et al., 1984), and decreased arterial pressure and cardiac output (Van Leeuwen et al., 1990). The effect of ketamine on the cardiac output of the rat has been variable (Idvall et al., 1980; Miller et al., 1980). In nonhuman primates, ketamine administration has resulted in an unchanged heart rate, mean arterial pressure, and rectal temperature (Reutlinger et al., 1980), or cardiodepression (Chimoskey et al., 1975; Ochsner, 1977).

Single IM injection of high doses of tiletamine in rabbits results in significant elevations in BUN and creatinine. At lower doses, there are no changes in serum chemistry values, but mild nephrosis is evident histologically in most animals (Doerning et al., 1992).

The respiratory effects of ketamine itself are relatively minor, although a dose-dependent suppression can be demonstrated. A characteristic apneustic pattern of breathing is seen commonly (Muir, 1985; Wright, 1982). In rhesus monkeys, normal respiratory variables are maintained, except for transient elevations in arterial PCO_2 and venous PO_2 (Reutlinger et al., 1980). Low doses of ketamine in the rabbit result in decreased respiratory rate and PO_2 (Dhasmana et al., 1984). Ketamine sympathomimetic actions promote bronchial muscle relaxation, and protective airway reflexes are generally maintained (Thurmon and Benson, 1987).

There are age and sex differences in the response of rats to ketamine (Waterman and Livingston, 1978). Ketamine sleeping time decreases as young rats mature from 1 to 3 weeks. This decrease in sleeping time seemed to be associated with the increased production of the cyclohexanone oxidation metabolite of ketamine, norketamine. After 3 weeks, females sleep longer in response to ketamine than males; which may be due to the greater ability of the male to produce the cyclohexanone oxidation metabolite. Older Sprague–Dawley rats have a decreased elimination of ketamine-xylazine (125 mg/kg–10 mg/kg IP) compared to younger rats (Veilleux-Lemieux et al., 2013).

Gerb et al. (2019) showed that repeated doses of ketamine produced tolerance to ketamine's anesthetic effects and, similarly, chronic morphine administration also produced tolerance.

Blood glucose levels following an IV glucose challenge are increased by ketamine (Aynsley-Green et al., 1973; Hsu and Hembrough, 1982; Reyes Toso et al., 1995).

Ketamine is traditionally considered to increase CBF and ICP (Wright, 1982), while CBF in the rabbit is increased without elevated PCO_2 (Dhasmana et al., 1984). However, direct cerebral vasodilation has not been a consistent finding, likely because many early studies were performed on spontaneously breathing subjects (Reich and Silvay, 1989). When ventilation is not controlled, ICP may rise following vasodilation secondary to hypercapnia (Pfenninger et al., 1985; Schwedler et al., 1982; Tranquilli et al., 1983). Using nuclear magnetic resonance perfusion imaging and electron paramagnetic resonance oximetry, Lei et al. (2001) found that in ventilated rats, ketamine at a dose of 50 mg/kg does not induce significant changes in CBF and increases cortical O_2 partial pressure.

In the human clinical setting, ketamine does not increase ICP when used under conditions of controlled ventilation, coadministration of a $GABA_A$ agonist, and without nitrous oxide (Himmelseher and Durieux, 2005). Compared with other anesthetics or sedatives, level II and III evidence (level II—evidence from at least one randomized clinical trial; level III—evidence from nonexperimental descriptive studies, such as comparative studies, correlation studies, and case-control studies) indicates that hemodynamic stimulation induced by ketamine may improve cerebral perfusion; this could make the drug a preferred choice after brain injury. In the laboratory, racemic ketamine has neuroprotective effects, and *S*(+)-ketamine has additional neuroregenerative effects, even when administered after the onset of a cerebral insult. However, improved outcomes were only reported in studies with brief recovery observation intervals. In developing animals, and in certain areas of the brain in adult rats without cerebral injury, neurotoxic effects were noted after administration of large doses of ketamine; these were prevented by coadministration of GABA receptor agonists (Himmelseher and Durieux, 2005).

Although ketamine and tiletamine have been reported to induce seizures in dogs and cats (Chen et al., 1969; Garmer, 1969; Wright, 1982), these agents raise the threshold to chemically or electrically induced seizures in rats and mice (Chen et al., 1969; Myslobodsky et al., 1981). Ketamine does not alter seizure threshold in epilepsy (Celesia et al., 1975), and induces excitatory activity in both the thalamus and limbic systems without evidence of spread to cortical areas (Ferrer-Allado et al., 1973). Thus, ketamine is unlikely to precipitate generalized convulsion even in the presence of preexisting seizure disorders. Myoclonic- and seizure-like activities may be observed; however, ketamine is considered to have anticonvulsant activity because EEG evidence of cortical epileptic activity is absent (Modica et al., 1990).

Tiletamine produces excitation in mice and rats at low doses; at higher doses, anesthesia may be produced in these species, but not in rabbits or guinea pigs (Chen et al., 1969). The classical stage 2 excitement phase, which occurs with subanesthetic concentrations of ketamine, may be associated with general stimulation of a variety of G-protein-linked receptors. The high-affinity states of dopamine D2 and D3 receptors, serotonin 5HT-2A receptors, β2-adrenoceptors, α2-1 and α2-2 adrenoceptors, opiate receptors, and muscarinic receptors are inhibited in vitro by clinical concentrations of ketamine; subanesthetic ketamine concentrations stimulate the incorporation of GTP into cloned dopamine D2 receptors (Seeman and Kapur, 2003).

Ketamine does not impair neutrophil function at clinically relevant concentrations (Nishina et al., 1998). Ketamine inhibits platelet aggregation in baboons (Atkinson et al., 1985) and humans, possibly due to suppressed formation of inositol 1,4,5-triphosphate and subsequent inhibition of cytosolic free calcium concentrations (Nakagawa et al., 2002). Small decreases in hematocrit and plasma protein, with a larger decrease in leukocyte (principally lymphocyte) count are observed, compared with values in manually restrained animals (Loomis et al., 1980).

Other reported pharmacologic effects of ketamine include the following: bronchodilatory activity as effective as halothane or enflurane in preventing experimentally induced bronchospasm in dogs (Hirshman et al., 1979); dose-dependent hypothermia in rats (Lin et al., 1978); maintained thermal balance in rhesus monkeys (Hunter et al., 1981); marked (normal) salivation response to hyperthermia, in contrast to five other anesthetic regimens

(Furuyama et al., 1989); increased serum renin activity (Pettinger et al., 1975); altered serum follicle-stimulating hormone, testosterone, and androstenedione in rats following decapitation (Nazian, 1988); resting myopia in humans and nonhuman primates, due largely to central parasympathetic neuronal tone (Crawford et al., 1990); enhancement of neuro-muscular blockade in humans (Reich and Silvay, 1989), and in rabbits (Bogdan et al., 1974) and monkeys (Tsai and Lee, 1989); teratologic effects in rats (Kochhar et al., 1986); muscle necrosis following IM injection of ketamine–xylazine in hamsters (Gaertner et al., 1987) and rabbits (Beyers et al., 1991); autoamputation of digits following ketamine–acepromazine injections in guinea pigs (Latt and Ecobichon, 1984).

6. Ketamine antagonists

Ketamine anesthesia is antagonized in mice by agonist drugs specifically targeting the metabotropic glutamate receptors 1 and 5 (Sou et al., 2006). Reich and Silvay (1989) discuss a number of agents that, based on the proposed mechanisms of action, should antagonize cyclohexamine effects. These agents include metaphit (1-(1-(3-isothiocyanatophenyl)-cyclohexyl-piperidine); acetylates NMDA receptors), naloxone (opioid antagonist), norepinephrine and serotonin receptor blockers, and anticholinesterase agents (e.g., 4-aminopyridine or physostigmine) (Reich and Silvay, 1989; Wright, 1982). GNE-5729, a pyridopyrimidinone-based GluN2A subunit-selective positive allosteric modulator of the NMDA receptor, works by enhancing the NMDA receptor response to its agonists and has been found to antagonize the effects of ketamine in a rat model (Li et al., 2020).

IV. Miscellaneous agents

A. Urethane

1. Pharmacokinetics and metabolism

Relatively little is known about urethane's mechanism of action, although it is apparent that it acts in ways unlike most other anesthetics; its effects on GABAergic neurotransmission are unclear (Hara and Harris, 2002). Urethane produces little or no enhancement (Maggi and Meli, 1986a; Shirasaka and Wasterlain, 1995), or inhibition (Accorsi-Mendonca et al., 2007) of GABAergic neurotransmission in the central and peripheral nervous systems. Sceniak and MacIver (2006) concluded that urethane acts by reducing the intrinsic excitability of neuronal membranes rather than affecting synaptic transmission. However, urethane reverses the antagonistic effect of bicuculline on GABA-induced depolarization in the isolated rat superior cervical ganglion (Bowery and Dray, 1978), and Hara and Harris (2002) found a variety of effects using recombinant neurotransmitter receptors expressed in *Xenopus* oocytes. Urethane, at presumed clinically effective concentrations, enhanced the function of $\alpha'_1\beta_2\gamma_{2S}$ $GABA_A$ and α'_1 glycine receptors (23% and 33%, respectively), inhibited the function of NR1a/NR2A NMDA and GluR1/GluR2 AMPA receptors (10% and 18%), and enhanced function of the nACh receptor (15%). These results are unusual, compared with other anesthetic agents, in that (1) most other agents do not have primary effects at more than one receptor type; (2) the magnitude of effect for urethane is less than that reported for other agents; and (3) other agents (e.g., isoflurane, ketamine, and thiopental) inhibit rather than enhance nACh function. This spectrum of action is similar only to that of ethanol.

2. Absorption

It was previously believed that the principal metabolic path for urethane was esterase-catalyzed hydrolysis to carbon dioxide, ammonia, and ethanol (Nomeir et al., 1989; Skipper et al., 1951). However, previous work has shown that more than 95% of urethane is metabolized via cytochrome P450, specifically CYP2E1, to vinyl carbamate, vinyl carbamate epoxide, and eventually CO_2 and NH_3. Knockout mice (Cyp2e1−/−) given ^{14}C-labeled urethane have a sixfold decrease in recovered $^{14}CO_2$ compared with wild-type mice, and a marked increase in half-life (22 vs. 0.8 h). Pretreatment of mice with 1-aminobenzotriazole (ABT), a universal P450 inhibitor, results in a similar metabolic pattern in both genotypes. Using a pharmacokinetic model production of CO_2 from urethane via esterase metabolism is negligible, accounting for less than 0.5% of an administered dose, compared with 96% via CYP2E1 and 3.2% for cytochromes P450 other than CYP2E1. CO_2 is a final end-product of urethane metabolism by each of these pathways, and 91%–93% of administered ^{14}C-urethane is recovered in expired CO_2 within 6 h (Hoffler et al., 2003). In both rats and mice given carbonyl-^{14}C-labeled urethane, there is almost complete recovery of radiolabel in expired CO_2, with small amounts found in feces or urine (Bryan et al., 1949). At low urethane doses, recovery of labeled CO_2 may approach 100% within 12 h. In vitro metabolism of CO_2 can be demonstrated in a variety of tissues, including the liver, plasma, brain, muscle, and kidney (Nomeir et al., 1989). Because urethane is a known carcinogen, there has been particular interest in its metabolism. Metabolic activation of the ethyl moiety is required for carcinogenic action, but the metabolic pathways leading to activation or detoxication remain incompletely characterized (Kurata et al., 1991). Neoplastic lesions are significantly reduced following 6-week urethane dosing in Cyp2e1−/− mice, indicating a central role of the CYP2E1 pathway, presumably via the formation of vinyl carbamate epoxide (Ganayem, 2007).

3. Distribution and fate

Urethane distributes evenly to most body tissues, except fat (Nomeir et al., 1989).

4. Preparation and route of administration

Urethane (ethyl carbamate) is the ethyl ester of carbamic acid. It is readily soluble in water, alcohol, and lipids. The frequent and continued use of urethane in neurophysiologic studies derives not only from its relatively minor effects on neurotransmission (Albrecht and Davidowa, 1989), but also from its ability to produce relatively long and stable anesthesia following a single administration (Flecknell, 1996). It is by no means an ideal anesthetic, as indicated by the variety of reported pharmacologic effects (below). Urethane differs from chloralose, especially in having analgesic properties sufficient to permit surgery in small rodents (Field and Lang, 1988; Flecknell, 1996; Maggi and Meli, 1986a). In discussing the pharmacologic effects of urethane, Maggi and Meli (1986c) stress the importance of dose and route of administration, and the need to distinguish between normal resting function during anesthesia and the degree of response to psychopharmacologic stimuli.

Urethane has been administered by most routes, including topical application in frogs (Strobel and Wollman, 1969). Following IV administration, urethane has a wide margin of safety and produces long-lasting narcosis (8−10 h) with minimal cardiovascular or respiratory depression and maintenance of spinal reflexes (Buelke-Sam et al., 1978).

As with other anesthetics, there are strain and sex differences in the dose of urethane needed to induce surgical levels of anesthesia. The threshold blood urethane concentration for narcosis in rats was determined by Boyland and Rhoden (1949) by injecting rats SQ with 1.0 g/kg urethane and measuring blood levels of urethane at various times. Rats with blood concentrations below 60 mg/100 mL are not anesthetized, while those with concentrations of at least 80 mg/100 mL (10 mM) are anesthetized for 8−12 h. A SQ dose of 1.6 g/kg urethane is required to surgically anesthetize male Sprague−Dawley rats (Braun et al., 1997), while female WU (WI) rats require a SQ urethane dose of 1.8 g/kg (Van Der Meer et al., 1975). In male Wistar Morini rats, 1.0 g/kg urethane SQ produces surgical levels of anesthesia in only 30% of the rats after 3 h and 90% after 6 h. In contrast, a dose of 1.2 g/kg SQ resulted in surgical anesthesia in 100% of the same rats after 3 h, with the anesthetic effect lasting at least 6 h (Maggi and Meli, 1986a).

The necessary IP urethane dose ranges from 0.8 to 1.2 g/kg. In male Wistar rats, a surgical level of anesthesia is achieved with 0.8 g/kg urethane IP (Pettinger et al., 1975). In female CD (Sprague−Dawley) rats, a surgical level of anesthesia is achieved with 0.8−1.0 g/kg urethane IP, although 1.2 g/kg is required to ensure anesthesia of all animals (Hamstra et al., 1984). Lincoln et al. (1973) reported that 1.1 g/kg IP provided anesthesia levels suitable for stereotaxic manipulation and neurosurgery for at least 8 h in female Wistar rats. Female WU (WI) rats require an IP dose of 1.0 g/kg to reach a surgical level of anesthesia (Van Der Meer et al., 1975).

5. Side effects

"Urethane is a potent multisite carcinogen capable of inducing tumors in various organs and animal species regardless of the route of administration" (Ganayem, 2007), and has been classified as "reasonably anticipated to be a human carcinogen" (National Toxicology Program (NTP), 2000). It is also a potent mutagen (Field and Lang, 1988; Ganayem, 2007). Before using urethane, alternative anesthetics should be considered whenever possible. Precautions suitable for handling a moderate carcinogen should be utilized, including the use of appropriate breathing masks, gloves, and fume hoods for preparing solutions from the powdered drug. Given its carcinogenic potential, urethane should not be used for recovery procedures (Flecknell, 1996), and most Institutional Animal Care and Use Committees strongly advise against its use entirely.

a. Nervous system effects

Urethane has slight depressant effects on autonomic reflexes and the activity of subcortical structures of the CNS. Basal activity of nigrostriatal dopamine-containing neurons in the rat is reduced as compared with unanesthetized paralyzed controls (Kelland et al., 1990). There is, in general, an activated sympathetic outflow from the CNS to peripheral organs (Maggi and Meli, 1986a). Cardiovascular stability with urethane is due in part to sustained sympathetic nervous system activity and is associated with high circulating catecholamine levels (Carruba et al., 1987). Urethane attenuates the expression of kindled seizures in rats, where brief, low-intensity, electrical stimulation is periodically applied to the amygdala, and may not be an appropriate anesthetic for the study of epileptiform phenomena (Cain et al., 1989). Steward et al. (2005) reviewed the effect of several anesthetics, including urethane, on neurotransmitter systems in the context of the rat BOLD contrast pharmacological MRI. Shumkova et al. (2021) recommended urethane as the anesthetic of choice in non-survival sensory evoked response recordings in the developing rat brain as it produced less prominent impairment of cortical neuronal activity in neonatal animals. Additionally, urethane−xylazine provided improved systemic physiologic conditions during anesthesia in mouse studies using the vestibular sensory evoked potential to evaluate peripheral vestibular function (Lee and Jones, 2018).

b. Cardiovascular effects

Blood pressure effects of urethane are dependent on the route of administration. IP injection of 1.2 g/kg in female Wistar rats decreases mean blood pressure to 95 mmHg, compared to 125 mmHg in unanesthetized animals, which persisted for at least 1 h after injection (Hillebrand et al., 1971); in some individual animals, pressure dropped below 80 mmHg. In contrast, IP injection of 1.2 g/kg urethane to male Wistar and Sprague–Dawley rats caused no change in mean arterial blood pressure and heart rate (Carruba et al., 1987). The fall in blood pressure after IP injection of 25% urethane at 1 g/kg can reportedly be reduced by slow injection and is absent if the dose is given rapidly intra-arterially (Van Der Meer et al., 1975).

When urethane was injected IV into male Wistar rats at a dose of 1.3 g/kg, blood pressure transiently dropped, but recovered to near baseline by 5 min after the infusion (Volicer and Loew, 1971); this was accompanied by a transient rise in heart rate, which also recovered. IV injection of 0.2–0.8 g/kg urethane also resulted in a 5–10 min drop in arterial pressure, followed by a progressive increase in pressure (Reinert, 1964).

Arterial pressure, cardiac output, and renal, hepatosplanchnic, and brain blood flow in rats were lowest with IP urethane anesthesia compared with four other anesthetic regimens, and lower than published values for the conscious rat (Gumbleton, 1989; Gumbleton et al., 1990a). Similar depressant effects on cardiac dynamics of the rat have been reported (Maggi et al., 1984; Wang et al., 1991), although others have found cardiorespiratory effects to be minimal (De Wildt et al., 1983; Folle and Levesque, 1976), especially when the IP route of administration is avoided and doses are kept to the minimum required (Maggi and Meli, 1986b). Heart rate and systolic pressure in rats are stable during prolonged (3-h) anesthesia, although pulse pressure is consistently elevated (due to decreased diastolic pressures) (Buelke-Sam et al., 1978). The baroreceptor reflex in rats is altered (Fluckiger et al., 1985; Wang et al., 1991). In a cellular model of simulated myocardial ischemia, diazoxide-induced cell protection of mitochondrial KATP channel activity was potentiated by urethane anesthesia (Zaugg et al., 2002).

c. Effect on ventilation

Respiratory effects of urethane anesthesia are minimal (Maggi and Meli, 1986c), although changes in blood gas values have been reported in the rabbit (Collado et al., 1987) and rat (Buelke-Sam et al., 1978; Folle and Levesque, 1976). Significant hypercapnia and hypoxia occur in the hamster (Reid et al., 1989). In contrast, Field et al. (1993) found that rats anesthetized with urethane had a severely depressed arterial pH, with an increased PaO_2 and decreased $PaCO_2$ suggestive of hyperventilation.

In decerebrate male Wistar rats, 750 mg/kg IV urethane has no effect on respiratory frequency or tidal volume, although blood pressure and heart rate decrease (Sapru and Krieger, 1979). In male Sprague–Dawley and Wistar rats, 1.2 g/kg urethane IP has minimal effects on blood gas parameters until 4 h after anesthesia (Carruba et al., 1987). There is a tendency for pH to decrease and arterial PO_2 and PCO_2 to rise during anesthesia. After 3–4 h under anesthesia, PCO_2 rises significantly from a baseline value of 40–49 mmHg, and PO_2 increases from 80 to 105 mmHg.

In Sprague–Dawley rats, where 1.2 and 1.5 g/kg IP provided sleep time in excess of 24 h, anesthesia was characterized by progressive acidosis, hypocapnia, hyperoxia, hypotension, and bradycardia (Field et al., 1993). In another study, male Sprague–Dawley rats were injected with 1.5 g/kg urethane IP, and blood gas parameters were measured under normothermic and hypothermic conditions (Alfaro and Palacios, 1992). If the rats were maintained at normal body temperature, changes in blood values were minimal. Arterial PO_2 and PCO_2 remained unchanged, while arterial pH dropped from 7.48 to 7.42. Bicarbonate levels decreased from 21.8 to 18.9 mmol/L, and arterial lactate increased from 0.89 to 2.78 mmol/L. If the rats were not warmed, their body temperature dropped from 37 to 30°C in 2 h. The hypothermic rats showed a progressive increase in PaO_2 over time, with an increase of 20–30 mmHg after 2 h. The changes in arterial bicarbonate, lactate, and pH in the hypothermic group were similar to those seen in the normothermic animals. It is suggested that the increase in arterial PO_2 seen in an earlier study (Carruba et al., 1987) might have been caused by hypothermia.

d. Effect on hematocrit and blood glucose levels

Urethane is known to affect hematocrit in rats. Rats injected with 1.5 g/kg urethane using a 50 wt% urethane solution show "marked hemoconcentration" after 8 h (Spriggs and Stockham, 1964). In a study investigating the effect of administration route on urethane-induced hemoconcentration, urethane was administered at doses sufficient to induce stage 4–5 anesthesia via four different routes: IP, SQ, PO, and IA. After 60 min, the hematocrit in the rats changed by the following respective amounts: +21.7%, +8.0%, −2.8%, and +1.5%. The substantial increase in hematocrit following IP injection was attributed to plasma loss to the peritoneal cavity. An approximately linear relationship between the dose of IP-injected urethane and the relative increase in hematocrit was also found, with a slope of 2.1% increase in hematocrit for every 0.1 g/kg increase in urethane dose (Van Der Meer et al., 1975). Severs et al. (1981) showed that IP urethane causes peritoneal fluid accumulation, hyperosmolality of body fluids, osmotic toxicity to the mesenteric vasculature, and increased plasma renin activity and aldosterone levels.

Urethane also has a profound effect on blood glucose levels. The blood glucose level of fasting rats increases from 58 to 168 mg/dL 1 h after IP injection of urethane at a dose of 1.25 g/kg (Reinert, 1964); similar findings were reported by Van Der Meer et al. (1975) and Braun et al. (1997). Van Der Meer et al. (1975) speculated that urethane induced hyperglycemia through "stimuli arising in the damaged tissues" at the injection site, although increased peripheral sympathetic activity and increased circulating catecholamine levels are a more plausible explanation (Carruba et al., 1987; Pettinger et al., 1975; Spriggs and Stockham, 1964). Elevated blood glucose also occurs in the rabbit (Collado et al., 1987) and rat, due at least in part to elevated catecholamine levels (Hinton, 1982; Maggi and Meli, 1986a).

e. Immune system effects

Urethane is immunosuppressive and has demonstrated antineoplastic effects. It is, however, more commonly recognized for its carcinogenic and mutagenic properties (Field and Lang, 1988; Iversen, 1991; Inai et al., 1991; Leithauser et al., 1990; Sotomayor and Collins, 1990).

In adult male HsdBrl:WH Wistar rats, urethane reduces splenic IL-1 β mRNA expression, while ketamine/xylazine, chloral hydrate, and pentobarbital all enhance the basal expression of IL-1β and IL-6 mRNA. Urethane, ketamine/xylazine, and TBE reduce basal TNFα mRNA levels, whereas TNFα mRNA expression is unaffected by chloral hydrate and pentobarbital (Bette et al., 2004).

f. Pathologic effects

Pathologic effects following IP administration of urethane have been reported in the rat (Gumbleton et al., 1988; Severs et al., 1981; Van der Meer et al., 1975). A toxic effect on the mesenteric vasculature results in peritoneal effusion and secondary impairment of renal function. The resulting hypovolemia may explain observed increases in serum renin (Severs et al., 1981). Hypertonic urethane administration in the rabbit, by either IV or IP routes, causes hemolysis, increases serum potassium, and prolongs clotting time (Bree and Cohen, 1965). Other reported pharmacologic effects of urethane include the following: depressed xenobiotic renal clearance in the rat (Gumbleton et al., 1990b); depressed antipyrine clearance, an indicator of intrinsic hepatic clearance in the rat (Gumbleton and Benet, 1991); blunted plasma GH response to GH-releasing hormone, due in part to enhanced somatostatin release from the hypothalamus (Hosoi et al., 1988); lowered basal gastric acid secretion, due in part to increased synthesis and release of endogenous (gastric) somatostatin (Yang et al., 1990); and rise in plasma β endorphin activity (Ramirez-Gonzalez et al., 1991).

V. Anesthetic combinations

Most of the individual drugs discussed above lack one or more of the properties of a practical and safe surgical anesthetic, such as hypnosis, analgesia, or muscle relaxation. This has resulted in attempts to improve the overall quality of injectable anesthesia by the combination of two or more drugs. Such balanced anesthesia also improves safety by reducing the dosage, and corresponding side effects of each component. The same goal may be achieved by total IV anesthesia, e.g., with propofol and an opioid (Bailey et al., 2000).

Following are general comments about common types of anesthetic combinations that have been used. The reader is referred to the sections on individual agents in this chapter, the species-specific chapters in this edition, as well as previous editions of this text, for practical information about their use. There is little information available on the biodisposition of anesthetic drugs when used in combination.

A. Ketamine combinations

The goals of ketamine combinations include improved analgesia, muscle relaxation and sedation, prolonged duration, and decreased side effects (Muir, 1985). The use of adjunctive agents alters the pharmacokinetics of ketamine, in general, leading to a potentiated and prolonged effect (Pascoe, 1992; Waterman, 1983, 1984). Ketamine has been combined with xylazine (Dittmar et al., 2004; Schwenke and Cragg, 2004; Wixson et al., 1987a–d), diazepam (Wixson et al., 1987a–d), midazolam (Gumbleton, 1989), azaperone (Olson and Renchko, 1988), guaifenesin (Olson et al., 1987), pentobarbital (Svendsen and Carter, 1985), chlorpromazine (Barzago et al., 1992), medetomidine (DiFilippo et al., 2004; Nevalainen et al., 1989; Taylor et al., 2000; Lee et al., 2010), dexmedetomidine (Fox et al., 2016), and xylazine–acepromazine (Arras et al., 2001; Welberg et al., 2006).

1. Ketamine–xylazine and ketamine/α-2 adrenergic receptor antagonists

Ketamine–xylazine mixtures have variable effects on blood pressure and cardiac output in rats and mice. In male Sprague–Dawley rats, an IP injection of 40/5 mg/kg ketamine/xylazine resulted in a 32.3% decrease in MAP (Wixson et al., 1987c). A dose of 60/7.5 mg/kg ketamine/xylazine decreased MAP by 26.7% or 30–35 mmHg. MAP remained decreased until recovery, which was more than 2 h at the high dose. IP injections of 40/5 and 60/7.5 mg/kg ketamine/xylazine decreased heart rate by 6% and 27%, respectively. In contrast, 50/5 mg/kg and 100/10 mg/kg ketamine/xylazine IM maintained mean arterial pressure around 110 mmHg for 90 min, and between 85 and 100 mmHg for 150 min, respectively, in male Sprague–Dawley rats (Taie et al., 1999).

An IM injection of 100/5 mg/kg ketamine/xylazine in BALB/c mice resulted in a decrease in MAP from 129 to 100 mmHg, a decrease of 22.5% (Erhardt et al., 1984). The heart rate decreased from 509 to 159 beats/min, and the respiratory rate dropped from 195 to 109 breaths/min. In comparison, 150/15 mg/kg ketamine/xylazine IP reduced heart rate in SvEv/Tac mice from 658 to 293 beats/min and cardiac output from 13.0 to 7.2 mL/min/g (Yang et al., 1999). Hemodynamic effects of ketamine/xylazine anesthesia were fully antagonized by the administration of the α2-antagonist atipamezole in CD-1, Swiss, and C57BL6 mice (Janssen et al., 2004). Atipamezole reversed the anesthetic effects of ketamine-dexmedetomidine (50 mg/kg–0.5 mg/kg IP) in female C57BL/6J mice without adversely affecting the analgesic effects of butorphanol or buprenorphine (Izer et al., 2014). Atipamezole (1 mg/kg IP) has also been shown to significantly lower the recovery time of male C57BL/6J mice anesthetized with ketamine-xylazine (80 mg/kg–8 mg/kg IP) as compared to yohimbine (1.5 mg/kg IP) or saline (Janssen et al., 2017).

Respiratory rates and SpO2 were significantly lower in male Wistar Han rats anesthetized with ketamine-dexmedetomidine (75 mg/kg–1 mg/kg IP) than those anesthetized with ketamine-xylazine (100 mg/kg–10 mg/kg IP); however, serum creatine kinase increases were acutely (3 h after dosing) more severe, and surface area of muscle necrosis at the injection site was larger in the ketamine-xylazine anesthetized rats (Wellington et al., 2013). Ketamine/xylazine mixtures also affect blood gas values in mice. IM injection of a 100/5 mg/kg mixture of ketamine/xylazine into BALB/c mice decreased arterial blood pH from 7.285 to 7.122, or 0.16 pH units (Erhardt et al., 1984). Arterial PCO_2 increased from 26.5 to 41.0 mmHg (55%), while PaO_2 decreased from 111.7 to 97.3 mmHg or about 13%.

In rodents, redosing of ketamine combinations is an important consideration of prolonged-duration anesthetic events or where redosing is important due to invasive procedures. Jaber et al. (2014) reviewed redosing male C57BL/6J mice during surgical planes of anesthesia or immediately after leaving the surgical plane, when the pedal withdrawal reflex returns, with various doses of ketamine or ketamine-xylazine after initial dosing with ketamine-xylazine-acepromazine (80 mg/kg–8 mg/kg–1 mg/kg IP). This study found that less than 100% of animals returned to a surgical plane of anesthesia after redosing with 0.25 (20 mg/kg IP) or 0.5 (40 mg/kg IP) of the original dose of ketamine alone, whereas 100% of animals returned to or maintained a surgical plane of anesthesia when redosed with an equal dose (80 mg/kg) of ketamine alone or 0.25 (20 mg/kg–2 mg/kg) or 0.5 (40 mg/kg–4mg/kg) of the original dose of ketamine-xylazine (Jaber et al., 2014). Larger percentages of these mice died when redosed during a surgical plane of anesthesia than they did if redosed immediately after leaving the surgical plane of anesthesia, once the pedal withdrawal reflex returned. Erickson et al. (2016) evaluated continuous-rate infusions of ketamine or ketamine-xylazine in C57BL/6J mice after induction of anesthesia with ketamine-xylazine (80 mg/kg–8 mg/kg IP) or ketamine-xylazine-acepromazine (80 mg/kg–8 mg/kg–0.1 or 0.5 mg/kg). Results were variable, but the groups with the longest continuous surgical plane of anesthesia and minimal mortality were 80 mg/kg/h ketamine administered after ketamine-xylazine-acepromazine (80 mg/kg–8mg/kg–0.1 mg/kg) and 40 mg/kg/h ketamine with 4 mg/kg/h xylazine after ketamine-xylazine-acepromazine (80 mg/kg–8 mg/kg–0.5 m/kg). Similarly, Heng et al. (2020) evaluated the delivery of alfaxalone as a CRI to Sprague–Dawley rats after induction with ketamine-xylazine (80 mg/kg–8 mg/kg SQ). Results showed that animals in the alfaxalone CRI group had a reliable surgical plane of anesthesia compared to those without additional anesthesia, but otherwise physiological changes were insignificant.

Age plays a role in the severity of effects from ketamine-xylazine anesthesia, with older rats more commonly experiencing cardiac depression and pulmonary edema and effusion at higher doses (Giroux et al., 2015).

Ketamine combined with xylazine can increase blood glucose levels. Blood glucose levels in male Sprague–Dawley rats injected with 50/10 mg/kg ketamine/xylazine mixture IP rose to 256 mg/dL, compared to 131 mg/dL in pentobarbital-injected rats (Kawai et al., 1997). In the 9L rat glioma, xylazine alone or in combination with ketamine resulted in hyperglycemia and intratumor pH acidification (Pavlovic et al., 1996).

Thompson et al. (2002) investigated the effects of anesthetic agents, including ketamine/xylazine, on hepatic and splenic injury in ICR mice. Injury to lymphocytes and to hepatic Kupffer and endothelial cells occurs within 3 h, as indicated by marked increases in apoptosis in splenic follicles and in hepatic Kupffer and endothelial cells, as well as by three to fourfold increase in serum aspartate transaminase. Ketamine/xylazine anesthesia enhances the basal expression of IL-1β and IL-6 mRNA and reduces basal TNFα mRNA in male Wistar rat spleen (Bette et al., 2004).

Sayce et al. (2020) reported that 55% of rabbits induced with ketamine-dexmedetomidine (20mg/kg–0.125 mg/kg IM) and maintained by ketamine-dexmedetomidine CRI

(343 μg/kg/min−1.6 μg/kg/min) showed no signs of laryngeal response (laryngospasm) during extended-duration nonsurvival laryngotracheal surgery. Historically, IP has been the most common route of administration for ketamine-xylazine, but Levin-Arama et al. (2016) found that 191.25/4.25 mg/kg of ketamine/xylazine administered SC to three common laboratory mouse strains was safe and effective for surgical anesthesia.

2. Ketamine–benzodiazepine

Ketamine-midazolam anesthesia (75 mg/kg−7.5 mg/kg IP) showed superior left ventricular systolic function in Sprague–Dawley rats compared with ketamine-medetomidine (75 mg/kg−0.5 mg/kg IP) or pentobarbital (40 mg/kg IP) anesthetized animals, although pentobarbital-anesthetized animals had higher heart rates (Sabatini et al., 2013). IP injections of mixtures of ketamine/diazepam result in modest decreases in MAP in rats. A dose of 40/5 mg/kg ketamine/diazepam decreased MAP by 12%. A higher dose of 60/7.5 mg/kg resulted in a transient decrease of 31%, but the MAP was back to its baseline value by 30–45 min after the injection (Wixson et al., 1987c). Neither mixture had significant effects on heart rate, with heart rate decreases of 9% and 12% at the two doses.

Ketamine/diazepam mixtures also affect blood gas values in rats (Wixson et al., 1987c). IP doses of 40/5 and 60/7.5 mg/kg decrease arterial pH in male Sprague–Dawley rats by about 0.05 and 0.08 pH units, respectively. The lower dose of ketamine/diazepam (40/5 mg/kg) results in a $PaCO_2$ increase of 20%–30%. The higher dose (60/7.5 mg/kg) transiently increases $PaCO_2$ by 4.9% (about 3–4 mmHg). The 40/5 and 60/7.5 mg/kg doses of ketamine/diazepam result in PaO_2 decreases of 23% and 11.5% (eight to nine mmHg), respectively.

3. Other ketamine combinations

Ambar et al. (2020) showed that ketamine-alfaxalone (20 mg/kg−4 mg/kg IM) produced a safe and effective protocol for brief, light anesthesia in naked mole rats (*Heterocephalus glaber*). Ketamine-xylazine (80 mg/kg−8 mg/kg SQ) followed by an alfaxalone CRI (10 mg/kg/hr IV) provided a safe and reliable surgical plane of anesthesia in Sprague–Dawley rats (Heng et al., 2020).

Ketamine-alfaxalone, ketamine-alfaxalone-dexmedetomidine, and alfaxalone-butorphanol-midazolam combinations were examined by Eshar and Beaufrere (2020) for anesthesia of five-striped palm squirrels (*Funambulus pennantii*). All tested protocols in this study were safe and effective for immobilization, but the surgical plane of anesthesia was more variable in the ketamine-alfaxalone group (Eshar and Beaufrere, 2020).

B. Tiletamine–zolazepam (telazol)

Telazol, a 1:1 combination of zolazepam and tiletamine, is indicated for inducing and maintaining anesthesia for short (about 30 min) surgical procedures. In an effort to improve effectiveness and reduce adverse side effects, Telazol has been combined with xylazine or medetomidine (Buchanan et al., 1998), and ketamine and xylazine (Ko et al., 1995).

Marked species differences in analgesic effectiveness, drug response, and rate of elimination, as well as substantial interanimal pharmacokinetic variability, are reported (Chen et al., 1969; Kumar et al., 2006). Although useful for surgical anesthesia in rats (Silverman et al., 1983), ferrets (Payton and Pick, 1989), gerbils (Hrapkiewicz et al., 1989), dogs and cats (Tracy et al., 1988), nociception is not eliminated in mice, hamsters (Silverman et al., 1983), guinea pigs, and rabbits (Ward et al., 1974), even at relatively high dosages associated with prolonged recumbency. Telazol does not produce analgesia in New Zealand White rabbits and is nephrotoxic at both 32 and 64 mg/kg (Brammer et al., 1991). Doerning et al. (1992) found pathologic lesions without azotemia in rabbits given 7.5 mg/kg tiletamine, in addition to azotemia with severe renal tubular necrosis in rabbits given 32 mg/kg tiletamine. For this reason, Telazol is not generally recommended for use in rabbits.

The pharmacology of Telazol has been reviewed (Lin et al., 1993). In domestic pigs, tiletamine level decreases faster than that of zolazepam (terminal elimination rate constant of 0.26/h for tiletamine vs. 0.11/h for zolazepam), with half-lives for tiletamine and zolazepam in the terminal elimination period phase of 3.7 and 8.4 h, respectively (Kumar et al., 2006). Semple et al. (2000) reported half-lives of 1.8 h for tiletamine and 1.2 h for zolazepam in the polar bear *Ursus maritimus*, with total clearance values of 2.1 and 1.1 L/h/kg for tiletamine and zolazepam, respectively. A 1-compartment model with first-order absorption and elimination best fits the time-series data for the drugs in serum during the immobilization period.

C. Propofol-dexmedetomidine-fentanyl

A combination of 100 mg/kg propofol, 0.1 mg/kg medetomidine, and 0.1 mg/kg fentanyl given IP to male Wistar rats provided safe and reliable surgical anesthesia for 25 min (Alves et al., 2010). Lower doses of both fentanyl and medetomidine were used to avoid severe cardiovascular depression. Atipamezole provides rapid recovery with the protection of analgesic effects. Likewise, 75/1/0.2 mg/kg of propofol/medetomidine/fentanyl administered IP to male CD1 mice provided surgical anesthesia for up to 15 min and restraint for up to 30 min (Alves et al., 2009).

D. Alfaxalone-dexmedetomidine-opioid

Since alfaxalone alone does not provide antinociception, its combination with dexmedetomidine and fentanyl can increase anesthetic duration and provide short-term analgesia. This combination does produce a marked decrease in heart rate since both dexmedetomidine and fentanyl can produce bradycardia (Virtanen, 1989; Laubie et al., 1974). 20/0.05/0.1 mg/kg alfaxalone/dexmedetomidine/fentanyl was administered IP to female Sprague−Dawley rats (60 mg/kg alfaxalone was given to male rats) and provided a more prolonged surgical anesthesia than alfaxalone alone (Arenillas and Gomez de Segura, 2018). Bradley et al. (2019) observed a synergistic effect in rabbits given 6/0.2 mg/kg alfaxalone/dexmedetomidine IM. When 0.3 mg/kg butorphanol was added, they did not see any effect on the duration of sedation but did see an influence on the response to an adverse stimulus (toe pinch). 15/0.25/0.05 mg/kg of alfaxalone/dexmedetomidine/buprenorphine administered SC to guinea pigs produced sedation of less than 90 min duration but did not result in general anesthesia (Doerning et al., 2018).

E. Alfaxalone-α-2 adrenergic receptor antagonists

Alfaxalone-xylazine may be a viable option for injectable surgical anesthesia in mice, but sex and strain differences were reported using various doses by Erickson et al. (2019).

West et al. (2020) evaluated various doses of alfaxalone alone or in combination with dexmedetomidine for anesthesia of Sprague−Dawley rats. The results of their study indicated that alfaxalone alone did not result in a surgical plane of anesthesia at any dose evaluated and that alfaxalone-dexmedetomidine (30 mg/kg−0.05 mg/kg IP) resulted in a surgical plane of anesthesia for female rats only.

VI. Injectable anesthetic delivery systems

Syringe pumps, or drivers, are used for controlled infusion of anesthetics, analgesics, or other high-potency drugs. Simple fixed-rate syringe drivers can be used for this purpose, but they place a considerable demand on the user to calculate and prepare drug dilutions and to closely monitor their operation. Instead, variable-rate, microprocessor-controlled syringe pumps are preferred. Such pumps are available from human and some veterinary medical suppliers as well as vendors of scientific equipment for biomedical research. For anesthesia use, the pump software should recognize the volume and concentration units used for drugs, and display infusion rates based on the selected units. The ability to deliver a user-programmable bolus of the drug is essential, as are alarms to warn of delivery line occlusion and an impending empty syringe. A display screen should indicate the infusion rate in appropriate units, the delivered and remaining volume, and the operating status of the pump. Pumps having these features are usually intended and labeled for use in anesthesia. Turner et al. (2011) provided a review of equipment considerations, including vascular access equipment, tethering and restraint equipment, and pumps, as well as formulation strategies. These considerations are all important parts of successful injectable anesthetic outcomes.

There is an increasing interest in human and veterinary medicine in total intravenous anesthesia (TIVA) and analgesia, although in many cases, inhalation agents are used concurrently. For human use, control algorithms have been developed based on the known pharmacodynamic and pharmacokinetic properties of some widely used IV anesthetic agents. These target-controlled infusion schemes are computer-controlled to vary the rate of administration over time, producing a more stable plane of anesthesia (Diba, 2005). For animals, the information needed is not available for many species, nor is the market sufficiently great to support development of the requisite control algorithms. The features and controls of anesthesia syringe pumps change with each new model and often with software updates. Those unfamiliar with these devices should research currently available models and seek advice from colleagues experienced in their use before purchasing them. For IV anesthesia, modern programmable syringe pumps are the equivalent to a precision vaporizer, with more complex user controls. Used equipment should be purchased with the same precautions discussed for used anesthesia machines.

CRI protocols provide a steady amount of drug that alleviates issues noted with administration of repeated boluses. CRI protocols like morphine-lidocaine-ketamine and propofol-fentanyl have been used in various species. Muir et al. (2003) concluded that a MLK CRI decreased the isoflurane MAC in dogs and was not associated with adverse hemodynamic effects. Most CRI's like MLK are used for their analgesic benefits, but some can be used for anesthetic administration. Since propofol as a sole agent is not a good analgesic, drugs labeled for analgesia should be administered for painful procedures. Davis et al. (2017) administered 5−10 ug/kg fentanyl to dogs, followed by induction with propofol (2 mg/kg followed by 1 mg/kg every 15 s to achieve intubation), and then maintained anesthesia with either propofol alone (0.5 mg/kg) or propofol (0.3−0.35 mg/kg) combined with fentanyl (0.1−0.2 ug/kg). With this protocol, the authors were able to decrease the propofol induction dose and the minimal infusion rate of propofol. Velázquez-Delgado et al. (2021), found that TIVA of propofol combined with fentanyl-lidocaine-ketamine produced adequate anesthesia but poor-quality recovery in goats undergoing abomasotomy.

References

Accorsi-Mendonca, D., Leao, R.M., Aguiar, J.F., Varanda, A.A., Machado, B.H., 2007. Urethane inhibits the GABAergic neurotransmission in the nucleus of the solitary tract of rat brain stem slices. Am. J. Physiol. Regul. Comp. Physiol. 292, R396–R402.

Adams, H.R., 1970. Prolongation of barbiturate anesthesia by chloramphenicol in laboratory animals. J. Am. Vet. Med. Assoc. 157, 1908–1913.

Adams, H.R., Dixit, B.N., 1970. Prolongation of pentobarbital anesthesia by chloramphenicol in dogs and cats. J. Am. Vet. Med. Assoc. 156, 902–905.

Aeschbacher, G., Webb, A.I., 1993a. Propofol in rabbits. 1. Determination of an induction dose. Lab. Anim. Sci. 43, 324–327.

Aeschbacher, G., Webb, A.I., 1993b. Propofol in rabbits 2. Long-term anesthesia. Lab. Anim. Sci. 43, 328–335.

Aisaka, K., Mitani, A., Kitajima, Y., Ohno, T., Ishihara, T., 1991. Difference in pressor responses to NG-monomethyl-l-arginine between conscious and anesthetized rats. Jpn. J. Pharmacol. 56, 245–248.

Akwa, Y., Baulieu, E.E., 1999. Neurosteroids: behavioral aspects and physiological implications. J. Soc. Biol. 193, 293–298.

Albrecht, D., Davidowa, H., 1989. Action of urethane on dorsal lateral geniculate neurons. Brain Res. Bull. 22, 923–927.

Aldridge, W.N., Parker, V.H., 1960. Barbiturates and oxidative phosphorylation. Biochem. J. 76, 47–56.

Alfaro, V., Palacios, L., 1992. Differential effects of hypothermia upon blood acid–base state and blood gases in sodium pentobarbital and urethane anesthetized rats. Gen. Pharmacol. 23, 677–682.

Allweiler, S., Leach, M.C., Flecknell, P.A., 2010. The use of propofol and sevoflurane for surgical anaesthesia in New Zealand White rabbits. Lab. Anim. 44 (2), 113–117.

Altura, B.M., Altura, B.T., Carella, A., Turlapaty, P.D.M.V., Weinburg, J., 1980. Vascular smooth muscle and general anesthetics. Fed. Proc. 39, 1584–1591.

Alves, H.N.C., da Silva, A.L.M., Olsson, I.A.S., Orden, J.M.G., Antunes, L.M., 2010. Anesthesia with intraperitoneal propofol, medetomidine, and fentanyl in rats. J. Am. Assoc. Lab. Anim. Sci. 49 (4), 454–459.

Alves, H.C., Valentim, A.M., Olsson, I.A.S., Antunes, L.M., 2009. Intraperitoneal anaesthesia with propofol, medetomidine and fentanyl in mice. Lab. Anim. 43, 27–33.

Ambar, N., Eshar, D., Shrader, T.C., Beaufrere, H., 2020. Anesthetic effects of intramuscular alfaxalone-ketamine in naked mole rats (*Heterocephalus glaber*). J. Am. Assn. Lab. An. Sci. 59, 539–545.

Andaluz, A., Tusell, J., Trasserres, O., Cristofol, C., Capece, B.P.S.C., Arboix, M., Garcia, F., 2003. Transplacental transfer of propofol in pregnant ewes. Vet. J. 166, 198–204.

Andress, J.L., Day, T.K., Day, D., 1995. The effects of consecutive day propofol anesthesia on feline red blood cells. Vet. Surg. 24, 277–282.

Antognini, J.F., Barter, L., Carstens, E., 2005. Overview movement as an index of anesthetic depth in humans and experimental animals. Comp. Med. 55, 413–418.

Arenillas, M., Gomez de Segura, I.A., 2018. Anaesthetic effects of alfaxalone administered intraperitoneally alone or combined with dexmedetomidine and fentanyl in the rat. Lab. Anim. 52 (6), 588–598.

Arras, M., Autenried, P., Rettich, A., Spaeni, D., Rulicke, T., 2001. Optimization of intraperitoneal injection anesthesia in mice: drugs, dosages, adverse effects, and anesthesia depth. Comp. Med. 51, 443–456.

Atkinson, P.M., Taylor, D.I., Chetty, N., 1985. Inhibition of platelet aggregation by ketamine hydrochloride. Thromb. Res. 40, 227–234.

Avila, M.Y., Carre, D.A., Stone, R.A., Civan, M.M., 2001. Reliable measurement of mouse intraocular pressure by a servo-null micropipette system. Invest. Ophthalmol. Vis. Sci. 42, 1841–1846.

Aynsley-Green, A., Biebuyck, J.F., Alberti, K.G., 1973. Anaesthesia and insulin secretion: the effects of diethyl ether, halothane, pentobarbitone sodium and ketamine hydrochloride on intravenous glucose tolerance and insulin secretion in the rat. Diabetologia 9, 274–281.

Azadegan, A., Johnson, D.W., Stowe, C.M., 1980. Influence of time interval between administration of chloramphenicol and thiamylal on the sleeping time of mice. Am. J. Vet. Res. 41, 976–977.

Bailey, K.M., Minter, L.J., Lewbart, G.A., Harms, C.A., Griffith, E.H., Posner, L.P., 2014. Alfaxalone as an intramuscular injectable anesthetic in koi carp (*Cyprinus carpio*). J. Zoo Wildl. Med. 45 (4), 852–859.

Bailey, P.L., Egan, T.D., Stanley, T.H., 2000. Intravenous opioid anesthetics. In: Miller, R.D. (Ed.), Anesthesia, fifth ed. Churchill Livingstone, Philadelphia, PA, pp. 273–376.

Banaszczyk, M.G., Carlo, A.T., Millan, V., Lindsey, A., Moss, R., Carlo, D.J., Hendler, S.S., 2002. Propofol phosphate, a water-soluble propofol prodrug: in vivo evaluation. Anesth. Analg. 95, 1285–1292.

Barzago, M.M., Bortolotti, A., Omarini, D., Aramayona, J.J., Bonati, M., 1992. Monitoring of blood gas parameters and acid–base balance of pregnant and non-pregnant rabbits (*Oryctolagus cuniculus*) in routine experimental conditions. Lab. Anim. 26, 73–79.

Batjer, H.H., 1993. Cerebral protective effects of etomidate: experimental and clinical aspects. Cerebrovasc. Brain Metab. Rev. 5, 17–32.

Beam, D.M., Neto-Neves, E.M., Stubblefield, W.B., Alves, N.J., Tune, J.D., Kline, J.A., 2015. Comparison of isoflurane and α-chloralose in an anesthetized swine model of acute pulmonary embolism producing right ventricular dysfunction. Comp. Med. 65 (1), 54–61.

Bellman, M.H., Pleuvry, B.J., 1981. Comparison of the respiratory effects of ICI 35 868 and thiopentone in the rabbit. Br. J. Anaesth. 53, 425–429.

Bette, M., Schlimme, S., Mutters, R., Menendez, S., Hoffmann, S., Schulz, S., 2004. Influence of different anaesthetics on pro-inflammatory cytokine expression in rat spleen. Lab. Anim. 38, 272–279.

Beyers, T.M., Richardson, J.A., Prince, M.D., 1991. Axonal degeneration and self-mutilation as a complication of the intramuscular use of ketamine and xylazine in rabbits. Lab. Anim. Sci. 41, 519–520.

Blake, D.W., Blombery, P.A., Korner, P.I., 1982. Effect of ketamine, althesin, and thiopentone on the Valsalva constrictor and heart rate reflexes of the rabbit. J. Auton. Nerv. Syst. 5, 291–301.

Blake, D.W., Jover, B., McGrath, B.P., 1988. Haemodynamic and heart rate reflex responses to propofol in the rabbit. Br. J. Anaesth. 61, 194–199.

Bloom, F.E., 2006. Neurotransmission and the central nervous system. In: Brunton, L.L., Lazo, J.S., Parker, K.L. (Eds.), Goodman and Gilman's Pharmacological Basis of Therapeutics, eleventh ed. McGraw-Hill Medical Publishing Division, New York, pp. 330–331.

Bogdan, L.G., Glisson, S.N., El-Etr, A.A., 1974. The effect of ketamine upon depolarizing and non-depolarizing neuromuscular blockade in rabbit. Naunyn-Schmiederberg's Arch. Pharmacol. 285, 223–231.

Booth, N.H., 1988. Intravenous and other parenteral anesthetics. In: Booth, N.H., McDonald, L.E. (Eds.), Veterinary Pharmacology and Therapeutics, sixth ed. Iowa State University Press, Ames, IA, pp. 212–274.

Borkowski, G.L., Danneman, P.J., Russell, G.B., Lang, C.M., 1990. An evaluation of three intravenous anesthetic regimens in New Zealand rabbits. Lab. Anim. Sci. 40, 270–276.

Boscan, P., Steffey, E.P., Farver, T.B., Mama, K.R., Huang, N.J., Harris, S.B., 2006. Comparison of high (5%) and low (1%) concentrations of micellar microemulsion propofol formulations with a standard (1%) lipid emulsion in horses. Am. J. Vet. Res. 67, 1476–1483.

Bowery, N.G., Dray, A., 1978. Reversal of the action of amino acid antagonists by barbiturates and anesthetic drugs. Br. J. Phamacol. 63, 197–215.

Boyland, E., Rhoden, E., 1949. The distribution of urethane in animal tissues, as determined by a microdiffusion method, and the effect of urethane treatment on enzymes. Biochem. J. 44, 528–531.

Bradley, M.P., Doerning, C.M., Nowland, M.H., Lester, P.A., 2019. Intramuscular administration of alfaxalone alone and in combination for sedation and anesthesia of rabbits (*Oryctolagus cuniculus*). J. Am. Assoc. Lab. Anim. Sci. 58 (2), 216–222.

Brammer, D.W., Doerning, B.J., Chrisp, C.E., Rush, H.G., 1991. Anesthetic and nephrotoxic effects of Telazol®in New Zealand white rabbits. Lab. Anim. Sci. 41, 432–435.

Branson, K.R., 2001. Injectable anesthetics. In: Adams, H.R. (Ed.), Veterinary Pharmacology and Therapeutics, eighth ed. Iowa State Press, Ames, IA, pp. 213–267.

Branson, K.R., Booth, N.H., 1995. Injectable anesthetics. In: Adams, H.R. (Ed.), Veterinary Pharmacology and Therapeutics, seventh ed. Iowa State University Press, Ames, IA, pp. 179–208.

Braun, R.D., Dewhirst, M.W., Hatchell, D.L., 1997. Quantification of erythrocyte flow in the choroid of the albino rat. Am. J. Physiol. 272, H1444–H1453.

Bree, M.M., Cohen, B.J., 1965. Effects of urethane anesthesia on blood and blood vessels in rabbits. Lab. Anim. Care 15, 254–259.

Bronley-DeLancey, A., McMillan, D.C., McMillan, J.M., Jollow, D.J., Mohr, L.C., Hoel, D.G., 2006. Application of cryopreserved human hepatocytes in trichloroethylene risk assessment: relative disposition of chloral hydrate to trichloroacetate and trichloroethanol. Environ. Health Perspect. 114, 1237–1242.

Bryan, C.E., Skipper, H.E., White, L., 1949. Carbamates in the chemotherapy of leucemia. IV. The distribution of radioactivity in tissues of mice following injection of carbonyl-labeled urethane. J. Biol. Chem. 177, 941–950.

Bu, X., Li, T., Wang, H., Xia, Z., Guo, D., Wang, J., Sun, Y., Yang, C., Liu, G., Ma, J., Yang, Z., Wang, G., 2020. Combination of isoflurane and propofol as general anesthesia during orthopedic surgery of perioperative cerebral hypoperfusion rats to avoid cognitive impairment. Front. Med. 7. https://doi.org/10.3389/fmed.2020.549081.

Buchanan, K.C., Burge, R.R., Ruble, G.R., 1998. Evaluation of injectable anesthetics for major survival procedures in Guinea pigs. Contemp. Top. Lab. Anim. Sci. 37, 58–63.

Buelke-Sam, J., Holson, J.F., Bazare, J.J., Young, J.F., 1978. Comparative stability of physiological parameters during sustained anesthesia in rats. Lab. Anim. Sci. 28, 157–162.

Buetow, B.S., Chen, L.I., Maggio-Price, L., Swisshelm, K., 1999. Peritonitis in nude mice in a xenograft study. Contemp. Top. Lab. Anim. Sci. 38, 47–49.

Bugman, A.M., Langer, P.T., Hadzima, E., Rivas, A.E., Mitchell, M.A., 2016. Evaluation of the anesthetic efficacy of alfaxalone in oscar fish (*Astronotus ocellatus*). Am. J. Vet. Res. 77 (3), 239–244.

Bunting, P., Ramsay, T.M., Pleuvry, B.J., 1989. An in-vitro study of the interactions between intravenous induction agents and the calcium antagonists verapamil and nifedipine. J. Pharm. Pharmacol. 41, 840–843.

Cain, D.P., Raithby, A., Corcoran, M.E., 1989. Urethane anesthesia blocks the development and expression of kindled seizures. Life Sci. 44, 1201–1206.

Caldwell, J.C., Keshava, N., 2006. Key issues in the modes of action and effects of trichloroethylene metabolites for liver and kidney tumorigenesis. Environ. Health Perspect. 114, 1457–1463.

Carmichael, F.J., Crawford, M.W., Khayyam, N., Saldivia, V., 1993. Effect of propofol infusion on splanchnic hemodynamics and liver oxygen consumption in the rat. Anesthesiology 79, 1051–1060.

Carruba, M.O., Bondiolotti, G., Picotti, G.B., Catteruccia, N., Da Prada, M., 1987. Effects of diethyl ether, halothane, ketamine and urethane on sympathetic activity in the rat. Eur. J. Pharmacol. 134, 15–24.

Celesia, G.G., Chen, R.C., Bamforth, B.J., 1975. Effects of ketamine in epilepsy. Neurology 25, 169–172.

Chang, T., Glazko, A.J., 1974. Biotransformation and disposition of ketamine. Int. Anesthesiol. Clin. 12, 157–177.

Chaplin, M.D., Roszkowski, A.P., Richards, R.K., 1973. Displacement of thiopental from plasma proteins by nonsteroidal anti-inflammatory agents. Proc. Soc. Exp. Biol. Med. 143, 667–671.

Charney, D.S., Mihic, S.J., Harris, R.A., 2006. Hypnotics and sedatives. In: Brunton, L.L., Lazo, J.S., Parker, K.L. (Eds.), Goodman & Gillman's the Pharmacological Basis of Therapeutics, eleventh ed. The McGraw-Hill Companies, Inc, New York, pp. 4404–4405.

Chen, G., Ensor, C.R., Bohner, B., 1969. The pharmacology of 2-(ethylamino)-2-(2-thienyl)-cyclohexanone_HCl (CI-634). J. Pharmacol. Exp. Therapeut. 168, 171–179.

Chimoskey, J.E., Huntsman, L.L., Gams, E., Flanagan, W.J., 1975. Effect of ketamine on ventricular dynamics of unanesthetized baboons. Cardiovasc. Res. Cent. Bull. (Houston) 14, 53–57.

Christensen, J., Fosse, R.T., Halvorsen, O.J., Morild, I., 1987. Comparison of various anesthetic regimens in the domestic fowl. Am. J. Vet. Res. 48, 1649–1657.

Coetzee, A., Fourie, P., Coetzee, J., Badenhorst, E., Rebel, A., Bolliger, C., Uebel, R., Wium, C., Lombard, C., 1989. Effect of various propofol plasma concentrations on regional myocardial contractility and left ventricular afterload. Anesth. Analg. 69, 473–483.

Cohen, M.L., Chan, S.-L., Way, W.L., Trevor, A.J., 1973. Distribution in the brain and metabolism of ketamine in the rat after intravenous administration. Anesthesiology (Hagerst.) 39, 370–376.

Collado, P.S., Pozo-Andrada, M.J., González, J., Jiménez, R., Esteller, A., 1987. Effect of pentobarbital or urethane on bile secretion and chemical composition of blood in the rabbit. Lab. Anim. 21, 11–17.

Collins Jr., T.B., Lott, D.F., 1968. Stock and sex specificity in the response of rats to pentobarbital sodium. Lab. Anim. Care 18, 192–194.

Commissaris, R.L., Semsyn, D.R., Rech, R.H., 1982. Dispositional without functional tolerance to the hypothermic effects of pentobarbital in the rat. J. Pharmacol. Exp. Therapeut. 220, 536–539.

Conney, A.H., Davison, C., Gastel, R., Burns, J.J., 1960. Adaptive increases in drug-metabolizing enzymes induced by phenobarbital and other drugs. J. Pharmacol. Exp. Therapeut. 130, 1–8.

Court, M.H., Duan, S.X., Hesse, L.M., Venkatakrishnan, K., Greenblatt, D.J., 2001. Cytochrome P-450 2B6 is responsible for interindividual variability of propofol hydroxylation by human liver microsomes. Anesthesiology 94, 110–119.

Court, M.H., Hay-Kraus, B.L., Hill, D.W., Kind, A.J., Greenblatt, D.J., 1999. Propofol hydroxylation by dog liver microsomes: assay development and dog breed differences. Drug Metab. Dispos. 27, 1293–1299.

Covert, R.F., Drummond, W.H., Gimotty, P.A., 1988. Chloralose alters circulatory response to a-receptor stimulation and blockade. Am. J. Physiol. 255, H419–H425.

Crawford, K., Gabelt, B.T., Kaufman, P.L., Bito, L.Z., 1990. Effects of various anesthetic and autonomic drugs on refraction in monkeys. Curr. Eye Res. 9, 525–532.

Cunliffe-Beamer, T.L., Freeman, L.C., Myers, D.D., 1981. Barbiturate sleeptime in mice exposed to autoclaved or unautoclaved wood beddings. Lab. Anim. Sci. 31, 672–675.

Cupples, W.A., Veress, A.T., Sonnenberg, H., 1982. Lack of effect of barbiturate and ketamine anesthesia on renal blood flow in chronically instrumented rats prepared for micropuncture. Can. J. Physiol. Pharmacol. 60, 204–205.

Dada, M.O., Campbell, G.T., Horacek, M.J., Blake, C.A., 1992. Intraperitoneal injection of chloral hydrate causes intra-abdominal adhesions and unilateral testicular atrophy in golden Syrian hamsters. Life Sci. 51, 29–35.

da Motta, P.G., Veiga, A.P., Francischi, J.N., Tatsuo, M.A., 2004. Evidence for participation of GABA(A) receptors in a rat model of secondary hyperalgesia. Eur. J. Pharmacol. 483, 233–239.

Davis, K., Griffin, B., 2003. Physiological responses of hybrid striped bass under sedation. Aquaculture 233, 531–548.

Daniel, F.B., DeAngelo, A.B., Stober, J.A., Olson, G.R., Page, N.P., 1992. Hepatocarcinogenicity of chloral hydrate, 2-chloroacetaldehyde, and dichloracetic acid in the male B6C3F1 mouse1. Fund. Appl. Toxicol. 19, 159–168.

Davis, C.A., Seddighi, R., Cox, S.K., Sun, X., Egger, C.M., Doherty, T.J., 2017. Effect of fentanyl on the induction dose and minimum infusion rate of propofol preventing movement in dogs. Vet. Anaesth. Analg. 44 (4), 727–737.

Davis, L.E., Davis, C.H., Baggot, J.D., 1973. Comparative pharmacokinetics in domesticated animals. In: Harmison, L.T. (Ed.), Research Animals in Medicine. U.S. Department of Health, Education, and Welfare, Bethesda MD, pp. 715–733. DHEW Publication No. (NIH) 72-333.

Dehuisser, V., Bosmans, T., Devreese, M., Gehring, R., Croubels, S., Duchateau, L., et al., 2019. Alfaxalone total intravenous anaesthesia in dogs: pharmacokinetics, cardiovascular data and recovery characteristics. Vet. Anaesth. Analg. 46 (5), 605–612.

De Paepe, P., Belpaire, F.M., Van Hoey, G., Boon, P.A., Buylaert, W.A., 1999. Influence of hypovolemia on the pharmacokinetics and the electroencephalographic effect of etomidate in the rat. J. Pharmacol. Exp. Therapeut. 290, 1048–1053.

De Wildt, D.J., Hillen, F.C., Rauws, A.G., Sangster, B., 1983. Etomidate-anaesthesia, with and without fentanyl, compared with urethane-anaesthesia in the rat. Br. J. Pharmacol. 79, 461–469.

Dewhirst, M.W., Ong, E., Rosner, G., Rehmus, S., Shan, S., Braun, R., Brizel, D., Secomb, T., 1996. Arteriolar oxygenation in tumor and subcutaneous arterioles: effects of inspired air oxygen content. Br. J. Cancer 74, S247–S251.

Dhasmana, K.M., Saxena, P.R., Prakash, O., Van Der Zee, H.T., 1984. A study on the influence of ketamine on systemic and regional haemodynamics in conscious rabbits. Arch. Int. Pharmacodyn. 269, 323–334.

Diba, A., 2005. Infusion equipment and intravenous anesthesia. In: Davy, A.J., Diba, A. (Eds.), Ward's Anaesthetic Equipment, fifth ed. Elsevier Saunders, Philadelphia, PA, pp. 409–426.

DiFilippo, S.M., Norberg, P.J., Suson, U.D., Savino, A.M., Reim, D.A., 2004. A comparison of xylazine and medetomidine in an anesthetic combination in New Zealand White rabbits. Contemp. Top. Lab. Anim. Sci. 43, 32–34.

Dittmar, M.S., Fehm, N.P., Vatankhah, B., Horn, M., 2004. Ketamine/xylazine anesthesia for radiologic imaging of neurologically impaired rats: dose response, respiratory depression, and management of complications. Comp. Med. 54, 652–655.

Dodam, J.R., Kruse-Elliott, K.T., Aucoin, D.P., Swanson, C.R., 1990. Duration of etomidate-induced adrenocortical suppression during surgery in dogs. Am. J. Vet. Res. 51, 786–788.

Doenicke, A., Roizen, M.F., Hoernecke, R., Mayer, M., Ostwald, P., Foss, J., 1997. Haemolysis after etomidate: comparison of propylene glycol and lipid formulations. Br. J. Anaesth. 79, 386–388.

Doerning, B.J., Brammer, D.W., Chrisp, C.E., Rush, H.G., 1992. Nephrotoxicity of tiletamine in New Zealand white rabbits. Lab. Anim. Sci. 42, 267–269.

Doerning, C.M., Bradley, M.P., Lester, P.A., Nowland, M.H., 2018. Effects of subcutaneous alfaxalone alone and in combination with dexmedetomidine and buprenorphine in Guinea pigs (*Cavia porcellus*). Vet. Anaesth. Analg. 45, 658–666.

Dos Santos, M., Bogan, J.A., 1974. The metabolism of pentobarbitone in sheep. Res. Vet. Sci. 17, 226–230.

D'Ovidio, D., Marino, F., Noviello, E., Lanaro, E., Monticelli, P., Adami, C., 2018. Sedative effects of intramuscular alfaxalone in pet Guinea pigs (*Cavia porcellus*). Vet. Anaesth. Analg. 45, 183–189.

Erhardt, W., Hebestedt, A., Aschenbrenner, G., Pichotka, B., Blümel, G., 1984. A comparative study with various anesthetics in mice (pentobarbitone, ketamine–xylazine, carfentanyl–etomidate). Res. Exp. Med. 184, 159–169.

Erickson, R.L., Blevins, C.E., Dyer, C.D., Marx, J.O., 2019. Alfaxalone-xylazine anesthesia in laboratory mice (*Mus musculus*). J. Am. Assn. Lab. Anim. Sci. 58, 30–39.

Erickson, R.L., Terzi, M.C., Jaber, S.M., Handenson, F.C., McKinstry-Wu, A., Kelz, M.B., Marx, J.O., 2016. Intraperitoneal continuous-rate infusion for the maintenance of anesthesia in laboratory mice (*Mus musculus*). J. Am. Assoc. Lab. Anim. Sci. 55 (5), 548–557.

Eshar, D., Beaufrere, H., 2020. Anesthetic effects of alfaxalone-ketamine, alfaxalone-ketamine-dexmedetomidine, and alfaxalone-butorphanol-midazolam administered intramuscularly in five-striped palm squirrels (Funambulus pennantii). J. Am. Assn. Lab. Anim. Sci. 59, 384–392.

Farry, T., Lau, C., Keates, H., McEwen, M., Woldeyohannes, S., Barnes, T., et al., 2019. Comparison of two formulations of alfaxalone in laboratory zebra fish (*Danio rerio*) for use in immersion anaesthesia. Vet. Anaesth. Analg. 46 (6), 831.e5–831.e6.

Ferrer-Allado, T., Brechner, V.L., Dymond, A., Cozen, H., Crandall, P., 1973. Ketamine-induced electroconvulsive phenomena in the human limbic and thalamic regions. Anesthesiology 38, 333–344.

Field, K.J., Lang, C.M., 1988. Hazards of urethane (ethyl carbamate): a review of the literature. Lab. Anim. 22, 255–262.

Field, K.J., White, W.J., Lang, C.M., 1993. Anaesthetic effects of chloral hydrate, pentobarbitone and urethane in adult male rats. Lab. Anim. 27, 258–269.

Fish, R.E., 1997. In: Kohn, D.F., Wixson, S.K., White, W.J., Benson, G.J. (Eds.), Anesthesia and Analgesia in Laboratory Animals, 1–28. Academic Press, San Diego, CA.

Flecknell, P., 1996. Laboratory Animal Anaesthesia, second ed. Academic Press, San Diego, CA.

Flecknell, P.A., 1987. Laboratory Animal Anaesthesia. Academic Press, San Diego, CA.

Flecknell, P.A., John, M., Mitchell, M., Shurey, C., Simpkin, S., 1983. Neuroleptanalgesia in the rabbit. Lab. Anim. 17, 104–109.

Fleischman, R.W., McCracken, D., Forbes, W., 1977. Adynamic ileus in the rat induced by chloral hydrate. Lab. Anim. Sci. 27, 238–243.

Fluckiger, J.-P., Sonnay, M., Boillat, N., Atkinson, J., 1985. Attenuation of the baroreceptor reflex by general anesthetic agents in the normotensive rat. Eur. J. Pharmacol. 109, 105–109.

Folle, L.E., Levesque, R.I., 1976. Circulatory, respiratory and acid–base balance changes produced by anesthetics in the rat. Acta Biol. Med. Ger. 35, 605–612.

Forman, S.A., Warner, D.S., 2011. Clinical and molecular pharmacology of etomidate. Anesthesiology 114 (3), 695–707.

Fox, L., Snyder, L.B.C., Mans, C., 2016. Comparison of dexmedetomidine-ketamine with isoflurane for anesthesia of chinchillas (*Chinchilla lanigera*). J. Am. Assoc. Lab. Anim. Sci. 55 (3), 312–316.

Freudenthal, R.I., Carroll, F.I., 1973. Metabolism of certain commonly used barbiturates. Drug Metab. Rev. 2, 265–278.

Friedman, J.J., 1959. Effect of Nembutal on circulating and tissue blood volumes and hematocrits of intact and splenectomized mice. Am. J. Physiol. 197, 399–402.

Frolich, M.A., Price, D.D., Robinson, M.E., Shuster, J.J., Theriaque, D.W., Heft, M.W., 2005. The effect of propofol onthermal pain perception. Anesth. Analg. 100, 481–486.

Furuyama, F., Ishida, Y., Furuyama, M., Hashitani, T., Isobe, Y., Sato, H., Ohara, K., Nishino, H., 1989. Thermal salivation in rats anesthetized with barbiturates, chloralose, urethane and ketamine. Comp. Biochem. Physiol. 94C, 133–138.

Gaertner, D.J., Boschert, K.R., Schoeb, T.R., 1987. Muscle necrosis in Syrian hamsters resulting from intramuscular injections of ketamine and xylazine. Lab. Anim. Sci. 37, 80–83.

Ganayem, B.I., 2007. Inhibition of urethane-induced carcinogenicity in *Cyp2e1-/-* in comparison to *Cyp2e1+/+* mice. Toxicol. Sci. 95, 331–339.

Gardner, D.J., Davis, J.A., Weina, P.J., Theune, B., 1995. Comparison of tribromoethanol, ketamine/acetylpromazine, Telazol/xylazine, pentobarbital, and methoxyflurane anesthesia in HSD:ICR mice. Lab. Anim. Sci. 45, 199–204.

Garmer, N.L., 1969. Effects of 2-ethylamino-2-(2-thienyl) cyclohexanone HCl (Cl-634) in cats. Res. Vet. Sci. 10, 382–388.

Garrett, K., Gan, J., 1998. Enhancement of gamma-aminobutyric acid-A receptor activity by alpha-chloralose. J. Pharmacol. Exp. Therapeut. 285, 680–686.

Gaumann, D.M., Yaksh, T.L., 1990. Alpha-chloralose anesthesia inhibits the somato-sympathetic reflex response in cats more effectively than halothane. J. Vet. Med. 37, 669–675.

Gerb, S.A., Cooke, J.E., Gochenauer, A.E., Young, C.S., Fulton, L.K., Grady, A.W., Freeman, K.B., 2019. Ketamine tolerance in Sprague-Dawley rats after chronic administration of ketamine, morphine, or cocaine. J. *Am. Assn. Lab. Anim. Sci.* 69, 29–34.

Gin, T., Yau, G., Jong, W., Tan, P., Leung, R.K., Chan, K., 1991. Disposition of propofol at caesarean section and in the postpartum period. Br. J. Anaesth. 67, 49–53.

Giroux, M.C., Helie, P., Burns, P., Vachon, P., 2015. Anesthetic and pathological changes following high doses of ketamine and xylazine in Sprague Dawley rats. Exp. Anim. 64 (3), 253–260.

Glen, J.B., 1980. Animal studies of the anaesthetic activity of ICI 35 868. Br. J. Anaesth. 52, 731–742.

Glen, J.B., Hunter, S.C., 1984. Pharmacology of an emulsion formulation of ICI 35 868. Br. J. Anaesth. 56, 617–625.

Goelz, M.F., 1994. Anesthetic and pathologic effects of tribromoethanol in mice. In: Toxicology Bibliographic Information (Toxline). Document Number CRISP/95/S22112-02. http://toxnet.nlm.nih.gov.

Green, C.J., 1979. Animal Anaesthesia: Laboratory Animal Handbooks 8. Laboratory Animals Ltd., London.

Green, C.J., Knight, J., Precious, S., Simpkin, S., 1981. Metomidate, etomidate and fentanyl as injectable anaesthetic agents in mice. Lab. Anim. 15, 171–175.

Gumbleton, M., 1989. Anaesthetic influences on brain haemodynamics in the rat and their significance to biochemical, neuropharmacological and drug disposition studies. Biochem. Pharmacol. 38, 2745–2748.

Gumbleton, M., Benet, L.Z., 1991. Drug metabolism and laboratory anesthetic protocols in the rat: examination of antipyrine pharmacokinetics. Pharm. Res. (N. Y.) 8, 544–546.

Gumbleton, M., Nicholls, P.J., Taylor, G., 1988. The renin-angiotensin system and intraperitoneal toxicity: possible basis to urethane anaesthesia-induced reductions in renal clearance in the rat. Arch. Int. Pharmacodyn. 294, 7–32.

Gumbleton, M., Nicholls, P.J., Taylor, G., 1990a. Differential influence of laboratory anaesthetic regimens upon renal and hepatosplanchnic haemodynamics in the rat. J. Pharm. Pharmacol. 42, 693–697.

Gumbleton, M., Nicholls, P.J., Taylor, G., 1990b. Differential effects of anesthetic regimens on gentamicin pharmacokinetics in the rat: a comparison with chronically catheterized conscious animals. Pharm. Res. (N. Y.) 7, 41–45.

Haberle, D.A., Davis, J.M., Kawabata, M., Metz, C., Wapler, P., Stachl, M., 1993. Renal and single-nephron function is comparable in thiobutabarbitone- and thiopentone-anaesthetised rats. Pflügers Archiv 424 (3–4), 224–230.

Hall, C.E., Ayachi, S., Hall, O., 1976. Differential sensitivity of spontaneously hypertensive (SHR) and control rats to various anaesthetic agents. Clin. Exp. Pharmacol. Physiol. 3, 83–86.

Hall, L.W., Clarke, K.W., Trim, C.M., 2001. General pharmacology of the injectable agents in anaesthesia. In: Veterinary Anesthesia, tenth ed. W. B Saunders, London, pp. 75–91. 113–132.

Hall, R., Murdoch, J., 1990. Brain protection: physiological and pharmacological considerations. Part II: the pharmacology of brain protection. Can. J. Anaesth. 37, 762–777.

Hamstra, W.N., Doray, D., Dunn, J.D., 1984. The effect of urethane on pituitary-adrenal function of female rats. Acta Endocrinol. 106, 362–367.

Hansen, M.K., Nymoen, U., Horsberg, T.E., 2003. Pharmacokinetic and pharmacodynamic properties of metomidate in turbot (*Scophthalmus max-imus*) and halibut (*Hippoglossus hippoglossus*). J. Vet. Pharmacol. Therapeut. 26, 95–103.

Hara, K., Harris, R.A., 2002. The anesthetic mechanism of urethane: the effects on neurotransmitter-gated ion channels. Anesth. Analg. 94, 313–318.

Hardman, J.G., Limbird, L.E., Molinoff, P.B., Ruddon, R.W., Gilman, A.G. (Eds.), 1996. Goodman and Gilmans' the Pharmacological Basis of Therapeutics, ninth ed. McGraw-Hill, New York.

Hart, C.Y., Burnett Jr., J.C., Redfield, M.M., 2001. Effects of avertin versus xylazine–ketamine anesthesia on cardiac function in normal mice. Am. J. Physiol. Heart Circ. Physiol. 281, H1938–H1945.

Haskins, S.C., 1992. Injectable anesthetics. Vet. Clin. North Am. Small Anim. Pract. 22, 245–260.

Hatch, R.C., 1973. Experiments on antagonism of barbiturate anesthesia with adrenergic, serotonergic, and cholinergic stimulants given alone and in combination. Am. J. Vet. Res. 34, 1321–1331.

Hatch, R.C., Kitzman, J.V., Zahner, J.M., Clark, J.D., 1984. Comparison of five preanesthetic medicaments in thiopental-anesthetized cats: antagonism by selected compounds. Am. J. Vet. Res. 45, 2322–2327.

Heavner, J.E., 1986. Anesthesia, analgesia, and restraint. In: Gay, W.I., Heavner, J.E. (Eds.), Methods of Animal Experimentation, vol. VII. Academic Press, Orlando, FL, pp. 1–35.

Hedenqvist, P., Hellebrekers, L.J., 2003. Laboratory animal analgesia, anesthesia, and euthanasia. In: Hau, J., Van Hoosier Jr., G.L. (Eds.), Handbook of Laboratory Animal Science, Vol. 1: Essential Principles and Practices. CRS Press, FL, pp. 413–455.

Heng, K., Marx, J.O., Jampachairsi, K., Huss, M.K., Pacharinsak, C., 2020. Continuous rate infusion of alfaxalone during ketmaine-xylazine anesthesia in rats. J. Am. Assn. Lab. Anim. Sci. 59, 170–175.

Hernandez, D.E., Meyer, R.E., Irving, P.E., Crane, S.W., 1987. Reversal of pentobarbital-induced narcosis by thyrotropin-releasing hormone (TRH) in dogs. Pharmacol. Res. Commun. 19, 567–577.

Heykants, J.J.P., Meuldermans, W.E.G., Michiels, L.J.M., Lewi, P.J., 1975. Distribution, metabolism and excretion of etomidate, a short-acting hypnotic drug, in the rat. Comparative study of (*R*)-(+) and (*S*)-(-)-etomidate. Arch. Int. Pharmacodyn. 216, 113–129.

Heys, S.D., Norton, A.C., Dundas, C.R., Eremin, O., Ferguson, K., Garlick, P.J., 1989. Anaesthetic agents and their effect on tissue protein synthesis in the rat. Clin. Sci. 77, 651–655.

Higashi, Y., Notoji, N., Yamajo, R., Yata, N., 1982. Effect of anesthesia on drug disposition in the rat. J. Pharm. Dyn. 5, 112–119.

Higuchi, S., Yamada, R., Hashimoto, A., Miyoshi, K., Yamashita, K., Ohsugi, T., 2016. Evaluation of a combination of alfaxalone with medetomidine and butorphanol for inducing surgical anesthesia in laboratory mice. Jpn. J. Vet. Res. 64 (2), 131–139.

Hill, J.V., Forster, M.E., 2004. Cardiovascular responses of Chinook salmon (*Oncorhynchus tshawytscha*) during rapid anaesthetic induction and recovery. Comp. Biochem. Physiol. C Toxicol. Pharmacol. 137, 167–177.

Hill, W.A., Tubbs, J.T., Carter, C.L., Czarra, J.A., Newkird, K.M., Sparer, T.E., Rohrbach, B., Egger, C.M., 2013. Repeated administration of tribromoethanol in C57BL/6NHsd mice. J. Am. Assn. Lab. Anim. Sci. 52, 176–179.

Hillebrand, A., Meer, C., Ariens, A.T., Wijnans, M., 1971. The effect of anesthetics on the occurrence of kidney lesions caused by hypotension. Eur. J. Pharmacol. 14, 217–237.

Himmelseher, S., Durieux, M.E., 2005. Revising a dogma: ketamine for patients with neurological injury? Anesth. Analg. 101, 524–534.

Hinton, B.T., 1982. Hyperglycemia in urethane-anesthetized rats: involvement of the adrenal gland. Lab. Anim. Sci. 32, 251–252.

Hirshman, C.A., Downes, H., Farbood, A., Bergman, N.A., 1979. Ketamine block of bronchospasm in experimental canine asthma. Br. J. Anaesth. 51, 713–718.

Hirshman, C.A., McCullough, R.E., Cohen, P.J., Weil, J.V., 1975. Hypoxic ventilatory drive in dogs during thiopental, ketamine, or pentobarbital anesthesia. Anesthesiology (Hagerst.) 43, 628–634.

Hobbs, B.A., Rolhall, T.G., Sprenkel, T.L., Anthony, K.L., 1991. Comparison of several combinations for anesthesia in rabbits. Am. J. Vet. Res. 52, 669–674.

Hoffler, U., El-Masri, H.A., Ghanayem, B.I., 2003. Cytochrome P450 2E1 (CYP2E1) is the principal enzyme responsible for urethane metabolism: comparative studies using CYP2E1-null and wild-type mice. J. Pharmacol. Exp. Therapeut. 305, 557–564.

Hogan, B., Costantini, F., Lacy, E., 1986. Manipulating the Mouse Embryo A Laboratory Manual. Cold Spring Harbor Laboratory, New York, 132, 137, 143, 271.

Holck, H.G.O., Kanân, M.A., Mills, L.M., Smith, E.L., 1937. Studies upon the sex-difference in rats in tolerance to certain barbiturates and to nicotine. J. Pharmacol. Exp. Therapeut. 60, 323–346.

Holzgrefe, H.H., Everitt, J.M., Wright, E.M., 1987. Alpha-chloralose as a canine anesthetic. Lab. Anim. Sci. 37, 587–595.

Hosoi, E., Saito, H., Yamasaki, R., Kimura, S., Saito, S., 1988. Influence of anesthetic agents on the release of growth hormone induced by growth hormone-releasing hormone in rats. Tokushima J. Exp. Med. 35, 85–90.

Hrapkiewicz, K.L., Stein, S., Smiler, K.L., 1989. A new anesthetic agent for use in the gerbil. Lab. Anim. Sci. 9, 338–341.

Hsu, W.H., Hembrough, F.B., 1982. Intravenous glucose tolerance test in cats: influenced by acetylpromazine, ketamine, morphine, thiopental, and xylazine. Am. J. Vet. Res. 43, 2060–2061.

Huang, L.Y., Barker, J.L., 1980. Pentobarbital: stereospecific actions of (+) and (-) isomers revealed on cultured mammalian neurons. Science 207, 195–197.

Huang, Q., Riviere, J.E., 2014. The application of allometric scaling principles to predict pharmacokinetic parameters across species. Expert Opin. Drug Metabol. Toxicol. 10 (9), 1241–1253.

Hughes, M.A., Glass, P.S., Jacobs, J.R., 1992. Context-sensitive half-time in multicompartment pharmacokinetic models for intravenous anesthetic drugs. Anesthesiology 76, 334–341.

Hunter, W.S., Holmes, K.R., Elizondo, R.S., 1981. Thermal balance in ketamine-anesthetized rhesus monkey *Macaca mulatta*. Am. J. Physiol. 241, R301–R306.

Huynh, M., Poumeyrol, S., Pignon, C., Le Teuff, G., Zilberstein, L., 2015. Intramuscular administration of alfaxalone for sedation in rabbits. Vet. Rec. 176 (10), 255–255.

Idvall, J., Aronsen, K.F., Stenberg, P., 1980. Tissue perfusion and distribution of cardiac output during ketamine anesthesia in normovolemic rats. Acta Anaesthesiol. Scand. 24, 257–263.

Ikbal, M., Tastekin, A., Dogan, H., Pirim, I., Ors, R., 2004. The assessment of genotoxic effects in lymphocyte cultures of infants treated with chloral hydrate. Mutat. Res. Genet. Toxicol. Environ. Mutagen. 564, 159–164.

Ilkiw, J.E., 1992. Advantages and guidelines for using ultrashort barbiturates for induction of anesthesia. Vet. Clin. North Am. Small Anim. Pract. 22, 261–265.

Ilkiw, J.E., Benthuysen, J.A., Ebling, W.F., McNeal, D., 1991. A comparative study of the pharmacokinetics of thiopental in the rabbit, sheep and dog. J. Vet. Pharmacol. Therapeut. 14, 134–140.

Ilkiw, J.E., Pascoe, P.J., 2003. Cardiovascular effects of propofol alone and in combination with ketamine for total intravenous anesthesia in cats. Am. J. Vet. Res. 64, 913–917.

Ilkiw, J.E., Pascoe, P.J., Haskins, S.C., Patz, J.D., 1992. Cardiovascular and respiratory effects of propofol administration in hypovolemic dogs. Am. J. Vet. Res. 12, 2323–2327.

Im, W.B., Blakeman, D.P., Davis, J.P., Ayer, D.E., 1990. Studies on the mechanism of interactions between anesthetic steroids and g-aminobutyric acidA receptors. Mol. Pharmacol. 37, 429–434.

Inai, K., Arihiro, K., Takeshima, Y., Yonehara, S., Tachiyama, Y., Khatun, N., Nishisaka, T., 1991. Quantitative risk assessment of carcinogenicity of urethane (ethyl carbamate) on the basis of long-term oral administration to B6C3F1 mice. Jpn. J. Cancer Res. 82, 380–385.

Ishikawa, N., Kallman, C.H., Sagawa, K., 1984. Rabbit carotid sinus reflex under pentobarbital, urethan, and chloralose anesthesia. Am. J. Physiol. 246, H696–H701.

Ishimaru, H., Takahashi, A., Ikarashi, Y., Maruyama, Y., 1995. Pentobarbital protects against CA1 pyramidal cell death but not dysfunction of hippocampal cholinergic neurons following transient ischemia. Brain Res. 673, 112–118.

Iversen, O.H., 1991. Urethan (ethyl carbamate) is an effective promoter of 7, 12-dimethylbenz[a]anthracene-induced carcinogenesis in mouse skin two-stage experiments. Carcinogenesis 12, 901–903.

Izer, J.M., Whitcomb, T.L., Wilson, R.P., 2014. Atipamezole reverses ketamine-dexmedetomidine anesthesia without altering the antinociceptive effects of butorphanol and buprenorphine in female C57BL/6J mice. J. Am. Assn. Lab. Anim. Sci. 53, 675–683.

Jaber, S.M., Hankenson, F.C., Heng, K., McKinstry-Wu, A., Kelz, M.B., Marx, J.O., 2014. Dose regimens, variability, and complications associated with using repeat-bolus dosing to extend a surgical plane of anesthesia in laboratory mice. J. Am. Assn. Lab. Anim. Sci. 53, 684–691.

Jackson Jr., W.L., 2005. Should we use etomidate as an induction agent for endotracheal intubation in patients with septic shock?: a critical appraisal. Chest 127 (3), 1031–1038.

Jackson, K.L., Dhaibar, H.A., Dayton, R.D., Cananzi, S.G., Mayhan, W.G., Glasscock, E., Klein, R.L., 2016. Severe respiratory changes at end stage in a FUS-induced disease state in adult rats. BMC Neurosci. 17, 69.

Janssen, B.J., DeCelle, T., Debets, J.J., Brouns, A.E., Callahan, M.F., Smith, T.L., 2004. Effects of anesthetics on systemic hemodynamics in mice. Am. J. Physiol. Heart Circ. Physiol. 287, H1618–H1624. Epub May 20.

Janssen, C.F., Maiello, P., Wright Jr., M.J., Kracinovsky, K.B., Newsome, J.T., 2017. Comparison of atipamezole with yohimbine for antagonism of xylazine in mice anesthetized with ketamine and xylazine. J. *Am. Assn. Lab. Anim. Sci.* 56, 142–147.

Jewett, B.A., Gibbs, L.M., Tarasiuk, A., Kendig, J.J., 1992. Propofol and barbiturate depression of spinal nociceptive neurotransmission. Anesthesiology 77, 1148–1154.

Johnson, K.B., Egan, T.D., Layman, J., Kern, S.E., White, J.L., McJames, S.W., 2003. The influence of hemorrhagic shock on etomidate: a pharmacokinetic and pharmacodynamic analysis. Anesth. Analg. 96, 1360–1368.

Johnson, R., Fowler, J.F., Zanelli, G.D., 1976. Changes in mouse blood pressure, tumor blood flow, and core and tumor temperatures following Nembutal or urethane anesthesia. Radiology 118, 697–703.

Jondorff, W.R., Maickel, R.P., Brodie, B.B., 1958. Inability of newborn mice and Guinea pigs to metabolize drugs. Biochem. Pharmacol. 1, 352–354.

Kawai, N., Keep, R.F., Betz, A.L., 1997. Hyperglycemia and the vascular effects of cerebral ischemia. Stroke 28, 149–154.

Kawaue, Y., Iriuchijima, J., 1984. Changes in cardiac output and peripheral flows on pentobarbital anesthesia in the rat. Jpn. J. Physiol. 34, 283–294.

Kazerani, H.R., Furman, B.L., 2006. Comparison of urethane/chloralose and pentobarbitone anaesthesia for examining effects of bacterial lipopolysaccharide in mice. Fundam. Clin. Pharmacol. 20, 379–384.

Kelland, M.D., Chiodo, L.A., Freeman, A.S., 1990. Anesthetic influences on the basal activity and pharmacological responsiveness of nigrostriatal dopamine neurons. Synapse 6, 207–209.

Kintz, K., Jamey, C., andMangin, P., 1996. Trichloroethanol is not a metabolite of alpha chloralose. Int. J. Leg. Med. 108, 191–193.

Klaassen, C.D., 1971. Biliary excretion of barbiturates. Br. J. Pharmacol. 43, 161–166.

Knotek, Z., 2017. Induction to inhalation anaesthesia in agamid lizards with alfaxalone. Vet. Med. 62 (1), 41–43.

Ko, J.C.H., Thurmon, J.C., Tranquilli, W.J., Benson, G.J., Olson, W.A., 1992. A comparison of medetomidine—propofol and medetomidine—midazolam—propofol anesthesia in rabbits. Lab. Anim. Sci. 42, 503–507.

Ko, J.C., Williams, B.L., Rogers, E.R., Pablo, L.S., McCaine, W.C., McGrath, C.J., 1995. Increasing xylazine dose-enhanced anesthetic properties of telazol–xylazine combination in swine. Lab. Anim. Sci. 45, 290–294.

Kochhar, M.M., Aykac, I., Davidson, P.P., Fraley, E.D., 1986. Teratologic effects of d, 1-2-(*o*-chlorophenyl)-2-(methylamino) cyclohexanone hydrochloride (ketamine hydrochloride) in rats. Res. Commun. Chem. Pathol. Pharmacol. 54, 413–416.

Kohro, S., Hogan, Q.H., Nakae, Y., Yamakage, M., Bosnjak, Z.J., 2001. Anesthetic effectsonmitochondrialATP-sensitive K channel. Anesthesiology 95, 1435–1440.

Kohrs, R., Durieux, M.E., 1998. Ketamine: teaching an old drug new tricks. Anesth. Analg. 87, 1186–1193.

Koizumi, T., Maeda, H., Hioki, K., 2002. Sleep-time variation for ethanol and the hypnotic drugs tribromoethanol, urethane, pentobarbital, and propofol within outbred ICR mice. Exp. Anim. 51, 119–124.

Krasowski, M.D., Harrison, N.L., 2000. The actions of ether, alcohol and alkane general anaesthetics on GABA-A and glycine receptors and the effects of TM2 and TM3 mutations. Br. J. Pharmacol. 129, 731–743.

Kumar, A., Mann, H.J., Remmel, R.P., 2006. Pharmacokinetics of tiletamine and zolazepam (Telazol) in anesthetized pigs. J. Vet. Pharmacol. Therapeut. 29, 587–589.

Kumar, R., Kumar, A., 1984. Ketamine with and without premedication in rats and rabbits. Indian Vet. J. 61, 372–376.

Kurata, N., Hurst, H.E., Benz, F.W., Kemper, R.A., Waddell, W.J., 1991. Studies on inhibition and induction of metabolism of ethyl carbamate by acetone and related compounds. Drug Metab. Dispos. 19, 388–393.

Larsson, J.E., Koskinen, L.O., Wahlstrom, G., 1996. Effects of TRH and atropine on induction and duration of anesthesia with propofol in rats. Peptides 17, 293–297.

Larsson, J.E., Wahlstrom, G., 1998. The influence of age and administration rate on the brain sensitivity to propofol in rats. Acta Anaesthesiol. Scand. 42, 987–994.

Lash, L.H., Fisher, J.W., Lipscomb, J.C., Parker, J.C., 2000. Metabolism of trichloroethylene. Environ. Health Perspect. 108, 177–200.

Latt, R.H., Ecobichon, D.J., 1984. Self-mutilation in Guinea pigs following the intramuscular injection of ketamine acepromazine. Lab. Anim. Sci. 34, 516.

Lau, C., Ranasinghe, M.G., Shiels, I., Keates, H., Pasloske, K., Bellingham, M.C., 2013. Plasma pharmacokinetics of alfaxalone after a single intraperitoneal or intravenous injection of Alfaxan in rats. J. Vet. Pharmacol. Therapeut. 36 (5), 516–520.

Laubie, M., Schmitt, H., Canella, J., Roquebert, J., Demichel, P., 1974. Centrally mediated bradycardia and hypotension induced by narcotic analgesics: dextromoramide and fentanyl. Eur. J. Pharmacol. 28, 66–75.

Laurent, Y., Wallemacq, P., Haufroid, V., Renkin, J., Liolios, A., Hantson, P., 2006. Electrocardiographic changes with segmental akinesia after chloral hydrate overdose. J. Emerg. Med. 30, 179–182.

Leary, S., Underwood, W., Anthony, R., Cartner, S., Corey, D., Grandin, T., Greenacre, C.B., Gwaltney-Bran, S., McCrackin, M.A., Meyer, R., Miller, D., Shearer, J., Yanong, R., 2020. AVMA Guidelines for the Euthanasia of Animals [Cited 2 September 2021]. Available at: https://www.avma.org/sites/default/files/2020-01/2020-Euthanasia-Final-1-17-20.pdf.

Lee, C., Jones, T.A., 2018. Effects of ketamine compared with urethane anesthesia on vestibular sensory evoked potentials and systemic physiology in mice. J. Am. Assoc. Lab. Anim. Sci. 57 (3), 268–277.

Lee, S.S., Girod, C., Valla, D., Geoffroy, P., Lebrec, D., 1985. Effects of pentobarbital sodium anesthesia on splanchnic hemodynamics of normal and portal-hypertensive rats. Am. J. Physiol. 249, G528–G532.

Lee, V.C., Moscicki, J.C., DiFazio, C.A., 1998. Propofol sedation produces dose-dependent suppression of lidocaine-induced seizures in rats. Anesth. Analg. 86, 652–657.

Lee, V.K., Flynt, K.S., Haag, L.M., Taylor, D.K., 2010. Comparison of the effects of ketamine, ketamine-medetomidine, and ketamine-midazolam on physiologic parameters and anesthesia-induced stress in rhesus (*Macaca mulatta*) and cynomolgus (*Macaca fascicularis*) macaques. J. Am. Assoc. Lab. Anim. Sci. 49 (1), 57–63.

Lei, H., Grinberg, O., Nwaigwe, C.I., Hou, H.G., Williams, H., Swartz, H.M., Dunn, J.F., 2001. The effects of ketamine—xylazine anesthesia on cerebral blood flow and oxygenation observed using nuclear magnetic resonance perfusion imaging and electron paramagnetic resonance oximetry. Brain Res. 913, 174–179.

Leithauser, M.T., Liem, A., Steward, B.C., Miller, E.C., Miller, J.A., 1990. 1, N6-ethenoadenosine formation, mutagenicity and murine tumor induction as indicators of the generation of an electrophilic eposide metabolite of the closely related carcinogens ethyl carbamate (urethane) and vinyl carbamate. Carcinogenesis 11, 463–473.

Levin-Arama, M., Abraham, L., Waner, T., Harmelin, A., Steinbery, D.M., Lahay, T., Harley, M., 2016. Subcutaneous compared with intraperitoneal ketamine-xylazine for anesthesia of mice. J. Am. Assoc. Lab. Anim. Sci. 55 (6), 794–800.

Lewi, P.J., Heykants, J.J.P., Janssen, P.A.J., 1976. Intravenous pharmacokinetic profile in rats of etomidate, a short-acting hypnotic drug. Arch. Int. Pharmacodyn. 220, 72–85.

Li, C., Yan, J., Tang, D., Zhu, J., Huang, C., Sun, Y., Hu, R., Wang, H., Fu, C., Chen, Y., Jiang, H., 2020. GluN2A-selective positive allosteric modulator-nalmefene-flumazenil reverses ketamine-fentanyl-dexmedetomidine-induced anesthesia and analgesia in rats. Sci. Rep. 10, 5265.

Li, L., Vlisides, P.E., 2016. Ketamine: 50 years of modulating the mind. Front. Hum. Neurosci. 10, 612.

Lieggi, C.C., Artwohl, J.E., Leszczynski, J.K., Rodriguez, N.A., Fickbohm, B.L., Fortman, J.D., 2005a. Efficacy and safety of stored and newly prepared tribromoethanol in ICR mice. Contemp. Top. Lab. Anim. Sci. 44, 17–22.

Lieggi, C.C., Fortman, J.D., Kleps, R.A., Sethi, V., Anderson, J.A., Brown, C.E., andArtwohl, J.E., 2005b. An evaluation of preparation methods and storage conditions of tribromoethanol. Contemp. Top. Lab. Anim. Sci. 44, 11–16.

Lin, H.C., 1996. Dissociative anesthetics. In: Thurmon, J.C., Tranquilli, W.J., Benson, G.J. (Eds.), Lumb and Jones' VeterinaryAnesthesia, third ed. Lippincott Williams and Wilkins, New York, pp. 241–296.

Lin, H.C., Thurmon, J.C., Benson, G.J., Tranquilli, W.J., 1993. Telazol—a review of its pharmacology and use in veterinary medicine. J. Vet. Pharmacol. Therapeut. 16, 383–418.

Lin, M.T., Chen, C.F., Pang, I.H., 1978. Effect of ketamine on thermoregulation in rats. Can. J. Physiol. Pharmacol. 56, 963–967.

Lincoln, D.W., Hill, A., Wakerley, J.B., 1973. The milk ejection reflex in the rat: an intermittent function not abolished by surgical levels of anesthesia. J. Endocrinol. 57, 459–476.

Lipscomb, J.C., Mahle, D.A., Brashear, W.T., Garrett, C.M., 1996. A species comparison of choral hydrate metabolism in blood and liver. Biochem. Biophys. Res. Commun. 227, 340–350.

Livingston, A., Waterman, A.E., 1978. The development of tolerance to ketaminein rats and the significance of hepatic metabolism. Br. J. Pharmacol. 64, 63–69.

Loomis, M.R., Henrickson, R.V., Anderson, J.H., 1980. Effects of ketamine hydrochloride on the hemogram of rhesus monkeys (*Macaca mulatta*). Lab. Anim. Sci. 30, 851–853.

Loop, T., Liu, Z., Humar, M., Hoetzel, A., Benzing, A., Pahl, H.L., Geiger, K.K., J Pannen, B.H., 2002. Thiopental inhibits the activation of nuclear factor kappaB. Anesthesiology 96, 1202–1213.

Löscher, W., Ganter, M., Fassbender, C.P., 1990. Correlation between drug and metabolite concentrations in plasma and anesthetic action of ketamine in swine. Am. J. Vet. Res. 51, 391–398.

Lovell, D.P., 1986a. Variation in pentobarbitone sleeping time in mice 1. Strain and sex differences. Lab. Anim. 20, 85–90.

Lovell, D.P., 1986b. Variation in pentobarbitone sleeping time in mice 2. Variables affecting test results. Lab. Anim. 20, 91–96.

Lovell, D.P., 1986c. Variation in barbiturate sleeping time in mice 3. Strain × environment interactions. Lab. Anim. 20, 307–312.

Lowson, S., Gent, J.P., Goodchild, C.S., 1990. Anticonvulsant properties of propofol and thiopentone: comparison using two tests in laboratory mice. Br. J. Anaesth. 64, 59–63.

Macdonald, R.L., McLean, M.J., 1986. Anticonvulsant drugs: mechanisms of action. Adv. Neurol. 44, 713–736.

Maggi, C.A., Manzinim, S., Parlani, M., Meli, A., 1984. An analysis of the effects of urethane on cardiovascular responsiveness to catecholamines in terms of its interference with Ca++. Experientia 40, 52–59.

Maggi, C.A., Meli, A., 1986a. Suitability of urethane anesthesia for physiopharmacological investigations in various systems. Part 1: general considerations. Experientia 42, 109–114.

Maggi, C.A., Meli, A., 1986b. Suitability of urethane anesthesia for physiopharmacological investigations in various systems. Part 2: cardiovascular system. Experientia 42, 292–297.

Maggi, C.A., Meli, A., 1986c. Suitability of urethane anesthesia for physiopharmacological investigations. Part 3: other systems and conclusions. Experientia 42, 531–537.

Manders, W.T., Vatner, S.F., 1976. Effects of sodium pentobarbital anesthesia on left ventricular function and distribution of cardiac output in dogs, with particular reference to the mechanism for tachycardia. Circ. Res. 39, 512–517.

Marietta, M.P., 1977. Characterization of ketamine induction of hepatic microsomal drug metabolism. Biochem. Pharmacol. 26, 2451–2453.

Marik, P.E., 2004. Propofol: therapeutic indications and side-effects. Curr. Pharmaceut. Des. 10, 3639–3649.

Marik, P.E., 2005. Propofol: an immunomodulating agent. Pharmacotherapy 25, 28S–33S.

Matthews, N.S., Brown, R.M., Barling, K.S., Lovering, S.L., Herrig, B.W., 2004. Repetitive propofol administration in dogs and cats. J. Am. Anim. Hosp. Assoc. 40, 255–260.

McIntosh, M.P., Schwarting, N., Rajewski, R.A., 2004. In vitro and in vivo evaluation of a sulfobutyl ether beta-cyclodextrin enabled etomidate formulation. J. Pharmacol. Sci. 93, 2585–2594.

McMillan, M.W., Leece, E.A., 2011. Immersion and branchial/transcutaneous irrigation anaesthesia with alfaxalone in a Mexican axolotl. Vet. Anaesth. Analg. 38 (6), 619–623.

Meyer, R.E., Braun, R.D., Dewhirst, M.W., 2002. Anesthetic considerations for the study of murine tumors. In: Teicher, B.A. (Ed.), Tumor Models in Cancer Research. Humana Press, Totowa, NJ, pp. 407–431.

Meyer, R.E., Fish, R.E., 2005. A review of tribromoethanol anesthesia for production of genetically engineered mice and rats. Lab. Anim. 34, 47–52.

Mihic, S.J., Mayfield, J., Harris, R.A., 2017. Hypnotics and sedatives. In: L Brunton, L., Hilal-Dandan, R., Knollman, B.C. (Eds.), Goodman and Gilman's the Pharmacologic Basis of Therapeutics, thirteenth ed. McGraw-Hill Medical Publishing Division, New York https://accessmedicine.mhmedical.com/content.aspx?bookid=2189§ionid=169518968.

Milde, L.N., Milde, J.H., Michenfelder, J.D., 1985. Cerebral functional, metabolic, and hemodynamic effects of etomidate in dogs. Anesthesiology 63, 371–377.

Miller, E.D., Kistner, J.R., Epstein, R.M., 1980. Whole-body distribution of radioactively labelled microspheres in the rat during anesthesia with halothane, enflurane, or ketamine. Anesthesiology 52, 296–302.

Minter, L.J., Bailey, K.M., Harms, C.A., Lewbart, G.A., Posner, L.P., 2014. The efficacy of alfaxalone for immersion anesthesia in koi carp (*Cyprinus carpio*). Vet. Anaesth. Analg. 41 (4), 398–405.

Mitterhauser, M., Wadsak, W., Wabnegger, L., Sieghart, W., Viernstein, H., Kletter, K., Dudczak, R., 2003.). In vivo and in vitro evaluation of [18F]FETO with respect to the adrenocortical and GABAergic system in rats. Eur. J. Nucl. Med. Mol. Imag. 30, 1398–1401. Epub 2003 Jul 3.

Modica, P.A., Tempelhoff, R., White, P.F., 1990. Pro- and anticonvulsant effects of anesthetics (Part II). Anesth. Analg. 70, 433–444.

Moon, P.F., 1994. Acute toxicosis in two dogs associated with etomidate-propylene glycol infusion. Lab. Anim. Sci. 44, 590–594.

Moon, P.F., 1997. Cortisol suppression in cats after induction of anesthesia with etomidate, compared with ketamine–diazepam combination. Am. J. Vet. Res. 58, 868–871.

Morey, T.E., Modell, J.H., Shekhawat, D., Grand, T., Shah, D.O., Gravenstein, N., McGorray, S.P., Dennis, D.M., 2006a. Preparation and anesthetic properties of propofol microemulsions in rats. Anesthesiology 104, 1184–1190.

Morey, T.E., Modell, J.H., Shekhawat, D., Shah, D.O., Klatt, B., Thomas, G.P., Kero, F.A., Booth, M.M., Dennis, D.M., 2006b. Anesthetic properties of a propofol microemulsion in dogs. Anesth. Analg. 103, 882–887.

Muir, W.W., 1985. Cyclohexanone drug mixtures: the pharmacology of ketamine and ketamine drug combinations. Proc. 2nd. Intl. Cong. Vet. Anes. 5–14.

Muir, W.W., Bednarski, L., Bednarski, R., 1991. Thiamylal- and halothane-sparing effect of diazepam in dogs. J. Vet. Pharmacol. Therapeut. 14, 46–50.

Muir, W.W., Hubbell, J.A.E., 1988. Cardiopulmonary and anesthetic effects of ketamine and its enantiomers in dogs. Am. J. Vet. Res. 49, 530–534.

Muir, W.W., Mason, D.E., 1989. Side effects of etomidate in dogs. J. Am. Vet. Med. Assoc. 194, 1430–1434.

Muir, W.W., Wiese, A.J., March, P.A., 2003. Effects of morphine, lidocaine, ketamine, and morphine-lidocaine-ketamine drug combination on minimum alveolar concentration in dogs anesthetized with isoflurane. Am. J. Vet. Res. 64 (9), 1155–1160.

Murthy, V.S., Zagar, M.E., Vollmer, R.R., Schmidt, D.H., 1982. Pentobarbital-induced changes in vagal tone and reflex vagal activity in rabbits. Eur. J. Pharmacol. 84, 41–50.

Myslobodsky, M.S., Golovchinsky, V., Mintz, M., 1981. Ketamine: convulsant or anti-convulsant? Pharmacol. Biochem. Behav. 14, 27–33.

Nair, A.B., Jacob, S., March 2016. A simple practice guide for dose conversion between animals and human. J. Basic Clin. Pharm. 7 (2), 27.

Nakagawa, T., Hirakata, H., Sato, M., Nakamura, K., Hatano, Y., Nakamura, T., Fukuda, K., 2002. Ketamine suppresses platelet aggregation possibly by suppressed inositol triphosphate formation and subsequent suppression of cytosolic calcium increase. Anesthesiology 96, 1147–1152.

National Toxicology Program (NTP), 2000. Report on Carcinogens, ninth ed. National Institute of Environmental Health Sciences, National Institutes of Health, Research Triangle Park, NC.

Nazian, S.J., 1988. Serum concentrations of reproductive hormones after administration of various anesthetics to immature and young adult male rats. Proc. Soc. Exp. Biol. Med. 187, 482–487.

Nevalainen, T., Pyhälä, L., Voipio, H., Virtanen, R., 1989. Evaluation of anaesthetic potency of medetomidine–ketamine combination in rats, Guinea-pigs and rabbits. Acta Vet. Scand. 85 (Suppl. 1.), 139–143.

Nishina, K., Akamatsu, H., Mikawa, K., Shiga, M., Maekawa, N., Obara, H., Niwa, Y., 1998. The inhibitory effects of thiopental, midazolam, and ketamine on human neutrophil functions. Anesth. Analg. 86, 159–165.

Nomeir, A.A., Ioannou, Y.M., Sanders, J.M., Matthews, H.B., 1989. Comparative metabolism and disposition of ethyl carbamate (urethane) in male Fisher 344 rats and male B6C3F1 mice. Toxicol. Appl. Pharmacol. 97, 203–215.

Norris, M.L., Turner, W.D., 1983. An evaluation of tribromoethanol (TBE) asananaesthetic agent in the Mongolian gerbil (*Meriones unguiculatus*). Lab. Anim. 17, 324–329.

Nunn, J.F., Utting, J.E., Brown Jr., B.R., 1989. Introduction. In: Nunn, J.F., Utting, J.E., Brown Jr., B.R. (Eds.), General Anaesthesia, fifth ed. Butterworths, London, pp. 1–6.

Ochsner, A.J., 1977. Cardiovascular and respiratory responses to ketamine hydrochloride in the rhesus monkey (*Macaca mulatta*). Lab. Anim. Sci. 27, 69–71.

Ogino, K., Hobara, T., Kobayashi, H., Iwamoto, S., 1990. Gastric mucosal injury induced by chloral hydrate. Toxicol. Lett. 52, 129–133.

Oguchi, K., Arakawa, K., Nelson, S.R., Samson, F., 1982. The influence of droperidol, diazepam, and physostigmine on ketamine-induced behavior and brain regional glucose utilization in rat. Anesthesiology 57, 353–358.

Olivar, T., Laird, J.M., 1999. Differential effects of *N*-methyl-d-aspartate receptor blockade on nociceptive somatic and visceral reflexes. Pain 79, 67–73.

Olson, M.E., McCabe, K., Walker, R.L., 1987. Guaifenesin alone or in combination with ketamine or sodium pentobarbital as an anesthetic in rabbits. Can. J. Vet. Res. 51, 383–386.

Olson, M.E., Renchko, P., 1988. Azaperone and azaperone–ketamine as a neuroleptic sedative and anesthetic in rats and mice. Lab. Anim. Sci. 38, 299–304.

Pablo, L.S., Bailey, J.E., Ko, J.C., 1997. Median effective dose of propofol required for induction of anaesthesia in goats. J. Am. Vet. Med. Assoc. 211, 86–88.

Papaioannou, V.E., Fox, J.G., 1993. Efficacy of tribromoethanol anesthesia in mice. Lab. Anim. Sci. 43, 189–192.

Parker, J.L., Adams, H.R., 1978. The influence of chemical restraining agents on cardiovascular function: a review. Lab. Anim. Sci. 28, 575–583.

Pascoe, P.J., 1992. The case for maintenance of general anesthesia with an injectable agent. Vet. Clin. North Am. Small Anim. Pract. 22, 275–276.

Pascoe, P.J., Ilkiw, J.E., Haskins, S.C., Patz, J.D., 1992. Cardiopulmonary effects of etomidate in hypovolemic dogs. Am. J. Vet. Res. 53, 2178–2182.

Pavlovic, M., Wroblewski, K., Manevich, Y., Kim, S., Biaglow, J.E., 1996. The importance of choice of anaesthetics in studying radiation effects in the 9L rat glioma. Br. J. Cancer Suppl. 27, S222–S225.

Payton, A.J., Pick, J.R., 1989. Evaluation of a combination of tiletamine and zolazepam as an anesthetic for ferrets. Lab. Anim. Sci. 39, 243–246.

Perrin, K.L., Bertelsen, M.F., 2017. Intravenous alfaxalone and propofol anesthesia in the bearded dragon (*Pogona vitticeps*). J. Herpetol. Med. Surg. 27 (3), 123–126.

Pettinger, W.A., Tanaka, K., Keeton, K., Campbell, W.B., Brooks, S.N., 1975. Renin release, an artifact of anesthesia and its implications in rats. Proc. Soc. Exp. Biol. Med. 148, 625–630.

Pfenninger, E., Dick, W., Ahnefeld, F.W., 1985. The influence of ketamine on both normal and raised intracranial pressure of artificially ventilated animals. Eur. J. Anaesthesiol. 2, 297–307.

Ponte, J., Sadler, C.L., 1989. Effect of thiopentone, etomidate and propofol on carotid body chemoreceptor activity in the rabbit and the cat. Br. J. Anaesth. 62, 41–45.

Pouget, P., Wattiez, N., Rivaud-Péchoux, S., Gaymard, B., 2010. Rapid development of tolerance to sub-anaesthetic dose of ketamine: an oculomotor study in macaque monkeys. Psychopharmacology 209 (4), 313–318.

Pozzi, A., Muir III, W.W., Traverso, F., 2006. J Prevention of central sensitization and pain by *N*-methyl-d-aspartate receptor antagonists. Am. Vet. Med. Assoc. 228, 53–60.

Preziosi, P., Vacca, M., 1988. Adrenocortical suppression and other endocrine effects of etomidate. Life Sci. 42, 477–489.

Quinn, G.P., Axelrod, J., Brodie, B.B., 1958. Species, strain, and sex differences in metabolism of hexobarbitone, amidopyrine, antipyrine and aniline. Biochem. Pharmacol. 1, 152–159.

Ramirez-Gonzalez, M.D., Barna, I., Wiegant, V.M., de Jong, W., 1991. Effect of anaesthetics on the release of beta-endorphin-immunoreactivity in rat plasma. Life Sci. 48, 1371–1377.

Reich, D.L., Silvay, G., 1989. Ketamine: an update on the first twenty-five years of clinical experience. Can. J. Anaesth. 36, 186–197.

Reid, W.C., Carmichael, K.P., Srinivas, S., Bryant, J.L., 1999. Pathologic changes associated with use of tribromoethanol (avertin) in the Sprague Dawley rat. Lab. Anim. Sci. 49, 665–667.

Reid, W.D., Davies, C., Pare, P.D., Pardy, R.L., 1989. An effective combination of anaesthetics for 6-h experimentation in the golden Syrian hamster. Lab. Anim. 23, 156–162.

Reinert, H., 1964. Urethane hyperglycaemia and hypothalamic activation. Nature 204, 889–891.

Reutlinger, R.A., Karl, A.A., Vinal, S.I., Nieser, M., 1980. Effects of ketamine HCl-xylazine HCl combination on cardiovascular and pulmonary values of the rhesus macaque (*Macaca mulatta*). Am. J. Vet. Res. 41, 1453–1457.

Reyes Toso, C.F., Linares, L.M., Rodriguez, R.R., 1995. Blood sugar concentrations during ketamine or pentobarbitone anesthesia in rats with or without alpha and beta adrenergic blockade. Medicina 55, 311–316.

Reynolds, J.E.F. (Ed.), 1982. Martindale: The Extra Pharmacopoeia, 29th ed. The Pharmaceutical Press, London, p. 760.

Rice, J.M., Diwan, B.A., Hu, H., Ward, J.M., Nims, R.W., Lubet, R.A., 1994. Enhancement of hepatocarcinogenesis and induction of specific cytochrome P450-dependent monooxygenase activities by the barbiturates allobarbital, aprobarbital, pentobarbital, secobarbital and 5-phenyl- and 5-ethylbarbituric acids. Carcinogenesis 15 (2), 395–402.

Rieg, T., Richter, K., Osswald, H., Vallon, V., 2004. Kidney function in mice: thiobutabarbital versus alpha-chloralose anesthesia. Naunyn-Schmiedeberg's Arch. Pharmacol. 370 (4), 320–323. Epub 2004 Sep. 30.

Robertson, S., 1992. Advantages of etomidate use as an anesthetic agent. Vet. Clin. North Am. Small Anim. Pract. 22, 277–280.

Rocchiccioli, C., Saad, M.A.A., Elghozi, J.-L., 1989. Attenuation of the baroreceptor reflex by propofol anesthesia in the rat. J. Cardiovasc. Pharmacol. 14, 631–635.

Rodrigues, S.F., de Oliveira, M.A., Martins, J.O., Sannomiya, P., de Cassia Tostes, R., Nigro, D., Carvalho, M.H.C., Fortes, Z.B., 2006.

Differential effects of chloral hydrate- and ketamine/xylazine-induced anesthesia by the s.c. route. Life Sci. 79, 1630–1637.

Rodrigo-Mocholí, D., Escudero, E., Belda, E., Laredo, F., Hernandis, V., Marín, P., July 4, 2018. Pharmacokinetics and effects of alfaxalone after intravenous and intramuscular administration to cats. N. Z. Vet. J. 66 (4), 172–177.

Rodríguez, J.M., Muñoz-Rascón, P., Navarrete-Calvo, R., Gómez-Villamandos, R.J., Pérez, J.M.D., Sarmiento, J.A.F., et al., 2012. Comparison of the cardiopulmonary parameters after induction of anaesthesia with alphaxalone or etomidate in dogs. Vet. Anaesth. Analg. 39 (4), 357–365.

Rodriguez-Lopez, J.M., Sanchez-Conde, P., Lozano, F.S., Nicolas, J.L., Garcia-Criado, F.J., Cascajo, C., Muriel, C., 2006. Laboratory investigation: effects of propofol on the systemic inflammatory response during aortic surgery. Can. J. Anaesth. 53, 701–710.

Roth, D.M., Swaney, J.S., Dalton, N.D., Gilpin, E.A., Ross Jr., J., 2002. Impact of anesthesia on cardiac function during echocardiography in mice. Am. J. Physiol. Heart Circ. Physiol. 282, H2134–H2140.

Rudolph, U., Mohler, H., 2004. Analysis of $GABA_A$ receptor function and dissection of the pharmacology of benzodiazepines and general anesthetics through mouse genetics. Annu. Rev. Pharmacol. Toxicol. 44, 475–498.

Rudy, D.C., Downie, J.W., McAndrew, J.D., 1991. Alpha-chloralose alters autonomic reflex function of the lower urinary tract. Am. J. Physiol. 261, R1560–R1567.

Ryder, S., Way, W.L., Trevor, A.J., 1978. Comparative pharmacology of the optical isomers of ketamine in mice. Eur. J. Pharmacol. 49, 15–23.

Sabatini, C.F., O'Sullivan, M.L., Valcour, J.E., Sears, W., Johnson, R.J., 2013. Effects of injectable anesthetic combinations on left ventricular function and cardiac morphology in Sprague-Dawley rats. J. Am. Assn. Lab. Anim. Sci. 52, 34–43.

Sapru, H.N., Krieger, A.J., 1979. Cardiovascular and respiratory effects of some anesthetics in the decerebrate rat. Eur. J. Pharmacol. 53, 151–158.

Saunders, P.A., Ho, I.K., 1990. Barbiturates and the $GABA_A$ receptor complex. Prog. Drug Res. 34, 261–286.

Sawyer, D.C., Lumb, W.V., Stone, H.L., 1971. Cardiovascular effects of halothane, methoxyflurane, pentobarbital, and thiamylal. J. Appl. Physiol. 30, 36–43.

Sayce, L.J., Powell, M.E., Kimball, E.E., Chen, P., Gartling, G.J., Rousseau, B., 2020. Continuous rate infusion of ketamine hydrochloride and dexmedetomidine for maintenance of anesthesia during laryngotracheal surgery in New Zealand white rabbits. J. Am. Assoc. Lab. Anim. Sci. 59 (2), 176–185.

Sceniak, M.P., MacIver, M.B., 2006. Cellular actions of urethane on rat visual cortical neurons in vitro. J. Neurophysiol. 95, 3865–3874.

Schaefer, C.F., Brackett, D.J., Biber, B., Lerner, M.R., Holaday, J.W., Wilson, M.F., Fagraeus, L., 1989. Respiratory and cardiovascular effects of thyrotropin-releasing hormone as modified by isoflurane, enflurane, pentobarbital and ketamine. Regul. Pept. 24, 269–282.

Scheelings, T.F., Baker, R.T., Hammersley, G., Hollis, K., Elton, I., Holz, P., 2011. A preliminary investigation into the chemical restraint with alfaxalone of selected Australian squamate species. J. Herpetol. Med. Surg. 21 (2–3), 63–67.

Schenkman, K.A., Yan, S., 2000. Propofol impairment of mitochondrial respiration in isolated perfused Guinea pig hearts determined by reflectance spectroscopy. Crit. Care Med. 28, 172–177.

Schiffer, T.A., Christensen, M., Gustafsson, H., Palm, F., 2018. The effect of inactin on kidney mitochondrial function and production of reactive oxygen species. PLoS One 13 (11), e0207728.

Schneemilch, C.E., Schilling, T., Bank, U., 2004. Effects of general anaesthesia on inflammation. Best Pract. Res. Clin. Anaesthesiol. 18, 493–507.

Schwartz, D.A., Horwitz, L.D., 1975. Effects of ketamine on left ventricular performance. J. Pharmacol. Exp. Therapeut. 194, 410–414.

Schwedler, M., Miletich, D.J., Albrecht, R.F., 1982. Cerebral blood flow and metabolism following ketamine administration. Can. Anaesth. Soc. J. 29, 222–226.

Schwenke, D.O., Cragg, P.A., 2004. Comparison of the depressive effects of four anesthetic regimens on ventilatory and cardiovascular variables in the Guinea pig. Comp. Med. 54, 77–85.

Sear, J.W., McGivan, J.D., 1981. Metabolism of alphaxalone in the rat: evidence for the limitation of the anaesthetic effect by the rate of degradation throught ehepatic mixed function oxygenase system. Br. J. Anaesth. 53 (4), 417–421.

Sear, J.W., 1996. Steroid anesthetics: old compounds, new drugs. J. Clin. Anesth. 8, 91S–98S.

Sebel, P.S., Lowdon, J.D., 1989. Propofol: a new intravenous anesthetic. Anesthesiology 71, 260–277.

Seeman, P., Kapur, S., 2003. Anesthetics inhibit high-affinity states of dopamine D2 and other G-linked receptors. Synapse 50, 35–40.

Semple, H.A., Goreck, D.K., Farley, S.D., Ramsay, M.A., 2000. Pharmacokinetics and tissue residues of Telazol in free-ranging polar bears. J. Wildl. Dis. 36, 653–662.

Severs, W.B., Keil, L.C., Klase, P.A., Deen, K.C., 1981. Urethane anesthesia in rats. Altered ability to regulate hydration. Pharmacology 22, 209–226.

Seyde, W.C., McGowan, L., Lund, N., Duling, B., Longnecker, D.E., 1985. Effects of anesthetics on regional hemodynamics in normovolemic and hemorrhaged rats. Am. J. Physiol. 249, H164–H173.

Sharma, R.P., Stowe, C.M., Good, A.L., 1970. Studies on the distribution and metabolism of thiopental in cattle, sheep, goats, and swine. J. Pharmacol. Exp. Therapeut. 172, 128–137.

Shimokawa, A., Kunitake, T., Takasaki, M., Kannan, H., 1998. Differential effects of anesthetics on sympathetic nerve activity and arterial baroreceptor reflex in chronically instrumented rats. J. Auton. Nerv. Syst. 72, 46–54.

Shirasaka, Y., Wasterlain, C.G., 1995. The effect of urethane anesthesia on evoked potentials in dentate gyrus. Eur. J. Pharmacol. 282, 11–17.

Shumkova, V., Sitdikova, V., Rechapov, I., Leukhin, A., Minlebaev, M., 2021. Effects of urethane and isoflurane on the sensory evoked response and local blood flow in the early postnatal rat somatosensory cortex. Sci. Rep. 11, 9567.

Short, T.G., Young, Y., 2003. Toxicity of intravenous anaesthetics. Best Pract. Res. Clin. Anaesthesiol. 17, 77–89.

Silverman, J., 2003. Protocol review. Anesthetics in GEM: does TBE make the grade? Lab. Anim. 32, 19–21.

Silverman, J., Huhndorf, M., Balk, M., Slater, G., 1983. Evaluation of a combination of tiletamine and zolazepam as an anesthetic for laboratory rodents. Lab. Anim. Sci. 33, 457–460.

Silverman, J., Muir III., W.W., 1993. A review of laboratory animal anesthesia with choloral hydrate and chloralose. Lab. Anim. Sci. 43, 210–216.

Skipper, H.E., Bennett Jr., L.L., Bryan, C.E., White Jr., L., Newton, M.A., Simpson, L., 1951. Carbamatesinthe chemotherapy of leukemiaVIII.

Overall tracer studies on carbonyl-labeled urethan, methylene-labeled urethan, and methylene-labeled ethyl alcohol. Cancer Res. 11, 46–51.

Sklar, G.E., 1997. Propofol and postoperative infections. Ann. Pharmacother. 31, 1521–1523.

Skolleborg, K.C., Grönbech, J.E., Grong, K., Åbyholm, F.E., Lekven, J., 1990. Distribution of cardiac output during pentobarbital versus midazolam/fentanyl/fluanisone anaesthesia in the rat. Lab. Anim. 24, 221–227.

Small, B.C., 2003. Anesthetic efficacy of metomidate and comparison of plasma cortisol responses to tricaine methanesulfonate, quinaldine, and clove oil-anesthetized channel catfish *Ictalurus punctatus*. Aquaculture 218, 177–185.

Soma, L.R., 1983. Anesthetic and analgesic considerations in the experimental animal. Ann. N. Y. Acad. Sci. 406, 32–47.

Sonner, J.M., Zhang, Y., Stabernack, C., Abaigar, W., Xing, Y., Laster, M.J., 2003. GABA(A) receptor blockade antagonizes the immobilizing action of propofol but not ketamine or isoflurane in a dose-related manner. Anesth. Analg. 96, 706–712.

Sotomayor, R.E., Collins, T.F., 1990. Mutagenicity, metabolism, and DNA interactions of urethane. Toxicol. Ind. Health 6, 71–108.

Sou, J.H., Chan, M.H., Chen, H.H., 2006. Ketamine, but not propofol, anaesthesia is regulated by metabotropic glutamate5receptors. Br. J. Anaesth. 96, 597–601. Epub 2006 Mar 10.

Spriggs, T.L.B., Stockham, M.A., 1964. Urethane anaesthesia and pituitary-adrenal function in the rat. J. Pharm. Pharmacol. 16, 603–610.

Stanley, T.H., 1973. Blood-pressure and pulse-rate responses to ketamine during general anesthesia. Anesthesiology 39, 648–649.

Steward, C.A., Marsden, C.A., Prior, M.J., Morris, P.G., Shah, Y.B., 2005. Methodological considerations in rat brain BOLD contrast pharmacological MRI. Psychopharmacology (Berl.) 180, 687–704. Epub 2005 Sep. 14.

Stoelting, R.K., Hillier, S.C., 2006. Pharmacology and Physiology in Anesthetic Practice, fourth ed. Lippincott Williams and Wilkins, Philadelphia, PA.

Storer, R.J., Butler, P., Hoskin, K.L., Goadsby, P.J., 1997. A simple method, using 2-hydroxypropyl-B-cyclodextrin, of administering a-chloralose at room temperature. J. Neurosci. Methods 77, 49–53.

Stowe, D.F., Bosnjak, Z.J., Kampine, J.P., 1992. Comparison of etomidate, ketamine, midazolam, propofol, and thiopental on function and metabolism of isolated hearts. Anesth. Analg. 74, 547–558.

Strigo, I.A., Duncan, G.H., Bushnell, M.C., Boivin, M., Wainer, I., Rodriguez Rosas, M.E., Persson, J., 2005. The effects of racemic ketamine on painful stimulation of skin and viscera in human subjects. Pain 113, 255–264.

Strobel, G.E., Wollman, H., 1969. Pharmacology of anesthetic agents. Fed. Proc. 28, 1386–1403.

Sutton, J.A., 1972. A brief history of steroid anaesthesia before Althesin (CT1341). Postgrad. Med. J. Suppl. 2, 9–13.

Suzdak, P.D., Schwartz, R.D., Skolnick, P., Paul, S.M., 1986. Ethanol stimulates g-aminobutyric acid receptor-mediated chloride transport in rat brain synaptoneurosomes. Proc. Natl. Acad. Sci. U.S.A. 83, 4071–4075.

Svendsen, P., Carter, A.M., 1985. Influence of injectable anaesthetic combinations on blood gas tensions and acid–base status in laboratory rats. Acta Pharmacol. Toxicol. 57, 1–7.

Taber, R., Irwin, S., 1969. Anesthesia in the mouse. Fed. Proc. 28, 1528–1532.

Taie, S., Leichtweis, S.B., Liu, K.J., Miyake, M., Grinberg, O., Demidenko, E., Swartz, H.M., 1999. Effects of ketamine/xylazine and pentobarbital anesthesia on cerebral tissue oxygen tension, blood pressure, and arterial blood gas in rats. Adv. Exp. Med. Biol. 471, 189–198.

Takahashi, Y., Yamato, K., Akiyama, H., Tsuji, K., Onishi, H., Machida, Y., 2005. Transdermal absorption of propofol in rats. Biol. Pharm. Bull. 28, 870–875.

Tan, P.C.P., Shyr, M.H., Yang, C.H., Kuo, T.B.J., Pan, W.H.T., Chan, S.H.H., 1993. Power spectral analysis of the electrencephalographic and hemo-dynamic correlates of propofol anesthesia in the rat: intravenous infusion. Neuroscience 160, 205–208.

Taniguchi, T., Yamamoto, K., 2005. Anti-inflammatory effects of intravenous anesthetics on endotoxemia. Mini Rev. Med. Chem. 5, 241–245.

Taniguchi, T., Kanakura, H., Yamamoto, K., 2002. Effects of post treatment with propofol on mortality and cytokine responses to endotoxin-induced shock in rats. Crit. Care Med. 30, 904–907.

Taniguchi, T., Yamamoto, K., Ohmoto, N., Ohta, K., Kobayashi, T., 2000. Effects of propofol on hemodynamic and inflammatory responses to endotoxemia in rats. Crit. Care Med. 28, 1101–1106.

Tarin, D., Sturdee, A., 1972. Surgical anaesthesia of mice: evaluation of tribromo-ethanol, ether, halothane and methoxyflurane and development of a reliable technique. Lab. Anim. 6, 79–84.

Taylor, R., Hayes, K.E., Toth, L.A., 2000. Evaluation of an anesthetic regimen for retroorbital blood collection from mice. Contemp. Top. Lab. Anim. Sci. 39, 14–17.

Teske, R.H., Carter, G.C., 1971. Effect of chloramphenicol on pentobarbital-induced anesthesia in dogs. J. Am. Vet. Med. Assoc. 159, 777–780.

The Merck Index, ninth ed., 1976. Merck and Co., Rahway, NJ, pp. 1234–1235.

Thompson, J.S., Brown, S.A., Khurdayan, V., Zeynalzadedan, A., Sullivan, P.G., Scheff, S.W., 2002. Early effects of tribromoethanol, ketamine/xylazine, pentobarbitol, and isoflurane anesthesia on hepatic and lymphoid tissue in ICR mice. Comp. Med. 52, 63–67.

Thurmon, J.C., 1985. Comparative pharmacokinetics of selected injectable anesthetic agents. Proc. 2nd Intl. Cong. Vet. Anes. 21–26.

Thurmon, J.C., Benson, G.J., 1987. Pharmacologic considerations in selection of anesthetics for animals. J. Am. Vet. Med. Assoc. 191, 1245–1251.

Ting, C.H., Arnott, R.H., Linkens, D.A., Angel, A., 2004. Migrating from target-controlled infusion to closed-loop control in general anaesthesia. Comput. Methods Progr. Biomed. 75, 127–139.

Tomemori, N., Shingu, K., Komatsu, T., Urabe, N., Mori, K., 1981. Antianalgesic action of thiamylal sodium in cats. Acta. Anaesthiol. Scand. Suppl. 25, 523–525.

Traber, D.L., Wilson, R.D., Priano, L.L., 1970. Blockade of the hypertensive effect to ketamine. Anesth. Analg. 49, 420–426.

Tracy, C.H., Short, C.E., Clark, B.C., 1988. Comparing the effects of intravenous and intramuscular administration of Telazol. Vet. Med. 104–111.

Tranquilli, W.J., Thurmon, J.C., Benson, G.J., 1983. Organ blood flow and distribution of cardiac output in hypocapnic ketamine-anesthetized swine. Am. J. Vet. Res. 44, 1578–1582.

Tsai, S.K., Lee, C., 1989. Ketamine potentiates nondepolarizing neuromuscular relaxants in a primate. Anesth. Analg. 68, 5–8.

Turner, D.M., Ransom, R.W., Yang, J.S.-J., Olsen, R.W., 1989. Steroid anesthetics and naturally occurring analogs modulate the g-aminobutyric acid receptor complex at a site distinct from barbiturates. J. Pharmacol. Exp.Ther. 248, 960–966.

Turner, P.V., Pekow, C., Vasbinder, M.A., Brabb, T., 2011. Administration of substances to laboratory animals: equipment considerations, vehicle selection, and solute preparation. J. Am. Assoc. Lab. Anim. Sci. 50, 614–627.

Turner, T.T., Howards, S.S., 1977. Hyperglycemia in the hamster anesthetized with Inactin®[5-ethyl-5-(1-methyl propyl)-2-thiobarbiturate]. Lab. Anim. Sci. 27, 380–382.

Ungemach, F.R., Heinritzi, K., Kersjes, C.M., Erhardt, W., 1997. Ban of the use of metomidate (Hypnodil) in swine. Background, consequences and alternatives. Tierarztl. Prax. Ausg. G. Grosstiere. Nutztiere. 25, 417–423.

Usenik, E.A., Cronkite, E.P., 1965. Effects of barbiturate anesthetics on leukocytes in normal and splenectomized dogs. Anesth. Analg. 44, 167–170.

Vachon, P., Faubert, S., Blais, D., Comtois, A., Bienvenu, J.G., 2000. A pathophysiological study of abdominal organs following intraperitoneal injections of chloral hydrate in rats: comparison between two anaesthesia protocols. Lab. Anim. 34, 84–90.

Van Leeuwen, A.F., Evans, R.G., Ludbrook, J., 1990. Effects of halothane, ketamine, propofol and alfentanil anaesthesia on circulatory control in rabbits. Clin. Exp. Pharmacol. Physiol. 17, 781–798.

Van Der Meer, C., Versluys-Broers, J.A.M., Tuynman, H.A.R.E., Buur, V.A., 1975. The effect of ethylurethane on hematocrit, blood pressure and plasma-glucose. Arch. Int. Pharmacodyn. Ther. 217, 257–275.

Vatner, S.F., Higgins, C.B., Patrick, T., Franklin, D., Braunwald, E., 1971. Effects of cardiac depression and of anesthesia on the myocardial action of a cardiac glycoside. J. Clin. Invest. 50, 2585–2595.

Veilleux-Lemieux, D., Castel, A., Carrier, D., Beaudry, F., Vachon, P., 2013. Pharmacokinetics of ketamine and xylazine in young and old Sprague-Dawley Rats. J. Am. Assn. Lab. Anim. Sci. 52, 562–570.

Velázquez-Delgado, P.I., Gutierrez-Blanco, E., Torres-Acosta, F.d.J., Ortega-Pacheco, A., Aguilar-Caballero, A.J., Dzikiti, B.T., 2021. Comparison of propofol or isoflurane anesthesia maintenance, combined with a fentanyl—lidocaine—ketamine constant-rate infusion in goats undergoing abomasotomy. Animals 11, 492.

Vesell, E.S., 1968. Factors affecting the responsiveness of micetohexobarbital. Pharmacology 1, 81–97.

Virtanen, R., 1989. Pharmacological profiles of medetomidine and its antagonist, atipamezole. Acta Vet. Scand. Suppl. 85, 29–37.

Volicer, L., Loew, C.G., 1971. The effect of urethane anesthesia on the cardiovascular action of angiotensin II. Pharmacology 6, 193–201.

Wafford, K.A., Macaulay, A.J., Fradley, R., O'Meara, G.F., Reynolds, D.S., Rosahl, T.W., 2004. Differentiating the role of gamma-aminobutyric acid typeA ($GABA_A$) receptor subtypes. Biochem. Soc. Trans. 32, 553–556.

Walker, L.A., Buscemi-Bergin, M., Gellai, M., 1983. Renal hemodynamics in conscious rats: effects of anesthesia, surgery, and recovery. Am. J. Physiol. 245, F67–F74.

Walker, L.A., Gellai, M., Valtin, H., 1986. Renal response to pentobarbital anesthesia in rats: effect of interrupting the renin-angiotensin system. J. Pharmacol. Exp. Therapeut. 236, 721–728.

Wang, Y., Zhou, T., Chua, T.C., Pang, C.C.Y., 1991. Effects of inhalation and intravenous anaesthetic agents on pressor response to NG-nitro-l-arginine. Eur. J. Pharmacol. 198, 183–188.

Ward, G.S., Johnson, D.O., Roberts, C.R., 1974. The use of CI 744 as an anesthetic for laboratory animals. Lab. Anim. Sci. 24, 737–742.

Warne, L.N., Beths, T., Whittem, T., Carter, J.E., Bauquier, S.H., 2015. A review of the pharmacology and clinical application of alfaxalone in cats. Vet. J. 203 (2), 141–148.

Waterman, A.E., 1983. Influence of premedication with xylazine on the distribution and metabolism of intramuscularly administered ketamine in cats. Res. Vet. Sci. 35, 285–290.

Waterman, A.E., 1984. The pharmacokinetics of ketamine administered intravenously in calves and the modifying effect of premedication with xylazine hydrochloride. J. Vet. Pharmacol. Therapeut. 7, 125–130.

Waterman, A.E., Livingston, A., 1978. Effects of age and sex on ketamine anaesthesia in the rat. Br. J. Anaesth. 50, 885–889.

Watney, G.C., Pablo, L.S., 1992. Median effective dosage of propofol for induction of anesthesia in dogs. Am. J. Vet. Res. 53, 2320–2322.

Wauquier, A., 1983. Profile of etomidate: a hypnotic, anticonvulsant, and brain protective compound. Anaesthesia 38 (Suppl. 1), 26–33.

Way, W.L., Trevor, A.J., 1986. Pharmacology of intravenous nonnar-cotic anesthetics. In: Miller, R.D. (Ed.), Anesthesia, second ed. Churchill Livingstone, New York, pp. 799–833.

Welberg, L.A.M., Kinkead, B., Thrivikraman, K.V., Huerkamp, M.J., Nemeroff, C.B., Plotsky, P.M., 2006. Ketamine—xylazine—acepromazine anesthesia and postoperative recovery in rats. J. Am. Assoc. Lab. Anim. Sci. 45, 13–20.

Wellington, D., Mikaelian, I., Singer, L., 2013. Comparison of ketamine-xylazine and ketamine-dexmedetomidine anesthesia and intraperitoneal tolerance in rats. J. Am. Assoc. Lab. Anim. Sci. 52, 481–487.

Wertz, E.M., Benson, G.J., Thurmon, J.C., Tranquilli, W.J., Davis, L.E., Koritz, G.D., 1990. Pharmacokinetics of etomidate in cats. Am. J. Vet. Res. 51, 281–285.

West, S.E., Lee, J.C., Johns, T.N., Nunamaker, E.A., 2020. Intraperitoneal alfaxalone and alfaxalone-dexmedetomidine anesthesia in Sprague-Dawley rats (*Rattus norvegicus*). J. Am. Assn. Lab. Anim. Sci. 59, 531–538.

Westenberg, I.S., Bolam, J.M., 1981. Lethal doses of pentobarbital sodium in albino versus pigmented rats: a within-strain comparison. Lab. Anim. Sci. 31, 360–361.

Westfall, B.A., Boulos, B.M., Shields, J.L., Garb, S., 1964. Sex differences in pentobarbital sensitivity in mice. Proc. Soc. Exp. Biol. Med. 115, 509–510.

Whelan, G., Flecknell, P.A., 1992. The assessment of depth of anaesthesia in animals and man. Lab. Anim. 26, 153–162.

White, K.L., Paine, S., Harris, J., 2017. A clinical evaluation of the pharmacokinetics and pharmacodynamics of intravenous alfaxalone in cyclodextrin in male and female rats following a loading dose and constant rate infusion. Vet. Anaesth. Analg. 44, 865–875.

White, P.F., 1989. Clinical uses of intravenous anesthetic and analgesic infusions. Anesth. Analg. 68, 161–171.

Whittem, T., Pasloske, K.S., Heit, M.C., Ranasinghe, M.G., 2008. The pharmacokinetics and pharmacodynamics of alfaxalone in cats after single and multiple intravenous administration of Alfaxan® at clinical and supraclinical doses. J. Vet. Pharmacol. Therapeut. 31 (6), 571–579.

Wixson, S.K., Smiler, K.L., 1997. Anesthesia and analgesia in rodents. In: Kohn, D.F., Wix-son, S.K., White, W.J., Benson, G.J. (Eds.), Anesthesia and Analgesia in Laboratory Animals. Academic Press, San Diego, CA, pp. 165–203.

Wixson, S.K., White, W.J., Hughes Jr., H.C., Lang, C.M., Marshall, W.K., 1987a. A comparison of pentobarbital, fentanyl–droperidol, ketamine– xylazine and ketamine–diazepam anesthesia in adult male rats. Lab. Anim. Sci. 37, 726–730.

Wixson, S.K., White, W.J., Hughes Jr., H.C., Marshall, W.K., Lang, C.M., 1987b. The effects of pentobarbital, fentanyl–droperidol, ketamine–xylazine and ketamine–diazepam on noxious stimulus perception in adult male rats. Lab. Anim. Sci. 37, 731–735.

Wixson, S.K., White, W.J., Hughes Jr., H.C., Lang, C.M., Marshall, W.K., 1987c. The effects of pentobarbital, fentanyl–droperidol, ketamine–xylazine and ketamine–diazepam on arterial blood pH, blood gases, mean arterial blood pressure and heart rate in adult male rats. Lab. Anim. Sci. 37, 736–742.

Wixson, S.K., White, W.J., Hughes Jr., H.C., Lang, C.M., Marshall, W.K., 1987d. The effects of pentobarbital, fentanyl–droperidol, ketamine–xylazine and ketamine–diazepam on core and surface body temperature regulation in adult male rats. Lab. Anim. Sci. 37, 743–749.

Wright, M., 1982. Pharmacologic effects of ketamine and its use in veterinary medicine. J. Am. Vet. Med. Assoc. 180, 1462–1471.

Yang, F.L., Li, C.H., Hsu, B.G., Tsai, N.M., Lin, S.Z., Harn, H.J., Chen, H.I., Liao, K.W., Lee, R.P., 2007. The reduction of tumor necrosis factor-alpha release and tissue damage by pentobarbital in the experimental endotoxemia model. Shock 28, 309–316.

Yang, H., Wong, H., Wu, V., Walsh, J.H., Taché, Y., 1990. Somatostatin monoclonal antibody immunoneutralization increases gastrin and gastric acid secretion in urethane-anesthetized rats. Gastroenterology 99, 659–665.

Yang, X.P., Liu, Y.H., Rhaleb, N.E., Kurihara, N., Kim, H.E., Carretero, O.A., 1999. Echocardiographic assessment of cardiac function in conscious and anesthetized mice. Am. J. Physiol. 277 (5 Pt. 2), H1967–H1974.

Ypsilantis, P., Mikroulis, D., Politou, M., Tsoukali, H., Pitiakoudis, M., Didilis, V., Theodoridis, G., Bougioukas, G., Simopoulos, C., 2006. Tolerance to propofol's sedative effect in mechanically ventilated rabbits. Anesth. Analg. 103, 359–365.

Zaugg, M., Lucchinetti, E., Spahn, D.R., Pasch, t., Garcia, C., Schaub, M.C., 2002. Differential effects of anesthetics on mitochondrial K (ATP) channel activity and cardiomyocyte protection. Anesthesiology 97, 15–23.

Zeller, W., Meier, G., Burki, K., Panoussis, B., 1998. Adverse effects of tribromoethanol as used in the production of transgenic mice. Lab. Anim. 32, 407–413.

Zhou, W., Fontenot, H.J., Wang, S.N., Kennedy, R.H., 1999. Propofol-induced alterations in myocardial beta-adrenoceptors binding and responsiveness. Anesth. Analg. 89, 604–608.

Zimpfer, M., Manders, W.T., Barger, A.C., Vatner, S.F., 1982. Pentobarbital alters compensatory neural and humoral mechanisms in response to hemorrhage. Am. J. Physiol. 243, H713.

Zimpfer, M., Sit, S.P., Vatner, S.F., 1981. Effects of anesthesia on the canine carotid chemoreceptor reflex. Circ. Res. 48, 400–406.

Further reading

Adam, H.K., Glen, J.B., Hoyle, P.A., 1980. Pharmacokinetics in laboratory animals of ICI 35 868, a new I.V. anaesthetic agent. Br. J. Anaesth. 52, 743–746.

Agostino, D., Cliffton, E.E., 1964. Anesthetic effect on pulmonary metastases in rats. Arch. Surg. 88, 735–739.

Badger, D.A., Smith, R.L., Bao, J., Kuester, R.K., Sipes, I.G., 2002. Disposition and metabolism of isoeugenol in the male Fischer 344 rat. Food Chem. Toxicol. 40, 1757–1765.

Belant, J.L., Seamans, T.W., 1999. Alpha-chloralose immobilization of rock doves in Ohio. J. Wildl. Dis. 35, 239–242.

Booker, J.L., Erickson, H.H., Fitzpatrick, E.L., 1982. Cardiodynamics in the macaque during dissociative anesthesia. Am. J. Vet. Res. 43, 671–675.

Boucher, M., Dubray, C., Li, J.H., Paire, M., Duchêne-Marullaz, P., 1991. Influence of pentobarbital and chloralose anesthesia on quinidine-induced effects on atrial refractoriness and heart rate in the dog. J. Cardiovasc. Pharmacol. 17, 199–206.

Box, P.G., Ellis, K.R., 1973. Use of CT1341 anaesthetic ('Saffan') in monkeys. Lab. Anim. 7, 161–170.

Britton, K.T., Page, M., Baldwin, H., Koob, G.F., 1991. Anxiolytic activity of steroid anesthetic alfaxalone. J. Pharmacol. Exp. Therapeut. 258, 124–128.

Brodin, P., Roed, A., 1984. Effects of eugenol on rat phrenic nerve and phrenic nerve-diaphragm preparations. Arch. Oral Biol. 29, 611–615.

Celleno, D., Capogna, G., Emanuelli, M., Varrassi, G., Muratori, F., Costantino, P., Sebastiani, M., 1993. Which induction drug for cesarean section? A comparison of thiopental sodium, propofol, and midazolam. J. Clin. Anesth. 5, 284–288.

Chappel, S.C., Barraclough, C.A., 1976. The effects of sodium pentobarbital or ether anesthesia on spontaneous and electrochemically-induced gonadotropin release. Proc. Soc. Exp. Biol. Med. 153, 1–6.

Cheney, D.H., Slogoff, S., Allen, G.W., 1974. Ketamine-induced stress ulcers in the rat. Anesthesiology 40, 531–535.

Child, K.J., English, A.F., Gilbert, H.G., Woollett, E.A., 1972b. An endocrinological evaluation of Althesin (CT 1341) with special reference to reproduction. Postgrad. Med. 51–55.

Child, K.J., Gibson, W., Harnby, G., Hart, J.W., 1972a. Metabolism and excretion of Althesin (CT 1341) in the rat. Postgrad. Med. 37–42.

Cockshott, I.D., Douglas, E.J., Plummer, G.F., Simons, P.J., 1992. The pharmacokinetics of propofol in laboratory animals. Xenobiotica 22, 369–375.

Cox, R.H., 1972. Influence of chloralose anesthesia on cardiovascular function in trained dogs. Am. J. Physiol. 223, 660–667.

Davis, D.W., Mans, A.M., Biebuyck, J.F., Hawkins, R.A., 1986. Regional brain glucose utilization in rats during etomidate anesthesia. Anesthesiology 64, 751–757.

De Paepe, P., Belpaire, F.M., Rosseel, M.T., Van Hoey, G., Boon, P.A., Buylaert, W.A., 2000. Influence of hypovolemia on the pharmacokinetics and the electroencephalographic effect of propofol in the rat. Anesthesiology 93, 1482–1490.

Dundee, J.W., Clarke, R.S.J., 1964. Clinical studies of induction agents IX: a comparative study of a new eugenol derivative, FBA.1420, with G.29.505 and standard barbiturates. Br. J. Anaesth. 36, 100–105.

Faber, J.E., 1989. Effects of althesin and urethane-chloralose on neurohumoral cardiovascular regulation. Am. J. Physiol. 256, R757–R765.

Ferre, P.J., Pasloske, K., Whittem, T., Ranasinghe, M.G., Lefebvre, H.P., 2006. Plasma pharmacokinetics of alfaxalone in dogs after an intravenous bolus of Alfaxan-CD RTU. Vet. Anaesth. Analg. 33, 229–236.

File, S.E., Simmonds, M.A., 1988. Myoclonic seizures in the mouse induced by alfaxalone and related steroid anaesthetics. J. Pharm. Pharmacol. 40, 57–59.

Getchell, R., Scott, D., Schroeter, J., Wandelear, N., Ramee, S., Blair, M., 2020. Safety of Aqui-S 20e (10% eugenol) as a sedative for striped bass. U.S. Fish and Wildlife Service. Drug Research Information Bulletin. No. 58.

Gilron, I., Coderre, T.J., 1996. Preemptive analgesic effects of steroid anesthesia with alfaxalone in the rat formalin test. Evidence for differential GABA(A) receptor modulation in persistent nociception. Anesthesiology 84, 572–579.

Guenette, S.A., Beaudry, F., Marier, J.F., Vachon, P., 2006. Pharmacokinetics and anesthetic activity of eugenol in male Sprague-Dawley rats. J. Vet. Pharmacol. Therapeut. 29, 265–270.

Guenette, S.A., Helie, P., Beaudry, F., Vachon, P., 2007. Eugenol for anesthesia of African clawed frogs (*Xenopus laevis*). Vet. Anaesth. Analg. 34, 164–170.

Heaton, J.T., Brauth, S.E., 1991. Effects of yohimbine as a reversing agent for ketamine–xylazine anesthesia in budgerigars. Lab. Anim. Sci. 42, 54–56.

Heldmann, E., Brown, D.C., Shofer, F., 1999. The association of propofol usage with postoperative wound infection rate in clean wounds: a retrospective study. Vet. Surg. 28, 256–259.

Hogan, B., Beddington, R., Costantini, F., Lacy, E., 1996. Manipulating the Mouse Embryo. Cold Spring Harbor Laboratory, New York.

Ingvast-Larsson, J.C., Axen, V.C., Kiessling, A.K., 2003. Effects of isoeugenol on in vitro neuromuscular blockade of rat phrenic nerve-diaphragm preparations. Am. J. Vet. Res. 64, 690–693.

Ishizuka, S., Sikdar, S.K., Yasui, S., Oyama, Y., Akaike, N., 1989. a-chloralose opens the chloride channel of frog isolated sensory neurons. Brain Res. 498, 181–184.

Jones, R.S., 1985. Steroid anaesthetics. Proc. 2nd Intl. Cong. Vet. Anes. 15, 17.

Keates, H., 2003. Induction of anaesthesia in pigs using a new alfaxalone formulation. Vet. Rec. 153, 627–628.

Keene, J.L., Noakes, D.L., Moccia, R.D., et al., 1998. The efficacy of clove oil as an anaesthetic for rainbow trout, *Oncorhynchus mykiss* (Walbaum). Aquacult. Res. 29, 89–101.

Kelbel, I., Koch, T., Weber, A., Schiefer, H.G., van Ackern, K., Neuhof, H., 1999. Alterations of bacterial clearance induced by propofol. Acta Anaesthesiol. Scand. 43, 71–76.

Kurz, H., Fichtl, B., 1981. Interrelation between plasma protein binding, rate of injection and the anaesthetic effect of thiopental. Biopharm. Drug Dispos. 2, 191–196.

Lafortune, M., Mitchell, M.A., Smith, J.A., 2001. Evaluation of medetomidine, clove oil, and propofol for anesthesia of leopard frogs, *Rana pipiens*. J. Herpetol. Med. Surg. 11, 13–18.

Langevin, P.B., Gravenstein, N., Doyle, T.J., Roberts, S.A., Skinner, S., Langevin, S.O., Gulig, P.A., 1999. Growth of *Staphylococcus aureus* in diprivan and intralipid: implications on the pathogenesis of infections. Anesthesiology (Hagerst.) 91, 1394–1400.

Lemm, C.A., 1993. Evaluation of Five Anesthetics on Striped Bass. Resource Publication 196. U.S Department of the Interior, Fish and Wildlife Service, Washington, DC.

Lögdberg, B., 1988. Alphaxolone–alphadolone for anesthesia of squirrel monkeys of different ages. J. Med. Primatol. 17, 163–167.

Mama, K.R., Gaynor, J.S., Harvey, R.C., Roberson, S.A., Koenig, R.L., Cozzi, E.M., 2013. Multicenter clinical evaluation of a multi-dose formulation of propofol in the dog. BMC Vet. Res. 9, 261.

Meyer, R.E., 2007. Pharmacokinetics and anesthetic activity of eugenol in male Sprague–Dawley rats. J. Vet. Pharmacol. Therapeut. 30, 265–270, 91.

Muir, W.W., Hubbell, J.A.E., 1985. Blood pressure response to acetylpromazine and lenperone in halothane anesthetized dogs. J. Am. Anim. Hosp. Assoc. 21, 285–289.

Mullenheim, J., Molojavyi, A., Preckel, B., Thamer, V., Schlack, W., 2001a. Thiopentone does not block ischemic preconditioningi n the isolated rat heart. Can. J. Anaesth. 48, 784–789.

Nadeson, R., Goodchild, C.S., 2001. Antinociceptive properties of neurosteroids III: experiments with alphadolone given intravenously, intraperitoneally, and intragastrically. Br. J. Anaesth. 86, 704–708.

Pachon, R.E., Scharf, B.A., Vatner, D.E., Vatner, S.F., 2015. Best anesthetics for assessing left ventricular systolic function by echocardiography in mice. Am. J. Physiol. Heart Circ. Physiol. 308 (12), H1525–H1529.

Pathirathna, S., Brimelow, B.C., Jagodic, M.M., Krishnan, K., Jiang, X., Zorumski, C.F., Mennerick, S., Covey, D.F., Todorovic, S.M., Jevtovic-Todorovic, V., 2005. New evidence that both T-type calcium channels and GABA-A channels are responsible for the potent peripheral analgesics effects of 5a-reduced neuroactive steroids. Pain 114, 429–443.

Peterson, S.L., 1989. Anticonvulsant profile of an anesthetic steroid. Neuropharmacology 28, 877–879.

Rank, J., Jensen, A.-G., 1989. The value of anaesthetic steroids alphaxolone-alphadolone in pregnant mice. Scand. J. Lab. Anim. Sci. 16, 115–117.

Sell, A.B., Carlini, E.A., 1976. Anesthetic action of methyleugenol and other eugenol derivatives. Pharmacology 14, 367–377.

Seymour, C., 1999. Caesarian section. In: Seymour, C., Gleed, R. (Eds.), Manual of Small Animal Anaesthesia and Analgesia, 217–222. British Small Animal Veterinary Association, Cheltenham, UK.

Shekarforoush, S., Fatahi, Z., Safari, F., 2016. The effects of pentobarbital, ketamine-pentobarbital and ketamine-xylazine anesthesia in a rat myocardial ischemic reperfusion injury model. Lab. Anim. 50 (3), 179–184.

Sladky, K.K., Swanson, C.R., Stoskopf, M.K., Loomis, M.R., Lewbart, G.A., 2001. Comparative efficacy of tricaine methanesulfonate and clove oil for use as anesthetics in red pacu (*Piaractus brachypomus*). Am. J. Vet. Res. 62, 337–342.

Soma, L.R., 1971. In: Soma, L.R. (Ed.), Textbook of Veterinary Anesthesia. Williams and Wilkins, Baltimore, MD, p. 147.

Soto, C.G., Burhanuddin, A.F., 1995. Clove oil as a fish anesthetic for measuring length and weight of rabbitfish (*Siganus lineatus*). Aquaculture 136, 149–152.

Taylor, J.M., Jenner, P.M., Jones, W.I., 1964. A comparison of the toxicity of some allyl, propenyl, and propyl compounds in the rat. Toxicol. Appl. Pharmacol. 6, 378–387.

Van Velzen, M., Dahan, A., 2014. Ketamine metabolomics in the treatment of major depression. Anesthesiology 121, 4–5.

Winter, L., Nadeson, R., Tucker, A.P., Goodchild, C.S., 2003. Antinocicep-tive properties of neurosteroids: a comparison of alphadolone and alphax-alone in potentiation of opioid antinociception. Anesth. Analg. 97, 798–805.

Chapter 5

Tranquilizers, sedatives, local anaesthetics and antimuscarinic agents

Chiara Adami[1], Alessandra Bergadano[2] and Daniela Casoni[3]

[1]*Department of Veterinary Medicine, University of Cambridge, Cambridge, United Kingdom;* [2]*Experimental Animal Center (EAC), University of Bern, Bern, Switzerland;* [3]*Experimental Surgical Facility, Experimental Animal Center (EAC), University of Bern, Bern, Switzerland*

Chapter outline

I. Tranquilizers and sedatives

The main action of tranquilizers is inducing a feeling of calmness or anxiolysis, while sedatives also reduce the overall response to external stimuli (Rankin, 2015). Analgesia is a feature of some sedatives, but not all. However, the distinction between tranquilizers and sedatives is often theoretical, and their actions tend to overlap. Moreover, due to differences between species, individuals, and doses, the same drug can be used as either a mild tranquilizer or a potent sedative. For simplicity, we will just refer to "sedation" for describing their action. Phenothiazines, butyrophenones, benzodiazepines, and α2-adrenergic receptor agonists can be injected alone or in combinations with opioids "neuroleptoanalgesia" (see Chapters 4, 6, and 7) or with hypnotics to induce sedation before and during anesthesia induction, reduce the sympathetic response to surgical stimulation, reduce anesthetic requirements, and promoting smooth induction and recovery.

A. Phenothiazines and butyrophenones

Phenothiazines (acepromazine, chlorpromazine) and butyrophenones (droperidol, azaperone, fluphenazine, and

Anesthesia and Analgesia in Laboratory Animals. https://doi.org/10.1016/B978-0-12-822215-7.00029-9

fluanisone) are major tranquilizers. In human medicine, phenothiazines and butyrophenones are used in the treatment of psychiatric disorders (i.e., schizophrenia), and sedation is an undesirable adverse effect. In veterinary medicine, these drugs are mostly used for their sedative action, to decrease anxiety and fear reactions, to improve the collaboration of the animal before a nonpainful manipulation, prior to a stressful event like transport, to decrease aggression, or as premedication to smooth the induction of and, depending on the duration of action, the recovery from anesthesia. The clinical efficacy is variable and species dependent. Tranquilizers do not have analgesic activity but work synergistically with opioids in neuroleptanalgesia combinations.

1. Pharmacology

a. Chemical structure

Phenothiazines Phenothiazines are a subgroup of thiazines in which the central nitrogen- and sulfur-containing thiazine ring carries two fused-on benzene rings. This three-ring structure is spatially planar, water-soluble, and must be kept protected from light. Chlorpromazine is the prototypical phenothiazine, but acepromazine is more commonly used based on the more intensive and long-acting clinical effect.

Butyrophenones Butyrophenones are synthetic agents containing a phenyl-1-butanone group. They are water-soluble and must be kept protected from light. The drugs currently used include azaperone and fluanisone. Droperidol and haloperidol are less commonly used.

b. Mechanisms of action

Phenothiazines and butyrophenones block a whole range of central and peripheral neurotransmitter receptors, including dopaminergic (D2), adrenergic (α1 and α2), serotoninergic (5HT2A), histamine (H1), acetylcholine (Ach), and muscarinic (M1) receptors (Table 5.1).

The calming and mood-altering antipsychotic effects are due to the antagonism of D2 receptors in the basal ganglia and mesolimbic portions of the forebrain. Sedation typically occurs at low doses; as the dose is increased, the dose-response curve quickly reaches a plateau after which sedation is merely prolonged and the incidence of adverse effects is increased (Tobin and Ballard, 1979). Overall, there is a decrease in spontaneous locomotion.

The dopaminergic antagonism within the chemoreceptor trigger zone is responsible for the antiemetic action, and at the hypothalamic level, it leads to a decoupling of central thermoregulation and hyperprolactinemia (Wieck and Haddad, 2003).

The antagonism of the peripheral α-1 adrenergic receptor relaxes the smooth muscle of the arterioles with a clinically relevant long-lasting hypotension and contributes largely to the hypothermia. They can have mild antiarrhythmic action.

The peripheral anticholinergic and central depressant effects result in decreased esophageal and gastrointestinal secretions, and decreased peristalsis.

TABLE 5.1 List of receptors, cellular mediators and their anatomic locations; diacylglycerol (DAG), inositol-3-phosphate (IP3), cyclic adenosine monophosphate (cAMP), norepinephrine (NE).

Receptor	Mediator	Cellular mechanism	Anatomic location	Tissue
α_1	DAG, IP_3	Blocks the synthesis of the G-protein- related phospholipase which blocks the release of inositol-3-phosphate (IP3) from the endoplasmic reticulum and calcium entrance with resultant relaxation of the smooth muscle of the arterioles	Postsynaptic	Smooth muscle, myocardium
α_2	cAMP ↓	Reduced adenyl cyclase activity resulting in decreased postsynaptic potassium conductance	Presynaptic	Feedback of NE release, smooth muscle
β_1	cAMP ↑	Activates a phosphatidylinositol-calcium second messenger system and Ca++ release	Cardiac	Myocardium
β_2	cAMP ↑	Activates a phosphatidylinositol-calcium second messenger system and Ca++ release	Vascular and bronchial smooth muscle	Myocardium, prejunctional on sympathetic nerves
D1	cAMP ↑	Activates a phosphatidylinositol-calcium second messenger system and Ca++ release	Smooth muscle of renal, splanchnic, coronary, cerebral vessels, inhibit tubular Na-reabsorption	
D2	cAMP ↓	Reduced adenyl cyclase activity resulting in reduced postsynaptic potassium conductance	Autonomic ganglia and sympathetic nerve endings, modulates aldosterone, thyroid, and prolactin	

The antagonism at H1 histamine receptors results in a weak antihistaminic action that further contributes to their sedative effects.

c. Biodistribution, metabolization, and excretion

Gastrointestinal absorption is good, but tranquilizers undergo extensive hepatic first-pass metabolism, reducing the oral bioavailability to 30%. They are highly plasma-protein bound and extensively metabolized in the liver, and excreted as glucuronide and nonglucuronide metabolites in the bile and urine (Plumb, 2018).

d. Routes of administration

They are mostly administered parenterally via the intraperitoneal (IP), subcutaneous (SC), intramuscular (IM), and intravenous (IV) route but can be also administered in the feed, though the clinical action is more variable by this route. For more accurate titration in very small animals, the injectable drug can be diluted in saline.

e. Adverse effects and toxicity

The most relevant adverse effects of the phenothiazines are prolonged hypothermia secondary to both the central uncoupling of thermoregulation and peripheral vasodilation, with increased heat loss and a dose-dependent, long-lasting significant hypotension in all species (Murison et al., 2003; Parry et al., 1982; Rangel et al., 2020). The hypotensive effects of the butyrophenones are less marked.

At high doses, acepromazine can affect the striatal area of the basal ganglia, causing extrapyramidal symptoms, such as muscle tremors, mild rigidity, and restlessness (Torre and Falorni, 2007). The extrapyramidal adverse effects are more common with the butyrophenones. Acepromazine lowers the stimulus threshold for seizures and increases intracranial pressure (Short et al., 1984).

Tranquilizers increase prolactin secretion and thus can lead to galactorrhea (Torre and Falorni, 2007).

There are no specific antagonists for phenothiazines, but they have a wide safety margin; overdoses and adverse effects are treated symptomatically.

2. *Clinical pharmacology*

a. Acepromazine

Acepromazine is the most commonly used phenothiazine in veterinary medicine, primarily administered SC or IM to achieve good sedation before general anesthesia, and is a valuable adjunct for achieving chemical restraint for difficult and fearful animals. Its clinical action and adverse effects are species-specific and dose-dependent: the sedative effect is dose-dependent but will plateau; however, the duration and magnitude of adverse effects do not plateau. It is thus meaningful to use the lowest effective dose or combine it with opioids to achieve a synergistic effect (neuroleptoanalgesia).

It is commonly used in dogs, horses, and small ruminants (Musk and Wilkes, 2018; Nishimura et al., 2017). In laboratory rodents, it is seldom used alone because of the limited clinical relevance of the achieved sedation and the risk of hypotensive and hypothermic side effects. Mostly, it is used as an adjunct to xylazine-ketamine anesthesia in mice (Arras et al., 2001; Buitrago et al., 2008; He et al., 2010) and rats (Welberg et al., 2006) to deepen and prolong the duration of surgical anesthesia but it delays the recovery from anesthesia also. In guinea pigs, it is used in association with ketamine to achieve surgical anesthesia (Radde et al., 1996; Shucard et al., 1975). In cats (Costa et al., 2021), rabbits (Lipman et al., 1990), and nonhuman primates (López et al., 2002) the adverse effects, especially hypothermia and hypotension, are very predominant and therefore not routinely used. In rabbits, its association with butorphanol can facilitate venous cannulation and blood sampling, as a result of sedation and vasodilation (Donovan and Brown, 1998). Acepromazine has limited action in pigs (personal communication) and azaperone is preferred.

Its use is contraindicated in extremes of age (neonates or geriatric models) or in the presence of comorbidities; neonates have a greater permeability of the blood-brain barrier, less mature hepatic microsomal enzyme systems, lower albumin concentrations, and a high body surface to weight ratio, exacerbating the adverse effects of acepromazine. In animals with hepatic or coagulation issues or an ASA status higher than three, i.e., animals with hypovolemia, acepromazine premedication is contraindicated. While some authors advise against using acepromazine in animals prone to seizures, there is no evidence of a proconvulsive effect in gerbils (Brown & Donnelly, 2011) and dogs (McConnell et al., 2007).

The influence on the experimental readouts, i.e., EEG recordings, blood pressure measurements, tear production (Ghaffari et al., 2009), or intradermal testing should be taken into account.

b. Azaperone

Azaperone is an approved drug for tranquilization or sedation of swine in Europe. It has a dose-dependent effect allowing to target a range of indications such as tranquilization before transport, reduction of interspecific aggression, and cannibalism. It has no analgesic action and should be used in combination with ketamine to provide anesthesia (Hoyt et al., 1986). It should not be used in the premedication of the sow for a C-section as it crosses the placenta and piglets are sedated at birth, which depresses deambulation and drinking (Clarke and Trim, 2013).

There has been renewed interest in the drug in the United States due to a combination known as BAM (butorphanol-azaperone-medetomidine), which is used to achieve chemical restraint in rhesus monkeys (Malinowski et al., 2019).

Azaperone provides long-lasting sedation and, in association with ketamine, anesthesia in mice and rats (Olson and Renchko, 1988).

B. Benzodiazepines

1. Chemical structure

The basic chemical structure of benzodiazepines consists of a seven-membered (diazepam) ring fused with an aromatic ring, with four main substituent groups, which can be modified without loss of activity. Diazepam is poorly water-soluble and is supplied in a solution for injection containing propylene glycol and ethanol. Midazolam is an imidazole-benzodiazepine of which a significant proportion exists in a ring-open form at a $pH < 4$, allowing the preparation of water-soluble salts.

2. Mechanism of action

Benzodiazepines act selectively on $GABA_A$ receptors, which mediate inhibitory synaptic transmission throughout the central nervous system. Benzodiazepines enhance the response to GABA by facilitating the opening of GABA-activated chloride channels. Indeed, they bind specifically to a regulatory site on the receptor, distinct from the GABA-binding sites, and act allosterically to increase the affinity of GABA for the receptor (Tan et al., 2011).

The $GABA_A$ receptor is a ligand-gated ion channel, consisting of a pentameric combination of subunits, the main ones being α, β, and γ, with a central pore. For each subunit, several subtypes are known. Benzodiazepines bind across the interface between the α and the γ subunits. The interaction with different subtypes of units has been linked to different behavioral effects of benzodiazepines (Tan et al., 2011). Both midazolam and diazepam attach to all the α units ($\alpha1-\alpha6$), therefore different behavioral effects can be observed in different subjects.

3. Compounds

Although more than 20 compounds are currently available on the market, only diazepam and midazolam are commonly used in veterinary anesthesia. In principle, a short-acting compound like midazolam should be preferentially used as sedative-hypnotic, while long-acting compounds like diazepam are more useful as anxiolytics and anticonvulsants.

a. Diazepam

Biodistribution, metabolism and excretion Diazepam is highly and rapidly absorbed when administered orally. Oral bioavailability in the range of 74%–100% has been reported in dogs (Loscher and Frey, 1981). As an anticonvulsant, the solution can be also administered rectally. Intranasal administration was investigated in rabbits and rats (Kaur and Kim, 2008), and brain uptake in rats was comparable to the uptake after IV injection. It binds strongly to plasma proteins, and due to its high lipid solubility, it tends to accumulate in fat. In most animal species, diazepam is converted into three metabolites, including nordiazepam (N-desmethyldiazepam), temazepam, and ultimately oxazepam, via phase I N-demethylation or hydroxylation reactions (van Beusekom et al., 2015). All three metabolites are pharmacologically active. Nordiazepam appears to be the principal metabolite of diazepam in men and dogs, and species-specific differences in the relative quantities of these metabolites have been observed (Chenery et al., 1987; Seddon et al., 1989; Vree et al., 1979). The half-life of diazepam is relatively short in dogs and humans: 3.2 h was reported in Greyhound dogs (KuKanich and Nauss, 2012) and 2.07 h in other breeds (Platt et al., 2000). The concentration of its active metabolites in dogs and men (nordiazepam and oxazepam) eventually exceeds diazepam concentration, and, due to a longer elimination half-life than diazepam, account for the tendency to produce cumulative effects. Two in vitro studies suggested that horses convert diazepam primarily to temazepam (Hayami et al., 2013; Nakayama et al., 2016). Diazepam is excreted primarily in urine.

Desired pharmacologic effects Benzodiazepines are used to elicit sedation, anxiolysis, anterograde amnesia (demonstrated in man), and as anticonvulsants. Due to its action on $GABA_A$ receptors in the spinal cord, diazepam reduces muscle tone, in the absence of appreciable loss of coordination (van Beusekom et al., 2015).

Adverse pharmacologic effects Intramuscular administration of diazepam is contraindicated due to severe tissue irritation. Pain at IV injection has been reported in humans, and thrombophlebitis, reported in humans, has been studied and confirmed in rats (Graham et al., 1977). Mild excitement and disorientation, due to disinhibition, can occasionally occur in several species (dogs, cats, goats, sheep, and humans). After repeated treatment, suddenly stopping administration can bring about withdrawal syndrome in rats (File, 1990).

b. Midazolam

Biodistribution, metabolism and excretion Midazolam is provided in a chemical preparation that produces little tissue irritation. Following injection into an environment of relatively neutral tissue pH, the chemical structure of midazolam shifts to a completely ring-closed form, which makes the drug highly lipophilic (Gerecke, 1983). Midazolam is metabolized by hepatic microsomes, but its pharmacological effects are largely due to the parent compound itself, while its metabolites are considered inactive (Pieri, 1983). Absorption of midazolam seems to be erratic after rectal administration, but a favorable profile has been shown for the IM route in men and dogs. In dogs, the time to peak concentration (Tmax) after IM administration was 7.8 ± 2.4 min with a bioavailability of $50 \pm 16\%$ (Schwartz et al., 2013). Other studies indicated a higher bioavailability (up to 115%) after IM injection of a higher dose of midazolam (Court and Greenblatt, 1992). Elimination half-life in dogs was shorter than 30 min after IM injection and 63.3 ± 28.5 min after IV injection in dogs. In juvenile pigs, elimination half-life after IV injection was 158 ± 127 min, comparable with half-life after intranasal administration. In horses, the half-life is longer and dose-dependent (Hubbell et al., 2012). After oral administration of the injectable solution, enteral availability is strongly influenced by pH in dogs and increases as pH increases (Zhang et al., 2002). Midazolam is excreted mostly through the urine.

Desired pharmacologic effects Desired effects are represented by: sedation, anxiolysis, anterograde amnesia (demonstrated in man), and anticonvulsant effect. Due to its action on $GABA_A$ receptors in the spinal cord, it reduces muscle tone, in absence of appreciable loss of coordination. In humans, it is considered a hypnotic, while in animals it has generally no hypnotic properties if used alone (Rankin, 2015). Midazolam is considered a reliable sedative in rabbits, although the depth of sedation can vary among individuals (Rousseau-Blass et al., 2021).

Adverse pharmacologic effects Ataxia and postural sway in the absence of sedation can occur in adult horses. Mild excitement and disorientation, instead of sedation, can occur in cats, dogs, and sheep. Excitation, hyperresponsiveness to noise, restlessness, change in handling behavior, aggression, ataxia, increased appetite, drooling, licking, chewing, and vocalization have been reported in dogs (Simon et al., 2014).

4. Clinical applications

Despite their favorable therapeutic index and their safe cardiovascular and respiratory profiles in horses, dogs, and pigs, benzodiazepines are an unpredictable sedative in several species. There is a risk of eliciting paradoxical excitation when midazolam is administered to healthy young adult or mature adult dogs (Simon et al., 2014). In horses, ataxia and myorelaxation in the absence of sedation have been reported (Hubbell et al., 2012). However, goats (Dzikiti et al., 2014), pigs, rabbits (Schroeder and Smith, 2011), mice and several species of birds (Doss et al., 2018) are well sedated after a midazolam injection. In swine, midazolam results in decreased respiratory rate, but blood gas values are maintained (Smith et al., 1991).

When given to smooth the recovery period, no advantage of administering midazolam IV versus saline was found when performing step-down titration of isoflurane anesthesia in pigs (Kleine et al., 2015). The intranasal administration of an injectable formulation resulted in tranquilization in pigs (Lacoste et al., 2000).

Benzodiazepines have been more widely used in combination to achieve deep sedation in rabbits (Raulic et al., 2021; Rousseau-Blass et al., 2021) and ferrets and as coinduction agents in several species used as animal models (Grint and Murison, 2008). Midazolam induces good sedation for 1h and enhances analgesia in association with dexmedetomidine in rats (Boehm et al., 2010). Midazolam also has a MAC-sparing effect on isoflurane in mice and dogs (Tsukamoto et al., 2015).

5. Antagonists

Competitive antagonists of benzodiazepines were first discovered in the 1980s. The best-known compound is flumazenil. It reverses the effects of midazolam, although, in human medicine, some effects as inverse agonist were hypothesized. Flumazenil acts quickly and effectively when administered by injection, but its action extends shorter than the one of benzodiazepine, therefore repetition of the injection might be necessary. When associations of midazolam-fentanyl and medetomidine were used in mice, antagonization of all three drugs was beneficial (Fleischmann et al., 2016), while in rabbits significant hypotension can occur (Baumgartner et al., 2010). When midazolam was administered alone in rabbits, flumazenil quickly and reliably reversed sedation. However, return of lateral recumbency or even loss of righting reflex was observed in some animals about 25 min after flumazenil administration (Rousseau-Blass et al., 2021). In rats, flumazenil enhances morphine-mediated antinociception (Holtman et al., 2003).

Another antagonist, sarmazenil, has been used as an antagonist in multiple species but is no longer commercially available.

C. α2-adrenergic receptor agonists

1. Chemical structure

Drugs identified as α2-adrenoreceptor (α2-receptor) agonists share a common mechanism of action, although they differ in their chemical structure. Indeed, xylazine is a thiazole drug structurally similar to the phenothiazines. It does not possess an imidazole ring, unlike romifidine, detomidine, medetomidine, and dexmedetomidine.

2. Mechanism of action

The α2-receptor is a transmembrane G protein-coupled receptor (Khan et al., 1999) found pre and post-synaptically scattered through the body, in neural tissues, most organs, and extrasynaptically in vascular tissue and platelets. Four different isoreceptors have been defined in terms of affinity for alpha adrenoreceptor ligands α2a, -2b, 2c, and 2d (Bylund, 1985; Trevor et al., 2015). The most important consequence of α2-receptor stimulation is the inhibition of adenylyl cyclase, resulting in decreased formation of cAMP, an important regulator of cellular function. The α2-receptor stimulation resulting in the inhibition of neurotransmitter release is mediated through a decrease in calcium ion conductance, involving direct regulation of calcium entry by voltage-gated calcium ion channels (Lipscombe et al., 1989). Some effects of detomidine, medetomidine, and dexmedetomidine are postulated as linked to their interactions with imidazoline receptors. These receptors, specifically recognizing the imidazoline or oxazoline chemical structure, have been classified into I1, found in the brain, and I2, found in the brain, kidney, and pancreas (Khan et al., 1999). Imidazoline receptor stimulation mediates a central hypotensive (I1) and antiarrhythmogenic action. Although dexmedetomidine can combine with noradrenergic imidazoline receptors (Hieble et al., 1995; Ruffolo et al., 1995), the clinical importance of this mechanism of action has not been elucidated.

The pharmacologic effects are discussed for the entire class of drugs, as they are common to all α2-adrenoreceptors agonists. However, for every compound, specific effects on specific systems will be reported below. The broad distribution of α2-receptors leads to a wide variety of physiologic effects when administered.

3. Desired pharmacologic effects

A study in rats suggested that the α2A and -2C subtypes are found mainly in the central nervous system, and stimulation of these receptor subtypes may be responsible for sedation, analgesia, muscle relaxation, and sympatholytic effects (Buerkle and Yaksh, 1998).

Analgesia results from agonists binding to α2-adrenergic receptors at various points in the nociceptive pathways. Receptors have been isolated in the dorsal horn of the spinal cord and in the brainstem. Afferent input into the dorsal horn from nociceptors in the periphery continues, but is modulated and dampened by the decrease in norepinephrine release (presynaptic inhibition) and occupancy of those receptors (postsynaptic inhibition). It has been postulated that analgesia results from a combination of direct activation of alpha2-adrenoceptors located within the spinal cord, and sedative-hypnotic effects activated by supraspinal α2-autoreceptors (α2-adrenoceptors on noradrenergic neurons) within the brainstem (Stenberg, 1989). However, it is believed that the spinal mechanism is primarily responsible for the analgesic action of α2 agonist drugs (Virtanen et al., 1988).

4. Adverse pharmacologic effects

Cardiovascular effects are the predominant adverse effect. Peripherally, they increase systemic vascular resistance (afterload). They exert centrally mediated effects on heart rate and afterload through decreased sympathetic nervous system activity. This results in decreased heart rate and cardiac output consistently across species, while blood pressure initially increases, but eventually decreases to baseline or slightly below baseline. The magnitude and duration of each effect are species-dependent, drug-dependent, and with limited dose-dependent. The hemodynamic effects of this class of drugs in dogs have typically been described as a biphasic blood pressure response with decreased heart rate and cardiac index, increased systemic vascular resistance index, and central venous pressure. This behavior has been interpreted as initially a primarily baroreceptor (vagal)-mediated reflex due to increased systemic vascular resistance. As vascular resistance returns to normal, bradycardia persists as the result of a continued decreased central sympathetic tone (Rankin, 2015). However, the mechanisms leading to these changes and the exact location and the specific receptors responsible for the central hypotensive effect and the bradycardia are still unknown (Murrell and Hellebrekers, 2005).

Current α2-adrenergic receptor agonists also have some impact on α1-adrenergic receptors, which results in excitation and increased motor activity in animals. The less selective for the α2-adrenergic receptor a drug is, the more likely in theory rigidity and/or paradoxical excitement may be noted. Variation in specificity for α2-and α1-adrenergic receptors may explain some of the clinical differences observed. In vitro, xylazine showed a α2/α1 receptor-binding ratio of 160:1. By contrast, the ratios for medetomidine, detomidine, and clonidine are 1620:1, 260:1, and 220:1 (Virtanen et al., 1988), respectively.

In dogs and cats, respiratory effects are usually minor, and normal blood gas parameters are generally maintained when using α2-adrenergic receptor agonists alone (Bloor et al., 1989; Lamont et al., 2001). When used in conjunction with other sedatives, opioids, or anesthetics respiratory depression may occur. In sheep, hypoxemia following the use of α2-adrenergic receptor agonists, likely a result of pulmonary edema secondary to pulmonary parenchymal damage has been reported (Uggla and Lindqvist, 1983). For an extended discussion of the topic, we refer to Kastner (2006).

5. Clinical applications

Reliable sedation, muscle relaxation, immobilization, and analgesia are expected after administration of α2-agonists in most species. Combinations with sedatives, opioids and ketamine are often used in laboratory animals to achieve different degrees of general anesthesia (from light to deep).

6. Compounds

a. Xylazine

Xylazine has a species-related potency therefore, different dosages must be used to obtain the same effect in different species. Among mammals, goats are very sensitive, while pigs are very resistant (Hall et al., 2001). Within the ruminants, the spectrum of sensitivity to the effects of xylazine is goats > cattle > sheep (Riebold, 2007). Birds are relatively resistant.

Onset of sedation and analgesia is rapid following IV and IM administration. In sheep, it has a short elimination half-life and is rapidly cleared from plasma after both IM and IV administration (Garcia-Villar et al., 1981). Hepatic metabolism includes oxidation of the aromatic moiety and cleavage of the heterocyclic ring; no active metabolites have been reported (Salonen et al., 1992a, 1992b). The elimination half-life of xylazine after IV administration is generally similar across studied species (dogs, horses, sheep, and calves) and is about 30 min. A high density of α2-receptors has been demonstrated in lamina II of the dorsal horn of the spinal cord of sheep (Bouchenafa and Livingston, 1987). This observation may explain processes of analgesia, which result from systemic and intrathecal administration of α2-agonists in ruminants. Analgesia following xylazine has been demonstrated in the rat and mouse (Browning et al., 1982; Schmitt et al., 1974), and the molecular mechanisms recently investigated (Zhao et al., 2019). Across species, following its administration, bradycardia and atrio-ventricular blocks are often recorded; initial hypertension is relatively brief, and subsequent hypotension frequently follows. With clinically used doses of xylazine, the respiratory rate usually decreases, but PaO2, PaCO2, and pH are typically unchanged. This is because tidal volume increases as respiratory rate falls, resulting in maintaining minute ventilation (Haskins et al., 1986; Lavoie et al., 1992).

Emesis in those species that vomit is a concern and is likely a result of central α2-adrenergic receptor stimulation, as pretreatment with yohimbine (α2-adrenergic receptor antagonist) limits this effect (Hikasa et al., 1992a, 1992b).

b. Medetomidine and dexmedetomidine

Medetomidine is an equal mixture of two optical enantiomers, the active isomer dexmedetomidine, and levomedetomidine. The latter is generally considered to be pharmacodynamically inactive (MacDonald et al., 1991). The selectivity of dexmedetomidine is greater for the α2-receptor than the α1-receptor, compared with the racemate (Aantaa et al., 1995).

In dogs, racemic medetomidine is quickly absorbed after IM administration, with peak plasma levels occurring in approximately 30 min. Elimination from the plasma is rapid, with reported half-lives varying between 0.96 and 1.28 h (Kuusela et al., 2000; Salonen et al., 1992a). After IV administration in isoflurane-anaesthetized rabbits, the elimination half-life in rabbits is 80 min (Bailey et al., 2017). Administration of medetomidine at 40 μg/kg IV and dexmedetomidine at 20 and 10 μg/kg IV produced peak sedation at 10−20 min in dogs (Kuusela et al., 2000).

Medetomidine is not routinely used alone in rats, as doses up to 250 mcg per rat do not produce satisfying sedation, while higher doses cause strong respiratory depression (Hauptman et al., 2003). In companion rats, IM medetomidine (50−100 mcg/kg) was seen producing reliable sedation alone or in combination, and HR and RR were affected in a dose-dependent manner (Bellini et al., 2014). Intravenous administration of a medetomidine bolus (0.05 mg/kg), combined with a subsequent continuous infusion (0.1 mg/kg/h), led to desirable anesthesia for functional MRI in rats, while SC administration or lower doses of medetomidine were not satisfactory (Sirmpilatze et al., 2019). Antinociceptive actions of medetomidine have been demonstrated in a variety of assays and species (Vainio et al., 1992), including SC formalin injection in rats (Pertovaara et al., 1990) and the acetic acid-induced writhing test in mice (Virtanen, 1986).

Medetomidine has significant effects on the stress response and tends to increase cortisol and glucose levels in ruminants (Carroll et al., 2005; Ranheim et al., 2000).

The reported cardiovascular effects of medetomidine and dexmedetomidine are very similar to those of other α2-agonists. Pypendop and collaborators (Pypendop and Verstegen, 1998) demonstrated a limited dose dependency of cardiovascular effects, while more recent work showed a dose dependency in the cardiovascular effects in the dose range studied in dogs (Kaartinen et al., 2010; Pascoe, 2015). In studies where blood pressure was measured, hypotension, the principle hemodynamic effect in humans (Khan et al., 1999) was not a concern in dogs (Ko et al., 2000; Kuusela et al., 2000, 2001). The same has been reported in sheep (Adam et al., 2018). When administered IV, dexmedetomidine can decrease blood pressure and heart rate in rabbits in a dose-dependent manner, but, interestingly, there was no effect on myocardial systolic and diastolic function (Ren et al., 2018).

In rabbits, dexmedetomidine alone decreased corticosteroid secretion, but in combination with ketamine, its effects were counteracted (Gonzalez-Gil et al., 2015).

In piglets with normal blood pressure, no significant changes in cerebral perfusion or oxygenation were seen in response to the addition of dexmedetomidine to the background anesthesia (Mikkelsen et al., 2017).

7. Antagonists

Central and peripheral antagonists: Atipamezole has replaced the antagonists yohimbine and tolazoline in small and exotic animal practices primarily because of the increasing use of highly specific agonists such as medetomidine and dexmedetomidine. Atipamezole is more effective compared to yohimbine, even when xylazine is used in small animals (Janssen et al., 2017; Mees et al., 2018). Administration of atipamezole reverses sedation but also antinociception when tested with nociceptive withdrawal reflex in experimental dogs (Siegenthaler et al., 2020). Atipamezole can antagonize the antinociceptive effect of butorphanol in Wistar rats (Interlandi et al., 2017), while it did not in B6 mice (Izer et al., 2014).

Peripheral antagonist: MK-467 (previously also known as L-659'066) and currently known as vatinoxan, is an α2-adrenoceptor antagonist that acts mainly on peripheral α2-adrenoceptors because of its limited ability to cross the blood-brain barrier, as demonstrated in rats and marmosets (Clineschmidt et al., 1988). In dogs sedated with IV dexmedetomidine, heart rate was higher and systemic vascular resistance lower when MK-467 was coadministered with a dose-dependent return to normotension (Honkavaara et al., 2011; Pagel et al., 1998). The desired central nervous system effects of α2-agonists, such as sedation, seem not to be affected (Honkavaara et al., 2008; Restitutti et al., 2011), whereas negative peripheral effects, such as cardiovascular depression, have been alleviated with both IV and IM administration of MK-467 (Honkavaara et al., 2011; Rolfe et al., 2012; Salla et al., 2014). In dogs, it seems that MK-467 influenced the early disposition of dexmedetomidine without obvious effects on the later plasma concentrations of the drug, while dexmedetomidine minimally affected the disposition of MK-467 (Honkavaara et al., 2017; Pypendop et al., 2016).

II. Local anesthetics

Local anesthetics provide effective and reliable analgesia in all species without major adverse effects and are increasingly used in laboratory animal anesthesia for preventive analgesia.

A. Pharmacology

1. Chemical structure

Most local anesthetics (LA) of clinical relevance are composed of an aromatic lipophilic end, an intermediate ester or amide linkage, and a hydrophilic portion. The lipophilic moiety is usually a substituted benzene ring, while the hydrophilic group is represented by a tertiary or quaternary amine. As a result of their chemical structure, LA are classified as either amino-esters (procaine, chloroprocaine, benzocaine, and tetracaine) or amino-amides (prilocaine, lidocaine, mepivacaine, bupivacaine/levobupivacaine, and ropivacaine).

2. Mechanisms of action

Local anesthetics are classified as ion channel blockers. They exert their anesthetic effect mostly by interrupting inward Na^+ currents through the voltage-gated Na^+ channels, thereby impeding axonal depolarization and, consequently, nerve excitation and conduction.

Local anesthetics are weak bases that exist in both charged (hydrophilic) and uncharged (hydrophobic) forms, the proportion of which varies based on specific drug pKa and local tissue pH. At physiological tissue pH (7.3–7.4), less than 50% of most LA agents exist in their uncharged, lipid-soluble form. Whilst uncharged LA are thought to reach their binding sites by crossing the lipophilic axonal membrane, LA in their charged form can only enter through the channel gate when the latter is open.

In general, lipid solubility and the pKa of LA determine their onset of action and potency, respectively. Additionally, increasing lipid solubility potentiates neural membrane penetration and partition of the drug at the target sites, which enhances the analgesic effects (Covino, 1986).

Neuraxial administration of LA may produce antinociception through mechanisms other than Na^+ blockade, namely inactivation of K^+ and Ca^{2+} channels at the level of the dorsal horn of the spinal cord, and modulation of various spinal neurotransmitters such as substance P-, N-methyl-D-aspartate (NMDA) and Ach (Furutani et al., 2010; Ku and Schneider, 2011; Li et al., 1995).

3. Biodistribution, metabolization, and excretion

The amino-esters are readily hydrolyzed by plasma esterases to produce the weakly active diethylaminoethanol and para-aminobenzoic acid. Following hydrolysis, these metabolites are excreted by the kidney, a process that can be enhanced by lowering urine pH (Feyh, 1993). The amino-amides undergo liver metabolism that includes *N*-dealkylation by cytochrome P450s and subsequent hydrolysis. These LA agents are extensively (55%–95%) bound to plasma proteins, mainly alpha1-acid glycoprotein; therefore, underlying conditions resulting in hypoproteinemia may increase their systemic toxicity. Lidocaine is dealkylated to monoethylglycinexylidide and glycinexylidide, both of which retain anesthetic activity; these metabolites require further hydrolyzation or sulfate-conjugation prior to urinary excretion.

4. Clinical pharmacology

a. Amino-esters

Procaine Procaine is used in veterinary medicine to perform infiltrations and nerve blocks for short procedures, owing to its quick onset and brief duration of effects (30–60 min), as it is rapidly hydrolyzed in blood. One of its metabolites, p-aminobenzoic acid (PABA), might cause allergic reactions (Cirstea et al., 1984).

Chloroprocaine The onset and duration of action of chloroprocaine are similar to that of procaine. Recently, chloroprocaine has been successfully used in piglets for continuous wound infusion after laparotomy (Allegri et al., 2017).

Benzocaine Benzocaine is fast-acting and short-lasting. It is available exclusively for topical use and for fish anesthesia as an additive to water. Methemoglobinemia has been reported as an adverse effect of benzocaine in several laboratory animal species (Davis et al., 1993; Guertler et al., 1992; Von Tungeln et al., 2011).

Tetracaine The chemical structure of tetracaine makes it exceptionally suitable for topical anesthesia thanks to its liposolubility; therefore, this LA is commonly included in solutions such as ophthalmologic drops as well as creams for cutaneous application. Ophthalmologic solutions have been used in neonatal mice, while topical tetracaine-based creams have been used to desensitize both the skin and the tympanic membrane of guinea pigs prior to pinprick and myringotomy, respectively (Gnuechtel et al., 2000; Rozette et al., 2014).

b. Amino-amides

Prilocaine Prilocaine is an LA of intermediate duration and low systemic toxicity, most common for topical use in animals. Although its intermediate metabolite o-toluidine, can induce methemoglobinemia, this side effect has never been described in the context of spinal anesthesia (Boyes, 1975).

Mepivacaine The pharmacologic profile of mepivacaine is very similar to that of lidocaine, with a duration of effect extending up to 2 h. Mepivacaine is commonly used for infiltration anesthesia in various animal species, including piglets, rats, and mice (Abendschon et al., 2020; Chiu et al., 2019; Katagiri et al., 2020).

Lidocaine Despite the increasing use of more modern LA in laboratory animal practice, lidocaine remains the most versatile and most widely used agent owing to its fast onset (2–5 min), moderate duration of effect (1–2 h), and relatively low risk (dose-related). Besides being used for locoregional and topical anesthesia, the relatively low risk (dose-related) of lidocaine makes it suitable for IV regional anesthesia as well as IV continuous infusions for non-anesthetic use. Some widely appreciated nonanesthetic effects of lidocaine in animals are the antiarrhythmic and intrinsic vasodilator properties, its antiinflammatory effects, and the prokinetic activity, which may prevent the development of postoperative ileus in susceptible animal species such as horses and rabbits (Caracas et al., 2009; Rosen et al., 1975; Schnellbacher et al., 2017; Torfs et al., 2009). Finally, systemically administered lidocaine is known to produce analgesia, presumably through a mechanism involving the Na^+, Ca^{2+}, and K^+ channels as well as the NMDA receptors at the level of the dorsal horns of the spinal cord (Ku and Schneider, 2011; Nagy and Woolf, 1996). Intravenous lidocaine produced effective analgesia in rats with the increase in the mechanical nociceptive threshold, but not in cats in a model of thermal nociception (Kurabe et al., 2016, 2017; Pypendop et al., 2006).

Bupivacaine and levobupivacaine These LA are highly lipophilic and their potency is about four times that of lidocaine, with a long duration of effect (4–8 h) and slow onset of action (20–30 min). Bupivacaine is suitable for infiltrations, neuraxial use, and peripheral nerve blocks. It is not used for topical anesthesia, and it is not recommended for IV regional anesthesia because of its high cardiotoxicity potential. Whilst bupivacaine is the racemic mixture of two enantiomers, levobupivacaine is the purified levo-isomer or S-enantiomer of bupivacaine. It has slightly less cardiotoxic potential and similar physicochemical properties and clinical indications as racemic bupivacaine. Both drugs are widely used in laboratory animals (Chang et al., 2018; Kim and Choi, 2019; Kluge et al., 2017; Korat and Kapupara, 2018).

Bupivacaine is used in all veterinary species as a 50:50 mixture with lidocaine to achieve fast onset and longer duration. To date there is a lack of scientific evidence supporting the combined use of lidocaine and other LA. Whilst anecdotal reports and small case series have been published, clear guidelines and prospective studies investigating the efficacy and toxicity of the combination are still missing.

Ropivacaine Chemically related to mepivacaine and bupivacaine, ropivacaine is formulated as the pure S-enantiomer in order to decrease the cardiotoxicity that is mostly associated with its R-enantiomer. Ropivacaine shares similar properties to bupivacaine regarding clinical use, onset, and duration of effects; however, compared to bupivacaine, it is reported to produce a marginally shorter onset and duration of sensory blockade (up to 6 h) in rats and dogs (Feldman and Covino, 1988) and a slightly lower degree of motor blockade at equipotent doses (Butterworth, 2009). As for other LA agents, at clinical doses ropivacaine affects vascular tone; at concentrations below 0.5% it exhibits vasoconstrictive properties, and at concentrations over 1% it acts as a vasodilator (Cederholm et al., 1992), which will affect reabsorption and duration of action.

5. Special formulations

A number of special formulations of LA have been developed to allow penetration of intact skin layers or to maintain high concentrations of the drug at the target site for longer.

Eutectic mixtures in the form of creams and lotions for topical use may be used to desensitize the intact skin prior to IV catheterization, tattooing, or similar minimally invasive procedures. The main pharmacological feature of eutectic mixtures is that they melt at lower temperatures than their individual components, which results in higher concentrations of LA available at the target site. Typical eutectic formulations are made of oil emulsified into the water, have a melting point of 18°C and contain a thickener, an emulsifier, and distilled water adjusted to a pH level usually above 7.3 (Kumar et al., 2015). After application in a thick layer to intact skin, it is advised to cover the area with an occlusive dressing (e.g., plastic wrap) to facilitate penetration through the stratum corneum. The application of EMLA cream, comprised of lidocaine and prilocaine, improved analgesia in rabbits undergoing ear tattooing and in mice during tail vein injections (David et al., 2014; Keating et al., 2012). In guinea pigs, the topical use of two in-house prepared eutectic mixtures (lidocaine-tetracaine and lidocaine-prilocaine) was effective in preventing pinprick response (Ohzeki et al., 2008).

A number of studies investigated the use of encapsulated liposomal LA in laboratory rodents and pigs, with the purpose of achieving longer-lasting analgesia compared to the plain compounds, possibly with fewer adverse effects owing to the decreased rate of systemic absorption of the drug (da Silva et al., 2017; Kang et al., 2017; Shaw et al., 2018; Zel et al., 2019). Liposomes are carriers capable of retaining the molecules they are associated with at the injection site for a longer time by means of a sustained release mechanism (Weiniger et al., 2010). In mice, liposomal 2% ropivacaine resulted in plantar hind paw desensitization, assessed with the von Frey filaments, which lasted up to 9 h, compared to 5 h with plain ropivacaine (da Silva et al., 2017). In a model of electrical nociception, SC infiltration of encapsulated liposomal bupivacaine in mice increased the duration of analgesia by more than 4 times that of plain bupivacaine (Grant et al., 2000). Liposomal bupivacaine was also successfully used in rats to attenuate postsurgical incisions in a model of mechanical and thermal hypersensitivity (Kang et al., 2017).

6. Additives

Additives may be added to enhance the local effects of LA by decreasing their systemic absorption or to act synergistically with the LA to reduce local tissue inflammation and edema. Epinephrine is commonly used as an adjuvant to promote local vasoconstriction and therefore delay the systemic absorption of the LA of short-duration of action as lidocaine, which results in increased drug concentration at the target tissue and consequently prolongation of the duration of the analgesic effect. The addition of epinephrine to levobupivacaine has been described in rats (Korat & Kapupara, 2017, 2018), whilst in mice, in a model of radiant heat nociception, the addition of epinephrine extended the duration of cutaneous anesthesia provided by bupivacaine (Smith, 1997). Recently, vasopressin was used in addition to mepivacaine as a vasoconstrictor, for SC tail infiltration in mice (Katagiri et al., 2020).

Nonsteroidal antiinflammatory drugs may be used in association with LAs and vasoconstrictors for surgical wound infiltration, with the purpose of decreasing local inflammation that, ultimately, contributes to nociception and pain. In rats, SC infiltration with levobupivacaine, ibuprofen, and epinephrine improved postlaparotomy analgesia, as assessed by rodent grimace scale scoring, as well as angiogenesis and tensile strength of the wound after 3 weeks of infiltration (Korat and Kapupara, 2017). The same combination was successfully used to decrease post-laparotomy pain in rats (Korat and Kapupara, 2018).

7. Routes of administration

Topical administration of LA refers to the application of the drugs on the intact skin or mucous membranes, and implies that the drug penetrates the stratum corneum of the epidermis or the mucosal layers, respectively. The topical use of LA has been addressed earlier in this chapter.

For neuraxial use, including both intrathecal and epidural administrations, LA is often combined with other classes of analgesics, such as opioids, alpha-2 adrenoreceptor agonists, and ketamine, which act synergistically with the LA agents, enhancing the sensory block.

Infiltrations of LA are commonly performed to provide perioperative analgesia in laboratory animal species. Various techniques have been described, including simple peri-incisional SC infiltrations, periodontal, intra-testicular, and intra-articular injections, as well as more targeted injections in the proximity of specific peripheral nerves (Adami et al., 2011; Grant et al., 2000; Haga and Ranheim, 2005; Kang et al., 2017; Smith, 1997; Waite et al., 2010).

Intratesticular injections of LA, either alone or combined with intrafunicular LA administration, have been successfully used to provide perioperative analgesia in piglets (Haga and Ranheim, 2005; Lomax et al., 2017).

Intra-articular injections are commonly used, especially before or after experimental stifle surgeries, and have been widely described in rabbits and small ruminants (Krohm et al., 2011; Shafford et al., 2004; Yazdi et al., 2014). However, based on the occurrence of microscopic alterations in the articular cartilage, characterized by mild inflammation followed by fibrosis on the longer term in a murine model, careful usage of intra-articular bupivacaine and levobupivacaine is recommended (Kurkcuoglu et al., 2014).

More targeted peripheral nerve blocks are becoming an increasingly popular means to provide analgesia to laboratory animals during experimental orthopaedic procedures. The sciatic nerve block with LA, either alone or combined with a femoral block, has been described in laboratory rodents, rabbits, small ruminants, and pigs undergoing stifle surgery (Adami et al., 2011; Kim and Choi, 2019; Kluge et al., 2017; Lee et al., 2020; Feldman and Covino, 1988). In rats, sciatic nerve block with levobupivacaine helped to prevent fentanyl-induced hyperalgesia as well as spinal upregulation of proinflammatory cytokines after plantar incision (Chang et al., 2018). In both goats and New Zealand White rabbits undergoing experimental stifle arthrotomy, combined sciatic-femoral nerve block reduced the requirement of systemic analgesics and improved postoperative pain scores (Adami et al., 2011; Kluge et al., 2017).

Finally, there is a body of literature on the use of LA to relieve dental and buccal pain in rabbits and rodents (de Almeida et al., 2019; Hashimoto et al., 2014; Ohkado et al., 2001). Simple infiltrations of maxillary molars and targeted infraorbital nerve blocks, with both lidocaine and ropivacaine have been described in rats (de Almeida et al., 2019; Tateno et al., 2008; Yamashiro et al., 2016).

8. Tachyphylaxis

Tachyphylaxis to LA is defined as a decreased duration and/or intensity of the regional block despite repeated administration of the drug (Kottenberg-Assenmacher and Peters, 1999). In human patients, neither the chemical properties of the drug nor the technique or route of administration seem to play a role in determining tachyphylaxis, as the latter can occur with different compounds and after either neuraxial or peripheral nerve blocks (Bromage et al., 1969). Regarding neuraxial anesthesia, factors that could predispose to tachyphylaxis include altered distribution of LA within the epidural space after repeated injections, and increased local blood flow that could accelerate clearance of the drug from the epidural space (Bromage et al., 1969). With respect to tachyphylaxis occurring after local and regional nerve blocks, decreased tissue pH, which could limit the migration of LA to the target nerve structures, has been hypothesized as a possible mechanism of action. However, one study conducted in rats failed to demonstrate an effect of tissue pH on the development of tachyphylaxis to bupivacaine (Baker et al., 1991).

Data from murine models showed that drugs that prevent spinal hyperalgesia, namely NMDA receptor antagonists and NO-synthase inhibitors, also decrease the likelihood to develop tachyphylaxis (Lee et al., 1994). Therefore, it has been suggested that a spinal nitric oxide pathway may be at the origin of tachyphylaxis to LA (Wang et al., 2001).

Longer intervals between subsequent LA administrations leading to fluctuating levels of analgesia, agent switching, and central hyperalgesia, as evidenced by studies in rats, also seem to be associated with the development of tachyphylaxis (Bromage et al., 1969; Lee et al., 1994).

9. Adverse effects and toxicity

The nonspecific molecular targets of the LA are at the origin of some of their adverse and toxic effects on various organ systems (Scholz, 2002). Local anesthetics interfere with axonal Na^+ channels preferentially, but not exclusively, with the potential to also block voltage-dependent K^+ and L-type Ca^{2+} channels, as well as Na^+ channels, in the brain and heart. As a result, most of the clinically relevant adverse effects of LA are produced in the central nervous and cardiovascular systems.

Systemic neurotoxicity increases with the potency and lipid solubility of the specific agent, and ranges from depression of the central nervous system, commonly seen at lower doses, to excitation, potentially escalating to seizures. In rats, peripheral administration of analgesic doses of LA resulted in detectable concentrations of free drug in the brain, which was deemed sufficient to affect measurements of brain function during neurophysiological studies (Ferrari et al., 2010). In rodents, the systemic neurotoxicity of lidocaine is enhanced by pregnancy (Xu et al., 2013). Besides their systemic neurotoxicity, LA can also alter the homeostasis of peripheral nerve endings and myocytes, an effect potentially enhanced by the addition of vasoconstrictors as adjuvants (Yang et al., 2011; Yu et al., 2019; Zink and Graf, 2004).

In general, greater doses of LA are necessary to produce cardiovascular toxicity than neurotoxicity. Cardiovascular toxicity is a function of specific LA potency, with bupivacaine being the most cardiotoxic in murine models (Lim and Sohn, 2019). The cardiovascular effects of LA are complex and nonlinear. At neurotoxic doses, lidocaine typically causes ventricular tachyarrhythmias potentially escalating to ventricular fibrillation (Feldman et al., 1989). However, higher doses profoundly inhibit cardiac conduction, which results in bradyarrhythmia characterized by prolonged PR and QRS intervals, ultimately culminating in cardiac arrest (Feldman et al., 1989) (Chang et al., 2000).

The occurrence of methemoglobinemia, which is more likely in neonates, has been associated with prilocaine, procaine, lidocaine, and topical use of benzocaine (Severinghaus et al., 1991; Taleb et al., 2013; Rosso et al., 2021).

Owing to their ability to alter vascular tone and the nonphysiological pH of most formulations, concerns have been raised that LA may delay surgical wound healing, predisposing to infections. However, in a model of murine ovariectomy, intradermal infiltration of both lidocaine and bupivacaine did not delay wound healing (Waite et al., 2010).

III. Muscarinic antagonists

Muscarinic receptor antagonists (otherwise called parasympatholytic drugs) are competitive antagonists of Ach on the muscarinic cholinergic receptors. Various compounds belong to this class of drugs, although only atropine and glycopyrrolate play a relevant role in modern veterinary anesthesia. Both drugs are used to counteract unwanted parasympathetic effects of anesthetics/analgesics, to prevent bradycardia, promote bronchodilation, and reduce airway secretion.

A. Chemical structure

All the muscarinic receptor antagonists contain ester and basic groups in the same relationship as Ach, but they have an aromatic group in place of the acetyl group. Atropine and scopolamine have a lipid-soluble tertiary amine structure that easily crosses the blood-brain and the blood-placenta barriers. Glycopyrrolate is a quaternary ammonium compound, poorly lipid-soluble and therefore lacks of central actions (Proakis and Harris, 1978).

B. Mechanism of action

Atropine and glycopyrrolate exert their effects by competitively antagonizing Ach at postganglionic muscarinic receptors in the parasympathetic nervous system. Muscarinic receptors are members of the G-coupled receptor family, having seven transmembrane sequences in their amino acid sequence. Five muscarinic receptors (M1-M5) have been cloned, though only M1, M2, and M3 are well characterized (Dale and Haylett, 2009).

Both atropine and glycopyrrolate are relatively unselective in binding to receptor subtypes. However, different tissues show different responses to clinical doses of these drugs (see desired pharmacologic effects).

C. Compounds

1. Atropine

a. Biodistribution, metabolism, and excretion

Atropine is a racemic mixture of L and D-hyoscyamine, with the L-isomer being responsible for the majority of the drug's activity. Atropine is highly bioavailable after IM administration, as well as after endobronchial administration in dogs and humans. The onset of action of atropine in dogs is 1 min after IV administration and 5 min after IM or endobronchial administration (Paret et al., 1999). In experimental pigs, after IV and intraosseous (IO) administration, atropine reached peak plasma concentration immediately and had a very rapid distribution with no apparent absorption phase for the IO way, while peak plasma concentration and time to reach peak concentration were both significantly lower after IM injection. Hypovolemia increased the absorption time of IM administration but not of IV and IO administration (Yost et al., 2015). In dogs and humans, atropine is rapidly cleared from the central compartment via hydrolysis to inactive metabolites, with some (up to 27%) excreted unchanged by the kidneys. Due to large amount of atropine, a plasma esterase, some strains of rabbits have the ability to rapidly metabolize atropine-like compounds, rendering typical clinical doses ineffective. However, not all rabbits possess large amounts of this enzyme, hence its efficacy in some animals (Harrison and McLoon, 2006). Atropine is well absorbed by the ocular mucosa, and in horses, repeated administrations at less than 3 h of distance lead to plasma accumulation over 24 h (Strom et al., 2021).

b. Desired pharmacologic effects

Atropine is mainly used in premedication to counteract unwanted parasympathetic effects of other anesthetics, in particular to prevent bradycardia, and promote bronchodilation, and reduce airway secretion (via antagonism on M2 and M3 receptors). In monogastric species, anticholinergics are effective antisialogogues (via antagonism on M3 receptors). Anticholinergic effects in the heart are mediated by antagonist effects on pre and postsynaptic M2 receptors located in the sinoatrial and atrioventricular nodes, and in the atrial myocardiocytes. Atropine typically leads to an increase in sinus rate and atrio-ventricular conduction. Dose-dependent tachycardia is expected after the administration of atropine in dogs (Hendrix and Robinson, 1997).

c. Adverse pharmacologic effects

Even at clinical doses, tachycardia and tachyarrhythmias can occur. In conscious dogs, an IV dose of 0.04 mg/kg is reported to increase heart rate by 50% (Hendrix and Robinson, 1997). However, in subjects with high vagal tone (young or athletes) "excess tachycardia" may be encountered.

A transient, self-limiting bradycardia (so-called paradoxical bradycardia) may occur immediately after anticholinergic administration. In humans, it has been postulated that rapid blockade of presynaptic M1 receptors takes place with inhibition of the feedback mechanism and transient increase of Ach release (Wellstein and Pitschner, 1988). In dogs, it has been associated with low IV doses, and IM or SC administration (Rishniw et al., 1996). In sheep, previously treated with neuromuscular blocking agents, the administration of atropine at a high dose (0.08 mg/kg) induced bradycardia (Clutton and Glasby, 2008).

In ruminants, rather than inhibition of salivation, atropine causes an increase in saliva viscosity that can be detrimental as it can obstruct the airways.

Atropine can significantly reduce tear production in dogs and cats (Arnett et al., 1984; Ludders and Heavner, 1979).

A reduction of gastric antral motility has been demonstrated in experimental dogs, partially resolved by the administration of metoclopramide or cisapride.

2. Glycopyrrolate

a. Biodistribution, metabolism, and excretion

The highly polar quaternary ammonium group of glycopyrrolate limits its passage across lipid membranes. Therefore, its onset of action is slightly slower than that of atropine. The PK profile of glycopyrrolate has been widely investigated in humans, but not in veterinary species, with the exception of horses (Rumpler et al., 2014).

b. Desired pharmacologic effects

Glycopyrrolate is used with the same indications that atropine has.

c. Adverse pharmacologic effects

Glycopyrrolate was introduced in the 1960s as a potent, long-acting anticholinergic agent with fewer adverse effects in humans than atropine (McCubbin et al., 1979). However, when administered to sedated dogs, atropine and glycopyrrolate produced very similar cardiovascular effects (Skues et al., 1989). Gastrointestinal motility is decreased in dogs for up to 30 min, with the duration being dose-dependent in horses.

d. Clinical applications (to prevent or to treat, indications and risks)

Atropine and glycopyrrolate are mostly used to prevent or treat bradycardia associated with anesthesia and to prevent excessive airway secretions. Atropine is commonly used before the administration of cholinergic drugs such as neostigmine and edrophonium when reversing neuromuscular blockade. Additionally, atropine has historically been recommended during cardiopulmonary-cerebral resuscitation (CPR).

The administration of an anticholinergic drug as part of a patient's premedication should be based on a thorough knowledge of the drug's benefits and risks, taking into account the drugs to be coadministered, species, age, and disease status of the patient, and the procedure being performed (Lerche, 2015).

When administered to counteract bradycardia after the administration of α2-adrenergic agonists, antimuscarinic drugs are often effective at increasing heart rate initially (also causing severe hypertension and potentially cardiac arrhythmias), but they are often less effective in the later phases. For an exhaustive review of the effects of antimuscarinics administered to dogs and cats with α-2 agonists, we refer the reader to (Sinclair et al., 2003).

IV. Conclusion

Sedatives, tranquilizers, local anesthetics, and antimuscarinics all contribute to multimodal and balanced anesthesia and analgesia and play an important role in the daily clinical and laboratory veterinary practice. The pharmacological information provided in this chapter should help the veterinarian and the interested reader to understand the species-specific clinical effects and adverse effects of these drugs and support the clinical decision-making in which is the right drug or drug combination for the animal to be anesthetized.

References

Aantaa, R., Marjamäki, A., Scheinin, M., August 1995. Molecular pharmacology of alpha 2-adrenoceptor subtypes. Ann. Med. 27 (4), 439–449. https://doi.org/10.3109/07853899709002452.

Abendschon, N., Senf, S., Deffner, P., Miller, R., Grott, A., Werner, J., Saller, A.M., Reiser, J., Weiss, C., Zablotski, Y., Fischer, J., Bergmann, S., Erhard, M.H., Baumgartner, C., Ritzmann, M., Zols, S., September 26, 2020. Local anesthesia in piglets undergoing castration-A comparative study to investigate the analgesic effects of four local anesthetics based on defensive behavior and side effects. Animals 10 (10). https://doi.org/10.3390/ani10101752.

Adam, M., Raekallio, M.R., Salla, K.M., Honkavaara, J.M., Mannikko, S., Scheinin, M., Kajula, M., Molsa, S.H., Vainio, O.M., September 2018. Effects of the peripherally acting alpha2-adrenoceptor antagonist MK-467 on cardiopulmonary function in sheep sedated by intramuscular administration of medetomidine and ketamine and reversed by intramuscular administration of atipamezole. Am. J. Vet. Res. 79 (9), 921–932. https://doi.org/10.2460/ajvr.79.9.921.

Adami, C., Bergadano, A., Bruckmaier, R.M., Stoffel, M.H., Doherr, M.G., Spadavecchia, C., April 2011. Sciatic-femoral nerve block with bupivacaine in goats undergoing elective stifle arthrotomy. Vet. J. 188 (1), 53–57. https://doi.org/10.1016/j.tvjl.2010.02.008.

Allegri, M., Bugada, D., De Gregori, M., Avanzini, M.A., De Silvestri, A., Petroni, A., Sala, A., Filisetti, C., Icaro Cornaglia, A., Cobianchi, L., 2017. Continuous wound infusion with chloroprocaine in a pig model of surgical lesion: drug absorption and effects on inflammatory response. J. Pain Res. 10, 2515–2524. https://doi.org/10.2147/JPR.S139856.

Arnett, B.D., Brightman 2nd, A.H., Musselman, E.E., July 15, 1984. Effect of atropine sulfate on tear production in the cat when used with ketamine hydrochloride and acetylpromazine maleate. J. Am. Vet. Med. Assoc. 185 (2), 214–215.

Arras, M., Autenried, P., Rettich, A., Spaeni, D., Rulicke, T., October 2001. Optimization of intraperitoneal injection anesthesia in mice: drugs, dosages, adverse effects, and anesthesia depth. Comp. Med. 51 (5), 443–456.

Bailey, R.S., Barter, L.S., Pypendop, B.H., July 2017. Pharmacokinetics of dexmedetomidine in isoflurane-anesthetized New Zealand White rabbits. Vet. Anaesth. Analg. 44 (4), 876–882. https://doi.org/10.1016/j.vaa.2017.01.003.

Baker, C.E., Berry, R.L., Elston, R.C., June 1991. Effect of pH of bupivacaine on duration of repeated sciatic nerve blocks in the albino rat. Local Anesthetics for Neuralgia Study Group. Anesth. Analg. 72 (6), 773–778. https://doi.org/10.1213/00000539-199106000-00010.

Baumgartner, C., Bollerhey, M., Ebner, J., Schuster, T., Henke, J., Erhardt, W., October 2010. Effects of medetomidine-midazolam-fentanyl IV bolus injections and its reversal by specific antagonists on cardiovascular function in rabbits. Can. J. Vet. Res. 74 (4), 286–298. https://www.ncbi.nlm.nih.gov/pubmed/21197229.

Bellini, L., Banzato, T., Contiero, B., Zotti, A., 2014. Evaluation of three medetomidine-based protocols for chemical restraint and sedation for non-painful procedures in companion rats (Rattus norvegicus). Vet. J. 200 (3), 456–458. https://doi.org/10.1016/j.tvjl.2014.03.024. https://www.sciencedirect.com/science/article/pii/S1090023314001245.

Bloor, B.C., Abdul-Rasool, I., Temp, J., Jenkins, S., Valcke, C., Ward, D.S., 1989. The effects of medetomidine, an alpha 2-adrenergic agonist, on ventilatory drive in the dog. Acta Vet. Scand. Suppl. 85, 65–70. https://www.ncbi.nlm.nih.gov/pubmed/2571280.

Boehm, C.A., Carney, E.L., Tallarida, R.J., Wilson, R.P., November 2010. Midazolam enhances the analgesic properties of dexmedetomidine in the rat. Vet. Anaesth. Analg. 37 (6), 550–556. https://doi.org/10.1111/j.1467-2995.2010.00565.x.

Bouchenafa, O., Livingston, A., May 1987. Autoradiographic localisation of alpha 2 adrenoceptor binding sites in the spinal cord of the sheep. Res. Vet. Sci. 42 (3), 382–386. https://www.ncbi.nlm.nih.gov/pubmed/2887016.

Boyes, R.N., February 1975. A review of the metabolism of amide local anesthetic agents. Br. J. Anaesth. 47 (Suppl. l), 225–230. https://www.ncbi.nlm.nih.gov/pubmed/1096919.

Bromage, P.R., Pettigrew, R.T., Crowell, D.E., 1969. Tachyphylaxis in epidural analgesia: I. Augmentation and decay of local anesthesia. J. Clin. Pharmacol. J. N. Drugs 9 (1), 30–38. https://www.ncbi.nlm.nih.gov/pubmed/5250310.

Brown, C., Donnelly, M., 2011. Disease Problems of Small Rodents. Ferrets, Rabbits, and Rodents, pp. 354–372.

Browning, S., Lawrence, D., Livingston, A., Morris, B., November 1982. Interactions of drugs active at opiate receptors and drugs active at alpha 2-receptors on various test systems. Br. J. Pharmacol. 77 (3), 487–491. https://doi.org/10.1111/j.1476-5381.1982.tb09322.x.

Buerkle, H., Yaksh, T.L., August 1998. Pharmacological evidence for different alpha 2-adrenergic receptor sites mediating analgesia and sedation in the rat. Br. J. Anaesth. 81 (2), 208–215. https://doi.org/10.1093/bja/81.2.208.

Buitrago, S., Martin, T.E., Tetens-Woodring, J., Belicha-Villanueva, A., Wilding, G.E., January 2008. Safety and efficacy of various combinations of injectable anesthetics in BALB/c mice. J. Am. Assoc. Lab. Anim. Sci. 47 (1), 11–17.

Butterworth, J.,F., 2009. Clinical pharmacology of local anesthetics. In: Cousins, M.J., Carr, D.B., Horlocker, T.T., Bridenbaugh, E. (Eds.), Cousins & Bridenbaugh's Neural Blockade in Clinical Anesthesia and Pain Medicine, fourth ed. Lippincott Williams & Wilkins, pp. 96–113.

Bylund, D.B., May 1985. Heterogeneity of alpha-2 adrenergic receptors. Pharmacol. Biochem. Behav. 22 (5), 835–843. https://doi.org/10.1016/0091-3057(85)90536-2.

Caracas, H.C., Maciel, J.V., Martins, P.M., de Souza, M.M., Maia, L.C., February 2009. The use of lidocaine as an anti-inflammatory substance: a systematic review. J. Dent. 37 (2), 93–97. https://doi.org/10.1016/j.jdent.2008.10.005.

Carroll, G.L., Hartsfield, S.M., Champney, T.H., Geller, S.C., Martinez, E.A., Haley, E.L., May 2005. Effect of medetomidine and its antagonism with atipamezole on stress-related hormones, metabolites, physiologic responses, sedation, and mechanical threshold in goats. Vet. Anaesth. Analg. 32 (3), 147–157. https://doi.org/10.1111/j.1467-2995.2005.00187.x.

Cederholm, I., Evers, H., Lofstrom, J.B., 1992. Skin blood flow after intradermal injection of ropivacaine in various concentrations with and without epinephrine evaluated by laser Doppler flowmetry. Reg. Anesth. 17 (6), 322–328. https://www.ncbi.nlm.nih.gov/pubmed/1286053.

Chang, D.H., Ladd, L.A., Wilson, K.A., Gelgor, L., Mather, L.E., September 2000. Tolerability of large-dose intravenous levobupivacaine in sheep. Anesth. Analg. 91 (3), 671–679. https://doi.org/10.1097/00000539-200009000-00033.

Chang, L., Ye, F., Luo, Q., Wang, Z., Wang, Y., Xia, Z., Shu, H., May 13, 2018. Effects of three forms of local anesthesia on perioperative fentanyl-induced hyperalgesia. Biosci Trends 12 (2), 177–184. https://doi.org/10.5582/bst.2018.01037.

Chenery, R.J., Ayrton, A., Oldham, H.G., Standring, P., Norman, S.J., Seddon, T., Kirby, R., 1987. Diazepam metabolism in cultured hepatocytes from rat, rabbit, dog, Guinea pig, and man. Drug Metab. Dispos. 15 (3), 312–317. https://www.ncbi.nlm.nih.gov/pubmed/2886305.

Chiu, C.C., Chen, J.Y., Chen, Y.W., Wang, J.J., Hung, C.H., October 5, 2019. Subcutaneous brompheniramine for cutaneous analgesia in rats. Eur. J. Pharmacol. 860, 172544. https://doi.org/10.1016/j.ejphar.2019.172544.

Cirstea, M., Suhaciu, G., Cirje, M., 1984. Spontaneous formation of immunogenic conjugates by 3-hydroxy-para-aminobenzoic acid—a biotransformation product of procaine and para-aminobenzoic acid. Physiologie 21 (1), 25–31. https://www.ncbi.nlm.nih.gov/pubmed/6424148.

Clarke, K., Trim, C.M., 2013. Veterinary Anaesthesia, 11th Edition - June 28, 2013 ed. Saunders.

Clineschmidt, B.V., Pettibone, D.J., Lotti, V.J., Hucker, H.B., Sweeney, B.M., Reiss, D.R., Lis, E.V., Huff, J.R., Vacca, J., April 1988. A peripherally acting alpha-2 adrenoceptor antagonist - L-659,066. J. Pharmacol. Exp. Therapeut. 245 (1), 32–40.

Clutton, R.E., Glasby, M.A., May 2008. Cardiovascular and autonomic nervous effects of edrophonium and atropine combinations during neuromuscular blockade antagonism in sheep. Vet. Anaesth. Analg. 35 (3), 191–200. https://doi.org/10.1111/j.1467-2995.2007.00374.x.

Costa, G.P., Monteiro, E.R., Marques É, J., Beck, R.C., Carneiro, R.K., da Costa, F.V., Valle, S.F., June 2021. Sedative effects of acepromazine in combination with nalbuphine or butorphanol, intramuscularly or intravenously, in healthy cats: a randomized, blinded clinical trial. J. Feline Med. Surg. 23 (6), 540–548. https://doi.org/10.1177/1098612x20962754.

Court, M.H., Greenblatt, D.J., December 1992. Pharmacokinetics and preliminary observations of behavioral changes following administration of midazolam to dogs. J. Vet. Pharmacol. Therapeut. 15 (4), 343–350. https://doi.org/10.1111/j.1365-2885.1992.tb01026.x.

Covino, B.G., July 1986. Pharmacology of local anesthetic agents. Br. J. Anaesth. 58 (7), 701–716. https://doi.org/10.1093/bja/58.7.701.

da Silva, C.M.G., Franz-Montan, M., Limia, C.E.G., Ribeiro, L.N.M., Braga, M.A., Guilherme, V.A., da Silva, C.B., Casadei, B.R., Cereda, C.M.S., de Paula, E., 2017. Encapsulation of ropivacaine in a combined (donor-acceptor, ionic-gradient) liposomal system promotes extended anesthesia time. PLoS One 12 (10), e0185828. https://doi.org/10.1371/journal.pone.0185828.

Dale, M.M., Haylett, D.G., 2009. Muscarinic receptors. In: Pharmacology Condensed, 2 ed. Elsevier (Churchill Livingstone).

David, J.M., Vogel, S.D., Longo, K., Sanchez, D., Lawson, G., November 2014. The use of eutectic mixture of lidocaine and prilocaine in mice (*Mus musculus*) for tail vein injections. Vet. Anaesth. Analg. 41 (6), 654–659. https://doi.org/10.1111/vaa.12177.

Davis, J.A., Greenfield, R.E., Brewer, T.G., August 1993. Benzocaine-induced methemoglobinemia attributed to topical application of the anesthetic in several laboratory-animal species. Am. J. Vet. Res. 54 (8), 1322–1326.

de Almeida, A.C.P., Pinto, L.M.A., Alves, G.P., Ribeiro, L.N.D., Santana, M.H.A., Cereda, C.M.S., Fraceto, L.F., de Paula, E., 2019. Liposomal-based lidocaine formulation for the improvement of infiltrative buccal anaesthesia. J. Liposome Res. 29 (1), 66–72. https://doi.org/10.1080/08982104.2018.1483947.

Donovan, J., Brown, P., 1998. Anesthesia. Curr. Protoc. Im. 27 (1). https://doi.org/10.1002/0471142735.im0104s27, 1.4.1–1.4.5.

Doss, G.A., Fink, D.M., Mans, C., December 2018. Assessment of sedation after intranasal administration of midazolam and midazolam-butorphanol in cockatiels (*Nymphicus hollandicus*). Am. J. Vet. Res. 79 (12), 1246–1252. https://doi.org/10.2460/ajvr.79.12.1246.

Dzikiti, T.B., Zeiler, G.E., Dzikiti, L.N., Garcia, E.R., August 19, 2014. The effects of midazolam and butorphanol, administered alone or combined, on the dose and quality of anaesthetic induction with alfaxalone in goats. J. S. Afr. Vet. Assoc. 85 (1), 1047. https://doi.org/10.4102/jsava.v85i1.1047.

Feldman, H.S., Arthur, G.R., Covino, B.G., December 1989. Comparative systemic toxicity of convulsant and supraconvulsant doses of IV ropivacaine, bupivacaine, and lidocaine in the conscious dog. Anesth. Analg. 69 (6), 794–801.

Feldman, H.S., Covino, B.G., 1988. Comparative motor-blocking effects of bupivacaine and ropivacaine, a new amino amide local anesthetic, in the rat and dog. Anesth. Analg. 67 (11), 1047–1052.

Ferrari, L., Crestan, V., Sabattini, G., Vinco, F., Fontana, S., Gozzi, A., February 15, 2010. Brain penetration of local anaesthetics in the rat: implications for experimental neuroscience. J. Neurosci. Methods 186 (2), 143–149. https://doi.org/10.1016/j.jneumeth.2009.11.005.

Feyh, L.S., 1993. The chemistry and pharmacology of local anesthetics. CRNA Clin. Forum Nurse Anesth. 4 (4), 161–169.

File, S.E., 1990, Summer. The history of benzodiazepine dependence: a review of animal studies. Neurosci. Biobehav. Rev. 14 (2), 135–146. https://doi.org/10.1016/s0149-7634(05)80214-3.

Fleischmann, T., Jirkof, P., Henke, J., Arras, M., Cesarovic, N., August 2016. Injection anaesthesia with fentanyl-midazolam-medetomidine in adult female mice: importance of antagonization and perioperative care. Lab. Anim. 50 (4), 264–274. https://doi.org/10.1177/0023677216631458.

Furutani, K., Koma, M., Ishii, H., Baba, H., Kohno, T., January 2010. Bupivacaine inhibits glutamatergic transmission in spinal dorsal horn neurons. Anesthesiology 112 (1), 138–143. https://doi.org/10.1097/01.anes.0000365964.97138.9a.

Garcia-Villar, R., Toutain, P.L., Alvinerie, M., Ruckebusch, Y., June 1981. The pharmacokinetics of xylazine hydrochloride: an interspecific study. J. Vet. Pharmacol. Therapeut. 4 (2), 87–92. https://doi.org/10.1111/j.1365-2885.1981.tb00715.x.

Gerecke, M., 1983. Chemical structure and properties of midazolam compared with other benzodiazepines. Br. J. Clin. Pharmacol. 16 (Suppl. 1), 11S–16S. https://doi.org/10.1111/j.1365-2125.1983.tb02266.x.

Ghaffari, M.S., Moghaddassi, A.P., Bokaie, S., 2009. Effects of intramuscular acepromazine and diazepam on tear production in rabbits. Vet. Rec. 164 (5), 147–148. https://doi.org/10.1136/vr.164.5.147.

Gnuechtel, M.M., Schenk, L.L., Postma, G.N., June 2000. Late effects of topical anesthetics on the healing of Guinea pig tympanic membranes after myringotomy. Arch. Otolaryngol. Head Neck Surg. 126 (6), 733–735. https://doi.org/10.1001/archotol.126.6.733.

Gonzalez-Gil, A., Villa, A., Millan, P., Martinez-Fernandez, L., Illera, J.C., May 2015. Effects of dexmedetomidine and ketamine-dexmedetomidine with and without buprenorphine on corticoadrenal function in rabbits. J. Am. Assoc. Lab. Anim. Sci. 54 (3), 299–303. https://www.ncbi.nlm.nih.gov/pubmed/26045456.

Graham, C.W., Pagano, R.R., Katz, R.L., 1977. Thrombophlebitis after IV diazepam–can it be prevented? Anesth. Analg. 56 (3), 409–413. https://doi.org/10.1213/00000539-197705000-00020.

Grant, G.J., Piskoun, B., Lin, A., Bansinath, M., 2000. An in vivo method for the quantitative evaluation of local anesthetics. J. Pharmacol. Toxicol. Methods 43 (1), 69–72. https://doi.org/10.1016/s1056-8719(00)00079-4.

Grint, N.J., Murison, P.J., March 2008. A comparison of ketamine-midazolam and ketamine-medetomidine combinations for induction of anaesthesia in rabbits. Vet. Anaesth. Analg. 35 (2), 113–121. https://doi.org/10.1111/j.1467-2995.2007.00362.x.

Guertler, A.T., Lagutchik, M.S., Martin, D.G., February 1992. Topical anesthetic-induced methemoglobinemia in sheep: a comparison of benzocaine and lidocaine. Fund. Appl. Toxicol. 18 (2), 294–298. https://doi.org/10.1016/0272-0590(92)90058-p.

Haga, H.A., Ranheim, B., January 2005. Castration of piglets: the analgesic effects of intratesticular and intrafunicular lidocaine injection. Vet. Anaesth. Analg. 32 (1), 1–9. https://doi.org/10.1111/j.1467-2995.2004.00225.x.

Hall, L.W., Clarke, K.W., Trim, C.M., 2001. General pharmacology of the injectable agents in anaesthesia. In: Saunders, W.B. (Ed.), Veterinary Anesthesia 10th Ed, 10 ed. Harcourt Publishers, pp. 75–91. 113–132.

Harrison, A.R., McLoon, L.K., May 29, 2006. Reduction in touch sensitivity and hyperinnervation in vesicant-injured rabbit eyelid by direct injection of corticotropin releasing factor. Neurosci. Lett. 400 (1–2), 30–34. https://doi.org/10.1016/j.neulet.2006.02.023.

Hashimoto, S., Yamashiro, M., Fujita, K., Yasuda, A., Sunada, K., September 2014. Effects of epinephrine on lidocaine pharmacokinetics and blood volume in the dental pulp. J. Endod. 40 (9), 1370–1374. https://doi.org/10.1016/j.joen.2014.02.029.

Haskins, S.C., Patz, J.D., Farver, T.B., March 1986. Xylazine and xylazine-ketamine in dogs. Am. J. Vet. Res. 47 (3), 636–641. https://www.ncbi.nlm.nih.gov/pubmed/3963565.

Hauptman, K., Jekl, V., Knotek, Z., December 2003. Use of medetomidine for sedation in the laboratory rats (*Rattus norvegicus*). Acta Vet. 72 (4), 583–591. https://doi.org/10.2754/avb200372040583.

Hayami, A., Darwish, W.S., Ikenaka, Y., Nakayama, S.M., Ishizuka, M., February 2013. In vitro diazepam metabolism in horses. Jpn. J. Vet. Res. 61 (Suppl. 1), S82–S84. https://www.ncbi.nlm.nih.gov/pubmed/23631163.

He, S., Atkinson, C., Qiao, F., Chen, X., Tomlinson, S., January 2010. Ketamine-xylazine-acepromazine compared with isoflurane for anesthesia during liver transplantation in rodents. J. Am. Assoc. Lab. Anim. Sci. 49 (1), 45–51.

Hendrix, P.K., Robinson, E.P., October 1997. Effects of a selective and a nonselective muscarinic cholinergic antagonist on heart rate and intestinal motility in dogs. J. Vet. Pharmacol. Therapeut. 20 (5), 387–395. https://doi.org/10.1046/j.1365-2885.1997.00084.x.

Hieble, J.P., Bondinell, W.E., Ruffolo Jr., R.R., September 1, 1995. Alpha- and beta-adrenoceptors: from the gene to the clinic. 1. Molecular biology and adrenoceptor subclassification. J. Med. Chem. 38 (18), 3415–3444. https://doi.org/10.1021/jm00018a001.

Hikasa, Y., Akiba, T., Iino, Y., Matsukura, M., Takase, K., Ogasawara, S., 1992a. Central alpha-adrenoceptor subtypes involved in the emetic pathway in cats. Eur. J. Pharmacol. 229 (2–3), 241–251.

Hikasa, Y., Ogasawara, S., Takase, K., 1992b. Alpha adrenoceptor subtypes involved in the emetic action in dogs. J. Pharmacol. Exp. Therapeut. 261 (2), 746–754.

Holtman Jr., J.R., Jing, X., Sloan, J.W., Wala, E.P., 2003. The effects of flumazenil on the antinociceptive actions of morphine in rats. Recept. Channel 9 (5), 325–328. https://doi.org/10.3109/713745175.

Honkavaara, J., Pypendop, B., Turunen, H., Ilkiw, J., January 2017. The effect of MK-467, a peripheral alpha2-adrenoceptor antagonist, on dexmedetomidine-induced sedation and bradycardia after IV administration in conscious cats. Vet. Anaesth. Analg. 44 (1), 42–51. https://doi.org/10.1111/vaa.12385.

Honkavaara, J.M., Raekallio, M.R., Kuusela, E.K., Hyvarinen, E.A., Vainio, O.M., September 2008. The effects of L-659,066, a peripheral alpha 2-adrenoceptor antagonist, on dexmedetomidine-induced sedation and bradycardia in dogs. Vet. Anaesth. Analg. 35 (5), 409–413. https://doi.org/10.1111/j.1467-2995.2008.00403.x.

Honkavaara, J.M., Restitutti, F., Raekallio, M.R., Kuusela, E.K., Vainio, O.M., August 2011. The effects of increasing doses of MK-467, a peripheral alpha(2)-adrenergic receptor antagonist, on the cardiopulmonary effects of intravenous dexmedetomidine in conscious dogs. J. Vet. Pharmacol. Therapeut. 34 (4), 332–337. https://doi.org/10.1111/j.1365-2885.2010.01242.x.

Hoyt Jr., R.F., Hayre, M.D., Dodd, K.T., Phillips, Y.Y., August 1986. Long-acting intramuscular anesthetic regimen for swine. Lab. Anim. Sci. 36 (4), 413–416.

Hubbell, J.A., Aarnes, T.K., Lerche, P., Bednarski, R.M., April 2012. Evaluation of a midazolam-ketamine-xylazine infusion for total IV anesthesia in horses. Am. J. Vet. Res. 73 (4), 470–475. https://doi.org/10.2460/ajvr.73.4.470.

Interlandi, C., Calapai, G., Nastasi, B., Mannucci, C., Morici, M., Costa, G.L., 2017. Effects of atipamezole on the analgesic activity of butorphanol in rats. J. Exot. Pet Med. 26 (4), 290–293. https://doi.org/10.1053/j.jepm.2017.07.001.

Izer, J.M., Whitcomb, T.L., Wilson, R.P., 2014. Atipamezole reverses ketamine-dexmedetomidine anesthesia without altering the antinociceptive effects of butorphanol and buprenorphine in female C57BL/6J mice. JAALAS 53 (6), 675–683.

Janssen, C.F., Maiello, P., Wright Jr., M.J., Kracinovsky, K.B., Newsome, J.T., 2017. Comparison of Atipamezole with Yohimbine for Antagonism of Xylazine in Mice Anesthetized with Ketamine and Xylazine. JAALAS 56 (2), 142–147.

Kaartinen, J., Pang, D., Moreau, M., Vainio, O., Beaudry, F., del Castillo, J., Lamont, L., Cuvelliez, S., Troncy, E., 2010, Spring. Hemodynamic effects of an intravenous infusion of medetomidine at six different dose regimens in isoflurane-anesthetized dogs. Vet. Therapeut. 11 (1), E1–E16. https://www.ncbi.nlm.nih.gov/pubmed/20949427.

Kang, S.C., Jampachaisri, K., Seymour, T.L., Felt, S.A., Pacharinsak, C., January 1, 2017. Use of liposomal bupivacaine for postoperative analgesia in an incisional pain model in rats (*Rattus norvegicus*). J. Am. Assoc. Lab .Anim. Sci. 56 (1), 63–68. https://www.ncbi.nlm.nih.gov/pubmed/28905717.

Kastner, S.B., March 2006. A2-agonists in sheep: a review. Vet. Anaesth. Analg. 33 (2), 79–96. https://doi.org/10.1111/j.1467-2995.2005.00243.x.

Katagiri, K., Hashimoto, S., Sunda, K., October 2020. Effect of vasopressin as a local anesthetic in mice. Odontology 108 (4), 626–635. https://doi.org/10.1007/s10266-020-00491-2.

Kaur, P., Kim, K., November 19, 2008. Pharmacokinetics and brain uptake of diazepam after intravenous and intranasal administration in rats and rabbits. Int. J. Pharm. 364 (1), 27–35. https://doi.org/10.1016/j.ijpharm.2008.07.030.

Keating, S.C.J., Thomas, A.A., Flecknell, P.A., Leach, M.C., September 7, 2012. Evaluation of EMLA cream for preventing pain during tattooing of rabbits: changes in physiological, behavioural and facial expression responses. PLoS One 7 (9). https://doi.org/10.1371/journal.pone.0044437.

Khan, Z.P., Ferguson, C.N., Jones, R.M., February 1999. alpha-2 and imidazoline receptor agonists. Their pharmacology and therapeutic role. Anaesthesia 54 (2), 146–165. https://doi.org/10.1046/j.1365-2044.1999.00659.x.

Kim, J.M., Choi, S.H., 2019. Reversing effect of insulin on local anesthetics-induced sciatic nerve block in rats. BioMed Res. Int. 2019, 4252349. https://doi.org/10.1155/2019/4252349.

Kleine, S.A., Quandt, J.E., Hofmeister, E.H., Peroni, J., April 2015. The effect of midazolam on the recovery quality, recovery time and the minimum alveolar concentration for extubation in the isoflurane-anesthetized pig. Lab. Anim. 49 (2), 111–116. https://doi.org/10.1177/0023677214556668.

Kluge, K., Larenza Menzies, M.P., Kloeppel, H., Pearce, S.G., Bettschart-Wolfensberger, R., Kutter, A.P., February 2017. Femoral and sciatic nerve blockades and incision site infiltration in rabbits undergoing stifle joint arthrotomy. Lab. Anim. 51 (1), 54–64. https://doi.org/10.1177/0023677215622734.

Ko, J.C.H., Fox, S.M., Mandsager, R.E., May 15, 2000. Sedative and cardiorespiratory effects of medetomidine, medetomidine-butorphanol, and medetomidine-ketamine in dogs. J. Am. Vet. Med. Assoc. 216 (10), 1578–1583. https://doi.org/10.2460/javma.2000.216.1578.

Korat, P.S., Kapupara, P., June 1, 2018. Analgesic effect of local infiltration of the surgical wound containing levobupivacaine, ibuprofen, and epinephrine in rats undergoing laparotomy. Folia Med. (Plovdiv) 60 (2), 254–260. https://doi.org/10.1515/folmed-2017-0096.

Korat, P.S., Kapupara, P.P., December 2017. Local infiltration of the surgical wound with levobupivacaine, ibuprofen, and epinephrine in postoperative pain: an experimental study. Biomed. Pharmacother. 96, 104–111. https://doi.org/10.1016/j.biopha.2017.09.131.

Kottenberg-Assenmacher, E., Peters, J., December 1999. Mechanisms of tachyphylaxis in regional anesthesia of long duration. Anasthesiol. Intensivmed. Notfallmed. Schmerzther. 34 (12), 733–742.

Krohm, P., Levionnois, O., Ganster, M., Zilberstein, L., Spadavecchia, C., July 2011. Antinociceptive activity of pre- versus post-operative intra-articular bupivacaine in goats undergoing stifle arthrotomy. Vet. Anaesth. Analg. 38 (4), 363–373. https://doi.org/10.1111/j.1467-2995.2011.00623.x.

Ku, W.H., Schneider, S.P., November 2011. Multiple T-type Ca2+ current subtypes in electrophysiologically characterized hamster dorsal horn neurons: possible role in spinal sensory integration. J. Neurophysiol. 106 (5), 2486–2498. https://doi.org/10.1152/jn.01083.2010.

KuKanich, B., Nauss, J.L., June 2012. Pharmacokinetics of the cytochrome P-450 substrates phenytoin, theophylline, and diazepam in healthy Greyhound dogs. J. Vet. Pharmacol. Therapeut. 35 (3), 275–281. https://doi.org/10.1111/j.1365-2885.2011.01316.x.

Kumar, M., Chawla, R., Goyal, M., 2015. Topical anesthesia. J. Anaesthesiol. Clin. Pharmacol. 31 (4), 450–456. https://doi.org/10.4103/0970-9185.169049.

Kurabe, M., Furue, H., Kohno, T., May 18, 2016. Intravenous administration of lidocaine directly acts on spinal dorsal horn and produces analgesic effect: an in vivo patch-clamp analysis. Sci. Rep. 6, 26253. https://doi.org/10.1038/srep26253.

Kurabe, M., Furue, H., Kohno, T., June 1, 2017. Corrigendum: IV administration of lidocaine directly acts on spinal dorsal horn and produces analgesic effect: an in vivo patch-clamp analysis. Sci. Rep. 7, 46814. https://doi.org/10.1038/srep46814.

Kurkcuoglu, B.S., Donmez, M., Altinel, S., Akinci, S.B., Saricaoglu, F., Aypar, U., 2014. Comparison of intraarticular bupivacaine and levobupivacaine injection in rat synovial inflammation. Turk. J. Med. Sci. 44 (4), 540–545. https://doi.org/10.3906/sag-1302-32.

Kuusela, E., Raekallio, M., Anttila, M., Falck, I., Molsa, S., Vainio, O., 2000. Clinical effects and pharmacokinetics of medetomidine and its enantiomers in dogs. J. Vet. Pharmacol. Therapeut. 23 (1), 15–20.

Kuusela, E., Raekallio, M., Vaisanen, M., Mykkanen, K., Ropponen, H., Vainio, O., July 2001. Comparison of medetomidine and dexmedetomidine as premedicants in dogs undergoing propofol-isoflurane anesthesia. Am. J. Vet. Res. 62 (7), 1073–1080. https://doi.org/10.2460/ajvr.2001.62.1073.

Lacoste, L., Bouquet, S., Ingrand, P., Caritez, J.C., Carretier, M., Debaene, B., January 2000. Intranasal midazolam in piglets: pharmacodynamics (0.2 vs 0.4 mg/kg) and pharmacokinetics (0.4 mg/kg) with bioavailability determination. Lab. Anim. 34 (1), 29–35. https://doi.org/10.1258/002367700780578073.

Lamont, L.A., Bulmer, B.J., Grimm, K.A., Tranquilli, W.J., Sisson, D.D., November 2001. Cardiopulmonary evaluation of the use of medetomidine hydrochloride in cats. Am. J. Vet. Res. 62 (11), 1745–1749. https://doi.org/10.2460/ajvr.2001.62.1745.

Lavoie, J.P., Pascoe, J.R., Kurpershoek, C.J., June 1992. Effects of xylazine on ventilation in horses. Am. J. Vet. Res. 53 (6), 916–920. https://www.ncbi.nlm.nih.gov/pubmed/1626781.

Lee, K.C., Wilder, R.T., Smith, R.L., Berde, C.B., November 1994. Thermal hyperalgesia accelerates and MK-801 prevents the development of tachyphylaxis to rat sciatic nerve blockade. Anesthesiology 81 (5), 1284–1293. https://doi.org/10.1097/00000542-199411000-00024.

Lee, M.G., Choi, S.U., Lim, J.K., Lee, M.J., Hong, J.S., Baek, M.O., Yoon, S.Z., Park, H.Y., Shin, H.J., August 2020. Ultrasound-guided sciatic nerve block at the midthigh level in a porcine model: a descriptive study. Vet. Med. Sci. 6 (3), 543–549. https://doi.org/10.1002/vms3.265.

Lerche, P., 2015. Anticholinergics. In: Grimm, K.A., Lamont, L.A., Tranquilli, W.J., Greene, S.A., Robertson, S.A. (Eds.), Veterinary Anaesthesia and Analgesia, the 5th Edition of Lumb and Jones. Wiley Blackwell, pp. 178–182.

Li, Y.M., Wingrove, D.E., Too, H.P., Marnerakis, M., Stimson, E.R., Strichartz, G.R., Maggio, J.E., January 1995. Local-anesthetics inhibit substance-P binding and evoked increases in intracellular Ca2+. Anesthesiology 82 (1), 166–173. https://doi.org/10.1097/00000542-199501000-00021.

Lim, D.H., Sohn, J.T., April 2019. Bupivacaine-induced cardiotoxicity and lipid emulsion. Hum. Exp. Toxicol. 38 (4), 494–495. https://doi.org/10.1177/0960327118819042.

Lipman, N.S., Marini, R.P., Erdman, S.E., July 1990. A comparison of ketamine/xylazine and ketamine/xylazine/acepromazine anesthesia in the rabbit. Lab. Anim. Sci. 40 (4), 395–398.

Lipscombe, D., Kongsamut, S., Tsien, R.W., August 24, 1989. Alpha-adrenergic inhibition of sympathetic neurotransmitter release mediated by modulation of N-type calcium-channel gating. Nature 340 (6235), 639–642. https://doi.org/10.1038/340639a0.

Lomax, S., Harris, C., Windsor, P.A., White, P.J., November 15, 2017. Topical anaesthesia reduces sensitivity of castration wounds in neonatal piglets. PLoS One 12 (11). https://doi.org/10.1371/journal.pone.0187988.

López, K.R., Gibbs, P.H., Reed, D.S., March 2002. A comparison of body temperature changes due to the administration of ketamine-acepromazine and tiletamine-zolazepam anesthetics in cynomolgus macaques. Contemp. Top. Lab. Anim. Sci. 41 (2), 47–50.

Loscher, W., Frey, H.H., December 1981. Pharmacokinetics of diazepam in the dog. Arch. Int. Pharmacodyn. Ther. 254 (2), 180–195. https://www.ncbi.nlm.nih.gov/pubmed/7337498.

Ludders, J.W., Heavner, J.E., September 15, 1979. Effect of atropine on tear formation in anesthetized dogs. J. Am. Vet. Med. Assoc. 175 (6), 585–586. https://www.ncbi.nlm.nih.gov/pubmed/511754.

MacDonald, E., Scheinin, M., Scheinin, H., Virtanen, R., November 1991. Comparison of the behavioral and neurochemical effects of the two optical enantiomers of medetomidine, a selective alpha-2-adrenoceptor agonist. J. Pharmacol. Exp. Therapeut. 259 (2), 848–854. https://www.ncbi.nlm.nih.gov/pubmed/1682487.

Malinowski, C.M., Cameron, A.I., Burnside, W.M., West, S.E., Nunamaker, E.A., 2019. Butorphanol-azaperone-medetomidine for the immobilization of rhesus macaques (*Macaca mulatta*). JAALAS 58 (3), 346–355. https://doi.org/10.30802/AALAS-JAALAS-18-000088.

McConnell, J., Kirby, R., Rudloff, E., 2007. Administration of acepromazine maleate to 31 dogs with a history of seizures. J. Vet. Emerg. Crit. Care 17 (3), 262–267. https://doi.org/10.1111/j.1476-4431.2007.00231.x.

McCubbin, T.D., Brown, J.H., Dewar, K.M., Jones, C.J., Spence, A.A., September 1979. Glycopyrrolate as a premedicant: comparison with atropine. Br. J. Anaesth. 51 (9), 885–889. https://doi.org/10.1093/bja/51.9.885.

Mees, L., Fidler, J., Kreuzer, M., Fu, J., Pardue, M.T., García, P.S., 2018. Faster emergence behavior from ketamine/xylazine anesthesia with atipamezole versus yohimbine. PLoS One 13 (10), e0199087. https://doi.org/10.1371/journal.pone.0199087.

Mikkelsen, M.L.G., Ambrus, R., Rasmussen, R., Miles, J.E., Poulsen, H.H., Moltke, F.B., Eriksen, T., May 3, 2017. The effect of dexmedetomidine on cerebral perfusion and oxygenation in healthy piglets with normal and lowered blood pressure anaesthetized with propofol-remifentanil total intravenous anaesthesia. Acta Vet. Scand. 59. https://doi.org/10.1186/s13028-017-0293-0.

Murison, P., Clutton, R., Blissitt, K., Funnell, O., 2003. Blood pressure and electrocardiographic effects of acepromazine in anaesthetized horses. Vet. Anaesth. Analg. 30 (2), 94–95. https://doi.org/10.1046/j.1467-2995.2003.00132_11.x.

Murrell, J.C., Hellebrekers, L.J., May 2005. Medetomidine and dexmedetomidine: a review of cardiovascular effects and antinociceptive properties in the dog. Vet. Anaesth. Analg. 32 (3), 117–127. https://doi.org/10.1111/j.1467-2995.2005.00233.x.

Musk, G.C., Wilkes, G.J., 2018. Sedation of sheep following the administration of acepromazine with buprenorphine or morphine is similar. Res. Vet. Sci. 118, 41–42. https://doi.org/10.1016/j.rvsc.2018.01.013.

Nagy, I., Woolf, C.J., January 1996. Lignocaine selectively reduces C fibre-evoked neuronal activity in rat spinal cord in vitro by decreasing N-methyl-D-aspartate and neurokinin receptor-mediated post-synaptic depolarizations; Implications for the development of novel centrally acting analgesics. Pain 64 (1), 59–70. https://doi.org/10.1016/0304-3959(95)00072-0.

Nakayama, S.M., Ikenaka, Y., Hayami, A., Mizukawa, H., Darwish, W.S., Watanabe, K.P., Kawai, Y.K., Ishizuka, M., October 2016. Characterization of equine cytochrome P450: role of CYP3A in the metabolism of diazepam. J. Vet. Pharmacol. Therapeut. 39 (5), 478–487. https://doi.org/10.1111/jvp.12303.

Nishimura, L.T., Villela, I.O.J., Carvalho, L.L., Borges, L.P.B., Silva, M.A.M., Mattos-Junior, E., 2017. The effect of acepromazine alone or in combination with methadone, morphine, or tramadol on sedation and selected cardiopulmonary variables in sheep. Vet. Med. Int. 2017. https://doi.org/10.1155/2017/7507616, 7507616-7507616.

Ohkado, S., Ichinohe, T., Kaneko, Y., 2001, Winter. Comparative study on anesthetic potency depending on concentrations of lidocaine and epinephrine: assessment of dental local anesthetics using the jaw-opening reflex. Anesth. Prog. 48 (1), 16–20. https://www.ncbi.nlm.nih.gov/pubmed/11495400.

Ohzeki, K., Kitahara, M., Suzuki, N., Taguchi, K., Yamazaki, Y., Akiyama, S., Takahashi, K., Kanzaki, Y., April 2008. Local anesthetic cream prepared from lidocaine-tetracaine eutectic mixture. Yakugaku Zasshi 128 (4), 611–616. https://doi.org/10.1248/yakushi.128.611.

Olson, M.E., Renchko, P., June 1988. Azaperone and azaperone-ketamine as a neuroleptic sedative and anesthetic in rats and mice. Lab. Anim. Sci. 38 (3), 299–304.

Pagel, P.S., Hettrick, D.A., Kersten, J.R., Warltier, D.C., September 1998. Dexmedetomidine produces similar alterations in the determinants of left ventricular afterload in conscious dogs before and after the development of pacing-induced cardiomyopathy. Anesthesiology 89 (3), 741–748. https://doi.org/10.1097/00000542-199809000-00026.

Paret, G., Mazkereth, R., Sella, R., Almog, S., Mayan, H., Lotan, D., Ben-Abraham, R., Barzilay, Z., Ezra, D., June 1999. Atropine pharmacokinetics and pharmacodynamics following endotracheal versus endobronchial administration in dogs. Resuscitation 41 (1), 57–62. https://doi.org/10.1016/s0300-9572(99)00031-3.

Parry, B.W., Anderson, G.A., Gay, C.C., November 1982. Hypotension in the horse induced by acepromazine maleate. Aust. Vet. J. 59 (5), 148–152. https://doi.org/10.1111/j.1751-0813.1982.tb02761.x.

Pascoe, P.J., July 2015. The cardiopulmonary effects of dexmedetomidine infusions in dogs during isoflurane anesthesia. Vet. Anaesth. Analg. 42 (4), 360–368. https://doi.org/10.1111/vaa.12220.

Pertovaara, A., Kauppila, T., Tukeva, T., April 25, 1990. The effect of medetomidine, an alpha 2-adrenoceptor agonist, in various pain tests. Eur. J. Pharmacol. 179 (3), 323–328. https://doi.org/10.1016/0014-2999(90)90172-3.

Pieri, L., 1983. Preclinical pharmacology of midazolam. Br. J. Clin. Pharmacol. 16 (Suppl. 1), 17S–27S. https://doi.org/10.1111/j.1365-2125.1983.tb02267.x.

Platt, S.R., Randell, S.C., Scott, K.C., Chrisman, C.L., Hill, R.C., Gronwall, R.R., June 2000. Comparison of plasma benzodiazepine concentrations following intranasal and IV administration of diazepam to dogs. Am. J. Vet. Res. 61 (6), 651–654. https://doi.org/10.2460/ajvr.2000.61.651.

Plumb, D.C., 2018. Plumb's Veterinary Drug Handbook: Desk, ninth ed. ed. Wiley-Blackwell.

Proakis, A.G., Harris, G.B., May 1978. Comparative penetration of glycopyrrolate and atropine across the blood–brain and placental barriers in anesthetized dogs. Anesthesiology 48 (5), 339–344. https://doi.org/10.1097/00000542-197805000-00007.

Pypendop, B.H., Honkavaara, J., Ilkiw, J.E., October 2016. Pharmacokinetics of dexmedetomidine, MK-467, and their combination following intravenous administration in male cats. J. Vet. Pharmacol. Therapeut. 39 (5), 460–468. https://doi.org/10.1111/jvp.12302.

Pypendop, B.H., Ilkiw, J.E., Robertson, S.A., January 2006. Effects of IV administration of lidocaine on the thermal threshold in cats. Am. J. Vet. Res. 67 (1), 16–20. https://doi.org/10.2460/ajvr.67.1.16.

Pypendop, B.H., Verstegen, J.P., 1998. Hemodynamic effects of medetomidine in the dog: a dose titration study. Vet. Surg. 27 (6), 612–622. https://doi.org/10.1111/j.1532-950X.1998.tb00539.x.

Radde, G.R., Hinson, A., Crenshaw, D., Toth, L.A., July 1996. Evaluation of anaesthetic regimens in guineapigs. Lab. Anim. 30 (3), 220–227. https://doi.org/10.1258/002367796780684935.

Rangel, J.P.P., Monteiro, E.R., Bitti, F.S., Junior, J.S.N., Campagnol, D., 2020. Hemodynamic, respiratory and sedative effects of progressively increasing doses of acepromazine in conscious dogs. Vet. Anaesth. Analg. 47 (4), 447–453. https://doi.org/10.1016/j.vaa.2020.02.007.

Ranheim, B., Horsberg, T.E., Soli, N.E., Ryeng, K.A., Arnemo, J.M., December 2000. The effects of medetomidine and its reversal with atipamezole on plasma glucose, cortisol and noradrenaline in cattle and sheep. J. Vet. Pharmacol. Therapeut. 23 (6), 379–387. https://doi.org/10.1046/j.1365-2885.2000.00291.x.

Rankin, D.C., 2015. Sedative and tranquillizers. In: Grimm, K.A., Lamont, L.A., Tranquilli, W.J., Greene, S.A., Robertson, S.A. (Eds.), Veterinary Anesthesia and Analgesia, the 5th of Lumb and Jones, fifth ed., vol. 1. Wiley-Blackwell, p. 1072.

Raulic, J., Leung, V.S., Doss, G.A., Graham, J.E., Keller, K.A., Mans, C., Sadar, M.J., Vergneau-Grosset, C., Pang, D.S., August 24, 2021. Development and testing of a sedation scale for use in rabbits (*Oryctolagus cuniculus*). J. Am. Assoc. Lab. Anim. Sci. 60, 549–555. https://doi.org/10.30802/aalas-jaalas-21-000002.

Ren, J., Li, C., Ma, S., Wu, J., Yang, Y., April 2018. Impact of dexmedetomidine on hemodynamics in rabbits. Acta Cir. Bras. 33 (4), 314–323. https://doi.org/10.1590/s0102-865020180040000003.

Restitutti, F., Honkavaara, J.M., Raekallio, M.R., Kuusela, E.K., Vainio, O.M., September 2011. Effects of different doses of L-659'066 on the bispectral index and clinical sedation in dogs treated with dexmedetomidine. Vet. Anaesth. Analg. 38 (5), 415–422. https://doi.org/10.1111/j.1467-2995.2011.00630.x.

Riebold, T.W., 2007. Ruminants. In: Tranquilli, W.G., Thurmonn, G.C., Green, K.A. (Eds.), Lumb's and Jones Veterinary Anaesthesia and Analgesia, fourth ed. Blackwell Publishing.

Rishniw, M., Tobias, A.H., Slinker, B.K., March 1996. Characterization of chronotropic and dysrhythmogenic effects of atropine in dogs with bradycardia. Am. J. Vet. Res. 57 (3), 337–341. https://www.ncbi.nlm.nih.gov/pubmed/8669765.

Rolfe, N.G., Kerr, C.L., McDonell, W.N., May 2012. Cardiopulmonary and sedative effects of the peripheral alpha2-adrenoceptor antagonist MK 0467 administered IVly or intramuscularly concurrently with medetomidine in dogs. Am. J. Vet. Res. 73 (5), 587–594. https://doi.org/10.2460/ajvr.73.5.587.

Rosen, M.R., Hoffman, B.F., Wit, A.L., April 1975. Electrophysiology and pharmacology of cardiac arrhythmias. V. Cardiac antiarrhythmic effects of lidocaine. Am. Heart J. 89 (4), 526–536. https://doi.org/10.1016/0002-8703(75)90162-3.

Rosso, C.D., Thomas, A., Hardy, N., Connelly, S., Davila, U., Pearce, J., Mazor, S., Burns, R., January 28, 2021. Pediatric toxidrome simulation curriculum: lidocaine-induced methemoglobinemia. Med EdPORTAL 17, 11089. https://doi.org/10.15766/mep_2374-8265.11089.

Rousseau-Blass, F., Cribb, A.E., Beaudry, F., Pang, D.S., May 1, 2021. A pharmacokinetic-pharmacodynamic study of intravenous midazolam and flumazenil in adult New Zealand white-californian rabbits (*Oryctolagus cuniculus*). J. Am. Assoc. Lab. Anim. Sci. 60 (3), 319–328. https://doi.org/10.30802/aalas-jaalas-20-000084.

Rozette, N.A., Matragoon, S., Sethi, S., Goei, S., Manasco, K.B., El-Remessy, A.B., 2014. Systemic effects of ophthalmic cyclopentolate on body weight in neonatal mice. Neonatology 106 (1), 37–41. https://doi.org/10.1159/000358228.

Ruffolo Jr., R.R., Bondinell, W., Hieble, J.P., September 15, 1995. Alpha- and beta-adrenoceptors: from the gene to the clinic. 2. Structure-activity relationships and therapeutic applications. J. Med. Chem. 38 (19), 3681–3716. https://doi.org/10.1021/jm00019a001.

Rumpler, M.J., Colahan, P., Sams, R.A., June 2014. The pharmacokinetics of glycopyrrolate in Standardbred horses. J. Vet. Pharmacol. Therapeut. 37 (3), 260–268. https://doi.org/10.1111/jvp.12085.

Salla, K., Restitutti, F., Vainionpaa, M., Junnila, J., Honkavaara, J., Kuusela, E., Raekallio, M., Vainio, O., November 2014. The cardiopulmonary effects of a peripheral alpha-2-adrenoceptor antagonist, MK-467, in dogs sedated with a combination of medetomidine and butorphanol. Vet. Anaesth. Analg. 41 (6), 567–574. https://doi.org/10.1111/vaa.12158.

Salonen, M., Onaivi, E.S., Maze, M., 1992a. Dexmedetomidine synergism with midazolam in the elevated plus-maze test in rats. Psychopharmacology (Berl) 108 (1–2), 229–234.

Salonen, M., Reid, K., Maze, M., 1992b. Synergistic interaction between alpha 2-adrenergic agonists and benzodiazepines in rats. Anesthesiology 76 (6), 1004–1011.

Schmitt, P., Eclancher, F., Karli, P., February 1974. Topographic analysis of areas of negative and positive reinforcement in the central grey matter of the rat (author's transl). Physiol. Behav. 12 (2), 271–279.

Schnellbacher, R.W., Divers, S.J., Comolli, J.R., Beaufrere, H., Maglaras, C.H., Andrade, N., Barbur, L.A., Rosselli, D.D., Stejskal, M., Barletta, M., Mayer, J., Rodriguez, P., Quandt, J.E., December 2017. Effects of IV administration of lidocaine and buprenorphine on gastrointestinal tract motility and signs of pain in New Zealand White rabbits after ovariohysterectomy. Am. J. Vet. Res. 78 (12), 1359–1371. https://doi.org/10.2460/ajvr.78.12.1359.

Scholz, A., July 2002. Mechanisms of (local) anaesthetics on voltage-gated sodium and other ion channels. Br. J. Anaesth. 89 (1), 52–61. https://doi.org/10.1093/bja/aef163.

Schroeder, C.A., Smith, L.J., March 2011. Respiratory rates and arterial blood-gas tensions in healthy rabbits given buprenorphine, butorphanol, midazolam, or their combinations. J. Am. Assoc. Lab. Anim. Sci. 50 (2), 205–211. https://www.ncbi.nlm.nih.gov/pubmed/21439214.

Schwartz, M., Munana, K.R., Nettifee-Osborne, J.A., Messenger, K.M., Papich, M.G., October 2013. The pharmacokinetics of midazolam after IV, intramuscular, and rectal administration in healthy dogs. J. Vet. Pharmacol. Therapeut. 36 (5), 471–477. https://doi.org/10.1111/jvp.12032.

Seddon, T., Michelle, I., Chenery, R.J., May 15, 1989. Comparative drug metabolism of diazepam in hepatocytes isolated from man, rat, monkey and dog. Biochem. Pharmacol. 38 (10), 1657–1665. https://doi.org/10.1016/0006-2952(89)90314-6.

Severinghaus, J.W., Xu, F.D., Spellman Jr., M.J., February 1991. Benzocaine and methemoglobin: recommended actions. Anesthesiology 74 (2), 385–387. https://doi.org/10.1097/00000542-199102000-00039.

Shafford, H.L., Hellyer, P.W., Turner, A.S., January 2004. Intra-articular lidocaine plus bupivacaine in sheep undergoing stifle arthrotomy. Vet. Anaesth. Analg. 31 (1), 20–26. https://doi.org/10.1111/j.1467-2995.2004.00126.x.

Shaw, K.A., Moreland, C., Jacobs, J., Hire, J.M., Topolski, R., Hoyt, N., Parada, S.A., Cameron, C.D., January 2018. Improved chondrotoxic profile of liposomal bupivacaine compared with standard bupivacaine after intra-articular infiltration in a porcine model. Am. J. Sports Med. 46 (1), 66–71. https://doi.org/10.1177/0363546517732558.

Short, C.E., Jones, R.S., Tintle, L.M., 1984. Anaesthetic management of major facial trauma in dogs. Br Vet. J. 140 (2), 169–180. https://doi.org/10.1016/0007-1935(84)90077-0. PMID: 6722504.

Shucard, D.W., Andrew, M., Beauford, C., March 1975. A safe and fast-acting surgical anesthetic for use in the Guinea pig. J. Appl. Physiol. 38 (3), 538–539. https://doi.org/10.1152/jappl.1975.38.3.538.

Siegenthaler, J., Pleyers, T., Raillard, M., Spadavecchia, C., Levionnois, O.L., July 2020. Effect of medetomidine, dexmedetomidine, and their reversal with atipamezole on the nociceptive withdrawal reflex in Beagles. Animals 10 (7). https://doi.org/10.3390/ani10071240.

Simon, B.T., Scallan, E.M., Siracusa, C., Henderson, A., Sleeper, M.M., Larenza Menzies, M.P., September 2014. Effects of acepromazine or methadone on midazolam-induced behavioral reactions in dogs. Can. Vet. J. 55 (9), 875–885. https://www.ncbi.nlm.nih.gov/pubmed/25183896.

Sinclair, M.D., O'Grady, M.R., Kerr, C.L., McDonell, W.N., October 2003. The echocardiographic effects of romifidine in dogs with and without prior or concurrent administration of glycopyrrolate. Vet. Anaesth. Analg. 30 (4), 211–219. https://doi.org/10.1046/j.1467-2995.2003.00122.x.

Sirmpilatze, N., Baudewig, J., Boretius, S., November 13, 2019. Temporal stability of fMRI in medetomidine-anesthetized rats. Sci. Rep. 9. https://doi.org/10.1038/s41598-019-53144-y.

Skues, M.A., Richards, M.J., Jarvis, A.P., Prys-Roberts, C., September 1989. Preinduction atropine or glycopyrrolate and hemodynamic changes associated with induction and maintenance of anesthesia with propofol and alfentanil. Anesth. Analg. 69 (3), 386–390. https://www.ncbi.nlm.nih.gov/pubmed/2505642.

Smith, A.C., Zellner, J.L., Spinale, F.G., Swindle, M.M., April 1991. Sedative and cardiovascular effects of midazolam in swine. Lab. Anim. Sci. 41 (2), 157–161. https://www.ncbi.nlm.nih.gov/pubmed/1658445.

Smith, F.L., 1997. Regional cutaneous differences in the duration of bupivacaine local anesthesia in mice. Life Sci. 60 (18), 1613–1621. https://doi.org/10.1016/s0024-3205(97)00128-8.

Stenberg, D., 1989. Physiological role of alpha 2-adrenoceptors in the regulation of vigilance and pain: effect of medetomidine. Acta Vet. Scand. Suppl. 85, 21–28. https://www.ncbi.nlm.nih.gov/pubmed/2571274.

Strom, L., Dalin, F., Domberg, M., Stenlund, C., Bondesson, U., Hedeland, M., Toutain, P.L., Ekstrand, C., April 7, 2021. Topical ophthalmic atropine in horses, pharmacokinetics and effect on intestinal motility. BMC Vet. Res. 17 (1), 149. https://doi.org/10.1186/s12917-021-02847-4.

Taleb, M., Ashraf, Z., Valavoor, S., Tinkel, J., October 2013. Evaluation and management of acquired methemoglobinemia associated with topical benzocaine use. Am. J. Cardiovasc. Drugs 13 (5), 325–330. https://doi.org/10.1007/s40256-013-0027-2.

Tan, K.R., Rudolph, U., Luscher, C., April 2011. Hooked on benzodiazepines: GABAA receptor subtypes and addiction. Trends Neurosci. 34 (4), 188–197. https://doi.org/10.1016/j.tins.2011.01.004.

Tateno, K., Inoue, K., Sato, T., Fukayama, H., August 2008. Differences in the degree of infiltration of local anesthesia according to the site of injection in rats. Oral Surg. Oral Med. Oral Pathol. Oral Radiol. Endod. 106 (2), E6–E10. https://doi.org/10.1016/j.tripleo.2008.03.034.

Tobin, T., Ballard, S., 1979. Pharmacology review - phenothiazine tranquilizers. J. Equine Med. Surg. 3 (10), 460–466.

Torfs, S., Delesalle, C., Dewulf, J., Devisscher, L., Deprez, P., 2009. Risk factors for equine postoperative ileus and effectiveness of prophylactic lidocaine. J. Vet. Intern. Med. 23 (3), 606–611. https://doi.org/10.1111/j.1939-1676.2009.0311.x.

Torre, D.L., Falorni, A., 2007. Pharmacological causes of hyperprolactinemia. Therapeut. Clin. Risk Manag. 3 (5), 929–951.

Trevor, A.J., Katzung, B.G., Kruidering-Hall, M., 2015. Adrenoceptor blockers. In: Katzung & Trevor's Pharmacology: Examination & Board Review. McGraw-Hill Education.

Tsukamoto, A., Iimuro, M., Sato, R., Yamazaki, J., Inomata, T., 2015. Effect of midazolam and butorphanol premedication on inhalant isoflurane anesthesia in mice. Exp. Anim. 64 (2), 139–145. https://doi.org/10.1538/expanim.14-0073.

Uggla, A., Lindqvist, A., July 9, 1983. Acute pulmonary oedema as an adverse reaction to the use of xylazine in sheep. Vet. Rec. 113 (2), 42. https://doi.org/10.1136/vr.113.2.42.

Vainio, O.M., Bloor, B.C., Kim, C., December 1992. Cardiovascular effects of a ketamine-medetomidine combination that produces deep sedation in Yucatan mini swine. Lab. Anim. Sci. 42 (6), 582–588. https://www.ncbi.nlm.nih.gov/pubmed/1479811.

van Beusekom, C.D., van den Heuvel, J.J., Koenderink, J.B., Russel, F.G., Schrickx, J.A., December 2015. Feline hepatic biotransformation of diazepam: differences between cats and dogs. Res. Vet. Sci. 103, 119–125. https://doi.org/10.1016/j.rvsc.2015.09.016.

Virtanen, R., 1986. Pharmacology of detomidine and other alpha 2-adrenoceptor agonists in the brain. Acta Vet. Scand. Suppl. 82, 35–46. https://www.ncbi.nlm.nih.gov/pubmed/2876607.

Virtanen, R., Savola, J.M., Saano, V., Nyman, L., May 20, 1988. Characterization of the selectivity, specificity and potency of medetomidine as an alpha 2-adrenoceptor agonist. Eur. J. Pharmacol. 150 (1–2), 9–14. https://doi.org/10.1016/0014-2999(88)90744-3.

Von Tungeln, L.S., Zhou, T., Woodling, K.A., Doerge, D.R., Greenlees, K.J., Beland, F.A., October 2011. Benzocaine-induced methemoglobinemia in an acute-exposure rat model. Food Chem. Toxicol. 49 (10), 2530–2535. https://doi.org/10.1016/j.fct.2011.06.048.

Vree, T.B., Baars, A.M., Hekster, Y.A., van der Kleijn, E., O'Reilly, W.J., April 11, 1979. Simultaneous determination of diazepam and its metabolies N-desmethyldiazepam, oxydiazepam and oxazepam in plasma and urine of man and dog by means of high-performance liquid chromatography. J. Chromatogr. 162 (4), 605–614. https://doi.org/10.1016/s0378-4347(00)81842-3.

Waite, A., Gilliver, S.C., Masterson, G.R., Hardman, M.J., Ashcroft, G.S., June 2010. Clinically relevant doses of lidocaine and bupivacaine do not impair cutaneous wound healing in mice. Br. J. Anaesth. 104 (6), 768–773. https://doi.org/10.1093/bja/aeq093.

Wang, C., Sholas, M.G., Berde, C.B., DiCanzio, J., Zurakowski, D., Wilder, R.T., September 2001. Evidence that spinal segmental nitric oxide mediates tachyphylaxis to peripheral local anesthetic nerve block. Acta Anaesthesiol. Scand. 45 (8), 945–953. https://doi.org/10.1034/j.1399-6576.2001.450805.x.

Weiniger, C.F., Golovanevski, M., Sokolsky-Papkov, M., Domb, A.J., 2010. Review of prolonged local anesthetic action. Exp. Opin. Drug Deliv. 7 (6), 737–752. https://doi.org/10.1517/17425241003767383.

Welberg, L.A., Kinkead, B., Thrivikraman, K., Huerkamp, M.J., Nemeroff, C.B., Plotsky, P.M., March 2006. Ketamine-xylazine-acepromazine anesthesia and postoperative recovery in rats. J. Am. Assoc. Lab. Anim. Sci. 45 (2), 13–20.

Wellstein, A., Pitschner, H.F., July 1988. Complex dose-response curves of atropine in man explained by different functions of M1- and M2-cholinoceptors. Naunyn-Schmiedeberg's Arch. Pharmacol. 338 (1), 19–27. https://doi.org/10.1007/bf00168807.

Wieck, A., Haddad, P.M., March 2003. Antipsychotic-induced hyperprolactinaemia in women: pathophysiology, severity and consequences. Selective literature review. Br. J. Psychiatry 182, 199–204. https://doi.org/10.1192/bjp.182.3.199.

Xu, F., Zhang, B.X., Li, T.Z., August 2013. The neurotoxicity of intrathecal lidocaine is enhanced in postpartum compared to virgin rats. Fund. Clin. Pharmacol. 27 (4), 427–433. https://doi.org/10.1111/j.1472-8206.2012.01034.x.

Yamashiro, M., Hashimoto, S., Yasuda, A., Sunada, K., 2016, Summer. Epinephrine affects pharmacokinetics of ropivacaine infiltrated into palate. Anesth. Prog. 63 (2), 71–79. https://doi.org/10.2344/0003-3006-63.2.71.

Yang, S., Abrahams, M.S., Hurn, P.D., Grafe, M.R., Kirsch, J.R., 2011. Local anesthetic Schwann cell toxicity is time and concentration dependent. Reg. Anesth. Pain Med. 36 (5), 444–451. https://doi.org/10.1097/AAP.0b013e318228c835.

Yazdi, H., Nimavard, B.T., Shokrgozar, M., Dehghan, M., Moayedi, R.J., Majidi, M., Mokhtari, T., December 2014. An evaluation of the delayed effect of intra-articular injections of lidocaine (2%) on articular cartilage: an experimental study in rabbits. Eur. J. Orthop. Surg. Traumatol. 24 (8), 1557–1561. https://doi.org/10.1007/s00590-014-1437-9.

Yost, J., Baldwin, P., Bellenger, S., Bradshaw, F., Causapin, E., Demotica, R., Livingston, M., Lee, C., Gegel, B., Burgert, J., Claessens, A., Johnson, D., Loughren, M., 2015. Autumn. The pharmacokinetics of intraosseous atropine in hypovolemic swine. Am. J. Disaster Med. 10 (3), 217–222. https://doi.org/10.5055/ajdm.2015.0204.

Yu, Z.Y., Geng, J., Li, Z.Q., Sun, Y.B., Wang, S.L., Masters, J., Wang, D.X., Guo, X.Y., Li, M., Ma, D., January 2019. Dexmedetomidine enhances ropivacaine-induced sciatic nerve injury in diabetic rats. Br. J. Anaesth. 122 (1), 141–149. https://doi.org/10.1016/j.bja.2018.08.022.

Zel, J., Hadzic, A., Cvetko, E., Seliskar, A., Damjanovska, M., Kuroda, M.M., Sega Jazbec, S., Stopar Pintaric, T., March 2019. Neurological and histological outcomes after subarachnoid injection of a liposomal bupivacaine suspension in pigs: a pilot study. Br. J. Anaesth. 122 (3), 379–387. https://doi.org/10.1016/j.bja.2018.10.025.

Zhang, J., Niu, S., Zhang, H., Streisand, J.B., April 2002. Oral mucosal absorption of midazolam in dogs is strongly pH dependent. J. Pharmacol. Sci. 91 (4), 980–982. https://doi.org/10.1002/jps.10079.

Zhao, J., Zhang, Y., Liu, W., Chen, Y., Chang, D., Zhang, X., Chang, T., Wang, Q., Liu, T., Gao, L., August 14, 2019. Molecular mechanisms of the sedation and analgesia induced by xylazine on Wistar rats and PC12 cell. Exp. Anim. 68 (3), 351–360. https://doi.org/10.1538/expanim.18-0167.

Zink, W., Graf, B.M., 2004. Local anesthetic myotoxicity. Reg. Anesth. Pain Med. 29 (4), 333–340. https://doi.org/10.1016/j.rapm.2004.02.008.

Chapter 6

Inhalant anesthetics and safety

Cholawat Pacharinsak[1], Patrick Sharp[2] and C. Tyler Long[3]

[1]*Department of Comparative Medicine, Stanford University, Stanford, CA, United States;* [2]*Office of Research and Economic Development, Merced, CA, United States;* [3]*BD Technology Innovation (BDTI), Durham, NC, United States*

Chapter outline

I. Veterinary pharmacology of inhalation anesthetics

A. Introduction

Inhalant gas anesthesia is an indispensable tool for veterinarians and animal researchers. Both rodent and large animal anesthesia rely heavily on the use of inhalants due to their unique chemical properties, physiology, delivery methods, and metabolism. Three of the most common inhalant anesthetics utilized in veterinary medicine are isoflurane, sevoflurane, and desflurane. These inhalants have all but replaced methoxyflurane (MOF) and halothane that were introduced in the 1960s but have since discontinued production in the United States. This chapter will focus on the use of isoflurane, sevoflurane, and desflurane in regards to pharmacology, anesthetic delivery systems, induction of anesthesia, and waste anesthetic gas (WAG) safety. Other inhalants will be briefly discussed for comparison.

Despite having many advantages to their use, some inherent disadvantages to the use of inhalants exist and must be considered when devising a patient's anesthetic protocol (Table 6.1). In certain instances, injectable anesthetics may be preferred for induction and maintenance of general anesthesia. For example, a pulmonary imaging

Anesthesia and Analgesia in Laboratory Animals. https://doi.org/10.1016/B978-0-12-822215-7.00011-1

TABLE 6.1 Pros and cons of inhalant anesthesia use in veterinary patients.

Pros	Cons
Accurate control of anesthetic depth	Not suitable as sole agent for large animal inductions
Rapid induction and recoveries	Rapid anesthetic depth changes can lead to complications
Ability to provide oxygen supplementation	Requires personnel training
Can be combined with injectable anesthetics and analgesics	Lack of analgesic properties
Allows for reproducible, accurate measurements for research purposes	Requires purchase and maintenance of expensive and bulky equipment (anesthesia machine, vaporizers, tanks, breathing circuits)
Constant infusion (inhalation) amenable to short and long procedures	Can be environmental pollutant and occupational health hazard if not scavenged properly

study may require patient breath holds, and therefore an appropriate level of anesthesia cannot be maintained with inhalants alone. In addition, if waste gas elimination is not possible or precise control of the anesthetic level is not needed then injectable anesthetics may be a more practical alternative. However, once the decision has been made to perform inhalant anesthesia, there are certain characteristics that make an "ideal" inhalant anesthetic and include (Eger, 2004; Jones, 1990):

1. Stable molecular structure making it resistant to physical and metabolic degradation. It should have a long shelf life and not react with alkali or soda lime.
2. Low solubility in blood and tissues as blood gas/solubility will determine rapid induction and recovery from anesthetic.
3. Nonflammable and nonexplosive with air, oxygen (O_2), or nitrous oxide (N_2O).
4. High potency allowing delivery with the administration of high concentrations of O_2.
5. Nonirritating to inhale and allow for smooth induction and recovery.
6. Cardiovascular and respiratory system side effects should be minimal, while central nervous system effects reversible and nonstimulating.
7. Compatible with other drugs.
8. Low acquisition cost and readily obtainable.
9. Easily delivered and able to be scavenged in a safe manner.

Regardless of anesthesia method, hypothermia and corneal desiccation develops rapidly requiring appropriate prevention with the prompt use of an exogenous heat source that circumvents burns and an eye lubricant application, respectively.

B. Chemical and physical properties

Several of the characteristics that make an inhalant "ideal" can be attributed to their chemical and physical properties, which are summarized in Table 6.2 for select inhalant anesthetics. All the inhalants listed in Table 6.2, except N_2O, are vapors which means they exist in a liquid state at room temperature and at sea level normal atmospheric pressure (760 mmHg). Therefore, they must be converted into gaseous form prior to delivery to the patient's alveoli. It is common practice to describe vapors and gases in terms of their percent concentration, as this is how vaporizers are calibrated for anesthetic delivery. A less common method is to quantify them by molecular weight.

1. Vapor pressure, maximum percent concentration, and molecular weight

Vapor pressure is a measure of the volatility of the gas or vapor and is defined as the maximum pressure that can be produced by the agent at a given temperature and pressure. Vapor pressure divided by atmospheric pressure gives the maximum percent concentration of anesthetic vapor that can be produced. For instance, sevoflurane has a vapor pressure of 160 mmHg at sea level, barometric pressure of 760 mmHg, and normal room temperature of 20°C. Sevoflurane's maximum percent concentration would then be 21% ($160/760 \times 100 = 21\%$), whereas MOF with a vapor pressure of 22.5 mmHg under similar conditions would have a maximum percent concentration of 3%. When using a bell jar or anesthetic chamber with liquid anesthetic, the partial pressure (concentration) of the anesthetic is at maximum percent concentration, which is why using highly potent inhalants with low blood/gas solubility, such as sevoflurane, in this setting can be very dangerous to the patient. On the other hand, since MOF has a much lower maximum percent concentration, its use would be less dangerous in terms of the percent concentration inhaled by the patient.

Since the more commonly used inhalants have similar molecular weights, the amount of vapor produced in 1 mL of liquid is also similar for sevoflurane, isoflurane, and desflurane. This allows us to determine how much liquid

TABLE 6.2 Chemical and physical properties of select inhalant anesthetics.

Property	Isoflurane	Sevoflurane	Desflurane	Enflurane	Halothane	Methoxyflurane	Ether	N_2O
Formula[a]	$C_3H_2ClF_5O$	$C_4H_3F_7O$	$C_3H_2F_6O$	$C_3H_2ClF_5O$	C_2HF_3Br	$C_3H_4Cl_2F_2O$	$(C_2H_5)_2O$	N_2O
Molecular weight[a]	184.5	200	168	184.5	197.4	165	74	44
Specific gravity	1.50	1.52	1.46	1.52	1.87	1.42	0.71	1.26
Boiling point[a] (°C)	48.5	58.5	23.5	56.5	50.2	105	36.5	−89
Vapor pressure at 20°C (mmHg)[a]	240	160	669	172	243	22.5	450	38,770
Maximum % concentration	31.5	21	88	22.6	32	3	49	100
MAC (dog)	1.39%	2.36%[b]	7.2%[c]	2.2%[d]	0.89%[b]	0.29%[e]	3.04%[f]	222%[e]
Odor[a]	Musty/mildly pungent	Sweet/minimally pungent	Pungent	Mildly sweet	Sweet	Fruity	Sweet/ Pungent	Mildly sweet
Biodegradation (% metabolized)[e,g]	0.17	3.0	<0.2	2.8	20.25	50.75	–	0.004
Stability in soda lime[g]	Yes	No	Yes	Yes	No	No	–	Yes
Flammable[a]	No	No	No	No	No	Yes	Yes, extremely	No
Preservatives	None	None	None	None	Thymol	Butylated hydroxytoluene	3% ethanol	None

Legend: *N_2O*, nitrous oxide.
[a]*National Institute of Health (2022).*
[b]*Kazama and Ikeda (1988).*
[c]*Doorley et al. (1988).*
[d]*Hall et al. (1987).*
[e]*Pawson and Forsyth (2008).*
[f]*Eger and Saidman (1965).*
[g]*Steffey et al. (2015).*

anesthetic is consumed during anesthesia. As an approximation, 1 mL of liquid anesthetic on vaporization produces 200 mL of its vapor for halothane, enflurane, isoflurane, and sevoflurane (Dhulkhed et al., 2013). This information can also be used to determine volume of liquid anesthetic to be added to a defined closed chamber space in order to operate at clinically usable inhalant ranges, Table 6.3. However, due to the lack of precise control of anesthetic delivered, a precision vaporizer should be used whenever possible. The advent of precision vaporizers allows the use of highly potent anesthetics in a controlled and adjustable manner; see later sections of this chapter on vaporizers and inhalant anesthetic induction.

2. *Minimum alveolar concentration*

Minimum alveolar concentration (MAC) of an anesthetic is the concentration at 1 atmosphere that produces immobility in 50% of patients exposed to a supramaximal noxious stimulus. MAC can be correlated to the ED_{50} of an anesthetic, where half the patients are appropriately anesthetized, and half are not (Steffey et al., 2015). MAC is a measure of anesthetic potency, where the lower the MAC, the more potent the anesthetic (Pawson and Forsyth, 2008).

TABLE 6.3 Approximate volume (mL) of isoflurane and sevoflurane required to fill enclosed chambers to produce anesthetic concentrations (%) in clinical useable ranges. Calculations assume 182.1 mL of isoflurane and 170.0 mL of sevoflurane formed from vaporization of 1 mL of liquid anesthetic. Calculations at 20°C, 273 K, and 760 mmHg.

	Internal volume of chamber (mL)		
Percent (%)	1000	2000	4000
Isoflurane			
1	0.05	0.11	0.22
2	0.11	0.22	0.44
3	0.16	0.33	0.66
4	0.22	0.44	0.88
5	0.27	0.55	1.10
Sevoflurane			
1	0.06	0.12	0.24
2	0.12	0.24	0.47
3	0.18	0.35	0.71
4	0.24	0.47	0.94
5	0.29	0.59	1.18
6	0.35	0.71	1.41

MAC also allows direct comparisons among different inhalant anesthetics and provides a method to maintain a patient at a measurable and stable depth of anesthesia. By knowing the MAC of different animal species and recording MAC during the anesthetic event of a patient, it can allow for a repeatable, smooth, and predictable anesthetic experience.

Determination of MAC generally involves the manual application of noxious stimulus with a large hemostat clamped to the tail or digit of the animal, or the application of an electric current to tissue (Quasha et al., 1980). First, the patient is allowed to equilibrate for 15 minutes at a measurable level of end-tidal anesthetic concentration. The noxious stimulus is then applied and the patient is monitored for gross purposeful movement. If no response is observed, the alveolar concentration is reduced by 20%, the patient is allowed to equilibrate for another 15 minutes, and the stimulus is repeated. This step-down procedure is repeated until gross purposeful movement is observed, and then the alveolar concentration is increased by 10% until the animal fails to respond to the noxious stimulus. For example, starting with an isoflurane concentration of 2%, after 15 minutes of steady state anesthesia, a hemostat is used to clamp the tail. If no response is noted, the alveolar concentration is reduced to 1.6% (20% decrease) for the same amount of time. If no response, then the concentration is lowered to 1.28% for another 15 minutes. If a response is noted then the concentration is reincreased to 1.41% (10% increase). If, after another 15 minutes, no response to the stimulus is noted at this concentration, the MAC would be 1.35% for this patient—halfway between the concentrations where the patient does and does not respond.

As stated previously, the MAC (ED_{50}) for the testing population is where 50% of the patients do not respond to stimulus. One standard deviation (SD) is about 10% of the MAC value, and 2 SDs indicate a MAC value corresponding to the dose where 95% of the patients will not move in response to noxious stimulation (ED_{95}) (Nguyen, 2014). The recorded MAC values of isoflurane and sevoflurane for different laboratory animal species are summarized in Table 6.4.

The use of MAC as a measurement of the animal's anesthetic level assumes that gases within the alveoli are in equilibrium with the blood exiting the lung. Thus, alveolar concentrations are assumed to represent the anesthetic concentration in the central nervous system. This is true if ventilation and perfusion are closely matched, and sufficient time has elapsed to allow equilibration between the alveolar gases and the pulmonary blood. Normally, ventilation and perfusion are equally matched in the lung, and alveolar gas is fully equilibrated with the blood. Ventilation/perfusion mismatching, where alveolar concentrations vary from the central nervous system and blood concentrations, is uncommon in healthy laboratory mammals

TABLE 6.4 Isoflurane and sevoflurane minimum alveolar concentrations (MAC) for select laboratory animal species.

MAC values of isoflurane and sevoflurane			
Species	**Isoflurane (MAC)**	**Sevoflurane (MAC)**	**References**
Mouse (C57Bl/6J)	1.85	3.25	Cesarovic et al. (2010)
Rat	1.12	1.97	Orliaguet et al. (2001)
Rabbit	2.05	3.70	Steffey et al. (2015)
Dog	1.39	2.36	Kazama and Ikeda (1988)
Cat	1.71	3.08	Shaughnessy and Hofmeister, (2014)
Pig	1.6–1.9	2.4.2.66	Clarke et al. (2014)
Monkey	1.46 (rhesus)	2.0 (cynos)	Rhesus-Steffey et al. (2015) Cynos-Soma et al. (1995)
Ferret	1.52	–	Murat and Housmans (1988)
Sheep	1.52 (pregnant Ewe) 1.92 (nonpregnant Ewe)	2.74	Okutomi et al. (2009), Columbano et al. (2018)
Goat	1.29	2.33	Hikasa et al. (1998)
Chicken	1.15	1.90	Velasco Gallego et al. (2021)
Pigeon	1.8	3.0	Botman et al. (2016a,b)
Captive thick-billed parrots	1.07	–	Mercado et al, (2008)
Peking duck	1.30	–	Ludders et al. (1990)
Quaker parrot	2.52	–	Zaheer et al. (2020)

weighing less than 50 kg but is more common in larger animals such as horses, pigs, and sheep. Other factors can affect MAC in a positive or negative manner and there are some physiological variables that do not affect MAC at all. The effects of different variables on MAC are summarized in Table 6.5.

3. Partition coefficients

Blood/gas solubility coefficients are a method for predicting the speed of anesthetic induction, recovery, and change of anesthetic depth (Steffey et al., 2015). The partition coefficients are expressed as ratios of the amounts of anesthetic in blood and tissue at equilibrium. The most important partition coefficient for inhaled anesthetics is the blood/gas partition coefficient (Table 6.6). Since blood is the first to equilibrate with alveolar anesthetic gases, the blood/gas coefficient is an indication of speed of onset. All other factors being equal, the greater the solubility of the anesthetic gas in blood, the longer the equilibration time. Although solubility varies among tissues, tissue components, temperature, and species, partition coefficients provide a consistent guideline for predicting how uptake

TABLE 6.5 Effect of different variables on minimum alveolar concentration (MAC).

Decrease MAC	Increase MAC	No effect on MAC
Hypothermia	Hyperthermia	Blood pressure changes (unless severe hypotension)
Age (older animal)	Hyperthyroidism	Sex
Hyponatremia	Hypernatremia	$PaO_2 > 40$ mmHg
Pregnancy	High activity time periods (circadian rhythm)	PCO_2 10–90 mmHg
CNS depressants/analgesics (benzodiazepines, opioids, local analgesics, NSAIDs)	CNS catecholamines	Type of stimulation
Severe anemia (PCV <13%)		Anesthetic duration

TABLE 6.6 Blood/gas and oil/gas partition coefficients for select inhalant anesthetics (Steffey et al., 2015).

Anesthetic	Blood/gas coefficient	Oil/gas coefficient
Methoxyflurane	15	970
Halothane	2.54	224
Enflurane	2.00	96
Desflurane	0.42	18.7
Sevoflurane	0.68	47
Isoflurane	1.46	91
N_2O	0.47	1.4

and elimination will occur when comparing anesthetics (Wollman and Smith, 1975). Inhalation anesthetics that are poorly soluble in blood and have low blood/gas partition coefficients produce more rapid induction, recovery, and change of anesthetic depth (Pawson and Forsyth, 2008).

The goal of using inhalant anesthetics is to depress the central nervous system function which is achieved by reaching a certain partial pressure of anesthetic in the brain to induce general anesthesia (Pawson and Forsyth, 2008). Because of the large amount of blood flow to the brain, equilibration rapidly occurs between anesthetic concentration in blood. N_2O, desflurane, and sevoflurane have exceptionally low blood/gas solubilities and are associated with rapid uptake and elimination (Eger, 1992; Jones, 1990).

Lipid solubility and potency of inhaled anesthetics have a direct relationship. Since the oil/gas partition coefficient is a measure of lipid solubility, the higher the oil/gas partition coefficient the more potent the anesthetic (Pawson and Forsyth, 2008). This means there is an inverse relationship between the oil/gas partition coefficient, and MAC, with a higher MAC correlating to a lower oil/gas partition coefficient and lower potency of the anesthetic (Table 6.6).

Tissue solubility is also important during the uptake and elimination of inhaled anesthetics. The higher the tissue solubility, the longer it will take to saturate the tissue with anesthetic and for the anesthetic to clear from the tissues. With other parameters being equal, anesthetics that are highly soluble in tissue will require longer inductions and recoveries (Steffey et al., 2015). The solubility of anesthetic gases in the delivery apparatus also can affect uptake and elimination. Absorption of gases into the rubber or plastic components of the anesthetic delivery apparatus slows the inhalation process, and hence induction. This can also delay patient recovery. Because isoflurane and sevoflurane have low rubber and plastic solubilities, uptake by the machine components is insignificant during induction and recovery.

4. Stability

Molecular stability of inhalants is closely correlated with lack of tissue toxicity. It is the metabolites of inhalant anesthetics that can cause tissue injury. Substitution of fluoride and bromide for chlorine in the newer volatile gas anesthetics has resulted in greater molecular stability and less toxic anesthetics. The percent level of biodegradation is summarized in Table 6.2 for select anesthetics. The low rate of biodegradation of isoflurane, sevoflurane, and desflurane has resulted in decreased potential for renal and hepatic injury in anesthetized animals, as well as in the personnel exposed to trace anesthetic levels (Njoku et al., 1997). Molecular stability is also important as it relates to the need for preservatives. For instance, ether, MOF, and halothane all require a preservative to prevent degradation during storage, whereas isoflurane, enflurane, desflurane, and sevoflurane do not require preservatives to prevent spontaneous oxidative decomposition.

5. Mode of action

The primary target sites for general anesthetics are not known. One hypothesis is that the ultimate target sites are ion channels in nerve membranes, influenced by proteins and/or lipids (Franks and Lieb, 1991; Jones, 1990). It is unknown whether gas anesthetics have a direct action on the lipid membrane to disrupt ion flow or whether a second messenger is involved. Inhaled anesthetics also bind proteins and can modulate function even in a nonlipid environment (Franks and Lieb, 1984; Steffey et al., 2015). In general, most inhalant anesthetics enhance the inhibitory neurotransmitter gamma-aminobutyric acid type A receptors ($GABA_A$) (Steffey et al., 2015). When activated, this channel causes an increase in the chloride permeability of neurons (Tanelian et al., 1993).

A solution to the mechanism of general anesthesia has not yet been found that fits the physical, chemical, and physiological factors associated with anesthetics. This is most likely due to the complexity of the neuronal networks involved in general anesthesia. A review of mechanisms of general anesthesia has been described elsewhere (Mashour et al., 2005; Son, 2010).

6. Uptake—Distribution—Elimination

The aim during anesthetic induction and maintenance is to raise the alveolar anesthetic concentration, which in turn, will raise the concentration in the brain to produce general anesthesia. Several factors affect alveolar concentrations of anesthetic, such as, alveolar ventilation, inspired anesthetic concentrations, solubility in blood and tissues, and cardiac output (Pawson and Forsyth, 2008). If unopposed by uptake, the alveolar concentration would rapidly equal the inspired concentration. Increasing ventilation increases alveolar anesthetic concentration, and likewise, decreasing ventilation will decrease alveolar concentration. Uptake into tissues also limits the rise in alveolar concentration. If more anesthetic is removed from the alveoli and taken up by the tissues and blood, the alveolar concentration will be lower relative to the inspired concentration. Anesthetics with high blood or tissue solubilities thus take longer for the alveolar concentrations to increase to the level required for anesthesia.

The higher the cardiac output, the larger the quantity of anesthetic removed from the lungs, and thus the lower the alveolar concentration. Induction is usually longer in patients that are excited and hypertensive and occurs more rapidly in patients suffering from hypovolemic conditions (Pawson and Forsyth, 2008). If lower cardiac output results in lower cerebral blood flow and thus slower equilibration of the brain and arterial anesthetic concentration, faster anesthetic equilibration is not achieved. However, cerebral blood flow is often preserved even when cardiac output decreases. This can potentially result in an anesthetic overdose in patients with low cardiac output but high cerebral blood flow. Therefore, to prevent this anesthetic overdosing, technically, if animals are sick or unhealthy (after procedural manipulation), surgical anesthesia plane can be achieved with a lower inhalant anesthetic concentration, reiterating the importance of appropriate anesthetic monitoring.

The metabolism of highly soluble anesthetics does not significantly affect recovery. The majority of anesthetic metabolism occurs after clinical anesthesia has been discontinued. Elimination of anesthetic occurs primarily through exhalation in the lungs. Anesthetics with high lipid solubilities have the slowest elimination from the lungs and the highest levels of hepatic metabolism. This is more important in terms of the production of toxic metabolites and their effects on the patient and personnel working with the anesthetic.

7. Inhalant anesthetics

a. Isoflurane

Due to a low blood/gas partition coefficient, induction, recovery, and the rate of change in anesthetic depth can occur rapidly with isoflurane use. However, the unpleasant odor makes it less optimal for mask inductions (Pawson and Forsyth, 2008). Isoflurane maintains cardiovascular functions better than previous generations of gas anesthetics. Isoflurane causes a dose-related depression of systemic arterial blood pressure (Peyton et al., 2011). The decreased blood pressure is due to a combination of myocardial depression and decreased systemic vascular resistance. Isoflurane has less of a depressant effect on myocardial contractility but causes greater vasodilatory effects when compared to halothane. Isoflurane, like MOF, desflurane, and sevoflurane, does not sensitize the heart to the arrhythmogenic effects of exogenously administered epinephrine (Eger, 1992).

Isoflurane has coronary vasodilatory effects with reported variable potency (Crystal et al., 1995). Isoflurane is commonly used in cardiovascular studies of mice due to minimal effects on the heart rate compared to other nonvolatile anesthetics (Hartley et al., 2007; Janssen et al., 2004). Like other inhalant anesthetics, isoflurane increases cerebral blood flow, but unlike other anesthetics, this can be mitigated by hyperventilating the patient prior to isoflurane administration (Boarini et al., 1984). For this reason, isoflurane is preferred in situations where cerebral blood flow must not increase.

Isoflurane is a ventilatory depressant, more so than halothane. Increasing concentrations produce a progressive decrease in tidal volume and a response to rising arterial carbon dioxide (CO_2) concentrations (Merin, 1993). CO_2 or spirometry should be used to determine the adequacy of ventilation during isoflurane anesthesia.

The high molecular stability of isoflurane results in a metabolism of less than 0.2% of the inspired dose. This reduces the potential for renal and hepatic injury (Fujita et al., 1991). Human exposure to trace amounts of isoflurane is less hazardous than exposure to MOF, halothane, or sevoflurane (Njoku et al., 1997). Low-flow delivery techniques and precision vaporizers should be used to minimize wastage and increase the control of delivered concentrations. The effects of inhalant anesthetics are summarized in Table 6.7.

b. Sevoflurane

Although less potent than isoflurane, sevoflurane has gained popularity in veterinary clinics because of its lower solubility in blood. This results in very rapid equilibration, enabling precise and rapid changes in anesthetic depth (Eger, 1992; Yasuda et al., 1990). The principal advantage is rapid induction and recovery which is most noticeable in large-sized animals, such as adult swine, cattle, and horses. This feature, along with a less pungent odor, makes it more suitable for mask induction versus isoflurane (Pawson and Forsyth, 2008). In addition, sevoflurane has been used as effectively as isoflurane in neonatal rats (Huss et al., 2016). Similar to isoflurane and desflurane, sevoflurane decreases systemic blood pressure and cardiac contractility in a dose-dependent manner and does not potentiate epinephrine-induced cardiac arrhythmias. Sevoflurane is a less potent coronary vasodilator than isoflurane (Ebert, 1996).

Sevoflurane is metabolized to about 3% in the liver. Degradation in the presence of soda lime and baralyme has raised concerns relating to the toxicity of the metabolites. Two degradation products have been reported, compound A and compound B, where only compound A is produced

TABLE 6.7 Effects of inhalant anesthetics on physiological systems.

	Halothane	Isoflurane	Sevoflurane	Desflurane	N_2O	Methoxyflurane
Cardiac output	↓↓↓	↓	↓	↓	–	↓↓
Arrhythmia	↑↑↑↑	↑	↑	↑	–	↑↑
Blood pressure	↓↓	↓↓↓	↓↓↓	↑↑	–	↓↓↓
Respiratory depression	↓	↓↓↓	↓↓	↓↓	–	↓↓↓
Hepatic blood flow	↓↓↓	↓↓	↓↓	↓↓	–	↓↓↓↓
Renal blood flow	↓↓	↓↓↓	↓↓	↓↓	–	↓↓↓
Cerebral blood flow	↑↑↑↑	↑↑	↑↑	↑↑	– or ↑	↑↑
Muscle relaxation	↑	↑↑	↑↑	↑↑	–	↑↑↑
Preservatives	Required	None	None	None	None	Required
Odor	–	Pungent	–	Pungent	–	Pungent
Stable in soda lime	No	Yes	No	Yes	Yes	Yes

↓ = decreased; ↑ = increased, "–" = no change.

in significant quantities. Baralyme, which is composed of more potassium hydroxide than soda lime, produces significantly higher concentrations of compound A (Bito and Ikeda, 1994). Absorbents which do not contain a strong base or cause anesthetic degradation and formation of toxic products have been suggested for use with sevoflurane (Kharasch et al., 2002). Studies have shown that clinically detectable nephrotoxicity and hepatoxicity do not occur with normal anesthetic delivery (Bito and Ikeda, 1994; Frink et al., 1994; Fukazawa and Lee, 2014). Agent-specific vaporizers must be used to deliver sevoflurane because of its unique vapor pressure.

c. Desflurane

Cardiorespiratory and hemodynamic effects of desflurane are similar to those of isoflurane (Warltier and Pagel, 1992). While both sevoflurane and desflurane provide rapid induction and recovery times, compared to sevoflurane, desflurane is less soluble in blood, is stable in soda lime, and undergoes the least amount of biodegradation of any volatile anesthetic (Steffey, 1992). Desflurane is more pungent and thus would not be recommended for mask inductions. Like isoflurane, hyperventilation can combat increases in cerebral blood flow if instituted prior to anesthetic delivery (Young, 1992). The low boiling point of desflurane requires a special heated vaporizer to control delivered concentrations. The high cost of specialized equipment and the limited need for faster anesthetic inductions or recoveries in animal research limit the use of desflurane in both animal clinical and research environments (Jones, 1990).

d. Methoxyflurane

The low volatility and high blood solubility of MOF made it safe for use in nonprecision systems. It is the most potent of the current inhaled anesthetics, with a MAC of less than 0.5% in dogs. Inexperienced researchers with limited anesthesia training preferred MOF because of the perceived safety associated with slow changes in anesthetic depth due to its high blood/gas partition coefficient and high lipid solubility (Fig. 6.1).

Methoxyflurane is extensively metabolized (Table 6.2), and renal toxicity was a significant complication with its use in people. Human exposure should be avoided. Metabolites include inorganic fluoride, oxalates, and trifluoroacetic acid, which are nephrotoxic (Brunson et al., 1979). Methoxyflurane has not been commercially available in the United States since 1999. There has been a resurgence in other countries with its use as an analgesic in the prehospital setting, where it can be self-administered with a hand-held inhaler (Ikeda, 2020).

e. Halothane

Halothane has good potency, low blood/gas solubility, and high volatility. It produces rapid anesthesia, where stable anesthetic levels are easily produced within 10 min. The high vapor pressure of halothane enables concentrations as high as 33% to be produced, which, combined with rapid equilibration, can quickly lead to lethal levels of anesthesia.

Halothane causes respiratory depression in a dose-dependent manner. At deep levels of anesthesia, ventilation becomes inadequate. Halothane also causes direct

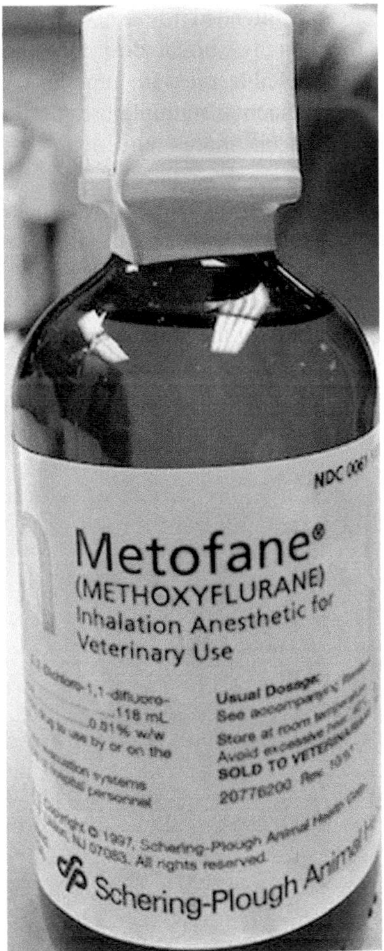

FIGURE 6.1 An example of an methoxyflurane bottle.

depression of myocardial muscle and relaxation of vascular smooth muscle. Myocardial contractility, cardiac output, and total peripheral resistance decrease upon exposure to halothane. Halothane also sensitizes the myocardium to endogenous and exogenously administered catecholamines.

Halothane increases cerebral blood flow due to direct vasodilation of vascular smooth muscle. This increased blood flow is not prevented by preanesthetic hyperventilation. Halothane is contraindicated in patients with increased intracranial pressure or intracranial hemorrhage.

The availability of alternate gas anesthetics with a lower metabolism and thus lower risk of toxicity for both animals and humans minimized the demand for this drug in North America. Halothane is still widely used in the developing world due to its low cost (Hudson et al., 2019).

f. Enflurane

The cardiovascular and respiratory characteristics of enflurane are like those of isoflurane. Enflurane increases cerebral blood flow similar to halothane; however, high concentrations are associated with seizure-like electroencephalogram activity. Like halothane and methoxyflurane, enflurane is no longer used in clinical practice in North America (Hudson et al., 2019).

g. Nitrous oxide

N_2O is the least potent of the inhaled anesthetics. As part of the second gas effect, rapid uptake of high concentrations of N_2O at induction of anesthesia produces an increase in alveolar concentrations of O_2 and the accompanying volatile anesthetic (Peyton et al., 2011). This effect is advantageous during veterinary patient anesthetic induction. N_2O must be inhaled when the other inhaled anesthetic is already present in the alveoli for the second gas effect to be effective, and higher N_2O concentrations are necessary due to its low potency.

When using N_2O, O_2 flow rates should be set based on the needs of the animal, with N_2O added to this base flow as the oxygen in N_2O is not available for cellular metabolism. A minimum of 20% of the inspired gases must be O2 (Dorsch and Dorsch, 2008c). Higher flow rates of N_2O result in increased heat loss from the patient and increase the costs associated with anesthesia. The amount of volatile anesthetic vaporized along with N_2O and O_2 increases proportionally to the increase in flow. Additional costs of using N_2O are related to the use of special flow meters and cylinder regulators.

N_2O can diffuse into gas-filled spaces much more readily than nitrogen (N_2) can diffuse out of these spaces. This results in N_2O accumulation in closed spaces. For this reason, it is relatively contraindicated in cases of intestinal obstruction and pneumothorax (Peyton et al., 2011; Reinelt et al., 2001). Due to its low blood/gas solubility, once the use of N_2O is discontinued, O_2 should be administered for approximately 5 min to ensure that the animal does not become hypoxic during the rapid exhalation of N_2O.

N_2O use can lead to drug abuse and other health-related issues in humans, including psychosis, reproductive disturbances, and vitamin B12 depletion, which can result in megaloblastic anemia, neurologic, and immune system disorders (National Institute of Health, 2022). Thus, effective scavenging systems, monitoring use, and adequate security should be employed to minimize occupational exposure and inappropriate use.

In summary, N_2O is a very weak anesthetic with minimal cardiovascular and respiratory depressive effects. It can be combined with O_2 and other volatile anesthetics as part of the second gas effect, but caution must be used to prevent increased heat loss and hypoxia in the patient. It requires the use of special equipment and care must be taken to prevent personnel abuse. The use of N_2O in animals does not produce the same effects seen in people and should not be included in research protocols for the sole reason of simulating human anesthetic protocols.

II. Single circuit and multi circuit design

A. Single circuit designs

It is possible to satisfactorily induce and maintain anesthesia in rodents and other small animals using any machine equipped with a nonrebreathing circuit. However, the term "rodent anesthesia machine" is usually understood to mean an anesthesia machine lacking all the components of a circle system and intended for use with a Mapleson-E circuit, or a functionally similar design, without a reservoir bag or an adjustable pressure limiting (APL) valve. Additional features, such as multiple breathing circuits and provision for one or more induction chambers, are common.

In the simplest form, a delivery system adequate for many rodent procedures consists of little more than a flowmeter, a vaporizer, a breathing circuit and mask, and some means of scavenging waste gas (Fig. 6.2). A means of delivering and controlling the pressure of fresh gas, either a central supply system or a tank and pressure regulator, is also needed. Without a frame to arrange the components on

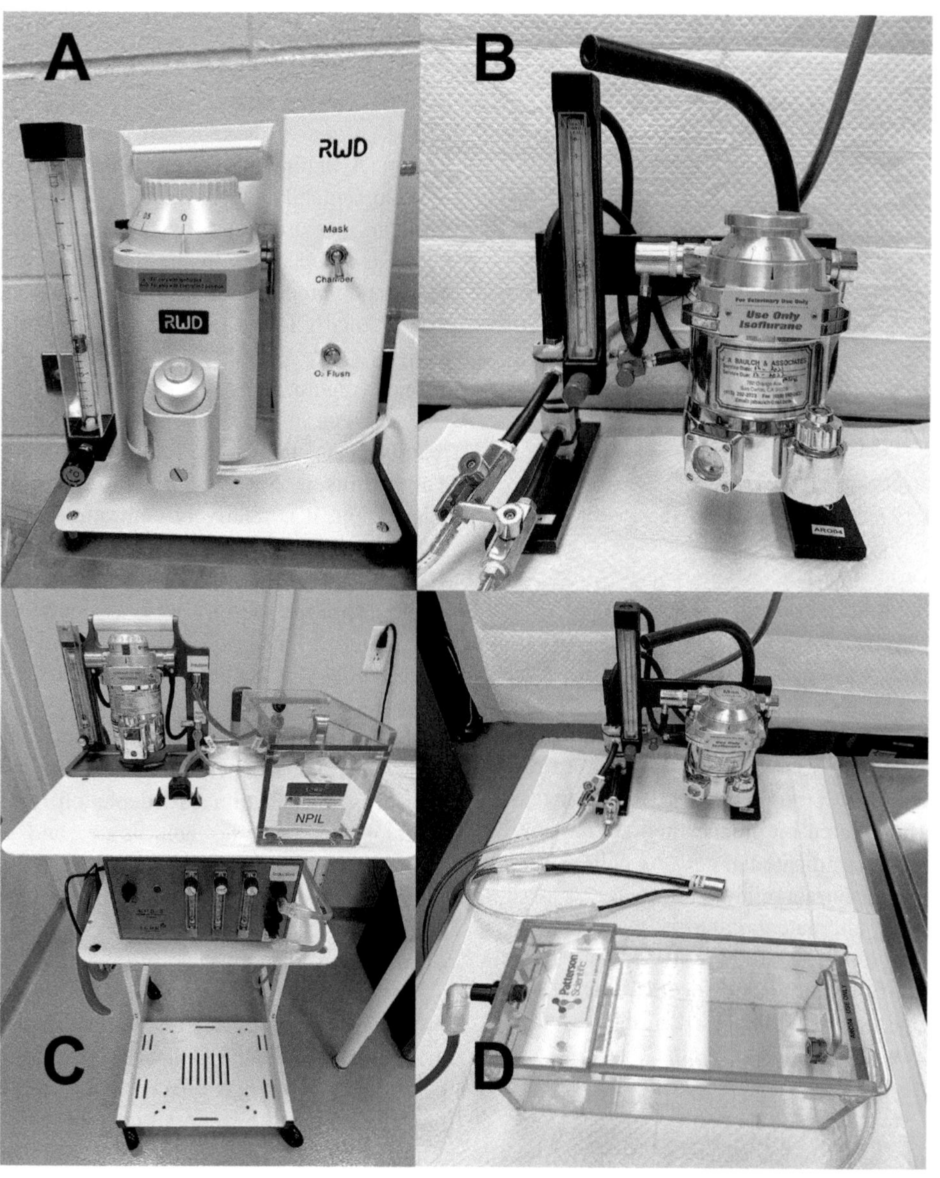

FIGURE 6.2 Portable (*table top*) rodent anesthesia machine ((A) from RWD and (B) from Summit, Tec 3 vaporizer). Somni (C) set up on a cart with wheels that has an induction box and a mask with an active scavenging system below. A complete set up with an induction chamber and a mask is shown in (D).

and to maintain the flowmeter and vaporizer upright and immobile when the controls are operated, such a "machine" will be inconvenient to use. Many small rodent machines are commercially available, usually equipped with gas supply connections to meet the user's needs, and often with an O_2 flush valve. The O_2 flush valve is intended to flush the induction chamber, in order to reduce pollution when the chamber is opened. The O_2 flush valve should never be used when an animal is connected to a nonrebreathing circuit. Inhalation anesthesia is often used for both induction and maintenance of laboratory rodents. The output of the vaporizer is frequently split in order to allow the use of an induction chamber as well as a breathing circuit, eliminating the need to disconnect one in order to use the other. Some machines use a Y-connection attached to the vaporizer output port and a two-way valve to divert the flow to the chamber or vaporizer leg, as desired, with a similar arrangement for the mask and chamber scavenging lines.

B. Multi circuit (multipatient) designs

Many rodent procedures are relatively brief and must be performed on groups of animals in a short time period, so multiple patient circuits are frequently needed. With the exception of a few machines, it is assumed that all of the patients can be adequately and safely anesthetized using the same fresh gas flow and agent concentration. Multi circuit designs may be inappropriate when a different anesthetic concentration is needed for each patient (i.e., healthy vs. unhealthy/manipulated patients). Several approaches are used to divide the vaporizer output.

A simple but cumbersome method is to subdivide the flow from the vaporizer using a sufficient number of sequential Y-connectors and tubing runs to form the needed number of patient circuits. Typically, tubing and connectors with an internal diameter of about 6.4 mm (0.25 inches) or somewhat greater are used. Simple on/off valves can be used to open or close individual patient circuits (Fig. 6.3B and C). The resistance to flow is directly proportional to the length and inversely proportional to the diameter of the tubing and connectors. For every patient to receive the same fresh gas flow, the fresh gas flow to the vaporizer must be adjusted to take into account the number of open circuits. If, for example, six circuits are in use and the desired flow to each is 0.5 L/min, the total flow would be 3 L/min. As the procedures are completed, if five of the

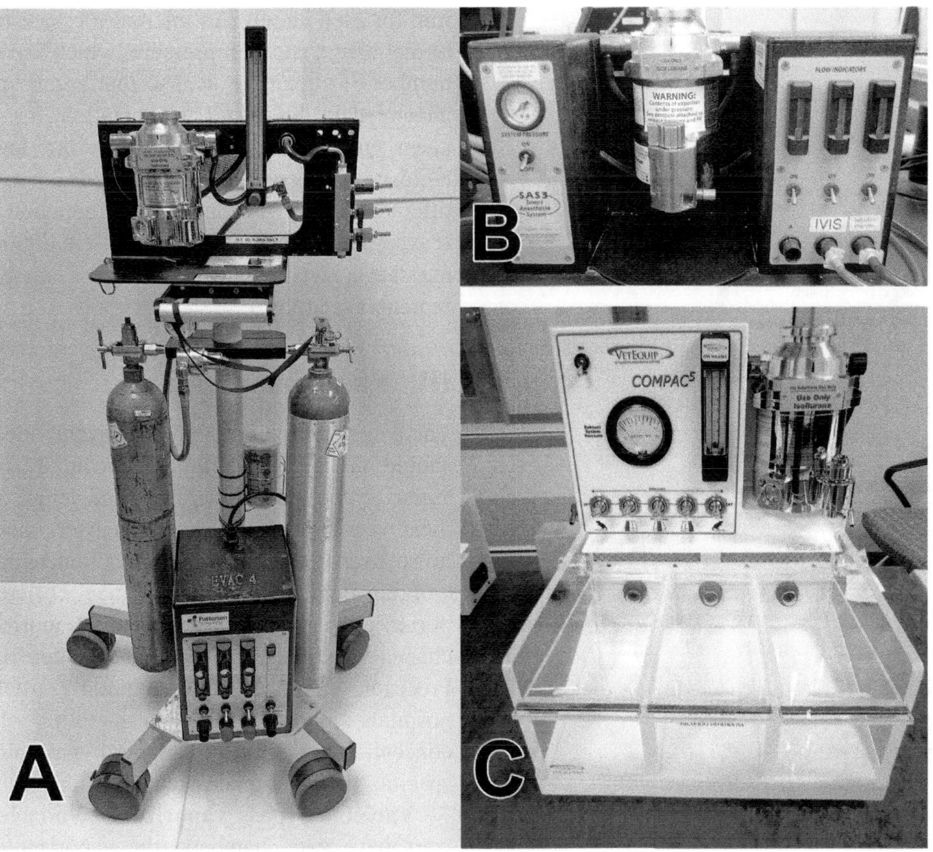

FIGURE 6.3 (A) Multistation anesthesia machine (for rodents) with flow meter and isoflurane vaporizer on top and active scavenging system down below (Evac 4 from Patterson Scientific). (B) This is Summit SAS3 anesthesia system—the control panel has three switches to independently control each of the breathing circuits. The large gauge on the left indicates system pressure. (C) This is VetEquip Compac5. A customized Tec 3 vaporizer is on the right—the control panel has five switches to independently control each of the breathing circuits and the three heated induction chambers. The large gauge indicates scavenging exhaust system pressure. For all of (A–C), multiple animals can be anesthetized at the same time.

circuits are closed without proportionately decreasing the total flow, the remaining animal would receive 3 L/min, an excessively high flow that might impede breathing. Occluding the unused ports will prevent gas leakage. Each patient circuit also requires appropriate scavenging connections, which ordinarily require wide-diameter tubing, 19 mm inner diameter (ID) or greater, to avoid back pressure, resistance to breathing, and leakage at the patient mask.

Multi circuit rodent machines are available that provide adjustable flowmeters to control the flow rate to each breathing circuit (Figs. 6.3A and C, and 6.4). These machines are commonly used for bioluminescence imaging. In this arrangement, the individual flowmeters are placed downstream of the vaporizer output, to separately control the flow to each mask. The total fresh gas to the vaporizer must be sufficient to allow further division of the vaporizer output for each individual patient circuit. Once this condition is met, individual circuits may be controlled by their respective flowmeters without further adjustment of the master flowmeter.

With almost all current multi circuit rodent anesthesia machines, the concentration of the anesthetic agent is set at the vaporizer and is the same for all patients (Fig. 6.3A and B). Some models may support multiple patients (up to six patient circuits) and allow the anesthetic agent concentration to be independently adjusted for each circuit. This is accomplished by selecting the desired flow and anesthetic concentration at the master flowmeter and vaporizer, respectively. Fresh gas flow from the vaporizer is equally divided between the patient stations in use, so that the flow set at the master flowmeter is the sum of the desired flows to each of the stations in use. To meet the linearity specifications for the vaporizer, a minimum total flow of 0.5 L/min on the master flowmeter is necessary. Each patient station has a secondary, or auxiliary O_2 flowmeter, which can be used to dilute the fresh gas flow from the vaporizer to a lower agent concentration determined by the user. Thus, in this design, the maximum agent concentration is set at the vaporizer, but lower concentrations can be obtained at each station at the discretion of the operator.

Some rodent anesthesia machines use flow restrictors in place of variable-area flowmeters. These machines offer multiple patient circuits controlled by simple pneumatic switches; the circuit is either on or off (Figs. 6.3B and C). The fresh gas flow rate is typically on the order of 0.5 L/min for each circuit. An internal pressure regulator is used to maintain a constant pressure, which varies little with the number of circuits in use, so that a constant fixed flow is generated in the circuit. In operation, the user selects the agent concentration on the vaporizer, and turns on the requisite number of circuits as needed. Various models are offered, some with integrated induction chambers and scavenging provisions. There is also a digital control rodent anesthesia available which can be easier to use for researchers (Fig. 6.5).

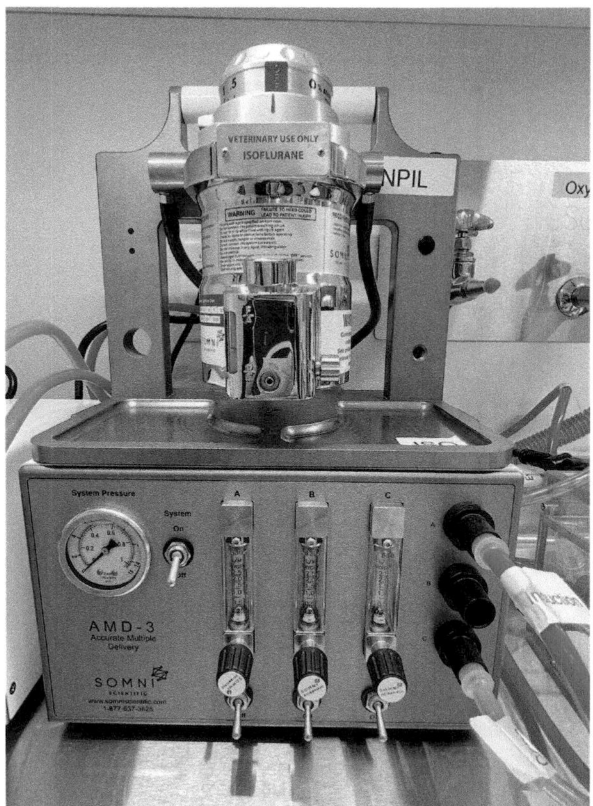

FIGURE 6.4 This portable anesthesia machine unit provides multiple delivery to 3 stations simultaneously (made by Somni AMD-3). It provides 3 fresh gas common outlets with color-coded (i.e., for a mask or induction chamber).

III. Vaporizers

There are many types of vaporizers. Ideally, vaporizers should deliver an accurate concentrations of anesthetic vapor at any carrier gas flow and temperature. Although ideal vaporizers do not exist, newer, modern vaporizers nowadays deliver an accurate concentration over the working flow or temperature range. Different types of vaporizers are shown in Table 6.8. Vaporizers are broadly characterized as either precision or nonprecision vaporizers. Precision vaporizers are commonly used in veterinary hospitals, including research facilities, characterized by concentration calibrated/variable bypass, flow over, agent-specific, thermocompensated, and high resistance.

Variable-bypass vaporizers—Variable-bypass vaporizers have two chambers (the vaporizer and the bypass chambers). When O_2 from a flowmeter enters the vaporizer, one portion of O_2 will flow into a vaporizer chamber to vaporize anesthetic gas, and the other O_2 portion will flow

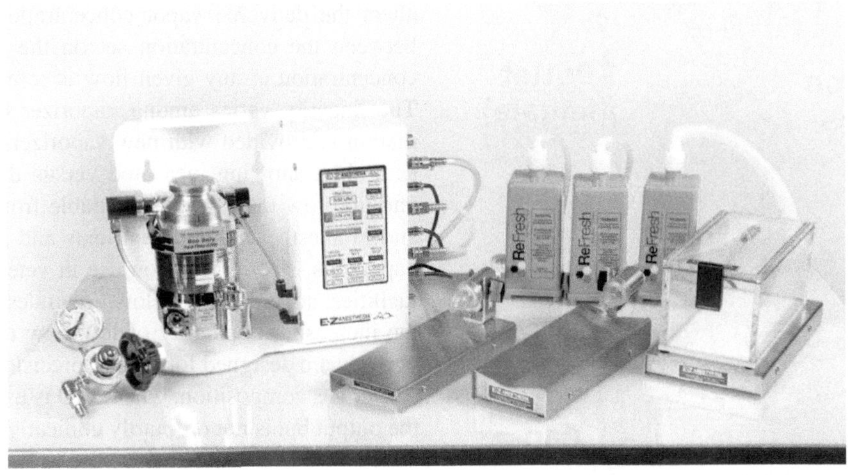

FIGURE 6.5 A digital control rodent anesthesia set up with Tec 3 vaporizer (AD-5000 digital anesthesia system by E-Z systems). This system includes digital control of an induction chamber, 2 breather ports, and warming surfaces. *Courtesy Paul Miller, E-Z Systems.*

TABLE 6.8 Classification characteristics of commonly used vaporizers in research facilities (Mosley, 2015).

Vaporizer	Method of output	Method of vaporization	Location	Temperature compensated	Resistance	Specificity
Tec 2	VBP CC	Flow-over wick	VOC	Yes	High	Yes
Tec 3	VBP CC	Flow-over wick	VOC	Yes	High	Yes
Vapor	VBP CC	Flow-over wick	VOC	Yes	High	Yes
Vapor 19.1	VBP CC	Flow-over wick	VOC	Yes	High	Yes

CC, concentration calibrated; *VBP*, variable bypass; VOC, vaporizer out of circuit.

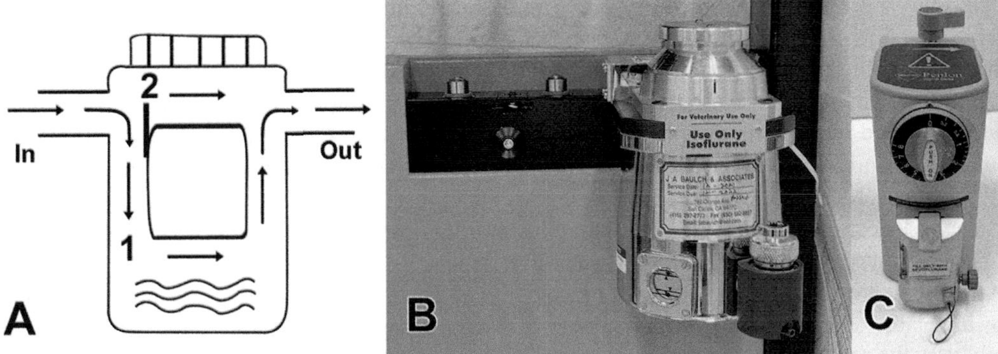

FIGURE 6.6 (A) Schematic diagram of variable bypass vaporizer with the flow to the vaporizing chamber (1) and bypass flow (2). (B) Variable bypass vaporizers for isoflurane, and (C) sevoflurane (Penlon Sigma Delta vaporizer made with aluminum) with mounting arrangements.

into a bypass chamber. Therefore, at the exit, these two portions of O_2 are mixed, and inhalant anesthetics will be delivered at the set concentration from the vaporizer dial setting (Fig. 6.6). Wicks are used to maximize the surface area for evaporation of the anesthetic agent in the chamber so that the fresh gas becomes saturated with the agent. The diverted gas, now saturated with vapor, leaves the chamber and joins the main flow before exiting the vaporizer. The ratio of diverted gas to total flow is determined by the vapor pressure of the agent and the desired concentration of the agent in the fresh gas. Thus, the vaporizer is agent specific. A dial or hand wheel is used to select the desired

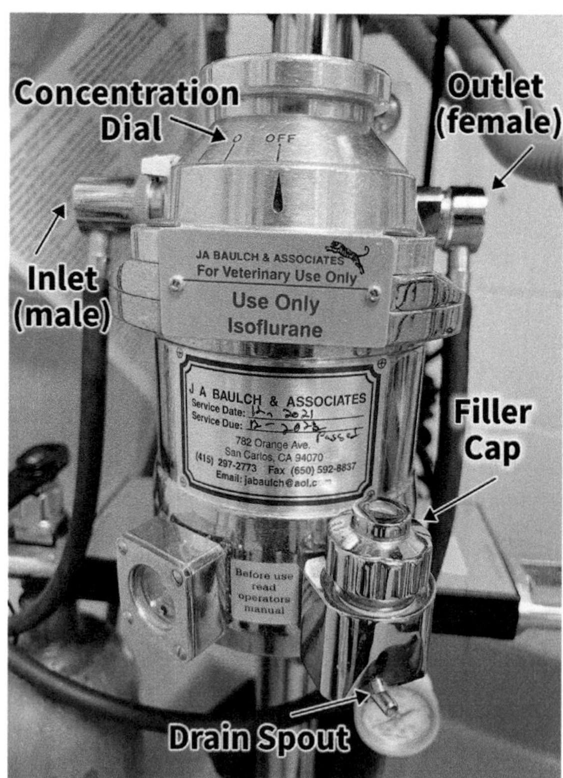

FIGURE 6.7 Apollo Tec 3 vaporizer. The filling port at the lower right is a funnel fill; the cap is reversed to fit the drain port. While this model is no longer in production, Tec 3 vaporizers for halothane, isoflurane, and sevoflurane remain popular.

concentration, and output is indicated in volume percent. Most modern vaporizers are equipped with a positive On/Off mechanical lock, usually, a button, which must be activated before the vaporizer can be turned on (Fig. 6.7). As with variable-area flowmeters, the first concentration on the dial is the first reliable reading. Some vaporizers will not deliver the agent below the first indicated value.

The output is affected by a number of physical factors, including temperature, pressure, fresh gas flow rate, and carrier gas composition. Modern vaporizers have mechanical, or in some cases, electronic means of compensating for the effects of temperature. Mechanical methods generally depend upon the thermal expansion or contraction of fluid-filled pistons, bimetallic strips, or mated metal surfaces to proportionately vary the resistance of the chamber outlet, to maintain a constant output. A notable feature of most vaporizers is their weight. Many vaporizers enclose the vaporizing chamber with a relatively large mass of metal to act as a heat sink and an additional buffer against temperature changes.

Pressure variations in the breathing circuit, as with mechanical ventilation, affect vaporizer output. This is also addressed in modern vaporizers by several methods to minimize the effect of back pressure. Flow dependency, the variation in output at different fresh gas flow rates, also alters the delivered vapor concentration. The relationship between the concentration set on the dial and the actual concentration at any given flow is referred to as *linearity*. The linearity varies among vaporizer models. This information is provided with new vaporizers, usually presented as a chart showing measured versus dial concentration at varying flow rates, and is available from the manufacturer and in anesthesia equipment texts and papers. Many older vaporizers, still in common use in veterinary and research facilities, are not linear below flow rates of 0.5 L/min. With the increasing popularity of low-flow techniques, new vaporizers are designed for greater precision at low flows. The carrier gas composition, when N_2O is used, has an effect on the output but is not ordinarily clinically significant (Davey, 2005).

In addition to the control wheel, vaporizers have a filling port, a sight glass to indicate fill level, a drain port, and a means of connecting to the gas supply and breathing circuit (Fig. 6.7). Many older vaporizers used funnel-filling ports. This style of filling port is more prone to spillage and personnel exposure to volatile agents, and allows filling with the wrong agent. In this event, the vaporizer must be drained and cleaned and may require service before further use. If funnel-style filling ports are used, a pouring adaptor for the agent bottle will increase control and reduce spillage during filling (Fig. 6.8). Keyed filling adaptors use a tube with an agent-specific connector for the vaporizer and bottle, greatly reducing the chance of misfiling, environmental contamination, and foreign material in the chamber. The sight glass is a window or a tube marked to show the maximum permissible filling level. Vaporizers should not be overfilled as this can result in the delivery of dangerously high anesthetic agent levels. In most cases, the vaporizer must be turned off and fresh gas flow discontinued during filling. Because this is an inconvenient process during anesthesia, the agent level should always be checked before the onset of a case (Table 6.9). Failure to secure the filling port cap before the carrier gas is turned on will result in a gas pressure forcing liquid agent out of the filling port, resulting in personnel hazard and wasting agent.

The drain port is used to empty the vaporizer chamber for storage and service. Few vaporizers are completely vapor-tight, and a small amount of agent will be lost over time. The vaporizer should be drained before storage, transport, or extended periods of disuse. By design, vaporizers are mounted and used in a vertical position. While some newer designs are relatively tolerant of tipping, many older designs are not, and will deliver high uncontrolled levels of anesthetic vapor if the control mechanism is wetted with the liquid agent.

Several different mounting arrangements are used to attach the vaporizer to the anesthetic machine. Most veterinary machines use the cage mount system (Fig. 6.6).

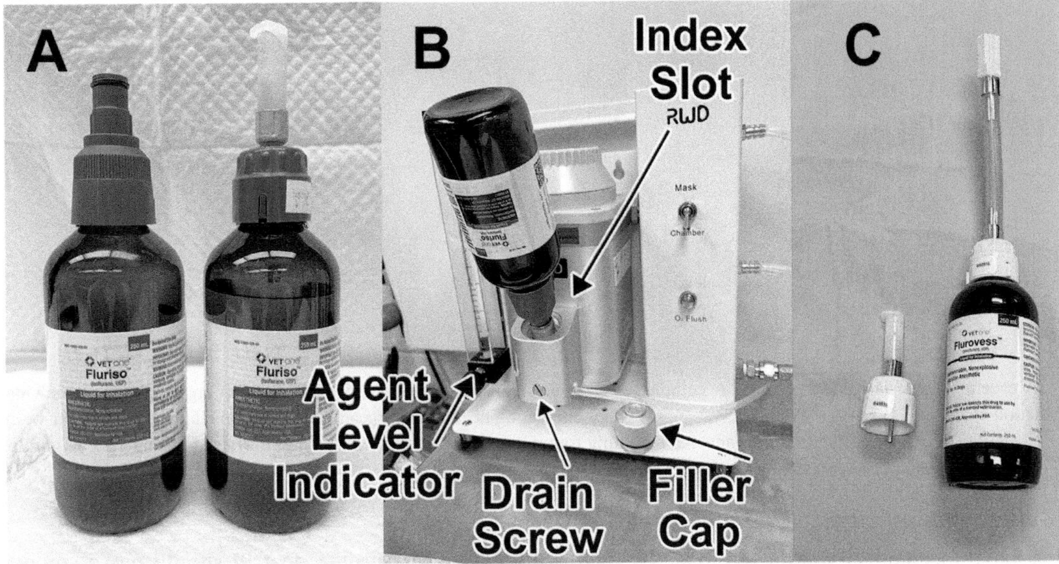

FIGURE 6.8 (A) Quick fill filler (*left*) and pouring adapter (*right*) for isoflurane to minimize spilling during filling of vaporizers. (B) A quick fill filler and vaporizer for sevoflurane (from RWD) with agent level indicator, drain screw, filler cap and index slot). (C) Example of a pouring adaptor (*left*) and keyed filling adaptor (*right*) for sevoflurane. They are color-coded and will fit only the correct bottle of anesthetic agents. The keys filling adaptor has keyed stainless steel fittings to fit the vaporizer and the anesthetic bottle, and provide the path for air to escape during filling.

TABLE 6.9 Summary recommendations of preanesthesia checklist (checkout) procedures.

Preinduction anesthetic machine check list • Patient name confirmed • Procedure confirmed • Intravenous catheter placed and patent • Airway equipment available and functioning • Endotracheal tube cuffs checked • Laryngoscope light working • Breathing system connected, leak free • APL valve opened
Anesthetic machine check list High-pressure system • adequate O_2 (N_2O, or medical grade air) in quantity and pressure (>50 psi) checked • backup O_2 (if needed) available • O_2 alarm working Low-pressure system • Flowmeters (O_2, N_2O, or medical grade air) working • Vaporizer attached and filled; filling port is tightly closed • Leak test • Turn on anesthesia system to confirm that AC is available • Scavenging system (proper connection between scavenging system and APL valve) checked • Check available required monitors including heating pads, cables, connectors, alarms, etc. • Check CO_2 absorbent is not exhausted • Breathing system pressure and leak testing • Equipment functioning and alarms are appropriately set • Emergency equipment and drugs (i.e., reversals), suction to clear the airway checked • Document completion of anesthetic machine checkout today

Modified from Association Veterinary Anaesthetists, (2014), Feldman et al. (2008), Mosley, (2015).

When two or more vaporizers are mounted on the same machine, lockout mechanisms should be used to prevent simultaneous use.

Other vaporizers—Because desflurane has an unusually high vapor pressure, boiling at 22.8°C, a conventional vaporizer cannot be used (Eger et al., 2002). The vaporizer is heated to a constant temperature to vaporize the agent. Electromechanical sensors and controls in the chamber and in the fresh gas flow paths act, in concert with the concentration dial, to proportionally alter the flow of agent vapor into the fresh gas pathway. A series of light emitting diode (LED) lights and a bar graph display vaporizer functional status and agent level in the vaporizer chamber. A specialized filling port is used to connect the agent bottle to the vaporizer chamber.

IV. Anesthesia machines and workstations

The recent trend toward building electronically controlled machines with integrated monitors, ventilators, and safety systems has resulted in a new class of anesthesia machines, often called anesthesia workstations.

Multiple flowmeters are the rule, including dual-tube O_2 flowmeters, as well as N_2O, an O_2 proportioning system, and often, medical air. In most cases, two or more vaporizers can be used with a lockout mechanism (Figs. 6.6 and 6.9). Pressure gauges for small tank yoke assemblies and often for the central gas supply system are located below the flowmeter block. In anticipation of a higher surgical caseload and lengthy procedures, dual canister absorber systems are frequently used. Many of these machines also include a mounting point for a nonrebreathing system

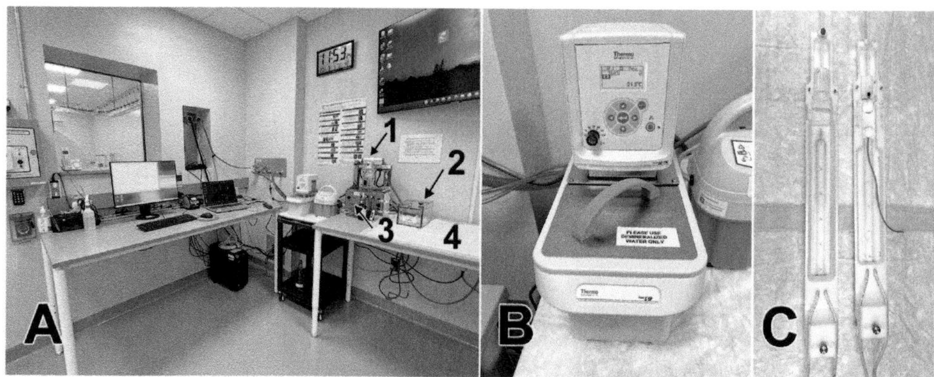

FIGURE 6.9 A rodent anesthesia workstation. (A) A complete set up for magnetic resonance imaging scanning area with (1) O_2 flowmeter and isoflurane; (2) induction chamber; (3) active scavenging system; (4) water circulating heating underneath the induction chamber. (B) Water warming system (ThermoFisher Scientific, Waltham, MA) that can connect to a holding tray (C) to warm the floor of the tray for rats (*left*) and mice (*right*). Note that the tray on the right has a respiratory pad connector (*blue*) used to monitor respiration.

adapter. Most have mechanical ventilators, made by or for the machine manufacturer. A ventilator selector switch may be included to facilitate changing from spontaneous or manually assisted ventilation to mechanical ventilation. Alarm warnings of fresh gas supply failure, high breathing circuit pressure, and ventilator function are also common.

Flat panel displays and touch-controlled screens allow the anesthetist to operate the machine and arrange and display critical patient and machine status information. A tiered system of alarms, warnings, and advisories are used to keep the operator aware of patient and machine status. Most of the familiar working components of the machine are concealed from the user, and the complexity of these machines is belied by a deceptively simple appearance. Except for emergency O_2, anesthesia workstations are dependent upon a steady power supply, and are often equipped with backup batteries. When the machine is turned on, it conducts a series of self-tests and checks, including prompts for needed corrective actions by the operator. Extensive training and familiarization are needed to operate workstations, and the procedures vary with each new model. Workstations require regular maintenance and service by a trained technician (Ehrenwerth et al., 2020).

A. Maintenance and testing

The anesthesia machine should be tested before use. The recommended steps vary with the machine and type of circuits to be used. Anesthesia equipment texts contain extensive descriptions of checkout procedures. With consistent use, the procedures can be accomplished in a reasonably short time and are an essential method of assuring patient and personnel safety.

The machine should be inspected to assure that breathing gas O_2 supplies are adequate, properly connected, and functioning. The flowmeters are turned on and off while observing the float. It should move smoothly as the flow is increased and decreased, and it should indicate zero flow in the off position.

With no fresh gas flow, the vaporizer is checked for an adequate fill level, ensuring that the filling port is closed and that the vaporizer is turned off. The low-pressure circuits are now checked using a suction bulb fitted with a valve and tubing terminating with a 15 mm connector to the common gas outlet. The bulb is compressed until it is empty, and observed for 10 seconds. If the bulb remains empty, the low-pressure circuitry is not significantly leaking. Again, with no gas flowing, the vaporizer is turned on, and the test is repeated to check for leaks in the vaporizer. For machines with multiple vaporizers, each is tested in turn. The fresh gas hose is reconnected to the fresh gas outlet.

The patient breathing circuit and reservoir bag are connected, and the APL valve is closed. The patient connector is occluded by hand, or more conveniently, an appropriately sized rubber stopper. Using the flowmeters or O_2 flush valve, the bag is filled to a pressure of 30–40 cm H_2O on the breathing system manometer. The pressure should not drop over a 10 seconds period (Dorsch and Dorsch, 2008b). Mason (1993) describes a similar test, but specifies a drop of less than 5 cm H_2O over a 30 second period. The pressure is released using the APL valve, allowing assessment of the valve and preventing dust from the absorber from being forced into the breathing circuit by sudden decompression. If a universal control arm is used, the mapleson circuits can be similarly assessed. However, coaxial versions of these systems, such as Bain circuits, must also be tested to assure that the inner fresh tube has not become disconnected. A disposable syringe plunger is used to occlude the inner fresh gas tube while the fresh gas is flowing. Suggested flow rates vary from 0.05 (Mason, 1993) to 2 L/min (Dorsch and Dorsch, 2008b). When the fresh gas supply tube is occluded, the flowmeter indicator should fall. A suggested anesthesia machine check list is provided in Table 6.9.

V. Induction chambers

Induction chambers are used as a means to induce anesthesia and avoid manual restraint. They are among the most common methods used to induce anesthesia in rodents, but are also used for aggressive or fearful larger animals. Ideally, this induction chamber should be performed in a fume hood or downdraft station. The chamber should allow enough space for the animal to assume a normally extended position as anesthesia is induced. A species-appropriate induction chamber helps ensure the volume is appropriate and not excessive, thereby minimizing induction time, and the volume of anesthetic gas released when opening the chamber, and reducing personnel exposure. A chamber may appear to be adequate for a conscious animal but might result in anatomical distortion and airway compromise as consciousness is lost.

Colorless, transparent chambers are preferred because they permit the anesthetist to observe the animal during induction. However, there are translucent (amber) induction chambers available to reduce environmental stimuli. Most commercially available chambers are plastic and meet these requirements. In facilities with access to a machine shop, custom plastic induction chambers are easily fabricated. However, inhalation agents are powerful solvents and aggressively degrade most plastics. The lid should fit tightly enough to prevent leaking and to foil escape attempts; many commercial designs use a gasket and locking mechanism to ensure a tight seal. While the chamber inlet diameter may vary, the diameter of the outlet should accommodate 19–30 mm tubing without significant restriction, in order to avoid resistance to flow and increased pressure in the chamber.

A connection to an anesthetic machine provides the ability to introduce O_2 and control the concentration of the anesthetic agent. The location of entry and exit ports for the gas varies widely, but in a study of carbon dioxide euthanasia, Golledge (2006) reported that introducing fresh gas at the top of the chamber ensured better mixing.

There is a relationship between the chamber volume and the fresh gas flow needed to achieve an anesthetic level in a given time. Using the time constant, tau, it is simple to predict the time needed to reach the desired anesthetic concentration in a chamber. Eq. (6.1) is a simplified version.

$$\text{Time Constant(tau)} = \frac{\text{Volume(liters)}}{\text{Flow(liters per minute)}} \quad (6.1)$$

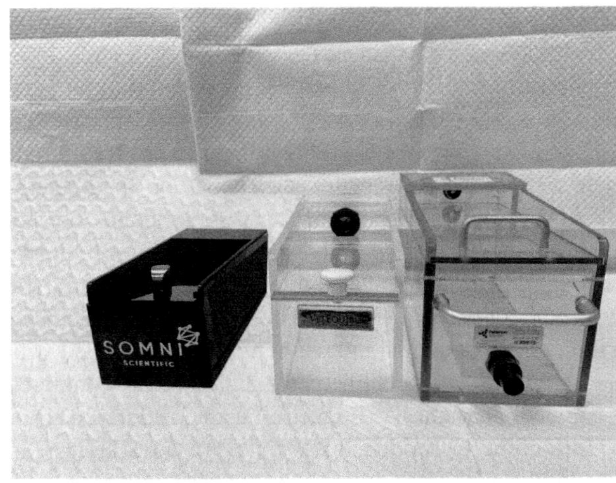

FIGURE 6.10 Anesthesia induction chambers that can be used with an active scavenging system from Somni Scientific (*left*), VetEquip (*middle*), and Patterson Scientific (vapor-vac hooded, *right*). These induction chambers simultaneously allow room air and waste gases to be drawn into a waste gas collection system.

The time constant, tau, is expressed in minutes to reach 95% of the concentration set on the vaporizer requires three time constants. The remaining 5% is negligible and well within the accuracy limits of vaporizers. At a fresh gas flow of 1 L/min into a 2-L chamber, tau is 2 min, and 3 tau is 6 minutes. In this example, doubling the fresh gas to 2 L halves the required time and illustrates a convenient relationship.

It is also obvious that very large (fish tank-size) chambers will require considerably more time, O_2, and anesthetic agents. Anesthesia flowmeters do not ordinarily exceed 10 L/min, and vaporizer output tends to drop off at high flows, so attempting to match the flow to the chamber volume is unrealistic in larger chambers.

Anesthesia induction chambers are major sources of pollution with waste gas, as discussed elsewhere in this text. Therefore, ideally, use induction chambers in a fume hood and/or with an active scavenging system. Actively scavenged chambers for rodents are available (Fig. 6.10).

VI. Choosing inhalants for research

Because there is no ideal inhalant, researchers should use an agent based on availability, what they want to accomplish, research aim(s), and/or the health and safety of the animal. Nowadays, isoflurane and sevoflurane are commonly used in research facilities. Although desflurane has a faster induction and recovery, because it must be used with specific heated vaporizers and it is expensive, it is not frequently used in research. Sevoflurane has been reported to be safe in neonatal rats compared to isoflurane or hypothermia (Huss et al., 2016). Most inhalants suppress the cardiopulmonary system, i.e., blood pressure, in a dose-dependent manner (for example, hypotension will be more severe at 2 MAC vs. 1 MAC) (Table 6.7). Heart rate may be increased with the use of isoflurane and sevoflurane while cardiac index remains the same for both agents (Ebert, 1996). Both isoflurane and sevoflurane do not sensitize the heart to catecholamine-induced arrhythmia. Although the arrhythmogenic threshold between isoflurane and sevoflurane seem to be similar, sevoflurane anesthesia in the swine myocardial infarction model is associated with less arrhythmia and better hemodynamic stability compared to isoflurane anesthesia (Regueiro-Purrinos et al., 2011).

Induction technique with inhalant anesthetics—In general, for most large animals, a sole mask induction with gas anesthetic is not recommended. Mask or chamber induction can significantly increase patients' stress, increase staff exposure to the gas anesthetic, increase induction time to patients compared to intravenous injectable anesthetics, and lengthen the period of unprotected airways, which may compromise airway patency. Due to the high gas anesthetic concentration needed especially if used as a sole agent, this technique can possibly lead to cardiorespiratory depression. However, after animals are premedicated with injectable drugs (i.e., ketamine/xylazine, acepromazine/morphine, etc.), mask induction with gas anesthetic could be done at a lower concentration. An alternative method of inhalant anesthetic induction is the use of injectable anesthetics such as propofol, ketamine/diazepam, alfaxalone, or etomidate, which are commonly performed in large animals. In rodents, an induction using gas anesthesia in an induction chamber commonly occurs. When possible, techniques minimizing human exposure to inhalant anesthetics should be used. These techniques can be, but are not limited to, turning off the gas anesthetic prior to opening an induction chamber or using an active scavenging system.

The mask induction technique should start with a mask that possesses a diaphragm supplied with 100% O_2 at 2–3 L/min for a few minutes (be careful with the patient's eyes). Then, an anesthetist can use an inhalant anesthetic, such as isoflurane or sevoflurane, at a lower concentration (0.5% for isoflurane; 1% for sevoflurane), then gradually increase to 2% for isoflurane; 3% for sevoflurane, within a few minutes, and finally increase to 3%–5% (isoflurane) or 6%–8% (sevoflurane) for a complete induction. This gradual technique minimizes the patient's excitement during anesthetic induction.

Maintenance with inhalant anesthetics—Inhalant anesthetics are the most commonly used anesthetic methodology, especially in North America. Although injectable anesthesia (i.e., propofol, etc.) can be used to maintain general anesthesia, gas anesthesia is much simpler to control the anesthetic depth. Additionally, the use of gas anesthesia via endotracheal tube (ET tube) protects the patient's airway, the ability to support and control respiration, and provides fast induction and recovery due to low blood/gas solubility. There are also some disadvantages, similar to other anesthetics in a dose-dependent manner, such as cardiorespiratory depression, vasodilation leading to hypotension, hypothermia, and arrhythmias. Usually, with premedication, inhalant anesthetics can be maintained at 1–1.5 MAC depending on the procedures, health status, and individual animals. Ideally, balanced anesthesia techniques should be used, for example, a combination of isoflurane with continuous rate infusion (CRI) of propofol or fentanyl. This balanced anesthesia reduces the dose requirement of each anesthetic.

Recovery from inhalant anesthetics—If gas anesthesia is used, fast recovery should be expected. One of the most common complications of prolonged recovery is hypothermia. Therefore, the patient's body temperature should be monitored throughout. If patient is intubated, typically, the ET tube should remain in place until a few strong swallow reflexes are noted. If premedication is used, a reversal agent may be needed. Note that if a reversal agent is used, analgesia (i.e., from dexmedetomidine) may be reversed. However, if the anesthesia is long or if a patient is hypothermic, the ET tube may be kept longer. After the ET tube is removed, patient should be closely monitored for airway patency or resedation after the reversal agent.

VII. Waste anesthetic gas

A. Introduction

WAG pollution awareness has steadily increased over the past half-century, and it is now accepted that volatile anesthetics release WAG into the environment. In fact, the estimated 250,000 healthcare professionals—including 50,000 veterinarians and veterinary technicians—are routinely exposed to trace WAG levels (Occupational Safety and Health Administration, 2000).

High WAG interest pertaining to veterinary anesthesia generally, and particularly laboratory animal anesthesia, has likewise increased. The first published works addressing WAG pollution in the veterinary setting occurred in 1976 (Sawyer, 1976a, 1976b), 1977 (Best and McGrath, 1977), and 1980 (Manley and McDonell, 1980a,b). Although these early commentaries created subject matter awareness, actual research studies were not conducted for several years. The first studies (Ruby et al., 1980; Wingfield et al., 1981) surveyed Colorado small-animal private practice veterinarians and indicated WAG exposure that occurred in private veterinary practice hospitals, was far less than the corresponding human literature. A similar study conducted in 1981 (Dreesen et al., 1981) assessed student, staff, and faculty WAG risk in a veterinary teaching hospital (University of Georgia), and concluded WAG exposure was present, but credited newly established scavenging systems with minimizing exposure. Ward and Byland (Ward and Byland, 1982a,b) reported on the use of a spectrophotometer device to monitor the real-time WAG exposure of veterinary personnel. This air sampling technique remains the gold standard for WAG monitoring. Milligan et al. (1982) reported real-time recovery room WAG monitoring results at a veterinary teaching hospital (Cornell University). This study showed postextubation methoxyflurane emissions were dependent on the anesthetic concentration delivered and that WAG could be emitted for up to 128 minutes. The first retrospective study published assessing veterinarians' reproductive outcomes with occupational exposure (Johnson et al., 1987) surveyed 1914 women US veterinary school graduates (1970–80). Although no direct correlations could be drawn, it was concluded that WAG employment advice and training should occur. These early veterinary facility environmental measurements indicated WAG exposures are an order of magnitude or more below the measured human surgical facility levels (Johnson et al., 1987). However, the low-level WAG exposure risk from laboratory animal anesthesia was unknown. The first laboratory animal anesthesia study demonstrated WAG pollution should also be expected when common rodent anesthetic techniques are employed (Smith and Bolon, 2002). Readers are directed to (Table 6.10) for a brief review of the key contributions to the veterinary literature described below.

Any WAG pollution discussion would be incomplete without including information on the U.S. government safety guidelines. Passage of the Occupational Safety and Health Act (1970) created two separate regulating bodies with different responsibilities to execute the provisions of the Act. The National Institute for Occupational Safety and Health (NIOSH) oversaw research, education, and rule-making, as they relate to occupational illnesses, while the Occupational Safety and Health Administration (OSHA) provided investigative, enforcement, and standard enacting responsibilities of the Act (Dorsch, 2008). To assist NIOSH in formulating its current criteria for a Recommended Standard document (National Institute for Occupational Safety and Health, 1977), the American Society of Anesthesiologists (ASA) joined forces with NIOSH. An ASA ad hoc committee was formed in 1974 with the charter of conducting a large U.S. epidemiological study of operating room personnel. The committee's first report was published in 1974, with the expectation of a follow-up study in 1978, measuring WAG-scavenging technique effectiveness. However, after the alleged incriminating data from the first study (1974), NIOSH withdrew its follow-up study support and proceeded to finalize its criteria document. Of note is the fact that this NIOSH Criteria Document (1977) (National Institute for Occupational Safety and Health, 1977) has never been adopted as a federal standard and thus is not officially enforceable by OSHA. However, lacking any further United States policy documents on this issue, these recommendations are still referred to today. A NIOSH Criteria Document summary, including its notorious recommended exposure levels (RELs) for halogenated agents, has been prepared for readers Table 6.11. After the NIOSH Criteria Document's was released, the ASA published "WAG in Operating Room Air: A Suggested Program to Reduce Personnel Exposure," written by its Ad Hoc Committee on Effects of Trace Anesthetic Agents on the Health of Operating Room Personnel (1981). This document has subsequently been revised to include more current standards and information. And in 1989, the American Conference of Governmental Industrial Hygienists (ACGIH) assigned a threshold limit value-time-weighted average (TLV-TWA) for N_2O, halothane, and enflurane of 50, 50, and 75 parts per million (ppm), respectively (for a normal 8-h workday). Table 6.12 provides WAG safety recommendations.

TABLE 6.10 Key contributions to WAG pollution in the veterinary literature.

Year	Authors	Contributions summary
1976	Sawyer (1976b)	Earliest mention of occupational WAG exposure hazards in veterinary industry
1980	Manley and McDonell (1980b)	Recommended employing gas-scavenging system to reduce WAG pollution
1980	Ruby et al. (1980)	First retrospective study—private practice
1981	Dreesen et al. (1981)	First retrospective study—veterinary school
1982	Ward and Byland (1982a)	Utilized infrared spectrophotometer equipment for real time WAG assessment
1982	Milligan et al. (1982)	Monitored anesthetic pollution in recovery rooms
1987	Johnson et al. (1987)	First retrospective study on reproductive outcomes
1990	Burkhart and Stobbe (1990)	Described mobile charcoal absorption device
2002	Smith and Bolon (2002)	Reported WAG emissions in rodent laboratory animal setting

TABLE 6.11 - Current NIOSH recommendation (NIOSH, 1977) summary relating to the laboratory.

- Issued recommended exposure levels (RELs) for both nitrous oxide and halogenated agents (including methoxyflurane, halothane, and enflurane).
- No worker should be exposed at ceiling concentrations greater than 2 ppm of any halogenated anesthetic agent over a sampling period not to exceed 1 h.
- The REL of nitrous oxide, when used as the sole inhaled anesthetic agent, is 25 ppm measured as a TWA.
- All anesthetic delivery machines should be equipped with WAG collection (scavenging) and removal (disposal) devices from the work environment.
- Anesthetic work practices should be utilized to obtain and maintain minimum WAG concentrations.
- Medical surveillance shall be made available to all employees subject to occupational WAG exposure.
- Employees shall be informed of the possible WAG exposure health effects.
- An air-monitoring program shall be implemented and supervised by knowledgeable personnel, with appropriate record keeping to follow.

TABLE 6.12 US WAG safety recommendation summaries.

Year	Action	Summary
1970	Passage of occupational health and safety Act[a]	NIOSH[b] and OSHA[c] agencies established
1974	ASA[d] ad hoc committee epidemiological study	Conducted national study of effects of WAG on health of operating room personnel
1977	Criteria document prepared by NIOSH[e]	Recommended permissible levels of exposure (REL) for halogenated anesthetic agents[f]
1981	ASA publication	ASA ad hoc committee results[g]
1983	Joint commission on accreditation of healthcare organizations	Recommend equipping all anesthesia machines with gas-scavenging devices
1987	ACGIH[h]	TLV-TWA recommendations[i]
1994	NIOSH alert[j]	Updates on N_2O usage and safety
1996	AVCA ad hoc committee	Veterinary anesthesia specialty recommendations[k]
1999	ASA document revision	Revised 1981 publication
2000	OSHA guidelines[l]	Established guidelines for use of halogenated agents in the workplace

[a]*Occupational Safety and Health Act of 1970, PL 91–596.*
[b]*National Institute for Occupational Safety and Health.*
[c]*Occupational Safety and Health Administration.*
[d]*ASA Ad Hoc Committee on Effects of Trace Anesthetic Agents on the Health of Operating Room Personnel.*
[e]*NIOSH Criteria for a Recommended Standard: Occupational Exposure to Waste Anesthetic Gases and Vapors, Publication No. 77–140 (1977).*
[f]*Summarized in Table 6.11.*
[g]*ASA Ad Hoc Committee on Effects of Trace Anesthetic Agents on the Health of Operating Room Personnel. Waste Anesthetic in Operating Room Air: A Suggested Program to Reduce Personnel Exposure (1981).*
[h]*American Conference of Governmental Industrial Hygienists.*
[i]*American Conference of Governmental Industrial Hygienists. TLV-TWA of 50 ppm for N_2O.*
[k]*ACVA, Ad Hoc Committee on Waste Anesthetic Gas Pollution and its Control. Commentary and recommendations on control of waste anesthetic gases in the workplace (1996).*
[l]*Occupational Safety and Health Association (OSHA). Guidelines for workplace exposures (2000).*

B. Potential health effects

1. *Historic perspectives*

Workplace environment WAG contamination is not a new phenomenon. Its medical literature discussion dates to the early 1900s, when a German surgeon connected the deleterious health effects to surgeons with constant anesthetic exposure (Kelling, 1918). In the 1920s, the idea of removing hazardous anesthetic gases from the operating room environment was discussed (Goerig and Pothmann, 2004). Early WAG pollution and health concerns in the literature were strictly anecdotal until the 1960s, when A.I.

Vaisman, a Russian anesthesiologist, published a now-historical epidemiological report correlating work conditions with the adverse health effects experienced by Russian anesthesiologists (Vaisman, 1967). Of particular concern in this notable study was the suspected link between WAG and increased spontaneous abortions. Sixteen similar studies were embarked upon during the following decade; most have now been criticized for their poor study design, statistical errors, under-powering, and poor result analysis. Nine of these studies connected WAG occupational exposure to deleterious health effects, while the remaining seven failed to make a statistically significant correlation (Sessler and Badgwell, 1998). One study was large epidemiological, undertaken jointly by the ASA and NIOSH, reporting an increased spontaneous abortion risk in exposed women and an increased congenital abnormalities risk in the offspring of exposed males; a 1.3–2-fold cancer occurrence increase (leukemia and lymphoma) in exposed females; a significant hepatic disease increase in all exposed women, and some exposed men; and a 1.2–1.4-fold renal disease increase in exposed women (Foley, 1993).

WAG studies after 1980 attempted to substantiate the earlier anecdotal studies' data. Laboratory investigations were conducted utilizing live animals, tissues, and cell cultures to provide sound scientific evidence supporting the earlier epidemiological data. Distinctions between trace and high WAG levels were also established after 1980 with the successful adoption of various scavenging techniques. Dorsch (2008) defined trace anesthetic gas levels as being far below the concentration needed for anesthesia, or levels detected by smell. To date, no studies link occupational exposure to trace WAG levels with any adverse health effects. The ASA Task Force (1999) noted that adverse health effects are associated with chronic exposure to high WAG levels, although these studies failed to demonstrate an association between trace WAG levels (such as those found in scavenged human/veterinary hospitals) and adverse health effects. The Task Force concluded that even at the maximum allowable isoflurane and halothane dose, there was no evidence of significant health damage and therefore no data to suggest WAG exposure is dangerous to hospital employees (including pregnant women) working in a properly scavenged environment.

In summary, controversy remains concerning the actual adverse health effects (discussed below) linked to occupational WAG exposure, as well as how much effort should be placed on risk mitigation. Initial veterinary literature concluded the WAG exposure levels of veterinarians and staff exposed were lower than the reported human hospital personnel exposures. Subsequent veterinary studies have shown this early premise may be incorrect (McKelvey and Hollingshead, 2003). However, these veterinary studies were not undertaken in a laboratory animal environment where common work practices and equipment (induction box use, high carrier-gas flow rates, face mask use, multiple patient delivery systems, high-throughput design, etc.) increase the likelihood of occupational WAG exposure (Smith and Bolon, 2002). Therefore, in the laboratory animal environment, continued vigilance is prudent to reduce occupational WAG exposure and is a high priority.

C. Health and safety

The majority of studies reporting potential adverse health effects of WAG exposure related to chronic or long-term exposure (weeks, months, and/or years). In the short-term setting (immediately following exposure), safety effects include drowsiness, irritability, depression, headache, nausea, and fatigue were reported (National Institute for Occupational Safety and Health, 1977). Anesthesiologists reported perceptual, cognitive, and motor skill deficits after high WAG exposure levels in unscavenged environments (Burm, 2003). While these effects usually dissipate soon after WAG exposure, they are concerning as they may impact the surgical success and compromise operating room staff safety and health. However, these short-term neurological effects are less likely when proper work practices (e.g., WAG scavenging) are employed (Dorsch and Dorsch, 2008a). Table 6.13 summarizes the published organ system effects.

TABLE 6.13 WAG organ system effects.

Organ system or condition	Author
Reproductive	McKelvey and Hollingshead (2003)
	Buring et al. (1985)
	Boivin (1997)
Liver	McKelvey and Hollingshead (2003)
	Byhahn et al. (2001)
	Dorsch and Dorsch (2008c)
Carcinogenicity	McKelvey and Hollingshead (2003)
	Hoerauf et al. (1999)
	Dorsch and Dorsch (2008c)
Other	Smith and Bolon (2003)
	Dorsch and Dorsch (2008c)

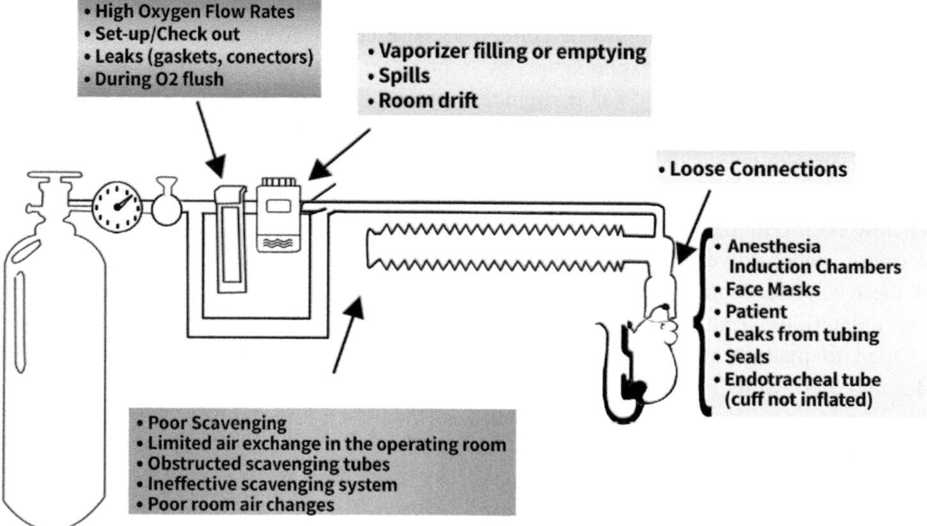

FIGURE 6.11 Schematic of common waste anesthetic gas leak sources.

D. Sources

Fig. 6.11 outlines the various WAG sources. Collectively, these comprise the anesthetic machine, the anesthetic environment, and the patient. Of particular concern in laboratory animal medicine are high O_2 flow rates, anesthetic induction chambers, poorly fitted face masks, and poor scavenging. Open-drop or bell-jar anesthetic techniques, commonly used in rodent anesthesia, employ an inhalant-anesthetic-soaked cotton ball may still be used, potentially yielding high WAG exposure and poorly controlled patient anesthesia. Taylor and Mook (2009) assessed WAG exposure using the open-drop method at 20 and 40 cm from the source opening to be at or near 0 ppm. Additionally, individuals may not provide themselves or small rodents with sufficient WAG protection or health protection by performing unscavenged gas anesthesia in fume hoods, type II A2 biosafety cabinets, or cage change stations. Fume hoods lack a biosecure environment for animals undergoing procedures while affording humans WAG protection. Type II A2 biosafety cabinets and cage change stations recirculate WAG within the room, providing potential WAG sources for humans and animals.

E. Exposure mitigation

WAG exposure mitigation includes the process of collecting the excess gases from the anesthetic delivery equipment, or the patient, and removing them from the working environment. Scavenging or evacuation systems utilize gas-capturing devices, interfaces, and gas-disposal systems to accomplish this important task.

The NIOSH Criteria Document (National Institute for Occupational Safety and Health, 1977) recommends WAG scavenging, work practices to reduce WAG pollution, WAG monitoring, and medical surveillance of all potentially exposed personnel. Of these recommendations, the most effective step in reducing WAG levels in the surgical environment is installing an effective scavenging system (McGregor, 2000). The Guide for the Care and Use of Laboratory Animals by the NRC (1996) states: "Exposure to anesthetic waste gases should be limited. This is usually accomplished by using various scavenging techniques."

In general, the N_2O and halothane concentrations reported in the anesthetist's breathing zone in a ventilated surgical suite (without scavenging) during the 1970s was 200–500 and 2–5 ppm, respectively. N_2O and halothane concentrations in unventilated, unscavenged surgical suites were as high as 7000 and 85 ppm, respectively (McKelvey and Hollingshead, 2003) The NIOSH Criteria Document (National Institute for Occupational Safety and Health, 1977) recommended human hospital scavenging systems capable of reducing halothane and N_2O concentrations to 0.2–0.5 and 15–35 ppm, respectively. In veterinary hospitals, applying scavenging techniques reduced isoflurane and halothane concentrations to 1–20 ppm and N_2O concentrations to 50–200 ppm (Gardner et al., 1991). Using scavenging techniques reduces WAG concentrations tenfold (Lecky, 1977), or by 90% (1996). However, even with the successful addition of WAG-scavenging systems, training and equipment-checking procedures are necessary. A study by Soontranan et al. (2002) showed 10/38 scavenging systems (26.3%) within a human teaching hospital were incorrectly installed. All problems were due to device assembly errors and could have been avoided with routine preuse equipment checks and regular maintenance.

1. Facility planning, design, and construction

Institutions should strongly consider employing computational fluid dynamics (CFD) in the design of various vivaria areas, including animal holding rooms, high-level containment facilities (e.g., A/BSL3), and areas where anesthetic gases will be employed. Using CFD, one can understand the likely air mixing and flow within an area, and with WAGs, one can optimize a layout to dilute WAGs, mitigate personnel exposure, etc. This is especially important considering (in the case of a surgical procedure) personnel WAG exposure may occur in multiple rooms throughout the facility, including the patient preparation area, operating room, postoperative/ICU facilities, and animal holding rooms. Using CFD to determine where the optimal placement of room air supply/exhaust elements would greatly facilitate WAG exposure while reducing exposure to personnel and animals. Placement of room air supply/exhaust elements would be of particular concern in procedure rooms (e.g., operating rooms, imaging), patient prep areas, postprocedure spaces, and animal holding rooms. Although numerous studies describe WAG pollution, very few specifically address patient exposure after they leave the surgical area. Recovery room and post-anesthesia care unit (PACU) personnel WAG exposure via exhalations of postoperative human and veterinary patients has been reported. Corbett and Ball (1971) measured methoxyflurane in the end-expired air of patients and anesthesiologist was detectable for 10–18 days and 30 hours after an anesthetic event, respectively. Bruce and Linde (1972), Byhahn et al. (2001), and Sessler and Badgwell (1998) measured human PACU halothane concentrations and found they exceeded current NIOSH recommendations; and Corbett and Ball (1971) reported increased fluoride concentrations in anesthesiologists' urine. In the veterinary literature, Milligan et al. (1982) reported canine methoxyflurane emissions for up to 128 minutes postextubation, while Smith and Bolon (2003) reported isoflurane emissions for 18 hours post-canine extubation. These studies confirm occupational WAG exposures, at levels exceeding trace amounts, occur in many human and veterinary hospital areas, and identify the patient as an exposure source. In the veterinary and laboratory animal settings, WAG exposure can be extended to research staff or animal owners. Therefore, anesthesia and recovery areas require appropriate planning, design, and construction considerations, including proper room ventilation and exhaust methods for controlling WAG.

Downdraft/back draft tables can provide a sound methodology to remove WAG while providing a heated surface to conduct anesthetic or surgical procedures (Fig. 6.12). An alternative or adjunct would be employing a moveable and pivoting "snorkel apparatus" (Fig. 6.13) to focally reduce WAG pollution via a partial vacuum at its inlet port.

Imaging equipment can be particularly troublesome for scavenging, especially the smaller, self-contained imaging devices such as those that provide radiographs and bioluminescence. These devices use inhalant anesthetics to immobilize animals for an otherwise nonpainful procedure. While the rooms may have the suggested 10–15 room air changes per hour, the ventilation rate in these contained devices is often significantly less.

2. Active scavenging equipment and techniques

Active scavenging uses a pump or fan to move anesthetic gases away from the patient and equipment, and into the

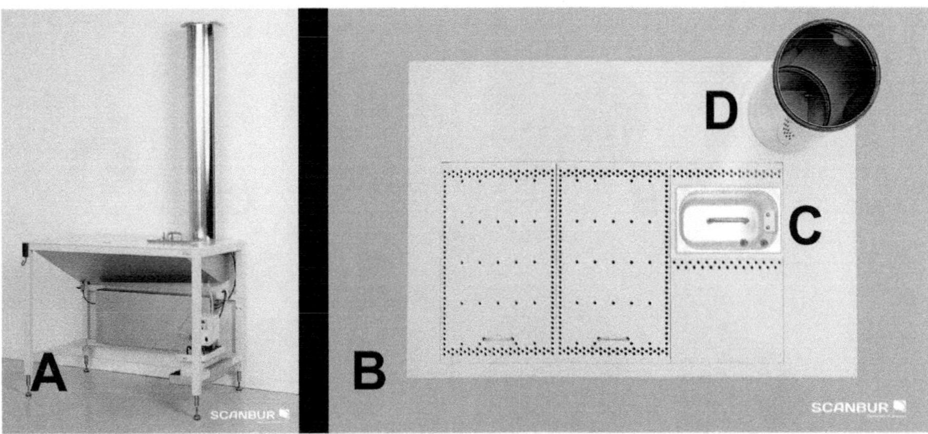

FIGURE 6.12 (A) A polymer operating downdraft table (front view, from Scanbur). This height-adjustable downdraft table has an easy to clean Corian surface, including a heated downdraft area for rodent procedures. (B) Top view of downdraft table demonstrating the heated downdraft surface, induction chamber (C) with adjacent downdraft ports, and (D) exhaust plenum. *Courtesy Janni Nielsen, Scanbur, Denmark.*

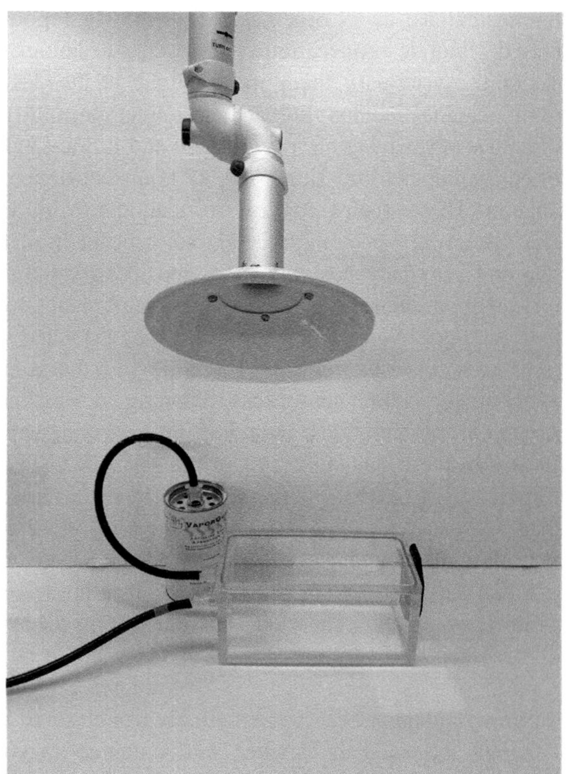

FIGURE 6.13 Example of simple "snorkel apparatus" for active WAG evacuation placed at the induction chamber opening. *Courtesy of Scanbur, Denmark.*

scavenging device. This is the most effective way to remove WAG. Many active scavenging systems are available in both human and veterinary settings (McKelvey and Hollingshead, 2003).

The "snorkel apparatus" is an active scavenging technique used in laboratory animal anesthesia (Fig. 6.13), consisting of corrugated plastic or stainless-steel tubing that directly vents to the heating, ventilation, and air-conditioning (HVAC) system (nonrecirculating air). The suction necessary to evacuate WAGs varies depending on the tubing diameter, the anesthetic carrier gas flow rates, and the existing facility design. Snorkel devices are generally placed around inhalant anesthetic delivery equipment areas where WAG emissions are the highest (vaporizer-filling port, induction box, animal, face-mask interface, charcoal absorption canister vents, etc.). Snorkel devices should not be placed so close to a patient that they diminish the anesthetic gas concentration delivered. Snorkel advantages include ease of use and flexibility in placement, while disadvantages include the initial expense of ducting these devices within the existing facility design and increased difficulty in cleaning and maintaining a sterile surgical environment. If active scavenging systems are used, coaxial masks (Fig. 6.14) are recommended.

3. *Passive scavenging equipment and techniques*

A passive WAG scavenging system utilizes the gas' positive pressure in the anesthetic machine to push WAG into the scavenging device. Different types of passive configurations can be used, which in the laboratory animal environment commonly include discharge tubing, room ventilation, and activated charcoal adsorption canisters.

Discharge tubing simply connects the anesthetic machine with the outside environment, usually through a hole in a wall. McKelvey and Hollingshead (2003) recommend

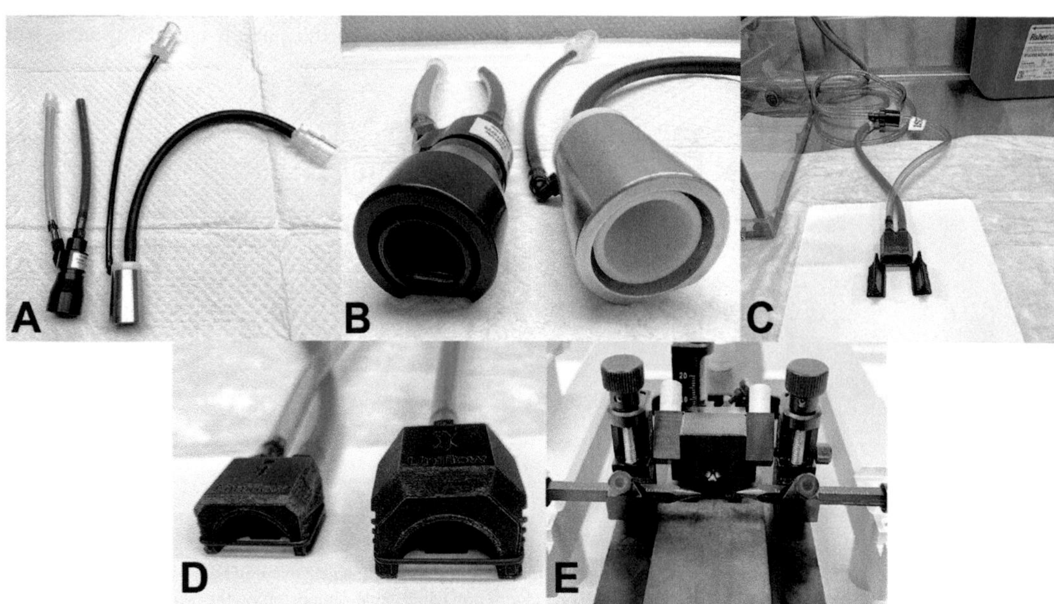

FIGURE 6.14 (A and B) Coaxial masks from Patterson Scientific, and (C and D) Somni Scientific [(D) A mask for mice (*left*) and rats (*right*)]. (E) A mouse gas anesthesia mask set up (Stoelting). The mask is mounted on a stereotaxic frame. The two tubes on either side are connected to fresh gas (i.e., O_2 and isoflurane) and scavenging system. This mask can be used with an active scavenging system.

a distance to the outside environment of less than 20 feet, making this method suitable only for externally adjacent rooms. The use of the room's nonrecirculating ventilation system is also a passive scavenging example. In this situation, the standard air changes per hour of the room's ventilation are employed to remove WAG and reduce their levels to acceptable standards. The American College of Veterinary Anesthesiologists (ACVA) (1996) recommends a nonrecirculating ventilation system, which can provide at least 12–15 air changes per hour.

In situations where other scavenging systems are unavailable, activated charcoal cannisters can be used to absorb volatile anesthetic agents from the waste gas. However, these devices cannot be used to remove N_2O. In the veterinary/laboratory animal setting, activated charcoal canister use is common due to their low cost, ease of use, and portability. Activated charcoal canisters should be weighed before and after use and changed based on the manufacturer's recommendations. Studies to qualify and quantify activated charcoal canister effectiveness in the laboratory animal setting (Smith and Bolon, 2002, 2003) found breakthrough WAG emissions; these should be expected when using these devices. Furthermore, their use resulted in WAG concentrations above the NIOSH RELs, illustrating the need for vigilant monitoring and the removal of such canisters when they have reached their manufacturer's suggested end of life or when breakthrough WAG emission occurs.

Active and passive scavenging techniques may be used alone or in combination. The latter option provides the most effective WAG scavenging and is recommended by the ACVA (1996) for veterinary and laboratory animal settings.

4. *Environmental impact of waste anesthetic gas evacuation*

Once proper WAG evacuation occurs, it is usually not reconsidered; however, halogenated agent pollution effects in the outside environment deserve discussion. The volatile anesthetics (halothane, enflurane, and isoflurane) are classified as halogenated chlorofluorocarbons (HCFCs); releasing fluorine, chlorine, and bromine into the atmosphere where these elements can damage the ozone layer. The newer volatile anesthetics, sevoflurane, and desflurane are not HCFCs, but rather fluorinated hydrocarbons, which contain only fluorine and thus are considered less damaging to the ozone layer (Marx, 1999). One recent study calculated that 25 million L of volatile anesthetics are released from German hospitals annually (Marx et al., 2001). To date, it has been considered the acceptable practice to vent or exhaust these agents directly to the outside. However, the Montreal Protocol on Substances That Deplete the Ozone Layer proposed HCFC release abolition into the atmosphere by the year 2030 (United Nations, 1987). The effect this will have on future volatile anesthetic use is unclear.

F. Detection methodologies

Various methodologies are available to detect and quantify WAGs and WAG exposure levels. It is important that these methodologies be employed with the institution's OSHE group to assess each research team's WAG Risk Mitigation Plan and to periodically assess personnel and environmental exposure according to an acceptable methodology. Researchers must include, among other pertinent items, their use of inhalant anesthetics, method of use (e.g., anesthetic machine, open drop bell jar), agent(s) used, and duration of procedures as part of their IACUC-approved protocol prior to initiating any research procedure. The OSHE group must give strong consideration to periodically assessing a research team's WAG exposure in conjunction with other relevant parties, including the attending veterinarian and the IACUC. Table 6.14 outlines the various sampling methodologies.

VIII. Summary and conclusions of waste anesthetic gas

Information gained over the past 50 years shows WAG would be emitted into the environment during volatile

TABLE 6.14 WAG sampling methodologies.

Methodology		Advantage	Disadvantage	References
Instantaneous air sampling	A sample of air from the anesthetic environment is quickly collected into a container (plastic or nylon bag) and transferred to a processing laboratory.	Quick Simple Inexpensive	Not real time	Dorsch and Dorsch (2008c)
Time-weighted average sampling	The TWA exposure during an 8–10 h workday Should not exceed 2 ppm over a period of no greater than 1 h Active and passive dosimetry	Ease of use	Not real time	National Institute for Occupational Safety and Health (1977) Dorsch (2008)
Continuous air sampling	Infrared spectrophotometry	Real time results	Equipment/ cost	Bruce and Linde (1972) Dorsch and Dorsch (2008c)

anesthetic agent use. Furthermore, research has shown this is likely within the laboratory animal research environment. However, work practices, training, and WAG-monitoring programs can be followed to decrease WAG environmental contamination, thereby leading to a safer work setting. Readers are referred to Table 6.11 for a summary of recommended work practices.

The laboratory animal worker is uniquely tasked with conducting anesthesia in a wide variety of species, many of which are small. Their small body size makes routine techniques used in human medicine (e.g., intubation) difficult. Therefore, an induction box, a face mask, and higher carrier-gas flow rates are often used. A further challenge facing the laboratory animal anesthetist is the current practice of high-throughput surgery, making multiple patient anesthesia events a common occurrence. These techniques increase WAG pollution in the laboratory animal setting.

Of the hundreds of studies published on WAG pollution, fewer than 25 were conducted specifically in the veterinary or laboratory animal environment. Although much of what has been written in the human literature can be extrapolated to the veterinary setting, more scientific studies specifically relating to this field should be undertaken. Such literature would lead to continued improvements in risk mitigation of the potential occupational hazards related to volatile anesthetic practices.

Acknowledgments

This book chapter was supported [in part] by the NIH Intramural Research Program, National Institute of Environmental Health Sciences. We thank Janis Atuk-Jones, Benjamin Franco, and Eden Alamaw for their kind assistance in manuscript formatting, sketches, and photo preparation, and Dr. Jieun Kim (Director, Neuroscience Preclinical Imaging Laboratory) for the anesthesia machine photos.

References

American College of Veterinary Anesthesiologists (Acva), 1996. Commentary and recommendations on control of waste anesthetic gases in the workplace. J. Am. Vet. Med. Assoc. 209, 75–77.

Association Veterinary Anaesthetists. 2014. Anaesthetic Safety Checklist. Jurox. http://https://www.jurox.com.au/wp-content/uploads/ANZ-Alfaxan-AVASafetyChecklistB-2014-08-DIGITAL.pdf/. (Accessed 7 April 2022).

Best, J.L., Mcgrath, C.J., 1977. Trace anesthetic gases: an overview. J. Am. Vet. Med. Assoc. 171, 1268–1269.

Bito, H., Ikeda, K., 1994. Long-duration, low-flow sevoflurane anesthesia using two carbon dioxide absorbents. Quantification of degradation products in the circuit. Anesthesiology 81, 340–345. https://doi.org/10.1097/00000542-199408000-00011.

Boarini, D.J., Kassell, N.F., Coester, H.C., Butler, M., Sokoll, M.D., 1984. Comparison of systemic and cerebrovascular effects of isoflurane and halothane. Neurosurgery 15, 400–409. https://doi.org/10.1227/00006123-198409000-00017.

Boivin, J.F., 1997. Risk of spontaneous abortion in women occupationally exposed to anaesthetic gases: a meta-analysis. Occup. Environ. Med. 54, 541–548. https://doi.org/10.1136/oem.54.8.541.

Botman, J., Dugdale, A., Gabriel, F., Vandeweerd, J.M., 2016a. Cardiorespiratory parameters in the awake pigeon and during anaesthesia with isoflurane. Vet. Anaesth. Analg. 43, 63–71. https://doi.org/10.1111/vaa.12262.

Botman, J., Gabriel, F., Dugdale, A.H., Vandeweerd, J.M., 2016b. Anaesthesia with sevoflurane in pigeons: minimal anaesthetic concentration (MAC) determination and investigation of cardiorespiratory variables at 1 MAC. Vet. Rec. 178, 560. Available at: https://doi.org/10.1136/vr.103654.

Bruce, D.L., Linde, H.W., 1972. Halothane content in recovery room air. Anesthesiology 36, 517–518. https://doi.org/10.1097/00000542-197205000-00024.

Brunson, D.B., Stowe, C.M., Mcgrath, C.J., 1979. Serum and urine inorganic fluoride concentrations and urine oxalate concentrations following methoxyflurane anesthesia in the dog. Am. J. Vet. Res. 40, 197–203.

Buring, J.E., Hennekens, C.H., Mayrent, S.L., Rosner, B., Greenberg, E.R., Colton, T., 1985. Health experiences of operating room personnel. Anesthesiology 62 (3), 325–330.

Burkhart, J.E., Stobbe, T.J., 1990. Real-time measurement and control of waste anesthetic gases during veterinary surgeries. Am. Ind. Hyg. Assoc. J. 51, 640–645. https://doi.org/10.1080/15298669091370284.

Burm, A.G., 2003. Occupational hazards of inhalational anaesthetics. Best Pract. Res. Clin. Anaesthesiol. 17, 147–161. https://doi.org/10.1053/bean.2003.0271.

Byhahn, C., Wilke, H.J., Westpphal, K., 2001. Occupational exposure to volatile anaesthetics: epidemiology and approaches to reducing the problem. CNS Drugs 15, 197–215. https://doi.org/10.2165/00023210-200115030-00004.

Cesarovic, N., Nicholls, F., Rettich, A., Kronen, P., Hassig, M., Jirkof, P., et al., 2010. Isoflurane and sevoflurane provide equally effective anaesthesia in laboratory mice. Lab. Anim. 44, 329–336. https://doi.org/10.1258/la.2010.009085.

Clarke, K.W., Trim, C.M., Hall, L.W. 2014. Anesthesia of the pig. In: Clarke, K.W., Trim, C.M., Hall, L.W. (Eds.), Veterinary Anesthesia, 11th ed. W.B. Saunders, New York, pp. 385–403.

Columbano, N., Scanu, A., Duffee, L., Melosu, V., Sotgiu, G., Driessen, B., 2018. Determination of the minimum alveolar concentration (MAC) and cardiopulmonary effects of sevoflurane in sheep. Vet. Anaesth. Analg. 45, 487–495. https://doi.org/10.1016/j.vaa.2018.01.007.

Corbett, T.H., Ball, G.L., 1971. Chronic exposure to methoxyflurane: a possible occupational hazard to anesthesiologists. Anesthesiology 34, 532–537. https://doi.org/10.1097/00000542-197106000-00012.

Crystal, G.J., Czinn, E.A., Silver, J.M., Salem, M.R., 1995. Coronary vasodilation by isoflurane. Abrupt versus gradual administration. Anesthesiology 82, 542–549. https://doi.org/10.1097/00000542-199502000-00024.

Davey, A.J., 2005. Vaporizers. In: Davey, A.J., Diba, A. (Eds.), Ward's Anaesthetic Equipment, fifth ed. Elsevier Saunders, Philadelphia, PA.

Dhulkhed, V., Shetti, A., Naik, S., Dhulkhed, P., 2013. Vapourisers: physical principles and classification. Indian J. Anaesth. 57, 455–463. https://doi.org/10.4103/0019-5049.120141.

Doorley, B.M., Waters, S.J., Terrell, R.C., Robinson, J.L., 1988. MAC of 1−653 in Beagle dogs and New Zealand white rabbits. Anesthesiology 69, 89−91. https://doi.org/10.1097/00000542-198807000-00013.

Dorsch, J.A., 2008. Controlling trace gas levels. In: Brown, B., Dernowski, N. (Eds.), Understanding Anesthesia Equipment, fifth ed. Lippincott, Williams & Wilkins, a Wolters Kluwer business, Philadelphia, PA, pp. 373−404.

Dorsch, J.A., Dorsch, S.E., 2008a. The breathing system: general principles, common components, and classifications. In: Brown, B., Dernowski, N. (Eds.), Understanding Anesthesia Equipment, fifth ed. Lippincott, Williams & Wilkins, a Wolters Kluwer business, Philadelphia, PA, pp. 191−209.

Dorsch, J.A., Dorsch, S.E., 2008b. Equipment checkout and maintenance. In: Brown, B., Dernowski, N. (Eds.), Understanding Anesthesia Equipment, fifth ed. Lippincott, Williams & Wilkins, a Wolters Kluwer business, Philadelphia, PA, pp. 931−955.

Dorsch, J.A., Dorsch, S.E., 2008c. Gas monitoring. In: Brown, B., Dernowski, N. (Eds.), Understanding Anesthesia Equipment, fifth ed. Lippincott, Williams & Wilkins, a Wolters Kluwer business, Philadelphia, PA.

Dreesen, D.W., Jones, G.L., Brown, J., Rawlings, C.A., 1981. Monitoring for trace anesthetic gases in a veterinary teaching hospital. J. Am. Vet. Med. Assoc. 179, 797−799.

Ebert, T.J., 1996. Cardiovascular and autonomic effects of sevoflurane. Acta Anaesthesiol. Belg. 47, 15−21.

Eger 2nd, E.I., 1992. Desflurane animal and human pharmacology: aspects of kinetics, safety, and MAC. Anesth. Analg. 75, S3−S7 discussion S8−S9.

Eger 2nd, E.I., 2004. Characteristics of anesthetic agents used for induction and maintenance of general anesthesia. Am. J. Emerg. Med. 61 (Suppl. 4), S3−S10. https://doi.org/10.1093/ajhp/61.suppl_4.S3.

Eger, 2nd, E.I, Saidman, L.J., 1965. Hazards of nitrous oxide anesthesia in bowel obstruction and pneumothorax. Anesthesiology 26, 61−66. https://doi.org/10.1097/00000542-196501000-00011.

Eger, E.I., Eisenkraft, J.B., Weiskopf, R.B., 2002. Pharmacology of Inhaled Anesthetics. P.8 Library of Congress Number TXV1-035635.

Ehrenwerth, J., Eisenkraft, J.B., Berry, J.M., 2020. The anesthesia machine and workstation. In: Ehrenwerth, J., Eisenkraft, J.B., Berry, J.M. (Eds.), Anesthesia Equipment Principles and Applications. Elsevier, St. Louis, MO, pp. 25−65.

Feldman, J.M., Olympio, M.A., Martin, D., Striker, A. 2008. New guidelines for pre-anesthesia checkout. Anesthesia Patient Safety Foundation. http://https://www.apsf.org/article/new-guidelines-available-for-pre-anesthesia-checkout/. (Accessed 7 April 2022).

Foley, K., 1993. AANA journal course: update for nurse anesthetists—occupational exposure to trace anesthetics: quantifying the risk. AANA J. (Am. Assoc. Nurse Anesth.) 61, 405−412 quiz 412.

Franks, N.P., Lieb, W.R., 1984. Do general anaesthetics act by competitive binding to specific receptors? Nature 310, 599−601. https://doi.org/10.1038/310599a0.

Franks, N.P., Lieb, W.R., 1991. Stereospecific effects of inhalational general anesthetic optical isomers on nerve ion channels. Science 254, 427−430. https://doi.org/10.1126/science.1925602.

Frink Jr., E.J., Isner, R.J., Malan Jr., T.P., Morgan, S.E., Brown, E.A., Brown Jr., B.R., 1994. Sevoflurane degradation product concentrations with soda lime during prolonged anesthesia. J. Clin. Anesth. 6, 239−242. https://doi.org/10.1016/0952-8180(94)90065-5.

Fujita, Y., Kimura, K., Hamada, H., Takaori, M., 1991. Comparative effects of halothane, isoflurane, and sevoflurane on the liver with hepatic artery ligation in the beagle. Anesthesiology 75, 313−318. https://doi.org/10.1097/00000542-199108000-00020.

Fukazawa, K., Lee, H.T., 2014. Volatile anesthetics and AKI: risks, mechanisms, and a potential therapeutic window. J. Am. Soc. Nephrol. 25, 884−892. https://doi.org/10.1681/asn.2013111215.

Gardner, R.J., Hampton, J., Causton, J.S., 1991. Inhalation anaesthetics–exposure and control during veterinary surgery. Ann. Occup. Hyg. 35, 377−388. https://doi.org/10.1093/annhyg/35.4.377.

Goerig, M., Pothmann, W., 2004. Anaesthetic gas pollution at the workplace-An "ancient" problem associated with inhalation anaesthesia. Anasthesiol. Intensivmed. 45, 572−577.

Golledge, H., 2006. Animal welfare aspects of carbon dioxide euthanasia. In: Presentation at the Charles River Laboratories 20th Annual Short Course. Newton, MA.

Hall, R.I., Szlam, F., Hug, C.C., Jr, 1987. The enflurane-sparing effect of alfentanil in dogs. Anesth. Analg 66, 1287−1291.

Hartley, C.J., Reddy, A.K., Madala, S., Michael, L.H., Entman, M.L., Taffet, G.E., 2007. Effects of isoflurane on coronary blood flow velocity in young, old and ApoE(-/-) mice measured by Doppler ultrasound. Ultrasound Med. Biol. 33, 512−521. https://doi.org/10.1016/j.ultrasmedbio.2006.11.002.

Hikasa, Y., Okuyama, K., Kakuta, T., Takase, K., Ogasawara, S., 1998. Anesthetic potency and cardiopulmonary effects of sevoflurane in goats: comparison with isoflurane and halothane. Can. J. Vet. Res. 62, 299−306.

Hoerauf, K., Lierz, M., Wiesner, G., Schroegendorfer, K., Lierz, P., Spacek, A., et al., 1999. Genetic damage in operating room personnel exposed to isoflurane and nitrous oxide. Occup. Environ. Med. 56, 433−437. https://doi.org/10.1136/oem.56.7.433.

Hudson, A.E., Herold, K.F., Hemmings Jr., H.C., 2019. Pharmacology of Inhaled Anesthetics. Pharmacology and Physiology for Anesthesia. Elsevier, pp. 217−240.

Huss, M.K., Chum, H.H., Chang, A.G., Jampachairsi, K., Pacharinsak, C., 2016. The physiologic effects of isoflurane, sevoflurane, and hypothermia used for anesthesia in neonatal rats (*Rattus norvegicus*). J. Am. Assoc. Lab. Anim. Sci. 55, 83−88.

Ikeda, S., 2020. The reincarnation of methoxyflurane. J. Anesth. Hist. 6, 79−83. https://doi.org/10.1016/j.janh.2019.07.001.

Janssen, B.J., De Celle, T., Debets, J.J., Brouns, A.E., Callahan, M.F., Smith, T.L., 2004. Effects of anesthetics on systemic hemodynamics in mice. Am. J. Physiol. Heart Circ. Physiol. 287, H1618−H1624. https://doi.org/10.1152/ajpheart.01192.2003.

Johnson, J.A., Buchan, R.M., Reif, J.S., 1987. Effect of waste anesthetic gas and vapor exposure on reproductive outcome in veterinary personnel. Am. Ind. Hyg. Assoc. J. 48, 62−66. https://doi.org/10.1080/15298668791384373.

Jones, R.M., 1990. Desflurane and sevoflurane: inhalation anaesthetics for this decade? Br. J. Anaesth. 65, 527−536. https://doi.org/10.1093/bja/65.4.527.

Kazama, T., Ikeda, K., 1988. Comparison of MAC and the rate of rise of alveolar concentration of sevoflurane with halothane and isoflurane in the dog. Anesthesiology 68, 435−437. https://doi.org/10.1097/00000542-198803000-00020.

Kelling, G., 1918. Uber die Beseitigung der Narkosedampfe aus dem Operationssaale. Zentralbi Chir 45, 602−606.

Kharasch, E.D., Powers, K.M., Artru, A.A., 2002. Comparison of Amsorb, sodalime, and Baralyme degradation of volatile anesthetics and formation of carbon monoxide and compound a in swine in vivo. Anesthesiology 96, 173−182. https://doi.org/10.1097/00000542-200201000-00031.

Lecky, J.H., 1977. The mechanical aspects of anesthetic pollution control. Anesth. Analg. 56, 769–774. https://doi.org/10.1213/00000539-197711000-00006.

Ludders, J.W., Mitchell, G.S., Rode, J., 1990. Minimal anesthetic concentration and cardiopulmonary dose response of isoflurane in ducks. Vet. Surg. 19, 304–307. https://doi.org/10.1111/j.1532-950x.1990.tb01193.x.

Manley, S.V., Mcdonell, W.N., 1980a. Anesthetic pollution and disease. J. Am. Vet. Med. Assoc. 176, 515–518.

Manley, S.V., Mcdonell, W.N., 1980b. Recommendations for reduction of anesthetic gas pollution. J. Am. Vet. Med. Assoc. 176, 519–524.

Marx, T., 1999. Global pollution—the anaesthetist's contribution. Anaesthesia 54, 301–302. https://doi.org/10.1046/j.1365-2044.1999.0811k.x.

Marx, T., Schmidt, M., Schirmer, U., Reinelt, H., 2001. Pollution of the environment and the workplace with anesthetic gases. Int. Anesthesiol. Clin. 39, 15–27. https://doi.org/10.1097/00004311-200104000-00004.

Mashour, G.A., Forman, S.A., Campagna, J.A., 2005. Mechanisms of general anesthesia: from molecules to mind. Best Pract. Res. Clin. Anaesthesiol. 19, 349–364. https://doi.org/10.1016/j.bpa.2005.01.004.

Mason, D.E., 1993. Anesthesia machine checkout and troubleshooting. In: Bednarski, R.M. (Ed.), Anesthetic Equipment, Seminars in Veterinary Medicine and Surgery (Small Animal), vol. 8. Saunders, Philadelphia, PA, pp. 104–108.

Mcgregor, D.G., 2000. Occupational exposure to trace concentrations of waste anesthetic gases. Mayo Clin. Proc. 75, 273–277. https://doi.org/10.4065/75.3.273.

Mckelvey, D., Hollingshead, K.W., 2003. Workplace safety. In: Mckelvey, D., Holilngshead, K.W. (Eds.), Veterinary Anesthesia and Analgesia. Mosby Elsevier Science, St. Louis, MO, pp. 217–237.

Mercado, J.A., Larsen, R.S., Wack, R.F., Pypendop, B.H., 2008. Minimum anesthetic concentration of isoflurane in captive thick-billed parrots (*Rhynchopsitta pachyrhyncha*). Am. J. Vet. Res. 69, 189–194. Available at: https://doi.org/10.2460/ajvr.69.2.189.

Merin, R., 1993. Are differences in cardiopulmonary effects among the inhalation agents clinically important. In: Proceedings of ASA Refresher Course Lectures, vol. 226. Lecture, Washington DC, pp. 1–6.

Milligan, J.E., Sablan, J.L., Short, C.E., 1982. Waste anesthetic gas concentrations in a veterinary recovery room. J. Am. Vet. Med. Assoc. 181, 1540–1541.

Mosley, C.A., 2015. Veterinary equipment. In: Grimm, K.A., Lamont, L.A., Tranquilli, W.J., Greene, S.A., Robertson, S.A. (Eds.), Veterinary anesthesia and analgesia: The fifth edition of Lumb and Jones, fifth ed. John Wiley & Sons, Inc, Ames, IA.

Murat, I., Housmans, P.R., 1988. Minimum alveolar concentrations (MAC) of halothane, enflurane, and isoflurane in ferrets. Anesthesiology 68, 783–786. https://doi.org/10.1097/00000542-198805000-00018.

National Institute for Occupational Safety and Health, 1977. Criteria for a Recommended Standard: Occupational Exposure to Waste Anesthetic Gases and Vapors. Centers for Disease Control and Prevention website. http://https://www.cdc.gov/niosh/docs/77-140/default.html/. (Accessed 16 March 2022).

National Institute of Health, 2022. PubChem. National Center for Biotechnology Information. https://pubchem.ncbi.nlm.nih.gov/. (Accessed 4 April 2022).

National Research Council (Nrc), 1996. Institutional Policies and Responsibilities. Guide for the Care and Use of Laboratory Aimals. National Academy Press, Washington, DC, pp. 8–20.

Nguyen, V., 2014. Minimum Alveolar Concentration. McGraw-Hill Eduction. http://https://accessanesthesiology.mhmedical.com/content.aspx?bookid=974§ionid=61587778/. (Accessed 16 March 2022).

Njoku, D., Laster, M.J., Gong, D.H., Eger 2nd, E.I., Reed, G.F., Martin, J.L., 1997. Biotransformation of halothane, enflurane, isoflurane, and desflurane to trifluoroacetylated liver proteins: association between protein acylation and hepatic injury. Anesth. Analg. 84, 173–178. https://doi.org/10.1097/00000539-199701000-00031.

Occupational Safety and Health Administration, 2000. Anesthetic Gases: Guidelines for Workplace Exposures. United States Department of Labor. http://https://www.osha.gov/waste-anesthetic-gases/workplace-exposures-guidelines/. (Accessed 17 March 2022).

Okutomi, T., Whittington, R.A., Stein, D.J., Morishima, H.O., 2009. Comparison of the effects of sevoflurane and isoflurane anesthesia on the maternal-fetal unit in sheep. J. Anesth. 23, 392–398. https://doi.org/10.1007/s00540-009-0763-2.

Orliaguet, G., Vivien, B., Langeron, O., Bouhemad, B., Coriat, P., Riou, B., 2001. Minimum alveolar concentration of volatile anesthetics in rats during postnatal maturation. Anesthesiology 95, 734–739. https://doi.org/10.1097/00000542-200109000-00028.

Pawson, P., Forsyth, S., 2008. Anesthetic agents. In: Maddison, J.E., Page, S.W., Church, D.B. (Eds.), Small Animal Clinical Pharmacology. Elsevier, Philadelphia, PA, pp. 83–112.

Peyton, P.J., Chao, I., Weinberg, L., Robinson, G.J., Thompson, B.R., 2011. Nitrous oxide diffusion and the second gas effect on emergence from anesthesia. Anesthesiology 114, 596–602. https://doi.org/10.1097/ALN.0b013e318209367b.

Quasha, A.L., Eger 2nd, E.I., Tinker, J.H., 1980. Determination and applications of MAC. Anesthesiology 53, 315–334. https://doi.org/10.1097/00000542-198010000-00008.

Regueiro-Purrinos, M., Fernandez-Vazquez, F., De Prado, A.P., Altonaga, J.R., Cuellas-Ramon, C., Ajenjo-Silverio, J.M., et al., 2011. Ventricular arrhythmias and mortality associated with isoflurane and sevoflurane in a porcine model of myocardial infarction. J. Am. Assoc. Lab. Anim. Sci. 50, 73–78.

Reinelt, H., Schirmer, U., Marx, T., Topalidis, P., Schmidt, M., 2001. Diffusion of xenon and nitrous oxide into the bowel. Anesthesiology 94, 475–477. https://doi.org/10.1097/00000542-200103000-00019 discussion 476A.

Ruby, D.L., Buchan, R.M., Gunter, B.J., 1980. Waste anesthetic gas and vapor exposures in veterinary hospitals and clinics. Am. Ind. Hyg. Assoc. J. 41, 229–231. https://doi.org/10.1080/15298668091424663.

Sawyer, D.C., 1976a. A personal hazard: O. R. environmental pollution. J. Am. Anim. Hosp. Assoc. 3, 73–77.

Sawyer, D.C., 1976b. A personal hazard: operating room environmental pollution. J. Am. Anim. Hosp. Assoc. 12, 214–217.

Senate and House of Representatives, 1970. Occupational Safety and Health Act of 1970. Public Law, 91–596.

Sessler, D.I., Badgwell, J.M., 1998. Exposure of postoperative nurses to exhaled anesthetic gases. Anesth. Analg. 87, 1083–1088. https://doi.org/10.1097/00000539-199811000-00019.

Shaughnessy, M.R., Hofmeister, E.H., 2014. A systematic review of sevoflurane and isoflurane minimum alveolar concentration in domestic cats. Vet. Anaesth. Analg. 41, 1–13. https://doi.org/10.1111/vaa.12083.

Smith, J.A., 1993. Anesthetic pollution and waste anesthetic gas scavenging. Semin. Vet. Med. Surg. Small Anim. 8, 90–103.

Smith, J.C., Bolon, B., 2002. Atmospheric waste isoflurane concentrations using conventional equipment and rat anesthesia protocols. Contemp. Top. Lab. Anim. Sci. 41, 10–17.

Smith, J.C., Bolon, B., 2003. Comparison of three commercially available activated charcoal canisters for passive scavenging of waste isoflurane during conventional rodent anesthesia. Contemp. Top. Lab. Anim. Sci. 42, 10–15.

Soma, L.R., Tierney, W.J., Hogan, G.K., Satoh, N., 1995. The effects of multiple administrations of sevoflurane to cynomolgus monkeys: clinical pathologic, hematologic, and pathologic study. Anesth. Analg. 81, 347–352. https://doi.org/10.1097/00000539-199508000-00024.

Son, Y., 2010. Molecular mechanisms of general anesthesia. Korean J. Anesthesiol. 59, 3–8. https://doi.org/10.4097/kjae.2010.59.1.3.

Soontranan, P., Lertakyamanee, J., Somprakit, P., Surachetpong, S., 2002. A survey of the anesthesia scavenging systems in a teaching hospital. J. Med. Assoc. Thai. 85 (Suppl. 3), S824–S829.

Steffey, E.P., 1992. Other new and potentially useful inhalational anesthetics. Vet. Clin. North Am. Small Anim. Pract. 22, 335–340. https://doi.org/10.1016/s0195-5616(92)50628-3.

Steffey, E.P., Khursheed, R.M., Brosnan, R.J., 2015. Inhalation anesthetics. In: Grimm, K.A., Lamont, L.A., Tranquilli, W.J., Greene, S.A., Sheilah, A.R. (Eds.), Veterinary Anesthesia and Analgesia, fifth ed. John Wiley & Sons, Inc., Ames, IA, pp. 297–331.

Tanelian, D.L., Kosek, P., Mody, I., Maciver, M.B., 1993. The role of the GABAA receptor/chloride channel complex in anesthesia. Anesthesiology 78, 757–776. https://doi.org/10.1097/00000542-199304000-00020.

Taylor, D.K., Mook, D.M., 2009. Isoflurane waste anesthetic gas concentrations associated with the open-drop method. J. Am. Assoc. Lab. Anim. Sci. 48, 61–64.

United Nations, 1987. The 1987 Montreal Protocols on Substances that Deplete the Ozone Layer. United Nations, New York. http://https://www.unido.org//. (Accessed 17 March 2022).

Vaisman, A.I., 1967. [Working conditions in the operating room and their effect on the health of anesthetists]. Eksp. Khir. Anesteziol. 12, 44–49.

Velasco Gallego, M.L., Martin Jurado, O., Hatt, J.-M., 2021. Effects of isoflurane and sevoflurane alone and in combination with butorphanol or medetomidine on the bispectral index in chickens. BMC Vet. Res. 17, 1–11.

Ward, G.S., Byland, R.R., 1982a. Concentration of halothane in veterinary operating and treatment rooms. J. Am. Vet. Med. Assoc. 180, 174–177.

Ward, G.S., Byland, R.R., 1982b. Concentrations of methoxyflurane and nitrous oxide in veterinary operating rooms. Am. J. Vet. Res. 43, 360–362.

Warltier, D.C., Pagel, P.S., 1992. Cardiovascular and respiratory actions of desflurane: is desflurane different from isoflurane? Anesth. Analg. 75, S17–S29 discussion S29–S31.

Wingfield, W., Ruby, D., Buchan, R., Gunther, B., 1981. Waste anesthetic gas exposures to veterinarians and animal technicians. J. Am. Vet. Med. Assoc. 178, 399–402.

Wollman, H., Smith, T.C., 1975. Uptake, Distribution, Elimination, and Administration of Inhalational Anesthetics. In: Goodman, L.S., Gilman, A. (Eds.), The Pharmacological Basis of Therapeutics, vol. 5. Macmillan, New York.

Yasuda, N., Targ, A.G., Eger 2nd, E.I., Johnson, B.H., Weiskopf, R.B., 1990. Pharmacokinetics of desflurane, sevoflurane, isoflurane, and halothane in pigs. Anesth. Analg. 71, 340–348. https://doi.org/10.1213/00000539-199010000-00004.

Young, W.L., 1992. Effects of desflurane on the central nervous system. Anesth. Analg. 75, S32–S37.

Zaheer, O.A., Sanchez, A., Beaufrère, H., 2020. Minimum anesthetic concentration of isoflurane and sparing effect of midazolam in Quaker parrots (*Myiopsitta monachus*). Vet. Anaesth. Analg. 47, 341–346. Available at: https://doi.org/10.1016/j.vaa.2020.01.005.

Chapter 7

Pharmacology of Analgesics

Lon V. Kendall[1], Vanessa L. Oliver[2,3] and Trinka W. Adamson[4]

[1]Laboratory Animal Resources, Colorado State University, Fort Collins, CO, United States; [2]Department of Comparative Biology and Experimental Medicine, Faculty of Veterinary Medicine, University of Calgary, Calgary, AB, Canada; [3]Animal Health Unit, University of Calgary, Calgary, AB, Canada; [4]Animal Resources Department, Salk Institute for Biological Studies, La Jolla, CA, United States

Chapter outline

I. Introduction

Pain is defined by the International Association for the Study of Pain as "an unpleasant sensory and emotional experience associated with, or resembling that associated with, actual or potential tissue damage" (Raja et al., 2020). Pain has been classified into three types: nociceptive pain, inflammatory pain, and pathologic pain (Woolf, 2010). Nociceptive and inflammatory pains provide a protective role. Nociceptive pain is a high-threshold pain used to sense noxious stimuli to prevent tissue damage. Inflammatory pain is initiated by the immune response to tissue damage and is one of the five hallmarks of inflammation: redness, heat, swelling, pain, and loss of function (Davies

Anesthesia and Analgesia in Laboratory Animals. https://doi.org/10.1016/B978-0-12-822215-7.00023-8

et al., 1984; Ricciotti and FitzGerald, 2011). Pathologic pain results from abnormal nervous system responses or disease states. These various classifications of pain explain why the effectiveness of analgesics varies depending upon the characteristics of pain (Woolf et al., 1998). For example, analgesic drugs effective against nociceptive pain may have limited effectiveness against neuropathic pain.

This chapter reviews the five main groups of analgesic drugs used in pain management: (1) nonsteroidal antiinflammatory drugs (NSAIDs), (2) opioids, (3) α_2-adrenergic agonists, (4) NMDA-receptor antagonists, and (5) gabapentinoids. General and local anesthetics will not be discussed here but can be used in pain management, especially in the perioperative period (see Chapters 5 and 6 for more details). In this chapter, we will briefly review the physiological mechanism of pain associated with each of these classes to provide an overview of their mechanism of actions, followed by a review of their pharmacology, route of administration, biodistribution, metabolism, excretion, pharmacologic effects, adverse effects, and clinical applications. The information provided below is a culmination from a variety of animal species, including humans, with important species differences noted throughout the sections. Species-specific applications will be reviewed in other chapters.

II. Nonsteroidal anti-inflammatory drugs

A. Overview

NSAIDs are one of the most commonly used analgesics in veterinary medicine; their advantages include high oral bioavailability, long duration of effect, lack of sedation, and minimal potential for abuse and development of tolerance. The details regarding the safety and efficacy of NSAIDs use in laboratory animals, from a clinical perspective, are becoming increasingly available. The NSAIDs have been classified based on their chemical structure (salicylates, propionic acid derivatives, arylacetic acid derivatives, oxicam derivates, pyrrolo-pyrrole derivatives, and indole derivatives) and their COX selectivity (nonselective cyclooxygenase (COX)) inhibitors, preferential COX-2 inhibitors, and selective COX-2 inhibitors (Table 7.1) (Bacchi et al., 2012). The classifications share a similar

TABLE 7.1 Classification of NSAIDs based on chemical structure and COX-2 activity.

NSAID classifications based on chemical structure:	NSAID classification based on COX inhibition:
Salicylates[a]	Nonselective
Aspirin	Aspirin
Salicylic acid	Salicylic acid
Para-aminophenol derivatives	Indomethacin
Acetaminophen	Diclofenac
Indole derivatives	Ketorolac
Indomethacin	Ibuprofen
Etodolac	Ketoprofen
Hetero-arylacetic acid derivatives	Naproxen
Diclofenac	Piroxicam
Ketorolac	Phenylbutazone
Robenacoxib	Dipyrone
Aryl-propionic acid derivatives	Flunixin
Ibuprofen	Nabumetone[a]
Ketoprofen	Preferential COX-2 activity
Flurbiprofen	Etodolac
Naproxen	Carprofen
Carprofen	Piroxicam
Anthranilic acids (Fenamates)	Meloxicam
Flunixin	Celecoxib
Enolic acids derivatives (oxicams)	Selective COX-2 activity
Piroxicam	Robenacoxib
Meloxicam	Rofecoxib[a]
Alkanones	
Nabumetone[a]	
Pyrazolidinediones	
Phenylbutazone	
Dipyrone	
Diarylheterocycles	
Celecoxib	
Rofecoxib[a]	

[a]*Use of these NSAIDs is limited in animals and are not discussed in the narrative.*
Adapted from Bacchi et al. (2012) and Green (2001).

mechanism of action for promoting analgesia by inhibiting COX activity during the arachidonic acid metabolic pathway.

Arachidonic acid is present in large amounts in the phospholipid membrane of cells and is the precursor to the active eicosanoids (Bacchi et al., 2012; Davies et al., 1984). Arachidonic acid is abundant in skeletal muscle, brain, liver, spleen, and retinal phospholipids (Hanna and Hafez, 2018). When cells are damaged, the phospholipid membrane releases arachidonic acid via phospholipase, which is metabolized into biologically active eicosanoids (Solomon and Goodson, 2007; Warner and Mitchell, 2004). This is mediated by the enzymatic activity of the COX enzymes (COX-1 and COX-2), also known as prostaglandin H synthetase. COX enzymes catalyze arachidonic acid through two sequential reactions. The first reaction is oxygenation within the COX active site to make the unstable endoperoxide intermediate, prostaglandin (PG) G_2 (PGG_2) (Blobaum and Marnett, 2007; Rao and Knaus, 2008). The second is a peroxidase reaction which reduces PGG_2 to PGH_2 (Brooks et al., 1999). PGH_2 is further metabolized to the bioactive prostanoids, which are determined based on tissue-specific synthases and isomerases (Fig. 7.1) (Atkinson and Collier, 1980; Rao and Knaus, 2008; Solomon and Goodson, 2007; Warner and Mitchell, 2004). These include thromboxane, prostaglandin D_2, E_2, $F_2\alpha$, and I_2, which possess diverse physiological functions acting as secondary messengers via G-protein-coupled receptors (Rao and Knaus, 2008).

The generation of PGE_2 is catalyzed by cytosolic PGE synthase (cPGES) and membrane-bound PGE synthases 1 and 2 (mPGES) (Patrignani and Patrono, 2015). The prostanoids act on the prostanoid receptors of cells to exert their effects (Chandrasekharan and Simmons, 2004; Warner and Mitchell, 2004). The PGD_2, $PGF_2\alpha$, PGE_2, PGI_2, and thromboxane act on the prostanoid receptors DP, FP, EP1-4, IP, and TP respectively, named based on their PG ligand, Table 7.2.

Some of the products, such as PGE_2, participate in the inflammatory process, resulting in fever, sensitivity to pain, proinflammatory mediator, and vasodilation. For example, PGE_2 and PGI_2 coupling to the EP and IP receptors results

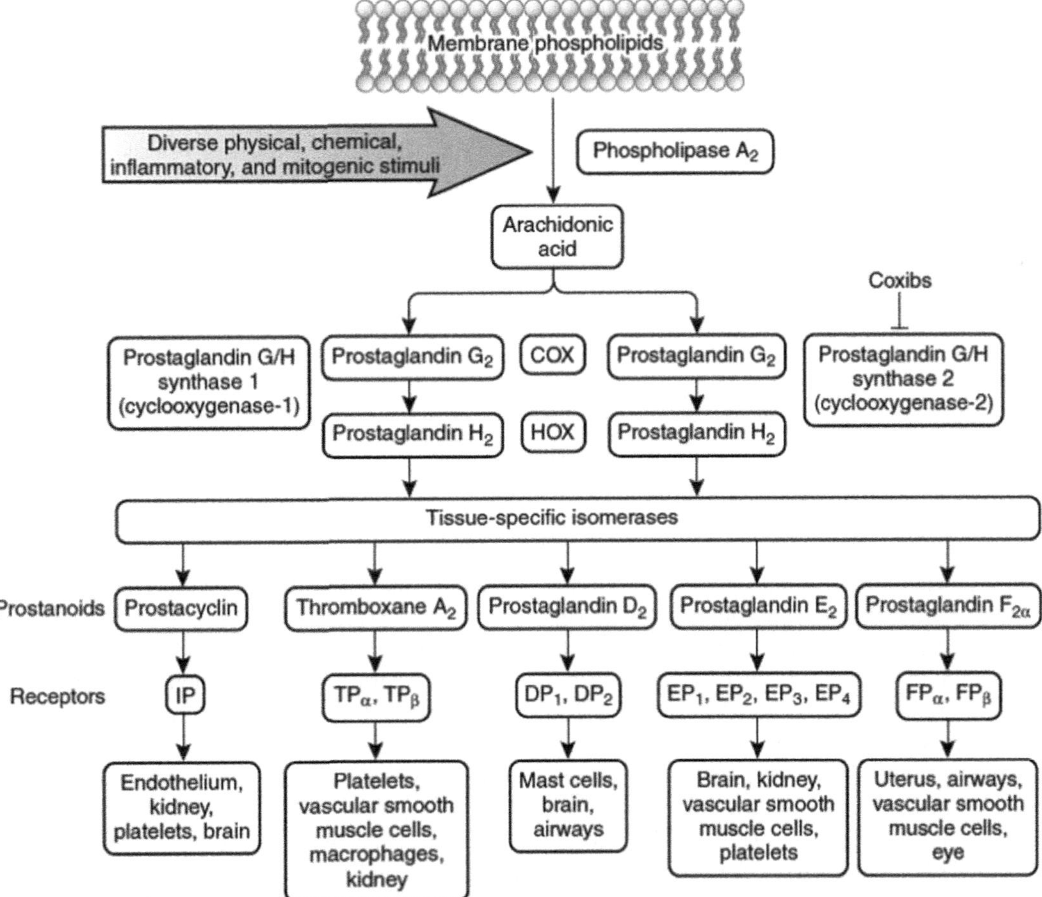

FIGURE 7.1 The receptor and tissue location of the prostanoids during arachidonic acid metabolism by COX enzymes. HOX-homeobox gene. *From Solomon and Goodson (2007) (Fig. 11.3, p 180)*

TABLE 7.2 Prostaglandin receptors and their proposed physiological effects.

Prostaglandin type	*Prostaglandin receptor*	*Function*
PGI_2	IP	Vasodilation Inhibit platelet aggregation Bronchodilation GI protection Renal homeostasis
PGE_2	EP_1	Bronchoconstriction GI tract smooth muscle contraction Regulation of blood pressure
	EP_2	Bronchodilation GI tract smooth muscle relaxation Vasodilation
	EP_3	↓ Gastric acid secretion ↑ Gastric mucus secretion Uterine contraction (when pregnant) GI tract smooth muscle contraction Lipolysis inhibition ↑ Autonomic neurotransmitters Fever generation Kidney reabsorption
	EP_4	Level and stability of COX-2 mRNA Neonatal adaptation of circulatory system
	Not specified	Inflammation Hyperalgesia Pyrogenic
$PGF_{2\alpha}$	FP	Uterine contraction Embryo implantation Bronchoconstriction Induces parturition Modulates intraocular pressure Inflammation
PGD_2	DP	Allergic responses Sleep-awake cycle
TXA_2	TP	Vascular homeostasis Thrombosis

GI, gastrointestinal; PG, prostaglandin; TXA, thromboxane. Prostaglandin receptors are termed DP, EP, FP, IP, and TP that relate to the receptor that ligates the corresponding prostanoid.
Adapted from Anderson (2008, Table 7.1, p. 916), and Brooks et al. (1999, Fig. 7.1, p782).

in sensitizing peripheral sensory nerve endings at the site of inflammation, which also has a bystander effect on adjacent tissues (Jang et al., 2020; Warner and Mitchell, 2004). This increase in neuronal activity is the result of lowering the activation threshold of sodium channels in the neurons (Patrignani and Patrono, 2015). Other PGs participate in physiological processes such as the maintenance of the integrity of the gastrointestinal (GI) mucosa, platelet function, ovulation, and renal function (Brooks et al., 1999; Chandrasekharan and Simmons, 2004; Rao and Knaus, 2008; Warner and Mitchell, 2004). For example, PGI_2 is the most common PG produced by the gastric mucosa and binding to the IP receptor provides a protective environment for the gastric mucosa with reduced acid secretions, increased bicarbonate and mucus secretions, and increased gastric blood flow (Russell, 1986; Wallace, 2000). $PGF_2\alpha$ binding of the FP receptor in the uterus facilitates parturition (Solomon and Goodson, 2007; Winchester et al., 2002). Thromboxane A_2 stimulates the activation of new platelets and increases platelet aggregation for hemostasis (Murray and FitzGerald, 1989). PGE_2 and PGD_2 made in the brain have opposite effects, with PGE_2 causing wakefulness and PGI_2 promoting sleep (Solomon and Goodson, 2007). While PGs contribute to inflammation, they also contribute to the resolution of inflammation and promote wound healing (Tallima and El

Ridi, 2018). Table 7.2 summarizes the physiological activities of the PGs (Brooks et al., 1999).

Arachidonic acid may also be metabolized by lipoxygenase (LOX) to form hydroperoxyeicosatetraenoic acids (HPETEs), which are the precursors to leukotrienes (Davies et al., 1984; Wang et al., 2021). Leukotrienes have potent biological activity including arterial constriction, negative inotropic effects on the heart, arrhythmogenic, and bronchoconstriction, implicating them as mediators of hypersensitivity reactions, myocardial infarction, and asthma (Needleman et al., 1986). Leukotrienes are also proinflammatory recruiting inflammatory cells to the tissues (Needleman et al., 1986; Rao and Knaus, 2008), have a role in nociception (Noguchi and Okubo, 2011), and play a role in resolving the inflammatory state (Serhan et al., 2008).

Both COX enzymes act on PGs. COX-1 has preferential activity with TXA synthase, PGF_2 synthase, and PGD_2 synthase to make TXA_2, $PGF_2\alpha$, and PGD_2, with a physiological impact on platelets, GI, and renal homeostasis. COX-2 has preferential activity with PGE_2 and PGI_2 synthase to form PGE_2 and PGI_2 with physiologic impact on the brain, renal perfusion, cardiovascular integrity, tracheal, and uterine functions (Hanna and Hafez, 2018; Ricciotti and FitzGerald, 2011; Wang et al., 2021).

The COX enzymes have varying degrees of expression and tissue localization. The COX enzymes are located on the endoplasmic reticulum and nuclear envelope (Rao and Knaus, 2008). COX-1 is constitutively expressed in cells such as endothelium, monocytes, platelets, renal tubules, and seminal vesicles (Rao and Knaus, 2008; Smith and Dewitt, 1996). It is relatively stable and is generally thought of as maintaining physiological functions, such as GI mucosal protection and hemostasis (Blobaum and Marnett, 2007; Brogan et al., 2019; Rouzer and Marnett, 2009). COX-1 is also expressed in inflammatory cells (Ricciotti and FitzGerald, 2011; Rouzer and Marnett, 2009), and likely plays a role in the acute phases of the inflammatory response (Patrignani and Patrono, 2015). Products of COX-1 regulate rapid physiological responses such as vascular hemostasis, gastric function, platelet activity, and renal function (Power, 2005). COX-2 is an immediate early gene inducible from a variety of cells (endothelium, osteoclasts, synovial endothelium, and monocytes) in response to cytokines, mitogens, endotoxins, and tumor promoters (Blobaum and Marnett, 2007; Rao and Knaus, 2008). It is expressed during inflammation and disease states (Brogan et al., 2019; Chandrasekharan and Simmons, 2004; Solomon and Goodson, 2007), and turns over rapidly due to instability sequences (Rouzer and Marnett, 2009). COX-2 is upregulated 20-fold during inflammation (Brooks et al., 1999), producing PGE_2 and PGI_2 promoting inflammation, vascular permeability, and edema (Rao and Knaus, 2008).

While these generalities exist, there are some exceptions. For example, COX-1 can be induced by stress in nervous tissue (O'Banion, 1999), and COX-2 is constitutively expressed in the kidney, central nervous system (CNS), and cardiovascular system (Blobaum and Marnett, 2007; Zeilhofer, 2007); and both COX-1 and COX-2 are constitutively expressed in some tissues, such as the dorsal root ganglion, spinal dorsal and ventral gray matter (Jang et al., 2020).

The two COX enzymes are 60% identical with similar mechanisms of action; however, they are structurally different at the inhibitor binding sites (Brooks et al., 1999). All vertebrates (fishes, birds, and mammals) have both COX genes, and they share 70%–95% amino acid identity and similar crystalline structure across species (Chandrasekharan and Simmons, 2004; Rao and Knaus, 2008).

Since COX-2 is more abundant during inflammation, it has been the target for the antiinflammatory effects of NSAIDs, to reduce the adverse effects of inhibiting COX-1 (Warner and Mitchell, 2004; Zeilhofer, 2007). This prompted the search for COX-2-selective drugs, which are made possible by a slightly larger active site in the COX-2 enzyme than in the COX-1 enzyme due to minor amino acid changes at the COX binding site (Rao and Knaus, 2008). This allows the development of COX-2-selective drugs that fit into the larger site (Brooks et al., 1999; Power, 2005).

The relative selectivity of drugs as inhibitors of COX-1 and COX-2 ranges from predominately selective for COX-1 (ketorolac) to purely selective for COX-2 (lumiracoxib) (Fig. 7.2) (Warner and Mitchell, 2004). The relative roles of COX-1 and COX-2 related to analgesia are still debatable and not completely understood. Some feel that the effects of COX-1 on analgesia are as important as those of COX-2, and selective COX-2 inhibitors can cause some side effects similar to those of COX-1 inhibitors, as the overall inhibition of PG synthesis via either COX enzyme induces gastric ulcers (Clark, 2006; Rouzer and Marnett, 2009). There is also variability in the relative degree of COX selectivity among species, which may be due to the differences in the methodology used to measure COX selectivity (Streppa et al., 2002).

COX-3 has been described in neural tissue, but its importance relative to COX-1 and COX-2 remains uncertain (Kis et al., 2005). COX-3 was identified in dogs as a splice variant of COX-1, which was selectively inhibited by acetaminophen, phenacetin, antipyrine, and dipyrone (Chandrasekharan et al., 2002). It has also been identified in the brain of patients suffering from Alzheimer's disease, as well as in mice and rats (Botting and Ayoub, 2005; Cui et al., 2004; Snipes et al., 2005). However, its role in the clinical treatment of pain and fever is debated based on dissimilarities in gene homology with COX-1 and COX-2 enzymes, a low expression level, and kinetic data (Kis et al., 2005). Its importance and status relative to COX-1

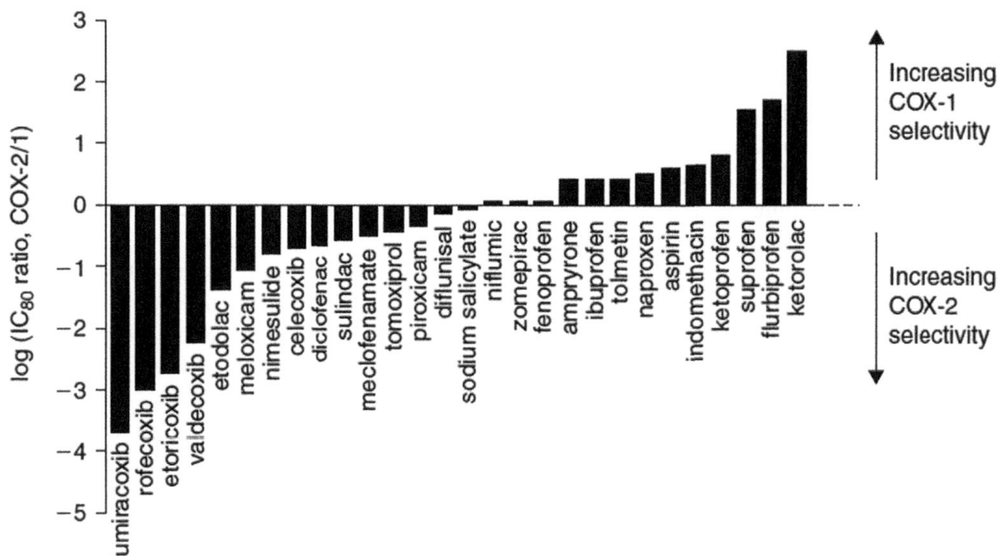

FIGURE 7.2 Relative selectivity of agents as inhibitors of human COX-1 and COX-2 displayed as the ratio of IC80 concentrations. Inhibitor curves for compounds against COX-1 and COX-2 were constructed in a human-modified whole blood assay and used to calculate IC80 concentration. The IC80 ratios are expressed logarithmically so that 0 represents the line of unity, i.e., compounds on this line are equiactive against COX-1 and COX-2. Compounds appearing above the line are COX-1 selective; those below the line COX-2 selective. *From Warner and Mitchell (2004, Fig. 7.2, p. 793).*

and COX-2 remain unresolved, and while labelled a COX enzyme, the COX-3 of rats and been found to have no COX-activity (Snipes et al., 2005).

B. Mechanism of action

All NSAIDs are thought to act by inhibiting COX (PGH synthase) enzyme activity during arachidonic acid metabolism, preventing the synthesis of bioactive PGs, prostacyclin, and thromboxane (Brogan et al., 2019; Warner and Mitchell, 2004). All NSAIDs inhibit COX-2, with varying degrees of COX-1 inhibition (Patrignani and Patrono, 2015). As an example, PGE_2 has a role in the perception of pain in the periphery and within the CNS. Thus, the effectiveness of analgesic-antipyretic and antiinflammatory drugs in acute pain conditions may be explained by their effects either at central sites or at peripheral sites (Warner and Mitchell, 2004).

There are two basic mechanisms of action of NSAIDs: (1) noncovalent binding at the catalytic site, which can further be characterized as (a) reversible binding, such as ibuprofen, or (b) rapid, low-affinity reversible binding followed by a time-dependent higher affinity slow reversible binding, such as indomethacin, and (2) inactivation through chemical structural changes, such as aspirin (Blobaum and Marnett, 2007; Rao and Knaus, 2008). The most potent NSAIDs form slow, tight, stable bonds (Rao and Knaus, 2008). The acidic nature of NSAIDs controls the distribution and pharmacological activity. The low dissociation constant is below the pH of most physiological environments, resulting in a small amount of unionized drugs. In inflamed tissues, the pH is reduced, resulting in a more unionized drug that diffuses through the cell membrane (Lucas, 2016). Nonacidic NSAIDs (usually selective COX-2 inhibitors) show enhanced binding to the altered active site of COX (Rao and Knaus, 2008). For example, diarylheterocycles, such as celecoxib are selective COX-2 inhibitors with structural features similar to phenylbutazone but have a distinct variation of the central heterocyclic ring and the 4-sulfonamido or 4-methylsulfonyl substation on the phenyl ring. In addition to their COX inhibitory effects, many NSAIDs have shown to have other mechanisms of action such as inhibition of the nuclear factor-kB (NF-kB), inhibition of leukocytes, inhibition of bradykinin, serotoninergic mechanisms, inhibition of NMDA receptor, activation of transient receptor potential ankyrin-1 (TRPA1), and activation of the arginine-nitric oxide cGMP.

Potential future analgesic targets are microsomal PGE syntase-1 (mPGES-1), in which inhibition results in antiinflammatory response with no cardiovascular effects as seen with selective COX-2 NSAIDs. Additionally, nitric oxide donor groups have been coupled with NSAIDs resulting in antiinflammatory response with decreased GI and cardiovascular effects due to the vasodilation and mucosal healing effects of nitric oxide. This has been demonstrated with nitric oxide coupled to aspirin, naproxen, and diclofenac. Finally, dual COX and LOX inhibitors, such as Licofelone, which leads to the reduction of PG as well as the proinflammatory leukotrienes show promise in analgesic efficacy (Bacchi et al., 2012; Rao and Knaus, 2008).

C. Desirable effects

NSAIDs reduce fever, pain, and inflammation through inhibition of the COX enzymes and their subsequent impact on PG synthesis, primarily PGE_2, and can impact both acute and chronic pain management (Bacchi et al., 2012; Patrignani and Patrono, 2015; Warner and Mitchell, 2004). As a class, NSAIDs are considered to be effective against pain of low-to-moderate intensity. However, it is important to consider the type and intensity of pain in assessing analgesic efficacy, as NSAIDs may be superior to opioid analgesics in some cases (Insel, 1991). These drugs are particularly effective in controlling the pain related to nociceptors that have been sensitized to normally painless mechanical, thermal, or chemical stimuli. COX-1 and COX-2 inhibition reduce the hyperalgesia effects of PGE_2 and PGI_2 on peripheral and central neurons, resulting in analgesia (Bacchi et al., 2012; Patrignani and Patrono, 2015). Similarly, the antiinflammatory effects of NSAIDs result in a decrease in vasodilation from PGE_2 and PGI_2 (Bacchi et al., 2012; Clark, 2006), and the antipyretic effects are due to reduced PGE_2 effects on the neurons controlling thermoregulation (Bacchi et al., 2012), presumably via preventing PGE_2 production in the hypothalamus, which regulates the set point at which the body temperature is maintained (Saper and Breder, 1994). Inhibition of PGE_2 production returns the set point to normal (Dascombe, 1985).

Some analgesic–antipyretic and antiinflammatory drugs also reversibly regulate neutrophil phagocytosis and secretion of lysosomal enzymes (beta-glucuronidase and acid protease), which could also contribute to their antiinflammatory properties and particular benefits in the treatment of osteoarthritis (Smith, 1977). This may be a COX-mediated effect through the stabilization of lysosomal membranes.

Although not a specific desirable effect as it relates to pain management, NSAIDs may also impact asthma and cancer growth. COX-2 is inducible in the epithelium and smooth muscle of the respiratory tract. This can result in smooth muscle proliferation and narrowing of the airway, particularly in asthmatic patients. Similarly, COX-2 is expressed at high levels in adenocarcinomas and inhibits apoptosis of cancerous cells. Inhibition of COX-2 can ameliorate these signs in asthma and cancer (Patrignani and Patrono, 2015; Rao and Knaus, 2008; Warner and Mitchell, 2004).

D. Adverse effects

The same COX inhibition that results in analgesia and antipyresis also causes adverse effects due to homeostasis associated with COX activity, and the common side effects are highlighted in Fig. 7.3. Nonselective NSAIDs, which act on both COX-1 and COX-2, typically lead to a greater risk of adverse effects than the selective COX-2 inhibitors (Bacchi et al., 2012). All NSAIDs have the potential for these common adverse effects. Other adverse effects associated with each drug are provided with their descriptions below.

Gastrointestinal. The most common adverse effect associated with NSAID use is GI toxicity including

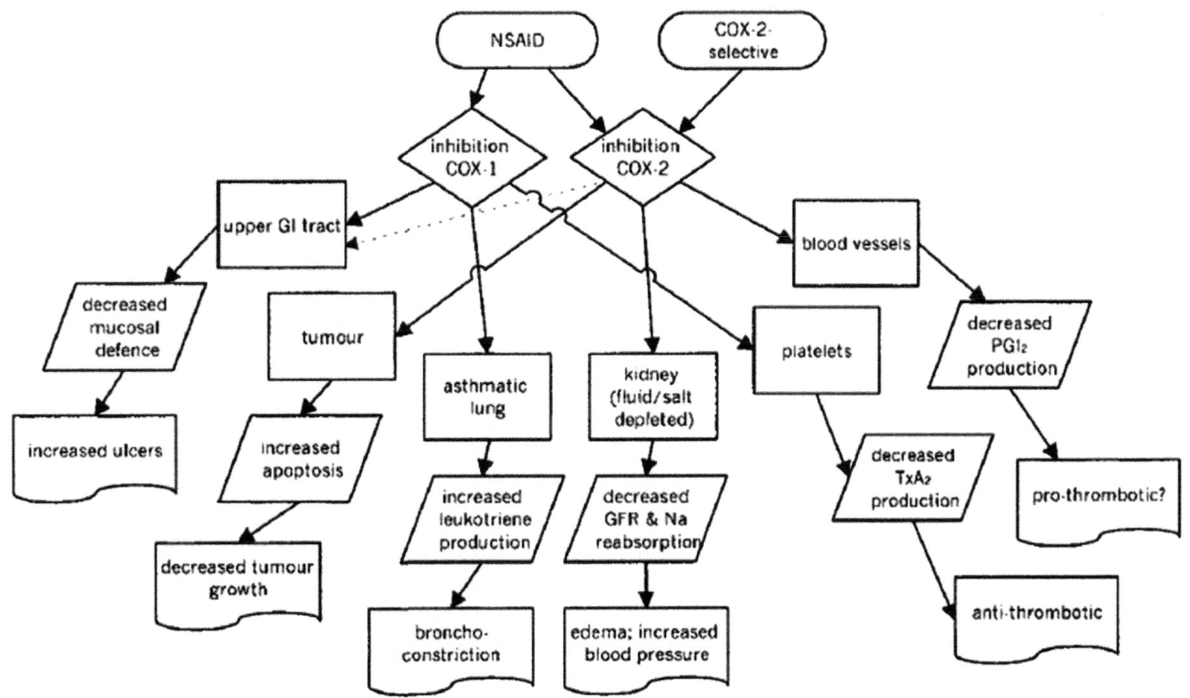

FIGURE 7.3 Schematic of adverse effects associated with COX inhibition. *From Warner and Mitchell (2004, Fig. 7.4, p. 795).*

perforation, ulcers, and bleeding (Brooks). PGE_2 and PGI_2 exhibit protective effects on the GI mucosa through reduced acid secretion, increase blood flow, mucus production, and epithelial proliferation (Patrignani and Patrono, 2015; Rao and Knaus, 2008). Within the acidic environment of the stomach, the NSAID migration to the gastric mucosa is favored, localizing the impacts on COX enzymes (Green, 2001). COX-1 inhibition counters the protective effects and is primarily responsible for gastric toxicity (Brooks et al., 1999) and associated clinical signs (nausea, vomiting, abdominal pain, and heartburn) (Sostres et al., 2010). However, COX-2 is also expressed to some degree in the GI mucosa of humans, rabbits, and dogs, and COX-2 may be induced following ulcer formation to facilitate healing (Rao and Knaus, 2008; Warner and Mitchell, 2004). Therefore, inhibition of COX-2 may delay the healing of gastric ulcers. Selective COX-2 NSAIDs were principally developed to have fewer GI side effects than nonselective NSAIDs (Bacchi et al., 2012). Gastric ulceration is enhanced by the impact of NSAIDs on platelet functions (Patrignani and Patrono, 2015).

Cardiovascular. COX-1 found in platelets is responsible for the formation of thromboxane A2 (TXA_2), which facilitates platelet aggregation. Inhibition of TXA_2 reduces the risk of thrombosis and is seen as cardioprotective (Rao and Knaus, 2008). COX-2 within the endothelium forms PGI_2, which causes vasodilation, prevents platelet aggregation, and is an endogenous antilipidemic agent (Rao and Knaus, 2008; Warner and Mitchell, 2004). Inhibition of PGI_2 reverses these cardioprotective effects. This is further enhanced given COX-2 inhibitors have minimal impact on TXA_2, resulting in a prothrombotic state and increasing the risk of cardiovascular disease associated with COX-2 inhibitors.

Platelet function. COX-1 is responsible for the formation of TXA_2, which facilitates platelet aggregation. Inhibition of TXA_2 can lead to bleeding diathesis due to impaired platelet aggregation (Awtry and Loscalzo, 2000; Rao and Knaus, 2008). Since aspirin irreversibly acetylates the active COX site, the effect on platelets lasts throughout the lifetime of platelets (5–11 days depending on the species) (Arif and Aggarwal, 2021; Tanaka et al., 2002). The effects of other nonselective NSAIDs on platelets are reversible (Brogan et al., 2019).

Kidney. COX-1 and COX-2 are found in the kidney and mediate PGE_2 and PGI_2 renal functions through the regulation of renin release, vascular tone, and tubular function (Awtry and Loscalzo, 2000; Bacchi et al., 2012; Green, 2001; Rao and Knaus, 2008; Solomon and Goodson, 2007). COX-1 is expressed in the vascular endothelium, collecting ducts, and loop of Henle; whereas COX-2 is expressed in the macula densa and ascending loop of Henle. Hence, COX-1 has a primary effect on renal homeostasis and perfusions, and COX-2 on diuretic and natriuretic effects. In normal patients, COX inhibition has minimal impact on renal function; however, NSAID use may lead to a transient imbalance in electrolytes and water. COX-2 inhibition can cause sodium and potassium retention in hyponatremic individuals. This could lead to hyperkalemia, which could be arrhythmogenic (Bacchi et al., 2012). In patients with compromised renal function, it can reduce glomerular filtration and urinary sodium excretion (Bacchi et al., 2012; Warner and Mitchell, 2004). In hypertensive patients, COX inhibition may result in elevated blood pressure and edema formation, which may also impact the cardiovascular system (Patrignani and Patrono, 2015; Warner and Mitchell, 2004).

Liver. NSAIDs are responsible for approximately 10% of the drug-induced hepatotoxicity (Bacchi et al., 2012). Other than aspirin, NSAIDs are metabolized by the liver and cause a transient increase in hepatic enzymes. The use of NSAIDs in patients with chronic liver disease may be contraindicated due to the increased risk of bleeding and further hepatic impairment (Green, 2001). The long-term use of NSAIDs should incorporate regular evaluation of renal and liver function.

Lung. COX activity inhibition using aspirin may result in aspirin-sensitive asthma (Green, 2001; Warner and Mitchell, 2004). This is due to an increase in leukotriene production exacerbating asthma symptoms.

Since NSAIDs are strongly protein-bound, they can impact the efficacy of other drugs, and this should be considered when administering NSAIDs (Green, 2001).

E. Pharmacokinetics

NSAIDs are weak acids and exist mostly in an ionized form. Most NSAIDs are completely and rapidly absorbed after oral administration with a peak plasma concentration within 2–3 h (Bacchi et al., 2012; Brogan et al., 2019). With the exception of aspirin, acetaminophen, and dipyrone, they are highly bound to plasma albumin with less than 10% unbound and pharmacologically active (Brogan et al., 2019; Solomon and Goodson, 2007). The binding to albumin can be saturated if the concentration of the NSAID exceeds the available albumin. The volume of distribution in extravascular tissues is small at 0.1–0.3 L per kg. They are primarily metabolized by the liver via cytochrome P450 and secreted in the urine or bile with little first-pass metabolism. NSAIDs can be divided into short-acting with a half-life less than 6 h, or long-acting with a half-life greater than 6 h, with the plasma half-life varying from 0.25 to 70 h. Table 7.3 provides a summary of key pharmacokinetic parameters (Bacchi et al., 2012; Solomon and Goodson, 2007).

TABLE 7.3 Summary of pharmacokinetic data for commonly used NSAIDs.

Drug[a]	Tmax	T1/2	Protein binding	Primary metabolite	Therapeutic plasma concentration
Acetaminophen	60	2–2.5	20%–50%	Sulfate and glucuronide conjugation	5–20 mg/mL
Indomethacin	90	5–10	90	Glucuronide conjugation and O-desmethylation and N-deacylation	0.5–3.0 mg/mL
Etodolac	60–120	6–8	99	Glucuronide conjugation and hydroxylation	2–5 mg/mL[b]
Diclofenac	10–40	1–2	99	Glucuronide conjugation and hydroxylation	0.1–0.5 mg/mL
Ketorolac	20–60	4–6	99	Glucuronide conjugation and hydroxylation	0.5–1.0 mg/mL[c]
Ibuprofen	60–120	2–2.5	99	Hydroxylation and carboxylation	0.01–0.05 mg/mL
Ketoprofen	20–70	2–4	99	Glucuronide conjugation	0.45–5.62 mg/mL
Flurbiprofen	60–180	3.5–5.5	99	Sulfate and glucuronide conjugation	>4 mg/mL
Naproxen	180	12–15	99	Glucuronide and sulfate conjugation	0.05 mg/mL
Carprofen[d]	60–180	10–20	99	Glucuronide conjugation and hydroxylation	20–24 mg/mL
Flunixin[e]	60–360	4–6	80	Hydroxylation	0.95 mg/mL
Piroxicam	120–240	40–50	99	Glucuronide and sulfate conjugation	3.9–5.6 mg/mL
Meloxicam[d]	300–360	15–20	99	Oxidation	390–911 mg/mL
Phenylbutazone[e]	240–360	50–105; 4–6[f]	98	Oxidation, hydroxylation	1–4 mg/mL
Dipyrone[e]	90–120	3–4	60[g]	Hydrolysis forms metabolically active compound	5–10 mg/mL
Celecoxib	120–240	6–12	97	Hydroxylation, carboxylation, glucuronide conjugation	0.25 mg/mL
Robenacoxib[d]	60–90	1	99	Oxidation and hydroxylation[h]	10 ng/mL

[a]*The information provided is based on human data, unless otherwise indicated, and should be interpreted with caution in veterinary species.*
[b]*Based on 400 mg dose in human with an effective duration of 4–6 h (Cayen et al., 1981).*
[c]*Based on plasma concentrations requiring redosing (Mroszczak et al., 1990).*
[d]*Based on dog and cat data.*
[e]*Based on horse data.*
[f]*Half-life in humans is significantly longer than in horses.*
[g]*Based on active metabolite (Levy et al., 1984).*
[h]*Based on metabolism of lumiracoxib in human (Mangold et al., 2004).*

1. *Para-aminophenol derivates*

Chemical structure of acetaminophen. https://pubchem.ncbi.nlm.nih.gov/compound/1983

a. Acetaminophen (also known as paracetamol)

Mechanism of action The exact mechanism of action of acetaminophen is still unclear, and several may not consider it an NSAID because of its weak antiinflammatory properties, but appears at least in part to involve COX inhibition (Anderson, 2008). Compared to other NSAIDs, acetaminophen has weak inhibition of both COX-1and COX-2 due to its low affinity for COX (Abbott and Hellemans, 2000), which accounts for fewer side effects such as antiplatelet and GI toxicity (Kis et al., 2005).

The central effects of acetaminophen predominant, with limited effects at the periphery (Anderson, 2008). It's been hypothesized that acetaminophen acts on the novel COX-3 identified from canine brains (Chandrasekharan et al., 2002). However, COX-3 sequences are very different than COX-1 and 2, and lack COX activity, questioning its clinical relevance (Kis et al., 2005; Rao and Knaus, 2008). There is evidence that acetaminophen inhibits COX-2, particularly in the CNS resulting in reduced PG synthesis and antipyretic effects (Botting and Ayoub, 2005; Kis et al., 2005). Rather than acting as a competitor for the COX site, acetaminophen inhibits COX by reducing the peroxidase enzyme back to its catalytically inactive state. This could explain the analgesic properties; however, within inflamed tissues there is a high level of peroxidase activity which is not overcome by acetaminophen, therefore it likely has little antiinflammatory effects (Aronoff et al., 2006; Kis et al., 2005). Additional proposed mechanism of action include: NMDA inhibition of the L-arginine-nitric oxide pathway, serotonergic pain pathways, and cannabinoid receptors (Aminoshariae and Khan, 2015; Anderson, 2008; Bonnefont et al., 2007; Ottani et al., 2006; Pickering et al., 2006). Acetaminophen and its metabolite, N-acetyl-p-benzo-quinone imine (NAPQI) which is hepatotoxic, have also been shown to activate TRPA1 resulting in analgesia acting at the CNS by inhibiting calcium and sodium voltage gates in sensory neurons, resulting in inhibition of C-fibre excitation (Anderson, 2008; Mallet et al., 2010).

Biodistribution, metabolism, and excretion Acetaminophen is absorbed from the small intestine with 90%–98% bioavailability and reaches peak concentrations within 1 h after oral administration (Aminoshariae and Khan, 2015; Raffa et al., 2014). An intravenous formation is also available with high bioavailability and onset of action of 5–10 min (Kerstenetzky, 2019; Mallinckrodt Pharmaceuticals, 2018). Unlike other NSAIDs, it has low protein binding (<25%) and is readily distributed in tissues with a therapeutic concentration of 5–20 μg/mL (Aminoshariae and Khan, 2015; Jackson et al., 1984). It has a plasma half-life of 1.5–2.5 h (Aminoshariae and Khan, 2015). The metabolism of acetaminophen occurs in the liver by glucuronidation and sulfate conjugation to inactive metabolites and a bioactive N-acylphenolamine compound (NAPQI) (Aronoff et al., 2006; Kennon-McGill and McGill, 2017; Mazaleuskaya et al., 2015). The glucuronidation, sulfation, and renal excretion eliminated up to 90% of the drug (Aminoshariae and Khan, 2015). In addition, deacetylation of acetaminophen yields p-aminophenol, which is nephrotoxic. This is a minor metabolic pathway (Aronoff et al., 2006).

Additional undesired pharmacologic effects Acute liver failure is the principle adverse effect associated with acetaminophen toxicity, which occurs at substantially higher than therapeutic doses in patients with normal hepatic function (Aminoshariae and Khan, 2015). This occurs through an accumulation of the bioactive NAPQI metabolite when the glutathione becomes saturated (Aminoshariae and Khan, 2015; Jackson et al., 1984). Hepatotoxicity in cats is higher than in other species because they lack glucuronyl transferase, resulting in excess NAPQI (Richardson, 2000). There have also been epidemiological reports of neurological, pulmonary, and developmental toxicities associated with acetaminophen use (Kennon-McGill and McGill, 2017). In addition to liver toxicity, methemoglobinemia is a common toxicity seen in dogs and cats (Richardson, 2000).

2. Indole derivatives

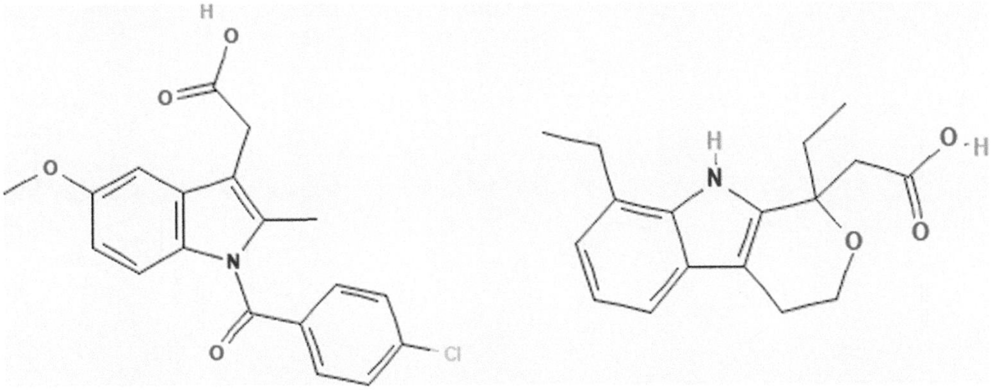

Chemical structure of indomethacin and etodolac. https://pubchem.ncbi.nlm.nih.gov/compound/3715; https://pubchem.ncbi.nlm.nih.gov/compound/3308

a. Mechanism of action

Indole derivative such as indomethacin are nonselective COX inhibitors that follow a two-step mode of inhibition in which the carboxylate of indomethacin forms a bridge and involves a conformational rather than chemical change through covalent bonds at the COX-1 site (Blobaum and Marnett, 2007; Prusakiewicz et al., 2004). Methyl ester or amide derivatives of indomethacin have more COX-2 selectivity due to their size and ability to form covalent bonds (Abdellatif et al., 2021; Blobaum and Marnett, 2007). Indomethacin has a demonstrated effect on modulating nitric oxide signaling and inhibiting vasodilation, particularly associated with headaches (Summ et al., 2021).

Indomethacin Indomethacin is available in oral formulations, including regular and sustained-release capsules, suspensions, as well as suppositories and injectables. Indomethacin is rapidly absorbed from the GI tract, with nearly 100% bioavailability with plasma concentrations within 1.5 h after administration. It is highly bound to plasma proteins with a therapeutic range of 0.5–3.0 μg/mL purported. It has a half-life of 5–10 h (Helleberg, 1981). Indomethacin is metabolized by the liver via conjugation with glucuronic acid as well as O-desmethylation and N-deacylation. The metabolites are inactive and eliminated in the urine, bile, and feces. Following excretion in the bile, indomethacin may be reabsorbed after hydrolysis, which can impact plasma levels. This may be responsible for the second peak plasma levels (Lucas, 2016).

b. Other undesired pharmacologic effects

Indomethacin has been associated with CNS effects such as headaches, tinnitus, ataxia, and tremors in people (Lucas, 2016).

Etodolac

Mechanism of action. Etodolac is thought to be a dual COX inhibitor with selectivity for COX-2. However, the data are inconsistent among studies (Clark, 2006). It may have more COX-2 selectivity in humans, but in dogs, it appears to be slightly selective for COX-1 (Streppa et al., 2002). Because of this, etodolac may have a narrower safety margin than other NSAIDs labelled for use in dogs, such as carprofen and meloxicam (Clark, 2006). Additional mechanism of action for etodolac is antiinflammatory by inhibiting neutrophil and macrophage chemotaxis, and bradykinin inhibition (Inoue et al., 1991).

Biodistribution, metabolism, and excretion. It is provided as a racemic mixture of the inactive R-enantiomer and active S-enantiomer. Etodolac is rapidly absorbed within 1–2 h following oral administration with an elimination half-life of 6–8 h. The S-enantiomer has less plasma protein binding than the R-enantiomer, which results in greater tissue distribution than most other NSAIDs (Brocks and Jamali, 1994). It is almost completely metabolized in the liver to 6- or 7-hydroxy etodolac, acyl-glucuronide, 8-1 hydroxyethyl etodolac, and 4-ureido-etodolac, which are excreted in the urine, and a small amount through the bile (Bellamy, 1997; Brocks and Jamali, 1994; Cayen et al., 1981).

3. Hetero-arylacetic acid derivates

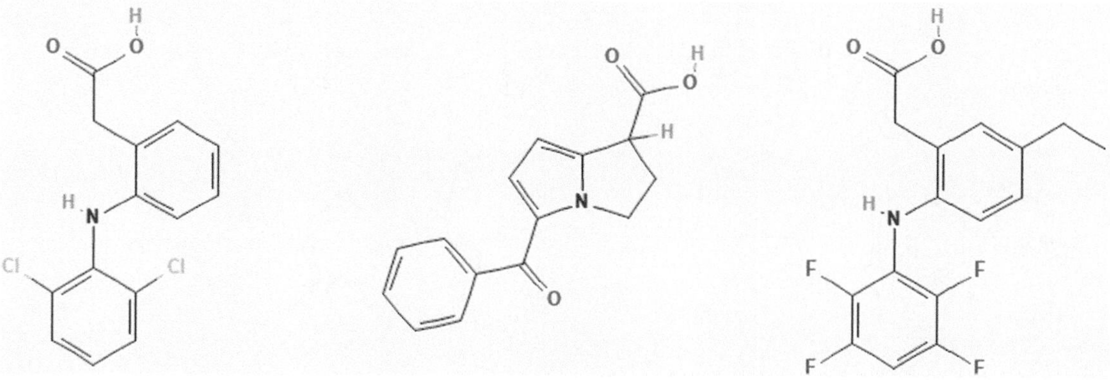

Chemical structure of diclofenac, ketorolac, and robenacoxib https://pubchem.ncbi.nlm.nih.gov/compound/3033; https://pubchem.ncbi.nlm.nih.gov/compound/3826; https://pubchem.ncbi.nlm.nih.gov/compound/6433107

a. Mechanism of action

Diclofenac and ketorolac bind the COX-2 active site inverted compared to other NSAIDs (Viegas et al., 2011). Diclofenac has additional potential mechanisms of action, including inhibition of substance P, inhibition of peroxisome proliferator-activated receptor gamma, inhibition of NMDA receptors, and altered IL-6 production (Gan, 2010). Diclofenac also inhibits lipoxygenase (LOX-5), with subsequent reduction in leukotrienes (Ku et al., 1986). Ketorolac activates the arginine-nitric oxide cGMP pathway producing nitric oxide inhibition of pain (Granados-Soto et al., 1995; Vadivelu et al., 2015). Robenacoxib is a potent COX-2 inhibitor that forms hydrogen bonds with COX-2 through the carboxylate group (King et al., 2009).

Diclofenac

Biodistribution, metabolism, and excretion. Diclofenac is available in tablets, capsules, sustained-release preparations, suspensions, suppositories, and topical gels. In humans, following oral administration, it is rapidly absorbed within 1 h. Oral administration results in 90% bioavailability, and 60% of the drug is systemically available following first-pass metabolism. In vitro therapeutic levels were determined to be 1–2 μg/mL (Giagoudakis and Markantonis, 2005), whereas in vivo therapeutic concentrations are 0.1–0.5 μg/mL (Davies and Anderson, 1997a). Gel formulations concentrate at the site of delivery but can be found systemically at lower concentrations within 2 h. The binding to albumin is reduced by using topical formulations. Diclofenac is metabolized by the liver by hydroxylation and conjugation with glucuronic acid and taurine. The 4-hydroxyl, 5-hydroxyl, and 4, 5-hydroxy metabolite is weakly biologically active (Wiesenberg-Boettcher et al., 1991). The metabolites are eliminated in the urine and bile. There is evidence of enterohepatic circulation resulting in increased levels. The majority of the drug is eliminated in 3–4 h, with a half-life of 1–2 h (Peris-Ribera et al., 1991).

Ketorolac

Biodistribution, metabolism, and excretion. Ketorolac tromethamine is a nonselective COX inhibitor and is composed of equal portions of (+) R and (−) S enantiomers, although the (−) S enantiomer is almost exclusively responsible for COX inhibition (Jett et al., 1999; Vadivelu et al., 2015). It is available as an oral, injectable, and intranasal spray formulation. It is absorbed in 20–60 min with 80%–100% bioavailable. It is more than 95% protein-bound with a low volume of distribution. Ketorolac is metabolized in the liver via glucuronidation and para-hydroxylation, and the majority of the inactive metabolites, glucuronide conjugated ketorolac and p-hydroxy ketorolac, and unchanged drugs (90%) are eliminated in the urine, and the rest in the feces (Brocks and Jamali, 1992). As an analgesic, ketorolac is more potent than other NSAIDs and is similar to that of morphine (Vadivelu et al., 2015), with peak analgesia in 2–4 h and a half-life of 4–6 h (Buckley and Brogden, 1990; Gillis and Brogden, 1997; Vadivelu et al., 2015).

Robenacoxib

Biodistribution, metabolism, and excretion. Robenacoxib is an exclusively veterinary NSAID developed for dogs and cats (Kongara and Chambers, 2018), but it has also been evaluated in trout (Raulic et al., 2021). It is available as an oral and injectable formulation. Robenacoxib is rapidly absorbed after oral administration reaching a maximum concentration in 1.5 h (King et al., 2009, 2010), and subcutaneous administration reaching a maximum concentration within

40 min (Pelligand et al., 2012) with a bioavailability of 84% −88%. It has a half-life of 0.6−0.9 h (Jung et al., 2010; King et al., 2010), and is eliminated in the urine and feces, presumably through hepatic metabolism and biliary excretion. Its metabolism is thought to be similar to lumiracoxib, a human drug, which was removed from the market (King and Jung, 2021; King et al., 2009). The therapeutic plasma concentration is 10 ng/mL (Jung et al., 2010; Pelligand et al., 2012), and it preferentially distributes to sites of inflammation delaying its elimination (King et al., 2009). Robenacoxib appears to have a wide margin of safety, as dogs dosed up to 40 mg/kg for 1 month, and up to 10 mg/kg for 6 months had no significant adverse effects (King et al., 2011).

4. Aryl-propionic acid derivatives

a. Mechanism of action

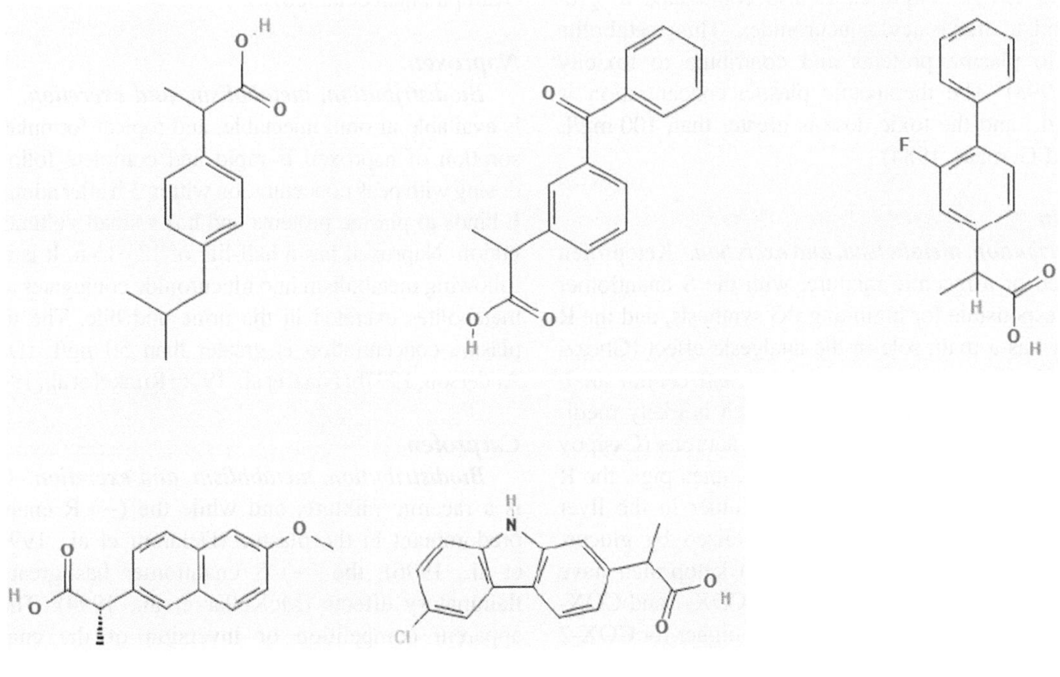

shown to inhibit proinflammatory cytokines by inhibiting the activation of NF-kB (Stuhlmeier et al., 1999). It also reduces neutrophil activation and oxidative phosphorylation (Evans, 2001). In addition to the COX pathway, ketoprofen also inhibits the LOX pathway, which reduces inflammation by inhibition of leukotrienes. It has also been demonstrated to inhibit the proinflammatory mediator bradykinin and reduce autolysis from lysosomes released from damaged cell membranes (Kantor, 1986). Some analgesic effects of ketoprofen may be mediated by serotonergic and noradrenergic mechanisms at the supraspinal and spinal levels (Díaz-Reval et al., 2004; Pinardi et al., 2001). Naproxen inhibits COX enzymes through a mixed inhibition, which exhibits an initial time-dependent loss in activity similar to slow, reversible, weakly bound inhibitors; however, it lacks a time-dependent inhibition of COX-1. This mechanism is similar to the inhibition effect of oxicams, with a greater effect on COX-2 (Blobaum and Marnett, 2007). In addition

Chemical structure of ibuprofen, ketoprofen, flurbiprofen, naproxen, and carprofen. https://pubchem.ncbi.nlm.nih.gov/compound/3672; https://pubchem.ncbi.nlm.nih.gov/compound/3825; https://pubchem.ncbi.nlm.nih.gov/compound/3394; https://pubchem.ncbi.nlm.nih.gov/compound/156391; https://pubchem.ncbi.nlm.nih.gov/compound/2581

Aryl-propionic acid derivatives are competitive, reversible inhibitors of COX. Ibuprofen COX inhibition is a single-step kinetics that is rapidly reversible. Structural analogues of ibuprofen, such as flurbiprofen, have a two-step mode of inhibition, resulting in an irreversible alteration of the COX enzyme complex. Similar to aspirin, ibuprofen has been

to COX-2 activity of carprofen, there is some inhibition of phospholipase A_2 (McKellar et al., 1994) and IL-6 (Armstrong and Lees, 2002). Flurbiprofen mechanism of action may include serotoninergic mechanisms but does not appear to be associated with L-arginine-nitric oxide or opioid systems (Hirakawa et al., 2022).

Ibuprofen

Biodistribution, metabolism, and excretion. Ibuprofen is available in oral, intravenous, intramuscular, and topical formulations. Ibuprofen is rapidly absorbed within 1–2 h after oral administration and 5–6 h with topical formulations. The half-life is 2 h (Albert and Gernaat, 1984). More than 99% of it is bound to plasma proteins and poorly distributed to the tissues. Ibuprofen is composed of equal portions of (−) R and (+) S enantiomers, with the majority of COX inhibition associated with the (+) S enantiomer. When given the racemic mixture, the (−) R enantiomer can be converted to the active (+) S enantiomer (Chen et al., 1991; Cheng et al., 1994; Davies, 1998; Evans, 2001). Both forms are extensively metabolized as conjugated hydroxy (2-hydroxyibuprofen) and carboxyibuprofen, and the biologically inactive metabolites are excreted in the urine and feces, with some enterohepatic circulation. Very small amounts are eliminated as unchanged drugs (Davies, 1998; Mills et al., 1973). Ibuprofen is also conjugated to glucuronic acid to make acyl glucuronides. This metabolite can bind to plasma proteins and contribute to toxicity (Davies, 1998). The therapeutic plasma concentration is 10–50 mg/L, and the toxic dose is greater than 100 mg/L (Albert and Gernaat, 1984).

Ketoprofen

Biodistribution, metabolism, and excretion. Ketoprofen is composed of a racemic mixture, with the S enantiomer primarily responsible for inhibiting PG synthesis, and the R enantiomer has a main role in the analgesic effect (Ghezzi et al., 1998). Ketoprofen has peripheral and central analgesic activity (Herrero et al., 1997), which is likely mediated by the R enantiomer through larger neurons (Ossipov et al., 2000). Other than in humans and guinea pigs, the R enantiomer is converted to the S enantiomer in the liver (Ghezzi et al., 1998) as well as metabolized by glucuronidation (Kantor, 1986). Metabolites of ketoprofen have also been shown to have activity against COX-1 and COX-2, and the selectivity of the metabolites is higher for COX-2 than the parent drug (Levoin et al., 2004). Ketoprofen is 20 times more potent than ibuprofen.

Ketoprofen is available in oral, injectable, and topical formulations. It is rapidly absorbed within 20–70 min with a peak concentration in 0.5–2.5 h (Upton et al., 1981), and greater than 90% is protein-bound (Ishizaki et al., 1980; Rençber et al., 2009). Ketoprofen has a half-life of 1–2 h. It is eliminated in the urine as a free drug and metabolites, ketoprofen glucuronide. The therapeutic plasma range is 0.45–5.62 ug/mL (Ishizaki et al., 1980; Kantor, 1986; Rençber et al., 2009).

Flurbiprofen

Biodistribution, metabolism, and excretion. - Flurbiprofen is provided as a racemic mixture of (+) S and (−) R enantiomers (Jamali et al., 1988). The S enantiomer has both antiinflammatory and analgesic effects, whereas the R enantiomer has primarily analgesic effects. Both enantiomers have a central analgesic effect, and the S enantiomer has additional peripheral analgesic effects (Geisslinger and Schaible, 1996). Flurbiprofen is completely absorbed within 1 h following oral administration, reaching peak plasma concentration within 3 h and a half-life of 3.5–5.5 h. There is little inversion of the R to the S enantiomer. The S enantiomer has a higher plasma concentration than the R enantiomer and the R enantiomer is more readily eliminated. Flurbiprofen is metabolized by oxidation, sulfate, and glucuronide conjugation. The major metabolite is fluoro-4-hydroxy-4-biphenylyl propionic acid (Davies, 1995; Kaiser et al., 1986; Maroof et al., 2015). The therapeutic plasma concentration is greater than 4 μg/mL (Kumpulainen et al., 2010).

Naproxen

Biodistribution, metabolism, and excretion. Naproxen is available in oral, injectable, and topical formulations. Absorption of naproxen is rapid and complete following oral dosing with peak concentration within 3 h after administration. It binds to plasma proteins and has a small volume of distribution. Naproxen has a half-life of 12–15 h. It is eliminated following metabolism into glucuronide conjugates and sulfate metabolites excreted in the urine and bile. The therapeutic plasma concentration is greater than 50 mg/L (Davies and Anderson, 1997b; Niazi et al., 1996; Runkel et al., 1972, 1973).

Carprofen

Biodistribution, metabolism, and excretion. Carprofen is a racemic mixture, and while the (−) R enantiomer is predominant in the plasma (Delatour et al., 1993; Taylor et al., 1996), the (+) S enantiomer has greater antiinflammatory effects (McKellar et al., 1994). There is no apparent competition or inversion of the enantiomers; however, the S enantiomer is more rapidly metabolized and eliminated (McKellar et al., 1994).

Carprofen is available in oral and injectable formulations. It is rapidly and completely absorbed with peak concentrations in 1–3 h (McKellar et al., 1994). While the terminal half-life is 10–20 h, there is an initial decline in 1 h. The principle metabolites are glucuronide and hydroxylated metabolites that are excreted in the urine and bile (Crevoisier, 1982; Ray and Wade, 1982; Rubio et al., 1980). The therapeutic plasma concentration is 20–24 μg/mL (Lees et al., 2004). Carprofen is a veterinary drug and not used in human medicine.

5. Anthranilic acids (Fenamates)

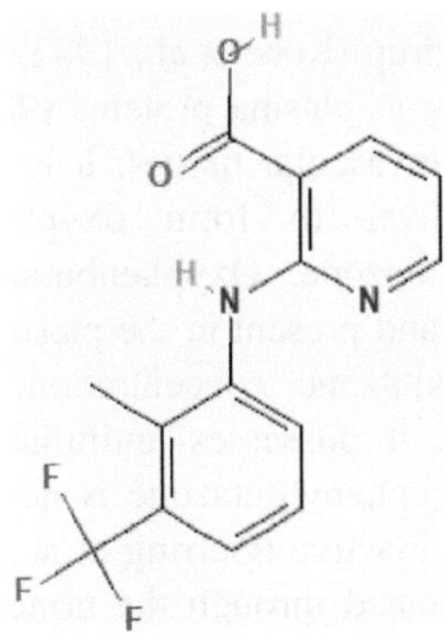

Chemical structure of flunixin. https://pubchem.ncbi.nlm.nih.gov/compound/38081

a. Flunixin

Biodistribution, metabolism, and excretion Flunixin is a veterinary NSAID approved for use in horses and cattle in the United States and also for use in dogs in other countries. It is usually formulated as flunixin meglumine. It is available in powder, pellet, and tablet form for oral administration and in liquid form for parenteral injection. In horses, it is readily absorbed with a peak concentration of 1–6 h depending on the species (Odensvik, 1995; Pairis-Garcia et al., 2013; Reppert et al., 2019). It is metabolized by hydroxylation to 5-OH flunixin and eliminated in the urine and feces (Knych et al., 2021). The half-life also varies among species with an average of 4–6 h (Baert and De Backer, 2002; Buur et al., 2006; Cheng et al., 1998; Elmas et al., 2006; Hardie et al., 1985; Horii et al., 2004; Königsson et al., 2003; Ogino et al., 2005). It has a therapeutic plasma level of 0.95 mg/mL (Toutain et al., 1994).

6. Enolic acids (oxicams)

a. Mechanism of action

Oxicams are preferential COX-2 inhibitors as the 4-hydroxyl group of the thiazine ring of the oxicams forms hydrogen bonds within COX, and an induced rotation creates an additional binding pocket. Some oxicams are potent inhibitors of mPGES-1, which is a necessary step in the formation of PGE_2, thereby inhibiting PGE_2 synthesis via a mechanism other than COX inhibition (Carty et al., 1980; Engelhardt, 1996; Engelhardt et al., 1996; Xu et al., 2014). In addition, the oxicams modulate cytokines with suppression of IL-1, IL-6, TNFα, and IFNγ (Herman et al., 1984; Rosenstein et al., 1994), and may inhibit NMDA receptor-mediated excitotoxicity (Mazumder and Borah, 2014).

Piroxicam

Biodistribution, metabolism, and excretion. Piroxicam is available as an oral, gel, and parenteral formulation which is readily absorbed with a peak concentration in 2–4 h. Like most NSAIDs, it is 99% protein-bound with a small volume of distribution (Verbeeck et al., 1986). Hepatic metabolism includes hydroxylation, cyclodehydration, amid hydrolysis, and glucuronide and sulfate conjugation, with no antiinflammatory properties. The metabolites are eliminated through the urine and feces (Brogden et al., 1984; Du, 2014; Lombardino, 1981; Mihalić et al., 1986; Xu et al., 2014). It has a half-life of 30–70 h (Ishizaki et al., 1980; Lee and Balfour, 1994). Prodrug formulations are available, such as ampiroxicam, droxicam, and pivoxicam, which reduce the GI toxicity. While the prodrugs are readily absorbed, the peak concentration is delayed (Olkkola et al., 1994). Conjugated formulations, such as piroxicam-β-cyclodextrin, similarly reduces the GI side effects but have a more rapid absorption with peak concentrations within 30 min (Lee). The therapeutic plasma concentration is 3.9–5.6 mg/L (Brogden et al., 1984).

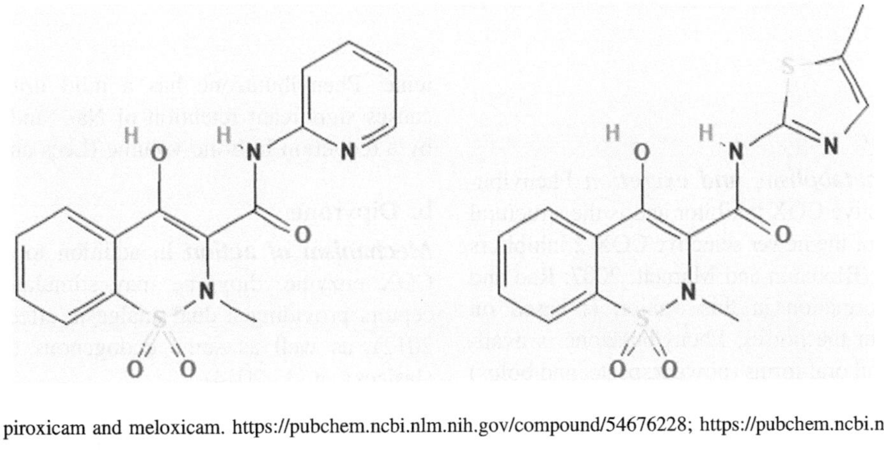

Chemical structure of piroxicam and meloxicam. https://pubchem.ncbi.nlm.nih.gov/compound/54676228; https://pubchem.ncbi.nlm.nih.gov/compound/54677470

Meloxicam

Biodistribution, metabolism, and excretion. Meloxicam is also available for oral or parenteral administration. It has a prolonged absorption reaching peak plasma levels in 5–6 h after administration, and is highly protein-bound. There is a second peak plasma level that occurs 12–14 h after administration due to enterohepatic recirculation. It is available in parenteral, oral, and rectal formulations. The drug has a prolonged, complete absorption with 99% plasma protein bound. It reaches peak plasma levels 5–6 h after administration, a second peak 12–14 h after enterohepatic recirculation. Meloxicam is metabolized primarily through oxidation to an inactive metabolite. There are no conjugated derivatives detected. The metabolites are excreted in urine and feces. The half-life of meloxicam is 15–20 h (Busch et al., 1998; Davies and Skjodt, 1999; Fleischmann et al., 2002; Gates et al., 2005; Türck et al., 1996). It has a therapeutic plasma concentration of 390–911 ng/mL in animals (Giraudel et al., 2005; Jeunesse et al., 2011).

7. Pyrazolidinediones

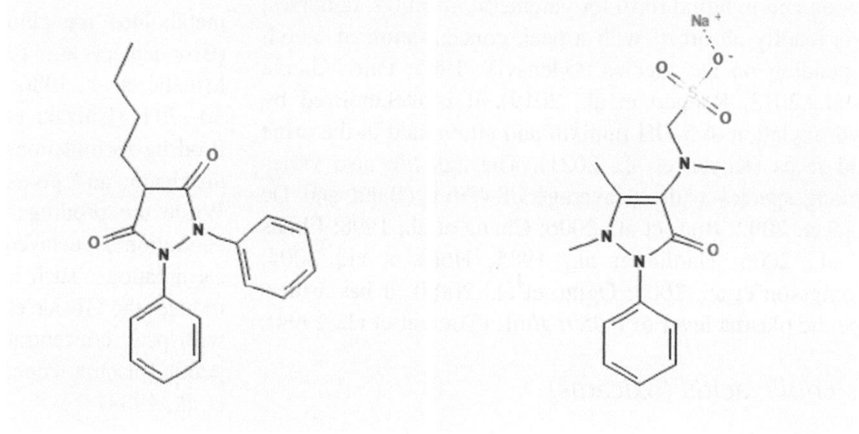

Chemical structure of phenylbutazone and dipyrone. https://pubchem.ncbi.nlm.nih.gov/compound/4781; https://pubchem.ncbi.nlm.nih.gov/compound/522325

a. Phenylbutazone

Biodistribution, metabolism, and excretion Phenylbutazone is a nonselective COX inhibitor and is the structural analogue for many of the newer selective COX-2 inhibitors as described above (Blobaum and Marnett, 2007; Rao and Knaus, 2008). Information in this section is based on studies performed in the horses. Phenylbutazone is available in parenteral and oral forms (powder, paste, and bolus) and is well absorbed following oral dosing (Lees and Toutain, 2013). The bioavailability is 69%–90%, with peak plasma concentrations in 4–6 h (Lees and Toutain, 2013; Rose et al., 1982). This can be impacted by the presence of food in the stomach, particularly fibrous foods which adsorb the drug (Rose et al., 1982). Phenylbutazone has a high binding to plasma proteins (98%) with limited distribution to extravascular tissues. It is primarily metabolized by the liver to form oxyphenbutazone and g-hydroxyphenylbutazone. Oxyphenbutazone is pharmacologically active and present in the plasma at 10% or less than the phenylbutazone concentration. Similar to the parent compound, it possesses antiinflammatory effects. Whereas g-hydroxyphenylbutazone is nearly undetectable in the plasma and inactive (Gerring et al., 1981). The metabolites are eliminated through the urine and bile, and a smaller portion of the unmetabolized drug is eliminated by renal excretion (Gerring et al., 1981; Lees and Toutain, 2013). The half-life is 4–6 h in horses with therapeutic plasma levels of 1–4 ug/mL (Lees and Toutain, 2013).

Additional undesired pharmacologic effects Phenylbutazone causes blood dyscrasias, including aplastic anemia, leukopenia, agranulocytosis, and thrombocytopenia. Its use in human medicine is limited due to its blood dyscrasias and phenylbutazone is principally used in veterinary medicine. Phenylbutazone has a mild uricosuric effect and causes significant retention of Na+ and Cl–accompanied by a reduction in urine volume (Lees and Toutain, 2013).

b. Dipyrone

Mechanism of action In addition to the effects on the COX enzyme, dipyrone may stimulate cannabinoid receptors providing a dual analgesic effect (Rogosch et al., 2012), as well as some endogenous opioidergic effects (Jasiecka et al., 2014).

Biodistribution, metabolism, and excretion Dipyrone is also known as metamizole. Dipyrone undergoes an initial hydrolysis to form 4-methylaminoantipyrine, which is rapidly absorbed within 2 h to achieve 85% bioavailability (Levy et al., 1984; Rogosch et al., 2012). Little is known about the biological activity of the metabolites, but they have been shown to inhibit TXA_2 formation in vitro (Levy et al., 1984) and PGE_2 synthesis in the brain, resulting in an antipyretic effect (Jasiecka et al., 2014; Shimada et al., 1994), but it is known that 4-methylaminoantipyrine functions as a nonselective COX inhibitor (Rogosch et al., 2012), with weak antiinflammatory effects (Jasiecka et al., 2014). The metabolites are poorly bound to plasma proteins (Zylber-Katz et al., 1992). The 4-methylaminoantipyrine is further metabolized in the liver to 4-aminoantipyrine (with subsequent metabolism to 4-acetylaminoantipyrine) and 4-formylaminoantipyrine (Levy et al., 1984; Volz and Kellner, 1980; Zylber-Katz et al., 1992). 4-acetylaminoantipyrine is the major form identified in the urine (Asmardi and Jamali, 1985). Dipyrone has a half-life of 3.5 h and the therapeutic plasma level of the active metabolite is 5–10 μg/mL (Levy et al., 1984).

Additional undesired pharmacologic effects Similar to phenylbutazone, dipyrone may cause blood dyscrasias (Rogosch et al., 2012), and for these reasons, it is not used in human medicine in the United States and several other countries. Dipyrone toxicity can result in impaired neurologic function, including coma and convulsions, cardiac arrhythmias, cardiogenic shock, and skin rashes (Brogden, 1986; Okonek and Reinecke, 1983).

8. *Diarylheterocycles*

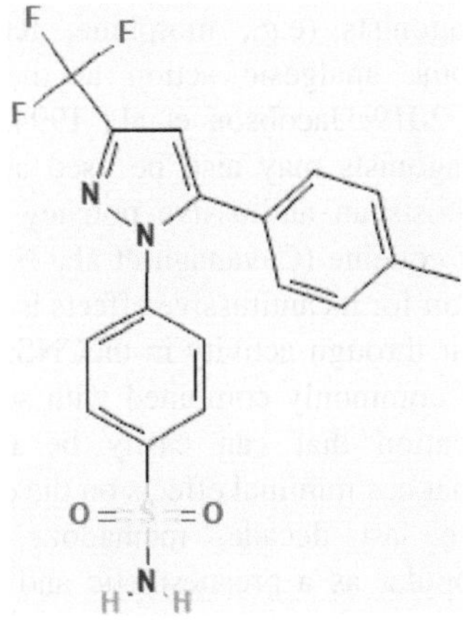

Chemical structure of celecoxib. https://pubchem.ncbi.nlm.nih.gov/compound/2662

a. Celecoxib

Mechanism of action Celecoxib exhibits an alternative binding pose with the insertion of their sulfur-containing substituent into a larger COX-2 specific side-pocket in addition to interactions with the main active site channel (Xu et al., 2014). In addition to the COX-2 inhibition, celecoxib has a proposed mechanism leading to apoptosis, cell cycle arrest, and angiogenesis. While these mechanisms have little analgesic or antiinflammatory properties, they do have anticancer properties, and celecoxib is used in patients with a high risk of colorectal cancer (Gong et al., 2012).

Biodistribution, metabolism, and excretion Celecoxib is the only selective COX-2 inhibitor of the diaryl-substituted furanones available for human use in the United States. Two other drugs in this chemical class, deracoxib, and firocoxib, are marketed in the United States for use in dogs to control pain and inflammation associated with osteoarthritis. These drugs are supplied as tablets for oral administration. After oral administration, absorption is high with peak plasma levels in 2–4 h. It is highly protein-bound and has a relatively high volume of distribution compared to other NSAIDs. It is metabolized through hydroxylation, carboxylation, and glucuronide conjugation and then eliminated in the feces and urine. It has a half-life of 11 h (Gong et al., 2012; Zeng et al., 2015). The therapeutic plasma level is 0.25 μg/mL (Angi et al., 2019).

III. Opioids

A. Overview

Opioids are powerful analgesics that are commonly used for managing acute pain in veterinary medicine due to their high efficacy and good safety margins. Their short half-lives and ability to be reversed allow clinicians to adjust doses based on patient response. Opioids are administered to relieve acute, chronic, and cancer pain, and as an immobilizing agent. Opioids with shorter half-lives (e.g., fentanyl, remifentanil) are commonly used to provide balanced anesthesia, e.g., an opioid, a hypnotic, and an amnesic agent combination. This group of analgesics can be administered alone or with other analgesics and local anesthetics for perioperative and intraoperative pain management. In addition to their analgesic properties, opioids may also be used therapeutically for sedation and chemical restraint, to suppress coughing, as well as decrease GI motility. They are available in a variety of different formulations, including oral, cutaneous, transdermal, and injectable, which may be administered through cutaneous, intravenous, subcutaneous, intramuscular, epidural, and intrathecal routes.

Opioid analgesics may be classified in several different ways, each providing useful distinguishing characteristics of the drugs. Classification schemes include mode of synthesis (naturally occurring alkaloids, semisynthetic, and synthetic compounds), chemical class (phenanthrene, benzomorphan, phenylpiperidine, and diphenylheptane), level of pain relief (mild, moderate, severe), and intrinsic effect at opioid receptors (full agonist, partial agonist, agonist-antagonist, or antagonist). A summary of common opioids used in laboratory animal medicine and their classification is provided in Table 7.4.

The term "narcotic", as used in a legal sense, includes opioids (as well as nonopioids, e.g., barbiturates), and the term generally has been used to refer to opioids. Thus, narcotic is derived from the word "narcosis", which refers to stupor or insensibility, obviously not usually the primary endpoint of opioid administration in most cases. The term narcotic is no longer a useful name for opioid analgesics in a pharmacological context. Opiate is a term once used to designate drugs derived from opium. Opioid is now used to designate those drugs plus all other drugs with morphine-like actions.

B. Mechanism of action

Opioids produce their effects by binding to transmembrane G-protein-coupled receptors distributed widely in the central and peripheral nervous systems. These receptors are also found in other tissues, such as the GI tract, cardiovascular, and immune systems. It is generally accepted that there are three different opioid receptors: μ (mu: M opioid peptide (OP)), δ (delta: DOP), and κ (kappa: KOP), each with variations in ligand activity (Borsodi et al., 2019; Cox et al., 2015; Dietis et al., 2011). Other receptors and receptor subtypes have been proposed (e.g., sigma, σ) but based on current literature and the clinical pharmacology community (Borsodi et al., 2019), are not presently recognized as opioid receptors. Depending on species, opioid receptors differ to varying degrees in their anatomic location and in the effect elicited when stimulated by an agonist; however, display similar cellular processes after activation. Opioid receptors can be activated by endogenous peptides (endorphins, enkephalins, and dynorphins) produced in response to noxious stimulation or exogenous agonists (morphine, fentanyl). Binding of an agonist, results in the activation of GTPase, leading to the conversion of guanosine diphosphate to guanosine triphosphate. Downstream signaling from this event leads to inhibition of adenylate cyclase, resulting in decreased cyclic adenosine monophosphate levels and modulation of synaptic plasticity and gene expression, as well as activation of potassium conductance and inhibition of calcium conductance (Al-Hasani and Bruchas, 2011; James and Williams, 2012; Riviere and Papich, 2018; Trescot et al., 2008). This change in conductance leads to hyperpolarization of the cell, reduced neurotransmitter release (Substance P), and ultimately, inhibition of neurons, which in turn inhibit spinal cord pain transmission.

As seen in Table 7.4, a given opioid may interact with multiple opioid receptor types; however, most clinically relevant opioid analgesics display activity at the μ receptor (James and Williams, 2012). Analgesia is thought to involve the activation of μ receptors (largely at supraspinal sites) and κ receptors (mainly in the spinal cord), while δ receptors may also be involved.

C. Desirable effects

The predominate analgesic action of opioids is through the μ and κ receptors. The level of analgesia and duration varies with the different opioids and are typically compared to the effects of morphine (Table 7.4). For example, oxymorphone and hydromorphone are used to treat mild to severe pain (Prommer, 2006). Fentanyl is commonly used for the control of postoperative pain, severe pain associated with chronic pain, as well as nonspecific, widespread pain. Methadone can be used as an analgesic to relieve moderate-to-severe pain. Methadone may also be an effective analgesic for chronic and neuropathic pain, where other opioids have provided little to no relief (Foley, 2003) or when mild pain is anticipated but a unimodal analgesic approach is planned (Murrell, 2011). Buprenorphine is commonly used as an analgesic for mild-to-moderate pain, as well as a preanesthetic agent. It may be preferred over full μ agonists due to its reduced adverse effects, wider safety margin, and lower potential for abuse, as reflected in its DEA classification as a schedule III drug. Partial agonists such as butorphanol and nalbuphine may be used to relieve mild-to-moderate pain. In some scenarios, butorphanol may be used as a reversal agent for the CNS and respiratory depression of μ opioid agonists (e.g., morphine, fentanyl) while maintaining some analgesic action at the κ receptors (Gomes et al., 2019; Jacobson et al., 1994; Mills et al., 1990). Partial agonists may also be used as antitussives. Butorphanol boosts an antitussive potency 100 times as great as that of codeine (Cavanagh et al., 1976). The specific site of action for its antitussive effects is unknown, but thought to occur through activity in theCNS.

Opioids are commonly combined with sedative agents as a premedication that can easily be reversed with naloxone and that has minimal effects on the cardiovascular system. In the last decade, methadone has become increasingly popular as a preanesthetic and postoperative analgesic, demonstrating improved efficacy over other opioids in some clinical settings (Raillard et al., 2017; Shah et al., 2018, 2019; Warne et al., 2013). The use of opioids as a preanesthetic agent reduces the requirements for inhalational anesthesia during surgery.

Species, strain, and sex differences in potency have been reported in rats, with higher potency observed in males (Bulka et al., 2004; Peckham and Traynor, 2006;

TABLE 7.4 Overview of commonly used opioids in laboratory animal medicine and their classification.

Substance	Controlled substance schedule	Mode of synthesis	Chemical class	Effect at opioid receptor	Pain category	μ	κ	δ	Other receptor activity
Morphine	II	Natural	Phenanthrene	Full agonist	Mild-to-severe	++	+		
Hydromorphone	II	Semisynthetic	Phenanthrene	Full agonist	Mild-to-severe	++			
Oxymorphone	II	Semisynthetic	Phenanthrene	Full agonist	Mild-to-severe	++		+	
Methadone	II	Synthetic	Diphenylheptane	Full agonist	Moderate-to-severe	++			NMDA inhibitor; α_2 agonist
Meperidine (Pethidine)	II	Synthetic	Phenylpiperidine	Full agonist	Mild-to-moderate	++			
Fentanyl	II	Synthetic	Phenylpiperidine	Full agonist	Moderate	++			
Remifentanil	II	Synthetic	Phenylpiperidine	Full agonist	Moderate	++			
Buprenorphine	III	Semisynthetic	Phenanthrene	Partial agonist	Mild-to-moderate	+	−		
Butorphanol	IV	Synthetic	Phenanthrene	Agonist-antagonist	Mild	+/−	++		
Nalbuphine	NS	Semisynthetic	Phenanthrene	Agonist-antagonist	Mild-to-moderate	−	++		
Tramadol	IV	Synthetic	Other	Opioid-like	Mild-to-moderate	+			Serotonin inhibitor; norepinephrine inhibitor; muscarinic inhibitor; α_2 agonist
Naloxone	NS	Synthetic	Phenanthrene	Antagonist	Reversal	−	−	−	GABA inhibitor
Naltrexone	NS	Synthetic	Phenanthrene	Antagonist	Reversal	−	−	−	
Nalmefene	NS	Synthetic	Phenanthrene	Antagonist	Reversal	−	−	−	

NS, not scheduled.
++ agonist; + submaximal agonist; − antagonist; /− agonist-antagonist.

Terner et al., 2003). Morphine does not appear to affect ruminant animals, the reason for which is still unknown (Davis, 1983).

D. Adverse effects

The adverse effects of opioids are exemplified by morphine. Morphine and morphine-related opioids produce respiratory depression, nausea, vomiting, dizziness, mental clouding, body temperature changes, increased pressure in the biliary tract, urinary retention, and hypotension (Barnhart et al., 2000; KuKanich et al., 2005; Riviere and Papich, 2018; Robertson and Taylor, 2004). Allergic reactions to opioids may occur, but they are not common (Aly et al., 2018). Excitatory behavior has been seen in dogs administered morphine (Robinson et al., 1988). Relatively large doses of morphine will cause a rage reaction in cats (i.e., 'morphine mania'), but lower doses can provide satisfactory analgesia.

Morphine suppresses respiration via a direct effect on the brain stem respiratory centers, primarily by reducing responsiveness to carbon dioxide (May et al., 2013). These drugs also suppress the cough reflex by a direct effect on the cough center in the medulla (Takahama and Shirasaki, 2007) and may induce nausea and vomiting by stimulation of the chemoreceptor trigger zone, cerebral cortex, vestibular apparatus of the brain, and GI tract (Porreca and Ossipov, 2009).

Morphine produces vasodilation and hypotension via histamine release but appears to have few cardiovascular effects (Chen and Ashburn, 2015). It inhibits baroreceptor reflexes (Szilagyi, 1987), and blunts the reflex vasoconstriction caused by increased P_{CO_2}.

Morphine can decrease hydrochloric acid secretion in the stomach. Relatively low doses of morphine decrease gastric motility, thereby prolonging gastric emptying time (Khansari et al., 2013). It also decreases biliary, pancreatic, and intestinal secretions. The amplitude of nonpropulsive rhythmic, segmental contractions of the small and large intestines is usually enhanced, but propulsive contractions are markedly decreased in the small and large intestines. The tone of the anal sphincter is greatly augmented, and the reflex relaxation response to rectal distention is reduced. These actions, together with the central actions of morphine, contribute to morphine-induced constipation. Morphine causes constriction of the sphincter of Oddi and pressure in the common bile duct to increase significantly (Wu et al., 2004). The fluid pressure in the gallbladder may also increase, producing signs that may vary from epigastric distress to biliary colic.

Morphine inhibits the urinary voiding reflex, and both the tone of the external sphincter and the volume of the bladder are increased (Herperger, 1998; Kona-Boun et al., 2003; Westerling and Andersson, 2007).

Short-term (<120 h) morphine administration has been shown to reduce natural killer (NK) activity (Bayer et al., 1990; Shavit et al., 1984), impair immunoglobulin production (Bussiere et al., 1992; Pruett et al., 1992), suppress phagocytic activity (Levier et al., 1993; Szabo et al., 1993), and induce thymic hypoplasia (Fuchs and Pruett, 1993). In monkeys and humans, the use of chronic morphine is known to suppress NK activity (Carr and France, 1993).

The other μ agonists have similar adverse effects. Hydromorphone has antitussive effects, causes respiratory depression, bradycardia, peripheral vasodilation and decreased peripheral resistance, sedation, euphoria, emesis, constipation, and urinary retention (Ambros et al., 2020; Guedes et al., 2007a, 2008; Kelly et al., 2014; KuKanich et al., 2008a; Wegner et al., 2004). Compared to morphine, hydromorphone appears to cause a similar level of sedation (Guedes et al., 2008), but less histamine release in dogs (Guedes et al., 2007b). Hyperthermia has been reported in cats postanesthesia for as long as 5h (Posner et al., 2007).

Oxymorphone also causes antitussive activity, sedation, euphoria, respiratory depression, emesis, physical dependence, mydriasis, pruritus, and constipation (Copland et al., 1987; Kelly et al., 2011; Krugner-Higby et al., 2009; KuKanich et al., 2008b; Siao et al., 2011a; Smith et al., 2004). In dogs and cats, it is noted to cause less emesis, nausea, and sedation than morphine and hydromorphone (Riviere and Papich, 2018). In addition, it appears to cause less histamine release than morphine in dogs (Robinson et al., 1988). The effects on the cardiovascular system are usually not clinically significant (Copland et al., 1987).

Sedation, panting, whining, mydriasis, and euphoria have been reported with methadone administration in cats and dogs (Ferreira et al., 2011; Ingvast-Larsson et al., 2010; Rohrer Bley et al., 2004). Methadone causes less nausea, vomiting, defecation, dysphoria, and histamine release than morphine. Respiratory and cardiovascular effects are minimal at clinical doses in both cats and dogs; however, bradycardia and bradypnea may occur when methadone is administered to anesthetized patients (Murrell, 2011).

Meperidine causes sedation, respiratory depression, cardiovascular changes, emesis, histamine release, physical dependence, and constipation. A study examining intravenous meperidine in horses described pacing, excitation, sedation, tremors, hives, pruritus, and decreased gut motility but no significant increases in respiratory rate (Hamamoto-Hardman et al., 2020). In dogs administered meperidine as a preanesthetic agent with acepromazine, one-third of dogs were reported to have vomited postoperatively (Vettorato and Bacco, 2011). Meperidine differs from morphine in that toxic doses can cause CNS excitation, leading to tremors, muscle twitching, and seizures (Schlick et al., 2015). The meperidine metabolite normeperidine is mainly responsible for these effects. The effects of meperidine on smooth muscle are less intense relative to its analgesic actions, as compared to morphine, and meperidine does not cause as much constipation.

The main adverse effects seen with fentanyl include dose-related respiratory and CNS depression, as well as changes in locomotor activity (Kamata et al., 2012). Cardiovascular effects appear to be minimal in healthy patients. Effects on the respiratory system can be seen immediately following intravenous administration. The use of transdermal formulations poses an occupational health and safety risk, as high concentrations of the drug can result in life-threatening respiratory depression if absorbed through the skin. In order to minimize personnel risk, it is recommended that personnel are appropriately trained, work in pairs, and don appropriate personal protective equipment (lab coat, safety glasses, and impermeable gloves). Additionally, since absorption and efficacy can be variable between patients, a rescue analgesia option should be available. Dermatologic reactions to these formulations have also been reported (Egger et al., 1998).

Remifentanil causes dose-dependent bradycardia, respiratory depression, and hypotension. Similar to other opioids, it has a ceiling effect, where increased doses do not enhance analgesia. In cats, hyperthermia, dysphoria, and increased activity may be noted.

The partial agonists, such as buprenorphine, have similar adverse effects that are typically associated with activity at the μ receptor. This includes sedation and respiratory depression. Other effects may include increased salivation, bradycardia, hypothermia, mydriasis, and vomiting. Buprenorphine has also been reported to cause pica on occasion in rats (Allen and Johnson, 2018; Bosgraaf et al., 2004; Clark et al., 1997). Some extended-release formulations may be associated with injection site reactions that are generally self-limiting and can be minimized by switching formulations (Carbone et al., 2012; Clark et al., 2014; Page et al., 2019; Thiede et al., 2014).

The mixed agonist-antagonist mostly have adverse effects associated with the μ receptor. This includes respiratory depression, sedation, dysphoria, mydriasis, nausea, anorexia, and diarrhea, as well as decreased GI motility and constipation with butorphanol use. Butorphanol does not cause histamine release like morphine (Pircio et al., 1976). A common adverse effect of nalbuphine is sedation (Costa et al., 2021; Lester et al., 2003). Nalbuphine causes minimal cardiovascular and respiratory effects (Gomes et al., 2018). At levels above clinical doses, excitation, dysphoria, vomiting, bradycardia, and a reduction in GI motility may be seen.

Repeated use of opioids may induce tolerance in some species. The development of tolerance will require adjustment of dosing to maintain efficacy. Tolerance develops at different rates to different pharmacologic effects. For example, tolerance to analgesia develops more rapidly than to respiratory depression, while tolerance to constipation develops very slowly, if at all. In general, opioid tolerance is not common in veterinary medicine, as most patients are administered opioids short term for durations less than a week.

Abuse of opioids and addiction to them are of major concern. This concern in laboratory animal medicine primarily relates to the diversion of drugs intended for patient administration to personnel having access to the drugs. Substantial effort in the development of opioids is aimed at reducing the abuse and addiction potential, as well as reducing the side effects such as respiratory depression and constipation. The abuse potential of opioids, the required permits to purchase and administer opioids, and the storage and record-keeping requirements imposed by federal and state governments often influence the decision of whether to administer these drugs to laboratory animals. Most opioids are classified as Schedule II narcotics according to U.S. Drug Enforcement Agency documents (DEA Form 225a). Details of federal and state classifications and regulations of narcotics will not be discussed here. More recently, there has also been an increase in the frequency of drug supply shortages, making some opioids difficult to procure. Supply shortages have been attributed to multiple factors, including manufacturing shortages, changes in compound regulations, and the opioid epidemic (Kogan et al., 2019). This variability in supply is an important factor to consider when developing an analgesic regime and may promote a multi-modal approach to pain relief.

E. Pharmacokinetics

1. *Opioid agonists*

a. Morphine

Chemical structure of morphine. https://pubchem.ncbi.nlm.nih.gov/compound/5288826

Biodistribution, metabolism, and excretion Morphine sulfate is commercially available as human-labelled products for oral use and injection. Oral formulations include solutions, tablets, and capsules. Rectal suppositories are also available. Extended-release capsules or tablets and liposomal extended-release injectables can provide a longer duration of action. Preservative-free solutions are intended for IV, epidural, or intrathecal injection. There are currently no veterinary-labelled products available.

Routes of administration in veterinary medicine include oral, intravenous, intramuscular, subcutaneous, epidural, and intraarticular. Parenteral administration of morphine offers rapid bioavailability, achieving therapeutic concentrations (Guedes et al., 2007a). In dogs administered a 0.5 mg/kg intravenous dose, the volume of distribution at steady state was 7.2 L/kg with a terminal half-life and clearance of 94.9 min and 85.2 mL/min/kg, respectively (Barnhart et al., 2000). Oral doses are subject to high (>80%) first-pass effects (Dohoo and Tasker, 1997), limiting the clinical effect in many species and requiring higher doses than parenteral routes. Rectal, transmucosal, and transdermal routes offer minimal absorption (Barnhart et al., 2000; Krotscheck et al., 2008; Pypendop et al., 2014), likely due to morphine's low lipophilicity. Compared with other more lipid-soluble opioids such as codeine, heroin, and methadone, morphine crosses the blood-brain barrier at a slow rate; only small quantities pass the blood-brain barrier in adults (Groenendaal et al., 2008). Morphine has moderate protein binding, and when unbound concentrates in the kidneys, liver, lungs, and to a lesser degree, the CNS. It crosses the placenta and can be present in the milk of lactating dams (DeVane et al., 1999; Gabrielsson and Paalzow, 1983; Welch and Findlay, 1981). Duration of analgesia is 2–6 h for most species (KuKanich et al., 2012). Elimination is primarily via glucuronidation of the parent drug into morphine-3-glucuronide (M3G) and morphine-6-glucuronide (M6G) in the liver. M3G has minimal analgesic effects and may be responsible for some of the adverse effects, whereas M6G provides analgesic effects more potent than the parent drug but is present in very low amounts that are unlikely to contribute to analgesia (Guedes et al., 2007a). In cats, their glucuronidation pathway deficiency creates sulfate conjugates as the primary metabolite and extends the drug half-life (Riviere and Papich, 2018; Yeh et al., 1971). Metabolites are eliminated from the body primarily via glomerular filtration in the kidneys.

b. Hydromorphone

Chemical structure of hydromorphone. https://pubchem.ncbi.nlm.nih.gov/compound/273032

Biodistribution, metabolism, and excretion Hydromorphone hydrochloride is commercially available as human-labelled products in the form of oral solutions and tablets, rectal suppositories, as well as injectable solutions for intravenous, intramuscular, and subcutaneous administration. Extended-release formulations are available as tablets and capsules commercially. A controlled-release liposome-encapsulated formulation has also been reported in the literature for use in rats, dogs, and macaques (Clark et al., 2004; Schmidt et al., 2011; Smith et al., 2008). There are currently no veterinary-labelled products available. Similar to other morphine-like agonists, hydromorphone has primary activity at μ receptors. Common routes of administration include intravenous, intramuscular, and subcutaneous. Most commonly, hydromorphone is administered parenterally, which results in immediate absorption. Its potency is 5–7× greater than morphine with a similar analgesic duration (i.e., 2–6 h, depending on species) (Riviere and Papich, 2018). Dogs administered 0.1 mg/kg hydromorphone intravenously were reported to have a mean steady state volume of distribution of 4.24 L/kg, a mean serum clearance of 106.3 mL/min/kg, and a mean half-life of 0.57 h (KuKanich et al., 2008a). Oral administration results in a significant decrease in bioavailability due to first-pass clearance (Chang et al., 1988). In humans, hydromorphone has been noted to distribute rapidly into breast milk (Edwards et al., 2003). Similar to morphine, hydromorphone has moderate protein binding and is primarily metabolized in the liver through glucuronidation. The primary route of elimination is through urine (Cone et al., 1977).

c. Oxymorphone

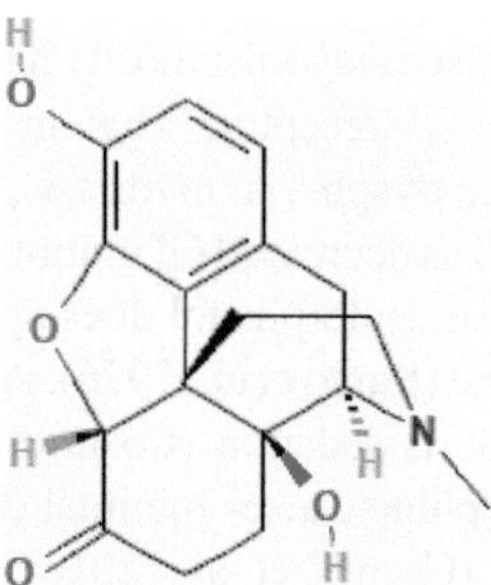

Chemical structure of oxymorphine. https://pubchem.ncbi.nlm.nih.gov/compound/5284604

Biodistribution, metabolism and excretion Oxymorphone hydrochloride is commercially available through human-labelled products, including injectable solutions, regular oral and extended-release tablets, as well as rectal suppositories. An extended-release formulation has been described in the literature in mice, rats, dogs, and rhesus macaques (Clark et al., 2004; Krugner-Higby et al., 2009; Smith et al., 2003, 2004, 2013). There are currently no veterinary-labelled products available. Common routes of administration include intravenous, intramuscular, subcutaneous, and epidural. Oxymorphone is a semisynthetic opioid substitute for morphine that has rapid absorption, a large volume of distribution, rapid clearance, and short half-life. Oxymorphone has primary activity at μ receptors, with some activity at δ receptors. It is 10 times more potent than morphine (Prommer, 2006). Bioavailability is significantly reduced when administered orally due to first-pass clearance. In dogs administered a 0.01 mg/kg intravenous dose, the mean steady state volume of distribution was 4.09 L/kg, with a mean clearance and half-life of 52.34 mL/min/kg and 0.82 h, respectively (KuKanich et al., 2008b). The drug is metabolized in the liver primarily through glucuronidation and the metabolites are excreted in the urine (Cone et al., 1983).

d. Methadone

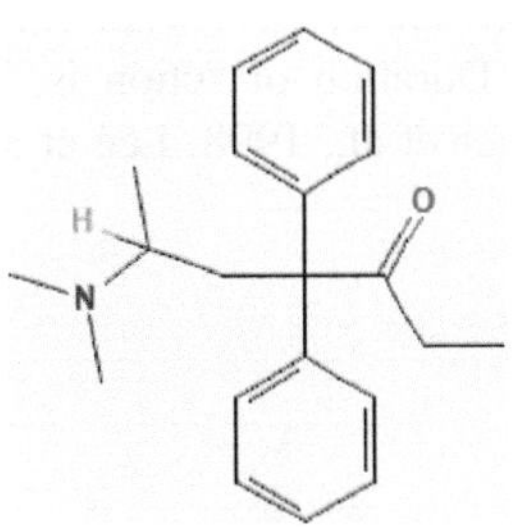

Chemical structure of methadone. https://pubchem.ncbi.nlm.nih.gov/compound/4095

Mechanism of action Methadone is a synthetic opioid that exists in the formulation as a racemic mixture (D- and L-methadone), with L-methadone primarily responsible for its opioid-like pharmacologic activity (Ferrari et al., 2004). It is considered to have similar or higher analgesic potency to morphine, providing relief for moderate-to-severe pain primarily by acting as a full agonist of the μ receptor. Methadone also has some activity at κ and σ receptors. Different from morphine, D- and L-methadone both have antagonist activity at NMDA receptors, which contributes to a reduction in central sensitization after tissue injury and is also thought to play a role in reducing the development of opioid tolerance in patients (Davis and Inturrisi, 1999; Holtman and Wala, 2007). In addition, methadone inhibits the reuptake of norepinephrine and serotonin (Codd et al., 1995), neurotransmitters involved in the provision of descending analgesia and ultimately, providing additional antinociceptive effects. In human medicine, it is commonly used to aid in the detoxification and treatment of opioid addiction.

Biodistribution, metabolism, and excretion Methadone hydrochloride is available through human-labelled injectable and oral formulations, including oral flavored concentrate, tablets for suspension, and oral tablets. Veterinary-labelled injectable formulations are available in the United Kingdom and Canada. Routes of administration include intravenous, intramuscular, subcutaneous, and epidural.

Information about the biodistribution, metabolism, and excretion of methadone is limited in veterinary medicine. Methadone is a lipophilic, weak base that is widely distributed and extensively protein-bound (60%–90%), making it prone to intracellular accumulation (Ferrari et al., 2004). When administered intravenously to dogs at 0.4 mg/kg, the steady state volume of distribution was 9.2 L/kg, and clearance and half-life 27.9 mL/kg/min and 3.9 h, respectively (Ingvast-Larsson et al., 2010). It is metabolized in the liver and eliminated through the kidneys. Elimination of methadone is slower than morphine (Ferrari et al., 2004), resulting in longer dosing intervals.

Oral administration of methadone in dogs has a short elimination half-life, rapid clearance, and low bioavailability (Kukanich et al., 2005). Subcutaneous administration provides a bioavailability of 80% and extended half-life relative to intravenous dosing (Ingvast-Larsson et al., 2010). In cats, oral transmucosal intravenous routes of administration appear to produce similar behavioral antinociceptive effects (Ferreira et al., 2011).

e. Meperidine (pethidine)

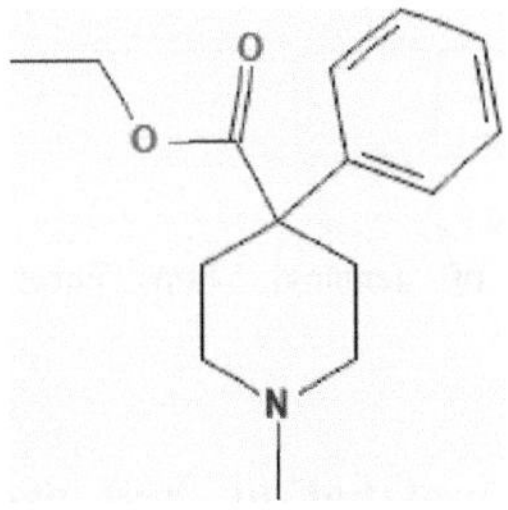

Chemical structure of meperidine. https://pubchem.ncbi.nlm.nih.gov/compound/4058

Biodistribution, metabolism, and excretion Meperidine hydrochloride is available through human-labelled products including injectable solutions and oral formulations consisting of tablets, syrups, or solutions. No veterinary-labelled products are currently available. Common routes of administration include intravenous, intramuscular, subcutaneous, and oral.

Meperidine is a synthetic opioid that is well absorbed by all routes but has relatively low (<25%) oral bioavailability after first-pass effects. Similar to morphine, meperidine has full μ agonist activity; however, its potency is less than morphine and typically requires higher doses. Following a 2 mg/kg intravenous bolus in dogs, the rates of distribution and elimination were 0.87 min^{-1} and 0.018 min^{-1}in young dogs (~2.8 years) and 0.40 min^{-1} and 0.011 min^{-1} in older dogs (~11.9 years), respectively (Waterman and Kalthum, 1989, 1990). Duration of action is variable depending on the route of administration and species, typically lasting 1–6 h. In dogs, mean half-life ranges from 52.5 to 62.7 min after intravenous administration in young and older dogs, respectively (Waterman and Kalthum, 1989, 1990). Meperidine has high protein-binding (60% –80%) and is metabolized in the liver, followed by excretion in the urine (Yeh, 1984). Meperidine is one of the more lipophilic opioids. It is known to cross the placenta (Lieberman et al., 1979), as well as enter the milk (Anonymous, 2021). Its use in pregnant and lactating animals is not recommended.

f. Fentanyl

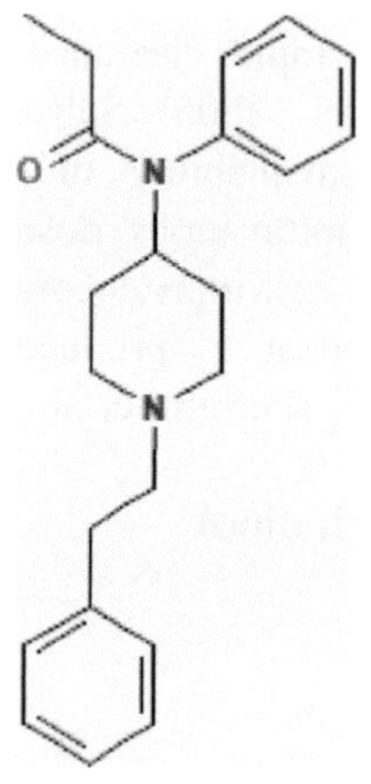

Chemical structure of fentanyl. https://pubchem.ncbi.nlm.nih.gov/compound/3345

Biodistribution, metabolism, and excretion Fentanyl citrate is available through human-labelled products, including injectable solutions, transdermal formulations (patches and extended-release solutions), nasal solutions or sprays, and oral formulations consisting of tablets, lozenges, soluble films, and sprays. A veterinary-labelled extended-release transdermal solution was available for dogs but appears to have been discontinued. In veterinary medicine, intravenous and transdermal routes of administration are commonly used due to their short duration of action. Epidural, intramuscular, and subcutaneous routes are also possible. Fentanyl is highly lipophilic (1000x more than morphine) and results in a rapid onset and diffusion of the drug into the CNS. Its high lipophilicity allows fentanyl to be successfully administered transdermally, bypassing first-pass hepatic metabolism. Fentanyl is a synthetic opioid with up to 100 times more potency than morphine at the μ opioid receptor. Fentanyl has a relatively high safety margin, where doses 300x the recommended amount do not result in apnea (Bailey et al., 1987). Fentanyl has moderate protein binding (60%) and undergoes primarily hydroxylation and dealkylation metabolism in the liver, followed by excretion in the urine.

In dogs administered a 10 μg/kg intravenous bolus, fentanyl was reported to rapidly distribute with a large volume of distribution (5 L/kg) (Sano et al., 2006). The terminal elimination half-life was reported to be approximately 45 min, and the total clearance was 78 mL/min/kg (Sano et al., 2006).

Administration of fentanyl using patches has yielded significant interpatient variability in the time to achieve therapeutic levels of the drug, as well as the plasma level of the drug achieved, where some animals may not achieve therapeutic levels (0.6–1 ng/mL) (Carlson et al., 2016; Egger et al., 1998). In dogs, it is recommended to apply the patch 12–24 h in advance of when it is needed, due to a lag time to achieve therapeutic levels. In cats, the lag time is shorter (6–12 h). Duration of action is 72 h in dogs and 120 h in cats (Egger et al., 1998; Lee et al., 2000).

g. Remifentanil

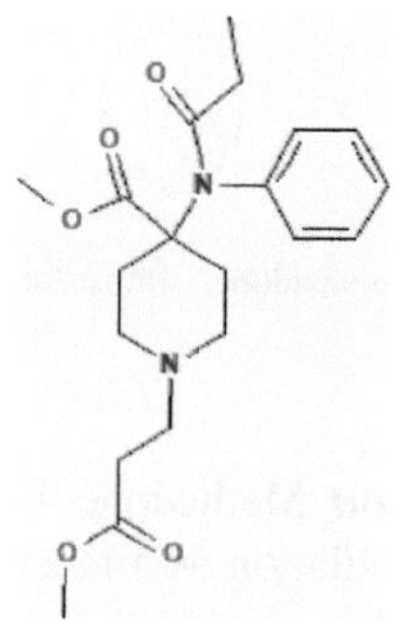

Chemical structure of remifentanil. https://pubchem.ncbi.nlm.nih.gov/compound/60815

Biodistribution, metabolism, and excretion Remifentanil hydrochloride is available through human-labelled products as an injectable solution for intravenous administration. No veterinary-labelled products are currently available. The primary route of administration is intravenous. Remifentanil has similar pharmacodynamic effects as fentanyl. Remifentanil is a synthetic opioid structurally related to fentanyl with full agonist activity at the μ opioid receptor. It has half the potency as fentanyl in dogs and is ultrashort acting in duration (Michelsen et al., 1996). This typically precludes the need for naloxone in the event of any adverse effects. It is rapidly distributed into the CNS and has high clearance (63 mL/min/kg in dogs, 766 mL/min/kg in cats), with a terminal half-life of 6 min in dogs (Feldman et al., 1991;

Hoke et al., 1997) and 17.4 min in cats (Pypendop et al., 2008). Different from fentanyl, it contains a methyl ester group that causes it to undergo rapid metabolism by blood and tissue (primarily muscle and intestinal) esterases (Chism and Rickert, 1996; Feldman et al., 1991). It is excreted in the urine.

2. Partial and mixed receptor opioids

a. Buprenorphine

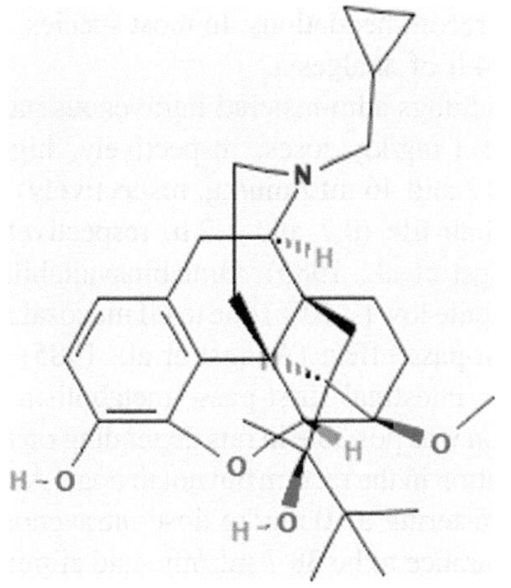

Chemical structure of buprenorphine. https://pubchem.ncbi.nlm.nih.gov/compound/644073

Biodistribution, metabolism, and excretion Buprenorphine hydrochloride is available through human-labelled products including injectable solutions, sublingual tablets, buccal films, subcutaneous implants, as well as transdermal patches and solutions. Veterinary-labelled formulations are available in injectable solutions, including extended-release formulations, and transdermal patches. Routes of administration may include intravenous, intramuscular, subcutaneous, buccal, and oral.

Bioavailability of buprenorphine after intravenous administration is very high. Buccal and oral bioavailabilities are quite a bit lower due to rapid clearance and first-pass metabolism. In cats, buccal and sublingual administrations were found to have an absorption rate of 30% and were associated with transient increases in thermal threshold in cats (Hedges et al., 2014). Absorption rates may be falsely reported higher if blood samples are taken from the jugular vein due to its anatomic proximity to the oral mucosa venous drainage. Buprenorphine is a partial agonist at the μ opioid receptor and an antagonist at the κ receptor. Its potency is 25–30 times higher than the morphine and it binds to the μ receptor with a higher affinity than many other opioids. This greater affinity can displace other opioids, but interestingly, this does not appear to impact analgesia (Kögel et al., 2005). This higher affinity is thought to play a role in buprenorphine's longer duration of analgesia, typically lasting 4–12 h depending on species and route of administration. Extended-release formulations can last 12–120 h after administration (Barletta et al., 2018; Carbone et al., 2012; Clark et al., 2014; Doodnaught et al., 2017; Johnson et al., 2017; Kendall et al., 2014; Levinson et al., 2021; Nunamaker et al., 2013; Oliver et al., 2017; Thiede et al., 2014; Walkowiak and Graham, 2015; Zullian et al., 2016). It is important to note that buprenorphine displays a ceiling effect for its analgesia and respiratory depression, where higher doses do not lead to increased pain relief or further respiratory changes.

In addition, the higher μ receptor affinity requires higher doses of naloxone for reversal.

Buprenorphine has a high lipophilicity with an extensive volume of distribution and rapid penetration through the blood-brain barrier. It is highly protein-bound and can cross the placenta, as well as be found in milk. It is metabolized to norbuprenorphine via N-dealkylation in the liver. Both buprenorphine and norbuprenorphine undergo glucuronidation to form inactive metabolites. The metabolites and drugs are primarily eliminated through the feces and to a lesser degree, excreted in the urine.

In dogs administered 0.015 mg/kg buprenorphine intravenously, the mean time of maximal serum drug concentration was 2.5 min, with a mean maximum serum drug concentration of 14 ng/mL achieved (Krotscheck et al., 2008). The mean clearance was 5.4 mL/min/kg and the mean half-life was 270 min. Similar values were seen in a different study administering a 0.02 mg/kg dose of buprenorphine intravenously in greyhounds (KuKanich and Allen, 2014). Another study examining a high-dose formulation of buprenorphine in dogs undergoing ovariohysterectomy yielded similar drug disposition and elimination to regular-dose buprenorphine after intravenous and intramuscular administration (Steagall et al., 2020). Subcutaneous administration of the higher-dose formulation has yielded mixed results (Hansford et al., 2021; Steagall et al., 2020). Other high-dose extended-release formulations have been found to provide antinociceptive effects up to 72 h after administration (Barletta et al., 2018).

b. Butorphanol

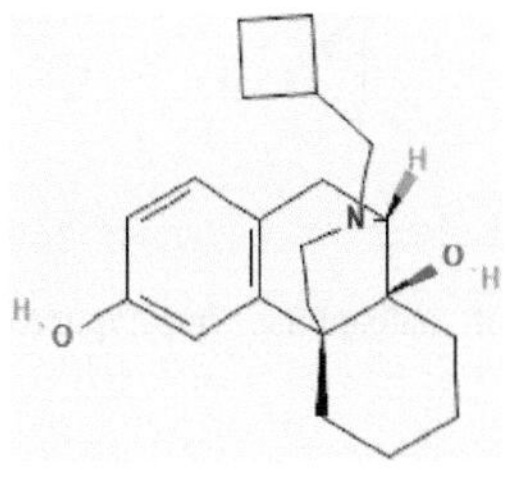

Chemical structure of butorphanol. https://pubchem.ncbi.nlm.nih.gov/compound/5361092

Biodistribution, metabolism, and excretion Butorphanol is commercially available as butorphanol tartrate in human-labelled products, including injectable solutions and nasal sprays, as well as in veterinary-labelled products such as injectable solutions and tablets. Routes of administration include intravenous, intramuscular, subcutaneous, epidural, oral, and transnasal. Butorphanol is rapidly absorbed after parenteral administration; however, will undergo significant first-pass effects if administered orally. Butorphanol is a synthetic mixed opioid with agonist activity at the μ and κ receptors, as well as partial antagonist activity at the μ receptor. It has 7 times greater potency than morphine (Tavakoli et al., 1976) and typically provides analgesia for 2 h in dogs and up to 6 h in cats (Pfeffer et al., 1980; Pypendop and Shilo-Benjamini, 2021; Wells et al., 2008). Butorphanol's analgesia displays a ceiling effect at higher doses, where analgesia is no longer enhanced and may be reduced. It is highly lipophilic, and protein-bound (80%) with good distribution to tissues, particularly the kidneys, liver, and intestine. It can also cross the placenta and be found in milk. In dogs administered a 0.25 mg/kg dose subcutaneously, the mean peak serum concentration was 29 ng/mL at mean times of 28 min (Pfeffer et al., 1980). Serum half-life was 1.62 h and clearance was 3.45 L/kg/h. Subcutaneous and intramuscular routes of administration are considered bioequivalent in dogs. Its terminal half-life ranges from 1 to 6 h depending on the species (Chiavaccini et al., 2015; Groenendaal et al., 2005; Pfeffer et al., 1980; Singh et al., 2011; Wells et al., 2008). Butorphanol is metabolized in the liver primarily by hydroxylation, and to a lesser degree N-dealkylation and conjugation (Pachter and Evens, 1985). Elimination occurs primarily in the urine, with a smaller amount excreted in the feces.

c. Nalbuphine

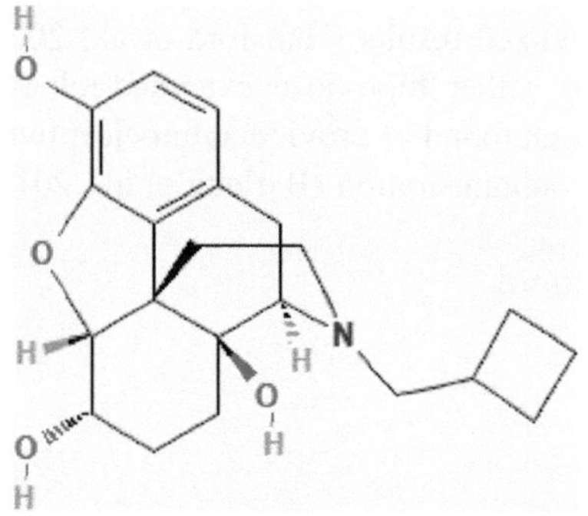

Chemical structure of nalbuphine. https://pubchem.ncbi.nlm.nih.gov/compound/5311304

Biodistribution, metabolism, and excretion Nalbuphine hydrochloride is available commercially, and it is not a DEA-controlled drug, through human-labelled injectable solutions for parenteral administration. There are currently no veterinary-labelled products available. Routes of administration include intravenous, intramuscular, subcutaneous, and topical.

There is not a lot of information on the pharmacokinetics of nalbuphine. Similar to butorphanol, nalbuphine is a κ agonist and μ receptor antagonist; however, its exact mechanism of action is unknown. Its potency and pharmacokinetics are similar to morphine, resulting in comparable dosing recommendations. In most species, nalbuphine provides 2–4 h of analgesia.

In rats and dogs administered intravenous nalbuphine at 2 mg/kg and 1 mg/kg doses, respectively, high systemic clearance (112 and 46 mL/min/kg, respectively) and a short elimination half-life (0.7 and 1.2 h, respectively) was reported (Aungst et al., 1985). Oral bioavailability was reported to be quite low ($<10\%$) due to GI mucosal metabolism and high first-pass effect (Aungst et al., 1985). Bypassing hepatic and intestinal first-pass metabolism by rectal administration was possible in rats depending on the location of administration in the rectum but not in dogs. Another study in rats administering a 10 mg/kg dose intravenously, found the mean clearance to be 38.7 mL/min and elimination half-life 56 min (Groenendaal et al., 2005), also indicating a high clearance and rapid elimination. Currently, the metabolic pathway has not been defined but is suspected to involve the liver. The route of elimination has yet to be determined.

3. *Opioid antagonists*

a. Mechanism of action

Naloxone is a short-acting opioid receptor antagonist with a high affinity for μ receptors where it causes the rapid removal of both endogenous and exogenous opioids bound to these receptors in a titratable fashion. It also has some activity at the κ and δ receptors. Naloxone has no analgesic activity and is primarily used to reverse the effects of respiratory and CNS depression due to high opioid doses. Naltrexone has also be used as an adjunctive therapy in animals with behavioral disorders (e.g., stereotypy) (Dodman et al., 1988; White, 1990).

b. Desirable effects

Opioid antagonists such as naloxone, naltrexone, and nalmefene are primarily used to reverse the CNS and respiratory depression induced by opioids. In order to titrate its reversal effects to minimize reversing analgesic effects, small increments of the dose should be administered over 30s periods until vocalization or signs of dysphoria stop. Opioids with longer durations of action than naloxone may require additional dosing of naloxone and supportive care. Naltrexone is a cyclopropyl derivative of oxymorphine. It is a pure opioid antagonist with activity at the μ, κ, and δ receptors, with the highest affinity to μ receptors. It competitively binds to opioid receptors to remove both endogenous and exogenous opioids. In many species, naltrexone is more potent and longer-acting than naloxone (Verebey and Mulé, 1975). The major advantage of nalmefene over naloxone is its longer duration of action; however, the relative potency of these two antagonists is reported to be similar (Glass et al., 1994).

c. Adverse effects

The most significant effect of using opioid antagonists is the reversal of the analgesic effects. Naloxone has a wide therapeutic window and does not have significant effects on patients, including those who have not taken opioids (Handal et al., 1983). It also acts on GABA receptors, which can elicit convulsions and seizures (Dingledine et al., 1978); however, this is usually not clinically relevant. It is important to remember that when it is administered to reverse the effects of opioids, it can also reverse the opioid's analgesic effects.

At clinical doses, naltrexone does not have significant adverse effects in nonopioid-dependent patients. Dysphoria, hyperexcitation, and extrapyramidal effects have been observed when naltrexone has been administered intravenously. In anesthetic emergency situations, it is recommended that ¼ of the dose be administered intravenously and ¾ administered intramuscularly to reduce the risk of adverse effects.

Naloxone

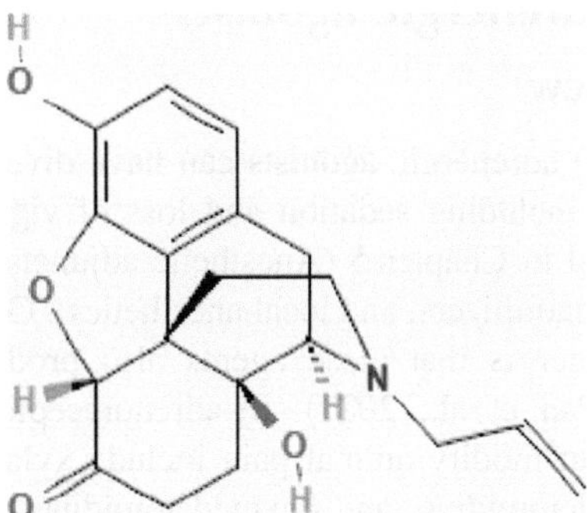

Chemical structure of naloxone. https://pubchem.ncbi.nlm.nih.gov/compound/5284596

Biodistribution, metabolism, and excretion. Naloxone hydrochloride is available commercially through human-labelled products, including injectable solutions for parenteral administration, as well as nasal sprays. There are currently no veterinary-labelled products available. Routes of administration include intravenous, intramuscular, subcutaneous, intraosseous, intraperitoneal, intranasal, and oral. Naloxone is rapidly absorbed after intravenous, intramuscular, and intranasal administration in dogs (Pace et al., 1979; Veng-Pedersen et al., 1995; Wahler et al., 2019), but displays poor absorption after oral administration and generally requires higher doses than parenteral administration. Intravenous administration results in a rapid onset of action typically within 1−2 min. Intramuscular administration has a slightly slower onset of activity at 5 min. Duration of action is 45−180 min. In dogs administered 0.04 mg/kg dose intravenously, the mean peak serum concentration was 18.8 ng/mL at mean times of 110 min (Wahler et al., 2019). The half-life was 37 min and clearance was 65 L/min/kg.

Naloxone is rapidly distributed throughout the body with high levels of the drug reaching the brain, heart, lungs, kidneys, spleen, and skeletal muscles. The drug is also able to cross the placenta (Wiegand et al., 2016) and the blood-brain barrier (Ngai et al., 1976). The drug is metabolized primarily through glucuronidation in the liver and excreted in the urine (Handal et al., 1983).

Naltrexone

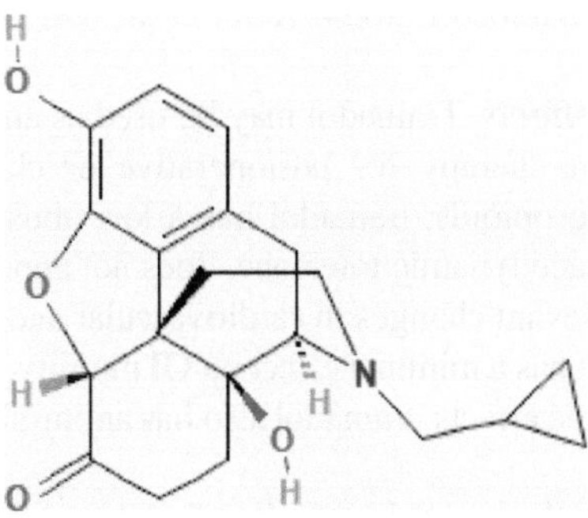

Chemical structure of naltrexone. https://pubchem.ncbi.nlm.nih.gov/compound/5360515

d. Biodistribution, metabolism, and excretion

Naltrexone hydrochloride is available commercially through human-labelled products including injectable solutions for intramuscular administration, oral tablets, and subcutaneous implants. A veterinary-labelled injectable solution is available. Naltrexone is well absorbed orally but undergoes significant first-pass metabolism such that 5%−40% reaches systemic circulation (Garrett and el-Koussi A el-D, 1985; Li et al., 1996). There is interspecies and interindividual variation in the extent and rate of absorption, in addition to the amount of drug entering circulation. It has moderate protein binding (20%−25%), and its ability to cross into the placenta or enter milk is currently unknown. The serum elimination half-life is approximately 78 min in dogs (Li et al., 1996); however, in humans, its duration of action ranges from 24 to 72 h. The drug is metabolized in the liver and excreted in the urine (Verebey and Mulé, 1975).

4. Other

a. Tramadol

Chemical structure of tramadol. https://pubchem.ncbi.nlm.nih.gov/compound/33741

Mechanism of action Tramadol acts centrally to provide multimodal analgesia via agonist activity at μ opioid receptors, inhibition of serotonin and noradrenergic reuptake, as well as antagonist activity at muscarinic receptors. It exists as a racemic (1:1) mixture of + enantiomers. Tramadol (+) is a weak μ agonist and serotonin uptake inhibitor, whereas tramadol (−) is a norepinephrine reuptake inhibitor with some analgesic activity through α_2 receptors (Grond and Sablotzki, 2004; Raffa et al., 1993).

Desirable effects Tramadol may be used as an alternative or adjunctive therapy for postoperative or chronic pain. Compared to opioids, tramadol has a low abuse potential, lacks pharmacodynamic tolerance, does not appear to cause clinically relevant changes in cardiovascular and respiratory systems, and has a minimal effect on GI motility. In addition to its analgesic effects, tramadol also has antitussive activity.

Undesired pharmacologic effects Adverse effects may include sedation, nausea, and vomiting. Changes in respiratory and heart rates have not been noted (McMillan et al., 2008). Tramadol has less of an effect on GI motility compared to opioid drugs (Topcu et al., 2006; Wilder-Smith and Bettiga, 1997; Wilder-Smith et al., 1999). In humans, it has been seen to cause seizures (Hassamal et al., 2018), so it should be used with caution in animals with preexisting seizure disorders.

When administered with other drugs that act through serotonergic mechanisms (tricyclic antidepressants, selective serotonin reuptake inhibitors, serotonin-norepinephrine reuptake inhibitors, meperidine), it can increase the risk of serotonin syndrome (Beakley et al., 2015; Hassamal et al., 2018; Takeshita and Litzinger, 2009).

Biodistribution, metabolism, and excretion Tramadol hydrochloride is commercially available through human formulations including injectable solutions, oral solutions, extended-release capsules, and tablets. Commercial veterinary formulations are available as injectable solutions and tablets. Routes of administration include intravenous, epidural, and oral.

Tramadol is highly lipophilic and soluble, making it suitable for both oral and intravenous administration. It is rapidly metabolized after both oral and intravenous administration in dogs (KuKanich and Papich, 2004). Oral bioavailability in dogs is similar to humans at 65%; however, marked interpatient variability has been noted (KuKanich and Papich, 2004). Rectal bioavailability in dogs has been reported to be 10% (Giorgi et al., 2009), and intranasal administration is variable between 3% and 21% (Di Salvo et al., 2020). Following a 4.4 mg/kg intravenous dose in dogs, the volume of distribution was 3.8 L/kg, clearance was 55 mL/kg/min, and the half-life was 1.7h (KuKanich and Papich, 2004). Metabolism occurs in the liver through glucuronidation or sulfation and results in >30 metabolites. The most important metabolite with respect to its pharmacological activity is O-desmethyltramadol, which is also referred to M1 metabolite, has a higher potency and greater affinity to the μ receptor than tramadol. The half-life, volume of distribution, and clearance of O-desmethyltramadol were reported to be 1 h, 2.8 K/kg, and 25 mL/kg/min, respectively (KuKanich and Papich, 2004). The duration of action in dogs is 6−7 h. Elimination of tramadol and its metabolites is through the urine. Excretion has been seen to be prolonged in middle-aged dogs (Itami et al., 2016).

IV. α_2-adrenergic agonists

A. Overview

Alpha-2 (α_2) adrenergic agonists can have diverse biological effects, including sedation and loss of vigilance, and are discussed in Chapter 5 (Anesthetic adjuncts, including sedatives, tranquilizers, and local anesthetics). Of relevance to this chapter is that these agents also produce potent analgesia (Pan et al., 2021). α_2-adrenoreceptor agonists used today to modify animal pain include xylazine, detomidine, medetomidine, and dexmedetomidine. Medetomidine is currently only available in the UK, Europe, Australia, and New Zealand.

B. Mechanism of action

The α_2-adrenergic receptors are located in tissues throughout the body. They exist presynaptically and postsynaptically in neuronal and nonneuronal tissues, and extrasynaptically in the vasculature. The endogenous ligands for these receptors are norepinephrine and epinephrine. In general, sedation and anxiolysis induced by α_2-adrenergic agonists occur by actions in a small group of neurons in the brain stem, the locus coeruleus (Lemke, 2004). The analgesic effects are mediated by the activation of receptors in the spinal cord dorsal gray matter (dorsal horn) (Valverde and Skelding, 2019). Descending modulation of nociceptive input due to α_2-receptor activation in the pons also plays a prominent role. Presynaptically, the α_2-adrenergic agonists selectively inhibit A-delta and C-fiber-evoked activity and suppress the release of substance P and glutamate. Postsynaptically, they hyperpolarize neurons in the dorsal horn, which modulates and decreases the transmission of ascending nociceptive information.

C. Desired effects

The α_2-adrenergic agonists are commonly used in laboratory animal medicine to achieve balanced anesthesia but also for their analgesic effects. When used as a premedication for surgery, epidurally, intrathecally, intraarticularly, or as an adjunct to local anesthetics, the desired effect is balanced anesthesia, decreased MAC of the inhalant being used, and enhanced pain control intraoperatively. α_2-adrenergic agonists are used in relatively large doses to induce sedation, analgesia, and immobilization. Their action is rapidly reversed by α_2-antagonists.

The analgesic action of α_2-adrenergic agonists is most clearly demonstrated following epidural or intrathecal injection. When administered systemically, they also have analgesic activity (e.g., inhibit acetic acid-induced writhing or tail-flick responses to heat). In rats, medetomidine was shown to reduce allodynia and mechanical and thermal hyperalgesia in a dose-dependent manner. This effect was more pronounced in animals with intact cerebral-spinal pathways than in animals that were spinalized (Molina and Herrero, 2006). In dogs, dexmedetomidine administered epidurally led to a prolonged analgesic effect at lower doses than what was required through IV administration (Sabbe et al., 1994). Clinically, the α_2-adrenergic agonists appear to have limited analgesic activity when used alone.

D. Adverse effects

Concerns regarding the hemodynamic effects of α_2-adrenergic agonists have historically led to reservations on their use in veterinary medicine (Pan et al., 2021). Low doses of these drugs decrease arterial blood pressure and heart rate and may produce atrioventricular conduction block. Heart rate continues to slow down as the dose increases, but blood pressure may increase. The effects on heart rate persist in dogs for approximately 6 h following administration (Väisänen et al., 2005). Similar cardiac effects are seen in the rhesus macaque (Capuano et al., 1999). In cats, medetomidine decreased cardiac index, stroke index, rate-pressure product, and right and left ventricular stroke work index, while systemic vascular resistance and central venous pressure increased. Arterial pressures, pH, oxygen, and carbon dioxide tensions were not affected (Lamont et al., 2001). In horses, medetomidine, detomidine, and xylazine caused atrioventricular block, slightly decreased heart rate, and significant decreases in cardiac index and stroke volume. Hypertension was seen initially, but then blood pressure decreased with most treatments (Yamashita et al., 2000). In general, bradycardia and transient hypertension may be seen in animals shortly after premedication with dexmedetomidine (Riviere and Papich, 2018). Anticholinergic premedication has been recommended to reduce cardiovascular side effects; however, the benefits of this are not clear (Sinclair, 2003).

Common side effects of α_2-adrenergic agonists include inhibition of insulin secretion and, hence, the production of hyperglycemia. The α_2-adrenergic agonists produce hypothermia and respiratory depression. They also produce emesis in a number of animal species (e.g., dog, cat). Other reported side effects of medetomidine/dexmedetomidine include mydriasis, increased urine volume, changes to endocrine function and uterine activity, decreased intestinal motility, decreased intraocular pressure, and muscle twitching (Hsu, 1981; Sinclair, 2003). Medetomidine increased the low-frequency EEG activity in dogs and decreased high-frequency activity (Itamoto et al., 2001). In rats, xylazine was shown to decrease seizure threshold and increase the length and severity of seizures at lower doses but had anticonvulsant activity at higher doses (Joy et al., 1983). In ferrets, medetomidine did not cause the elevations in pituitary and adrenocortical hormones normally seen with isoflurane anesthesia (Schoemaker et al., 2003).

Because of the wide range of effects of α_2-adrenergic agonists, there is potential for them to interact with many other drugs. The doses of barbiturates, inhalational anesthetics, and dissociative anesthetics should be reduced when given along with α_2-adrenergic agonists. It is common to administer α_2-adrenergic agonists with other drugs to take advantage of synergistic interactions (e.g., along with local anesthetics via epidural or subarachnoid routes, or with ketamine or opioids via IV or IM routes).

E. Pharmacokinetics

1. α_2-adrenergic agonists

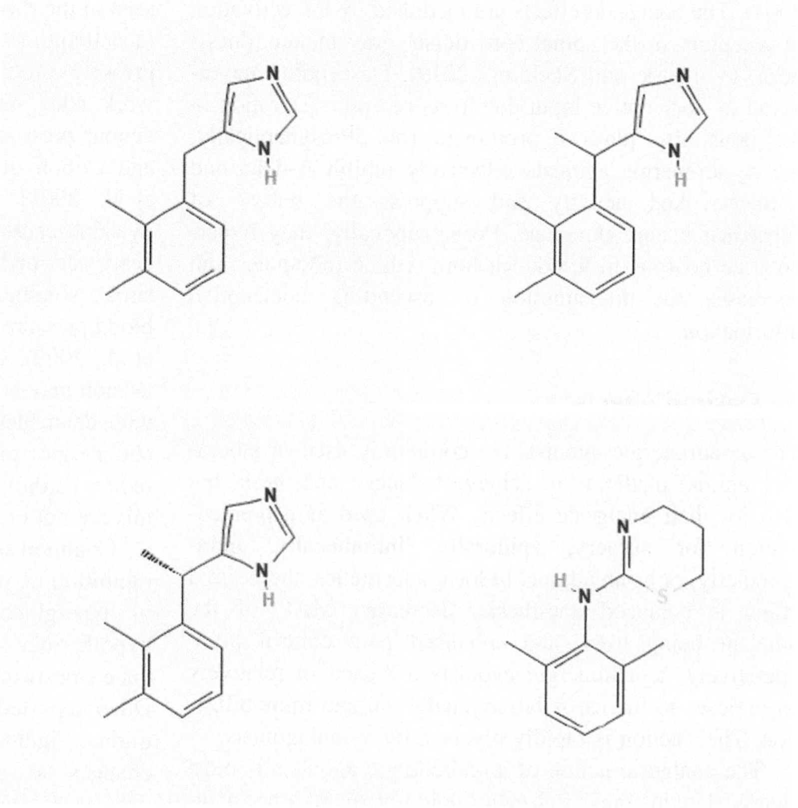

Chemical structure of detomidine, medetomidine, dexmedetomidine, and xylazine. https://pubchem.ncbi.nlm.nih.gov/compound/56032; https://pubchem.ncbi.nlm.nih.gov/compound/68602; https://pubchem.ncbi.nlm.nih.gov/compound/5311068; https://pubchem.ncbi.nlm.nih.gov/compound/5707

a. Biodistribution, metabolism, and excretion

Detomidine and medetomidine are closely related to imidazole derivatives, and xylazine is a thiazole. Medetomidine occurs as two stereoisomers, with only the D-isomer (dexmedetomidine) being active. Dexmedetomidine may also be called (S)-medetomidine or (+)-medetomidine.

The systemic availability of detomidine, medetomidine, dexmedetomidine, and xylazine by the oral route is low. Studies on the bioavailability of detomidine, medetomidine, dexmedetomidine, and xylazine following IM administration reveal species variability (e.g., bioavailability is good for detomidine in cattle and horses, good for xylazine in dogs but not in horses).

The α_2-adrenergic agonists are lipophilic and hence are readily distributed into tissues. Approximately 94% of dexmedetomidine, 85% of detomidine and medetomidine, and about 70% of xylazine are bound to plasma proteins.

Generally, all four are eliminated relatively rapidly in all animal species. The half-life of elimination varies between 0.5 and 1.5 h (Kastner et al., 2003, 2006). In patients with hypoalbuminemia, both prolonged and shortened elimination half-lives have been reported for dexmedetomidine (Weerink et al., 2017) more than likely due to differences in hepatic blood flow. The effects on allodynia and hyperalgesia in rats were greatly reduced within 1 h of administration (Molina and Herrero, 2006). In goats, recumbency is seen within 1.5 min of IV administration and persisted for at least 2 h (Carroll et al., 2005). Medetomidine sedation in rabbits lasts up to 30 min longer than xylazine when used in combination with ketamine and buprenorphine (Difilippo et al., 2004).

All four of the agonists are biotransformed primarily by the liver and then the metabolites are excreted in the urine. Renal clearance of the unchanged drug is insignificant.

2. α_2-adrenergic antagonists

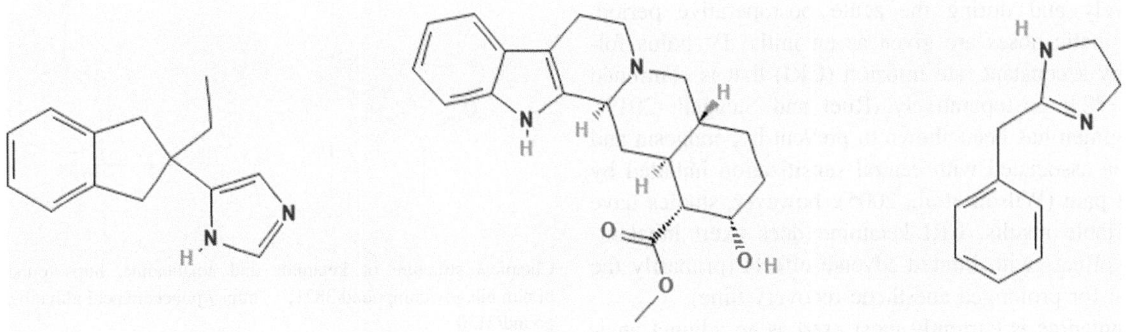

Chemical structure of atipamezole, yohimbine, and tolazoline. https://pubchem.ncbi.nlm.nih.gov/compound/71310; https://pubchem.ncbi.nlm.nih.gov/compound/8969; https://pubchem.ncbi.nlm.nih.gov/compound/5504

The α_2-adrenergic antagonist most often used clinically is atipamezole; however, yohimbine and tolazoline may also be used. They should be used with caution in horses due to the potential agitation, excitement, and stress they may cause. Atipamezole, yohimbine, and tolazoline are approved for veterinary use in the United States. Vatinoxan (also known as L-659, 066 or MK 0467) is a peripheral α_2 antagonist that can attenuate the cardiovascular effects of dexmedetomidine while sparing its sedative effects (Valverde and Skelding, 2019).

The obvious value of antagonists is to reverse overdose or hasten recovery from the sedative effects of α_2-adrenergic agonists; however, their effect on analgesia has not been studied directly.

V. N-methyl-D-aspartate receptor antagonists

A. Overview

The discovery of the N-methyl-D-aspartate (NMDA) receptor and its role in pain perception increased interest in NMDA-receptor antagonists as potential analgesic agents. Current NMDA-receptor antagonists used in veterinary medicine for their analgesic properties include ketamine and amantadine. Ketamine was produced in the 1960s as a safer alternative to phencyclidine (PCP), and its analgesic properties were discovered shortly after (Niesters et al., 2014). Amantadine was first prescribed for influenza treatment in the 1960s (it targets the M2 ion channel protein of influenza A viruses), and its NMDA receptor binding ability was discovered in 1989 (Danysz et al., 2021). NMDA-receptor antagonists are also discussed in Chapter 4 (Injectable anesthetics) because some are used to produce "dissociative" anesthesia, which may be caused by pharmacologic activity other than or in addition to NMDA-receptor antagonism. Details below are specifically related to their use as analgesics.

B. Mechanism of action

NMDA receptors are activated by glycine and glutamate (excitatory neurotransmitters) for baseline sensory synaptic transmission; however, their activation is heightened at times of sustained nociception (Ruel and Steagall, 2019). They are primarily involved with the induction of various forms of synaptic plasticity, including the medium- and long-term changes observed in the transition from acute to chronic pain (Aiyer et al., 2018). Examples of these include "wind-up" facilitation, central sensitization, and long-term potentiation, i.e., maladaptive and not necessarily nociceptive pain (Cousins and Power, 1999). Ketamine binds noncompetitively to the PCP binding site of NMDA receptors, blocking the stimulating effects of glutamate. Instead of blocking glutamate activity directly, amantadine binding accelerates and stabilizes channel closure (Aiyer et al., 2018), thereby exerting the same effect (decreasing glutamate's activity on the receptor).

C. Desirable effects

When administered perioperatively, the goal is to inhibit the excessive activation of NMDA receptors observed during times of sustained painful stimuli. Excessive activation of these receptors leads to increased glutamate release, upregulation of the number and function of glutamate receptors, and decreased clearance of glutamate. Inhibition of these changes decreases hyperalgesia, allodynia, and spontaneous pain associated with tissue inflammation and/or nerve injury (Aiyer et al., 2018).

Ketamine is commonly used as an adjunct to opioid therapy (as well as local blocks and NSAIDs) intraoperatively and during the acute postoperative period. Subanesthetic doses are given as an initial IV bolus followed by a constant rate infusion (CRI) that is continued for 24–72 h postoperatively (Ruel and Steagall, 2019). This regimen has been shown to prevent hyperalgesia and allodynia associated with central sensitization initiated by surgical pain (Wilson et al., 2005); however, studies have had variable results. CRI ketamine does exert inhalant-sparing effects with limited adverse effects (primarily the potential for prolonged anesthetic recovery time).

Amantadine is currently most used as an adjunct analgesic in cats, typically in combination with opioids. In animals experiencing chronic pain, depending on the species, NSAIDs and gabapentin are likely on board as well. It would be a recommended addition to a multimodal protocol that suddenly stops working or is not achieving the level of pain management desired. There is a lack of data to support current dosing regimens; however, studies suggest that twice-daily dosing may be more effective than once-a-day dosing in dogs and cats (Brigham et al., 2018; Chen et al., 2012; KuKanich, 2013; Lascelles et al., 2008; Shipley et al., 2021; Siao et al., 2011b). To decrease the central sensitization occurring with chronic pain, a treatment plan of at least 3 weeks is recommended, and treatment may need to be extended for life.

D. Adverse effects

Ketamine's most common undesired pharmacologic effects across species include hallucinations and/or mood changes (Nowacka and Borczyk, 2019). These effects have been termed "dissociative anesthesia", and they typically wear off within a couple of hours. While ketamine has a wide margin of safety, when used alone it may cause seizures, and when given in high doses can cause respiratory depression, emesis, convulsions, and cardiac arrest (Plumb, Donald C, 2018). In humans, there have been reports of abnormal liver function tests postketamine administration as well as drug-induced liver injury (Niesters et al., 2014). Given the short duration of ketamine administration, the risk is minimal; however, monitoring liver values would be recommended in animals with hepatic dysfunction or if repeat high-dose ketamine infusions are needed. In animals with impaired renal function, the effect of the drug may be prolonged due to delayed excretion (Ruel and Steagall, 2019).

Little is known about amantadine's adverse effect profile. GI effects seem to be most likely, particularly in dogs (Plumb 2018a, 2018b). Restlessness and agitation/anxiety after administration may indicate toxicity.

E. Pharmacokinetics

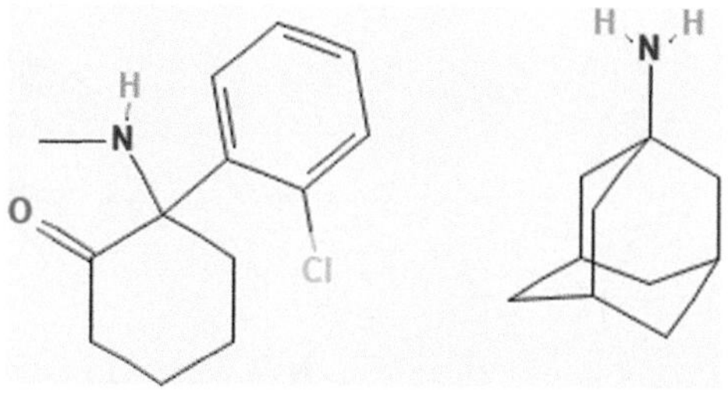

Chemical structure of ketamine and amantadine. https://pubchem.ncbi.nlm.nih.gov/compound/3821; https://pubchem.ncbi.nlm.nih.gov/compound/2130

1. Ketamine

a. Biodistribution, metabolism, and excretion

Ketamine is a phenylpiperidine derivative, structurally related to PCP (Niesters et al., 2014). It occurs in two enantiomers (S)-(+) and (R)-(−)-2(2-chlorophenyl)-2-(methylamino) cyclohexanone (Nowacka and Borczyk, 2019). Ketamine products available and commonly used in veterinary medicine are a racemic mixture of both enantiomers. The S (+) enantiomer is approximately 4 times more potent than the R (−).

For analgesic purposes, ketamine can be administered intranasally, orally, transdermally, rectally, subcutaneously, intramuscularly, and intravenously. IV injection leads to a rapid onset of action, while peak concentrations occur around 5–10 min following IM injection (Nowacka and Borczyk, 2019). Oral bioavailability is poor; however, intranasal administration seems effective. Approximately 30%–50% becomes bound to plasma proteins, and in most species, approximately 80% of ketamine is metabolized in the liver to norketamine. This is an active metabolite with approximately 1/3–1/5 the potency of ketamine. Cats do not metabolize ketamine and excrete it unchanged in the urine. Most animals excrete ketamine, norketamine, and other hydroxylated derivatives in the urine or feces, with the rat reportedly excreting the compounds via the bile duct (Ireland and Livingston, 1980).

b. Antagonists

There is no specific reversal agent for ketamine; however, benzodiazepines could be administered to help with aggression or agitation that may be seen in hyperresponsive animals. It has also been suggested that yohimbine with 4-aminopyridine can be used as a partial antagonist in cats (Plumb, 2018C).

2. *Amantadine*

a. Biodistribution, metabolism, and excretion

There are two amantadine salts available on the market: amantadine hydrochloride and amantadine sulfate. Amantadine sulfate has a longer duration of effect after oral treatment, due to lower solubility and slower absorption. However, amantadine HCl is the formulation most used in veterinary medicine.

The drug has a large volume of distribution after both IV and oral administration with peak concentrations occurring between 2 and 5 h (Bleidner et al., 1965; Brigham et al., 2018; Siao et al., 2011b). There is very little metabolism of amantadine in mice and monkeys; however, a fraction is converted to N-methyl derivatives in the dogs (Bleidner et al., 1965). The major route of excretion is through the kidneys.

VI. Gabapentinoids

A. Overview

Gabapentinoids, such as gabapentin and pregabalin, have become standard drugs for the treatment of neuropathic pain in human and veterinary medicine (Davis et al., 2020; Domon et al., 2018; Kim et al., 2020). They inhibit the release of excitatory neurotransmitters (for example, glutamate, norepinephrine, substance P, and calcitonin gene-related peptide), resulting in anticonvulsant, anxiolytic, and analgesic effects.

B. Mechanism of action

As indicated by their name, gabapentinoids are GABA (gamma-aminobutyric acid) analogs. Lipophilic groups were added to the carbon backbone of GABA to allow penetration of the blood-brain barrier and increase bioavailability. They are branched-chain amino acids and are similar in structure to the essential amino acid leucine (Bockbrader et al., 2010).

Even though these drugs were initially developed to mimic GABA, they do not bind to GABA receptors. They bind to the α2δ-1 and α2δ-2 subunits of voltage-gated calcium channels (VGCC), inhibiting the calcium influx at nerve terminals and preventing the release of excitatory neurotransmitters. The α2δ-1 subunit is concentrated in the dorsal root ganglion and plays a role in the development of chronic neuropathic pain (Kim et al., 2021). It is significantly upregulated at presynaptic sites following neuronal injury (Taylor and Harris, 2020), and gabapentinoids decrease their accumulation and subsequently reduce the response to painful stimuli in animal models (Bauer et al., 2010). The α2δ-2 subunit is found primarily in the Purkinje cells of the cerebellum, and binding in this location explains many of the side effects (sleepiness and gait disturbances) commonly encountered with gabapentin or pregabalin treatment. It should be noted that a novel gabapentinoid, mirogabalin, is in development in humans, and while it still binds to both the α2δ-1 and α2δ-2 subunits, it has a significantly higher affinity for and slower dissociation from the α2δ-1 subunit (extending its therapeutic efficacy) and a lower affinity and faster dissociation time from the α2δ-2 subunit (decreasing the adverse side effects of the drug). As of 2021, mirogabalin is not available in the US (Kim et al., 2021).

Recently, several publications have outlined a compelling case for other proposed mechanisms of action. These include stimulation of glutamate uptake by extracellular excitatory amino acid transporters, inhibition of descending serotonergic facilitation, inhibition of thrombospondin-mediated processes extracellularly, antiinflammatory effects, and influencing the affective component of pain (Chincholkar, 2018, 2020; Kim et al., 2021). It's been discovered that beyond the α2δ-1 subunit's connection to the calcium channel pore, it also interacts with a variety of other proteins, including certain NMDA-sensitive glutamate receptors, neurexin-1α, and thrombospondin, and these interactions likely also contribute to the analgesic properties of gabapentinoids (Taylor and Harris, 2020).

C. Desirable effects

Gabapentinoids are well-known anticonvulsants and anxiolytics, which is mediated through inhibition of the α2δ-1 subunit of VGCCs in the dorsal root ganglia. However, relevant to this chapter is their ability to curb chronic pain, such as that experienced with neuropathies, arthritis, cancer, hyperalgesia, and/or allodynia. While they have been used in conjunction with other analgesics (NSAIDs and opioids) to treat acute pain (such as postsurgical pain), studies have been inconclusive and suggest gabapentin may not be beneficial in this context (Davis et al., 2020; Pypendop et al., 2010; Wagner et al., 2010). Given that acute pain is not often neuropathic pain, these mixed results are not surprising. However, the doses used in these studies may have been too low to be effective, and in humans, appropriate dosing is very patient-specific. It's therefore critical for a clinician to attempt different dosing regimens before giving up on its adjunct therapy potential. They do, however, seem to amplify the analgesic effects of NSAIDs and opioids (Jokinen et al., 2016), and this may be the reasoning behind adding them to a variety of analgesic therapy regimens. There are no gabapentinoid antagonists, and gabapentin and pregabalin have a wide margin of safety (Plumb, 2018a, 2018b).

D. Undesirable effects

Sedation and ataxia are the most common acute adverse effects (Davis et al., 2020) with humans reporting variable rates of dizziness, visual blurring, confusion, impaired concentration, euphoria, and relaxation as well. These effects are most notable when first starting treatment and tend to diminish after a week or so of administration. Respiratory depression has been noted when given in conjunction with opioids, and weight gain is a common long-term side effect of gabapentin and/or pregabalin treatment. While less frequent, GI upset, such as diarrhea and vomiting, has also been reported (Chincholkar, 2020; Esteban et al., 2018).

Though gabapentinoids are not metabolized by the liver, drug-induced hepatotoxicity has been reported in humans (Jackson et al., 2018). In veterinary medicine, the primary toxicity of concern is renal. In animals with renal disease, a lower starting dose is recommended as well as a slower dose escalation.

Pregabalin is DEA class V and fairly expensive, therefore gabapentin is almost exclusively used in veterinary practice.

E. Pharmacokinetics

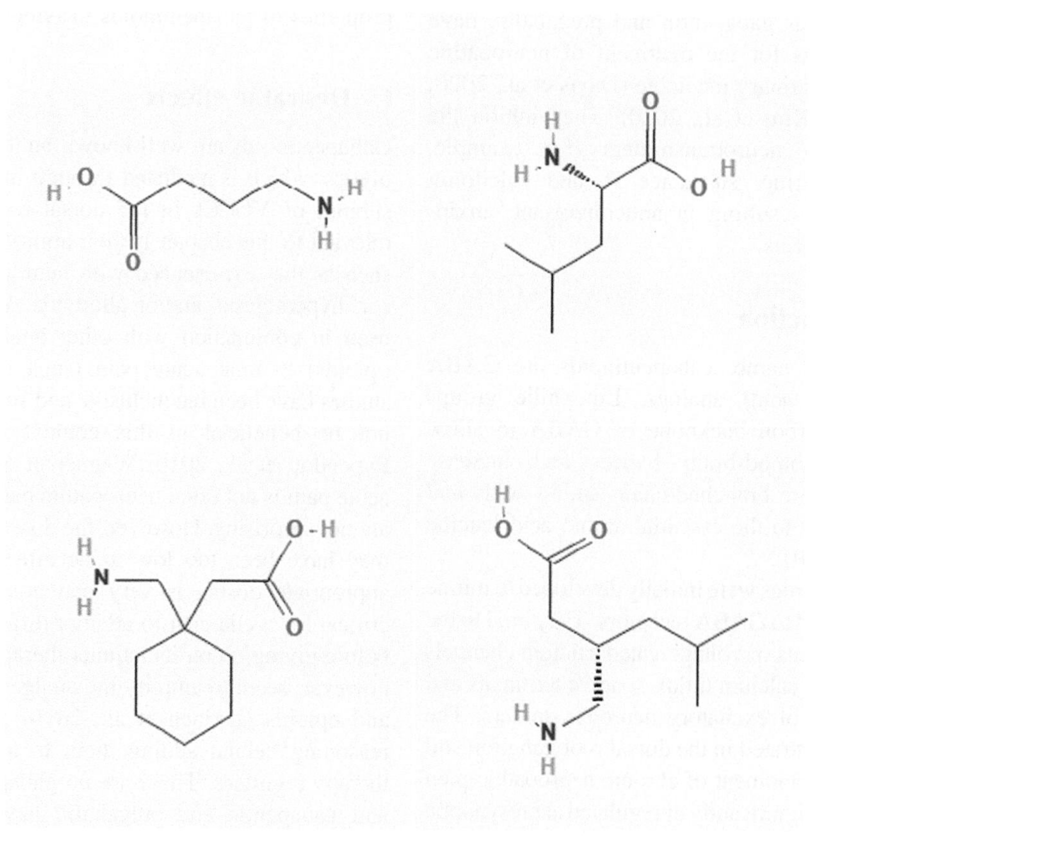

Chemical structure of gamma-aminobutyric acid, L-leucine, gabapentin, and pregabalin. https://pubchem.ncbi.nlm.nih.gov/compound/119; https://pubchem.ncbi.nlm.nih.gov/compound/6106; https://pubchem.ncbi.nlm.nih.gov/compound/3446; https://pubchem.ncbi.nlm.nih.gov/compound/5486971

1. Biodistribution, metabolism, and excretion

Gabapentin and pregabalin are well absorbed in the small intestine by system L-amino acid transporters (LAT) (Bockbrader et al., 2010; Chincholkar, 2020). In species studied (mice, rats, rabbits, and humans), gabapentin absorption is solely dependent on this route, and there is dose-limited absorption due to saturation of this mechanism (del Amo et al., 2008). Pregabalin is also absorbed in the proximal colon by an additional unknown pathway and shows a nonsaturable rate of absorption and a linear pharmacokinetic profile. This results in a faster absorption time, with peak plasma concentrations occurring approximately 1 h after oral intake versus 3 h with gabapentin (Kim et al., 2020). They do not bind to plasma proteins, and peak cerebrospinal fluid concentrations occur at approximately 8 h.

In general, they are not metabolized by the liver, with very little biotransformation seen in mice, rats, monkeys, and humans. Dogs are the one known exception, showing significant formation of N-methyl metabolite after administration (Radulovic et al., 1995; Vollmer et al., 1986). Elimination is almost exclusively via the kidneys. In most species, 100% of gabapentin and >90% of pregabalin is excreted unchanged with elimination half-lives of approximately 6 h (Chincholkar, 2020).

VII. Future prospects

Continued efforts in four areas of research will strongly influence the management of pain in laboratory animals in the future. These areas are: (1) understanding of pain mechanisms; (2) advances in optimization of alternative routes of drug administration, especially transmucosal, transcutaneous, epidural, and spinal; (3) improved methods for pain assessment; and (4) improved methods for assuring optimal dosing regimens, e.g., simple, rapid measurement of drug concentration in blood. The reader is referred to other chapters in this book that address several of these areas.

References

Abbott, F.V., Hellemans, K.G.C., 2000. Phenacetin, acetaminophen and dipyrone: analgesic and rewarding effects. Behav. Brain Res. 112, 177–186. https://doi.org/10.1016/S0166-4328(00)00179-0.

Abdellatif, K.R.A., Abdelall, E.K.A., Elshemy, H.A.H., El-Nahass, E.-S., Abdel-Fattah, M.M., Abdelgawad, Y.Y.M., 2021. New indomethacin analogs as selective COX-2 inhibitors: synthesis, COX-1/2 inhibitory activity, anti-inflammatory, ulcerogenicity, histopathological, and docking studies. Arch. Pharmazie 354, 2000328. https://doi.org/10.1002/ardp.202000328.

Aiyer, R., Mehta, N., Gungor, S., Gulati, A., 2018. A systematic review of NMDA receptor antagonists for treatment of neuropathic pain in clinical practice. Clin. J. Pain 34, 450–467. https://doi.org/10.1097/AJP.0000000000000547.

Al-Hasani, R., Bruchas, M.R., 2011. Molecular mechanisms of opioid receptor-dependent signaling and behavior. Anesthesiology 115, 1363–1381. https://doi.org/10.1097/ALN.0b013e318238bba6.

Albert, K.S., Gernaat, C.M., 1984. Pharmacokinetics of ibuprofen. Am. J. Med. 77, 40–46. https://doi.org/10.1016/S0002-9343(84)80017-0.

Allen, M., Johnson, R.A., 2018. Evaluation of self-injurious behavior, thermal sensitivity, food intake, fecal output, and pica after injection of three buprenorphine formulations in rats (*Rattus norvegicus*). Am. J. Vet. Res. 79, 697–703. https://doi.org/10.2460/ajvr.79.7.697.

Aly, M., Ibrahim, A., Farrag, W., Abdelsalam, K., Mohamed, H., Tawfik, A., 2018. Pruritus after intrathecal morphine for cesarean delivery: incidence, severity and its relation to serum serotonin level. Int. J. Obstet. Anesth. 35, 52–56. https://doi.org/10.1016/j.ijoa.2018.02.004.

Ambros, B., Knych, H.K., Sadar, M.J., 2020. Pharmacokinetics of hydromorphone hydrochloride after intravenous and intramuscular administration in Guinea pigs (*Cavia porcellus*). Am. J. Vet. Res. 81, 361–366. https://doi.org/10.2460/ajvr.81.4.361.

Aminoshariae, A., Khan, A., 2015. Acetaminophen: old drug, new issues. J. Endod. 41, 588–593. https://doi.org/10.1016/j.joen.2015.01.024.

Anderson, B.J., 2008. Paracetamol (Acetaminophen): mechanisms of action. Pediatr. Anesth. 18, 915–921. https://doi.org/10.1111/j.1460-9592.2008.02764.

Angi, R., Solymosi, T., Erdősi, N., Jordán, T., Kárpáti, B., Basa-Dénes, O., Ujhelyi, A., McDermott, J., Roe, C., Mair, S., et al., 2019. Preparation, pre-clinical and clinical evaluation of a novel rapidly absorbed celecoxib formulation. AAPS PharmSciTech 20, 90. https://doi.org/10.1208/s12249-018-1270-2.

Anonymous, 2021. Meperidine.

Arif, H., Aggarwal, S., 2021. Salicylic acid (aspirin). In: StatPearls (Treasure Island (FL). StatPearls Publishing.

Armstrong, S., Lees, P., 2002. Effects of carprofen (R and S enantiomers and racemate) on the production of IL-1, IL-6 and TNF-α by equine chondrocytes and synoviocytes. J. Vet. Pharmacol. Therapeut. 25, 145–153. https://doi.org/10.1046/j.1365-2885.2002.00397.

Aronoff, D., Oates, J., Boutaud, O., 2006. New insights into the mechanism of action of acetaminophen: its clinical pharmacologic characteristics reflect its inhibition of the two prostaglandin H2 synthases. Clin. Pharmacol. Therapeut. 79, 9–19. https://doi.org/10.1016/j.clpt.2005.09.009.

Asmardi, G., Jamali, F., 1985. Pharmacokinetics of dipyrone in man; role of the administration route. Eur. J. Drug Metab. Pharmacokinet. 10, 121–125. https://doi.org/10.1007/BF03189705.

Atkinson, D.C., Collier, H.O.J., 1980. Salicylates: molecular mechanism of therapeutic action. In: Garattini, S., Goldin, A., Hawking, F., Kopin, I.J., Schnitzer, R.J. (Eds.), Advances in Pharmacology. Academic Press, pp. 233–288.

Aungst, B.J., Lam, G., Shefter, E., 1985. Oral and rectal nalbuphine bioavailability: first-pass metabolism in rats and dogs. Biopharm. Drug Dispos. 6, 413–421. https://doi.org/10.1002/bdd.2510060407.

Awtry, E.H., Loscalzo, J., 2000. Aspirin. Circulation 101, 1206–1218. https://doi.org/10.1161/01.CIR.101.10.1206.

Bacchi, S., Palumbo, P., Sponta, A., Coppolino, M.F., 2012. Clinical pharmacology of non-steroidal anti-inflammatory drugs: a review. Antiinflamm. Antiallergy Agents Med Chem 11, 52–64. https://doi.org/10.2174/187152312803476255.

Baert, K., De Backer, P., 2002. Disposition of sodium salicylate, flunixin and meloxicam after intravenous administration in broiler chickens. J. Vet. Pharmacol. Therapeut. 25, 449–453. https://doi.org/10.1046/j.1365-2885.2002.00441.

Bailey, P.L., Port, J.D., McJames, S., Reinersman, L., Stanley, T.H., 1987. Is fentanyl an anesthetic in the dog. Anesth. Analg. 66, 542–548.

Barletta, M., Ostenkamp, S.M., Taylor, A.C., Quandt, J., Lascelles, B.D.X., Messenger, K.M., 2018. The pharmacokinetics and analgesic effects of extended-release buprenorphine administered subcutaneously in healthy dogs. J. Vet. Pharmacol. Therapeut. 41, 502–512. https://doi.org/10.1111/jvp.12497.

Barnhart, M.D., Hubbell, J.A., Muir, W.W., Sams, R.A., Bednarski, R.M., 2000. Pharmacokinetics, pharmacodynamics, and analgesic effects of morphine after rectal, intramuscular, and intravenous administration in dogs. Am. J. Vet. Res. 61, 24–28. https://doi.org/10.2460/ajvr.2000.61.24.

Bauer, C.S., Rahman, W., Tran-Van-Minh, A., Lujan, R., Dickenson, A.H., Dolphin, A.C., 2010. The anti-allodynic α2δ ligand pregabalin inhibits the trafficking of the calcium channel α2δ-1 subunit to presynaptic terminals in vivo. Biochem. Soc. Trans. 38, 525–528. https://doi.org/10.1042/BST0380525.

Bayer, B.M., Daussin, S., Hernandez, M., Irvin, L., 1990. Morphine inhibition of lymphocyte activity is mediated by an opioid dependent mechanism. Neuropharmacology 29, 369–374. https://doi.org/10.1016/0028-3908(90)90096-a.

Beakley, B.D., Kaye, A.M., Kaye, A.D., 2015. Tramadol, pharmacology, side effects, and serotonin syndrome: a review. Pain Physician 18, 395–400.

Bellamy, N., 1997. Etodolac in the management of pain: a clinical review of a multipurpose analgesic. Inflammopharmacology 5, 139–152. https://doi.org/10.1007/s10787-997-0023-8.

Bleidner, W.E., Harmon, J.B., Hewes, W.E., Lynes, T.E., Hermann, E.C., 1965. Absorption, distribution and excretion of amantadine hydrochloride. J. Pharmacol. Exp. Therapeut. 150, 484–490.

Blobaum, A.L., Marnett, L.J., 2007. Structural and functional basis of cyclooxygenase inhibition. J. Med. Chem. 50, 1425–1441. https://doi.org/10.1021/jm0613166.

Bockbrader, H.N., Wesche, D., Miller, R., Chapel, S., Janiczek, N., Burger, P., 2010. A comparison of the pharmacokinetics and pharmacodynamics of pregabalin and gabapentin. Clin. Pharmacokinet. 49, 661–669. https://doi.org/10.2165/11536200-000000000-00000.

Bonnefont, J., Daulhac, L., Etienne, M., Chapuy, E., Mallet, C., Ouchchane, L., Deval, C., Courade, J.-P., Ferrara, M., Eschalier, A., et al., 2007. Acetaminophen recruits spinal p42/p44 MAPKs and GH/IGF-1 receptors to produce analgesia via the serotonergic system. Mol. Pharmacol. 71, 407–415.

Borsodi, A., Bruchas, M., Caló, G., Chavkin, C., Christie, M.J., Civelli, O., Connor, M., Cox, B.M., Devi, L.A., Evans, C., et al., 2019. Opioid Receptors (Version 2019.4) in the IUPHAR/BPS Guide to Pharmacology Database. GtoPdb CITE. https://doi.org/10.2218/gtopdb/F50/2019.4.

Bosgraaf, C.A., Suchy, H., Harrison, C., Toth, L.A., 2004. What's your diagnosis? Respiratory distress in rats. Lab. Anim. 33, 21–22. https://doi.org/10.1038/laban0304-21.

Botting, R., Ayoub, S.S., 2005. COX-3 and the mechanism of action of paracetamol/acetaminophen. Prostagl. Leukot. Essent. Fat. Acids 72, 85–87. https://doi.org/10.1016/j.plefa.2004.10.005.

Brigham, E.F., Johnston, T.H., Brown, C., Holt, J.D.S., Fox, S.H., Hill, M.P., Howson, P.A., Brotchie, J.M., Nguyen, J.T., 2018. Pharmacokinetic/pharmacodynamic correlation analysis of amantadine for levodopa-induced Dyskinesia. J. Pharmacol. Exp. Therapeut. 367, 373–381. https://doi.org/10.1124/jpet.118.247650.

Brocks, D.R., Jamali, F., 1992. Clinical pharmacokinetics of ketorolac tromethamine. Clin. Pharmacokinet. 23, 415–427. https://doi.org/10.2165/00003088-199223060-00003.

Brocks, D.R., Jamali, F., 1994. Etodolac clinical pharmacokinetics. Clin. Pharmacokinet. 26, 259–274. https://doi.org/10.2165/00003088-199426040-00003.

Brogan, S.E., Mandyam, S., Odell, D.W., 2019. 19 - nonopioid analgesics. In: Hemmings, H.C., Egan, T.D. (Eds.), Pharmacology and Physiology for Anesthesia, second ed. Elsevier, Philadelphia, pp. 369–389.

Brogden, R.N., 1986. Pyrazolone derivatives. Drugs 32 (Suppl. 4), 60–70. https://doi.org/10.2165/00003495-198600324-00006.

Brogden, R.N., Heel, R.C., Speight, T.M., Avery, G.S., 1984. Piroxicam. Drugs 28, 292–323. https://doi.org/10.2165/00003495-198428040-00002.

Brooks, P., Emery, P., Evans, J.F., Fenner, H., Hawkey, C.J., Patrono, C., Smolen, J., Breedveld, F., Day, R., Dougados, M., et al., 1999. Interpreting the clinical significance of the differential inhibition of cyclooxygenase-1 and cyclooxygenase-2. Rheumatology 38, 779–788. https://doi.org/10.1093/rheumatology/38.8.779.

Buckley, M.M.-T., Brogden, R.N., 1990. Ketorolac. Drugs 39, 86–109. https://doi.org/10.2165/00003495-199039010-00008.

Bulka, A., Kouya, PF., Bottiger, Y., Svensson, J., Xu, X., Wiesenfeld-Hallin, Z., 2004. Comparison of the antinociceptive effect of morphine, methadone, buprenorphine and codeine in two substrains of Sprague–Dawley rats. Eur. J. Pharmacol. 492, 27–35. https://doi.org/10.1016/j.ejphar.2004.03.041.

Busch, U., Schmid, J., Heinzel, G., Schmaus, H., Baierl, J., Huber, C., Roth, W., 1998. Pharmacokinetics of meloxicam in animals and the relevance to humans. Drug Metab. Dispos. 26, 576–584.

Bussiere, J.L., Adler, M.W., Rogers, T.J., Eisenstein, T.K., 1992. Differential effects of morphine and naltrexone on the antibody response in various mouse strains. Immunopharmacol. Immunotoxicol. 14, 657–673. https://doi.org/10.3109/08923979209005416.

Buur, J.L., Baynes, R.E., Smith, G., Riviere, J.E., 2006. Pharmacokinetics of flunixin meglumine in swine after intravenous dosing. J. Vet. Pharmacol. Therapeut. 29, 437–440. https://doi.org/10.1111/j.1365-2885.2006.00788.

Capuano, S.V. III, Lerche, N.W., Valverde, C.R., 1999. Cardiovascular, respiratory, thermoregulatory, sedative, and analgesic effects of intravenous administration of medetomidine in rhesus macaques (*Macaca mulatta*). Lab. Anim. Sci. 49, 537–544.

Carbone, E.T., Lindstrom, K.E., Diep, S., Carbone, L., 2012. Duration of action of sustained-release buprenorphine in 2 strains of mice. J. Am. Assoc. Lab. Anim. Sci. 51, 815–819.

Carlson, A.M., Kelly III, R., Fetterer, D.P., Rico, P.J., Bailey, E.J., 2016. Pharmacokinetics of 2 formulations of transdermal fentanyl in cynomolgus macaques (*Macaca fascicularis*). JAALAS 55, 436–442.

Carr, D.J., France, C.P., 1993. Immune alterations in morphine-treated rhesus monkeys. J. Pharmacol. Exp. Therapeut. 267, 9–15.

Carroll, G.L., Hartsfield, S.M., Champney, T.H., Geller, S.C., Martinez, E.A., Haley, E.L., 2005. Effect of medetomidine and its antagonism with atipamezole on stress-related hormones, metabolites, physiologic responses, sedation, and mechanical threshold in goats. Vet. Anaesth. Analg. 32, 147–157. https://doi.org/10.1111/j.1467-2995.2005.00187.

Carty, T.J., Stevens, J.S., Lombardino, J.G., Parry, M.J., Randall, M.J., 1980. Piroxicam, a structurally novel anti-inflammatory compound. Mode of prostaglandin synthesis inhibition. Prostaglandins 19, 671–682. https://doi.org/10.1016/0090-6980(80)90166-5.

Cavanagh, R.L., Gylys, J.A., Bierwagen, M.E., 1976. Antitussive properties of butorphanol. Arch. Int. Pharmacodyn. Ther. 220, 258–268.

Cayen, M.N., Kraml, M., Ferdinandi, E.S., Greselin, E., Dvornik, D., 1981. The metabolic disposition of etodolac in rats, dogs, and man. Drug Metabol. Rev. 12, 339–362. https://doi.org/10.3109/03602538108994036.

Chandrasekharan, N., Simmons, D.L., 2004. The cyclooxygenases. Genome Biol. 5, 241. https://doi.org/10.1186/gb-2004-5-9-241.

Chandrasekharan, N.V., Dai, H., Roos, K.L.T., Evanson, N.K., Tomsik, J., Elton, T.S., Simmons, D.L., 2002. COX-3, a cyclooxygenase-1 variant inhibited by acetaminophen and other analgesic/antipyretic drugs: cloning, structure, and expression. Proc. Natl. Acad. Sci. USA 99, 13926–13931. https://doi.org/10.1073/pnas.162468699.

Chang, S.F., Moore, L., Chien, Y.W., 1988. Pharmacokinetics and bioavailability of hydromorphone: effect of various routes of administration. Pharm. Res. (N. Y.) 5, 718–721. https://doi.org/10.1023/a:1015959912021.

Chen, A., Ashburn, M.A., 2015. Cardiac effects of opioid therapy. Pain Med. 16, S27–S31. https://doi.org/10.1111/pme.12915.

Chen, C.-S., Shieh, W.-R., Lu, P.-H., Harriman, S., Chen, C.-Y., 1991. Metabolic stereoisomeric inversion of ibuprofen in mammals. Biochim. Biophys. Acta Protein Struct. Mol. Enzymol. 1078, 411–417. https://doi.org/10.1016/0167-4838(91)90164-U.

Chen, Y.-W., Shieh, J.-P., Chen, Y.-C., Leung, Y.-M., Hung, C.-H., Wang, J.-J., 2012. Cutaneous analgesia after subcutaneous injection of memantine and amantadine and their systemic toxicity in rats. Eur. J. Pharmacol. 693, 25–30. https://doi.org/10.1016/j.ejphar.2012.07.037.

Cheng, H., Rogers, J.D., Demetriades, J.L., Holland, S.D., Seibold, J.R., Depuy, E., 1994. Pharmacokinetics and bioinversion of ibuprofen enantiomers in humans. Pharm. Res. (N. Y.) 11, 824–830. https://doi.org/10.1023/A:1018969506143.

Cheng, Z., McKeller, Q., Nolan, A., 1998. Pharmacokinetic studies of flunixin meglumine and phenylbutazone in plasma, exudate and transudate in sheep. J. Vet. Pharmacol. Therapeut. 21, 315–321. https://doi.org/10.1046/j.1365-2885.1998.00144.

Chiavaccini, L., Claude, A.K., Lee, J.H., Ross, M.K., Meyer, R.E., Langston, V.C., 2015. Pharmacokinetics and pharmacodynamics comparison between subcutaneous and intravenous butorphanol administration in horses. J. Vet. Pharmacol. Therapeut. 38, 365–374. https://doi.org/10.1111/jvp.12191.

Chincholkar, M., 2018. Analgesic mechanisms of gabapentinoids and effects in experimental pain models: a narrative review. Br. J. Anaesth. 120, 1315–1334. https://doi.org/10.1016/j.bja.2018.02.066.

Chincholkar, M., 2020. Gabapentinoids: pharmacokinetics, pharmacodynamics and considerations for clinical practice. Br. J. Pain 14, 104–114. https://doi.org/10.1177/2049463720912496.

Chism, J.P., Rickert, D.E., 1996. The pharmacokinetics and extra-hepatic clearance of remifentanil, a short acting opioid agonist, in male beagle dogs during constant rate infusions. Drug Metab. Dispos. 24, 34–40.

Clark, T., 2006. The clinical pharmacology of cyclooxygenase- 2-selective and dual inhibitors. Vet. Clin. Small Anim. Pract. 36, 1061–1085.

Clark, J.A., Myers, P.H., Goelz, M.F., Thigpen, J.E., Forsythe, D.B., 1997. Pica behavior associated with buprenorphine administration in the rat. Lab. Anim. Sci. 47, 300–303.

Clark, M.D., Krugner-Higby, L., Smith, L.J., Heath, T.D., Clark, K.L., Olson, D., 2004. Evaluation of liposome-encapsulated oxymorphone hydrochloride in mice after splenectomy. Comp. Med. 54, 558–563.

Clark, T.S., Clark, D.D., Hoyt, R.F., 2014. Pharmacokinetic comparison of sustained-release and standard buprenorphine in mice. J. Am. Assoc. Lab. Anim. Sci. 53, 387–391.

Codd, E.E., Shank, R.P., Schupsky, J.J., Raffa, R.B., 1995. Serotonin and norepinephrine uptake inhibiting activity of centrally acting analgesics: structural determinants and role in antinociception. J. Pharmacol. Exp. Therapeut. 274, 1263–1270.

Cone, E.J., Phelps, B.A., Gorodetzky, C.W., 1977. Urinary excretion of hydromorphone and metabolites in humans, rats, dogs, Guinea pigs, and rabbits. J. Pharmacol. Sci. 66, 1709–1713. https://doi.org/10.1002/jps.2600661213.

Cone, E.J., Darwin, W.D., Buchwald, W.F., Gorodetzky, C.W., 1983. Oxymorphone metabolism and urinary excretion in human, rat, Guinea pig, rabbit, and dog. Drug Metab. Dispos. 11, 446–450.

Copland, V.S., Haskins, S.C., Patz, J.D., 1987. Oxymorphone: cardiovascular, pulmonary, and behavioral effects in dogs. Am. J. Vet. Res. 48, 1626–1630.

Costa, G.P., Monteiro, E.R., Marques, É.J., Beck, R.C., Carneiro, R.K., da Costa, F.V., Valle, S.F., 2021. Sedative effects of acepromazine in combination with nalbuphine or butorphanol, intramuscularly or intravenously, in healthy cats: a randomized, blinded clinical trial. J. Feline Med. Surg. 23, 540–548. https://doi.org/10.1177/1098612X20962754.

Cousins, M., Power, I., 1999. Acute and postoperative pain. In: Textbook of Pain. Churchill Livingstone, Edinburgh, pp. 447–491.

Cox, B.M., Christie, M.J., Devi, L., Toll, L., Traynor, J.R., 2015. Challenges for opioid receptor nomenclature: IUPHAR Review 9: challenges for opioid receptor nomenclature. Br. J. Pharmacol. 172, 317–323. https://doi.org/10.1111/bph.12612.

Crevoisier, C., 1982. Pharmacokinetic properties of carprofen in humans. Eur. J. Rheumatol. Inflamm. 5, 492–502.

Cui, J.-G., Kuroda, H., Chandrasekharan, N.V., Pelaez, R.P., Simmons, D.L., Bazan, N.G., Lukiw, W.J., 2004. Cyclooxygenase-3 gene expression in Alzheimer Hippocampus and in stressed human neural cells. Neurochem. Res. 29, 1731–1737. https://doi.org/10.1023/B:NERE.0000035809.70905.8a.

Danysz, W., Dekundy, A., Scheschonka, A., Riederer, P., 2021. Amantadine: reappraisal of the timeless diamond—target updates and novel therapeutic potentials. J. Neural. Transm. 128, 127–169. https://doi.org/10.1007/s00702-021-02306-2.

Dascombe, M.J., 1985. The pharmacology of fever. Prog. Neurobiol. 25, 327–373. https://doi.org/10.1016/0301-0082(85)90019-X.

Davies, N.M., 1995. Clinical pharmacokinetics of flurbiprofen and its enantiomers. Clin. Pharmacokinet. 28, 100–114. https://doi.org/10.2165/00003088-199528020-00002.

Davies, N.M., 1998. Clinical pharmacokinetics of ibuprofen. Clin. Pharmacokinet. 34, 101–154. https://doi.org/10.2165/00003088-199834020-00002.

Davies, N.M., Anderson, K.E., 1997a. Clinical pharmacokinetics of diclofenac. Clin. Pharmacokinet. 33, 184–213. https://doi.org/10.2165/00003088-199733030-00003.

Davies, N.M., Anderson, K.E., 1997b. Clinical pharmacokinetics of naproxen. Clin. Pharmacokinet. 32, 268–293. https://doi.org/10.2165/00003088-199732040-00002.

Davies, N.M., Skjodt, N.M., 1999. Clinical pharmacokinetics of meloxicam. Clin. Pharmacokinet. 36, 115–126. https://doi.org/10.2165/00003088-199936020-00003.

Davies, P., Bailey, P.J., Goldenberg, M.M., Ford-Hutchinson, A.W., 1984. The role of arachidonic acid oxygenation products in pain and inflammation. Annu. Rev. Immunol. 2, 335–357. https://doi.org/10.1146/annurev.iy.02.040184.002003.

Davis, A.M., Inturrisi, C.E., 1999. d-Methadone blocks morphine tolerance and N-methyl-D-aspartate-induced hyperalgesia. J. Pharmacol. Exp. Therapeut. 289, 1048–1053.

Davis, L.E., 1983. Species differences in drug disposition as factors in alleviation of pain. In: Kitchell, R.L., Erickson, H.H. (Eds.), Animal Pain. American Physical Society, Bethesda, MD, pp. 161–178.

Davis, L.V., Hellyer, P.W., Downing, R.A., 2020. Retrospective study of 240 dogs receiving gabapentin for chronic pain relief. J. Vet. Med. Res. 7 (4), 1194.

del Amo, E.M., Urtti, A., Yliperttula, M., 2008. Pharmacokinetic role of L-type amino acid transporters LAT1 and LAT2. Eur. J. Pharmaceut. Sci. 35, 161–174. https://doi.org/10.1016/j.ejps.2008.06.015.

Delatour, P., Benoit, E., Bourdin, M., Gobron, M., Moysan, F., 1993. Comparative enantioselectivity of the disposition of two non-steroidal anti-inflammatory agents, ketoprofen and carprofen, in man and animals. Bull. Acad. Natl. Med. 177, 515–526 discussion 526-7.

DeVane, C.L., Simpkins, J.W., Boulton, D.W., Laizure, S.C., Miller, R.L., 1999. Disposition of morphine in tissues of the pregnant rat and foetus following single and continuous intraperitoneal administration to the mother. J. Pharm. Pharmacol. 51, 1283–1287. https://doi.org/10.1211/0022357991776859.

Di Salvo, A., Conti, M.B., Nannarone, S., Bufalari, A., Giorgi, M., Moretti, G., Marenzoni, M.L., Della Rocca, G., 2020. Pharmacokinetics and analgesic efficacy of intranasal administration of tramadol in dogs after ovariohysterectomy. Vet. Anaesth. Analg. 47, 557–566. https://doi.org/10.1016/j.vaa.2019.12.011.

Dietis, N., Rowbotham, D.J., Lambert, D.G., 2011. Opioid receptor subtypes: fact or artifact? Br. J. Anaesth. 107, 8–18. https://doi.org/10.1093/bja/aer115.

Difilippo, S.M., Norberg, P.J., Suson, U.D., Savino, A.M., Reim, D.A., 2004. A comparison of xylazine and medetomidine in an anesthetic combination in New Zealand White Rabbits. Contemp. Top. Lab. Anim. Sci. 43, 32–34.

Dingledine, R., Iversen, L.L., Breuker, E., 1978. Naloxone as a GABA antagonist: evidence from iontophoretic, receptor binding and convulsant studies. Eur. J. Pharmacol. 47, 19–27. https://doi.org/10.1016/0014-2999(78)90369-2.

Díaz-Reval, M.I., Ventura-Martínez, R., Déciga-Campos, M., Terrón, J.A., Cabré, F., López-Muñoz, F.J., 2004. Evidence for a central mechanism of action of S-(+)-ketoprofen. Eur. J. Pharmacol. 483, 241–248. https://doi.org/10.1016/j.ejphar.2003.10.036.

Dodman, N.H., Shuster, L., White, S.D., Court, M.H., Parker, D., Dixon, R., 1988. Use of narcotic antagonists to modify stereotypic self-licking, self-chewing, and scratching behavior in dogs. J. Am. Vet. Med. Assoc. 193, 815–819.

Dohoo, S.E., Tasker, R.A., 1997. Pharmacokinetics of oral morphine sulfate in dogs: a comparison of sustained release and conventional formulations. Can. J. Vet. Res. 61, 251–255.

Domon, Y., Arakawa, N., Inoue, T., Matsuda, F., Takahashi, M., Yamamura, N., Kai, K., Kitano, Y., 2018. Binding characteristics and analgesic effects of mirogabalin, a novel ligand for the α2δ subunit of voltage-gated calcium channels. J. Pharmacol. Exp. Therapeut. 365, 573–582. https://doi.org/10.1124/jpet.117.247551.

Doodnaught, G.M., Monteiro, B.P., Benito, J., Edge, D., Beaudry, F., Pelligand, L., Steagall, P., 2017. Pharmacokinetic and pharmacodynamic modelling after subcutaneous, intravenous and buccal administration of a high-concentration formulation of buprenorphine in conscious cats. PLoS One 12, e0176443. https://doi.org/10.1371/journal.pone.0176443.

Du, J., 2014. Piroxicam. In: Handbook of Metabolic Pathways of Xenobiotics. John Wiley & Sons, Ltd, pp. 1–2.

Edwards, J.E., Rudy, A.C., Wermeling, D.P., Desai, N., McNamara, P.J., 2003. Hydromorphone transfer into breast milk after intranasal administration. Pharmacotherapy 23, 153–158. https://doi.org/10.1592/phco.23.2.153.32081.

Egger, C.M., Duke, T., Archer, J., Cribb, P.H., 1998. Comparison of plasma fentanyl concentrations by using three transdermal fentanyl patch sizes in dogs. Vet. Surg. 27, 159–166. https://doi.org/10.1111/j.1532-950x.1998.tb00114.

Elmas, M., Yazar, E., Uney, K., Karabacak, A., 2006. Pharmacokinetics of flunixin after intravenous administration in healthy and endotoxaemic rabbits. Vet. Res. Commun. 30, 73–81. https://doi.org/10.1007/s11259-005-3227-7.

Engelhardt, G., 1996. Pharmacology of meloxicam, A new non-steroidal anti-inflammatory drug with an improved safety profile through preferential inhibition of COX-2. Rheumatology 35, 4–12. https://doi.org/10.1093/rheumatology/35.suppl_1.4.

Engelhardt, G., Bögel, R., Schnitzler, C., Utzmann, R., 1996. Meloxican: influence on arachidonic acid metabolism: Part II. In vivo findings. Biochem. Pharmacol. 51, 29–38. https://doi.org/10.1016/0006-2952(95)02110-8.

Esteban, M.A., Dewey, C.W., Schwark, W.S., Rishniw, M., Boothe, D.M., 2018. Pharmacokinetics of single-dose oral pregabalin administration in normal cats. Front. Vet. Sci. 5, 136. https://doi.org/10.3389/fvets.2018.00136.

Evans, A.M., 2001. Comparative pharmacology of S (+)-Ibuprofen and (RS)-Ibuprofen. Clin. Rheumatol. 20, 9–14. https://doi.org/10.1007/BF03342662.

Feldman, P.L., James, M.K., Brackeen, M.F., Bilotta, J.M., Schuster, S.V., Lahey, A.P., Lutz, M.W., Johnson, M.R., Leighton, H.J., 1991. Design, synthesis, and pharmacological evaluation of ultrashort- to long-acting opioid analgetics. J. Med. Chem. 34, 2202–2208. https://doi.org/10.1021/jm00111a041.

Ferrari, A., Coccia, C.P.R., Bertolini, A., Sternieri, E., 2004. Methadone–metabolism, pharmacokinetics and interactions. Pharmacol. Res. 50, 551–559. https://doi.org/10.1016/j.phrs.2004.05.002.

Ferreira, T.H., Rezende, M.L., Mama, K.R., Hudachek, S.F., Aguiar, A.J.A., 2011. Plasma concentrations and behavioral, antinociceptive, and physiologic effects of methadone after intravenous and oral transmucosal administration in cats. Am. J. Vet. Res. 72, 764–771. https://doi.org/10.2460/ajvr.72.6.764.

Fleischmann, R., Iqbal, I., Slobodin, G., 2002. Meloxicam. Expert Opin. Pharmacother. 3, 1501–1512. https://doi.org/10.1517/14656566.3.10.1501.

Foley, K.M., 2003. Opioids and chronic neuropathic pain. N. Engl. J. Med. 348, 1279–1281. https://doi.org/10.1056/NEJMe030014.

Fuchs, B.A., Pruett, S.B., 1993. Morphine induces apoptosis in murine thymocytes in vivo but not in vitro: involvement of both opiate and glucocorticoid receptors. J. Pharmacol. Exp. Therapeut. 266, 417–423.

Gabrielsson, J.L., Paalzow, L.K., 1983. A physiological pharmacokinetic model for morphine disposition in the pregnant rat. J. Pharmacokinet. Biopharm. 11, 147–163. https://doi.org/10.1007/BF01061846.

Gan, T.J., 2010. Diclofenac: an update on its mechanism of action and safety profile. Curr. Med. Res. Opin. 26, 1715–1731. https://doi.org/10.1185/03007995.2010.486301.

Garrett, E.R., el-Koussi, A.D., 1985. Pharmacokinetics of morphine and its surrogates V: naltrexone and naltrexone conjugate pharmacokinetics in the dog as a function of dose. J. Pharmacol. Sci. 74, 50–56. https://doi.org/10.1002/jps.2600740114.

Gates, B.J., Nguyen, T.T., Setter, S.M., Davies, N.M., 2005. Meloxicam: a reappraisal of pharmacokinetics, efficacy and safety. Expert Opin. Pharmacother. 6, 2117–2140. https://doi.org/10.1517/14656566.6.12.2117.

Geisslinger, G., Schaible, H.-G., 1996. New insights into the site and mode of antinociceptive action of flurbiprofen enantiomers. J. Clin. Pharmacol. 36, 513–520. https://doi.org/10.1002/j.1552-4604.1996.tb05041.

Gerring, E.L., Lees, P., Taylor, J.B., 1981. Pharmacokinetics of phenylbutazone and its metabolites in the horse. Equine Vet. J. 13, 152–157. https://doi.org/10.1111/j.2042-3306.1981.tb03472.

Ghezzi, P., Melillo, G., Meazza, C., Sacco, S., Pellegrini, L., Asti, C., Porzio, S., Marullo, A., Sabbatini, V., Caselli, G., et al., 1998. Differential contribution of R and SIsomers in ketoprofen anti-inflammatory activity: role of cytokine modulation. J. Pharmacol. Exp. Therapeut. 287, 969–974.

Giagoudakis, G., Markantonis, S.L., 2005. Relationships between the concentrations of prostaglandins and the nonsteroidal antiinflammatory drugs indomethacin, diclofenac, and ibuprofen. Pharmacotherapy 25, 18–25. https://doi.org/10.1592/phco.25.1.18.55618.

Gillis, J.C., Brogden, R.N., 1997. Ketorolac. Drugs 53, 139–188. https://doi.org/10.2165/00003495-199753010-00012.

Giorgi, M., Del Carlo, S., Saccomanni, G., Łebkowska-Wieruszewska, B., Kowalski, C.J., 2009. Pharmacokinetics of tramadol and its major metabolites following rectal and intravenous administration in dogs.

N. Z. Vet. J. 57, 146–152. https://doi.org/10.1080/00480169.2009.36894.

Giraudel, J.M., Diquelou, A., Laroute, V., Lees, P., Toutain, P.-L., 2005. Pharmacokinetic/pharmacodynamic modelling of NSAIDs in a model of reversible inflammation in the cat. Br. J. Pharmacol. 146, 642–653. https://doi.org/10.1038/sj.bjp.0706372.

Glass, P.S., Jhaveri, R.M., Smith, L.R., 1994. Comparison of potency and duration of action of nalmefene and naloxone. Anesth. Analg. 78, 536–541. https://doi.org/10.1213/00000539-199403000-00021.

Gomes, V.H., Oliveira, R.L., Marques, J.L., Coelho, C.M., Silva, M.F., 2018. Comparison of the sedative effects of nalbuphine and butorphanol, alone or in combination with acepromazine in dogs. Vet. Anaesth. Analg. 45, 68–72. https://doi.org/10.1016/j.vaa.2017.08.003.

Gomes, V.H., Barcellos, M.C., Lima, V.C., de Moura, R.A., de Freitas, J.B., da Silva, M.F., 2019. Effect of three doses of nalbuphine on reversal of sedation and cardiopulmonary effects of morphine-acepromazine in healthy dogs. Vet. Anaesth. Analg. 46, 429–434. https://doi.org/10.1016/j.vaa.2019.03.001.

Gong, L., Thorn, C.F., Bertagnolli, M.M., Grosser, T., Altman, R.B., Klein, T.E., 2012. Celecoxib pathways: pharmacokinetics and pharmacodynamics. Pharmacogenetics Genom. 22, 310–318. https://doi.org/10.1097/FPC.0b013e32834f94cb.

Granados-Soto, V., Flores-Murrieta, F.J., Castañeda-Hernández, G., López-Muñoz, F.J., 1995. Evidence for the involvement of nitric oxide in the antinociceptive effect of ketorolac. Eur. J. Pharmacol. 277, 281–284. https://doi.org/10.1016/0014-2999(95)00123-3.

Green, G.A., 2001. Understanding NSAIDs: from aspirin to COX-2. Clin. Cornerstone 3, 50–59. https://doi.org/10.1016/S1098-3597(01)90069-9.

Groenendaal, D., Blom-Roosemalen, M.C.M., Danhof, M., Lange, E.C.M., 2005. High-performance liquid chromatography of nalbuphine, butorphanol and morphine in blood and brain microdialysate samples: application to pharmacokinetic/pharmacodynamic studies in rats. J. Chromatogr. B Anal. Technol. Biomed. Life Sci. 822, 230–237. https://doi.org/10.1016/j.jchromb.2005.06.008.

Groenendaal, D., Freijer, J., Rosier, A., de Mik, D., Nicholls, G., Hersey, A., Ayrton, A.D., Danhof, M., de Lange, E.C.M., 2008. Pharmacokinetic/pharmacodynamic modelling of the EEG effects of opioids: the role of complex biophase distribution kinetics. Eur. J. Pharmaceut. Sci. 34, 149–163. https://doi.org/10.1016/j.ejps.2008.03.003.

Grond, S., Sablotzki, A., 2004. Clinical pharmacology of tramadol. Clin. Pharmacokinet. 43, 879–923. https://doi.org/10.2165/00003088-200443130-00004.

Guedes, A.G.P., Papich, M.G., Rude, E.P., Rider, M.A., 2007a. Pharmacokinetics and physiological effects of two intravenous infusion rates of morphine in conscious dogs. J. Vet. Pharmacol. Therapeut. 30, 224–233. https://doi.org/10.1111/j.1365-2885.2007.00849.

Guedes, A.G.P., Papich, M.G., Rude, E.P., Rider, M.A., 2007b. Comparison of plasma histamine levels after intravenous administration of hydromorphone and morphine in dogs. J. Vet. Pharmacol. Therapeut. 30, 516–522. https://doi.org/10.1111/j.1365-2885.2007.00911.

Guedes, A.G.P., Papich, M.G., Rude, E.P., Rider, M.A., 2008. Pharmacokinetics and physiological effects of intravenous hydromorphone in conscious dogs. J. Vet. Pharmacol. Therapeut. 31, 334–343. https://doi.org/10.1111/j.1365-2885.2008.00966.

Hamamoto-Hardman, B.D., Steffey, E.P., McKemie, D.S., Kass, P.H., Knych, H.K., 2020. Meperidine pharmacokinetics and effects on physiologic parameters and thermal threshold following intravenous administration of three doses to horses. BMC Vet. Res. 16, 368. https://doi.org/10.1186/s12917-020-02564-4.

Handal, K.A., Schauben, J.L., Salamone, F.R., 1983. Naloxone. Ann. Emerg. Med. 12, 438–445. https://doi.org/10.1016/s0196-0644(83)80343-6.

Hanna, V.S., Hafez, E.A.A., 2018. Synopsis of arachidonic acid metabolism: a review. J. Adv. Res. 11, 23–32. https://doi.org/10.1016/j.jare.2018.03.005.

Hansford, J., Henao-Guerrero, N., Machado, M.L., Pypendop, B.H., 2021. Pharmacokinetics of a high-concentration formulation of buprenorphine (Simbadol) in male dogs. Vet. Anaesth. Analg. 48, 509–516. https://doi.org/10.1016/j.vaa.2021.04.003.

Hardie, E.M., Hardee, G.E., Rawlings, C.A., 1985. Pharmacokinetics of flunixin meglumine in dogs. Am. J. Vet. Res. 46, 235–237.

Hassamal, S., Miotto, K., Dale, W., Danovitch, I., 2018. Tramadol: understanding the risk of serotonin syndrome and seizures. Am. J. Med. 131, 1382. https://doi.org/10.1016/j.amjmed.2018.04.025.

Hedges, A.R., Pypendop, B.H., Shilo-Benjamini, Y., Stanley, S.D., Ilkiw, J.E., 2014. Pharmacokinetics of buprenorphine following intravenous and buccal administration in cats, and effects on thermal threshold. J. Vet. Pharmacol. Therapeut. 37, 252–259. https://doi.org/10.1111/jvp.12084.

Helleberg, L., 1981. Clinical pharmacokinetics of indomethacin. Clin. Pharmacokinet. 6, 245–258. https://doi.org/10.2165/00003088-198106040-00001.

Herman, J.H., Appel, A.M., Khosla, R.C., Kelch, K.S., Hess, E.V., 1984. Cytokine modulation of chondrocyte metabolism-in vivo and in vitro effects of piroxicam. Inflammation 8, S125–S137. https://doi.org/10.1007/BF00915721.

Herperger, L.J., 1998. Postoperative urinary retention in a dog following morphine with bupivacaine epidural analgesia. Can. Vet. J. 39, 650–652.

Herrero, J.F., Parrado, A., Cervero, F., 1997. Central and peripheral actions of the NSAID ketoprofen on spinal cord nociceptive reflexes. Neuropharmacology 36, 1425–1431. https://doi.org/10.1016/S0028-3908(97)00120-2.

Hirakawa, H., Taguchi, K., Murakawa, S., Asano, M., Noguchi, S., Kikkawa, S., Harada, K., Adachi, N., Ueyama, T., Hide, I., et al., 2022. Effects of flurbiprofen on the functional regulation of serotonin transporter and its misfolded mutant. J. Pharmacol. Sci. 148, 187–195. https://doi.org/10.1016/j.jphs.2021.11.006.

Hoke, J.F., Cunningham, F., James, M.K., Muir, K.T., Hoffman, W.E., 1997. Comparative pharmacokinetics and pharmacodynamics of remifentanil, its principle metabolite (GR90291) and alfentanil in dogs. J. Pharmacol. Exp. Therapeut. 281, 226–232.

Holtman, J.R., Wala, E.P., 2007. Characterization of the antinociceptive and pronociceptive effects of methadone in rats. Anesthesiology 106, 563–571. https://doi.org/10.1097/00000542-200703000-00022.

Horii, Y., Ikenaga, M., Shimoda, M., Kokue, E., 2004. Pharmacokinetics of flunixin in the cat: enterohepatic circulation and active transport mechanism in the liver. J. Vet. Pharmacol. Therapeut. 27, 65–69. https://doi.org/10.1111/j.1365-2885.2004.00551.

Hsu, W.S., 1981. Xylazine-induced depression and its antagonism by a_2-adrenergic blocking agents. J. Pharmacol. Exp. Ther. 218, 188–192.

Ingvast-Larsson, C., Holgersson, A., Bondesson, U., Lagerstedt, A.-S., Olsson, K., 2010. Clinical pharmacology of methadone in dogs. Vet. Anaesth. Analg. 37, 48–56. https://doi.org/10.1111/j.1467-2995.2009.00476.

Inoue, K., Motonaga, A., Nishimura, T., Yokota, M., Miki, N., Fujisawa, H., Ueda, F., Shibata, Y., Kimura, K., 1991. Mechanism of anti-inflammatory action of etodolac. Arzneimittelforschung 41, 235–239.

Insel, P.A., 1991. Analgesic-antipyretics and anti-inflammatory agents; drugs employed in the treatment of rheumatoid arthritis and gout. In: Gilman, A.G., Rall, T.W., Nies, A.S. Taylor P. (Eds.), The Pharmacological Basis of Therapeutics. Pergamon, New York, pp. 638–681.

Ireland, S.J., Livingston, A., 1980. Effect of biliary excretion on ketamine anaesthesia in the rat. Br. J. Anaesth. 52, 23–28. https://doi.org/10.1093/bja/52.1.23.

Ishizaki, T., Sasaki, T., Suganuma, T., Horai, Y., Chiba, K., Watanabe, M., Asuke, W., Hoshi, H., 1980. Pharmacokinetics of ketoprofen following single oral, intramuscular and rectal doses and after repeated oral administration. Eur. J. Clin. Pharmacol. 18, 407–414. https://doi.org/10.1007/BF00636794.

Itami, T., Saito, Y., Ishizuka, T., Tamura, J., Umar, M.A., Inoue, H., Miyoshi, K., Yamashita, K., 2016. Comparison of pharmacokinetics of tramadol between young and middle-aged dogs. J. Vet. Med. Sci. 78, 1031–1034. https://doi.org/10.1292/jvms.15-0638.

Itamoto, K., Taura, Y., Wada, N., Taga, A., Takuma, T., Matsumura, H., Miyara, T., 2001. Effect of medetomidine on electroencephalography and use of a quantitative electroencephalograph for evaluating sedation levels in dogs. J. Vet. Med. A Physiol. Pathol. Clin. Med. 48, 525–535. https://doi.org/10.1046/j.1439-0442.2001.00381.

Jackson, C.H., MacDonald, N.C., Cornett, J.W., 1984. Acetaminophen: a practical pharmacologic overview. Can. Med. Assoc. J. 131, 25–37.

Jackson, C.D., Clanahan, M.J., Joglekar, K., Decha-Umphai, S.T., 2018. Hold the gaba: a case of gabapentin-induced hepatotoxicity. Cureus 10, e2269. https://doi.org/10.7759/cureus.2269.

Jacobson, J.D., McGrath, C.J., Smith, E.P., 1994. Cardiorespiratory effects of four opioid-tranquilizer combinations in dogs. Vet. Surg. 23, 299–306. https://doi.org/10.1111/j.1532-950x.1994.tb00488.

Jamali, F., Berry, B.W., Tehrani, M.R., Russell, A.S., 1988. Stereoselective pharmacokinetics of flurbiprofen in humans and rats. J. Pharmaceut. Sci. 77, 666–669. https://doi.org/10.1002/jps.2600770805.

James, A., Williams, J., 2012. Basic opioid pharmacology — an update. Br. J. Pain 7, 11–16.

Jang, Y., Kim, M., Hwang, S.W., 2020. Molecular mechanisms underlying the actions of arachidonic acid-derived prostaglandins on peripheral nociception. J. Neuroinflammation 17, 30. https://doi.org/10.1186/s12974-020-1703-1.

Jasiecka, A., Maślanka, T., Jaroszewski, J.J., 2014. Pharmacological characteristics of metamizole. Pol. J. Vet. Sci. 17, 207–214. https://doi.org/10.2478/pjvs-2014-0030.

Jett, M.-F., Ramesha, C.S., Brown, C.D., Chiu, S., Emmett, C., Voronin, T., Sun, T., O'Yang, C., Hunter, J.C., Eglen, R.M., et al., 1999. Characterization of the analgesic and anti-inflammatory activities of ketorolac and its enantiomers in the rat. J. Pharmacol. Exp. Therapeut. 288, 1288–1297.

Jeunesse, E.C., Bargues, I.A., Toutain, C.E., Lacroix, M.Z., Letellier, I.M., Giraudel, J.M., Toutain, P.L., 2011. Paw inflammation model in dogs for preclinical pharmacokinetic/pharmacodynamic investigations of nonsteroidal anti-inflammatory drugs. J. Pharmacol. Exp. Therapeut. 338, 548–558. https://doi.org/10.1124/jpet.110.178350.

Johnson, R.J., Kerr, C.L., Enouri, S.S., Modi, P., Lascelles, B.D.X., Del Castillo, J.R.E., 2017. Pharmacokinetics of liposomal encapsulated buprenorphine suspension following subcutaneous administration to cats. J. Vet. Pharmacol. Therapeut. 40, 256–269. https://doi.org/10.1111/jvp.12357.

Jokinen, V., Lilius, T.O., Laitila, J., Niemi, M., Rauhala, P.V., Kalso, E.A., 2016. Pregabalin enhances the antinociceptive effect of oxycodone and morphine in thermal models of nociception in the rat without any pharmacokinetic interactions. Eur. J. Pain 20, 297–306. https://doi.org/10.1002/ejp.728.

Joy, R.M., Stark, L.G., Albertson, T.E., 1983. Dose-dependent proconvulsant and anticonvulsant actions of the alpha2 adrenergic agonist, xylazine, on kindled seizures in the rat. Pharmacol. Biochem. Behav. 19, 345–350. https://doi.org/10.1016/0091-3057(83)90063-1.

Jung, M., Lees, P., Seewald, W., 2010. Analytical determination and pharmacokinetics of robenacoxib in the dog. Le Nouveau Praticien Vétérinaire Canine - Féline 12–13.

Kaiser, D.G., Brooks, C.D., Lomen, P.L., 1986. Pharmacokinetics of flurbiprofen. Am. J. Med. 80, 10–15. https://doi.org/10.1016/0002-9343(86)90104-X.

Kamata, M., Nagahama, S., Kakishima, K., Sasaki, N., Nishimura, R., 2012. Comparison of behavioral effects of morphine and fentanyl in dogs and cats. J. Vet. Med. Sci. 74, 231–234. https://doi.org/10.1292/jvms.10-0565.

Kantor, T.G., 1986. Ketoprofen: a review of its pharmacologic and clinical properties. Pharmacotherapy. J. Human Pharmacol.Drug Ther. 6, 93–102. https://doi.org/10.1002/j.1875-9114.1986.tb03459.

Kelly, K.R., Pypendop, B.H., Grayson, J.K., Stanley, S.D., Christe, K.L., Summers, L.M., Lerche, N.W., 2011. Pharmacokinetics of oxymorphone in titi monkeys (Callicebus spp.) and rhesus macaques (*Macaca mulatta*). J. Am. Assoc. Lab. Anim. Sci. 50, 212–220.

Kastner, S.B.R., Pakarinen, S.M., Ramela, M.P., Kutter, A.P.N., Boller, J., Huhtinen, M.K., 2006. Comparative pharmacokinetics of medetomidine enantiomers in goats and sheep during sevoflurane anaesthesia. J. Vet. Pharmacol. Ther. 29, 63–66. https://doi.org/10.1111/j.1365-2885.2006.00701.x.

Kastner, S.B.R., Wapf, P., Feige, K., Demuth, D., Bettschart-Wolfensberger, R., Akens, M.K., Huhtinen, M., 2003. Pharmacokinetics and sedative effects of intramuscular medetomidine in domestic sheep. J. Vet. Pharmacol. Ther. 26, 271–276. https://doi.org/10.1046/j.1365-2885.2003.00492.x.

Kelly, K.R., Pypendop, B.H., Christe, K.L., 2014. Pharmacokinetics of hydromorphone after intravenous and intramuscular administration in male rhesus macaques (*Macaca mulatta*). J. Am. Assoc. Lab. Anim. Sci. 53, 512–516.

Kendall, L.V., Hansen, R.J., Dorsey, K., Kang, S., Lunghofer, P.J., Gustafson, D.L., 2014. Pharmacokinetics of sustained-release analgesics in mice. J. Am. Assoc. Lab. Anim. Sci. 53, 478–484.

Kennon-McGill, S., McGill, M.R., 2017. Extrahepatic toxicity of acetaminophen: critical evaluation of the evidence and proposed mechanisms. J. Clin. Transl. Res. 3, 297–310.

Kerstenetzky, L., 2019. Acetaminophen. In: Abd-Elsayed, A. (Ed.), Pain: A Review Guide. Springer International Publishing, Cham, pp. 231–235.

Khansari, M., Sohrabi, M., Zamani, F., 2013. The useage of opioids and their adverse effects in gastrointestinal practice: a review. Middle East J. Dig. Dis. 5, 5–16.

Kim, K.H., Lim, S.H., Shim, C.R., Park, J., Song, W.H., Kwon, M.C., Lee, J.H., Park, J.S., Choi, H.-G., 2020. Development of a novel controlled-release tablet of pregabalin: formulation variation and pharmacokinetics in dogs and humans. Drug Des. Dev. Ther. 14, 445–456. https://doi.org/10.2147/DDDT.S222505.

Kim, J.-Y., Abdi, S., Huh, B., Kim, K.-H., 2021. Mirogabalin: could it be the next generation gabapentin or pregabalin? Korean J. Pain 34, 4–18. https://doi.org/10.3344/kjp.2021.34.1.4.

King, J.N., Jung, M., 2021. Determination of the route of excretion of robenacoxib (Onsior™) in cats and dogs: a pilot study. J. Vet. Pharmacol. Therapeut. 44. https://doi.org/10.1111/jvp.12973.

King, J.N., Dawson, J., Esser, R.E., Fujimoto, R., Kimble, E.F., Maniara, W., Marshall, P.J., O'byrne, L., Quadros, E., Toutain, P.L., et al., 2009. Preclinical pharmacology of robenacoxib: a novel selective inhibitor of cyclooxygenase-2. J. Vet. Pharmacol. Therapeut. 32, 1–17. https://doi.org/10.1111/j.1365-2885.2008.00962.

King, J.N., Rudaz, C., Borer, L., Jung, M., Seewald, W., Lees, P., 2010. In vitro and ex vivo inhibition of canine cyclooxygenase isoforms by robenacoxib: a comparative study. Res. Vet. Sci. 88, 497–506. https://doi.org/10.1016/j.rvsc.2009.11.002.

King, J.N., Arnaud, J.P., Goldenthal, E.I., Gruet, P., Jung, M., Seewald, W., Lees, P., 2011. Robenacoxib in the dog: target species safety in relation to extent and duration of inhibition of COX-1 and COX-2. J. Vet. Pharmacol. Therapeut. 34, 298–311. https://doi.org/10.1111/j.1365-2885.2010.01209.

Kis, B., Snipes, J.A., Busija, D.W., 2005. Acetaminophen and the cyclooxygenase-3 puzzle: sorting out facts, fictions, and uncertainties. J. Pharmacol. Exp. Therapeut. 315, 1–7. https://doi.org/10.1124/jpet.105.085431.

Knych, H.K., Finno, C.J., Baden, R., Arthur, R.M., McKemie, D.S., 2021. Identification and characterization of the enzymes responsible for the metabolism of the non-steroidal anti-inflammatory drugs, flunixin meglumine and phenylbutazone, in horses. J. Vet. Pharmacol. Therapeut. 44, 36–46. https://doi.org/10.1111/jvp.12891.

Kogan, L., Hellyer, P., Rishniw, M., Schoenfeld-Tacher, R., 2019. The US opioid epidemic and its impact on US general practice veterinarians. Front. Vet. Sci. 6. https://doi.org/10.3389/fvets.2019.00222.

Kögel, B., Christoph, T., Straßburger, W., Friderichs, E., 2005. Interaction of μ-opioid receptor agonists and antagonists with the analgesic effect of buprenorphine in mice. Eur. J. Pain 9. https://doi.org/10.1016/j.ejpain.2005.02.002, 599–599.

Kona-Boun, J.-J., Pibarot, P., Quesnel, A., 2003. Myoclonus and urinary retention following subarachnoid morphine injection in a dog. Vet. Anaesth. Analg. 30, 257–264. https://doi.org/10.1046/j.1467-2995.2003.00076.

Kongara, K., Chambers, J.P., 2018. Robenacoxib in the treatment of pain in cats and dogs: safety, efficacy, and place in therapy. Vet. Med. 9, 53–61. https://doi.org/10.2147/VMRR.S170893.

Königsson, K., Törneke, K., Engeland, I., Odensvik, K., Kindahl, H., 2003. Pharmacokinetics and pharmacodynamic effects of flunixin after intravenous, intramuscular and oral administration to dairy goats. Acta Vet. Scand. 44, 153. https://doi.org/10.1186/1751-0147-44-153.

Krotscheck, U., Boothe, D.M., Little, A.A., 2008. Pharmacokinetics of buprenorphine following intravenous administration in dogs. Am. J. Vet. Res. 69, 722–727. https://doi.org/10.2460/ajvr.69.6.722.

Krugner-Higby, L., KuKanich, B., Schmidt, B., Heath, T.D., Brown, C., Smith, L.J., 2009. Pharmacokinetics and behavioral effects of an extended-release, liposome-encapsulated preparation of oxymorphone in rhesus macaques. J. Pharmacol. Exp. Therapeut. 330, 135–141. https://doi.org/10.1124/jpet.108.150052.

Ku, E.C., Lee, W., Kothari, H.V., Scholer, D.W., 1986. Effect of diclofenac sodium on the arachidonic acid cascade. Am. J. Med. 80, 18–23. https://doi.org/10.1016/0002-9343(86)90074-4.

KuKanich, B., 2013. Outpatient oral analgesics in dogs and cats beyond nonsteroidal antiinflammatory drugs: an evidence-based approach. Vet. Clin. Small Anim. Pract. 43, 1109–1125. https://doi.org/10.1016/j.cvsm.2013.04.007.

KuKanich, B., Allen, P., 2014. Comparative pharmacokinetics of intravenous fentanyl and buprenorphine in healthy greyhound dogs. J. Vet. Pharmacol. Therapeut. 37, 595–597. https://doi.org/10.1111/jvp.12129.

KuKanich, B., Papich, M.G., 2004. Pharmacokinetics of tramadol and the metabolite O-desmethyltramadol in dogs. J. Vet. Pharmacol. Therapeut. 27, 239–246. https://doi.org/10.1111/j.1365-2885.2004.00578.

KuKanich, B., Lascelles, B.D.X., Papich, M.G., 2005a. Assessment of a von Frey device for evaluation of the antinociceptive effects of morphine and its application in pharmacodynamic modeling of morphine in dogs. Am. J. Vet. Res. 66, 1616–1622. https://doi.org/10.2460/ajvr.2005.66.1616.

Kukanich, B., Lascelles, B.D.X., Aman, A.M., Mealey, K.L., Papich, M.G., 2005b. The effects of inhibiting cytochrome P450 3A, p-glycoprotein, and gastric acid secretion on the oral bioavailability of methadone in dogs. J. Vet. Pharmacol. Therapeut. 28, 461–466. https://doi.org/10.1111/j.1365-2885.2005.00681.

KuKanich, B., Hogan, B.K., Krugner-Higby, L.A., Smith, L.J., 2008a. Pharmacokinetics of hydromorphone hydrochloride in healthy dogs. Vet. Anaesth. Analg. 35, 256–264. https://doi.org/10.1111/j.1467-2995.2007.00379.

KuKanich, B., Schmidt, B.K., Krugner-Higby, L.A., Toerber, S., Smith, L.J., 2008b. Pharmacokinetics and behavioral effects of oxymorphone after intravenous and subcutaneous administration to healthy dogs. J. Vet. Pharmacol. Therapeut. 31, 580–583. https://doi.org/10.1111/j.1365-2885.2008.00987.

KuKanich, B., Bidgood, T., Knesl, O., 2012. Clinical pharmacology of nonsteroidal anti-inflammatory drugs in dogs. Vet. Anaesth. Analg. 39, 69–90. https://doi.org/10.1111/j.1467-2995.2011.00675.

Kumpulainen, E., Välitalo, P., Kokki, M., Lehtonen, M., Hooker, A., Ranta, V.-P., Kokki, H., 2010. Plasma and cerebrospinal fluid pharmacokinetics of flurbiprofen in children. Br. J. Clin. Pharmacol. 70, 557–566. https://doi.org/10.1111/j.1365-2125.2010.03720.

Lamont, L.A., Bulmer, B.J., Grimm, K.A., Tranquilli, W.J., Sisson, D.D., 2001. Cardiopulmonary evaluation of the use of medetomidine hydrochloride in cats. Am. J. Vet. Res. 62, 1745–1749. https://doi.org/10.2460/ajvr.2001.62.1745.

Lascelles, B.D.X., Gaynor, J.S., Smith, E.S., Roe, S.C., Marcellin-Little, D.J., Davidson, G., Boland, E., Carr, J., 2008. Amantadine in a multimodal analgesic regimen for alleviation of refractory osteoarthritis pain in dogs. J. Vet. Intern. Med. 22, 53–59. https://doi.org/10.1111/j.1939-1676.2007.0014.

Lee, C.R., Balfour, J.A., 1994. Piroxicam-β-Cyclodextrin. Drugs 48, 907–929. https://doi.org/10.2165/00003495-199448060-00007.

Lee, D.D., Papich, M.G., Hardie, E.M., 2000. Comparison of pharmacokinetics of fentanyl after intravenous and transdermal administration in cats. Am. J. Vet. Res. 61, 672–677. https://doi.org/10.2460/ajvr.2000.61.672.

Lees, P., Toutain, P.-L., 2013. Pharmacokinetics, pharmacodynamics, metabolism, toxicology and residues of phenylbutazone in humans and horses. Vet. J. 196, 294–303. https://doi.org/10.1016/j.tvjl.2013.04.019.

Lees, P., Landoni, M.F., Giraudel, J., Toutain, P.L., 2004. Pharmacodynamics and pharmacokinetics of nonsteroidal anti-inflammatory drugs in species of veterinary interest. J. Vet. Pharmacol. Therapeut. 27, 479–490. https://doi.org/10.1111/j.1365-2885.2004.00617.

Lemke, K.A., 2004. Perioperative use of selective alpha-2 agonists and antagonists in small animals. Can. Vet. J. 45, 475–480.

Lester, P.A., Gaynor, J.S., Hellyer, P.W., Mama, K., Wagner, A.E., 2003. The sedative and behavioral effects of nalbuphine in dogs. Contemp. Top. Lab. Anim. Sci. 42, 27–31.

Levier, D.G., Brown, R.D., McCay, J.A., Fuchs, B.A., Harris, L.S., Munson, A.E., 1993. Hepatic and splenic phagocytosis in female B6C3F1 mice implanted with morphine sulfate pellets. J. Pharmacol. Exp. Therapeut. 267, 357–363.

Levinson, B.L., Leary, S.L., Bassett, B.J., Cook, C.J., Gorman, G.S., Coward, L.U., 2021. Pharmacokinetic and histopathologic study of an extended-release, injectable formulation of buprenorphine in Sprague-Dawley rats. J. Am. Assoc. Lab. Anim. Sci. 60, 462–469. https://doi.org/10.30802/AALAS-JAALAS-20-000149.

Levoin, N., Blondeau, C., Guillaume, C., Grandcolas, L., Chretien, F., Jouzeau, J.-Y., Benoit, E., Chapleur, Y., Netter, P., Lapicque, F., 2004. Elucidation of the mechanism of inhibition of cyclooxygenases by acyl-coenzyme A and acylglucuronic conjugates of ketoprofen. Biochem. Pharmacol. 68, 1957–1969. https://doi.org/10.1016/j.bcp.2004.07.015.

Levy, M., Flusser, D., Zylber-Katz, E., Granit, L., 1984. Plasma kinetics of dipyrone metabolites in rapid and slow acetylators. Eur. J. Clin. Pharmacol. 27, 453–458. https://doi.org/10.1007/BF00549594.

Li, H., Zhao, S.F., Wang, N., Ge, Z.H., 1996. Pharmacokinetics of naltrexone hydrochloride and naltrexone glucuronide in the dog. Yao Xue Xue Bao 31, 254–257.

Lieberman, B.A., Rosenblatt, D.B., Belsey, E., Packer, M., Redshaw, M., Mills, M., Caldwell, J., Notarianni, L., Smith, R.L., Williams, M., et al., 1979. The effects of maternally administered pethidine or epidural bupivacaine on the fetus and newborn. Br. J. Obstet. Gynaecol. 86, 598–606. https://doi.org/10.1111/j.1471-0528.1979.tb10820.

Lombardino, J.G., 1981. Synthesis and antiinflammatory activity of metabolites of piroxicam. J. Med. Chem. 24, 39–42. https://doi.org/10.1021/jm00133a009.

Lucas, S., 2016. The pharmacology of indomethacin. J. Headache Face Pain 56, 436–446. https://doi.org/10.1111/head.12769.

Mallet, C., Barrière, D.A., Ermund, A., Jönsson, B.A.G., Eschalier, A., Zygmunt, P.M., Högestätt, E.D., 2010. TRPV1 in brain is involved in acetaminophen-induced antinociception. PLoS One 5, e12748. https://doi.org/10.1371/journal.pone.0012748.

Mallinckrodt Pharmaceuticals, 2018. OFIRMEV (Acetaminophen) Injection.

Mangold, J.B., Gu, H., Rodriguez, L.C., Bonner, J., Dickson, J., Rordorf, C., 2004. Pharmacokinetics and metabolism of lumiracoxib in healthy male subjects. Drug Metab. Dispos. 32, 566–571. https://doi.org/10.1124/dmd.32.5.566.

Maroof, K., Zafar, F., Ali, H., Naveed, D.S., 2015. Flurbiprofen: a potent pain reliever. Bioequiv. Bioavaila. 7, 026–029. https://doi.org/10.4172/jbb.1000214.

May, W.J., Henderson, F., Gruber, R.B., Discala, J.F., Young, A.P., Bates, J.N., Palmer, L.A., Lewis, S.J., 2013. Morphine has latent deleterious effects on the ventilatory responses to a hypoxic-hypercapnic challenge. Open J. Mol. Integr. Physiol. 3, 134–145. https://doi.org/10.4236/ojmip.2013.33019.

Mazaleuskaya, L.L., Sangkuhl, K., Thorn, C.F., FitzGerald, G.A., Altman, R.B., Klein, T.E., 2015. PharmGKB summary: pathways of acetaminophen metabolism at the therapeutic versus toxic doses. Pharmacogenetics Genom. 25, 416–426. https://doi.org/10.1097/FPC.0000000000000150.

Mazumder, M.K., Borah, A., 2014. Piroxicam inhibits NMDA receptor-mediated excitotoxicity through allosteric inhibition of the GluN2B subunit: an in silico study elucidating a novel mechanism of action of the drug. Med. Hypotheses 83, 740–746. https://doi.org/10.1016/j.mehy.2014.09.031.

McKellar, Q.A., Delatour, P., Lees, P., 1994. Stereospecific pharmacodynamics and pharmacokinetics of carprofen in the dog. J. Vet. Pharmacol. Therapeut. 17, 447–454. https://doi.org/10.1111/j.1365-2885.1994.tb00276.

McMillan, C.J., Livingston, A., Clark, C.R., Dowling, P.M., Taylor, S.M., Duke, T., Terlinden, R., 2008. Pharmacokinetics of intravenous tramadol in dogs. Can. J. Vet. Res. 72, 325–331.

Michelsen, L.G., Salmenperä, M., Hug, C.C., Szlam, F., VanderMeer, D., 1996. Anesthetic potency of remifentanil in dogs. Anesthesiology 84, 865–872. https://doi.org/10.1097/00000542-199604000-00014.

Mihalić, M., Hofman, H., Kuftinec, J., Krile, B., Čaplar, V., Kajfež, F., Blažević, N., 1986. Piroxicam. In: Florey, K. (Ed.), Analytical Profiles of Drug Substances. Academic Press, pp. 509–531.

Mills, R.F.N., Adams, S.S., Cliffe, E.E., Dickinson, W., Nicholson, J.S., 1973. The metabolism of ibuprofen. Xenobiotica 3, 589–598. https://doi.org/10.3109/00498257309151547.

Mills, C.A., Flacke, J.W., Flacke, W.E., Bloor, B.C., Liu, M.D., 1990. Narcotic reversal in hypercapnic dogs: comparison of naloxone and nalbuphine. Can. J. Anaesth. 37, 238–244. https://doi.org/10.1007/BF03005476.

Molina, C., Herrero, J.F., 2006. The influence of the time course of inflammation and spinalization on the antinociceptive activity of the α2-adrenoceptor agonist medetomidine. Eur. J. Pharmacol. 532, 50–60. https://doi.org/10.1016/j.ejphar.2005.12.030.

Mroszczak, E.J., Jung, D., Yee, J., Bynum, L., Sevelius, H., Massey, I., 1990. Ketorolac tromethamine pharmacokinetics and metabolism after intravenous, intramuscular, and oral administration in humans and animals. Pharmacotherapy 10, 33S–39S. https://doi.org/10.1002/j.1875-9114.1990.tb03578.x.

Murray, R., FitzGerald, G.A., 1989. Regulation of thromboxane receptor activation in human platelets. Proc. Natl. Acad. Sci. USA 86, 124–128. https://doi.org/10.1073/pnas.86.1.124.

Murrell, J., 2011. Clinical use of methadone in cats and dogs. UK Vet. Companion Anim. 16, 56–61. https://doi.org/10.1111/j.2044-3862.2011.00077.

Needleman, P., Truk, J., Jakschik, B.A., Morrison, A.R., Lefkowith, J.B., 1986. Arachidonic acid metabolism. Annu. Rev. Biochem. 55, 69–102. https://doi.org/10.1146/annurev.bi.55.070186.000441.

Ngai, S.H., Berkowitz, B.A., Yang, J.C., Hempstead, J., Spector, S., 1976. Pharmacokinetics of naloxone in rats and in man: basis for its potency and short duration of action. Anesthesiology 44, 398–401. https://doi.org/10.1097/00000542-197605000-00008.

Niazi, S.K., Alam, S.M., Ahmad, S.I., 1996. Dose dependent pharmacokinetics of naproxen in man. Biopharm Drug Dispos. 17, 355–361. https://doi.org/10.1002/(SICI)1099-081X(199605).

Niesters, M., Martini, C., Dahan, A., 2014. Ketamine for chronic pain: risks and benefits. Br. J. Clin. Pharmacol. 77, 357–367. https://doi.org/10.1111/bcp.12094.

Noguchi, K., Okubo, M., 2011. Leukotrienes in nociceptive pathway and neuropathic/inflammatory pain. Biol. Pharm. Bull. 34, 1163–1169. https://doi.org/10.1248/bpb.34.1163.

Nowacka, A., Borczyk, M., 2019. Ketamine applications beyond anesthesia – a literature review. Eur. J. Pharmacol. 860, 172547. https://doi.org/10.1016/j.ejphar.2019.172547.

Nunamaker, E.A., Halliday, L.C., Moody, D.E., Fang, W.B., Lindeblad, M., Fortman, J.D., 2013. Pharmacokinetics of 2 formulations of buprenorphine in macaques (*Macaca mulatta* and *Macaca fascicularis*). JAALAS 52, 48–56.

Odensvik, K., 1995. Pharmacokinetics of flunixin and its effect on prostaglandin F2 alpha metabolite concentrations after oral and intravenous administration in heifers. J. Vet. Pharmacol. Therapeut. 18, 254–259. https://doi.org/10.1111/j.1365-2885.1995.tb00589.

Ogino, T., Mizuno, Y., Ogata, T., Takahashi, Y., 2005. Pharmacokinetic interactions of flunixin meglumine and enrofloxacin in dogs. Am. J. Vet. Res. 66, 1209–1213. https://doi.org/10.2460/ajvr.2005.66.1209.

Okonek, S., Reinecke, H.J., 1983. Acute toxicity of pyrazolones. Am. J. Med. 75, 94–98. https://doi.org/10.1016/0002-9343(83)90238-3.

Oliver, V.L., Athavale, S., Simon, K.E., Kendall, L.V., Nemzek, J.A., Lofgren, J.L., 2017. Evaluation of pain assessment techniques and analgesia efficacy in a female Guinea pig (*Cavia porcellus*) model of surgical pain. J. Am. Assoc. Lab. Anim. Sci. 56, 425–435.

Olkkola, K.T., Brunetto, A.V., Mattila, M.J., 1994. Pharmacokinetics of oxicam nonsteroidal anti-inflammatory agents. Clin. Pharmacokinet. 26, 107–120. https://doi.org/10.2165/00003088-199426020-00004.

Ossipov, M.H., Jerussi, T.P., Ren, K., Sun, H., Porreca, F., 2000. Differential effects of spinal (R)-ketoprofen and (S)-ketoprofen against signs of neuropathic pain and tonic nociception: evidence for a novel mechanism of action of (R)-ketoprofen against tactile allodynia. Pain 87, 193–199. https://doi.org/10.1016/S0304-3959(00)00280-3.

Ottani, A., Leone, S., Sandrini, M., Ferrari, A., Bertolini, A., 2006. The analgesic activity of paracetamol is prevented by the blockade of cannabinoid CB1 receptors. Eur. J. Pharmacol. 531, 280–281. https://doi.org/10.1016/j.ejphar.2005.12.015.

O'Banion, M.K., 1999. Cyclooxygenase-2: molecular biology, pharmacology, and neurobiology. CRN 13. https://doi.org/10.1615/CritRevNeurobiol.v13.i1.30.

Pace, N.L., Parrish, R.G., Lieberman, M.M., Wong, K.C., Blatnick, R.A., 1979. Pharmacokinetics of naloxone and naltrexone in the dog. J. Pharmacol. Exp. Therapeut. 208, 254–256.

Pachter, I.J., Evens, R.P., 1985. Butorphanol. Drug Alcohol Depend. 14, 325–338. https://doi.org/10.1016/0376-8716(85)90065-1.

Page, C.D., Sarabia-Estrada, R., Hoffman, R.J., Lo, C.-P., Gades, N.M., 2019. Lack of absorption of a sustained-release buprenorphine formulation administered subcutaneously to athymic nude rats. JAALAS 58, 597–600. https://doi.org/10.30802/AALAS-JAALAS-19-000013.

Pairis-Garcia, M.D., Karriker, L.A., Johnson, A.K., Kukanich, B., Wulf, L., Sander, S., Millman, S.T., Stalder, K.J., Coetzee, J.F., 2013. Pharmacokinetics of flunixin meglumine in mature swine after intravenous, intramuscular and oral administration. BMC Vet. Res. 9, 165. https://doi.org/10.1186/1746-6148-9-165.

Pan, S.-Y., Liu, G., Lin, J.-H., Jin, Y.-P., 2021. Efficacy and safety of dexmedetomidine premedication in balanced anesthesia: a systematic review and meta-analysis in dogs. Animals 11, 3254. https://doi.org/10.3390/ani11113254.

Patrignani, P., Patrono, C., 2015. Cyclooxygenase inhibitors: from pharmacology to clinical read-outs. Biochim. Biophys. Acta Mol. Cell Biol. Lipids 1851, 422–432. https://doi.org/10.1016/j.bbalip.2014.09.016.

Peckham, E.M., Traynor, J.R., 2006. Comparison of the antinociceptive response to morphine and morphine-like compounds in male and female Sprague-Dawley rats. J. Pharmacol. Exp. Ther. 316, 1195–1201. https://doi.org/10.1124/jpet.105.094276.

Pelligand, L., King, J.N., Toutain, P.L., Elliott, J., Lees, P., 2012. Pharmacokinetic/pharmacodynamic modelling of robenacoxib in a feline tissue cage model of inflammation. J. Vet. Pharmacol. Therapeut. 35, 19–32. https://doi.org/10.1111/j.1365-2885.2011.01288.

Peris-Ribera, J.-E., Torres-Molina, F., Garcia-Carbonell, M.C., Aristorena, J.C., Pla-Delfina, J.M., 1991. Pharmacokinetics and bioavailability of diclofenac in the rat. J. Pharmacokinet. Biopharm. 19, 647–665. https://doi.org/10.1007/BF01080872.

Pfeffer, M., Smyth, R.D., Pittman, K.A., Nardella, P.A., 1980. Pharmacokinetics of subcutaneous and intramuscular butorphanol in dogs. J. Pharmacol. Sci. 69, 801–803. https://doi.org/10.1002/jps.2600690715.

Pickering, G., Loriot, M.-A., Libert, F., Eschalier, A., Beaune, P., Dubray, C., 2006. Analgesic effect of acetaminophen in humans: first evidence of a central serotonergic mechanism. Clin. Pharmacol. Therapeut. 79, 371–378. https://doi.org/10.1016/j.clpt.2005.12.307.

Pinardi, G., Sierralta, F., Miranda, H.F., 2001. Interaction between the antinociceptive effect of ketoprofen and adrenergic modulatory systems. Inflammation 25, 233–239. https://doi.org/10.1023/A:1010923820109.

Pircio, A.W., Gylys, J.A., Cavanagh, R.L., Buyniski, J.P., Bierwagen, M.E., 1976. The pharmacology of butorphanol, a 3,14-dihydroxymorphinan narcotic antagonist analgesic. Arch. Int. Pharmacodyn. Ther. 220, 231–257.

Plumb, D.C., 2018a. Gabapentin. In: Plumb's Veterinary Drug Handbook. Wiley-Blackwell, Ames, IA, pp. 731–734.

Plumb, D.C., 2018b. Pregabalin. In: Plumb's Veterinary Drug Handbook. Wiley-Blackwell, Ames, IA, pp. 1363–1365.

Plumb, D.C., 2018c. Ketamine. In: Plumb's Veterinary Drug Handbook. Wiley-Blackwell, Ames, IA, pp. 905–914.

Porreca, F., Ossipov, M.H., 2009. Nausea and vomiting side effects with opioid analgesics during treatment of chronic pain: mechanisms, implications, and management options. Pain Med. 10, 654–662. https://doi.org/10.1111/j.1526-4637.2009.00583.

Posner, L.P., Gleed, R.D., Erb, H.N., Ludders, J.W., 2007. Post-anesthetic hyperthermia in cats. Vet. Anaesth. Analg. 34, 40–47. https://doi.org/10.1111/j.1467-2995.2006.00287.

Power, I., 2005. Recent advances in postoperative pain therapy. Br. J. Addiction Br. J. Anaesth. 95, 43–51. https://doi.org/10.1093/bja/aei037.

Prommer, E., 2006. Oxymorphone: a review. Support. Care Cancer 14, 109–115. https://doi.org/10.1007/s00520-005-0917-1.

Pruett, S.B., Han, Y.C., Fuchs, B.A., 1992. Morphine suppresses primary humoral immune responses by a predominantly indirect mechanism. J. Pharmacol. Exp. Therapeut. 262, 923–928.

Prusakiewicz, J.J., Felts, A.S., Mackenzie, B.S., Marnett, L.J., 2004. Molecular basis of the time-dependent inhibition of cyclooxygenases by indomethacin. Biochemistry 43, 15439–15445. https://doi.org/10.1021/bi048534q.

Pypendop, B.H., Shilo-Benjamini, Y., 2021. Pharmacokinetics of butorphanol in male neutered cats anesthetized with isoflurane. J. Vet. Pharmacol. Therapeut. 44, 883–887. https://doi.org/10.1111/jvp.13014.

Pypendop, B.H., Brosnan, R.J., Siao, K.T., Stanley, S.D., 2008. Pharmacokinetics of remifentanil in conscious cats and cats anesthetized with isoflurane. Am. J. Vet. Res. 69, 531–536. https://doi.org/10.2460/ajvr.69.4.531.

Pypendop, B.H., Siao, K.T., Ilkiw, J.E., 2010. Thermal antinociceptive effect of orally administered gabapentin in healthy cats. Am. J. Vet. Res. 71, 1027–1032. https://doi.org/10.2460/ajvr.71.9.1027.

Pypendop, B.H., Ilkiw, J.E., Shilo-Benjamini, Y., 2014. Bioavailability of morphine, methadone, hydromorphone, and oxymorphone following buccal administration in cats. J. Vet. Pharmacol. Therapeut. 37, 295–300. https://doi.org/10.1111/jvp.12090.

Radulovic, L.L., Türck, D., von Hodenberg, A., Vollmer, K.O., McNally, W.P., DeHart, P.D., Hanson, B.J., Bockbrader, H.N., Chang, T., 1995. Disposition of gabapentin (neurontin) in mice, rats, dogs, and monkeys. Drug Metab. Dispos. 23, 441–448.

Raffa, R.B., Friderichs, E., Reimann, W., Shank, R.P., Codd, E.E., Vaught, J.L., Jacoby, H.I., Selve, N., 1993. Complementary and synergistic antinociceptive interaction between the enantiomers of tramadol. J. Pharmacol. Exp. Therapeut. 267, 331–340.

Raffa, R.B., Pergolizzi, J.V., Taylor, R., Decker, J.F., Patrick, J.T., 2014. Acetaminophen (paracetamol) oral absorption and clinical influences. Pain Pract. 14, 668–677. https://doi.org/10.1111/papr.12130.

Raillard, M., Michaut-Castrillo, J., Spreux, D., Gauthier, O., Touzot-Jourde, G., Holopherne-Doran, D., 2017. Comparison of medetomidine-morphine and medetomidine-methadone for sedation, isoflurane requirement and postoperative analgesia in dogs undergoing laparoscopy. Vet. Anaesth. Analg. 44, 17–27. https://doi.org/10.1111/vaa.12394.

Raja, S.N., Carr, D.B., Cohen, M., Finnerup, N.B., Flor, H., Gibson, S., Keefe, F.J., Mogil, J.S., Ringkamp, M., Sluka, K.A., et al., 2020. The revised International Association for the Study of Pain definition of pain: concepts, challenges, and compromises. Pain 161, 1976–1982. https://doi.org/10.1097/j.pain.0000000000001939.

Rao, P., Knaus, E.E., 2008. Evolution of nonsteroidal anti-inflammatory drugs (NSAIDs): cyclooxygenase (COX) inhibition and beyond. J. Pharm. Pharmaceut. Sci. 11, 81s–110s. https://doi.org/10.18433/J3T886.

Raulic, J., Beaudry, F., Beauchamp, G., Jalenques, M., Summa, N., Lair, S., Youcef, W.A., Vergneau-Grosset, C., 2021. Pharmacokinetic, pharmacodynamic, and toxicology study of robenacoxib in rainbow trout (*Oncorhynchus mykiss*). Zamd 52, 529–537. https://doi.org/10.1638/2020-0130.

Ray, J.E., Wade, D.N., 1982. The pharmacokinetics and metabolism of 14C-carprofen in man. Biopharm. Drug Dispos. 3, 29–38. https://doi.org/10.1002/bdd.2510030105.

Rençber, S., Karavana, S.Y., Özyazici, M., 2009. Bioavailability File: Ketoprofen, vol 14.

Reppert, E.J., Kleinhenz, M.D., Montgomery, S.R., Bornheim, H.N., Magnin, G., Sidhu, P.K., Zhang, Y., Joo, H., Coetzee, J.F., 2019. Pharmacokinetics and pharmacodynamics of intravenous and transdermal flunixin meglumine in meat goats. J. Vet. Pharmacol. Therapeut. 42, 309–317. https://doi.org/10.1111/jvp.12756.

Ricciotti, E., FitzGerald, G.A., 2011. Prostaglandins and inflammation. Arterioscler. Thromb. Vasc. Biol. 31, 986–1000. https://doi.org/10.1161/ATVBAHA.110.207449.

Richardson, J.A., 2000. Management of acetaminophen and ibuprofen toxicoses in dogs and cats. J. Vet. Emerg. Crit. Care 10, 285–291. https://doi.org/10.1111/j.1476-4431.2000.tb00013.

Riviere, J.E., Papich, M.G., 2018. Veterinary Pharmacology and Therapeutics. John Wiley & Sons.

Robertson, S.A., Taylor, P.M., 2004. Pain management in cats–past, present and future. Part 2. Treatment of pain–clinical pharmacology. J. Feline Med. Surg. 6, 321–333. https://doi.org/10.1016/j.jfms.2003.10.002.

Robinson, E.P., Faggella, A.M., Henry, D.P., Russell, W.L., 1988. Comparison of histamine release induced by morphine and oxymorphone administration in dogs. Am. J. Vet. Res. 49, 1699–1701.

Rogosch, T., Sinning, C., Podlewski, A., Watzer, B., Schlosburg, J., Lichtman, A.H., Cascio, M.G., Bisogno, T., Di Marzo, V., Nüsing, R., et al., 2012. Novel bioactive metabolites of dipyrone (metamizol). Bioorg. Med. Chem. 20, 101–107. https://doi.org/10.1016/j.bmc.2011.11.028.

Rohrer Bley, C., Neiger-Aeschbacher, G., Busato, A., Schatzmann, U., 2004. Comparison of perioperative racemic methadone, levo-methadone and dextromoramide in cats using indicators of post-operative pain. Vet. Anaesth. Analg. 31, 175–182. https://doi.org/10.1111/j.1467-2987.2004.00148.

Rose, R.j., Kohnke, J.r., Baggot, J.D., 1982. Bioavailability of phenylbutazone preparations in the horse. Equine Vet. J. 14, 234–237. https://doi.org/10.1111/j.2042-3306.1982.tb02404.

Rosenstein, E., Kunicka, J., Kramer, N., Goldstein, G., 1994. Modification of cytokine production by piroxicam. J. Rheumatol. 21, 901–904.

Rouzer, C.A., Marnett, L.J., 2009. Cyclooxygenases: structural and functional insights. J. Lipid Res. 50, S29–S34. https://doi.org/10.1194/jlr.R800042-JLR200.

Rubio, F., Seawall, S., Pocelinko, R., Debarbieri, B., Benz, W., Berger, L., Morgan, L., Pao, J., Williams, T.H., Koechlin, B., 1980. Metabolism of carprofen, a nonsteroidal anti-inflammatory agent, in rats, dogs, and humans. J. Pharmaceut. Sci. 69, 1245–1253. https://doi.org/10.1002/jps.2600691104.

Ruel, H.L.M., Steagall, P.V., 2019. Adjuvant analgesics in acute pain management. Vet. Clin. Small Anim. Pract. 49, 1127–1141. https://doi.org/10.1016/j.cvsm.2019.07.005.

Runkel, R., Chaplin, M., Boost, G., Segre, E., Forchielli, E., 1972. Absorption, distribution, metabolism, and excretion of naproxen in various laboratory animals and human subjects. J. Pharmaceut. Sci. 61, 703–708. https://doi.org/10.1002/jps.2600610507.

Runkel, R., Forchielli, E., Boost, G., Chaplin, M., Hill, R., Sevelius, H., Thompson, G., Segre, E., 1973. Naproxen-metabolism, excretion and comparative pharmacokinetics. Scand. J. Rheumatol. 2, 29–36. https://doi.org/10.3109/03009747309097093.

Russell, R.I., 1986. Protective effects of the prostaglandins on the gastric mucosa. Am. J. Med. 81, 2–4. https://doi.org/10.1016/S0002-9343(86)80002-X.

Sabbe, M.B., Penning, J.P., Ozaki, G.T., Yaksh, T.L., 1994. Spinal and systemic action of the alpha 2 receptor agonist dexmedetomidine in dogs. Antinociception and carbon dioxide response. Anesthesiology 80, 1057–1072. https://doi.org/10.1097/00000542-199405000-00015.

Sano, T., Nishimura, R., Kanazawa, H., Igarashi, E., Nagata, Y., Mochizuki, M., Sasaki, N., 2006. Pharmacokinetics of fentanyl after single intravenous injection and constant rate infusion in dogs. Vet. Anaesth. Analg. 33, 266–273. https://doi.org/10.1111/j.1467-2995.2005.00266.

Saper, C.B., Breder, C.D., 1994. The neurologic basis of fever. N. Engl. J. Med. 330, 1880–1886.

Schlick, K.H., Hemmen, T.M., Lyden, P.D., 2015. Seizures and meperidine: overstated and underutilized. Ther. Hypothermia Temp. Manag. 5, 223–227. https://doi.org/10.1089/ther.2015.0013.

Schmidt, J.R., Krugner-Higby, L., Heath, T.D., Sullivan, R., Smith, L.J., 2011. Epidural administration of liposome-encapsulated hydromorphone provides extended analgesia in a rodent model of stifle arthritis. J. Am. Assoc. Lab. Anim. Sci. 50, 507–512.

Schoemaker, N.J., Mol, J.A., Lumeij, J.T., Thijssen, J.H.H., Rijnberk, A., 2003. Effects of anaesthesia and manual restraint on the plasma concentrations of pituitary and adrenocortical hormones in ferrets. Vet. Rec. 152, 591–595. https://doi.org/10.1136/vr.152.19.591.

Serhan, C.N., Chiang, N., Van Dyke, T.E., 2008. Resolving inflammation: dual anti-inflammatory and pro-resolution lipid mediators. Nat. Rev. Immunol. 8, 349–361. https://doi.org/10.1038/nri2294.

Shah, M.D., Yates, D., Hunt, J., Murrell, J.C., 2018. A comparison between methadone and buprenorphine for perioperative analgesia in dogs undergoing ovariohysterectomy. J. Small Anim. Pract. 59, 539–546. https://doi.org/10.1111/jsap.12859.

Shah, M., Yates, D., Hunt, J., Murrell, J., 2019. Comparison between methadone and buprenorphine within the QUAD protocol for perioperative analgesia in cats undergoing ovariohysterectomy. J. Feline Med. Surg. 21, 723–731. https://doi.org/10.1177/1098612X18798840.

Shavit, Y., Lewis, J.W., Terman, G.W., Gale, R.P., Liebeskind, J.C., 1984. Opioid peptides mediate the suppressive effect of stress on natural killer cell cytotoxicity. Science 223, 188–190. https://doi.org/10.1126/science.6691146.

Shimada, S.G., Otterness, I.G., Stitt, J.T., 1994. A study of the mechanism of action of the mild analgesic dipyrone. Agents Actions 41, 188–192. https://doi.org/10.1007/BF02001915.

Shipley, H., Flynn, K., Tucker, L., Wendt-Hornickle, E., Baldo, C., Almeida, D., Allweiler, S., Guedes, A., 2021. Owner evaluation of quality of life and mobility in osteoarthritic cats treated with amantadine or placebo. J. Feline Med. Surg. 23, 568–574. https://doi.org/10.1177/1098612X20967639.

Siao, K.T., Pypendop, B.H., Stanley, S.D., Ilkiw, J.E., 2011a. Pharmacokinetics of oxymorphone in cats. J. Vet. Pharmacol. Therapeut. 34, 594–598. https://doi.org/10.1111/j.1365-2885.2011.01271.

Siao, K.T., Pypendop, B.H., Stanley, S.D., Ilkiw, J.E., 2011b. Pharmacokinetics of amantadine in cats. J. Vet. Pharmacol. Therapeut. 34, 599–604. https://doi.org/10.1111/j.1365-2885.2011.01278.

Sinclair, M.D., 2003. A review of the physiological effects of α2-agonists related to the clinical use of medetomidine in small animal practice. Can. Vet. J. 44, 885–897.

Singh, P.M., Johnson, C., Gartrell, B., Mitchinson, S., Chambers, P., 2011. Pharmacokinetics of butorphanol in broiler chickens. Vet. Rec. 168, 588. https://doi.org/10.1136/vr.d1191.

Smith, R.J., 1977. Modulation of phagocytosis by and lysosomal enzyme secretion from Guinea-pig neutrophils: effect of nonsteroid anti-inflammatory agents and prostaglindins. J. Pharmacol. Exp. Therapeut. 200, 647–657.

Smith, W.L., Dewitt, D.L., 1996. Prostaglandin endoperoxide H synthases-1 and -2. In: Dixon, F.J. (Ed.), Advances in Immunology. Academic Press, pp. 167–215.

Smith, L.J., Krugner-Higby, L., Clark, M., Wendland, A., Heath, T.D., 2003. A single dose of liposome-encapsulated oxymorphone or morphine provides long-term analgesia in an animal model of neuropathic pain. Comp. Med. 53, 280–287.

Smith, L.J., Krugner-Higby, L., Trepanier, L.A., Flaska, D.E., Joers, V., Heath, T.D., 2004. Sedative effects and serum drug concentrations of oxymorphone and metabolites after subcutaneous administration of a liposome-encapsulated formulation in dogs. J. Vet. Pharmacol. Therapeut. 27, 369–372. https://doi.org/10.1111/j.1365-2885.2004.00582.

Smith, L.J., KuKanich, B., Hogan, B.K., Brown, C., Heath, T.D., Krugner-Higby, L.A., 2008. Pharmacokinetics of a controlled-release liposome-encapsulated hydromorphone administered to healthy dogs. J. Vet. Pharmacol. Therapeut. 31, 415–422. https://doi.org/10.1111/j.1365-2885.2008.00974.

Smith, L.J., Kukanich, B.K., Krugner-Higby, L.A., Schmidt, B.H., Heath, T.D., 2013. Pharmacokinetics of ammonium sulfate gradient loaded liposome-encapsulated oxymorphone and hydromorphone in healthy dogs. Vet. Anaesth. Analg. 40, 537–545. https://doi.org/10.1111/vaa.12042.

Snipes, J.A., Kis, B., Shelness, G.S., Hewett, J.A., Busija, D.W., 2005. Cloning and characterization of cyclooxygenase-1b (putative cyclooxygenase-3) in rat. J. Pharmacol. Exp. Therapeut. 313, 668–676. https://doi.org/10.1124/jpet.104.079533.

Solomon, D.H., Goodson, N.J., 2007. Osteoarthritis a companion to rheumatology. In: Sharma, L., Berenbaum, F. (Eds.), Osteoarthritis A Companion to Rheumatology. Elsevier, pp. 178–201.

Sostres, C., Gargallo, C.J., Arroyo, M.T., Lanas, A., 2010. Adverse effects of non-steroidal anti-inflammatory drugs (NSAIDs, aspirin and coxibs) on upper gastrointestinal tract. Best Pract. Res. Clin. Gastroenterol. 24, 121–132. https://doi.org/10.1016/j.bpg.2009.11.005.

Steagall, P.V., Ruel, H.L.M., Yasuda, T., Monteiro, B.P., Watanabe, R., Evangelista, M.C., Beaudry, F., 2020. Pharmacokinetics and analgesic effects of intravenous, intramuscular or subcutaneous buprenorphine in dogs undergoing ovariohysterectomy: a randomized, prospective, masked, clinical trial. BMC Vet. Res. 16, 154. https://doi.org/10.1186/s12917-020-02364-w.

Streppa, H.K., Jones, C.J., Budsberg, S.C., 2002. Cyclooxygenase selectivity of nonsteroidal anti-inflammatory drugs in canine blood. Am. J. Vet. Res. 63, 91–94. https://doi.org/10.2460/AJVR.2002.63.91.

Stuhlmeier, K.M., Li, H., Kao, J.J., 1999. Ibuprofen: new explanation for an old phenomenon. Biochem. Pharmacol. 57, 313–320. https://doi.org/10.1016/S0006-2952(98)00301-3.

Summ, O., Andreou, A.P., Akerman, S., Holland, P.R., Hoffmann, J., Goadsby, P.J., 2021. Differential actions of indomethacin: clinical relevance in headache. Pain 162, 591–599. https://doi.org/10.1097/j.pain.0000000000002032.

Szabo, I., Rojavin, M., Bussiere, J.L., Eisenstein, T.K., Adler, M.W., Rogers, T.J., 1993. Suppression of peritoneal macrophage phagocytosis of Candida albicans by opioids. J. Pharmacol. Exp. Therapeut. 267, 703–706.

Szilagyi, J.E., 1987. Opioid modulation of baroreceptor reflex sensitivity in dogs. Am. J. Physiol. Heart Circ. Physiol. 252, H733–H737. https://doi.org/10.1152/ajpheart.1987.252.4.H733.

Takahama, K., Shirasaki, T., 2007. Central and peripheral mechanisms of narcotic antitussives: codeine-sensitive and -resistant coughs. Cough 3, 8. https://doi.org/10.1186/1745-9974-3-8.

Takeshita, J., Litzinger, M.H., 2009. Serotonin syndrome associated with tramadol. Prim. Care Companion J. Clin. Psychiatry 11, 273. https://doi.org/10.4088/PCC.08l00690.

Tallima, H., El Ridi, R., 2018. Arachidonic acid: physiological roles and potential health benefits – a review. J. Adv. Res. 11, 33–41. https://doi.org/10.1016/j.jare.2017.11.004.

Tanaka, R., Murota, A., Nagashima, Y., Yamane, Y., 2002. Changes in platelet life span in dogs with mitral valve regurgitation. J. Vet. Intern. Med. 16, 446–451. https://doi.org/10.1111/j.1939-1676.2002.tb01263.

Tavakoli, M., Corssen, G., Caruso, F.S., 1976. Butorphanol and morphine: a double-blind comparison of their parenteral analgesic activity. Anesth. Analg. 55, 394–401. https://doi.org/10.1213/00000539-197605000-00025.

Taylor, C.P., Harris, E.W., 2020. Analgesia with gabapentin and pregabalin may involve N-Methyl-d-Aspartate receptors, neurexins, and thrombospondins. J. Pharmacol. Exp. Therapeut. 374, 161–174. https://doi.org/10.1124/jpet.120.266056.

Taylor, P.M., Delatour, P., Landont, F.M., Deal, C., Pickett, C., Aliabadi, F.S., Foot, R., Lees, P., 1996. Pharmacodynamics and enantioselective pharmacokinetics of carprofen in the cat. Res. Vet. Sci. 60, 144–151. https://doi.org/10.1016/S0034-5288(96)90009-0.

Terner, J.M., Lomas, L.M., Smith, E.S., Barrett, A.C., Picker, M.J., 2003. Pharmacogenetic analysis of sex differences in opioid antinociception in rats. Pain 106, 381–391.

Thiede, A.J., Garcia, K.D., Stolarik, D.F., Ma, J., Jenkins, G.J., Nunamaker, E.A., 2014. Pharmacokinetics of sustained-release and transdermal buprenorphine in Gottingen minipigs (*Sus scrofa* domestica). JAALAS 53, 692–699.

Topcu, I., Ekici, N.Z., Isik, R., Sakarya, M., 2006. The effects of tramadol and fentanyl on gastrointestinal motility in septic rats. Anesth. Analg. 102, 876–881. https://doi.org/10.1213/01.ane.0000196506.28780.94.

Toutain, P.L., Autefage, A., Legrand, C., Alvinerie, M., 1994. Plasma concentrations and therapeutic efficacy of phenylbutazone and flunixin meglumine in the horse: pharmacokinetic/pharmacodynamic modelling. J. Vet. Pharmacol. Therapeut. 17, 459–469. https://doi.org/10.1111/j.1365-2885.1994.tb00278.

Trescot, A.M., Datta, S., Lee, M., Hansen, H., 2008. Opioid pharmacology. Pain Physician 11, S133–S153.

Türck, D., Roth, W., Busch, U., 1996. A review of the clinical pharmacokinetics of meloxicam. Rheumatology 35, 13–16. https://doi.org/10.1093/rheumatology/35.suppl_1.13.

Upton, R.A., Williams, R.L., Guentert, T.W., Buskin, J.N., Riegelman, S., 1981. Ketoprofen pharmacokinetics and bioavailability based on an improved sensitive and specific assay. Eur. J. Clin. Pharmacol. 20, 127–133. https://doi.org/10.1007/BF00607149.

Vadivelu, N., Gowda, A.M., Urman, R.D., Jolly, S., Kodumudi, V., Maria, M., Taylor Jr., R., Pergolizzi Jr., J.V., 2015. Ketorolac tromethamine – routes and clinical implications. Pain Pract. 15, 175–193. https://doi.org/10.1111/papr.12198.

Väisänen, M.A.M., Vainio, O.M., Raekallio, M.R., Hietanen, H., Huikuri, H.V., 2005. Results of 24-hour ambulatory electrocardiography in dogs undergoing ovariohysterectomy following premedication with medetomidine or acepromazine. J. Am. Vet. Med. Assoc. 226, 738–745. https://doi.org/10.2460/javma.2005.226.738.

Valverde, A., Skelding, A.M., 2019. Alternatives to opioid analgesia in small animal anesthesia. Vet. Clin. Small Anim. Pract. 49, 1013–1027. https://doi.org/10.1016/j.cvsm.2019.07.010.

Veng-Pedersen, P., Wilhelm, J.A., Zakszewski, T.B., Osifchin, E., Waters, S.J., 1995. Duration of opioid antagonism by nalmefene and naloxone in the dog: an integrated pharmacokinetic/pharmacodynamic comparison. J. Pharmacol. Sci. 84, 1101–1106. https://doi.org/10.1002/jps.2600840913.

Verbeeck, R.K., Richardson, C.J., Blocka, K.L., 1986. Clinical pharmacokinetics of piroxicam. J. Rheumatol. 13, 789–796.

Verebey, K., Mulé, S.J., 1975. Naltrexone pharmacology, pharmacokinetics, and metabolism: current status. Am. J. Drug Alcohol Abuse 2, 357–363. https://doi.org/10.3109/00952997509005661.

Vettorato, E., Bacco, S., 2011. A comparison of the sedative and analgesic properties of pethidine (meperidine) and butorphanol in dogs. J. Small Anim. Pract. 52, 426–432. https://doi.org/10.1111/j.1748-5827.2011.01085.

Viegas, A., Manso, J., Corvo, M.C., Marques, M.M.B., Cabrita, E.J., 2011. Binding of ibuprofen, ketorolac, and diclofenac to COX-1 and COX-2 studied by saturation transfer difference NMR. J. Med. Chem. 54, 8555–8562. https://doi.org/10.1021/jm201090k.

Vollmer, K.O., von Hodenberg, A., Kölle, E.U., 1986. Pharmacokinetics and metabolism of gabapentin in rat, dog and man. Arzneimittelforschung 36, 830–839.

Volz, M., Kellner, H.M., 1980. Kinetics and metabolism of pyrazolones (propyphenazone, aminopyrine and dipyrone). Br. J. Clin. Pharmacol. 10 (Suppl. 2), 299S–308S. https://doi.org/10.1111/j.1365-2125.1980.tb01813.

Wagner, A.E., Mich, P.M., Uhrig, S.R., Hellyer, P.W., 2010. Clinical evaluation of perioperative administration of gabapentin as an adjunct for postoperative analgesia in dogs undergoing amputation of a forelimb. J. Am. Vet. Med. Assoc. 236, 751–756. https://doi.org/10.2460/javma.236.7.751.

Wahler, B.M., Lerche, P., Ricco Pereira, C.H., Bednarski, R.M., KuKanich, B., Lakritz, J., Aarnes, T.K., 2019. Pharmacokinetics and pharmacodynamics of intranasal and intravenous naloxone hydrochloride administration in healthy dogs. Am. J. Vet. Res. 80, 696–701. https://doi.org/10.2460/ajvr.80.7.696.

Walkowiak, K.J., Graham, M.L., 2015. Pharmacokinetics and antinociceptive activity of sustained-release buprenorphine in sheep. J. Am. Assoc. Lab. Anim. Sci. 54, 763–768.

Wallace, J.L., 2000. The arachidonic acid pathway. In: Gaginella, T.S., Guglietta, A. (Eds.), Drug Development: Molecular Targets for GI Diseases. Humana Press), Totowa, NJ, pp. 1–20.

Wang, B., Wu, L., Chen, J., Dong, L., Chen, C., Wen, Z., Hu, J., Fleming, I., Wang, D.W., 2021. Metabolism pathways of arachidonic acids: mechanisms and potential therapeutic targets. Signal Transduct. Targeted Ther. 6, 1–30. https://doi.org/10.1038/s41392-020-00443-w.

Warne, L.N., Beths, T., Holm, M., Bauquier, S.H., 2013. Comparison of perioperative analgesic efficacy between methadone and butorphanol in cats. J. Am. Vet. Med. Assoc. 243, 844–850. https://doi.org/10.2460/javma.243.6.844.

Warner, T.D., Mitchell, J.A., 2004. Cyclooxygenases: new forms, new inhibitors, and lessons from the clinic. Faseb. J. 18, 790–804. https://doi.org/10.1096/fj.03-0645rev.

Waterman, A.E., Kalthum, W., 1989. Pharmacokinetics of intramuscularly administered pethidine in dogs and the influence of anaesthesia and surgery. Vet. Rec. 124, 293–296. https://doi.org/10.1136/vr.124.12.293.

Waterman, A.E., Kalthum, W., 1990. Pharmacokinetics of pethidine administered intramuscularly and intravenously to dogs over 10 years old. Res. Vet. Sci. 48, 245–248.

Weerink, M.A.S., Struys, M.M.R.F., Hannivoort, L.N., Barends, C.R.M., Absalom, A.R., Colin, P., 2017. Clinical pharmacokinetics and pharmacodynamics of dexmedetomidine. Clin. Pharmacokinet. 56, 893–913. https://doi.org/10.1007/s40262-017-0507-7.

Wegner, K., Robertson, S.A., Kollias-Baker, C., Sams, R.A., Muir, W.W., 2004. Pharmacokinetic and pharmacodynamic evaluation of intravenous hydromorphone in cats. J. Vet. Pharmacol. Therapeut. 27, 329–336. https://doi.org/10.1111/j.1365-2885.2004.00593.

Welch, R.M., Findlay, J.W., 1981. Excretion of drugs in human breast milk. Drug Metab. Rev. 12, 261–277. https://doi.org/10.3109/03602538108994032.

Wells, S.M., Glerum, L.E., Papich, M.G., 2008. Pharmacokinetics of butorphanol in cats after intramuscular and buccal transmucosal administration. Am. J. Vet. Res. 69, 1548–1554. https://doi.org/10.2460/ajvr.69.12.1548.

Westerling, D., Andersson, K.-E., 2007. Opioids and bladder pain/function. In: Schmidt, R.F., Willis, W.D. (Eds.), Encyclopedia of Pain. Springer, Berlin, Heidelberg, pp. 1573–1579.

White, S.D., 1990. Naltrexone for treatment of acral lick dermatitis in dogs. J. Am. Vet. Med. Assoc. 196, 1073–1076.

Wiegand, S.L., Swortwood, M.J., Huestis, M.A., Thorp, J., Jones, H.E., Vora, N.L., 2016. Naloxone and metabolites quantification in cord blood of prenatally exposed newborns and correlations with maternal concentrations. AJP Rep. 6, e385–e390. https://doi.org/10.1055/s-0036-1593993.

Wiesenberg-Boettcher, I., Pfeilschifter, J., Schweizer, A., Sallmann, A., Wenk, P., 1991. Pharmacological properties of five diclofenac metabolites identified in human plasma. Agents Actions 34, 135–137. https://doi.org/10.1007/BF01993259.

Wilder-Smith, C.H., Bettiga, A., 1997. The analgesic tramadol has minimal effect on gastrointestinal motor function. Br. J. Clin. Pharmacol. 43, 71–75. https://doi.org/10.1111/j.1365-2125.1997.tb00035.

Wilder-Smith, C.H., Hill, L., Osler, W., O'Keefe, S., 1999. Effect of tramadol and morphine on pain and gastrointestinal motor function in patients with chronic pancreatitis. Dig. Dis. Sci. 44, 1107–1116. https://doi.org/10.1023/a:1026607703352.

Wilson, J.A., Garry, E.M., Anderson, H.A., Rosie, R., Colvin, L.A., Mitchell, R., Fleetwood-Walker, S.M., 2005. NMDA receptor antagonist treatment at the time of nerve injury prevents injury-induced changes in spinal NR1 and NR2B subunit expression and increases the sensitivity of residual pain behaviours to subsequently administered NMDA receptor antagonists. Pain 117, 421–432. https://doi.org/10.1016/j.pain.2005.07.005.

Winchester, S.K., Imamura, T., Gross, G.A., Muglia, L.M., Vogt, S.K., Wright, J., Watanabe, K., Tai, H.-H., Muglia, L.J., 2002. Coordinate regulation of prostaglandin metabolism for induction of parturition in mice. Endocrinology 143, 2593–2598. https://doi.org/10.1210/endo.143.7.8926.

Woolf, C.J., 2010. What is this thing called pain? J. Clin. Invest. 120, 3742–3744. https://doi.org/10.1172/JCI45178.

Woolf, C.J., Bennett, G.J., Doherty, M., Dubner, R., Kidd, B., Koltzenburg, M., Lipton, R., Loeser, J.D., Payne, R., Torebjork, E., 1998. Towards a mechanism-based classification of pain? Pain 77, 227–229. https://doi.org/10.1016/S0304-3959(98)00099-2.

Wu, S.-D., Zhang, Z.-H., Jin, J.-Z., Kong, J., Wang, W., Zhang, Q., Li, D.-Y., Wang, M.-F., 2004. Effects of narcotic analgesic drugs on human Oddi's sphincter motility. World J. Gastroenterol. 10, 2901–2904. https://doi.org/10.3748/wjg.v10.i19.2901.

Xu, S., Rouzer, C.A., Marnett, L.J., 2014. Oxicams, a class of NSAIDs and beyond. IUBMB Life 66, 803–811. https://doi.org/10.1002/iub.1334.

Yamashita, K., Tsubakishita, S., Futaoka, S., Ueda, I., Hamaguchi, H., Seno, T., Katoh, S., Izumisawa, Y., Kotani, T., Muir, W.W., 2000. Cardiovascular effects of medetomidine, detomidine and xylazine in horses. J. Vet. Med. Sci. 62, 1025–1032. https://doi.org/10.1292/jvms.62.1025.

Yeh, S.Y., 1984. Metabolism of meperidine in several animal species. J. Pharmacol. Sci. 73, 1783–1787. https://doi.org/10.1002/jps.2600731231.

Yeh, S.Y., Chernov, H.I., Woods, L.A., 1971. Metabolism of morphine by cats. J. Pharmacol. Sci. 60, 469–471. https://doi.org/10.1002/jps.2600600330.

Zeilhofer, H.U., 2007. Prostanoids in nociception and pain. Biochem. Pharmacol. 73, 165–174. https://doi.org/10.1016/j.bcp.2006.07.037.

Zeng, C., Wei, J., Li, H., Yang, T., Gao, S., Li, Y., Xiong, Y., Xiao, W., Luo, W., Yang, T., et al., 2015. Comparison between 200 mg QD and 100 mg BID oral celecoxib in the treatment of knee or hip osteoarthritis. Sci. Rep. 5, 10593. https://doi.org/10.1038/srep10593.

Zullian, C., Lema, P., Lavoie, M., Dodelet-Devillers, A., Beaudry, F., Vachon, P., 2016. Plasma concentrations of buprenorphine following a single subcutaneous administration of a sustained release formulation of buprenorphine in sheep. Can. J. Vet. Res. 80, 250–253.

Zylber-Katz, E., Granit, L., Levy, M., 1992. Formation and excretion of dipyrone metabolites in man. Eur. J. Clin. Pharmacol. 42, 187–191. https://doi.org/10.1007/BF00278482.

Chapter 8

Neuromuscular blocking agents

Manuel Martin Flores[1] and Bhupinder Singh[2]
[1]Department of Clinical Sciences, College of Veterinary Medicine, Cornell University, Ithaca, NY, United States; [2]Comparative Medicine Resources, Rutgers University, Piscataway, NJ, United States

Chapter outline

I. Introduction

The discovery and use of curare (extracted from tropical American plants such as *Strychnos* spp. and *Chondrodendron* spp.) by South American indigenous people as arrow poisons, caught the attention of European explorers and physicians. In 1596, Sir Walter Raleigh mentioned curare in his book titled "*The Discovery of the Large, Rich, and Beautiful Empire of Guiana*". For centuries, the actual ingredients of the "poison" were kept a secret and known only to tribal medicine men. The name "curare" originated from the Guyana Macushi word *wurari*, also known among indigenous people as *ourara*, *urali*, *urare*, *wourali*, and *woorari*.

Sir Benjamin Brodie used samples of crude curare (brought by physician Edward Bancroft from South America) in early 19th century to demonstrate that animals injected with curare could be kept alive by ventilating their lungs. A few years later, Claude Bernard's experiments in frogs revealed that curare acted at neuromuscular junctions. The role of acetylcholine (Ach) in neuromuscular transmission was first discovered by Sir Henry Dale (1934), leading him to win a Nobel Prize (Physiology or Medicine) in 1936. Curare was used for the first time in human clinical medicine in 1942 by Dr. Harold Randall Griffith and his resident, Dr. Enid Johnson, during anesthesia to a patient undergoing appendectomy (Gillies and Wynands, 1986). The studies by Drs. John Halton and Cecil Gray at the University of Liverpool with tubocurarine in 1946 (Gray and Halton, 1946) laid the foundation work for development of the Liverpool anesthetic technique—the first concept of balanced general anesthesia, which included a hypnotic agent, an analgesic, and a neuromuscular blocker. Since then, advances in pharmacology have led to the development of several compounds, such as gallamine and succinylcholine, by Daniel Bovet, and later pancuronium, atracurium, and vecuronium. Both vecuronium and atracurium remain as commonly used agents in veterinary medicine. These drugs and new agents, such as cisatracurium and rocuronium, are used ubiquitously when humans are anesthetized. New agents are still being developed, which also include modern ways to reverse neuromuscular block. However, in addition to the study of new drugs, research has also facilitated the development of

Anesthesia and Analgesia in Laboratory Animals. https://doi.org/10.1016/B978-0-12-822215-7.00010-X

clinical monitors that allow the assessment of neuromuscular function. The combination of modern agents with fewer side effects, and quantitative monitoring has greatly improved the overall safety of these drugs.

II. Indications for use of neuromuscular blocking agents

The NMBA are used in various clinical situations, including but not limited to:

- Skeletal muscle relaxation for select surgical procedures
- Facilitate mechanical ventilation when the animal is resisting or is in asynchrony.
- Uncontrolled convulsions despite administration of usual anticonvulsant agents, for example, sometimes during strychnine poisoning
- Facilitate endotracheal intubation:
  - Species that are challenging to intubate due to laryngospasm.
  - When faster intubation is needed in animals with severe respiratory compromise (for example, diaphragmatic hernia), or those with a high risk of vomiting.

III. Contraindications for use of NMBA

- Hypersensitivity reaction: the presence of the quaternary ammonium ion in NMBA can cause IgE-mediated hypersensitivity reactions (Claudius et al., 2009).
- Liver disease and renal failure: the NMBA that depend on liver metabolism or renal excretion are likely to have prolonged clearance, so those drugs should be avoided in these conditions.
- Pig breeds susceptible to malignant: depolarizing NMBA (e.g., succinylcholine) must not be used in these animals as it can trigger MH (Short et al., 1976; Iaizzo and Wedel, 1994).

IV. Welfare implications of using neuromuscular blocking agents

Because NMBAs produce paralysis of skeletal muscles (diaphragm included) without loss of consciousness or analgesia, their use must always be accompanied by general anesthesia to ensure the animal is unconscious. The use of NMBAs in laboratory animals should be approved by the Institutional Animal Care and Use Committee and must have scientific justification for their use. The investigator must have a plan for appropriate physiologic monitoring, which usually includes (at a minimum) monitoring of heart rate (HR) and blood pressure (BP). It should be noted that common clinical indicators of anesthetic depth, such as eye position or jaw (muscle) tone, are devoid of any meaning when the animal is paralyzed. The "Guide for the Care and Use of Laboratory Animals" states that "if paralyzing agents are to be used, the appropriate amount of anesthetic should first be defined based on results of a similar procedure using the anesthetic without a blocking agent" (Council, 2011). Before administration of an NMBA, endotracheal intubation and controlled ventilation should be initiated, except in cases when the NMBA is specifically used to facilitate placement of the tracheal tube. The general anesthetic and analgesic(s) must be used for the entire duration of neuromuscular blockade and should be appropriate for the level of expected pain during the procedure. If a surgical procedure is to be performed, baseline HR and BP values should be obtained before the initiation of the skin incision. An increase from a baseline of more than 20% in any of these parameters, without other explanation, usually indicates nociception or inadequate anesthetic depth and should be corrected immediately. Other parameters, such as oxygen saturation, mucous membrane color, capillary refill time, and end-tidal CO_2, should also be monitored. It should be kept in mind that some NMBAs may have cardiovascular effects, and thus affect the HR and BP values. The administration of pancuronium causes a 22%–26% increase in HR and 8%–9% increase in MAP in humans (Kelman and Kennedy, 1971), and causes tachycardia in Lewis rats (Kandukuri et al., 2018). These effects should be considered during the monitoring of cardiovascular variables under anesthesia so that changes specific to the action of the NMBA can be considered within a new baseline value. The monitoring of bispectral index or electroencephalography can also be useful for tracking changes in the depth of anesthesia, but the impact of NMBAs on these variables should be considered. It must be ensured that neuromuscular function has recovered before discontinuing the use of the ventilator or stopping the administration of anesthesia.

V. Neuromuscular junction anatomy and physiology

Motor nerves supplying striated muscle travel from the ventral horn of the spinal cord (where the motor neuron cell bodies are located) to the muscles. As the nerve reaches the muscle fibers, it loses its myelin sheath, branches, and divides into many presynaptic boutons. These nerve terminals synthesize and store the neurotransmitter ACh in vesicles called quanta. The arrival of an action potential opens voltage-gated calcium channels that trigger a process of mobilization and excretion of large quantities of ACh into the synaptic cleft. The motor (postsynaptic) cell is densely populated with nicotinic ACh receptors (nAChR). The binding of ACh molecules to the two alpha subunits of these pentameric receptors results in a conformational change that allows an influx of sodium and the generation and transmission of action potentials to the muscle membrane, which is carried along the muscle fiber by transverse tubules. This triggers a cascade of events that ultimately results in the contraction of the muscle cells. The interaction between ACh and nAChR is very brief. Any ACh molecules released from the presynaptic cell that did not interact immediately with a receptor, or those released after binding to the receptors, are hydrolyzed almost instantly by acetylcholinesterase (AChE) present in synaptic/junctional cleft. This enzyme is very efficient; approximately half of the ACh released from the presynaptic cell is hydrolyzed even before it reaches the receptors. The products of ACh hydrolysis are choline and acetate. Choline is taken up by the nerve terminal and used for the synthesis of ACh.

Presynaptic nAChR has also been identified. These receptors mediate feedback loops that regulate the transport of reserve ACh vesicles to the membrane in preparation for exocytosis. Blockades of both postsynaptic and presynaptic receptors occurs when NMBAs are administered (Brown et al., 1981; Slater, 2017; Hirsch, 2007; Jones et al., 2017; Martyn et al., 2009).

More quanta than necessary are released by the presynaptic cell, and more receptors than necessary are available to trigger a response resulting in muscle contraction. This redundancy confers the NMJ with a large margin of safety to perform this function. As a result, a large number of receptors need to be occupied by the NMBA before an effect occurs.

VI. Mechanism of action of NMBA

The NMBA are quaternary ammonium compounds that produce their effects by binding to the nAChR receptors. These drugs can be classified into two types according to their mechanism of action: depolarizing and nondepolarizing agents.

A. Depolarizing agents

These are agonists to the nAChRs and mimic the effects of ACh to cause membrane depolarization. These drugs cause initial disorganized muscle contractions, known as fasciculations, followed by relaxation, as the membrane remains depolarized and unresponsive to further stimulation (Burns and Paton, 1951). Depolarizing agents are not susceptible to hydrolysis by the AChE enzyme, so they are not eliminated from the synaptic cleft promptly. Only when plasma concentrations are lower due to the activity of the plasma pseudocholinesterase (PChE) enzyme, does the concentration at the synaptic cleft decrease. This process is the main determinant of the duration of the neuromuscular block.

1. Succinylcholine

Succinylcholine is the only drug in this group in clinical use for human anesthesia. Succinylcholine has the fastest onset and shortest duration of any NMBA in use; these qualities make it an ideal candidate for emergency intubation and are the reason why the agent remains in clinical use for people, despite its well-described side effects. Succinylcholine is a bis-choline ester of succinic acid, and structurally it is two molecules of Ach bound together. The difference in levels of PChE between animal species leads to significant differences in dose requirements and the duration of action of this drug. Species like dogs, sheep, and cattle are very sensitive and paralyzed by small doses, whereas cats, pigs, and horses are relatively resistant (Clarke, 2013). Equine plasma has 8–10 times higher PChE levels as compared to cows, so horses recover much faster from succinylcholine (Stowe et al., 1958). Dogs have a lower level of PChE than horses, and hence, the duration of action is prolonged in this species (Hall et al., 1953). Succinylcholine is a known trigger for malignant hyperthermia and should be avoided in animals with mutations in ryanodine receptor 1 (RYR1), the gene encoding the skeletal muscle calcium release channel (some breeds of pig, dog, cat, and horse), which makes them susceptible to this disease. This drug causes spastic paralysis in young chicks with the extension of the neck and limbs (Ranendra Kumar et al., 2005).

Multiple side effects including cardiac arrhythmias and changes in BP are noted with this drug as it may interact with other nicotinic and muscarinic ACh receptors located outside of the NMJ. Fasciculations from succinylcholine can release potassium and increase the plasma concentration of this electrolyte. This could lead to dangerous concentrations of potassium in animals with muscular dystrophies, extensive muscular injuries, or burns.

Any drug (e.g., procaine) or compound (e.g., organophosphates) which inhibits PChE will potentially prolong the duration of action of succinylcholine. It should also be noted that PChE level is decreased in certain disease conditions such as liver disease, malnutrition, and chronic anemia, thus prolonging the duration of action of succinylcholine. The use of this drug should be avoided in animals in which increase in intraocular, intracranial, and intragastric pressure is undesirable. With the availability of newer short-acting NMBA with reliable and quick reversal, the use of succinylcholine has very limited application in veterinary medicine.

B. Nondepolarizing agents

These drugs are competitive antagonists to the nAChR and prevent the binding of ACh to this receptor, thereby impairing neurotransmission. Only one of both alpha subunits of the nAChR needs to be blocked by these compounds in order to exert their action. Unlike succinylcholine, nondepolarizing agents are used frequently in veterinary anesthesia. They fall into three different classes based on their structure—the aminosteroids, the benzylisoquinolines, and the asymmetric mixed-onium chlorofumarates.

1. *Aminosteroids*

As a group, aminosteroid compounds are characterized for cardiovascular stability (except for pancuronium), and hepatic and renal metabolism, and excretion. These agents do not result in histamine release upon injection.

a. Pancuronium

It has a slow onset time and a long duration of action. Pancuronium is primarily excreted by the kidneys, with 10%–40% of the drug metabolized by the liver. Therefore, it should be used cautiously in animals with liver or kidney disease. It binds to muscarinic receptors in the heart, resulting in vagolysis causing tachycardia and hypertension; it was demonstrated in guinea pigs that pancuronium is an antagonist for M2 and M3 muscarinic receptors (Okanlami et al., 1996).

Pancuronium is considered a long-lasting NMBA. In dogs, this drug has a dose-dependent onset of approximately 5 minutes and duration of action up to 60 minutes (Gleed and Jones, 1982). A study in cats showed that after prolonged administration, the initial rapid decrease in plasma concentration after infusion termination was followed by a plateau phase from which the decline was very slow (Henning et al., 1993). Because of its long duration of action, the use of pancuronium has largely been replaced by intermediate-acting agents, such as vecuronium or rocuronium, which are more easily reversed and less likely to result in the residual block after anesthesia.

b. Vecuronium

It is a monoquaternary analogue of pancuronium with an intermediate duration of action. It undergoes both hepatic metabolism and renal elimination and has higher biliary elimination due to its increased lipid solubility. Higher or multiple doses should be avoided in animals with liver or kidney disease to prevent prolonged recovery. The major advantage of vecuronium compared to pancuronium is that even large doses of this drug have minimal cardiovascular effects (Morris et al., 1983).

In a dose-finding study in healthy dogs, an initial dose of 0.1 mg/kg produced a period of paralysis of 25 minutes, and a further six doses (0.04 mg/kg) were noncumulative and without any side effects (Jones and Seymour, 2008).

c. Rocuronium

It is a 2-morpholino, 3-desacetyl, 16-*N*-allyl-pyrrolidino derivative of vecuronium and lacks the acetyl ester found in pancuronium and vecuronium. It has a rapid onset and intermediate duration of action (Bartkowski et al., 1993). Like vecuronium, this drug does not cause a significant change in plasma histamine level or have any significant cardiovascular side effects (Hudson et al., 1998; Naguib et al., 1995). Metabolism is primarily hepatic, with significant biliary excretion, and a small portion is eliminated via the kidneys (Proost et al., 2000) (Proost et al., 2000).

2. *Benzylisoquinolines*

These compounds are characterized by alternate pathways of metabolism that do not rely on liver or renal function and have a potential to release histamine upon injection.

a. Atracurium

Atracurium is an intermediate-acting competitive NMBA. It has a dose-dependent speed of onset and duration of action. This drug is metabolized via Hofmann elimination, ester hydrolysis, and other unspecified pathways. Hofmann elimination is a temperature- and pH-dependent process and is slowed by acidosis and hypothermia. Consequently, the presence of hypothermia has a significant effect on the offset time of atracurium (Playfor et al., 2000b); (Diefenbach et al., 1992). These pathways of biotransformation make it a suitable agent for use in animals with liver or kidney disease. The use of repeated doses is usually not cumulative, making it a suitable agent for administration via a constant-rate infusion (Playfor et al., 2000a).

Atracurium has the potential to cause histamine release. However, this requires several times the ED_{95} (effective dose producing a 95% reduction in twitch height) before significant amounts of histamine are released, making side effects such as hypotension and tachycardia uncommon in clinical cases (Hackett et al., 1989). The potential for histamine release is largely reduced by small doses and slow administration (over 75 seconds) (Scott et al., 1986).

A major metabolite of Hofmann elimination of atracurium is laudanosine, which does not have any neuromuscular blocking activity (Colin and Singlas, 1985). Unlike atracurium, laudanosine is both hepatically metabolized and renally excreted. Therefore, the presence of hepatic disease or renal failure causes a prolonged elimination half-life and the potential for accumulation (Fodale and Santamaria, 2002). Laudanosine can cross the blood-brain barrier and cause CNS stimulation if sufficient levels are achieved. This, however, does not occur with clinically used doses of atracurium in healthy animals.

b. Cisatracurium

This is one of the 10 isomers of atracurium. It is approximately three times more potent and produces less histamine release than atracurium, the reason why it has widely replaced atracurium for use in humans in many countries. Cisatracurium is metabolized primarily by Hofmann elimination. The presence of portosystemic shunt did not affect the rate of onset or duration of action of cisatracurium in dogs (initial dose 0.1 mg/kg; additional dose 0.03 mg/kg when at least one twitch of the TOF was noted) (Adams et al., 2006). It is in general slower acting than atracurium, but more cardiovascular stable.

c. Mivacurium

This drug is unique amongst the benzylisoquinolines in that it is metabolized mostly by PChE and minimally by AChE, so interspecies differences in PChE explain its variable duration of action between species. It is a short-acting NMBA in humans (15–20 minutes); however, the duration of effect is markedly prolonged in dogs, where a dose of 0.05 mg/kg resulted in rapid onset (1.63 ± 0.25 minutes) with minimal hemodynamic changes and duration of effect up to 151.0 ± 38.50 minutes (Smith et al., 1999). Clinical observations in cats suggest that mivacurium has a shorter duration of action compared to that in dogs. The agent is currently unavailable.

d. Doxacurium

It is a long-acting NMBA with a slow onset of action. It is excreted unchanged in the urine and via biliary pathways. The elimination is significantly decreased in renal failure and is unaffected in hepatic failure, so the duration of action is likely to be prolonged in renal disease patients (Faulds and Clissold, 1991). A study in dogs showed that a 3.5 μg/kg IV dose approximates an ED_{90} with a long duration of action (108 ± 31 minutes) with high individual variations (Martinez et al., 1998). The dose of 0.008 mg/kg in dogs was effective for a long duration (until reversed at 120 minutes) without any significant cardiovascular effects in isoflurane-anesthetized dogs (Martinez et al., 1997).

3. *Asymmetric mixed-onium chlorofumarates*

Agents of this family, with a range of durations from ultrashort to intermediate, are being studied. These agents are degraded in the plasma by pH-sensitive chemical hydrolysis and inactivation by cysteine adduction; they do not undergo Hofmann elimination. Exogenous cysteine can be administered to accelerate recovery. Only preclinical data are available for these agents at the time that this chapter was prepared.

a. Dosing and species extrapolation

Doses for currently used agents in several species are summarized in Table 8.1. It is important to acknowledge that important species differences exist regarding the potency and duration of these drugs. For example, the dose of vecuronium used in dogs is similar to that for humans and produces paralysis lasting approximately 30 minutes, also similar to humans (Engbaek et al., 1984; Kariman and Clutton, 2008). By contrast, only a quarter of that dose is sufficient to produce paralysis in sheep (Martin-Flores et al., 2012), and doses 8–12 times higher than those in dogs (that is, 30–45 times higher than for sheep) might be used in pigs (Grong et al., 2015). In horses, vecuronium produces a neuromuscular block lasting substantially longer than in other domestic species, that could be difficult to reverse pharmacologically (Martin-Flores et al., 2012); however, this is not observed with atracurium or rocuronium. Such magnitude of differences in potency and duration highlights that care must be exercised before extrapolating doses from one species to another. This is particularly important given the paucity of species-specific information regarding the potency of many agents.

VII. Clinical use and monitoring

As previously described, NMBAs are used to facilitate muscle relaxation as part of balanced anesthesia protocols for a variety of procedures. Neuromuscular block produces profound skeletal muscle relaxation that may be useful during reduction of fractures, thoracic and abdominal surgeries (including laparoscopy), or simply to decrease the concentration of volatile anesthetics, since the alveolar concentration of an anesthetic required to prevent all movement is higher than that required to produce unconsciousness (Hofmeister et al., 2008; Seddighi et al., 2012). NMBAs can also be used to facilitate tracheal intubation. This technique is used ubiquitously in people, as intubation with paralysis is easier to perform and results in less laryngeal trauma (Lundstrom et al., 2009, 2017). The inclusion of NMBAs during intubation in veterinary medicine is not routine practice but has been used in cats (Doodnaught and Pang, 2017; Moreno-Sala et al., 2013; Sakai et al., 2018). Paralysis during intubation not only prevents laryngospasm, a prominent reflex in cats, but may also prevent vomiting in animals at risk.

Regardless of the reason for inclusion of these agents in an anesthetic protocol, the most important clinical implications of their use are that NMBAs do not provide any anesthetic or analgesic effect, and that spontaneous ventilation will be impaired or absent. Thus, the anesthesia provider must ensure that appropriate levels of anesthesia

TABLE 8.1 Doses.

Agent	Species	Dose (in mg/kg)	Duration	References
Pancuronium	Rabbits Pig Cat NHP (Rhesus monkey)	1.1 1.1–0.5 0.12 0.007 (ED80) 0.05	Approx. 60 minutes – 60–100 minutes 15 minutes (50% recovery) 110 minutes (50% recovery)	Diaz et al. (2014) Veres-Nyéki et al. (2012) Miller et al. (1979) Durant et al. (1980)
Vecuronium	Rats Pig Cat Dogs Sheep Horse NHP (M. fascicularis)	0.33 (ED95) 0.14 (ED90) 0.4–0.6 + 0.2–0.3 mg/kg/h 0.02 (ED90) 0.03 (ED90) 0.05–0.1 0.01–0.025 0.1 0.05 + 0.1 mg/kg/h	93 minutes to 25% T1 10 minutes – – 13 minutes 30–40 minutes 40 minutes >140 minutes –	Sunaga et al. (2006) Muir & Marshall (1987) Grong et al. (2015) Michalek-Sauberer et al. (2000) Sutherland et al. (1983), Wastila et al. (1996) Lorenzutti et al. (2019) Clutton & Glasby (1998) Martin-Flores et al. (2012) Forte et al. (2002)
Rocuronium	Rabbits Pig Cat Dog Horse NHP (Macaca mulatta) (Japanese macaque)	0.056 (ED50) 1.2 3 + 0.7–1.8 mg/k/h 0.09 (ED90) 0.3–0.6 0.3–0.6 0.2–0.6 0.3 0.6 mg/kg/h	– 40 minutes – Approx. 5 minutes 15–20 minutes 20–30 minutes 20–65 minutes – –	Kim et al. (1999) Loughren et al. (2014) Madsen et al. (2015) Michalek-Sauberer et al. (2000) Auer and Mosing (2006), Martin-Flores et al. (2016) Auer (2007) Auer et al. (2007) Wang et al. (2015) Miwa et al. (2021)
Atracurium	Rabbit Pig Cat Dog Sheep Horse NHP (C. jacchus)	0.1–0.3 2.0 (ED90) 0.12 (ED90) 0.1–0.3 0.5 0.07–0.15 0.5 + 0.75 mg/kg/h	– – 15 minutes 40–60 30 minutes 40–110 minutes –	Adami et al. (2019) Pittet et al. (1990) Sutherland et al. (1983), Wastila et al. (1996) Kastrup et al. (2005) Clutton & Glasby (1998) Hildebrand and Arpin (1988) Scherrer and Hopster (2021) Freret et al. (2008)
Cisatracurium	Rabbits Pig Cat Dog Horse NHP (Macaca mulatta)	0.04 (ED95) 0.3–0.5 + 0.4–1.0 mg/kg/h 1.0 0.06 (ED95) 0.15 0.1–0.16 (ED95) 0.15 0.05–0.1 0.15 + 0.18 mg/kg/h	40 minutes – 60 minutes 12 minutes 20–30 35–50 35 minutes 12–33 minutes –	Diaz et al. (2014) Tutunaru et al. (2017) Aguilar et al. (2019) Wastila et al. (1996) Van Wijnsberghe et al. (2022) Chen et al. (2020) Ida et al. (2020) Tutunaru et al. (2019) Uhrig et al. (2018)

and analgesia are reached and that positive pressure ventilation is used. Moreover, since reflexive movements in response to noxious stimuli are absent during neuromuscular block, and some common subjective signs of depth of anesthesia, such as eye position or muscle (jaw) tone (which rely on functioning muscular activity) cannot be evaluated, assessment of anesthetic depth is limited, and the risk of a completely paralyzed but only partially unconscious animal is a real concern. Awareness under anesthesia is a rare but tragic complication reported in humans, and its incidence increases when NMBAs are used (Bergman et al., 2002). Therefore, while NMBAs may be included as part of a balanced anesthetic protocol, they do not replace anesthetic and analgesic agents.

All skeletal muscles will be paralyzed if a sufficient NMBA dose is administered; positive pressure ventilation is mandatory when these agents are used. However, the potency of NMBAs in different muscle groups varies. In general, the diaphragm shows more resistance to the effects of these drugs than other muscle groups, which explains why spontaneous ventilation returns early during recovery from the neuromuscular block, producing the well-known “curare cleft” in the capnographic waveform, and why animals may take occasional spontaneous breaths when paralysis is incomplete. Unlike the diaphragm, extraocular muscles are particularly sensitive to the effects of NMBAs, lower doses might be used to provide relaxation of the ocular globe. This distinction between muscle groups must be considered during the monitoring of neuromuscular function.

VIII. Monitoring of neuromuscular function

Monitoring neuromuscular function is essential to the safe use of NMBAs, and it should be performed with a neurostimulator. Monitoring allows the anesthetist to maintain a desired depth of muscle relaxation as required by the procedure and redose when required. It also guides the decision as to whether pharmacological reversal can be attempted, and to assess whether neuromuscular function has recovered to adequate levels before discontinuation of anesthesia at the end of a procedure. The latter is fundamental for the prevention of residual neuromuscular block—the inadvertent presence of partial blockade following anesthesia.

Residual neuromuscular block, also called postoperative residual curarization (PORC), is a common complication with the use of NMBAs. Signs of PORC in people range from mild discomfort and diplopia (double vision) to more generalized weakness, an inability to maintain a patent upper airway, and hypoxia (Murphy, 2006; Murphy et al., 2008). Even mild degrees of residual weakness, which are not easily detected without quantitative monitoring, may contribute to laryngeal dysfunction and aspiration (Eriksson et al., 1997; Sundman et al., 2000). These adverse effects might be augmented by the presence of residual anesthetic drugs, hypothermia, or the use of postoperative opioid analgesics. It should be noticed that these complications arise during a particularly vulnerable period; the early recovery from anesthesia, when monitoring and oxygen supplementation are typically reduced (if present at all). Therefore, despite the paucity of data regarding the consequences of a residual block in animals, current best practices suggest that all efforts should be made to avoid partial neuromuscular block at recovery.

Despite substantial data supporting the use of neuromuscular monitoring, the technique is not yet widely adopted in veterinary anesthesia (Martin-Flores et al., 2018). When neuromuscular monitoring is not available, clinicians often rely on other surrogates to assess the return of neuromuscular function. Commonly, the return of spontaneous ventilation has been used for this purpose. As mentioned before, the diaphragm is relatively resistant to the effects of NMBAs, and observations made on that muscle should not be extrapolated to the entire animal. In other words, the return of spontaneous ventilation does not imply that neuromuscular function is adequate in other muscle groups. In dogs, spontaneous ventilation recovers substantially earlier than neuromuscular function measured at the limbs (Martin-Flores et al., 2014). Therefore, return of spontaneous ventilation, even to baseline values for tidal volume or inspiratory pressure, should not be used to assume that recovery from neuromuscular block is complete. Relying on the expected duration of a neuromuscular block to avoid residual weakness is also an unreliable practice. Duration of block varies with agents and doses, and several external factors, such as body temperature, electrolyte concentrations, type, and dose of anesthetic agent, and concurrent use of other drugs including (but not limited to) aminoglycoside antibiotics. Moreover, there is substantial interindividual variation within a species and variation between species. Hence, the actual duration of action of a given agent may easily surpass expectations (Kopman and Sinha, 2003; Martin-Flores et al., 2008), and substantial residual block might go undetected after emergence from anesthesia.

A. Neuromuscular stimulation

Nondepolarizing NMBAs interrupt the transmission at the NMJ. Consequently, neuromuscular monitoring evaluates the status of that transmission by stimulating a motor nerve and evaluating the evoked response to those stimuli. Traditionally, the ulnar or peroneal nerves are stimulated, and the flexion of the carpus or tarsus is evaluated. The simplest method to evaluate the response is to observe the magnitude of the evoked muscle contraction, or “twitch”.

This technique is subjective and, as such, limited in the information that it can provide, as mild changes in muscle contractions cannot be appreciated by simple observation.

Objective monitoring involves measuring the evoked twitches. While mechanomyography (the measurement of isometric force of contraction) is widely considered the gold standard, that methodology is difficult to implement in the clinical setting and mostly used during research. Unlike mechanomyography, acceleromyography (AMG) measures the acceleration of a free-moving extremity. An acceleration-sensitive crystal is secured (taped) to, typically, a paw, and the peak acceleration of each twitch is measured. This technique is user-friendly and easily implemented in a clinical setting, and thus, has gained popularity for both clinical and research use (Claudius and Viby-Mogensen, 2008). Unlike the subjective observation of evoked twitches, AMG allows the quantification of neuromuscular transmission, so that residual block can be prevented. Indeed, the use of AMG in people is linked with a lower incidence of PORC (Murphy et al., 2011; Murphy et al., 2008), and it has been shown to detect residual block that was undetected by subjective visual exams in horses and dogs (Martin-Flores et al., 2008, 2019). Several hand-held AMG devices are currently available (Fig. 8.2).

During neuromuscular stimulation, stimuli of short duration are used; 0.2–0.3 msec. Short stimuli are used in order to avoid direct muscle stimulation that bypasses the NMJ and produces erroneous results (the goal is to stimulate the motor nerve and assess transmission through the NMJ, the target site for NMBAs). Typically, the supramaximal current is used during neuromuscular stimulation. That is, a current above that which results in a stimulus that recruits all muscle fibers innervated. However, it should be noted that supramaximal currents can be painful. Under certain circumstances (see below), submaximal currents may be used. Electrical stimuli can be applied in a variety of patterns. Single twitches, consisting of isolated stimuli, separated by 10 seconds (0.1 Hz), are used during research into the potency of NMBAs. The absolute magnitude of the evoked response is measured, and the percentage decrease in that magnitude following different doses of the NMBA is measured. From that information, dose-response curves can be constructed. The dose which decreases the response by 95% of its baseline magnitude is referred to as the effective dose 95 (ED95), and it is commonly used to guide the clinical use of these agents. Commonly, a multiple of this dose (for example, 2 × ED95) is administered in a clinical setting. Single twitch has little value as a clinical tool, as it requires an accurate baseline measurement against which all subsequent values are compared and, most importantly, because it is not sensitive for detecting residual block.

The limitations of subjective monitoring and single twitch monitoring, can be overcome by using the train-of-four (TOF) pattern. The TOF consists of four stimuli delivered every 0.5 seconds (2 Hz), with each TOF separated by 12–15 seconds. When an NMBA is administered, the magnitude of each twitch of the TOF decreases; if a sufficient dose is used (>ED95), all four responses are

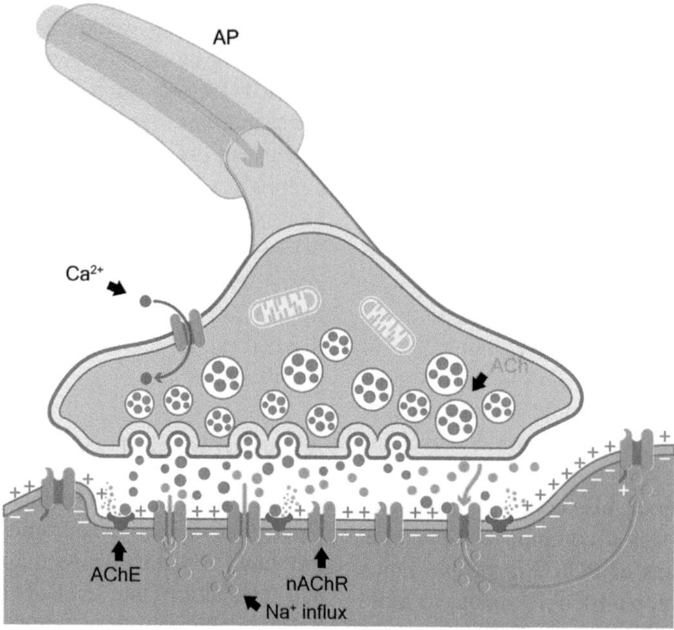

FIGURE 8.1 Representation of the neuromuscular junction. The presynaptic (motor neuron) cell releases acetylcholine (ACh) into the neuromuscular cleft, upon the arrival of an action potential. ACh interacts with the nicotinic acetylcholine receptor (nAChR) in the postsynaptic (skeletal muscle) cell and induces a conformational change that results in an influx of sodium and depolarization. A cascade of events that follow results in the contraction of the skeletal muscle cells. Free ACh in the clef is rapidly hydrolyzed by the acetylcholinesterase enzyme.

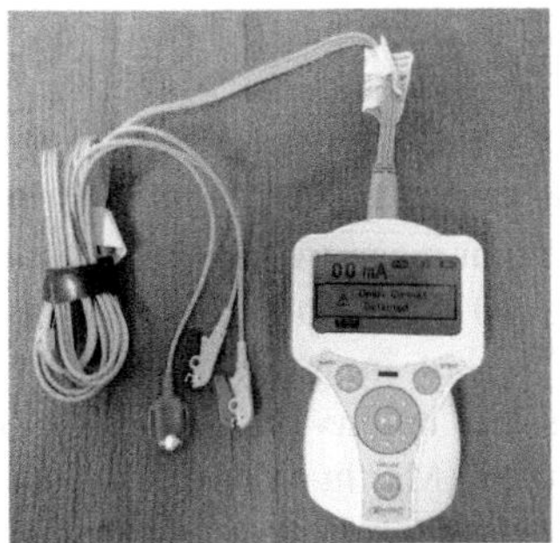
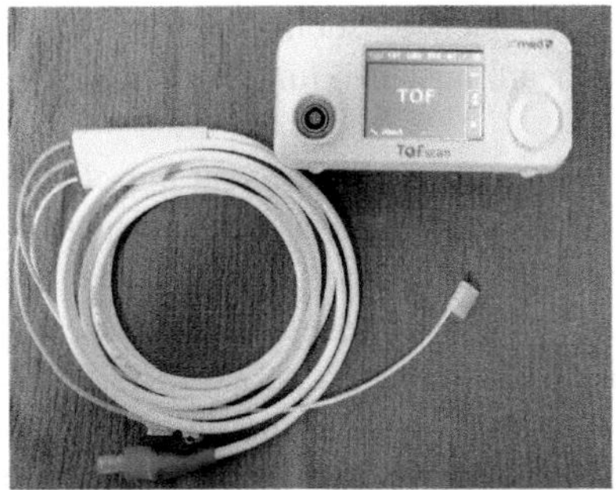

FIGURE 8.2 Two hand-held acceleromyography monitors; the Stimpod NMS 450X (Xavant technology; *left*) and the ToFScan (Drager; *right*). Both monitors measure peak acceleration during evoked muscular twitches and can report the train-of-four ratio, among other patterns of stimulation.

ablated. During recovery from the nondepolarizing block, all four twitches of the TOF return in order from the first (T1) to last (T4) twitch. The speed of recovery for each twitch also occurs in that order, that is, the recovery of T1 occurs faster than that of T4. As a result, during recovery from the neuromuscular block, a "fade" in the magnitude of four consecutive responses can be appreciated (Fig. 8.3). This fade in the magnitude of evoked responses is the result of a progressive decay in the release of ACh during repetitive stimulation, mediated by the actions of NMBAs on presynaptic nAChRs.

Fade during TOF stimulation can be quantified as the ratio of T4:T1, known as the TOF ratio. The TOF ratio is the most useful tool to quantify neuromuscular transmission in a clinical setting and to detect and avoid the residual block. Because the magnitude of fade is quantified within each train (T4:T1), there is no need for a baseline value as each train acts as its own control. Neuromuscular transmission can be confirmed prior to extubation without having established a baseline value. In the absence of block, the TOF ratio is usually 1.0−1.2; ratios >1.0 can be observed (called reverse fade) with AMG and are likely the result of the extremity not returning to the exact same position between twitches. Hence, a TOF ratio <1.0 indicate the presence of partial neuromuscular block (incomplete neuromuscular transmission). During recovery from block, it is recommended that T4:T1 ratios >0.9 are documented to ensure that neuromuscular function is adequate, as ratios <0.9 have been associated with impaired functions, including swallowing and an increase in ventilation in response to hypoxia (Eriksson et al., 1997; Sundman et al., 2000). It is important to notice that while the substantial neuromuscular block can be observed with subjective evaluation (TOF ratios <0.5), weakness is difficult to appreciate by observation once the ratio exceeds 0.5. That is to say, mild to moderate residual block (TOF ratio >0.5 but <0.9) cannot be reliably detected by subjective means (Martin-Flores et al., 2019).

Unlike single twitch, where supramaximal stimulation is mandatory, submaximal currents have been used with TOF to detect partial (residual) blocks in people. As long as the submaximal current is sufficient to elicit four twitches in response to TOF stimulation, this technique is reliable (Brull et al., 1990; Silverman et al., 1992) while producing

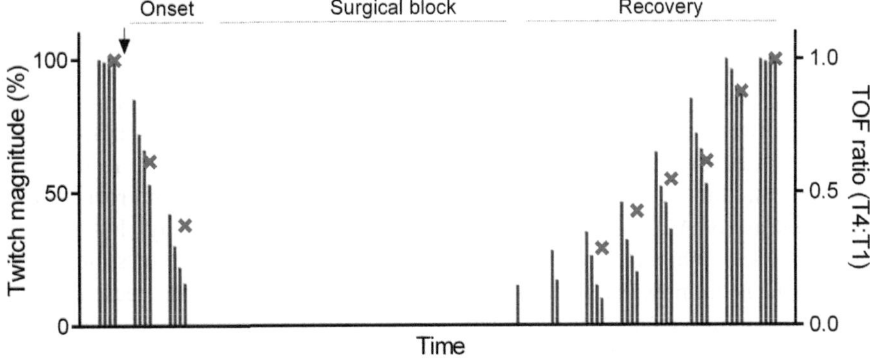

FIGURE 8.3 Representation of train-of-four (TOF) monitoring with acceleromyography. The magnitude (peak acceleration; also called "twitch height") of each response of the TOF, displayed as blue vertical lines is shown on the left Y-axis, and expressed as a percentage value of the baseline (preblock) response. The TOF ratio (T4:T1) is shown as red Xs and referenced in the right Y-axis. The onset is the period between NMBA administration (black arrow) and the maximal response, in this case, complete neuromuscular block. The period of surgical block is the time with zero or one responses to TOF, and it is followed the recovery period, which is characterized by the presence of a fade during TOF. Complete recovery is achieved when the magnitude of each twitch has returned to baseline levels, with no measurable fade between the fourth and first twitches.

substantially less discomfort. Hence, submaximal TOF might be useful to assess neuromuscular function during recovery from anesthesia.

As mentioned before, the sensitivity of different muscle groups to the effects of NMBAs varies. This is an important observation, since neuromuscular monitoring is only carried out on few peripheral motor nerves/muscles; those results must be extrapolated with care to the entire individual. For example, it has been shown in dogs that neuromuscular block at some laryngeal muscles may extend beyond the duration measured at the limbs, where monitoring is typically performed (Sakai et al., 2017). Because neuromuscular monitoring can only be carried in some peripheral muscles, the anesthetist needs to be familiar with these differences between muscle groups and consider that recovery of laryngeal function in dogs may require a few more minutes than the extremities. These authors recommend that complete recovery of neuromuscular transmission measured at the limbs (TOF ratio $\geq$1.0) be documented for at least 15 minutes before tracheal extubation is performed.

IX. Clinical pharmacology and use of reversal agents

Reversal of neuromuscular block does not occur through direct receptor antagonism as it may be achieved with other agents, such as opioids (naloxone) or alpha-2 adrenoceptor agonists (atipamezole). Instead, recovery from block can be accelerated by the use of cholinesterase inhibitors, namely neostigmine or edrophonium. These agents inhibit the activity of the AChE enzyme, responsible for the hydrolysis of ACh (Fig. 8.1). As this enzyme is inhibited, the concentration of local ACh increases as it accumulates in the NMJ. It is this increased concentration of ACh, and not the reversal agent itself, that competes against the NMBAs for the nicotinic receptor. While their mechanism of action is similar, neostigmine is more potent and produces more inhibition of enzymatic function than edrophonium. As a result, it is typically considered a more reliable reversal agent, but with more intense cardiovascular side effects.

There are important consequences of this indirect mechanism: first, the concentration of ACh that can be reached is limited by the release of ACh from the presynaptic cell, even when complete inhibition of AChE is achieved. Hence, the profound neuromuscular block cannot be reversed with neostigmine or edrophonium because not enough ACh will be available to compete with high plasma (and NMJ) concentrations of the NMBA. It is therefore recommended that some evidence of the spontaneous return of function, indicative of a lower concentration of NMBA at the NMJ, is documented before the reversal agent is administered. Typically, the return of at least T1 of the TOF should occur before the reversal is performed. Predictably, the speed and efficacy of recovery increases if the reversal agent is given at more shallow levels of partial block; that is to say, reversal is faster and more predictable if performed when four responses are present rather than one (Lorenzutti et al., 2014). Second, the increase in the concentration of ACh is not immediate. In dogs, 5–10 minutes may be necessary before the full effect of neostigmine can be observed (Martin-Flores et al., 2017). Third, once all activity of the enzyme has been inhibited, further doses of neostigmine or edrophonium will have no effect on the speed of recovery. For example, if reversal was attempted during a complete block (no responses to TOF) and recovery did not occur within a few minutes, additional doses of reversal agents will be ineffective. In that case, monitoring should continue until some evidence of spontaneous recovery occurs (at a minimum return of one to two responses to TOF), and only then should reversal be attempted again. Fourth, the systemic concentration of ACh (at sites outside the NMJ) also increases after the administration of neostigmine or edrophonium (albeit less with the latter). Unwanted cholinergic effects, mainly bradycardia but also potentially bronchoconstriction, could occur and can be prevented by administering atropine or glycopyrrolate prior to the reversal agent. The combination of neostigmine with atropine/glycopyrrolate is typically used in clinical practice.

An alternate method to reverse neuromuscular block is now available. Sugammadex is the first selective relaxant binding agent (SRBA) introduced to clinical practice. Sugammadex was specifically developed to interact with the aminosteroid NMBA rocuronium. It binds to rocuronium and encapsulates it, creating a stable, irreversible bond. The sugammadex-rocuronium complex is devoid of neuromuscular blocking effects and is eliminated through urine (Bom et al., 2002; Bom et al., 2002, 2009). As sugammadex binds to rocuronium, the concentration of free rocuronium in plasma decreases abruptly. This creates a favorable gradient that allows rocuronium to "move" out of the NMJ, restoring neuromuscular function. As long as sufficient sugammadex is administered, rocuronium will continue to be bound as it moves from the NMJ to the systemic circulation. As a result, even deep levels of neuromuscular block from rocuronium can be reversed promptly, and without any cholinergic effects when these agents are used. Because of structural similarities, sugammadex can also reverse vecuronium blockade (Mosing et al., 2010, 2012).

A. Strategies to minimize the risk of residual block

Prevention of residual block is of paramount importance when providing anesthesia involving the use of NMBAs, as is the provision of adequate hypnosis and analgesia. Several strategies can be used, sometimes in combination, to reduce the risk of PORC. Short-or-intermediate acting agents should be used preferably to long-lasting drugs. For this reason, the use of pancuronium has decreased substantially and is largely replaced by intermediate-acting agents. Repeating small doses to prolong duration might be preferred over administering large doses with less frequency, as the progression of recovery is slowed down after large doses (Lorenzutti et al., 2019). This is particularly beneficial for modern agents, for which the cumulative effects are minimized in healthy animals, and although possibly impractical, it could be safer than constant-rate infusions. Constant-rate infusions of NMBA carry a risk of overdosing, as the effect of any unnecessary administration of the NMBA beyond that which causes complete paralysis (TOF ratio 0) cannot be measured. If an infusion is to be used, it is probably advantageous to titrate the rate in order to keep one response to TOF (i.e., T1) present.

Neuromuscular monitoring should always be performed. If objective monitoring is available, then a TOF ratio >0.9, or preferably ≥ 1.0 should be targeted for recovery. If only subjective monitoring is available, then reversal with neostigmine or edrophonium should be performed once the block is intermediate; that is, when two to four twitches can be elicited. Reversal of rocuronium-induced block with sugammadex might be performed at deeper levels of the block, providing a sufficient dose of sugammadex is administered. Lastly, it is probably wise to document that neuromuscular transmission has been restored for several minutes before the trachea is extubated, instead of making that decision on a single, isolated measurement obtained at emergence. Particularly in species in which laryngeal muscles are more sensitive to the effects of NMBA than the limbs.

X. Future and upcoming agents

Technological advances in pharmacology are creating exciting new possibilities in the use of neuromuscular blocking agents (NMBAs). The relaxant-binding agent sugammadex is now available and licensed for use in many countries. A nonselective binding agent, calabadion, is being researched. This molecule can bind to NMBAs of different chemical structures (and with other agents besides NMBAs) and may have a role in the near future (Haerter et al., 2015; Hoffmann et al., 2013; Lim and Landsittel, 2016).

A new family of compounds for the neuromuscular blockade is being developed. These agents are susceptible to cysteine inactivation; administration of cysteine has shown to promptly reverse neuromuscular block without side effects. Several compounds are promising, ranging from fast, ultra-short-acting drugs to others of intermediate duration (Heerdt et al., 2016; Kaullen et al., 2018; Lien, 2011; Lien et al., 2009; Savarese et al., 2018; Sunaga et al., 2016). All are susceptible to cysteine inactivation, which results in prompt reversal and restoration of neuromuscular function, upon administration. Gantacurium, a short-acting compound was evaluated in cats, resulting in a fast and short block that could facilitate tracheal intubation (Martin-Flores et al., 2015). An intermediate-acting molecule was also successfully used in rabbits (Diaz et al., 2014). This new family of agents will increase the versatility and safety of clinical neuromuscular block.

References

Adami, C., Sanchez, R.F., Monticelli, P., 2019. Use of atracurium and its reversal with neostigmine in 14 pet rabbits undergoing ophthalmic surgery: a retrospective study. Vet. Rec. 184 (14), 443. https://doi.org/10.1136/vr.105266.

Adams, W.A., Mark Senior, J., Jones, R.S., Williams, J.M., Gleed, R.D., 2006. cis-Atracurium in dogs with and without porto-systemic shunts. Vet. Anaesth. Analg. 33 (1), 17–23. https://doi.org/10.1111/j.1467-2995.2005.00231.x.

Aguilar, A., Moll, X., García, F., Andaluz, A., 2019. Neuromuscular block monitoring after the administration of 1 mg/kg intravenous cis-atracurium in the anaesthetized pig. J. Vet. Pharmacol. Therapeut. 42 (1), 67–73. https://doi.org/10.1111/jvp.12707.

Auer, U., 2007. Clinical observations on the use of the muscle relaxant rocuronium bromide in the dog. Vet. J. 173 (2), 422–427. https://doi.org/10.1016/j.tvjl.2005.11.014.

Auer, U., Mosing, M., 2006. A clinical study of the effects of rocuronium in isoflurane-anaesthetized cats. Vet. Anaesth. Analg. 33 (4), 224–228. https://doi.org/10.1111/j.1467-2995.2005.00262.x.

Auer, U., Uray, C., Mosing, M., 2007. Observations on the muscle relaxant rocuronium bromide in the horse–a dose-response study. Vet. Anaesth. Analg. 34 (2), 75–81. https://doi.org/10.1111/j.1467-2995.2006.00298.x.

Bartkowski, R.R., Witkowski, T.A., Azad, S., Lessin, J., Marr, A., 1993. Rocuronium onset of action: a comparison with atracurium and vecuronium. Anesth. Analg. 77 (3), 574–578. https://doi.org/10.1213/00000539-199309000-00025.

Bergman, I.J., Kluger, M.T., Short, T.G., 2002. Awareness during general anaesthesia: a review of 81 cases from the Anaesthetic Incident Monitoring Study. Anaesthesia 57 (6), 549–556. https://doi.org/10.1046/j.1365-2044.2002.02565.x.

Bom, A., Bradley, M., Cameron, K., Clark, J.K., Van Egmond, J., Feilden, H., Zhang, M.Q., 2002a. A novel concept of reversing neuromuscular block: chemical encapsulation of rocuronium bromide by a cyclodextrin-based synthetic host. Angew Chem. Int. Ed. Engl. 41 (2), 266–270.

Bom, A., Clark, J.K., Palin, R., 2002b. New approaches to reversal of neuromuscular block. Curr. Opin. Drug Discov. Dev 5 (5), 793–800.

Bom, A., Hope, F., Rutherford, S., Thomson, K., 2009. Preclinical pharmacology of sugammadex. J. Crit. Care 24 (1), 29–35. https://doi.org/10.1016/j.jcrc.2008.10.010.

Brown, M.C., Holland, R.L., Hopkins, W.G., 1981. Motor nerve sprouting. Annu. Rev. Neurosci. 4, 17–42. https://doi.org/10.1146/annurev.ne.04.030181.000313.

Brull, S.J., Ehrenwerth, J., Silverman, D.G., 1990. Stimulation with submaximal current for train-of-four monitoring. Anesthesiology 72 (4), 629–632. https://doi.org/10.1097/00000542-199004000-00009.

Burns, B.D., Paton, W.D., 1951. Depolarization of the motor end-plate by decamethonium and acetylcholine. J. Physiol. 115 (1), 41–73. https://doi.org/10.1113/jphysiol.1951.sp004652.

Chen, I.Y., Liang, Y.Y., Chen, K.S., Lee, W.M., Wang, H.C., 2020. Comparison of the neuromuscular blocking effects of cisatracurium during isoflurane or propofol anesthesia in dogs. Vet. Anaesth. Analg. 47 (4), 454–462. https://doi.org/10.1016/j.vaa.2020.03.002.

Clarke, K.W.H.L.W.T.C.M., 2013. Veterinary anaesthesia.

Claudius, C., Garvey, L.H., Viby-Mogensen, J., 2009. The undesirable effects of neuromuscular blocking drugs. Anaesthesia 64 (s1), 10–21. https://doi.org/10.1111/j.1365-2044.2008.05866.x.

Claudius, C., Viby-Mogensen, J., 2008. Acceleromyography for use in scientific and clinical practice: a systematic review of the evidence. Anesthesiology 108 (6), 1117–1140. https://doi.org/10.1097/ALN.0b013e318173f62f.

Clutton, R.E., Glasby, M.A., 1998. A comparison of the neuromuscular and cardiovascular effects of vecuronium, atracurium and mivacurium in sheep. Res. Vet. Sci. 64 (3), 233–237.

Colin, J.N., Singlas, E., 1985. Metabolism and pharmacokinetics of atracurium. Ann. Fr. Anesth. Reanim. 4 (6), 465–470. https://doi.org/10.1016/s0750-7658(85)80242-2.

Council, N.R., 2011. Guide for the Care and Use of Laboratory Animals, eighth ed. The National Academies Press. https://doi.org/10.17226/12910.

Dale, H., 1934. Chemical transmission of the effects of nerve impulses. BMJ Br. Med. J. (Clin. Res. Ed.) 3827, 835–841. https://doi.org/10.1136/bmj.1.3827.835.

Diaz, L.L., Zhang, J., Heerdt, P.M., 2014. Comparative pharmacodynamics of pancuronium, cisatracurium, and CW002 in rabbits. J. Am. Assoc. Lab. Anim. Sci. 53 (3), 283–289.

Diefenbach, C., Abel, M., Buzello, W., 1992. Greater neuromuscular blocking potency of atracurium during hypothermic than during normothermic cardiopulmonary bypass. Anesth. Analg. 75 (5), 675–678. https://doi.org/10.1213/00000539-199211000-00004.

Doodnaught, G.M., Pang, D.S., 2017. Intubation following high-dose rocuronium in a cat with protracted laryngospasm. JFMS Open Rep. 3. https://doi.org/10.1177/2055116917733642, 2055116917733642.

Durant, N.N., Houwertjes, M.C., Crul, J.F., 1980. Comparison of the neuromuscular blocking properties of ORG NC 45 and pancuronium in the rat, cat and rhesus monkey. Br. J. Anaesth. 52 (8), 723–730. https://doi.org/10.1093/bja/52.8.723.

Engbaek, J., Ording, H., Pedersen, T., Viby-Mogensen, J., 1984. Dose-response relationships and neuromuscular blocking effects of vecuronium pancuronium during ketamine anaesthesia. Br. J. Anaesth. 56 (9), 953–957. https://doi.org/10.1093/bja/56.9.953.

Eriksson, L.I., Sundman, E., Olsson, R., Nilsson, L., Witt, H., Ekberg, O., Kuylenstierna, R., 1997. Functional assessment of the pharynx at rest and during swallowing in partially paralyzed humans: simultaneous videomanometry and mechanomyography of awake human volunteers. Anesthesiology 87 (5), 1035–1043.

Faulds, D., Clissold, S.P., 1991. Doxacurium. A review of its pharmacology and clinical potential in anaesthesia. Drugs 42 (4), 673–689. https://doi.org/10.2165/00003495-199142040-00009.

Fodale, V., Santamaria, L.B., 2002. Laudanosine, an atracurium and cisatracurium metabolite. Eur. J. Anaesthesiol. 19 (7), 466–473. https://doi.org/10.1017/s0265021502000777.

Forte, J., Peirce, J.W., Kraft, J.M., Krauskopf, J., Lennie, P., 2002. Residual eye-movements in macaque and their effects on visual responses of neurons. Vis. Neurosci. 19 (1), 31–38. https://doi.org/10.1017/s0952523801191030.

Freret, T., Bouet, V., Toutain, J., Saulnier, R., Pro-Sistiaga, P., Bihel, E., Touzani, O., 2008. Intraluminal thread model of focal stroke in the non-human primate. J. Cerebr. Blood Flow Metabol. 28 (4), 786–796. https://doi.org/10.1038/sj.jcbfm.9600575.

Gillies, D., Wynands, J.E., 1986. Harold Randall Griffith. The pioneer of the use of muscle relaxants in anaesthesia. Br. J. Anaesth. 58 (9), 943–945. https://doi.org/10.1093/bja/58.9.943.

Gleed, R.D., Jones, R.S., 1982. Observations on the neuromuscular blocking action of gallamine and pancuronium and their reversal by neostigmine. Res. Vet. Sci. 32 (3), 324–326.

Gray, T.C., Halton, J., 1946. A milestone in anaesthesia? Anesthesiology 7 (6), 679–680. https://doi.org/10.1097/00000542-194611000-00018.

Grong, K., Salminen, P.R., Stangeland, L., Dahle, G.O., 2015. Haemodynamic differences between pancuronium and vecuronium in an experimental pig model. Vet. Anaesth. Analg. 42 (3), 242–249. https://doi.org/10.1111/vaa.12198.

Hackett, G.H., Jantzen, J.P., Earnshaw, G., 1989. Cardiovascular effects of vecuronium, atracurium, pancuronium, metocurine and RGH-4201 in dogs. Acta Anaesthesiol. Scand. 33 (4), 298–303. https://doi.org/10.1111/j.1399-6576.1989.tb02912.x.

Haerter, F., Simons, J.C., Foerster, U., Duarte, I.M., Diaz-Gil, D., Ganapati, S., Eikermann, M., 2015. Comparative effectiveness of calabadion and sugammadex to reverse non-depolarizing neuromuscular-blocking agents. Anesthesiology. https://doi.org/10.1097/aln.0000000000000868.

Hall, L.W., Lehmann, H., Silk, E., 1953. Response in dogs to relaxants derived from succinic acid and choline. Br. Med. J. 1 (4802), 134–136.

Heerdt, P.M., Sunaga, H., Owen, J.S., Murrell, M.T., Malhotra, J.K., Godfrey, D., Lien, C.A., 2016. Dose-response and cardiopulmonary side effects of the novel neuromuscular-blocking drug CW002 in man. Anesthesiology 125 (6), 1136–1143. https://doi.org/10.1097/aln.0000000000001386.

Henning, R.H., Houwertjes, M.C., Scaf, A.H., den Hertog, A., Agoston, S., 1993. Prolonged paralysis after long-term, high-dose infusion of pancuronium in anaesthetized cats. Br. J. Anaesth. 71 (3), 393–397. https://doi.org/10.1093/bja/71.3.393.

Hildebrand, S.V., Arpin, D., 1988. Neuromuscular and cardiovascular effects of atracurium administered to healthy horses anesthetized with halothane. Am. J. Vet. Res. 49 (7), 1066–1071.

Hirsch, N.P., 2007. Neuromuscular junction in health and disease. Br. J. Anaesth. 99 (1), 132–138. https://doi.org/10.1093/bja/aem144.

Hoffmann, U., Grosse-Sundrup, M., Eikermann-Haerter, K., Zaremba, S., Ayata, C., Zhang, B., Eikermann, M., 2013. Calabadion: a new agent to reverse the effects of benzylisoquinoline and steroidal neuromuscular-blocking agents. Anesthesiology 119 (2), 317–325. https://doi.org/10.1097/ALN.0b013e3182910213.

Hofmeister, E.H., Brainard, B.M., Sams, L.M., Allman, D.A., Cruse, A.M., 2008. Evaluation of induction characteristics and hypnotic potency of isoflurane and sevoflurane in healthy dogs. Am. J. Vet. Res. 69 (4), 451–456. https://doi.org/10.2460/ajvr.69.4.451.

Hudson, M.E., Rothfield, K.P., Tullock, W.C., Firestone, L.L., 1998. Haemodynamic effects of rocuronium bromide in adult cardiac surgical patients. Can. J. Anaesth. 45 (2), 139–143. https://doi.org/10.1007/bf03013252.

Iaizzo, P.A., Wedel, D.J., 1994. Response to succinylcholine in porcine malignant hyperthermia. Anesth. Analg. 79 (1), 143–151. https://doi.org/10.1213/00000539-199407000-00027.

Ida, K.K., Van-Wijnsberghe, A.S., Tutunaru, A., Limpens, V., Sauvage, A., Serteyn, D., Sandersen, C., 2020. Onset and duration of cis-atracurium neuromuscular block during fentanyl and lidocaine infusions in isoflurane-anaesthetised dogs. Vet. Rec. 187 (5), e33. https://doi.org/10.1136/vr.105522.

Jones, R., Seymour, C., 2008. Clinical observation on the use of vecuronium as a muscle relaxant in the dog. J. Small Anim. Pract. 26, 213–218. https://doi.org/10.1111/j.1748-5827.1985.tb02103.x.

Jones, R.A., Harrison, C., Eaton, S.L., Llavero Hurtado, M., Graham, L.C., Alkhammash, L., Gillingwater, T.H., 2017. Cellular and molecular anatomy of the human neuromuscular junction. Cell Rep. 21 (9), 2348–2356. https://doi.org/10.1016/j.celrep.2017.11.008.

Kandukuri, D.S., Phillips, J.K., Tahmindjis, M., Hildreth, C.M., 2018. Effect of anaesthetic and choice of neuromuscular blocker on vagal control of heart rate under laboratory animal experimental conditions. Lab. Anim 52 (3), 280–291. https://doi.org/10.1177/0023677217725365.

Kariman, A., Clutton, R.E., 2008. The effects of medetomidine on the action of vecuronium in dogs anaesthetized with halothane and nitrous oxide. Vet. Anaesth. Analg. 35 (5), 400–408. https://doi.org/10.1111/j.1467-2995.2008.00401.x.

Kastrup, M.R., Marsico, F.F., Ascoli, F.O., Becker, T., Soares, J.H., Gomez de Segura, I.A., 2005. Neuromuscular blocking properties of atracurium during sevoflurane or propofol anaesthesia in dogs. Vet. Anaesth. Analg. 32 (4), 222–227. https://doi.org/10.1111/j.1467-2995.2005.00240.x [doi].

Kaullen, J.D., Owen, J.S., Brouwer, K.L.R., Heerdt, P.M., Lien, C.A., Savarese, J.J., Schmith, V.D., 2018. Pharmacokinetic/pharmacodynamic model of CW002, an investigational intermediate neuromuscular blocking agent, in healthy volunteers. Anesthesiology 128 (6), 1107–1116. https://doi.org/10.1097/aln.0000000000002157.

Kelman, G.R., Kennedy, B.R., 1971. Cardiovascular effects of pancuronium in man. Br. J. Anaesth. 43 (4), 335–338. https://doi.org/10.1093/bja/43.4.335.

Kim, K.S., Shim, J.C., Jun, J.H., Lee, K.H., Chung, C.W., 1999. Rabbits treated with chronic isepamicin are resistant to mivacurium and rocuronium. Anesth. Analg. 88 (3), 654–658. https://doi.org/10.1097/00000539-199903000-00034.

Kopman, A.F., Sinha, N., 2003. Acceleromyography as a guide to anesthetic management: a case report. J. Clin. Anesth. 15 (2), 145–148. https://doi.org/10.1016/s0952-8180(02)00518-4.

Lien, C.A., 2011. Development and potential clinical impairment of ultra-short-acting neuromuscular blocking agents. Br. J. Anaesth. 107 (Suppl. 1), i60–i71. https://doi.org/10.1093/bja/aer341.

Lien, C.A., Savard, P., Belmont, M., Sunaga, H., Savarese, J.J., 2009. Fumarates: unique nondepolarizing neuromuscular blocking agents that are antagonized by cysteine. J. Crit. Care 24 (1), 50–57. https://doi.org/10.1016/j.jcrc.2008.11.001.

Lim, G., Landsittel, D.P., 2016. Effectiveness versus efficacy of calabadion and sugammadex for nondepolarizing neuromuscular blocking agent reversal. Anesthesiology 124, 1417. https://doi.org/10.1097/aln.0000000000001097.

Lorenzutti, A.M., Martin-Flores, M., Baldivieso, J.M., Himelfarb, M.A., Litterio, N.J., 2014. Evaluation of neostigmine antagonism at different levels of vecuronium-induced neuromuscular blockade in isoflurane anesthetized dogs. Can. Vet. J. 55 (2), 156–160.

Lorenzutti, A.M., Zarazaga, M.P., Sakai, D.M., Nejamkin, P., Rosetti, V., Duran, V., Martin-Flores, M., 2019. Context-sensitive recovery of neuromuscular function from vecuronium in dogs: effects of dose and dosing protocol. Vet. J. 248, 14–17. https://doi.org/10.1016/j.tvjl.2019.04.004.

Loughren, M., Banks, S., Naluan, C., Portenlanger, P., Wendorf, A., Johnson, D., 2014. Onset and duration of intravenous and intraosseous rocuronium in swine. West. J. Emerg. Med. 15 (2), 241–245. https://doi.org/10.5811/westjem.2013.9.14484.

Lundstrom, L.H., Duez, C.H., Norskov, A.K., Rosenstock, C.V., Thomsen, J.L., Moller, A.M., Wetterslev, J., 2017. Avoidance versus use of neuromuscular blocking agents for improving conditions during tracheal intubation or direct laryngoscopy in adults and adolescents. Cochrane Database Syst. Rev. 5, Cd009237. https://doi.org/10.1002/14651858.CD009237.pub2.

Lundstrom, L.H., Moller, A.M., Rosenstock, C., Astrup, G., Gatke, M.R., Wetterslev, J., 2009. Avoidance of neuromuscular blocking agents may increase the risk of difficult tracheal intubation: a cohort study of 103,812 consecutive adult patients recorded in the Danish Anaesthesia Database. Br. J. Anaesth. 103 (2), 283–290. https://doi.org/10.1093/bja/aep124.

Madsen, M.V., Donatsky, A.M., Jensen, B.R., Rosenberg, J., Hammelev, K.P., Gätke, M.R., 2015. Influence of intense neuromuscular blockade on surgical conditions during laparotomy: a pig model. J. Anesth. 29 (1), 15–20. https://doi.org/10.1007/s00540-014-1877-8.

Martin-Flores, M., Campoy, L., Ludders, J.W., Erb, H.N., Gleed, R.D., 2008. Comparison between acceleromyography and visual assessment of train-of-four for monitoring neuromuscular blockade in horses undergoing surgery. Vet. Anaesth. Analg. 35 (3), 220–227. https://doi.org/10.1111/j.1467-2995.2007.00380.x.

Martin-Flores, M., Cheetham, J., Campoy, L., Sakai, D.M., Heerdt, P.M., Gleed, R.D., 2015. Effect of gantacurium on evoked laryngospasm and duration of apnea in anesthetized healthy cats. Am. J. Vet. Res. 76 (3), 216–223. https://doi.org/10.2460/ajvr.76.3.216.

Martin-Flores, M., Lorenzutti, A.M., Litterio, N.J., Rossetti, V.L., Zarazaga, M.P., Bonetto, C.C., Aguirre, G.E., 2017. Speed of reversal of vecuronium neuromuscular block with different doses of neostigmine in anesthetized dogs. Vet. Anaesth. Analg. 44 (1), 28–34. https://doi.org/10.1111/vaa.12395.

Martin-Flores, M., Pare, M.D., Adams, W., Campoy, L., Gleed, R.D., 2012a. Observations of the potency and duration of vecuronium in isoflurane-anesthetized horses. Vet. Anaesth. Analg. 39, 385–389.

Martin-Flores, M., Pare, M.D., Campoy, L., Gleed, R.D., 2012b. The sensitivity of sheep to vecuronium: an example of the limitations of extrapolation. Can. J. Anaesth. 59 (7), 722–723. https://doi.org/10.1007/s12630-012-9707-7.

Martin-Flores, M., Sakai, D.M., Campoy, L., Gleed, R.D., 2018. Survey of how different groups of veterinarians manage the use of neuromuscular blocking agents in anesthetized dogs. Vet. Anaesth. Analg. https://doi.org/10.1016/j.vaa.2018.03.002.

Martin-Flores, M., Sakai, D.M., Portela, D.A., Borlle, L., Campoy, L., Gleed, R.D., 2016. Prevention of laryngospasm with rocuronium in cats: a dose-finding study. Vet. Anaesth. Analg. 43 (5), 511–518. https://doi.org/10.1111/vaa.12342.

Martin-Flores, M., Sakai, D.M., Tseng, C.T., Gleed, R.D., Campoy, L., 2019. Can we see fade? A survey of anesthesia providers and our ability to detect partial neuromuscular block in dogs. Vet. Anaesth. Analg. 46 (2), 182–187. https://doi.org/10.1016/j.vaa.2019.01.002.

Martin-Flores, M., Saki, D.M., Campoy, L., Gleed, R.D., 2014. Recovery from neuromuscular block in dogs: restoration of spontaneous ventilation does not exclude residual blockade. Vet. Anaesth. Analg. https://doi.org/10.1111/vaa.12109.

Martinez, E.A., Wooldridge, A.A., Hartsfield, S.M., Mealey, K.L., 1998. Neuromuscular effects of doxacurium chloride in isoflurane-anesthetized dogs. Vet. Surg. 27 (3), 279–283. https://doi.org/10.1111/j.1532-950x.1998.tb00127.x.

Martinez, E.A., Wooldridge, A.A., Mercer, D.E., Slater, M.R., Hartsfield, S.M., 1997. Cardiovascular effects of doxacurium chloride in isoflurane-anaesthetised dogs. J. Vet. Anaesth. 24 (1), 10–13. https://doi.org/10.1111/j.1467-2995.1997.tb00261.x.

Martyn, J.A., Fagerlund, M.J., Eriksson, L.I., 2009. Basic principles of neuromuscular transmission. Anaesthesia 64 (Suppl. 1), 1–9. https://doi.org/10.1111/j.1365-2044.2008.05865.x.

Michalek-Sauberer, A., Gilly, H., Steinbereithner, K., Vizi, E.S., 2000. Effects of vecuronium and rocuronium in antagonistic laryngeal muscles and the anterior tibial muscle in the cat. Acta Anaesthesiol. Scand. 44 (5), 503–510.

Miller, R.D., Agoston, S., van der Pol, F., Booij, L.H., Crul, J.F., 1979. Effect of different anesthetics on the pharmacokinetics and pharmacodynamics of pancuronium in the cat. Acta Anaesthesiol. Scand. 23 (3), 285–290. https://doi.org/10.1111/j.1399-6576.1979.tb01453.x.

Miwa, Y., Komatsu, H., Shinojima, A., Oda, A., Inagaki, M., Usami, K., Kobayashi, Y., 2021. Bilateral cataract surgery in a Japanese macaque (*Macaca fuscata*): a case report. Clin. Case Rep. 9, e05112. https://doi.org/10.1002/ccr3.5112. © 2021 The Authors. Clinical Case Reports published by John Wiley & Sons Ltd.

Moreno-Sala, A., Ortiz-Martinez, R., Valdivia, A.G., Torres-de-Moreno, M.G., Martinez, A., 2013. Use of neuromuscular blockade with rocuronium bromide for intubation in cats. Vet. Anaesth. Analg. 40 (4), 351–358. https://doi.org/10.1111/vaa.12028.

Morris, R.B., Cahalan, M.K., Miller, R.D., Wilkinson, P.L., Quasha, A.L., Robinson, S.L., 1983. The cardiovascular effects of vecuronium (ORG NC45) and pancuronium in patients undergoing coronary artery bypass grafting. Anesthesiology 58 (5), 438–440. https://doi.org/10.1097/00000542-198305000-00008.

Mosing, M., Auer, U., Bardell, D., Jones, R.S., Hunter, J.M., 2010. Reversal of profound rocuronium block monitored in three muscle groups with sugammadex in ponies. Br. J. Anaesth. 105 (4), 480–486. https://doi.org/10.1093/bja/aeq172.

Mosing, M., Auer, U., West, E., Jones, R.S., Hunter, J.M., 2012. Reversal of profound rocuronium or vecuronium-induced neuromuscular block with sugammadex in isoflurane-anaesthetised dogs. Vet. J. 192 (3), 467–471. https://doi.org/10.1016/j.tvjl.2011.08.034.

Muir, A.W., Marshall, R.J., 1987. Comparative neuromuscular blocking effects of vecuronium, pancuronium, Org 6368 and suxamethonium in the anaesthetized domestic pig. Br. J. Anaesth. 59 (5), 622–629.

Murphy, G.S., 2006. Residual neuromuscular blockade: incidence, assessment, and relevance in the postoperative period. Minerva Anestesiol. 72 (3), 97–109.

Murphy, G.S., Szokol, J.W., Avram, M.J., Greenberg, S.B., Marymont, J.H., Vender, J.S., Gupta, D.K., 2011. Intraoperative acceleromyography monitoring reduces symptoms of muscle weakness and improves quality of recovery in the early postoperative period. Anesthesiology 115 (5), 946–954. https://doi.org/10.1097/ALN.0b013e3182342840.

Murphy, G.S., Szokol, J.W., Marymont, J.H., Greenberg, S.B., Avram, M.J., Vender, J.S., 2008a. Residual neuromuscular blockade and critical respiratory events in the postanesthesia care unit. Anesth. Analg. 107 (1), 130–137. https://doi.org/10.1213/ane.0b013e31816d1268.

Murphy, G.S., Szokol, J.W., Marymont, J.H., Greenberg, S.B., Avram, M.J., Vender, J.S., Nisman, M., 2008b. Intraoperative acceleromyographic monitoring reduces the risk of residual neuromuscular blockade and adverse respiratory events in the postanesthesia care unit. Anesthesiology 109 (3), 389–398. https://doi.org/10.1097/ALN.0b013e318182af3b.

Naguib, M., Samarkandi, A.H., Bakhamees, H.S., Magboul, M.A., el-Bakry, A.K., 1995. Histamine-release haemodynamic changes produced by rocuronium, vecuronium, mivacurium, atracurium and tubocurarine. Br. J. Anaesth. 75 (5), 588–592. https://doi.org/10.1093/bja/75.5.588.

Okanlami, O.A., Fryer, A.D., Hirshman, C., 1996. Interaction of non-depolarizing muscle relaxants with M2and M3Muscarinic receptors in Guinea pig lung and heart. Anesthesiology 84 (1), 155–161. https://doi.org/10.1097/00000542-199601000-00018.

Pittet, J.F., Tassonyi, E., Schopfer, C., Morel, D.R., Mentha, G., Fathi, M., Benakis, A., 1990. Plasma concentrations of laudanosine, but not of atracurium, are increased during the anhepatic phase of orthotopic liver transplantation in pigs. Anesthesiology 72 (1), 145–152.

Playfor, S.D., Thomas, D.A., Choonara, I., 2000a. Duration of action of atracurium when given by infusion to critically ill children. Paediatr. Anaesth. 10 (1), 77–81. https://doi.org/10.1046/j.1460-9592.2000.00436.x.

Playfor, S.D., Thomas, D.A., Choonara, I., 2000b. The effect of induced hypothermia on the duration of action of atracurium when given by infusion to critically ill children. Paediatr. Anaesth. 10 (1), 83–88. https://doi.org/10.1046/j.1460-9592.2000.00437.x.

Proost, J.H., Eriksson, L.I., Mirakhur, R.K., Roest, G., Wierda, J.M.K.H., 2000a. Urinary, biliary and faecal excretion of rocuronium in humans. Br. J. Anaesth. 85 (5), 717–723. https://doi.org/10.1093/bja/85.5.717.

Proost, J.H., Wierda, J.M., Houwertjes, M.C., Roggeveld, J., Meijer, D.K., 2000b. Structure-pharmacokinetics relationship of series of amino-steroidal neuromuscular blocking agents in the cat. J. Pharmacol. Exp. Therapeut. 292 (3), 861–869.

RanendraKumar, R., Ray, N.M., Das, A.K., 2005. Skeletal muscle relaxant effect of Chonemorpha macrophylla in experimental animals. Indian J. Pharmacol. 37 (2), 37. https://doi.org/10.4103/0253-7613.15113 (ISSN: 0253-7613).

Sakai, D.M., Martin-Flores, M., Romano, M., Tseng, C.T., Campoy, L., Gleed, R.D., Cheetham, J., 2017. Recovery from rocuronium-induced neuromuscular block was longer in the larynx than in the pelvic limb of anesthetized dogs. Vet. Anaesth. Analg. 44 (2), 246–253. https://doi.org/10.1016/j.vaa.2016.04.001.

Sakai, D.M., Zornow, K.A., Campoy, L., Cable, C., Appel, L.D., Putnam, H.J., Martin-Flores, M., 2018. Intravenous rocuronium 0.3 mg/kg improves the conditions for tracheal intubation in cats: a randomized, placebo-controlled trial. J. Feline Med. Surg. 20 (12), 1124–1129. https://doi.org/10.1177/1098612x18754425.

Savarese, J.J., Sunaga, H., McGilvra, J.D., Belmont, M.R., Murrell, M.T., Jeannotte, E., Heerdt, P.M., 2018. Preclinical pharmacology in the rhesus monkey of CW 1759-50, a new ultra-short acting nondepolarizing neuromuscular blocking agent, degraded and antagonized by L-cysteine. Anesthesiology 129 (5), 970–988. https://doi.org/10.1097/aln.0000000000002408.

Scherrer, N.M., Hopster, K., 2021. Neuromuscular blockade with atracurium for ophthalmic surgery in horses-effects on surgical and anesthetic characteristics and recovery quality. Vet. Ophthalmol. 24 (5), 442–446. https://doi.org/10.1111/vop.12922.

Scott, R.P., Savarese, J.J., Basta, S.J., Embree, P., Ali, H.H., Sunder, N., Hoaglin, D.C., 1986. Clinical pharmacology of atracurium given in high dose. Br. J. Anaesth. 58 (8), 834–838. https://doi.org/10.1093/bja/58.8.834.

Seddighi, R., Egger, C.M., Rohrbach, B.W., Hobbs, M., Doherty, T.J., 2012. Effect of nitrous oxide on the minimum alveolar concentration for sevoflurane and the minimum alveolar concentration derivatives that prevent motor movement and autonomic responses in dogs. Am. J. Vet. Res. 73 (3), 341–345. https://doi.org/10.2460/ajvr.73.3.341.

Short, C.E., Paddleford, R.R., McGrath, C.J., Williams, C.H., 1976. Preanesthetic evaluation and management of malignant hyperthermia in the pig experimental model. Anesth. Analg. 55 (5).

Silverman, D.G., Connelly, N.R., O'Connor, T.Z., Garcia, R., Brull, S.J., 1992. Accelographic train-of-four at near-threshold currents. Anesthesiology 76 (1), 34–38. https://doi.org/10.1097/00000542-199201000-00005.

Slater, C.R., 2017. The structure of human neuromuscular junctions: some unanswered molecular questions. Int. J. Mol. Sci. 18 (10). https://doi.org/10.3390/ijms18102183.

Smith, L.J., Moon, P.F., Lukasik, V.M., Erb, H.N., 1999. Duration of action and hemodynamic properties of mivacurium chloride in dogs anesthetized with halothane. Am. J. Vet. Res. 60 (9), 1047–1050.

Stowe, C.M., Bieter, R.N., Roepke, M.H., 1958. The relationship between cholinesterase activity and the effects of succinylcholine chloride in the horse and cow. Cornell Vet. 48 (3), 241–259.

Sunaga, H., Kaneko, M., Amaki, Y., 2006. The efficacy of intratracheal administration of vecuronium in rats, compared with intravenous and intramuscular administration. Anesth. Analg. 103 (3), 601–607. https://doi.org/10.1213/01.ane.0000229720.13815.73.

Sunaga, H., Savarese, J.J., McGilvra, J.D., Heerdt, P.M., Belmont, M.R., Van Ornum, S.G., Carnathan, G.W., 2016. Preclinical pharmacology of CW002: a nondepolarizing neuromuscular blocking drug of intermediate duration, degraded and antagonized by l-cysteine-additional studies of safety and efficacy in the anesthetized rhesus monkey and cat. Anesthesiology 125 (4), 732–743. https://doi.org/10.1097/aln.0000000000001254.

Sundman, E., Witt, H., Olsson, R., Ekberg, O., Kuylenstierna, R., Eriksson, L.I., 2000. The incidence and mechanisms of pharyngeal and upper esophageal dysfunction in partially paralyzed humans: pharyngeal videoradiography and simultaneous manometry after atracurium. Anesthesiology 92 (4), 977–984.

Sutherland, G.A., Squire, I.B., Gibb, A.J., Marshall, I.G., 1983. Neuromuscular blocking and autonomic effects of vecuronium and atracurium in the anaesthetized cat. Br. J. Anaesth. 55 (11), 1119–1126.

Tutunaru, A., Dupont, J., Gougnard, A., Ida, K., Serteyn, D., Sandersen, C., 2019. Retrospective evaluation of clinical use of cis-atracurium in horses. PLoS One 14 (8), e0221196. https://doi.org/10.1371/journal.pone.0221196.

Tutunaru, A., Dupont, J., Huberty, V., Ibrahim, M., Serteyn, D., Sandersen, C., 2017. Use of cis-atracurium to maintain moderate neuromuscular blockade in experimental pigs. Vet. Anaesth. Analg. 44 (4), 910–914. https://doi.org/10.1016/j.vaa.2016.09.006.

Uhrig, L., Sitt, J.D., Jacob, A., Tasserie, J., Barttfeld, P., Dupont, M., Jarraya, B., 2018. Resting-state dynamics as a cortical signature of anesthesia in monkeys. Anesthesiology 129 (5), 942–958. https://doi.org/10.1097/aln.0000000000002336.

Van Wijnsberghe, A.S., Ida, K.K., Dmitrovic, P., Tutunaru, A., Sandersen, C., 2022. Neuromuscular blockade effects of cisatracurium in 11 cats undergoing ophthalmological surgery anaesthetised with isoflurane. J. Feline Med. Surg. 24 (4), 402–406. https://doi.org/10.1177/1098612x211021829.

Veres-Nyéki, K.O., Rieben, R., Spadavecchia, C., Bergadano, A., 2012. Pancuronium dose refinement in experimental pigs used in cardiovascular research. Vet. Anaesth. Analg. 39 (5), 529–532. https://doi.org/10.1111/j.1467-2995.2012.00732.x.

Wang, Z.M., Yang, Z.J., Zhao, F., Wang, B., Wang, X.C., Qu, P.R., Liu, P.N., 2015. Auditory rehabilitation in rhesus macaque monkeys (*Macaca mulatta*) with auditory brainstem implants. Chin. Med. J. (Engl) 128 (10), 1363–1369. https://doi.org/10.4103/0366-6999.156783.

Wastila, W.B., Maehr, R.B., Turner, G.L., Hill, D.A., Savarese, J.J., 1996. Comparative pharmacology of cisatracurium (51W89), atracurium, and five isomers in cats. Anesthesiology 85 (1), 169–177.

Section III

Anesthetic equipment and monitoring

Chapter 9

Anesthesia delivery systems

Petra Seebeck[1] and Stephan Zeiter[2]

[1]*Zurich Integrative Rodent Physiology (ZIRP), University of Zurich, Zurich, ZH, Switzerland;* [2]*AO Research Institute Davos (ARI), Davos, GR, Switzerland*

Chapter outline

I. Introduction

Inhalation anesthesia offers responsive and consistent control of the onset, depth, and duration of general anesthesia. Subject of this chapter is the delivery equipment associated with inhalation anesthesia. Within the first section, the anesthesia machine, the different components of the breathing circuit, carrier gas supply, flow and scavenging devices, as well as ventilators will be presented. The following section focuses on the patient interface, explaining airway management devices (e.g., endotracheal tubes and supraglottic airway devices (SADs)), laryngoscopes, and stylets for intubation, as well as face masks and nose cones. Vaporizer systems will be discussed in Chapter 6.

Two important aspects need to be taken into account when choosing the breathing systems: dead space and resistance to breathing.

Dead space is the volume of ventilated air that does not participate in gas exchange. The two types of dead space are anatomical or physiologic dead space and apparatus dead space. Anatomical dead space is represented by the volume of air that fills the conducting airways, where there is no potential for gas exchange, i.e., nose, trachea, and

Anesthesia and Analgesia in Laboratory Animals. https://doi.org/10.1016/B978-0-12-822215-7.00013-5

bronchi (Intagliata et al., 2022). In the intact lung, anatomical dead space is equivalent to physiological dead space, but in lung disease, the physiological dead space might be increased due to diffusion problems.

Apparatus dead space means the part of the breathing circuit with bidirectional gas flow, i.e., fresh gas and expired gas. The apparatus dead space is the internal volume of the patient interface (see paragraph III). Various components of the anesthesia machine, like connectors or adaptors, can significantly increase dead space. The apparatus dead space should be kept as low as possible—if the dead space is too large, a significant amount of exhaled, carbon dioxide-rich gas is reinhaled, leading to an increase in blood carbon dioxide over time.

The different types of rebreathing systems vary in the amount of resistance they produce to breathing. This resistance to breathing can make it difficult for smaller patients to ventilate. A system with an inappropriate resistance to breathing for the animal's size will result in depressing respiration due to fatigue of the respiratory muscle. Therefore, rebreathing systems should not be used for rodents or other small animals with a body weight below 2 kg.

While the open mask system is the most commonly used breathing system for small laboratory rodents, more complex systems are available. Over the years, these anesthesia machines have evolved into an advanced care-station with advanced electronics, software, and technology to offer extensive capabilities for ventilation, monitoring, inhaled agent delivery, or low-flow anesthesia (Patil et al., 2013; Romero-Ávila et al., 2021).

II. Anesthesia machine

In its simplest form, an anesthetic machine must control fresh gas flow, provide a means of delivering the fresh carrier gas to the patient (breathing circuit), and control the concentration of anesthetic vapor delivered. A method of disposing of waste anesthetic gas may be incorporated into the machine or may be added as a separate component. A large number of different breathing circuits have been invented and described. Fortunately, only a few types of breathing circuits are needed to accomplish a wide range of anesthetic tasks. A detailed description and examples of different anesthesia machines are beyond the scope of this chapter. It is essential that the user clearly understand the function, operation, and limitations of their machine. Therefore, this section aims to provide the general principles of the most commonly used types of circuits. More in-depth information can be found in the textbooks recommended for additional reading in Section IV.

Terms such as *open*, *closed*, *semi-open*, and *semi-closed*, among others, have been used in a variety of classification schemes. Various authors understand these terms differently, and the result is a confusing array of classification schemes. The most important differentiation is between rebreathing and nonrebreathing systems.

A. Rebreathing systems—the circle system

1. General principle—the breathing circuit

The conventional circle system remains the most commonly used breathing circuit for larger patients. In this circuit, the gases coming from the patient are recycled (Baum, 1990; Hylani, 1986). As the patient uses oxygen and produces carbon dioxide, these gases must be replenished and removed, respectively. Removal of carbon dioxide and recirculation of the remaining gases reduce the consumption of volatile anesthetic agents and fresh gas. With moderate flows, some heat and moisture are also retained. The most important part of a conventional circle system, the breathing circuit, is shown and explained below (Fig. 9.1).

The breathing circuit is connected via the Y-piece with the patient interface (e.g., endotracheal tube or face mask, see paragraph III). Disposable systems are commercially available mainly in human medicine. In veterinary clinical and research use, disposable circuits are frequently cleaned and reused. It is essential to avoid irritating or toxic residues left by the cleaning method. A thorough rinsing of all components to eliminate cleaning agent and disinfectant residues is needed, in addition to compliance with any sterilization guidelines for the method used.

2. Unidirectional valves

Unidirectional valves direct the flow of gases to prevent rebreathing of expired gases. Valves are thin discs made of light materials to reduce resistance to breathing. They are arranged horizontally and clearly labeled to indicate their proper connection to the breathing hoses. Clear plastic domes cover the valves to allow inspection during anesthesia and testing (Fig. 9.2). Gases entering the valve force the disc up, permitting flow through the port. Flow in the opposite direction forces the disc onto the seat, sealing the port. Thus, for the inspiratory valve, when the patient inhales, pressure is reduced across the valve, and the valve rises, allowing gas to flow. At the same time, the drop in pressure across the expiratory valve causes the disc valve to close, stopping the flow of gas. Upon exhalation, pressures in the circuit are reversed, sealing the inhalation valve and opening the exhalation valve.

Breathing valves are subject to accumulated moisture and debris and should be cleaned regularly to prevent valves from sticking. Care is needed during reassembly. Correct valve function should be observed when the machine is checked and tested before use and during anesthesia.

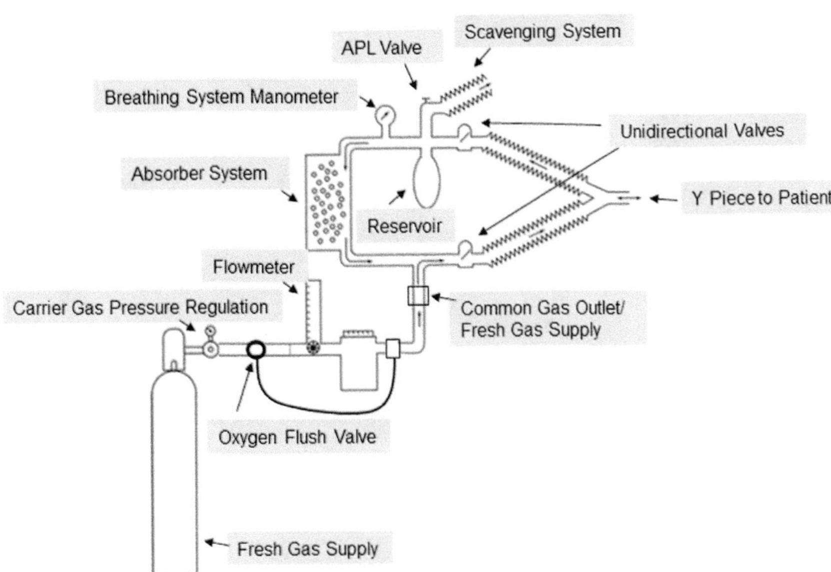

FIGURE 9.1 Schematic drawing of an anesthesia delivery system with the example of a rebreathing system displaying all components being discussed in this chapter.

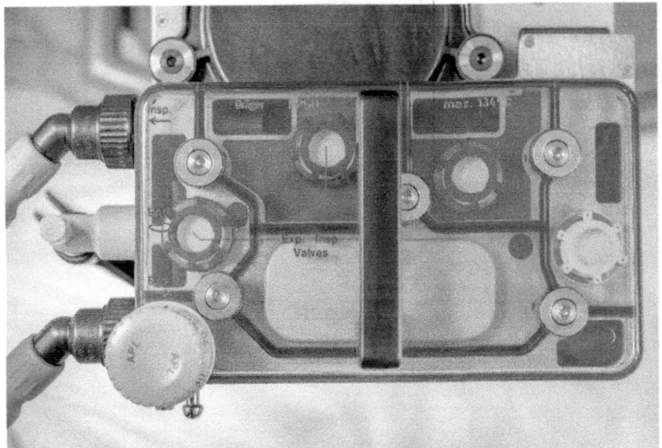
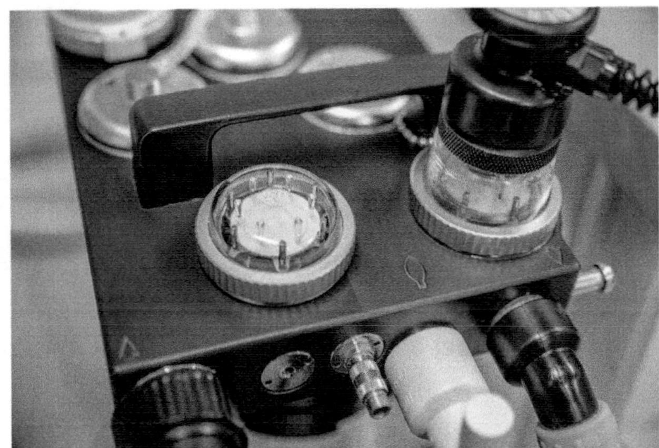

FIGURE 9.2 Different types of unidirectional valves (F. Gantenbein).

3. Adjustable pressure-limiting valve

The pressure in the breathing system is controlled by the adjustable pressure-limiting (APL) ("pop-off") valve (Fig. 9.3). The APL releases anesthetic gases into the scavenging system and provides pressure control in the breathing circuit. It ensures that the pressure within the system is not too high to cause lung damage. Although the specific design varies with the manufacturer, all APL valves can be gradually adjusted from fully open to fully closed, imposing progressive resistance to gas escape. During spontaneous breathing, the APL valve usually is fully open. Partially closing the valve during spontaneous or assisted ventilation adds continuous positive airway pressure or positive end-expiratory pressure to the circuit. A completely closed APL valve means that all the exhaled gases except carbon dioxide are returned to the patient. The system becomes an entirely closed one, which can be used with flows as low as 250–500 mL—termed as a low-flow system.

4. Breathing system manometer

The pressure in the breathing circuit is usually expressed in centimeters of water, measured by a manometer located in the breathing circuit. The manometer is an important safety component, used not only to assure appropriate inflation pressures during assisted or positive pressure ventilation but also to detect or avoid dangerously high pressures due to operator error or mechanical malfunction. The manometer indicates negative as well as positive pressure, i.e., it indicates pressure below atmospheric pressure, as when a patient attempts to inspire in the presence of an empty reservoir bag, or a malfunction in certain active waste gas scavenging systems. The indicator needle should move smoothly in response to pressure changes and should

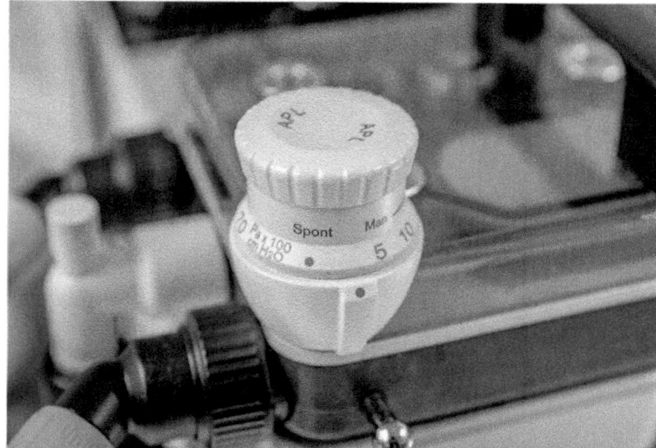

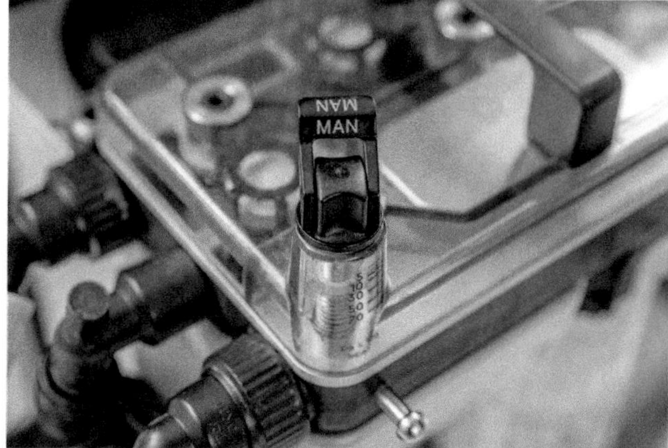

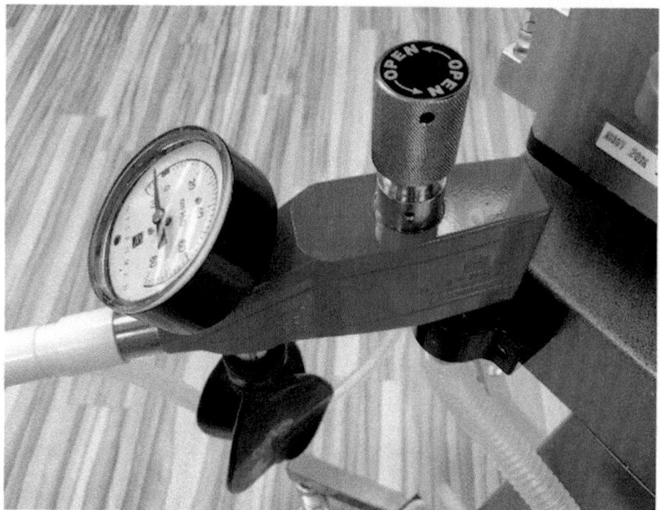

FIGURE 9.3 Different types of adjustable pressure limiting (APL) valves (*top,* F. Gantenbein, *bottom,* D. Pang).

indicate zero pressure when the breathing circuit is not in use. Time and exposure to pressure extremes can result in a loss of calibration, which should be corrected before continued use.

5. Fresh gas supply (common gas outlet)

Fresh gases (typically oxygen and inhalational anesthetic agents) are delivered to the breathing system/circuit through the common gas outlet. The entry point for fresh gases can be close to the patient (allowing a faster impact on patient anesthesia) or further away in the circle (better to retain heat and moisture within the system). All components regarding the (fresh) carrier gas are discussed in part C.

6. Reservoir bag

At the beginning of inspiration, very high temporary gas flows are needed; for larger patients, the flows required could exceed the flowmeter limits of the machines. The reservoir bag serves as a volume reservoir to meet this high flow demand during the early part of the inspiration. This reservoir function also allows for lower, and more economical fresh gas flows to be used. Most reservoir bags are elastic. Up to a certain point, the gas volume will continue to increase, but with no substantial increase in pressure (Davis and Kenny, 2003). This feature provides a degree of protection against high breathing circuit pressures. However, as the upper limit of the reservoir bag volume is approached, pressure increases quickly, and this pressure is transmitted to the patient, risking trauma. The maximum pressure reached for small breathing bags of up to 1.5 L is 50 cm H_2O at four times the nominal volume; for bags greater than 1.5 L, the pressure limit is 60 cm H_2O, but these pressures may be exceeded, if noncompliant bags are used (Davey and Diba, 2011; Dorsch and Dorsch, 2007). To minimize the risk of barotrauma, highly compliant reservoir bags (e.g., DN-3) are recommended, and bags should be prestretched before first use (Ambrisko et al., 2021). Both reusable and disposable reservoir bags are available in a variety of sizes. While the reservoir bag must at least accommodate the demands of a single tidal breath, in practice larger bags are used. The tidal volume is the amount delivered in a single breath. For veterinary patients, Lerche et al. (2000a) recommended using reservoir bags of 3–5 times the tidal volume of the patient. Fig. 9.4 gives an overview of tidal volumes and respiratory rates of common laboratory species.

Bags, intended to be disposable are thinner, lighter than reusable bags, and reasonably durable. With time, reservoir bags deteriorate and tear; they rank high on the list of the usual suspects when the machine fails a pressure test.

7. Absorber systems

Absorber systems are used with circle breathing circuits to remove carbon dioxide from exhaled breathing gases, so that they may be reused, reducing fresh gas requirements, and conserving volatile anesthetic agents, moisture, and heat. Absorbents are granular materials, typically comprising calcium hydroxide and water with small amounts of potassium, sodium, or barium hydroxide to speed up the uptake of carbon dioxide. A small amount of water is essential for the absorbent to function properly. Carbon dioxide is removed by an exothermic chemical reaction with the formation of calcium carbonate. A color change, indicated by pH-sensitive dyes, signals that the absorbent is exhausted and needs to be changed.

Sevoflurane is known to degrade in the presence of conventional soda lime to produce a product called Compound A, which has been found to have nephrotoxic effects at high levels in animals (Kharasch et al., 2005; Van Bocxlaer and Mortier, 2004). However, nowadays, preparations are available that generate no Compound A at all, regardless of the degree of humidity (Struys et al., 2014).

General recommendations emphasize measures to avoid drying absorbents, changing all absorbents when the indicator changes color, and changing absorbents regardless of color indicator if it has not been used for some time (Coppens et al., 2006).

The configuration of absorber assemblies varies in detail, but in all designs, the exhaled gas is directed through the assembly by way of the unidirectional valves (described earlier). The fresh gas inlet for the circle system is located near or on the assembly, usually adjacent to the outflow side.

Absorbents are sold in several forms: as sealed packages designed for one filling, prefilled canister inserts to fit many common absorber canisters, and in bulk containers. While bulk supplies are less expensive per unit weight, they are more difficult to seal and are best used in facilities with

Species (and typical adult body weight)	Respiratory rate (breathes/minute)	Tidal volume (ml) of an adult animal or mk/kg of bodyweight)
Mini-Pig, Dog (20kg)	15-25	150
Pig (>20kg), Sheep (>20kg)	10-15	8-10ml/kg
Primates (>5kg)	20-30	8-10ml/kg
Marmosets (500g)	40-50	4-5ml
Rabbit (3kg)	25-40	20-30
Guinea pig (1kg)	50-80	8-10
Rat (250g)	60-100	2-2.5
Mouse (30g)	80-120	0.25-0.3

FIGURE 9.4 Tidal volumes and respiratory rates of common laboratory animals (P. Flecknell).

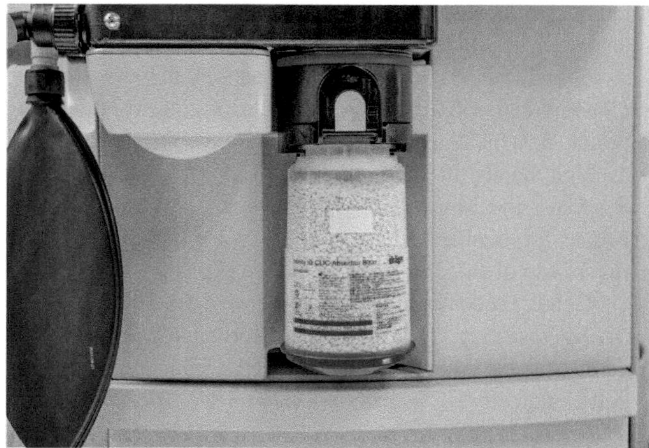
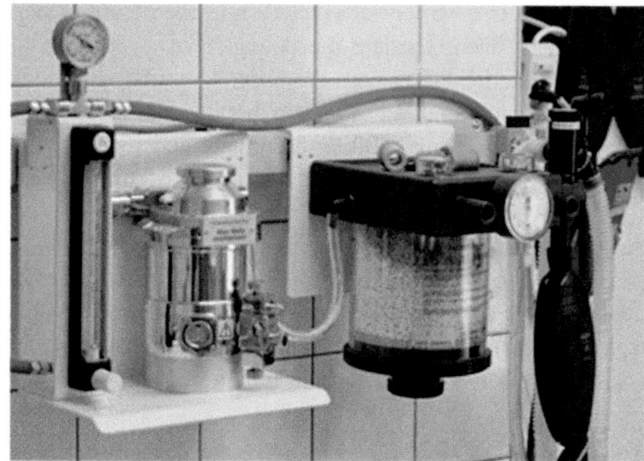

FIGURE 9.5 Disposable canister with absorbent (*left*, F. Gantenbein), refillable system (*right*, Rothacher medical).

relatively high workloads. Absorbers should be cleaned when they are refilled to remove dust and caked absorbent. In order to minimize leaks, absorbent granules and dust should be removed from the canister rim and seals before closing the canister. Disposable absorber systems are used on some veterinary and human machines. They are available in a number of configurations (Fig. 9.5).

B. Nonrebreathing systems

A number of systems have been described and also classified (Kaul and Mittal, 2013; Mapleson, 1998). Although called nonrebreathing systems, the amount of rebreathing that occurs is largely dependent upon the fresh gas flow. While these circuits differ somewhat in their characteristics, in general, the higher the fresh gas flow, the less rebreathing is liable to occur. On the other hand, elevated respiratory rates may increase the risk of rebreathing.

In contrast to the rebreathing system, the parts of the breathing circuits differ from one type to the other. Nonrebreathing systems are useful, especially for small patients, and they are extensively used for rodent anesthesia. The simplest nonrebreathing system is the open mask system. The most frequently used systems are described below. Many of these circuits are available as preassembled disposable units.

One advantage of these systems is that changes in vaporizer settings are rapidly reflected in these breathing circuits, as most of these circuits deliver fresh gas close to the endotracheal tube or mask connection. For example, in the Bain modification (described in more detail below) the flow is directly in line with the patient connection. If a rapid change in inhaled concentration is needed, altering the vaporizer setting and increasing the fresh gas flow at the flowmeter will suffice.

On the other hand, there is a serious risk of barotrauma in activating the oxygen flush valve, when the patient is connected to these systems. The flush valve should not be used in this situation. Nonrebreathing systems also have a limited volume compared with circle systems, so the pressure in the breathing circuit can rise rapidly when the APL valve is partially closed, as it is when manually assisting ventilation. The anesthetist must be scrupulous in returning the APL valve to the open position after delivering a breath. A distracted or inattentive anesthetist can be unpleasantly surprised at the speed with which the breathing circuit pressure rises to dangerous levels. A unique modification of the APL valve, the Humphrey valve, allows greater efficiency in the use of Mapleson-A, -E, and -D circuits (described in more detail below) in terms of convenience and fresh gas flow requirements (Davey and Diba, 2011; Dorsch and Dorsch, 2007).

1. Open mask circuit

In the open mask circuit, the exhaled gases are removed by the arriving fresh gas flow, which pushes these gases out of the mask. Care has to be taken to have a gas flow high enough to avoid breathing room air leading to a decrease in the depth of anesthesia. Besides relatively high costs due to the high gas flow rates, the main disadvantage is that patient's ventilation cannot be assisted. Also, this setup requires a separate scavenging system (such as an active suction system placed near the head) to avoid workplace pollution.

2. Magill circuit (Mapleson-A)

Fig. 9.6A depicts a configuration called the Magill circuit, to be used for patients heavier than 10 kg. The fresh gas enters near the reservoir bag, flows toward the patient through a corrugated tube, and exits via a relief valve adjacent to the mask or endotracheal tube. The direction of gas flow, which forces expired gas out of the circuit very close to the patient connection, makes it very efficient for spontaneous breathing because alveolar gas is eliminated early during expiration (Conway, 1985). It is less efficient for assisted or controlled ventilation and should not be used with some mechanical ventilators (Dorsch and Dorsch, 2007). The circuit is somewhat clumsy to use because of the location of the relief valve and the scavenging tubing near the patient's head.

The Lack system is another variation of the Mapleson-A system in which the relief valve is located adjacent to the fresh gas entry point, improving convenience and scavenging connections. Originally presented as a coaxial circuit, the design has undergone further modifications. It is now available in both coaxial and parallel versions. The performance is similar to that of the Magill system. Walsh and Taylor compared a miniature parallel Lack circuit to a Jackson-Reese modified Mapleson-F circuit for use in cats and found the miniature Lack circuit to be more efficient, requiring a markedly lower fresh gas flow to prevent rebreathing (Walsh and Taylor, 2004). The Lack circuit is popular in the United Kingdom and elsewhere, but appears to be unavailable in the United States.

3. Bain circuit (Mapleson-D)

Both coaxial and parallel forms of the circuit are available (Fig. 9.6D). The coaxial version, or Bain circuit, is perhaps the most common configuration used in research institutions. In this version, fresh gas enters at the end of the circuit distal from the patient and is conducted to the patient end by a small-diameter tube contained within the large-diameter exhalation limb. The parallel circuit is similar, except that the fresh gas supply tube is outside the exhalation limb, entering the circuit near the patient connection. The circuit can be used by attaching a bag with a pressure relief valve and scavenger connection to the distal end, resulting in a somewhat cumbersome assembly. It is much more convenient to use a Mapleson-D control arm (Bain block), or universal control arm. The control arm incorporates a manometer, an APL valve and scavenging port, and a mount for the reservoir bag. Mapleson-D control arms carry the risk of inadvertent barotrauma due to a failure to open the APL valve after delivering a breath (McMurphy et al., 1995). Systems (Bain and circle) now increasingly use quick-release APL valves, which can be simply depressed to be closed and spring open when released, avoiding the need to turn them closed and risk of forgetting to open them (Fig. 9.3, bottom).

Functionally, coaxial and parallel systems have similar performance. In terms of the fresh gas flow needed to limit rebreathing, Mapleson-D circuits are less efficient than Mapleson-A circuits during spontaneous breathing. During assisted or controlled ventilation, it is generally considered that moderate fresh gas flows in conjunction with adequate minute ventilation will avoid hypercapnia (Davey and Diba, 2011; Dorsch and Dorsch, 2007; Lerche et al., 2000b).

Fresh gas flows of 100−130 mL/kg/minute, with a minimum flow of 0.5 L/minute (liters per minute) (or the lowest flow marked on the flowmeter), have been recommended for small animals, although higher flows may be needed in patients with increased respiration rates to avoid rebreathing (Bain and Spoerel, 1979; Grimm et al., 2015; Sasse et al., 1979).

4. Mapleson-E circuits

Mapleson-E circuits (Fig. 9.6E) perform much like Mapleson-D circuits but lack a reservoir bag. The expiratory end of the circuit is open or, if inhalant anesthesia is used, connected to a scavenging interface. Without a reservoir bag, the circuit is not well suited to assisted ventilation. Some rodent anesthesia machines use a parallel or coaxial Mapleson-D circuit, omitting the reservoir bag and APL valve. In this form, it is a Mapleson-E circuit.

5. Jackson-Rees/Ayre's T-piece circuits (Mapleson-F)

The Ayre's T-piece (Fig. 9.6F) is the classic example but, in its simplest form, is seldom used for inhalation anesthesia (Oswald et al., 2018). The Jackson-Rees modification is commonly used. The modified circuit is similar to the Mapleson-E, but a reservoir bag is added with provision for scavenging at the distal end of the bag (tail), alongside an adjustable pressure relief valve (Fukunaga, 2019). It offers a simple, cheap lightweight design but requires high fresh gas flow adding to cost and environmental pollution. Arnold and colleagues discuss the pros and cons, possible indications and limitations for the T-Piece are discussed together with alternative strategies (Arnold and Kaufmann, 2022).

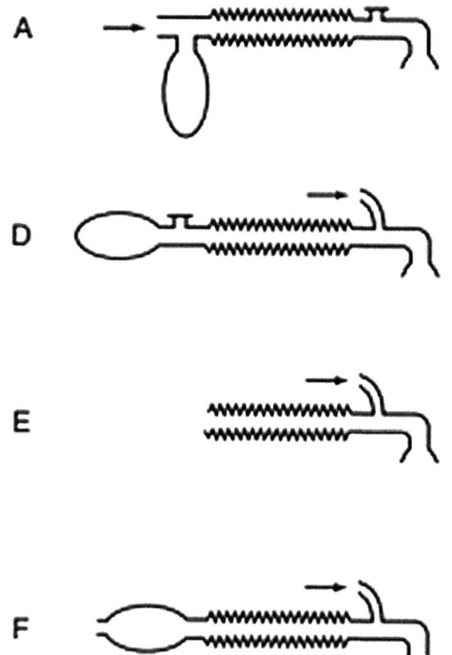

FIGURE 9.6 Drawings of different Mapleson circuits. Redraw with permission of the British Journal of Anaesthesia and Dr. W. Mapleson

C. Carrier gas supply, flow and scavenging

1. Supply

The compressed gases most commonly used in laboratory animal anesthesia are oxygen and medical air. The manufacture of compressed gases, cylinders, and associated delivery equipment is regulated by governmental agencies. Medical gases are treated as drugs, and their composition, manufacture, and identification are further regulated by appropriate national entities. Gases and gas mixtures intended for industrial use may contain toxic contaminants and hence should not be used for medical purposes.

a. Tanks

Medical gas cylinders are color-coded. Although color codes are helpful in identifying cylinder contents, the label should always be read to ensure the correct gas is being used. Gas cylinders are identified by a series of numbers and symbols stamped into the metal near the neck. These markings specify the type and manufacturing standard for the cylinder, the maximum service pressure, the maker or owner, the serial number, the test date, and inspector's identification. The user should ensure that the label clearly and legibly describes the contents. Cylinders with missing or defaced labels should be returned to the vendor, and should not be used.

Safety Precautions: Compressed gas cylinders are potentially hazardous; all those who handle, connect, or use cylinders should be aware of the danger and be trained in safe handling practices (Davey and Diba, 2011; Dorsch and Dorsch, 2007). A few elements of safe practice are summarized below:

1. Cylinders should be stored in a manner that prevents exposure to extremes of temperature, weather, and chemicals or fumes that can cause corrosion of valves and caps.
2. Cylinders should never be subjected to rough or careless handling. Cylinder carriers or carts should always be used for moving cylinders. Cylinders in use or in storage should be properly secured.
3. Cylinders should be inspected before use. Damaged cylinders or valve components should be tagged and the cylinder returned to the filler. No attempt to repair a cylinder should be made by the user.
4. Cylinder labels should be legible and the contents clearly identified. Regardless of color code, the cylinder should not be used if the label is illegible.
5. Cylinder valves should be opened slowly to avoid damage or explosion caused by sudden temperature and pressure increases. Before connecting cylinders to yokes, manifolds, or regulators, the valve should be slightly opened to clear dust and debris from the port, then closed again for attachment.
6. Cylinder valves, connections, and regulators must be kept free of foreign materials. Never attempt to lubricate a gas fitting, and avoid exposing any fitting to oils, greases, or any other flammable substance.
7. Connection to regulators, manifolds, and yokes should never be forced. Connection hardware is designed to prevent the connection of incompatible gases and equipment. Failure to connect easily indicates incompatible or damaged fittings and represents a potential safety hazard.

Small tanks ("E cylinders") are mounted on the anesthetic machine or attached to a separate regulator by means of a yoke assembly. The cylinder valve port forms a flush connection with the yoke, using the Pin Index Safety System (PISS) specific to a particular gas, preventing the wrong gas from being connected to the yoke. Damaged or missing pins can defeat the safety system, and care should be taken to inspect the yoke each time a fresh cylinder is mounted to assure that the pins are intact and the yoke is in good condition.

A gasket is used to assure a gas-tight seal between the cylinder and the yoke. E cylinders are usually supplied with a fresh gasket fitted over the port and covered by a plastic seal. The gasket should be replaced each time a fresh tank is mounted. If both the cylinder port and the yoke are in good repair, only a single gasket is needed. In case of a leaky connection, the yoke should be repaired if needed, or the cylinder should be labeled and returned to the supplier.

Special cylinder wrenches, or handles, are made to fit small tank valves. These valves incorporate a pressure relief device opposite the outlet port and below the conical depression for the yoke retaining screw. The pressure relief device is designed to release the tank contents at unsafe levels of pressure, temperature, or both.

Large tanks are used to supply small central piping systems, or to directly supply gas to an anesthetic machine. The valve assembly includes a hand wheel, so a wrench is not needed to open or close the valve. The threaded protective cap that covers the valve assembly during shipping should remain in place until the tank is in use. Tank valves are not pressure regulators. For safe use, a pressure regulator is necessary, either for individual tanks or as part of a manifold supply system. Large tank outlet ports use specific styles and patterns of threaded connections to minimize the risk of unsafe connections with regulators or manifolds. As with small cylinders, a safety relief device is incorporated into the valve assembly.

b. Medical gas piping systems

Central medical gas supply systems offer considerable advantages in terms of safety and convenience. In various configurations, such systems supply medical gases, medical vacuum, and, in most cases, central waste anesthetic scavenging connections to surgical and medical support sites.

Outlets for central gas piping systems are configured as wall connections, ceiling drops, or more elaborate fixed or retractable utility drops incorporating the required gases, vacuum, and scavenging services, as well as electrical outlets. The reduction in the need to routinely transport cylinders to and from the surgical areas greatly enhances the safety, sanitation, and convenience of surgical and procedural areas. There are several common styles of outlets, including several proprietary "quick disconnect" designs, all intended to prevent misconnections.

c. Oxygen concentrators

Oxygen concentrators are typically used as stationary sources to provide long-term oxygen therapy to patients at home. These continuous-flow oxygen regulators consist of wheeled cabinets housing the compressor and filters and could be connected to the anesthesia machine via tubing. They come in different sizes, with the common ones delivering flow rates of up to 5 L/minute of 92%–96% pure oxygen and only a few concentrators being capable of delivering flow rates of up to 10 L/minute. They can be equipped with a humidifier or nebulizer to moisten the inhaled air and offer a safe and convenient lightweight and mobile alternative to heavy static gas tanks during anesthesia. They need no pressure regulators and are increasingly used with rodent anesthesia machines.

Oxygen concentrators typically separate oxygen from the principal component of air, nitrogen, via a pressure swing adsorption mechanism. Following compression, the air passes through a series of valves balancing the flow through several sieve beds containing an adsorbent. This absorbent is typically silica and/or aluminum-based zeolite, which binds the gas components in the air depending on their properties, such as molecular size, polarity, and electrochemical properties (Friesen et al., 1999; Friesen, 1992). Typical adsorbents bind most strongly with nitrogen, carbon dioxide, water vapor, and other gases with a strong dipole moment, and weakly with oxygen and monoatomic gases such as argon. Following adsorption, the product gas is then passed through an oxygen analyzer to confirm the output of an adequate product—the current standard for oxygen concentrators is the delivery of a product gas containing between 90% and 96% oxygen. Factors that may reduce the output of an oxygen concentrator include high altitude and high ambient humidity (Bunel et al., 2016; Friesen et al., 1999; Friesen, 1992).

It is not recommended to use fresh gas flows of less than 0.5 L/minute with an oxygen concentrator since argon can accumulate during closed-circuit anesthesia, leading to a displacement of oxygen. This is especially relevant when the inspired oxygen fraction is less than 50% (Parker and Snowdon, 1988; Dorsch and Dorsch, 2007). Care should be taken to ensure that adequate oxygen is being supplied to patients, including inspired oxygen monitoring (Parker and Snowdon, 1988). However, the produced argon does not interfere with conventional gas monitoring techniques or the function of modern vaporizers or precision flowmeters (Friesen et al., 1999; Friesen, 1992).

In large animal anesthesia, most oxygen concentrators are incapable of supplying oxygen at the rates needed in order to provide even low-flow anesthesia (Carter et al., 1985). Practitioners should be familiar with the capabilities of any oxygen concentrator units in use. Additionally, many oxygen concentrators may be unable to generate sufficient pressure to supply gas-driven ventilators, requiring a pipeline pressure of approximately 50 psi. However, piston-driven ventilators do not have this requirement (Carter et al., 1985; Dobson, 1992). Regular service is required, which may include the replacement or cleaning of filters.

2. *Carrier gas pressure regulation*

Gas pressure in anesthetic machines is conventionally divided into three zones: high, intermediate, and low-pressure systems.

The high-pressure system refers to those components connected directly to gas cylinders. Cylinder pressure is too high for patient safety, difficult to regulate at the relatively low flows required, and variable, dropping as the cylinder contents are used. Pressure reduction valves are used to lower the pressure to a safer, more constant, and more easily controlled level (Davey and Diba, 2011; Dorsch and Dorsch, 2007). When connected to a cylinder, pressure gauges give an accurate estimation of the amount remaining for gases such as oxygen. As gas is withdrawn, gauge pressure decreases proportionally. The reduction valves can be one-stage valves—with one gauge indicating the tank pressure and a defined outlet flow, or two-stage pressure valves—possessing one gauge for the tank pressure and one for variably adjusting the working pressure (Fig. 9.7). The second gauge can indicate pressure (bar or PSI) or flow (LPM, sometimes also designed as a flowmeter).

The intermediate pressure zone comprises gases entering the machine at reduced pressure from central pipelines or from cylinders equipped with pressure regulators. This system supplies gas to the flowmeter assembly, flush valve, ventilator drive, and auxiliary gas power outlets. Pressure is further reduced as breathing gases pass through the flowmeters and to the patient breathing circuit, forming the low-pressure zone of the machine.

3. Flowmeters

The gas flow to the patient's breathing circuit is controlled by flowmeters. Many different designs exist including the "classical" mechanical flowmeters with a clear glass or plastic tube as well as the use of flow restrictors or electronic flowmeters.

The tubes of mechanical flowmeters have a gradually tapered bore narrower at the bottom and wider at the top. The bore contains a float that is driven up the tube by the force of the gas flow and stops when the weight of the float equals the force of the gas. Because the space between the walls of the bore and the float increases toward the top, the height of the float increases with increasing flow. This design is called a variable-area or variable-orifice flowmeter or a Thorpe tube. A scale indicates the flow rate in liters per minute. Ball floats are read at the center of the float, cylindrical floats (bobbins) are read at the top. Bobbins vary somewhat in design, but characteristically have a flat top, a cylindrical body, and a conical base. Both ball and bobbin should not be adjusted to be lower than the lowest marked gradation on the flowmeter, to avoid providing an unknown flow of gas.

The arrangement of flowmeters is not internationally standardized (Davey and Diba, 2011).

Flow is controlled by a needle valve. On new equipment, the valves are usually equipped with positive stops to prevent damage to the needle and seat due to overtightening on closure. Valves without positive stops remain common on older veterinary machines, and care is needed not to overtighten and damage the valves.

Some older human anesthetic machines do not permit oxygen flow to be turned off completely; rather, a continuous minimum flow of oxygen is established once the machine is connected to the pipeline supply or when the small tanks are opened. This should not be mistaken for a faulty valve: it is a safety feature intended to prevent hypoxia.

It is important to note that flowmeter tubes are individually calibrated for a specific gas. Thus, tubes will not read correctly for other gases, and the tubes and floats are not interchangeable. Damaged tubes should be replaced as a unit (Dorsch and Dorsch, 2007). Unless specifically designed otherwise, flowmeters must be vertical to operate correctly; if the float contacts the side of the tube, friction will cause erroneous readings. Dirt, debris, and static electricity can also interfere with the free movement of the float. Needle valves are subject to wear and require periodic adjustment, or replacement. Valve replacement does not require the replacement of the flowmeter tube.

Flow restrictors are often used for mobile emergency medical oxygen supplies. Essentially, a small orifice is interposed between the pressure regulator and the gas outlet; constant pressure produces constant flow. In this application, flow restrictors usually employ a rotating

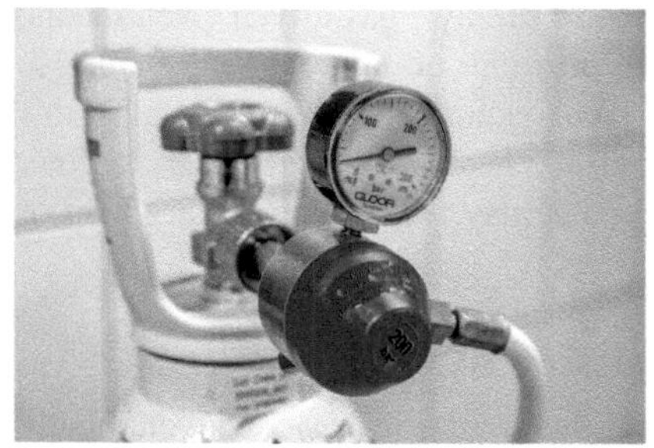

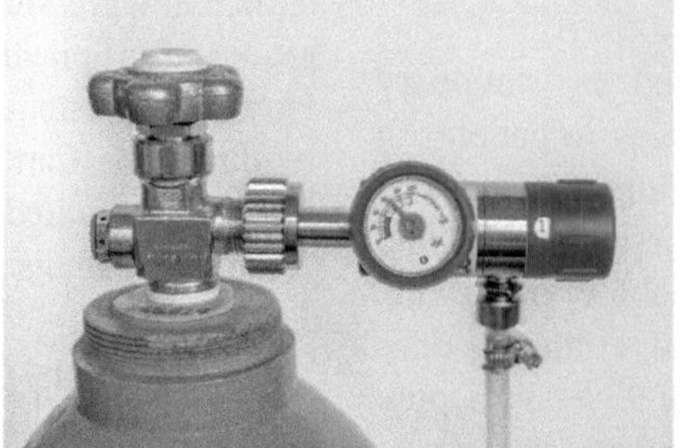

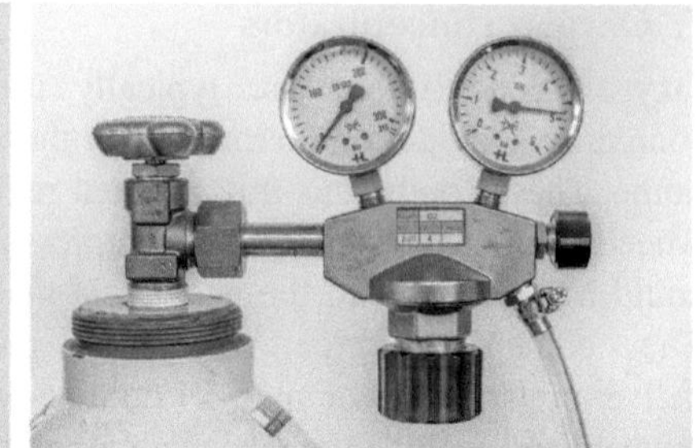

FIGURE 9.7 Different types of pressure reduction valves: one-stage with fixed reduction, the manometer indicating the tank pressure (*left*), one stage with adjustable flow via a turning knob (*middle*) and two stage with adjustable flow via a second manometer (on the *right*), the *left* manometer indicating the tank pressure (*right*) (all pictures F. Gantenbein).

cylinder with a sequence of orifices of increasing size, allowing the user to select a suitable flow rate from a range of discrete settings. Flow restrictors will function in any orientation making them well-suited for emergency and field applications.

Flow restrictors are also used in machines designed specifically to support multiple patient circuits for rodent procedures. Because these machines are intended for relatively brief, repetitive procedures on small rodents, a predetermined fixed flow rate can be used for each patient circuit. Pressure regulators in the machine maintain constant pressure so that each patient circuit can be switched on or off independently of the others (see also part E).

Gas flow can be sensed and controlled *electronically* using microprocessors to detect and control flow, and to prevent the use of hypoxic mixtures. Some machines may depend entirely upon electronic detection and control, displaying only "virtual" flowmeters on a monitor. Other models, bowing to convention and familiarity, include a single variable-area flowmeter to indicate and allow adjustment of the total flow of gas to the breathing circuit. Solenoids can be used to control fresh gas supplies by opening valves to release fresh gases to the vaporizer and breathing system. The amount of gas is determined by the frequency and duration of valve opening, yielding an accurate average flow. The specific arrangements used vary with the manufacturer and model of the machine. In general, such electronic control systems provide better accuracy than conventional variable-area flowmeters, as well as the opportunity to include additional sophisticated safety and control functions (Fig. 9.8).

4. Oxygen fail-safe and proportioning systems

Failure of the oxygen supply can be catastrophic. Ideally, anesthesia machines are equipped with alarms to warn the anesthetist of oxygen supply failure, when pressure falls below a predetermined minimum pressure (Dorsch and Dorsch, 2007). Unfortunately, oxygen failure alarms are not commonly included with all anesthesia machines. If these alarms are missing, the responsibility to monitor the supply status is placed on the user. Proportioning systems are intended to prevent hypoxic oxygen:nitrous oxide ratios. These systems may use mechanical linkages, pneumatic systems, or electronic sensors. They operate to prevent the oxygen content of the mixture from falling below a safe level, usually about 25%. On some machines, loss of normal oxygen pressure will interrupt or proportionately reduce nitrous oxide flow.

5. Oxygen flush valve

The oxygen flush valve is usually located on the front of the machine and is provided with some form of protection against accidental activation. When the valve is activated, fresh oxygen is delivered to the common gas outlet at the rate of 35–75 L/minute (varying according to supply pressure), bypassing the flowmeters and vaporizer. Flush valves are usually spring-loaded and close as soon as pressure on the button is released.

Activating the flush valve will result in rapid dilution of the anesthetic gases in the patient circuit. Although the volume of the absorber assembly and breathing tubing usually acts to buffer pressure changes, a dangerous increase in breathing circuit pressure may still occur. The APL valve, or "pop-off" valve, should be fully open when the flush valve is activated. To avoid the risk of high circuit pressures being transmitted to the patient, it is considered best practice to detach the breathing system hoses from the patient before activating the flush valve (the patient end of the hoses is occluded by the anesthetist's palm/thumb to prevent workplace pollution by directing excess gas into the scavenging system, via the open APL valve). When there is a less urgent need to lower anesthetic agent levels in the circuit, this can be achieved by turning down the

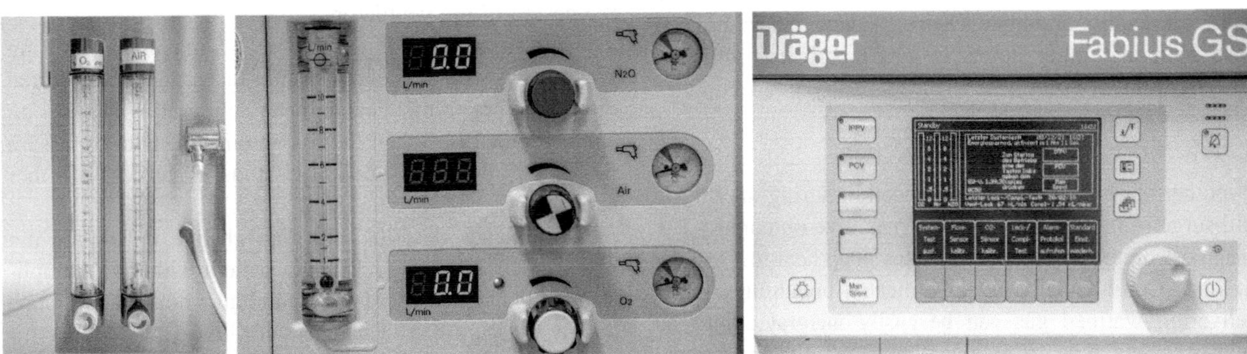

FIGURE 9.8 Different types of flowmeters: (*Left*) in a traditional flowmeter, flow is mechanically controlled (needle valve) and displayed (glass tube with ball), (*middle*) in a transitional flowmeter, flow is mechanically controlled (needle valve) and electronically displayed (bar graph on computer screen), (*right*) in electronic flowmeters, the gas mixer electronically controls flow of all gas and vapor to the patient, and these are displayed on a monitor screen (all pictures F. Gantenbein).

vaporizer and temporarily increasing fresh gas flows using the flowmeter.

6. Common gas outlet

The common gas outlet is the point at which the mixture of breathing gas and anesthetic agent exits the machine and, by means of a connecting hose, enters the breathing circuit. Depending upon the manufacturer, model, and intended use, common gas outlet appearance and labeling may vary considerably.

7. Scavenging systems

Scavenging systems are used to avoid health risks for staff exposed to waste anesthetic gases and comprise collection devices, interfaces, and disposal systems (Figueiredo et al., 2021). The most common collection device is the APL valve, used for circle systems, and some types of nonrebreathing circuit adaptors. In other nonrebreathing circuits, waste gas is conducted directly from the circuit or reservoir bag to the interface.

Charcoal canisters are often used for nonrebreathing systems to scavenge anesthetic gases from the working environment. These canisters contain activated carbon, which adsorbs all organic gases extremely efficiently. They can be used either passively or in combination with active scavenging units to scavenge anesthetic gases from the working environment. Active scavenging makes use of a fan or pump to provide continuous low pressure at the scavenging interface, drawing the waste gas into the disposal system. Vacuum systems use narrow gauge tubing to conduct gas to a central suction system, and generate a large pressure differential. Fan-driven duct systems operate at much lower pressure differences and employ wide-gauge tubing and ducts to remove a high volume of gas. Active scavenging systems ordinarily have an additional valve to regulate the suction from the vacuum or duct system. Passive scavenging uses the pressure generated in the breathing circuit to drive gas to the interface. Scavenging interfaces require periodic cleaning to remove accumulated dust, hair, and other debris to avoid problems with the scavenging interfaces.

8. Warmed breathing circuit

Hypothermia is a common complication during anesthesia and surgery, increasing the risk of negative outcomes. The usage of compressed gases facilitates body heat loss via the airways. Commercially available heated breathing circuits delivering warmed gas can be easily integrated into an anesthesia machine. Bowling et al. (2021) demonstrated that a heated breathing circuit had a significant positive effect on perianesthetic body temperature in rhesus macaques, with a faster return to baseline temperature and higher body temperatures during a 2-hour anesthetic procedure. Heated anesthesia breathing circuits are a significant refinement to thermal support anesthesia, especially for longer-lasting procedures.

D. Ventilators

Mechanical ventilators are an integral part of most modern anesthesia workstations and are used to free the anesthetist from the task of manually assisting ventilation (Jain and Swaminathan, 2013). In terms of both physiology and technology, the subject of positive pressure ventilation is complex. Readers unfamiliar with the subject should consult anesthesia and respiratory therapy texts for thorough discussions. The following is a greatly simplified overview of the terminology and technology used in positive pressure ventilation. There are substantial differences in ventilator designs; a careful reading of the operating manual for the ventilator is essential to understand the controls, abilities, and limitations of each specific model. More in-depth information can be found in the textbooks recommended for additional reading in Section IV.

It is useful to define a few of the terms used in describing ventilator functions and controls before discussing individual examples. The minute volume is the total amount of gas delivered to the patient in 1 minute. The minute volume equals the tidal volume multiplied by the respiratory rate. The inspiratory flow rate is the rate at which the gas enters the airways and is, in effect, the speed at which a tidal volume is delivered. The inspiratory flow phase is the time from the beginning of inspiratory flow to the beginning of expiratory flow, including an inspiratory pause, if present. The period from the end of the inspiratory flow phase until the beginning of the next inspiratory flow phase is the expiratory phase time. The inspiratory and expiratory phase time ratio, or I:E ratio, is fixed at about 1:2 on some ventilators, but can be altered on others. Because these variables are interrelated, they may be set directly or indirectly using a combination of controls, and vary with the design of the ventilator.

Maximum inspiratory pressure, or maximum working pressure, is the highest pressure that can be generated during the breathing cycle and can be preset by the user on some ventilators. When the maximum inspiratory pressure is reached, the inspiratory flow stops, regardless of other settings.

Compliance describes the unit change in volume per unit change in pressure. Thus, a patient with high compliance will have a greater increase in lung volume at the same airway pressure than a patient with low compliance. Animals with compliant chest walls, such as rabbits, maybe over-distended and suffer lung damage at pressures safe, or even necessary for a larger and less compliant patient, such as a pig. Patients are not the only source of compliance;

equipment compliance due to distensible circuits and other machine components can reduce the volume the patient receives from the ventilator. Although this is not ordinarily a problem with large tidal volumes, it should be considered when small tidal volumes are used.

Positive end-expiratory pressure (PEEP) maintains a controlled minimum pressure in the airways at the end of expiration, preventing complete collapse of the small airways during positive pressure ventilation. A discussion of the indications for using PEEP is beyond the scope of this chapter, but it is mentioned because anesthesia machines may have an integrated PEEP valve. PEEP can also be applied by interposing a PEEP valve in the expiratory limb of the breathing circuit, usually attached to the expiratory unidirectional valve. Reusable PEEP valves are sold individually or in sets, including a range of pressures indicated in centimeters of water.

The basic ventilation mode for most anesthesia ventilators is intermittent positive pressure ventilation (IPPV). The ventilator delivers a breath at the frequency determined directly or indirectly by the control settings, and exhalation is passive. However, the patient can also breathe independently of the ventilator. The inspiratory phase can be terminated based on time, pressure, volume, or flow rate. Most veterinary anesthesia ventilators are volume- or pressure-cycled (and may also include a maximum allowable time for the inspiratory phase), and most have a control to limit the maximum inspiratory pressure. The mode of ventilation refers to the breathing pattern, usually based on delivered volume or pressure. Some anesthesia ventilators may offer the user a choice of ventilation modes. For example, the ventilator may be able to monitor spontaneous breathing and match it to deliver a desired tidal volume. A number of different ventilation modes are used and are described differently by various manufacturers (Davey and Diba, 2011).

Ventilators suitable for use with magnetic resonance imaging equipment are available in models suitable for patients ranging in size from adult humans to mice.

Positive pressure anesthesia ventilators require a source of compressed gas as bellows, pistons, or valves directly controlling the high-pressure gas are used to direct the tidal volume to the patient. In the following section, they are referred to as bellows, piston, and pneumatic ventilators, although the latter description is not strictly accurate.

1. *Bellows ventilators*

The most common design of veterinary anesthesia ventilator uses bellows housed in a transparent housing. The bellows are intermittently compressed by high-pressure gas admitted into the surrounding housing. This design, which separates the drive gas in the housing from the breathing gas in the bellows, is called a dual circuit. The tidal volume can be controlled by limiting the excursion of the bellows with a mechanical stop; in that case, the bellows are completely emptied with each breath. Alternatively, and more commonly, the tidal volume may be determined by precisely limiting the volume of drive gas entering the housing. Because the bellows are emptied proportionately to the amount of drive gas entering the housing, the bellows may not be completely emptied. A ventilator exhaust valve releases the drive gas in the housing during exhalation (the breathing system APL valve is usually closed when a mechanical ventilator is in use).

The pressure generated in the breathing circuit is primarily a function of the volume of gas delivered by the bellows. However, the fresh gas flow can also affect delivered pressure and volume. In new ventilators, this is addressed by fresh gas decoupling, which prevents the interaction between the ventilator, oxygen flush valve, and fresh gas flow. Excess gas in the patient circuit is exhausted by a relief valve, or spill valve, after the bellows are refilled. A spill valve is needed because, in most cases, the APL valve is closed or isolated from the breathing circuit during positive pressure ventilation. Tidal volume, maximum inspiratory pressure, and rate are adjusted to achieve the desired ventilation pattern. The breathing system manometer indicates pressure in the breathing system.

For many ventilators, interchangeable pediatric bellows assemblies are available. If the ventilator is integrated into the anesthesia machine, a selector switch is used to isolate the APL valve and reservoir bag and open a connection between the ventilator and the breathing circuit. Otherwise, the APL valve is closed, and the reservoir bag is removed and replaced with the ventilator hose.

2. *Piston ventilators*

Piston ventilators use an electrically driven piston to deliver a preset volume to the breathing circuit. The volume is determined by the diameter of the cylinder and the stroke of the piston. In many models, interchangeable cylinder assemblies are available to provide a range of tidal volumes. The stroke is controlled either by electronic or, more typically, by a mechanical linkage to alter the swept volume of the cylinder. The selection of tidal volume is usually based upon the patient weight, taken from a nomogram or chart, or derived from experience (ideally, capnography should be used to guide minute ventilation). The assumption is that all patients are typical or normal. In piston ventilators, all of the tidal volume is delivered to the patient regardless of the airway pressure. Therefore, implementing an airway manometer into the breathing circuit can help to prevent, or at least diagnose, the risk for barotrauma.

Conversely, if an oral endotracheal tube is used in rodents, the lack of a cuff will result in a variable amount of leakage around the tube. In this case, the selected tidal volume represents the total of the desired tidal volume and the additional volume needed to compensate for the leak, which may account for some of the diverse ventilator settings reported in the literature (see also paragraph III).

Piston ventilators are generally rugged and reliable, but they do require maintenance. Cleaning and proper lubrication are essential for proper performance, as is the replacement of worn components.

3. Pneumatic ventilators

If the gas delivery pressure is known, a selected volume of gas can be delivered by timing the opening and closing of a valve controlling the inspiratory flow. Alternatively, the pressure in the breathing circuit can be measured and the inspiratory valve closed at a predetermined pressure setting. Both of these means are used to regulate tidal volumes in some of the ventilators previously described. Rodent ventilators are available, which allow for volume- or pressure-limited modes using valves connected directly to the patient breathing circuit.

4. Jet ventilation and high-frequency ventilation

Briefly, a jet ventilator is a small-diameter tube inserted into the trachea through which oxygen is supplied at relatively high pressures. The technique, also called transtracheal ventilation, is used in situations where an endotracheal tube cannot be used and a tracheotomy is not desired, such as in some head and neck procedures, during bronchoscopy, or in emergencies when an airway cannot be secured. In a situation where the patient cannot be intubated and cannot be ventilated by mask, a catheter is inserted percutaneously into the trachea and connected to the common gas outlet of the anesthesia machine. The techniques and equipment are described in Davey and Diba (2011).

High-frequency ventilation is characterized by very high respiration rates and very small tidal volumes. The technique is used to maintain perfusion and oxygenation in a collapsed lung during surgery, or to ventilate patients with some types of lung disease. It may also be used with jet ventilation. High-frequency positive-pressure ventilation is possible with some current anesthesia ventilators, and special ventilators are made for high-frequency jet ventilation. During high-frequency oscillatory ventilation, normal respiratory excursions cease and only a slight vibration is seen. While initially disconcerting, the lack of gross movement may be an advantage in some surgical procedures.

E. Anesthesia systems for batches of animals

Many rodent procedures are relatively brief and are performed on groups of animals in a short time period. Anesthesia systems for batches of animals permit multiple animals to be anesthetized with one anesthesia system while using only one vaporizer/gas supply. These systems are commonly used for rodents, where batches of animals undergo an identical procedure, e.g., within imaging equipment or certain types of longitudinal sampling under anesthesia. The gas flow is adjusted centrally so that all of the patients can be adequately and safely anesthetized using the same fresh gas flow and anesthetic agent concentration. Several approaches are used to divide the flow from the vaporizer.

A simple method is to subdivide the flow from the vaporizer using a sufficient number of sequential Y-connectors and tubings to form the needed number of patient circuits. Simple on/off valves can be used to open or close individual patient circuits. The resistance to flow is directly proportional to the length and inversely proportional to the diameter of the tubing and connectors. For every patient to receive the same fresh gas flow, each leg of the assembly, measured from the vaporizer outlet to the patient mask, should be of equal length. The fresh gas flow to the vaporizer must be adjusted to take into account the number of open circuits. If, for example, six circuits are in use and the desired flow to each is 0.5 L/minute, the total flow would be 3.0 L/minute. As the procedures are completed, if five of the circuits are closed without proportionately decreasing the total flow, the remaining animal would receive 3.0 L/minute, an excessively high flow that might impede breathing. Leaving an unoccupied circuit open avoids the need to adjust the flowmeter, but further contributes to pollution with anesthetic gas and hence is not an acceptable practice. Each patient circuit also requires appropriate scavenging connections. Several commercial machines using this basic system are available. Alternatively, this type of multi-circuit design can be easily assembled onsite. However, as more circuits are added, the proliferation of tubing, connectors, and valves becomes difficult to keep track of and promotes operator error.

Additionally, multi-circuit rodent machines are available that provide adjustable flowmeters to control the flow rate to each breathing circuit. In this arrangement, the individual flowmeters are placed downstream of the vaporizer output, to separately control the flow to each mask. The total fresh gas to the vaporizer must be sufficient to allow further division of the vaporizer output for each individual patient circuit. Once this condition is met, individual circuits may be controlled by their respective flowmeters without further adjustment of the master flowmeter. An overpressure relief valve or a secondary low-pressure regulator is used to prevent excessive pressure and damage to the vaporizer and master flowmeter should the circuit flowmeters be turned off without turning off the master flowmeter.

So-called manifolds allow for the convenient arrangement and proper gas distribution for a number of rodents that need to be anesthetized for an identical procedure at the same time, e.g., during high-throughput imaging procedures (Fig. 9.9).

There are systems allowing the anesthetic agent concentration to be independently adjusted for each circuit. This is accomplished by selecting the desired flow and anesthetic concentration at the master flowmeter and vaporizer, respectively. Fresh gas flow from the vaporizer is equally divided between the patient stations in use so that the flow set at the master flowmeter is the sum of the desired flows to each of the stations in use. Each patient station has a secondary, or auxiliary oxygen flowmeter, which can be used to dilute the fresh gas flow from the vaporizer to a lower agent concentration determined by the user. Thus, in this design, the maximum agent concentration is set at the vaporizer, but lower concentrations can be obtained at each station, at the discretion of the operator.

A relatively new class of rodent anesthesia machines uses flow restrictors in place of variable-area flowmeters. These machines offer multiple patient circuits controlled by simple pneumatic switches; the circuit is either on or off. An internal pressure regulator is used to maintain a constant pressure, which varies little with the number of circuits in use, so that a constant fixed flow is generated in the circuit. In operation, the user selects the agent concentration on the vaporizer and turns on the requisite number of circuits as needed.

F. Maintenance and testing

Maintenance of anesthetic machines is essential to assure safety and performance. While the operator's manual is usually the best source for information concerning user maintenance, cleanliness is a universal recommendation. Operating rooms are not a friendly environment for anesthesia machines. Many cleaning agents, intravenous fluids,

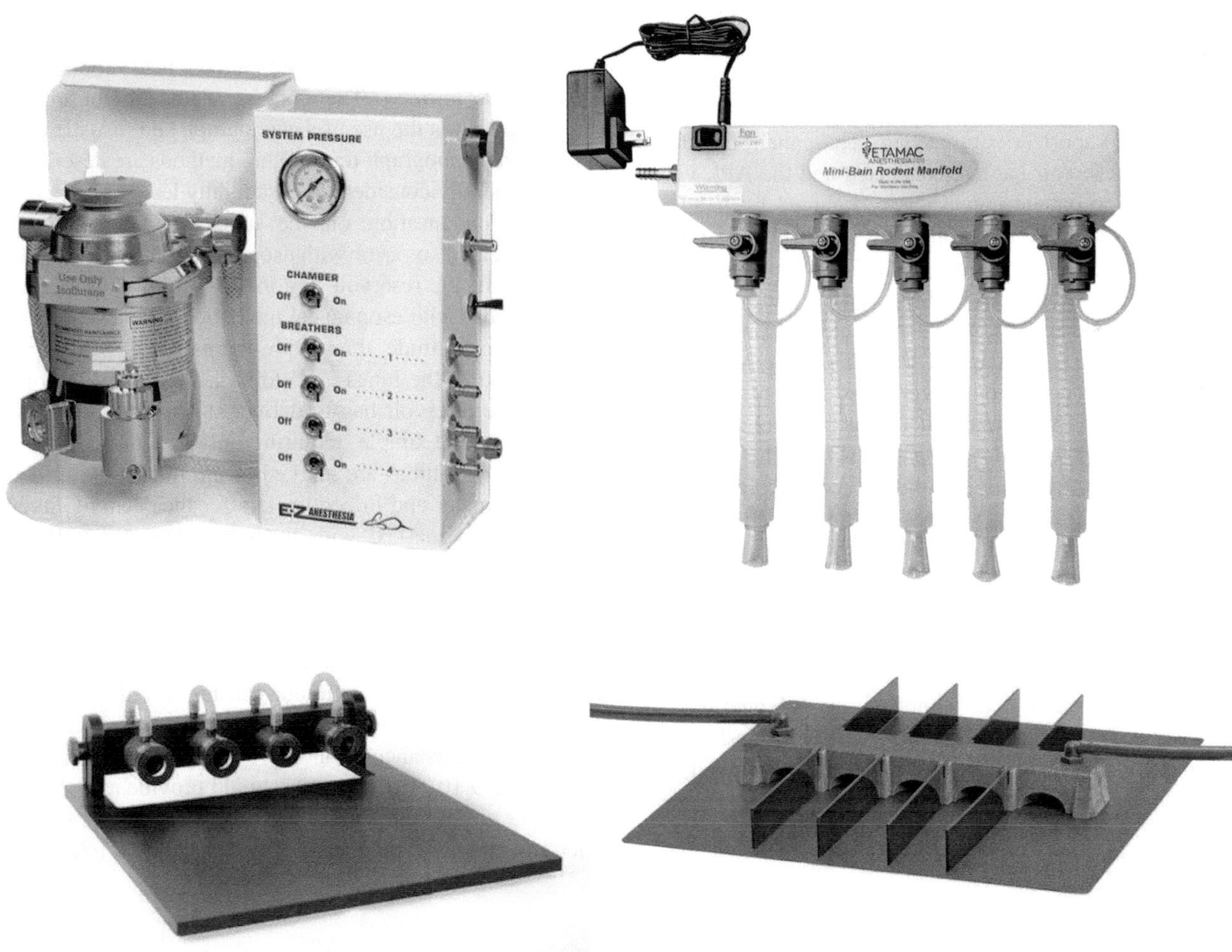

FIGURE 9.9 Different types of anesthesia systems and manifolds for anesthetizing multiple animals at the same time (from *top left to bottom right*: E-Z systems, vetamac, Orchid Scientific, Somni Scientific).

and disinfectants attack metal surfaces, especially on prolonged contact. Dust and hair accumulate on all exposed surfaces; if allowed to infiltrate the control mechanisms of flowmeters, vaporizers, and APL valves, debris can cause premature failure. The anesthesia machine should be always tested before use. A few basic elements of checkout procedures are described below. Modification of the procedures may be needed for specific machines (Dorsch and Dorsch, 2007). With consistent use, the procedures can be accomplished in a reasonably short time and are an essential method of assuring patient and personnel safety. It is strongly recommended that users develop and implement a regular schedule of checkout procedures. Circuit leak tests are typically recommended before each anesthetic with more complete testing once daily/weekly depending on frequency of use, or each time a machine is moved to a different location.

The machine should be inspected to assure that breathing gas oxygen supplies are adequate, properly connected, and functioning. The flowmeters are turned on and off while observing the float. It should move smoothly as the flow is increased and decreased, and it should indicate zero flow in the off position.

With no fresh gas flow, the vaporizer is checked for adequate fill level, ensuring that the filling port is closed and that the vaporizer is turned off. The patient breathing circuit and reservoir bag are connected and the APL valve is closed. The patient connector is occluded by hand or, more conveniently, an appropriately sized rubber stopper. Using the flowmeters or oxygen flush valve, the bag is filled to a pressure of 30–40 cm H_2O on the breathing system manometer. The pressure should not drop over a 10 second period (Dorsch and Dorsch, 2007). Mason describes a similar test, but specifies a drop of less than 5 cm H_2O over a 30 second period. The pressure is released using the APL valve, allowing assessment of the valve and preventing dust from the absorber from being forced into the breathing circuit by sudden decompression. If a universal control arm is used, the Mapleson circuits can be similarly assessed. However, coaxial versions of these systems, such as Bain circuits, must also be tested to assure that the inner fresh tube has not become disconnected (a relatively common occurrence and cause of increased mechanical dead space). A disposable syringe plunger is used to occlude the inner fresh gas tube while the fresh gas is flowing. When the fresh gas supply tube is occluded, the flowmeter indicator should fall. Disconnection of the fresh gas tube can convert the entire circuit into apparatus dead space.

III. Patient interface

A. Airway management device

Airway management devices (endotracheal tubes, supraglottic airway devices = SADs) are used to provide oxygen and to deliver anesthetic breathing mixtures. Using an airway management device in combination with a breathing system enables better control and support of respiratory function. When combined with monitoring systems and positive pressure ventilation, physiological variables such as arterial carbon dioxide concentrations can be maintained within normal limits.

1. Endotracheal tubes

Endotracheal tubes are passed through the larynx and into the trachea. Many modified and specialty endotracheal tubes are available for nasal intubation, endobronchial intubation, laser surgery, respiratory gas sampling, and other special applications. They are well described, illustrated, and discussed in current anesthesia equipment texts, and in numerous published papers (Dorsch and Dorsch, 2007).

The correct placement of the endotracheal tube should always be confirmed. The gold standard for confirming tube placement is the use of a capnograph and visualization of a normal capnograph trace. Other methods are described, but are generally considered substantially less sensitive and specific. Condensation on the tube can be deceiving, because it can also occur with esophageal placement. Also, excursions of the reservoir bag in synchrony with respiration can occur with esophageal intubation, albeit usually in a smaller magnitude than with intratracheal placement. Auscultation of the lungs and stomach while briskly compressing the reservoir bag to deliver short small breaths is more certain and simple, requiring only a stethoscope.

Commercial tubes are marked in millimeters with their internal diameter and in centimeters for their length. Some tubes are also marked with the outer diameter (OD) in millimeters. Tubes can be purchased in a range of different diameters (2 mm upwards). While the size of the tube is known, tracheal diameter is estimated based on anesthetist experience. The tube diameter should be small enough to pass through the larynx without causing any damage, but large enough to fill most of the trachea in order to reduce leakage and resistance to airflow. Tubes can be plain or cuffed (Fig. 9.10). Cuffed tubes should provide a good seal when the cuff is inflated. An endotracheal tube should extend from the tip of the nose to the thoracic inlet. The

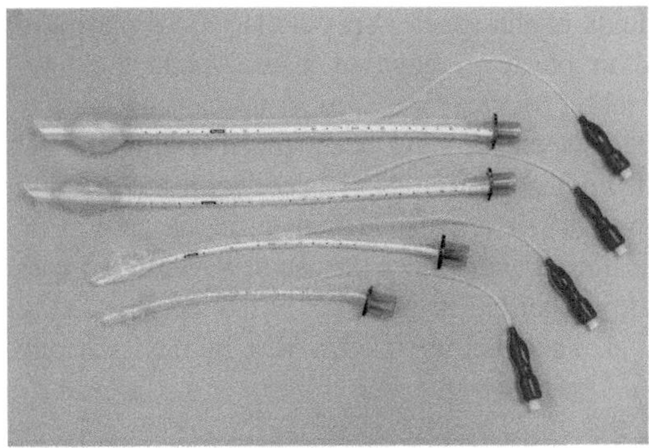
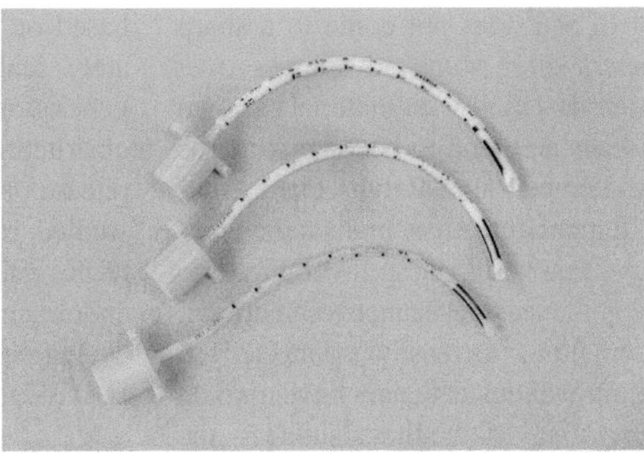
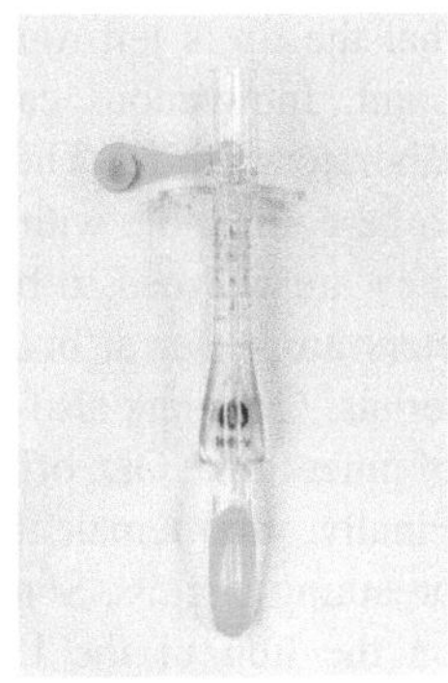

FIGURE 9.10 Different types and sizes of endotracheal tubes with (*left*) and without cuff (*middle*), V-gel airway devices are available for rabbits and cats (*right*, all pictures F. Gantenbein).

length of the tube extending beyond the patient's mouth does add to equipment dead space, and may contribute significantly to rebreathing in small patients, therefore, tubes should be cut to fit.

Most endotracheal tubes have a preformed curve. The curve increases visualization of the laryngeal opening when intubation is performed using a conventional laryngoscope. The distal end is beveled and may have a small opening opposite the bevel called a Murphy eye, intended to provide an additional path for gas if the bevel is occluded. A radiopaque marker is often present to help with the radiographic assessment of the tube position.

The tubes most commonly encountered are made of polyvinyl chloride (PVC), polyurethane (PU), silicone rubber, and red rubber tubes. In general, PVC tubes are less expensive, lighter than silicone or red rubber tubes, transparent, and offer a good balance of wall thickness to internal diameter. While PVC tubes are somewhat rigid at room temperature, they soften as they warm to body temperature. PU tubes are softer than PVC tubes, but offer many of the same advantages, although at a higher price. Silicone tubes are soft and are translucent rather than transparent. They are thick-walled in comparison with PVC tubes. However, silicone tubes are relatively resistant to kinking and can be autoclaved. The use of red rubber tubes has decreased because they are opaque, subject to deterioration, use low volume-high pressure cuffs (associated with increased risk of tracheal wall damage), and are allergenic for those with latex allergies.

Cuff pressure needs only to be sufficient to minimize leakage during manual or positive pressure ventilation and to limit aspiration of oral secretions or gastric contents. Excessive cuff pressure can impede blood flow to the tracheal mucosa. The resulting damage becomes apparent in the postanesthesia period, ranging from transient partial airway obstruction and dyspnea to persistent severe airway strictures. Low-volume, high-pressure cuffs require a higher inflation pressure and provide a narrow seal at the tracheal wall. Therefore, they are usually somewhat easier to insert but associated with a greater risk of tracheal damage. High-volume, low-pressure cuffs have a greater area of tracheal contact but require less pressure to attain it. Frequently, the balloon has a short extension terminating in a one-way valve fitted with a female Luer connection. If a one-way valve is not present or is incompetent, a three-way stopcock is often used to provide for easy inflation and adjustment. Cuff pressure can change during anesthesia and should be periodically reassessed. Silicone is especially permeable to gases, and may slowly lose pressure during extended anesthesia.

Especially with high-volume, low-pressure cuffs, palpating the pilot balloon to determine cuff pressure is insensitive and unreliable. With these cuffs, pressure is best measured using a cuff manometer made for the purpose. The manometer will not work with high-pressure low-volume designs because the pressure needed to expand the cuff to any degree is considerable and does not indicate contact with the tracheal wall. A less convenient but effective alternative is to use the breathing circuit manometer to perform an airway seal test; the cuff is slowly inflated until no audible leak is detected during a positive pressure inspiration (up to 15–20 cm H_2O). Because the cuff pressure needed to prevent leakage depends to a large degree on peak airway pressure, large patients generally require a higher pressure than small patients, for which lower ventilation pressures are commonly used. For small patients, when a cuffed tube cannot be used, uncuffed tubes are available in very small sizes for human neonates.

Tubes for rodents are usually made by adapting "over-the-needle" catheters or flexible gavage needles. In adult rats, 14G or 16G catheters are usually suitable, although a smaller catheter may be needed for juvenile animals. As with other animals, the tube size is limited not by the tracheal diameter, but rather by the smaller diameter of the larynx adjacent to the tracheal opening. The tip of the catheter may be trimmed to create a bevel of approximately 40° to facilitate passage into the trachea. When trimming a tube or catheter to create a bevel, it is essential that the tip is left rounded, and does not come to a sharp point. Intravenous catheters offer some advantages over laboratory tubing. They are designed with materials known to be compatible with tissues and tend to become softer as they are warmed to body temperature. Polyurethane catheters are softer at body temperature than many other materials. Catheters also have thin walls and a favorable ratio of inner to the OD, offering the least resistance to breathing. Finally, the female Luer fitting is easily connected to breathing circuits. Some intravenous catheters have a notch on the hub of the Luer fitting to facilitate suturing the catheter in place, and equally useful for tying the tube over the nose with tape or, in mice, sutures. In mice, 20G catheters are often used (Brown et al., 1999). Another option is to use PE-90 polyethylene tubing to make an endotracheal tube for mice weighing 20–25 g. The tubing has an OD of 1.27 mm, about 20% larger than a 20G catheter. Ideally, the rule of using the largest endotracheal tube that can be placed without causing trauma should also apply to rodents, but a more limited selection of catheter and tubing sizes complicates the issue.

2. Supraglottic airway devices (SADs)—laryngeal mask airway

SADs are designed as an alternative to endotracheal intubation. In patients where endotracheal intubation is not possible, SADs can provide a secure and open airway and enable intermittent positive pressure ventilation. SADs are placed in the oropharynx so that they are positioned over the laryngeal opening. An inflatable cuff helps to seal the device over the larynx and to maintain its correct position. Laryngeal masks can be inserted blindly or under direct vision using a laryngoscope.

In human medicine, SADs rapidly replaced endotracheal intubation and face masks in >40% of general anesthesia cases due to their versatility and ease of use (Ramachandran and Kumar, 2014).

In veterinary medicine, SADs have become more popular, especially in cats, rodents, rabbits, and pigs (Goldmann et al., 2005). However, experience with their use is limited and, especially in smaller animals, not entirely satisfactory (Bateman et al., 2005; Brietzke and Mair, 2001). For example, in dogs, they are more difficult to use due to breed and anatomical variances (Reed and Iff, 2012). It has been observed that the laryngeal mask is working properly when the patient is breathing spontaneously, but that it should be carefully used for positive-pressure ventilation, because there is the risk of anesthetic gases passing into the stomach, with the increased possibility of regurgitation or active vomiting.

Veterinary laryngeal masks of different sizes are available for rabbits and cats with body weights of approximately 1 kg upwards. Their design and dimensions are based on molds of the species-specific larynx, proportionately scaled to create a range of sizes. While the first-generation rabbit device was prone to causing airway obstruction, this seems to have been solved with the recent release of the updated design, but has not yet independently studied to assess performance (Engbers et al., 2017). A recent publication demonstrates the use of V-gel to aid with endotracheal intubation in rabbits (Fusco et al., 2021). Cheong et. al. successfully used SADs in rats (Cheong et al., 2013).

3. Laryngoscope/stylets

Laryngoscopes are used to obtain a clear view of the larynx so that an endotracheal tube may be passed easily and atraumatically. Direct visualization of the caudal oropharynx is also useful to visually assess the larynx and surrounding area, alerting the anesthetist to damage, swelling, hemorrhage, secretions, and foreign materials (Engbers et al., 2016). A variety of different shapes and sizes of blades are available commercially which are suitable for use in animals with body weights from approximately 500 g to >100 kg. Intubation of animals such as cats and dogs can be accomplished relatively easily without a laryngoscope. In other species, including swine, small ruminants, and often nonhuman primates, a laryngoscope is essential for rapid and minimally traumatic intubation. A firm practical knowledge of airway anatomy, careful preparation of the patient and equipment, attention to patient positioning, and gentle technique are required for consistent minimally traumatic intubation. When intubating small rodents, either a modified otoscope or a purpose-made laryngoscope blade, or other specialized equipment can be used.

The classic laryngoscope consists of a cylindrical handle housing one or more batteries for an integrated light source with a connection for a detachable blade. A standard hook-on connection is used, and with some exceptions, the blades are interchangeable among handles. Handles are available in several styles. Small handles are convenient for small blades, which tend to be overbalanced on larger handles. For the same reason, larger blades are more easily controlled when an appropriately large handle is used. A disposable laryngoscope may be preferred when sterilization of the intubation equipment is essential, as with use in biohazard facilities.

Laryngoscope blades are typically divided into straight or curved styles, each style requiring a somewhat different technique in use. Curved blades are designed to lift the epiglottis indirectly by advancing the tip into the vallecula, the depression formed at the base of the tongue and epiglottis. Gently depressing the base of the tongue with the blade, in combination with slight retraction, will further lower the epiglottis and improve the view of the laryngeal opening. This technique avoids the potential for damaging the epiglottis by direct contact and pressure. Straight blades can be placed over the epiglottis to depress it directly, but may also be used in the same manner as a curved blade.

The Macintosh blade is one of the most popular blades used for humans, and works equally well in many nonhuman primates and other species with similar oral anatomy. Typical straight blades include the Miller/Foregger and Wisconsin patterns. Straight blades are especially useful in animals with a long oropharynx e.g., pigs and sheep. On many laryngoscope blades, a flange is used to control and deflect the tongue. However, for patients with a restricted mouth opening, blades in which the flange is reduced or absent are preferred. The Wisconsin, Robertshaw, and Macintosh blades are flanged. The flange is reduced or absent in the Miller, Phillips, and Choi blades. For some designs, laryngoscope blades are available and equipped with a port to supply oxygen during intubation, a useful feature for critically ill patients, or when a difficult and prolonged intubation is anticipated (Figs. 9.11 and 9.12).

A limited number of human blades are available with a reversed light position. When the blade is held with the hook-on connector facing up, the light is ordinarily on the left side. For left-handed human anesthetists, as well as right-handed anesthetists whose patients are in sternal recumbency, the light is more conveniently placed on the right of the blade.

Although similar to flexible fiber-optic endoscopes, flexible fiber-optic laryngoscopes are adapted to the needs of the anesthetist. They are used when airway access is anticipated to be difficult or complicated by anatomical or pathological conditions. These devices are usually configured for direct viewing by the operator via a lens or small screen. They can be used in a variety of ways, but often, the endotracheal tube is placed over the fiber-optic bundle, which is directed into the trachea. The endotracheal tube is then advanced, using the fiber-optic bundle as a guide. The fiber-optic bundles are somewhat delicate and should be handled with care, especially to protect the bundle from being bitten by the patient. Other small diagnostic endoscopes can be used similarly.

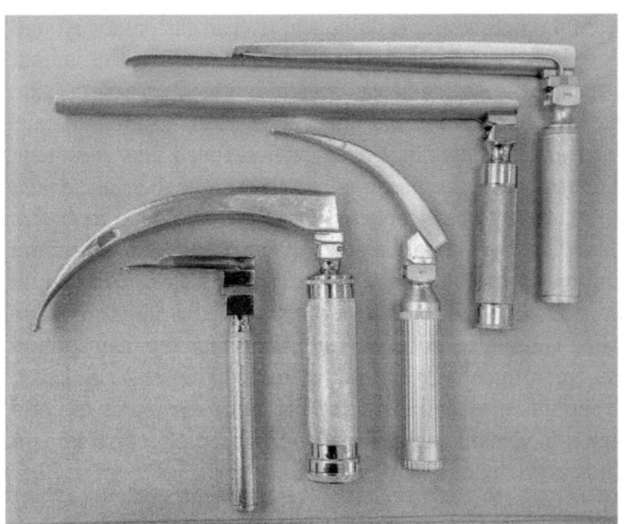

FIGURE 9.11 Different types of laryngoscopes (F. Gantenbein).

Endotracheal tube introducers, intubation guides, intubation stylets, and bougies, all refer to rigid or malleable rods or wires used to adjust the curve of an endotracheal tube in order to make insertion into the trachea easier. They are sufficiently rigid to pass into the trachea, but smooth and flexible enough to avoid injury. Used this way, in order to avoid airway trauma, the stylet should not extend beyond the tip of the tube. Many types of stylets are sold for this purpose, usually coated with smooth plastic to make withdrawal from the tube easier and reduce the risk of airway trauma, and often having an adjustable stop mechanism to limit their working length. Alternatively, the malleable stylet can be bent sharply at the tube connector to accomplish the same end. Lighted, malleable stylets are available.

Intubation guides are used when vision is limited, and the endotracheal tube would obscure the tracheal opening as it is advanced. They can be used in several ways. If the view of the tracheal opening is very limited, or if the tracheal opening is very small, an intubation guide can be directed into the trachea under direct vision and held in place while an endotracheal tube is threaded over it. This technique is sometimes referred to as railroading the tube. In rodents, a Seldinger guidewire is sometimes used as an intubation aid. For convenient use, the guide wire should be relatively short, but because Seldinger guide wires consist of a spring encircling a stiffer inner wire, they cannot easily be shortened simply by cutting them. Alternatively, the guide can be placed within the lumen of the tube to extend a desired distance beyond the tip and held in place while the guide and endotracheal tube are advanced as a single unit. This technique is often useful in pigs, small ruminants, and other species in which the view is likely to be obscured by the endotracheal tube as it approaches the tracheal opening.

Methods and equipment for endotracheal intubation of mice and rats have been described by numerous authors (Das et al., 2013; Nelson et al., 2020; Struys et al., 2014). The methods involve blind intubation, intubation using direct light, and intubation using indirect light. Blind intubation is feasible, but difficult to learn and prone to result in trauma in inexperienced hands. Direct illumination alone, or in combination with laryngoscopes, lighted stylets, or mouth gags is a common approach to endotracheal intubation in rodents. Transillumination is simple in terms of equipment, and relatively easy to perform, but positioning the light to gain the best view is sometimes difficult.

Species	Body weight	Endotracheal tube diameter	Laryngoscope
Cat	0.5–1.5 kg	2.0–3 mm O/D[a]	MacIntosh size 1
	>1.5 kg	3–4.5 mm O/D	
Dog	0.5–5 kg	2–5 mm O/D	MacIntosh size 1–4
	>5 kg	4.0–15 mm O/D	
Guinea pig	400–1000 g	16–12 gauge plastic cannula	Purpose-made laryngoscope[b] Otoscope
Hamster	120 g	1.5 mm	Purpose-made laryngoscope[b]
Mouse	25–35 g	1.0 mm	Purpose-made laryngoscope[b]
Primate	0.35–20 kg	2–8 mm O/D (or purpose-made tube for smallest animals)	MacIntosh or Wisconsin size 1–3
Pig	1–10 kg	2–6 mm O/D	Soper or Wisconsin size 1–4
	10–200 kg	6–15 mm O/D	
Rabbit	1–3 kg	2–3 mm O/D	Wisconsin size 0–1 or Otoscope
	3–7 kg	3–6 mm O/D	
Rat	200–400 g	18–12 gauge plastic cannula	Purpose-made laryngoscope[b] Otoscope
Sheep	10–90 kg	5–15 mm O/D	MacIntosh size 2–4

[a]O/D, Outside diameter.
[b]see text.

FIGURE 9.12 Tube sizes and suggested laryngoscopes for different laboratory species (P. Flecknell).

Rigid stylets, or guides, are problematic and likely to cause trauma if not used with care. Flexible intubation guides, such as guide wires, avoid the problem of the endotracheal tube blocking the view as the laryngeal entrance is approached, and are less likely to cause trauma than rigid stylets. However, their flexibility can make them more difficult to control. Positioning aids, such as intubation stands, make the process much more comfortable for the user but, because most depend upon intact upper incisors, they cannot be used in animals with abnormal dentition. Some systems are available commercially (Fig. 9.13).

B. Face masks and nose cones

Face masks or nose cones are the most common means of maintaining inhalational anesthesia in rodents. In larger animals, endotracheal intubation or SADs are preferred though face masks may be used to provide oxygen during anesthetic induction and recovery. To work efficiently and safely, a face mask must have a tight seal to the patient and minimal dead space (Smith and Bolon, 2006).

Face masks can be used for small animals like dogs, cats, and species of similar size and conformation for very short procedures (<15−20 minutes). The larger sizes are also suitable for domestic swine. Masks intended for use with human pediatric and neonatal patients could be useful for nonhuman primates. For rodents, a variety of masks with or without diaphragms is available, examples are shown in Fig. 9.14.

The mask is connected directly to the fresh gas supply from the anesthetic machine and excess gas passes around the animal's face and exits the mask. When the animal breathes out, exhaled gas which contains carbon dioxide passes into the mask and flows out around the animal's face as fresh gas blows in. Fresh gas flows (and thus anesthetic agent consumption) need to be relatively high to make sure all exhaled gases are blown out of the mask and to ensure that when the animal breathes in, only fresh gases from the anesthetic machine are inhaled. Thus, gas flow rates should be maintained at three times the estimated minute volume (tidal volume x respiratory rate—assuming the tidal volume is approximately 10−15 mL/kg of body mass). In addition, it should be ensured that the mask fits closely to the animal's face, reducing space where expired gas could remain and be reinhaled ("equipment dead space").

Coaxial, actively scavenged nose cones do not use a diaphragm. The animal's head is placed in the inner tube,

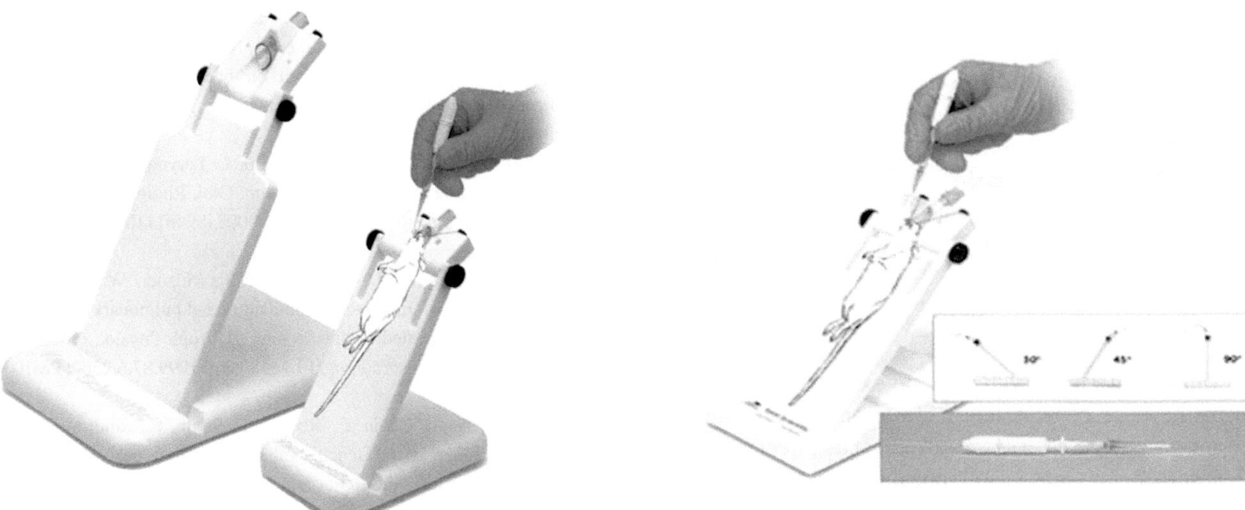

FIGURE 9.13 Intubation stand for rats and mice (Kent Scientific Corporation).

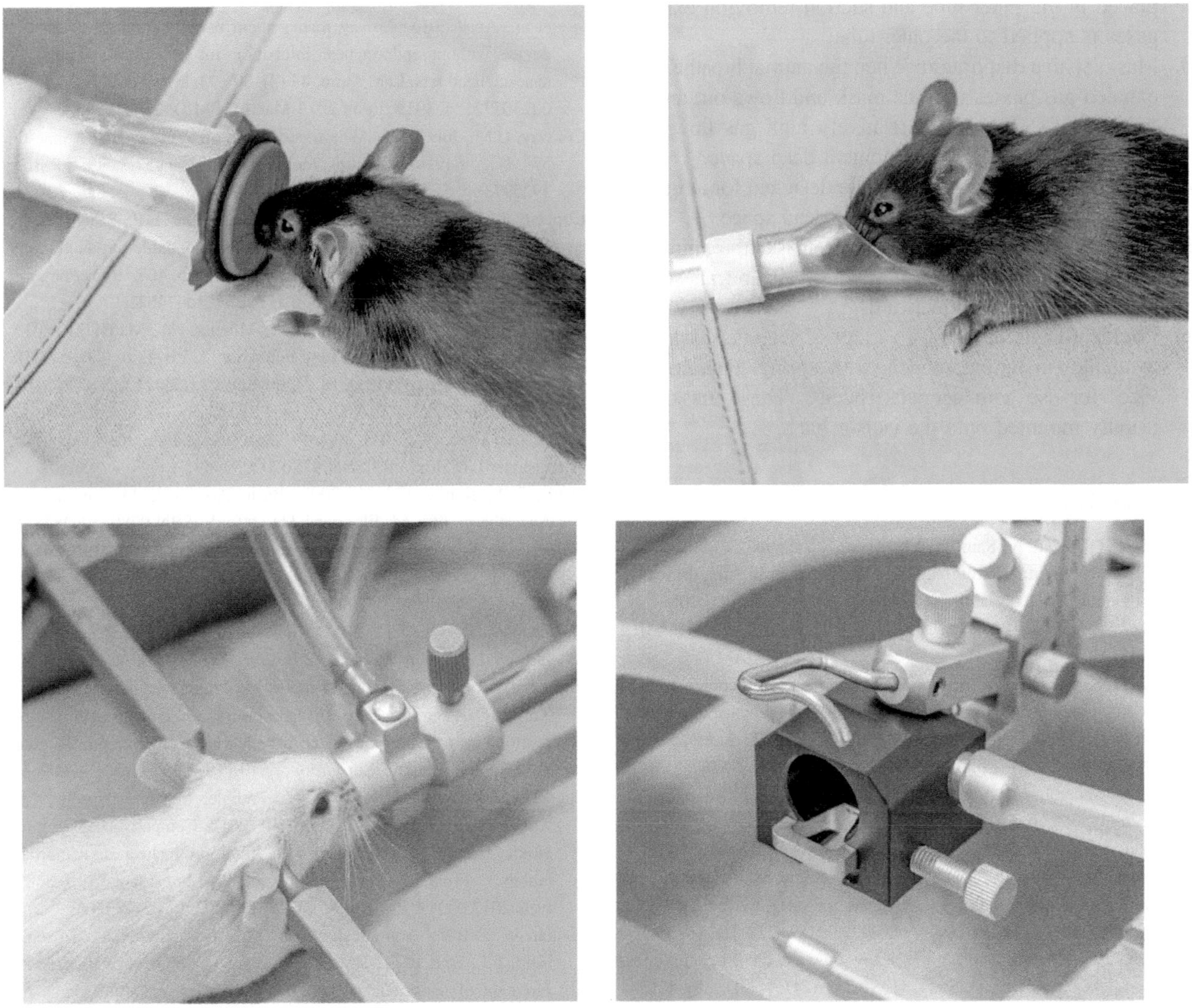

FIGURE 9.14 Different types of face masks: with diaphragm (*top left*) or without (*top right*), special solutions are available e.g., integrated into stereotaxic frames (*bottom*, all pictures F. Gantenbein).

which is connected to the fresh gas outlet of the anesthesia machine. The inner tube is surrounded by a larger outer tube connected to a suction source for rodents have been described by several authors (Glen et al., 1980; Henry and Casto, 1989; Hunter et al., 1984; Levy et al., 1980; Li et al., 2001; McGarrick and Thexton, 1979).

In order to reduce personnel exposure to anesthetic gases, the gases delivered to the mask need to be safely removed. In either case, the scavenging flow needed is high in comparison with fresh gas flow. A number of different systems are available:

1. Simple nose cone with separate exhaust openings next to the nose cone: Using a simple nose cone, air and anesthetic gases are removed and directed to an absorber through lateral openings next to the nose cone, often used for manifolds or with imaging devices when imaging batches of animals.
2. Concentric mask systems, where the inner tube is surrounded by a larger outer tube. The animal's nose is placed in the inner tube and suction removing exhaled gases is applied to the outer tube.
3. Masks with a diaphragm: When the animal breathes out, exhaled gas passes into the mask and flows out around the animal's face, needs relatively high gas flow rate, and might have a large equipment dead space.
4. Low-profile anesthesia masks are designed for a tight fit and thus have a small equipment dead space.
5. Downdraft tables: Using a simple mask, the animal is placed on a downdraft table, where air and anesthetic gases are removed downwards.
6. For stereotaxic devices, a variety of specific masks are available, including models with special restraint devices for use with neonatal rodents. These masks are usually mounted onto the incisor bar.

References

Ambrisko, T.D., Gal, A., Sarol Jr., J.N., Mitek, A., Braun, C., March 2021. Quantification of reservoir bags as airway pressure-limiting devices in a nonrebreathing system. Vet. Anaesth. Analg. 48 (2), 205–212. https://doi.org/10.1016/j.vaa.2020.11.004. Epub 2020 Dec 11. PMID: 33431268.

Arnold, P., Kaufmann, J., February 2022. Going around in circles. Is there a continuing need to use the T-piece circuit in the practice of pediatric anesthesia? Paediatr. Anaesth. 32 (2), 273–277. https://doi.org/10.1111/pan.14331. Epub 2021 Nov 16. PMID: 34752679.

Bain, J.A., Spoerel, W.E., January 1979. Bain circuit. Can. Anaesth. Soc. J. 26 (1), 65–66. PMID: 761119.

Bateman, L., Ludders, J.W., Gleed, R.D., Erb, H.N., September 2005. Comparison between facemask and laryngeal mask airway in rabbits during isoflurane anesthesia. Vet. Anaesth. Analg. 32 (5), 280–288. https://doi.org/10.1111/j.1467-2995.2005.00169.x. PMID: 16135209.

Baum, J., 1990. Clinical applications of low flow and closed circuit anesthesia. Acta Anaesthesiol. Belg. 41 (3), 239–247. PMID: 2260429.

Bowling, P.A., Bencivenga, M.A., Leyva, M.E., Grego, B.E., Cornelius, R.N., Cornelius, E.M., et al., November 2021. Effects of a heated anesthesia breathing circuit on body temperature in anesthetized Rhesus Macaques (*Macaca mulatta*). J. Am. Assoc. Lab. Anim. Sci.

Brietzke, S.E., Mair, E.A., September 2001. Laryngeal mask versus endotracheal tube in a ferret model. Ann. Otol. Rhinol. Laryngol. 110 (9), 827–833. https://doi.org/10.1177/000348940111000905. PMID: 11558758.

Brown, R.H., Walters, D.M., Greenberg, R.S., Mitzner, W., December 1999. A method of endotracheal intubation and pulmonary functional assessment for repeated studies in mice. J. Appl. Physiol. (1985) 87 (6), 2362–2365. https://doi.org/10.1152/jappl.1999.87.6.2362. PMID: 10601190.

Bunel, V., Shoukri, A., Choin, F., Roblin, S., Smith, C., Similowski, T., et al., December 2016. Bench evaluation of four portable oxygen concentrators under different conditions representing altitudes of 2438, 4200, and 8000 m. High Alt. Med. Biol. 17 (4), 370–374.

Carter, J.A., Baskett, P.J., Simpson, P.J., June 1985. The 'Permox' oxygen concentrator. Its mode of action, performance and potential application. Anaesthesia 40 (6), 560–565. PMID: 4025751.

Cheong, S.H., Lee, J.H., Kim, M.H., Cho, K.R., Lim, S.H., Lee, K.M., et al., April 2013. Airway management using a supraglottic airway device without endotracheal intubation for positive ventilation of anaesthetized rats. Lab. Anim. 47 (2), 89–93. https://doi.org/10.1177/0023677212473919. Epub 2013 Mar 14. PMID: 23492512.

Conway, C.M., July 1985. Anaesthetic breathing systems. Br. J. Anaesth. 57 (7), 649–657. https://doi.org/10.1093/bja/57.7.649. PMID: 3925973.

Coppens, M.J., Versichelen, L.F., Rolly, G., Mortier, E.P., Struys, M.M., May 2006. The mechanisms of carbon monoxide production by inhalational agents. Anaesthesia 61 (5), 462–468. https://doi.org/10.1111/j.1365-2044.2006.04536.x. PMID: 16674622.

Das, S., MacDonald, K., Chang, H.Y., Mitzner, W., March 21, 2013. A simple method of mouse lung intubation. J. Vis. Exp. (73), e50318. https://doi.org/10.3791/50318. PMID: 23542122; PMCID: PMC3639692.

Davey, A., Diba, A., 2011. Ward's Anaesthetic Equipment, sixth ed. Elsevier LTD Oxford, ISBN 9780702030949.

Davis, P.D., Kenny, G.N.C., 2003. Basic Physics & Measurement in Anaesthesia, fifth ed. Elsevier LTD Oxford, ISBN 9780750648288.

Dobson, M.B., April 1992. Oxygen concentrators for the smaller hospital—a review. Trop. Doct. 22 (2), 56–58. https://doi.org/10.1177/004947559202200204. PMID: 1604716.

Dorsch, J.A., Dorsch, S.E., 2007. Understanding Anesthesia Equipment, fifth ed. Lippincott Williams & Wilkins, ISBN 978-0-7817-7603-5.

Engbers, S., Larkin, A.E., Jonnalagadda, M., Prebble, M.,N., Rousset, N., Knight, C., Pang, D., 2016. Difficult orotracheal intubation in a rabbit resulting from the presence of faecal pellets in the oropharynx. Vet. Rec. Case Rep. 4, e000265. https://doi.org/10.1136/vetreccr-2015-000265.

Engbers, S., Larkin, A., Rousset, N., Prebble, M., Jonnalagadda, M., Knight, C.G., Pang, D.S.J., April 10, 2017. Comparison of a supraglottic airway device (v-gel) with blind orotracheal intubation in rabbits. Front. Vet. Sci. 4, 49. https://doi.org/10.3389/fvets.2017.00049. PMID: 28443290; PMCID: PMC5385366.

Figueiredo, D.B.S., Aun, A.G., Lara, J.R., Garofalo, N.A., Teixeira-Neto, F.J., Braz, L.G., Braz, M.G., September–October 2021. Measurement of anesthetic pollution in veterinary operating rooms for small animals: isoflurane pollution in a university veterinary hospital. Braz. J. Anesthesiol. 71 (5), 517–522. https://doi.org/10.1016/j.bjane.2021.02.007. Epub 2021 Feb 3. PMID: 33685758.

Friesen, R.M., May 1992. Oxygen concentrators and the practice of anaesthesia. Can. J. Anaesth. 39 (5 Pt 2), R80–R89. English, French. PMID: 1600576.

Friesen, R.M., Raber, M.B., Reimer, D.H., December 1999. Oxygen concentrators: a primary oxygen supply source. Can. J. Anaesth. 46 (12), 1185–1190. https://doi.org/10.1007/BF03015531. PMID: 10608216.

Fukunaga, A., April 2019. The F breathing circuit, a universal single-limb breathing circuit: brief historical perspective. J. Anesth. 33 (2), 317–320. https://doi.org/10.1007/s00540-019-02622-8. Epub 2019 Mar 11. PMID: 30859365; PMCID: PMC6443618.

Fusco, A., Douglas, H., Barba, A., Hopster, K., Stefanovski, D., Sinder, B., et al., August 10, 2021. V-Gel guided endotracheal intubation in rabbits. Front. Vet. Sci. 8, 684624. https://doi.org/10.3389/fvets.2021.684624. PMID: 34447802; PMCID: PMC8383107.

Glen, J.B., Cliff, G.S., Jamieson, A., July 1980. Evaluation of a scavenging system for use with inhalation anaesthesia techniques in rats. Lab. Anim. 14 (3), 207–211. https://doi.org/10.1258/002367780780937553. PMID: 7431835.

Goldmann, K., Kalinowski, M., Kraft, S., September 2005. Airway management under general anaesthesia in pigs using the LMA-ProSeal: a pilot study. Vet. Anaesth. Analg. 32 (5), 308–313. https://doi.org/10.1111/j.1467-2995.2005.00248.x. PMID: 16135212.

Grimm, K.A., Lamont, L.A., Tranquilli, W.J., Greene, S.A., Robertson, S.A., 2015. Lumb and Jones Veterinary Anesthesia and Analgesia. Wiley-Blackwell, ISBN 978-1-118-52623-1.

Henry, R.T., Casto, R., September 1989. Simple and inexpensive delivery of halogenated inhalation anesthetics to rodents. Am. J. Physiol. 257 (3 Pt 2), R668–R671. https://doi.org/10.1152/ajpregu.1989.257.3.R668. PMID: 2782468.

Hunter, S.C., Glen, J.B., Butcher, C.J., January 1984. A modified anaesthetic vapour extraction system. Lab. Anim. 18 (1), 42–44. https://doi.org/10.1258/002367784780864965. PMID: 10628786.

Hylani, M.A., October 1986. Closed circuit anesthesia. Middle East J. Anaesthesiol. 8 (6), 505–510. PMID: 3785100.

Jain, R.K., Swaminathan, S., September 2013. Anaesthesia ventilators. Indian J. Anaesth. 57 (5), 525–532. https://doi.org/10.4103/0019-5049.120150. PMID: 24249886; PMCID: PMC3821270.

Intagliata, S., Rizzo, A., Gossman, W., January 2022. Physiology, lung dead space [Updated 2021 Oct 18]. In: StatPearls. StatPearls Publishing, Treasure Island (FL). Available from: https://www.ncbi.nlm.nih.gov/books/NBK482501/.

Kaul, T.K., Mittal, G., September 2013. Mapleson's breathing systems. Indian J. Anaesth. 57 (5), 507–515. https://doi.org/10.4103/0019-5049.120148. PMID: 24249884; PMCID: PMC3821268.

Kharasch, E.D., Schroeder, J.L., Sheffels, P., Liggitt, H.D., December 2005. Influence of sevoflurane on the metabolism and renal effects of compound A in rats. Anesthesiology 103 (6), 1183–1188. https://doi.org/10.1097/00000542-200512000-00012. PMID: 16306730.

Lerche, P., Muir 3rd, W.W., Bednarski, R.M., August 15, 2000a. Rebreathing anesthetic systems in small animal practice. J. Am. Vet. Med. Assoc. 217 (4), 485–492. https://doi.org/10.2460/javma.2000.217.485. PMID: 10953709.

Lerche, P., Muir 3rd, W.W., Bednarski, R.M., August 15, 2000b. Nonrebreathing anesthetic systems in small animal practice. J. Am. Vet. Med. Assoc. 217 (4), 493–497. https://doi.org/10.2460/javma.2000.217.493. PMID: 10953710.

Levy, D.E., Zwies, A., Duffy, T.E., October 1980. A mask for delivery of inhalation gases to small laboratory animals. Lab. Anim. Sci. 30 (5), 868–870. PMID: 7431871.

Li, W., Tse, J.Y., James, A.E., Lik-Wang, L., Chi-Kwan, Y., Man-Po, C., Chung, S.C., August 2001. Delivery and scavenging system for small animal inhalational anesthesia. J. Surg. Res. 99 (2), 175–178. https://doi.org/10.1006/jsre.2001.6107. PMID: 11469884.

Mapleson, W.W., February 1998. The elimination of rebreathing in various semi-closed anaesthetic systems. 1954. Br. J. Anaesth. 80 (2), 263–269. https://doi.org/10.1093/bja/80.2.263. PMID: 9602602.

McGarrick, J., Thexton, A., April 1979. A safer open-circuit anaesthetic system for administering halothane to rats [proceedings]. J. Physiol. 289, 15P–16P. PMID: 458646.

McMurphy, R.M., Hodgson, D.S., Cribb, P.H., July–August 1995. Modification of a nonrebreathing circuit adapter to prevent barotrauma in anesthetized patients. Vet. Surg. 24 (4), 352–355. https://doi.org/10.1111/j.1532-950x.1995.tb01342.x. PMID: 7571388.

Nelson, A.M., Nolan, K.E., Davis, I.C., March 27, 2020. Repeated orotracheal intubation in mice. J. Vis. Exp. (157). https://doi.org/10.3791/60844. PMID: 32281980.

Oswald, L., Smith, E.J., Mathew, M., Goonasekera, C., August 2018. The Ayre's T-piece turns 80: a 21st century review. Paediatr. Anaesth. 28 (8), 694–696. https://doi.org/10.1111/pan.13408. Epub 2018 Jun 7. PMID: 29882229.

Parker, C.J., Snowdon, S.L., October 1988. Predicted and measured oxygen concentrations in the circle system using low fresh gas flows with oxygen supplied by an oxygen concentrator. Br. J. Anaesth. 61 (4), 397–402. https://doi.org/10.1093/bja/61.4.397. PMID: 2973341.

Patil, V.P., Shetmahajan, M.G., Divatia, J.V., September 2013. The modern integrated anaesthesia workstation. Indian J. Anaesth. 57 (5), 446–454. https://doi.org/10.4103/0019-5049.120139. PMID: 24249877; PMCID: PMC3821261.

Ramachandran, S.K., Kumar, A.M., June 2014. Supraglottic airway devices. Respir. Care 59 (6), 920–931. https://doi.org/10.4187/respcare.02976. Discussion 931–2. PMID: 24891199.

Reed, F., Iff, I., March 2012. Use of a laryngeal mask airway in a brachycephalic dog with masticatory myositis and trismus. Can. Vet. J. 53 (3), 287–290. PMID: 22942446; PMCID: PMC3280784.

Romero-Ávila, P., Márquez-Espinós, C., Cabrera Afonso, J.R., March–April 2021. Historical development of the anesthetic machine: from Morton to the integration of the mechanical ventilator. Braz. J. Anesthesiol. 71 (2), 148–161. https://doi.org/10.1016/j.bjane.2021.02.017. Epub 2021 Feb 10. PMID: 33894858.

Sasse, F.J., Flemming, D.C., Hoff, B., Smith, N.T., Rampil, I.J., September 1979. The "D circle": closed-circuit operation of the Bain circuit. Can. Anaesth. Soc. J. 26 (5), 420–423. https://doi.org/10.1007/BF03006458. PMID: 290406.

Smith, J.C., Bolon, B., April 2006. Isoflurane leakage from nonrebreathing rodent anaesthesia circuits: comparison of emissions from conventional and modified ports. Lab. Anim. 40 (2), 200–209. https://doi.org/10.1258/002367706776318999. PMID: 16600080.

Struys, M.M., Bouche, M.P., Rolly, G., Vandevivere, Y.D., Dyzers, D., Goeteyn, W., et al., April 5, 2014. Endotracheal intubation in mice via direct laryngoscopy using an otoscope. J. Vis. Exp. (86), 50269. https://doi.org/10.3791/50269. PMID: 24747695; PMCID: PMC4162455.

Van Bocxlaer, J.F., Mortier, E.P., June 2004. Production of compound A and carbon monoxide in circle systems: an in vitro comparison of two carbon dioxide absorbents. Anaesthesia 59 (6), 584–589. https://doi.org/10.1111/j.1365-2044.2004.03704.x. PMID: 15144299.

Walsh, C.M., Taylor, P.M., July 2004. A clinical evaluation of the 'mini parallel Lack' breathing system in cats and comparison with a modified Ayre's T-piece. Vet. Anaesth. Analg. 31 (3), 207–212. https://doi.org/10.1111/j.1467-2987.2004.00172.x. PMID: 15268692.

Further reading

Cooley, K.G., Johnson, R.A., 2018. Veterinary Anesthetic and Monitoring Equipment. Wiley-Blackwell, ISBN 9781119277156.

Duke-Novakovski, T., de Vries, M., Seymour, C., 2016. BSAVA Manual of Canine and Feline Anaesthesia and Analgesia, third ed. Wiley-Blackwell, ISBN 978-1-905-31961-9.

Ehrenwerth, J., Eisenkraft, J.B., Berry, J.M., 2020. Anesthesia Equipment Principles and Application, third ed. Saunders, ISBN 978-0-323-67279-5. https://doi.org/10.1016/C2017-0-04059-4.

Flecknell, P., 2015. Laboratory Animal Anaesthesia, fourth ed. Elsevier LTD Oxford, ISBN 9780128000366.

Chapter 10

Monitoring of anesthesia

Debra L. Hickman[1] **and Kathleen R. Pritchett-Corning**[2,3]

[1]*Department of Comparative Pathobiology, Purdue University, West Lafayette, IN, United States;* [2]*Office of Animal Resources, Harvard University Faculty of Arts and Sciences, Cambridge, MA, United States;* [3]*Department of Comparative Medicine, University of Washington, Seattle, WA, United States*

Chapter outline

I. Introduction

Anesthesia will affect a patient's normal homeostasis and may have unpredictable effects, particularly in sick patients or those undergoing complex or invasive procedures. These effects register as changes in the body's normal physiologic states and provide the basis of anesthetic monitoring. Anesthetic monitoring allows recognition of the extent of compromise to each body system during the course of a procedure and adjustments in the anesthetic protocol to prevent untoward short- and long-term effects on the animal.

Many variations can be expected in the way a patient will respond to anesthetic agents. These variations are affected by the patient's health/pathology, metabolism, and uptake/distribution of the anesthetic agents being delivered. In order for anesthetic monitoring to be successful, three basic processes should occur: early recognition of homeostatic disturbances, the correct interpretation of changes, and appropriate intervention.

The first principle of anesthetic monitoring is to assure that the level of anesthesia is consistent with the welfare of the animal. If the level of anesthesia is insufficient to prevent the animal from experiencing potential pain or distress, this can create a negative welfare experience for the animal. Likewise, with an excessive depth of anesthesia, an animal may become significantly compromised because of the direct depressant effects of particular anesthetic drugs on the cardiovascular or respiratory systems. Therefore, monitoring anesthetic influence on the central

Anesthesia and Analgesia in Laboratory Animals. https://doi.org/10.1016/B978-0-12-822215-7.00008-1

nervous system (CNS), more commonly referred to as the depth of anesthesia, is critically important. Ideally, anesthetic depth will be titrated to the procedure being performed, with the desirable level of anesthesia correlating with stage 3 of anesthesia (Table 10.1). During the induction of anesthesia, adverse effects can occur acutely as a result of drug effects. During the maintenance phase of anesthesia, cardiovascular, respiratory, and neurological depression may be insidious and go unnoticed until a critical event occurs (e.g., apnea, cardiac arrest) unless appropriate monitoring is performed. Monitoring these parameters should allow for early recognition of negative trends while physiologic disturbances are still reversible.

The second principle of anesthetic monitoring involves the correct interpretation of the observed physiologic changes, including the limitations associated with the monitoring techniques that are utilized. When an animal is anesthetized, its physiologic processes are altered by the anesthetic itself, the surgery being performed, and/or the research manipulations required by the study. If an animal appears compromised during a procedure, one must be able to determine quickly the likely cause of the problem in order to choose the appropriate steps to correct it. A thorough knowledge of the anticipated effects of different anesthetic drugs on each physiological parameter will make this interpretation of cause and effect much easier. The reader is referred to other chapters in this text in which the specific pharmacology and expected physiological effects of each anesthetic agent are discussed in detail. In addition to pharmacologically induced complications, physiologic status may be further compromised by complications related to procedural manipulations (i.e., severe blood loss and nerve injury).

TABLE 10.1 Stages of anesthesia.

Stage	Description
Stage of voluntary movement (I)	From initial administration of the drug *to loss of consciousness;* may see a strong, rapid heartbeat, struggling, and dilation of the pupils; progresses to ataxia
Stage of involuntary movement (II)	Lasts from *loss of consciousness* to onset of a regular pattern of breathing; may see reflex struggling, prominent reflexes, and hyperventilation
Stage of surgical anesthesia (III)	Characterized by progressive depression of reflexes; may see muscle relaxation with slow and regular breathing; *desired for survival procedures*
Extreme central nervous system depression (IV)	Cessation of breaths and heartbeats, delay in capillary refill times, death quickly follows unless anesthetic is withdrawn

Modified from Haskins (2015).

The third principle of anesthetic monitoring involves intervention. Because regular anesthetic monitoring indicates deterioration of the patient before it becomes irreversible, the anesthetist is able to make adjustments in the anesthetic level, provide supportive therapy, or institute drug therapy that can positively affect outcome. The appropriate intervention is based on interpretation of the cause of the underlying problem.

II. Monitoring of the anesthetized patient

A. Core components

The American College of Veterinary Anesthesia and Analgesia (ACVAA) has developed a set of guidelines for anesthetic monitoring in small animal veterinary patients (ACVAA, 2009). These guidelines include monitoring of circulation, oxygenation, and ventilation, as well as the use of an anesthetic record and appropriate personnel training. Although not applicable to all laboratory animals, these guidelines are a good starting point for building monitoring paradigms.

B. Observation and evaluation

The techniques used in monitoring range from the use of sophisticated electronic equipment to simple visual and tactile observation. Mechanical and electronic devices enhance patient monitoring and are very useful in the laboratory setting, where the anesthetist often has other duties, including that of a surgeon. Further, some parameters can only be monitored using sophisticated equipment and these become especially important in high-risk patients or procedures. This equipment can also provide numerical data, which may be necessary for the interpretation of research results. Despite all the advantages of such sophisticated equipment, it is crucial that anesthetists not neglect their senses (touch, sight, and hearing) as well as clinical observations. The senses are simple and reliable, supplement, and complement the use of monitors, and do not need an emergency backup power generator. However, as with many components of the medical evaluation of patients, practice makes perfect, and regular practice is required to maintain the skills required for the successful interpretation of the information obtained by the senses. In addition, the efficacy of anesthetic monitoring depends on the choice of physiologic variables that are studied. Certain parameters, such as withdrawal response to a toe pinch, are not very sensitive indicators of patient status. While the presence of a withdrawal in response to a toe pinch would indicate that the depth of anesthesia is insufficient (too light) for surgery, the absence of a withdrawal does not distinguish between a depth of anesthesia sufficient for surgery or an excessive depth of anesthesia (with an increased risk of physiologic compromise). Alternatively, quantitative variables like arterial blood pressure (ABP) give numerical information that can be easily compared to previous readings to indicate trends in patient status. It is also important that an anesthetist never rely on just one single parameter to monitor patient status. A single parameter, such as respiratory rate, may allow one to recognize trends during anesthesia; however, it can often be misleading when it comes to the correct interpretation of cause and effect, therefore resulting in inappropriate treatment measures.

C. Vital signs

In the anesthetized patient, vital signs are considered as those basic elements that can be easily monitored by the anesthetist's senses. Although specialized equipment can serve as an adjunct to monitoring vital signs, a trained anesthetist should be able to rely on their own senses to assess the anesthetized patient. The vital signs that should be monitored during anesthesia in larger laboratory animals include heart rate (HR) and rhythm, pulse pressure, capillary refill time (CRT), mucus membrane color, blood loss, respiratory rate, and temperature (Pollock et al., 2020). For smaller laboratory animals (like rodents), the adaptation of these techniques may be necessary.

D. Thermoregulation

Most anesthetic agents cause a depression of the hypothalamic thermoregulatory mechanism, predisposing animals to hypothermia. This is an even greater problem in small laboratory animal species (Skorupski et al., 2017). These animals have a very large surface area relative to their body mass, which causes a correspondingly faster loss of body heat. This is further compounded by the removal of hair and wetting the remaining hair coat during the aseptic preparation of the surgical site. When this small, damp animal is then placed on a cold metal surface, the result can be fatal hypothermia. Opening a body cavity will further accelerate the loss of body heat. Body temperature is best monitored using a small thermistor placed rectally or into the esophagus to the level of the heart. This will provide a closer indication of the core body temperature than other methods (Haskins, 2015). Clinical thermometers do not register a continuous decrease in body temperature and thus are not recommended unless recordings are taken at regular intervals. Hypothermia can be minimized by thorough preparation before the procedure, by ensuring that everything is prepared before the anesthetic is initiated, and by utilizing prewarming to slow the onset of hypothermia. During the procedure, additional measures such as the warming of surgical preparation solutions, insulating the patient from both cool ambient temperatures and a cold procedural surface, using warm fluids if supplemental fluids are provided, warming inspired gases, and using supplemental heat provided by a circulating water blanket or forced air warming systems (i.e., Bair Hugger) can help to preserve body temperature. Active warming should be initiated with the induction of anesthesia as hypothermia is difficult to slow or reverse once present. Electric heating pads and heating lamps should be avoided as they can cause serious thermal burns and even hyperthermia (Rembert et al., 2004). Electric recirculating water blankets should be checked for performance to ensure that they are heating evenly as well. Anesthetic-induced hyperthermia can be seen in some breeds of pigs (MacLennan and Phillips, 1992). Because both hypo-and hyperthermia can enhance the effects of central depressant drugs, as well as confound experimental data, monitoring the body temperature of the patient is particularly important in laboratory animals.

E. Anesthetic depth

The single most important concept of anesthetic monitoring is the assurance that the depth of anesthesia is consistent with the welfare of the patient. The depth of anesthesia required for an animal is determined by the type of procedure being performed and the response of the patient to the surgical stimulus. The type of procedure will determine the intensity of the stimulation. In general, high-intensity painful procedures, such as joint capsule incision, periosteal stimulation, fracture manipulation, visceral or peritoneal traction, diaphragmatic stimulation, corneal manipulation, or the manipulation of inflamed tissue will require a deeper level of anesthesia with special consideration of analgesia administration than less painful procedures. Because different pain intensities occur within a procedure as different tissues are manipulated, the anesthetist must frequently reassess and adjust the depth of anesthesia and provision of additional analgesia as appropriate. Experience with a procedure will allow the anesthetist to anticipate necessary changes in the depth of anesthesia. Observational techniques that help indicate the depth of anesthesia include the level of muscle relation, reflex activities, and physiologic responses to surgical stimulation (Pollock et al., 2020).

A good assessment of muscle relaxation can be made by monitoring jaw tone in certain species. The ease of monitoring jaw muscle tone varies with species due to the differences in jaw size and masseter muscle strength. Jaw tone is easily assessed in certain small animal species, such as dogs and cats. It is much more difficult to evaluate in rodents, sheep, and swine. Although it is usually desirable to maintain some degree of muscle tone during anesthesia, if an animal demonstrates resistance to opening its mouth when gentle traction is placed on the mandible during a procedure, more anesthesia is generally needed.

The purposeful movement has traditionally been thought of as an indication that anesthesia is too light, and the animal is responding to a painful stimulus. However, purposeful movement in response to surgical manipulation must be differentiated from the spontaneous movement, which can be seen with certain anesthetic agents such as ketamine, opioids, enflurane, and methoxyflurane and which does not occur in response to a surgical stimulus. The pedal withdrawal reflex is commonly used to help determine the level of surgical anesthesia in small laboratory animals. The pinnae of rabbits or rodents are often tested in a similar manner, looking for head shaking in response to a painful stimulus. However, reliance on the presence or absence of spontaneous movement as a sole indicator of the depth of anesthesia should be avoided (Antognini, et al., 2005; Shafer and Stanski, 2008).

The ocular reflexes can be used to indicate anesthetic depth. These include palpebral response, ocular position, and corneal reflex. The palpebral response is the blinking that occurs when the edge of the eyelid is lightly touched. There is species variation in this response under anesthesia. Most animals lose the palpebral response fairly early in surgical anesthesia; however, rabbits may maintain a palpebral response even at deeper planes of anesthesia. The intensity of the palpebral response is also influenced by the particular anesthetic agent used. The palpebral response is lost early with barbiturates and most inhalation agents; however, it is well maintained with ketamine.

Ocular position is generally a reliable sign of changing anesthetic depth in many species. As anesthesia is induced and in light planes of anesthesia the eyeball remains central in the orbit, and the palpebral response is present. Nystagmus and lacrimation are also indications of a light plane of surgical anesthesia. When a surgical plane of anesthesia is reached, the globe rotates ventromedialy. As anesthesia deepens (and muscle relaxation continues to increase), the globe will again rotate upward and return to a central position in the orbit. A centrally located globe during a deep plane of anesthesia can be distinguished from the centrally located globe of light anesthesia by the absence of the palpebral response during increased anesthetic depth. The corneal reflex is another ocular reflex that changes with the changing depth of anesthesia. To determine the presence of a corneal reflex, the surface of the cornea is lightly touched with a clean cotton bud, and the presence or absence of a blinking response is noted. A brisk corneal reflex is found in awake animals and its intensity begins to diminish as the plane of anesthesia deepens. Certain species, such as ruminants, will maintain a corneal reflex during a surgical plane of anesthesia, whereas the reflex is often absent at a deep surgical plane in other species, such as dogs or cats.

Various physiologic responses to stimuli are also used to assess the level of surgical anesthesia. Increases in HR, BP, and/or respiratory rate (RR) or depth can be seen in response to surgical stimulation, and often precedes purposeful movement. Changes in HR, BP, and RR are also affected by the specific drugs given and the physiologic state of the animal. An accurate interpretation of the cause of such autonomic responses requires an understanding of predicted cardiopulmonary responses to the pharmacologic agents being used in the animal, combined with an evaluation of anesthetic depth based on CNS signs. Again, no single parameter that can be monitored is solely adequate to pinpoint accurately the plane of anesthesia in an anesthetized animal. All of the above information on anesthetic depth should be considered when formalizing a proper anesthetic monitoring plan to assure the best possible anesthetic outcome (Shafer and Stanski, 2008).

F. Monitoring techniques

The key body systems responsible for the short-term wellbeing of an animal during anesthesia and surgery are the cardiovascular, respiratory, and CNS. These systems' normal homeostatic mechanisms are affected by anesthetic administration. Patient monitoring allows for the recognition of the extent of compromise to each body system during the course of a procedure and lets the anesthetist make adjustments in the anesthetic protocol to prevent untoward long-term effects in the animal (Dorsch and Dorsch, 2008a). Specialized monitoring equipment is available to supplement routine observational skills. Physiologic data relating to the cardiovascular, respiratory, and CNS can be collected and recorded using common monitoring equipment (Fig. 10.1).

G. Cardiovascular system monitoring

Most anesthetic agents cause a dose-dependent depression of the cardiovascular system. Therefore, monitoring of this system provides not only an assessment of overall circulatory function and any potential compromise but also additional information on the depth of anesthesia.

H. Heart rate

Monitoring HR is important because of its effects on overall cardiac output (CO), which directly relates to the delivery of oxygen to tissues. CO is the product of HR and stroke volume. HR may be influenced by the depth of anesthesia, such that bradycardia frequently occurs as the anesthetic plane deepens and tachycardia occurs when the anesthetic plane lightens. The definition of bradycardia and

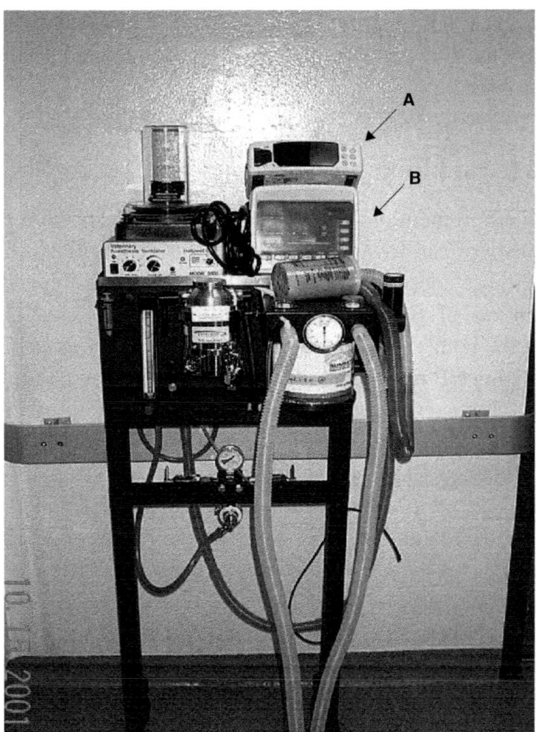

FIGURE 10.1 Typical anesthesia monitoring equipment used in the laboratory environment. (A) Pulse oximetry, ECG, and capnography. (B) NIBP and HR.

tachycardia is species-dependent, so at the start of anesthesia, the anesthetist should be aware of the normal range of HR for the species being studied. Stethoscopes and other cardiac monitoring equipment can be useful in assessing the heartbeat, but cardiac function should be assessed in conjunction with measures of blood pressure (BP), capillary refill times, and palpation of peripheral pulses. The importance of not relying solely on one parameter while monitoring is well illustrated by understanding physiologic parameters that can cause changes in HR. Tachycardia can be caused by painful surgical stimulation in a lightly anesthetized animal, and deepening the plane of anesthesia or providing additional analgesia is often indicated in this case. However, hypotension, hypovolemia, hypoxia, hyperthermia, and hypercarbia are also potential causes of elevated HR, and increasing the level of anesthesia would be contraindicated. Determination of the actual cause of tachycardia requires examination of other monitored information and normalization of HR may require treatment of any derangements found. Bradycardia may be caused by too deep a plane of anesthesia, certain specific anesthetic drugs (i.e., opioids and alpha-2-agonists), reflex activity (i.e., mesenteric traction, intubation, oculocardiac reflex, and hypertension), hypothermia, hyperkalemia, or cardiac conduction disturbances. If anesthetic depth is determined to be appropriate, bradycardia may be treated by anticholinergics. Anticholinergics would be the treatment of choice for bradycardia caused by opioids, alpha-2 agonists, vagal reflex activity, and certain cardiac conduction disturbances, but the assessment of ABP in conjunction with HR can be used to guide the necessity for intervention in these cases. Bradycardia secondary to hypothermia is unresponsive to anticholinergics and requires rewarming of the animal for improvement. Bradycardia as a result of hyperkalemia represents a serious disturbance in cardiac conduction, and emergency steps to reduce serum potassium need to be instituted.

I. Pulse

Pulse strength and regularity are usually determined by digital palpation of the pulse from an accessible site (i.e., femoral artery, lingual artery, auricular artery, or tail artery). Pulse strength may be impossible to palpate in some smaller species. Palpation of the pulse is helpful in assessing the mechanical activity of the heart. Palpation can reveal the presence of an arrhythmia and, based on the subjective assessment of the pulse strength, can provide some information relating to the adequacy of CO. It is important to realize when interpreting pulse strength that the perceived intensity of the palpated pulse is a function of the magnitude of the pulse pressure. Pulse pressure is the numerical difference between the systolic and the diastolic ABP. The larger the systolic/diastolic difference, the stronger the pulse feels. A large systolic/diastolic difference resulting in good pulse strength does not always indicate adequate tissue perfusion. Once again, relying only on a single parameter—in this case, the pulse strength—could be misleading, and therefore other parameters should be used to confirm adequate cardiovascular function. Although a good pulse is not always an absolute indication that all is going well during anesthesia, the absence of a palpable pulse should always be considered an indicator of an emergency as well as a sign of inadequate cardiovascular function.

J. Capillary refill time

CRT is defined as the time it takes for mucous membrane (MM) color to return to normal after a blanching digital pressure is applied to the membrane and released. Normal CRT should be less than 2.5 seconds. CRT is considered an indicator of peripheral perfusion, and a prolonged CRT is seen during hypotension or low CO states. It is important to realize, however, that CRT is markedly influenced by arteriolar tone. A number of conditions causing peripheral arterial vasoconstriction will prolong CRT even though overall tissue perfusion is likely adequate. Pain, excitement, hypothermia, and certain drugs (i.e., alpha-2 agonists) induce vasoconstriction and can increase CRT above the acceptable upper limit. On detecting a prolonged CRT, other monitoring parameters must be examined in order to determine its significance.

K. Electrocardiography

Electrocardiography (ECG/EKG) is a technique that provides important information during the course of anesthesia. ECG monitoring during anesthesia is possible in most large species. Specialized units that are capable of counting HRs greater than 300 bpm are available and can be used with smaller laboratory animal species. Many ECG monitors also provide a continuous readout of HR. When attached to a recording device, ECG monitors allow the continuous or intermittent accumulation of HR and rhythm data at different stages of an experiment. In addition, an ECG is the only way to diagnose arrhythmias that might occur as a result of anesthesia or surgical manipulations. The major shortcoming of the ECG as a monitoring tool is that it represents only cardiac electrical activity and does not provide an assessment of the CO or tissue perfusion, which are the critical functional aspects of cardiovascular performance.

The ECG of most species consists of a set of waves, including the P wave that indicates atrial depolarization and the T wave that represents ventricular repolarization. The shape, size, and timing of each of these waves are dependent on the species and the particular lead system that is being used. For diagnostic purposes in an individual with suspected cardiac disease, a multilead system (12 lead) is frequently used. During monitoring of anesthesia, the ECG mostly serves as an HR and rhythm monitor, and therefore a three-lead system (i.e., lead II with reference electrodes attached at the right forelimb and left hind limb) is often used. In small laboratory animal species, the electrical signal is small (low millivoltage), as are the amplitudes of the ECG waves. In addition, the HR is relatively rapid, sometimes making it difficult to discern anything other than the QRS complex on the ECG. Therefore, it is critical to ensure that the equipment that is being utilized was designed for the species that is being evaluated. Despite this situation, the ECG can still be useful in these smaller species as an indicator of HR, and an irregular PR interval, or changes in the shape of the QRS complex can be a useful indicator of the development of arrhythmias (Fig. 10.2). The recognition of the type of arrhythmia usually determines the appropriate treatment; consultation of a comprehensive cardiology text is recommended (Santilli et al., 2018).

L. Arterial blood pressure

The measurement of ABP can be helpful in determining the adequacy of cardiovascular function during anesthesia. The majority of anesthetic agents will cause a dose-dependent depression of BP through their effects on CO, vascular tone, or both, and, therefore, a trend of progressively decreasing BP may be an indication of excessive anesthetic depth. However, to accurately interpret the significance of changes, the anesthetist must consider the varied factors that influence BP. Factors that contribute most notably to BP are CO, peripheral vascular resistance (PVR), and blood volume. If CO and/or PVR increase, so will arterial BP. If CO decreases by way of direct anesthetic depression of the myocardium or decreased filling pressures due to loss of blood volume, without a compensatory increase in arteriolar tone (this response is depressed by many anesthetics), the BP will fall.

The practical significance of arterial BP is that it is a determinant of tissue blood flow. The upstream (arterial) pressure must significantly exceed the downstream (venous) pressure to drive flow through tissue capillary beds. The perfusion pressure should be greater than 60 mmHg for adequate tissue perfusion. Therefore, in monitoring arterial BP, a mean BP less than 60 mmHg is considered unacceptable for maintaining tissue blood flow. Mean BP is not the mathematical mean of systolic and diastolic BP. Rather, it can be estimated from the measured systolic and diastolic pressures by the following equation:

$$\text{mean BP} = \text{diastolic BP} + 0.3\,(\text{systolic BP} - \text{diastolic BP}).$$

The gold standard of BP measurement is via the direct arterial cannulation and connection to a pressure transducer. This allows for the determination of accurate, beat-by-beat, systolic, diastolic, and mean BP. Because of the invasive nature of this technique, the difficulty in placing arterial catheters in many species, and the expense of the electronic monitor, direct ABP monitoring is infrequently performed. There are, however, two reasonable noninvasive alternatives for indirect BP monitoring: the oscillometric monitor and the Doppler ultrasonic BP monitor (Skelding and Valverde, 2020). Although both of these devices are versatile and very

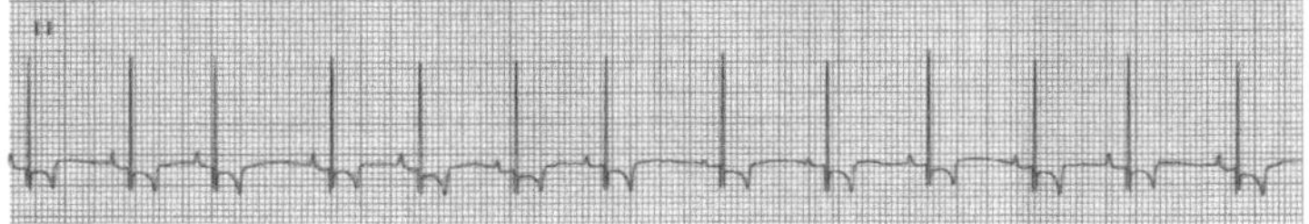

FIGURE 10.2 Sample ECG from a dog with a mild sinus arrhythmia with wandering pacemaker. *Photo credit is Daniel Hogan, DVM, DCVIM-Cardiology, College of Veterinary Medicine, Purdue University, West Lafayette, IN.*

useful in the clinical setting, there are some limitations to their use. Small patient size, extremes of HR (<40 or >200 bpm), significant hypotension, and hypothermia (through peripheral vasoconstriction) may all interfere with the accuracy of the pressures obtained with either of these methods. Additionally, oscillometric monitors vary in their accuracy and reliability between manufacturers (Skelding and Valverde, 2020). However, Wilde et al. (2017) report useful adaptations to oscillometric BP monitors for use in the laboratory animal setting, although limitations to this method are acknowledged.

Oscillometric monitors generally report a measured systolic and mean BP and extrapolate a diastolic BP. Some oscillometric devices also report HR, which can be used as an index of the accuracy of the reported pressures. Pressure values reported by equipment should be questioned when monitor readings are accompanied by a reported HR that varies more than 10% from the actual HR as determined by auscultation or palpation of pulses.

A Doppler ultrasonic monitor is used with a sphygmomanometer and cuff to measure BP. The value generated approximates the systolic BP in dogs and rabbits, and mean BP in cats. As a rule, a systolic BP > 100 mmHg is accompanied by adequate tissue perfusion. A major advantage of the Doppler monitor is that it also transmits a pulse of sound signal through a speaker device. This audible signal can be used to count HR and indicates that there is functional cardiac activity adequate enough to generate a peripheral pulse. In addition, although subjective, changes in the intensity of the audible signal correlate with changes in CO. If the audible Doppler signal becomes diminished, one should quickly examine other parameters of hemodynamic status. Doppler monitors are useful in virtually all species, although in small species they are primarily used as pulse monitors, with the probe placed on the chest wall directly over the cardiac apex (Stypmann, 2007).

M. Central venous pressure

Central venous pressure (CVP) is measured directly by insertion of a catheter through the anterior vena cava to the level of the right atrium. This catheter is then connected to a fluid manometer, where the pressure reading can be read. Thus, the CVP value reflects the pressure in the right atrium and is an index of cardiac filling pressure (Magder, 2005). The CVP value allows the anesthetist to assess how well the blood is returning to the heart, which is helpful in right-sided heart failure patients. The factors that influence the CVP are the volume of the blood in the central veins, the compliance of the right atrium during filling, central vein vascular tone, and intrathoracic pressure. Monitoring CVP is an insensitive measure of volume status and has been largely superseded by assessments of responses to delivering a fluid bolus and dynamic measures (such as pulse pressure variation).

N. Pulmonary artery pressures and cardiac output

The standard method of obtaining CO data during anesthesia is through measurements of pulmonary blood flow by thermodilution. The pulmonary artery (Swan-Ganz) catheter is a balloon-tipped, flow-directed device equipped with a thermistor tip for measuring the change in blood temperature after injection of a cold solution. This device is passed into the pulmonary artery (PA) via the jugular vein-right atrium-right ventricle route, and confirmation of correct placement is usually made by observation of characteristic changes in the pressure waveform during its passage (Rodriguez Ziccardi and Khalid, 2021). The PA catheter allows measurement of CO, systolic, diastolic, and mean PA pressures, as well as PA occlusion pressure (PAOP, also called "wedge" pressure), which is obtained upon inflation of the balloon tip, impeding PA blood flow, and reflecting left atrial pressure. Normal values in many species for PA pressures are: systolic, 20–40 mmHg; mean, 10–20 mmHg; diastolic, 5–10 mmHg; and PAOP, 3–8 mmHg. PA catheters are indicated for mixed venous blood gas sampling, measurement of CO, and pulmonary hemodynamics. Because much of the hemodynamic data obtained from PA catheters involve the calculation of derived variables (i.e., vascular resistances and ventricular stroke work index), PA catheters are used more often in the experimental setting for the collection of study-specific data rather than for anesthetic monitoring per se; however, the information gained from the catheter is often useful for making real-time anesthetic determinations during these studies. Additional, less invasive, methods include the use of lithium dilution or the pulse contour analysis for CO.

O. Respiratory system monitoring

The major function of the respiratory system is to act as a gas exchange organ. The lung is responsible for the introduction of oxygen into the arterial blood (oxygenation), and the elimination of carbon dioxide (CO_2) from the body (ventilation), and the uptake and elimination of gas anesthetics when inhalation anesthesia is used. To evaluate respiratory function, both oxygenation and ventilation must be assessed. It is important to monitor the respiratory system during anesthesia not only because of its life-sustaining importance but also because many anesthetic agents suppress respiratory control mechanisms; respiratory arrest usually precedes cardiovascular collapse from excess anesthetic. Direct observation allows the anesthetist to assess respiratory frequency, rhythm, and volume as well as MM color. Each of these parameters alone provides little information about the adequacy of ventilation and oxygenation. However, when viewed collectively, these parameters accurately report the state of respiratory function.

P. Respiratory rate

The RR can be determined by visual observation of the animal for chest wall motion, by auscultation of the thorax, or by observing the rebreathing bag on the anesthetic machine. There are significant species variations in the range of normal respiratory rates, and the anesthetist should know relevant values prior to anesthetizing any animal. In particular, in smaller laboratory animal species (rodents), it can be difficult to visually assess RR. Usually, the higher the basal metabolic rate (and CO_2 production) of the animal, the higher the resting RR. Most anesthetics are respiratory depressants, and, as a general rule, the RR decreases with increasing anesthetic depth.

Q. Mucous membrane color

Cyanosis is the bluish or purplish discoloration of MM, peripheral extremities, or skin that results from reduced hemoglobin in the blood. Cyanosis may be central, which occurs when deoxygenated hemoglobin in the arteries is above 5 g/dL with oxygen saturation below 85% (Adeyinka and Kondamudi, 2022). Peripheral cyanosis results from a difference in the saturation between the arterial and venous blood. This occurs as a result of increased oxygen extraction by the peripheral tissue in the capillary bed and can occur in hypothermia and low CO. In anemic states, when the blood hemoglobin concentration is low, hypoxemia can be quite severe even though cyanosis is not evident. Therefore, the appearance of cyanotic MM indicates hypoxemia, but a lack of visible cyanosis does not mean that the animal is adequately oxygenated. Identifying cyanosis by MM color is insensitive and should not be used in place of pulse oximetry (or arterial blood gas analysis, where available) (Comroe and Botelho, 1947).

R. Tidal volume

The amount of gas entering the respiratory tract during one respiratory cycle is called the tidal volume. An average tidal volume for most species is about 10–15 mL/kg; however, there can be wide variations among species. Monitoring tidal volume is usually subjective and based on the degree of chest wall motion with each breath or the amount of movement in the rebreathing bag of an anesthetic machine. It is important to realize that monitoring chest wall motion alone tells little about the actual volume of gas inhaled, as an animal with an airway obstruction or restrictive pulmonary disease often has marked chest wall motion with little air movement, since the chest wall motion reflects difficulty in breathing. In certain species, such as ruminants, rabbits, and guinea pigs, which have the potential to develop abdominal distension secondary to gas accumulation in their gastrointestinal tract, close attention should be paid to respiratory effort and tidal volume because abdominal distension can be a significant cause of respiratory insufficiency. Evaluation of other parameters, such as the concurrent change of volume in the rebreathing bag, can be beneficial to help confirm adequate tidal volume. The volume of gas in each respiratory cycle can be measured by attaching an instrument called a respirometer to the endotracheal tube.

S. Minute ventilation

Minute ventilation is a measurement of the amount of air that enters the lungs per minute. Minute ventilation is the product of RR and tidal volume. The adequacy of ventilation is judged by the effectiveness of the lung in removing CO_2 from the pulmonary capillary blood and is directly linked to minute ventilation. The partial pressure of carbon dioxide ($PaCO_2$) in the arterial blood is inversely proportional to minute ventilation, such that if metabolism (CO_2 production) remains constant, doubling the minute ventilation decreases $PaCO_2$ by one-half. The $PaCO_2$ in arterial blood is the major stimulus for ventilation in the respiratory control center in the brain, where anesthetics exert their respiratory depressant effect (increased threshold and decreased sensitivity to CO_2) (Rocco and Zin, 2002). Decreasing minute ventilation during anesthesia may reflect a decrease in CO_2 production (often seen with hypothermia) or it may reflect increased depression of the respiratory control centers from the anesthetic drugs. An elevation in $PaCO_2$ (above 60 mmHg) indicates the need for increased minute ventilation, through an increase in respiratory rate, volume, or both, and may also indicate the need to decrease anesthetic depth.

T. Capnography

The concentration of CO_2 in the inspired and expired gas can be continuously measured from the airway using capnography. The capnograph samples airway gas from a port located either at the endotracheal tube/breathing circuit interface or from a site at the distal end of the endotracheal tube. The capnograph measures the CO_2 in the inspired and expired air that passes through the monitor and displays it in graph form (the capnograph). Inspired gas should contain virtually no CO_2. As an animal exhales and alveolar emptying occurs, CO_2 appears in the exhaled gas. The peak of expired (end-tidal) CO_2 is a reflection of the $PaCO_2$ in alveolar gas, which is equilibrated with arterial blood (Lafferty and Pollock, 2018). Therefore increased values suggest hypoventilation, whereas low end-tidal CO_2 suggests hyperventilation. The end-tidal CO_2 may underestimate the $PaCO_2$ because the gas sampling flow rate of the machine is high enough that gas (containing virtually no CO_2) is entrained from the breathing circuit, diluting the end-tidal sample (Dorsch and Dorsch, 2008b). In addition to ventilatory information, a capnograph can be useful in the rapid detection of endotracheal tube malfunctions, such as disconnection from the circuit or a kinked or obstructed tube. Capnographs have also proven to be sensitive early indicators of the development of malignant hyperthermia in susceptible species (primarily swine), in which a rapid rise in end-tidal CO_2 reflects the marked metabolic increase in CO_2 production that precedes the often fatal increase in body temperature (Rosenberg et al., 2015).

U. Pulse oximetry

A pulse oximeter is an instrument that, by means of a light source and photodetector, measures the light absorbance of tissues and indicates the level of oxygen saturation of hemoglobin (SaO_2) in the arterial blood (Duke-Novakovski, 2017). The selection of a monitor that utilizes low-noise cabled technology can aid in superior performance under conditions where the patient is potentially experiencing vasoconstriction secondary to alpha-2 agonists or weak pulses. Oxygen saturation of hemoglobin is related to the partial pressure of oxygen (PaO_2) in arterial blood such that for each value of PaO_2 there is a corresponding percentage of hemoglobin that is saturated with oxygen. Adequate arterial oxygenation requires a minimum PaO_2 value greater than 60 mmHg (and ideally >90 mmHg). A PaO_2 of 60 mmHg corresponds to a 90% saturation of the hemoglobin in the arterial blood. Using a pulse oximeter, changes in hemoglobin saturation can be monitored continuously. When the O_2 saturation value falls below 90%, the animal is hypoxemic and steps should be taken to improve oxygenation, such as administering 100% oxygen, endotracheal intubation, and/or assisted ventilation as indicated. There are also a number of conditions that produce erroneously low oximeter values. Because the pulse oximeter is highly dependent on good peripheral perfusion, hypotension and hypothermia will impair accuracy. Motion artifacts (i.e., patient movement or shivering) and bright external light sources (i.e., fluorescent lights, surgery lights, and heat lamps) will interfere with the probe's ability to detect the signal, and pigmented tissue may change light absorbance values, resulting in inaccurate readings (Chan et al., 2013). In addition to reporting SaO_2, the pulse oximeter often gives a value for HR. If the HR value, as reported, varies significantly from the actual HR obtained by palpation, then the accuracy of the reported SaO_2 should be questioned. Pulse oximeter probes in animals work best when placed on nonpigmented, hairless tissues such as the tongue or the tail.

V. Blood gas analysis

Although the abovementioned techniques can provide the anesthetist with respiratory system information, the only absolute way to effectively judge the adequacy of ventilation and oxygenation in any animal is through arterial blood gas analysis, although noninvasive measurements of pulmonary gas exchange are gaining traction in human medicine (Prisk and West, 2021). This analysis is carried out on an arterial blood sample, which must be stored on ice and analyzed within 2 hours of collection. The $PaCO_2$ in arterial blood should fall between 35 and 45 mmHg. A $PaCO_2 < 35$ mmHg is defined as hyperventilation, which most often occurs iatrogenically in animals that are being ventilated. A $PaCO_2 > 45$ mmHg is, by definition, hypoventilation and, depending on the experimental conditions, may also indicate the need for assisted ventilation. If an animal has a $PaCO_2$ above 60 mmHg during anesthesia, steps should be taken immediately to improve ventilation, which may include endotracheal intubation, manual or mechanical ventilation, or decreasing the level of anesthesia as indicated. A PaO_2 in the arterial blood >90 mmHg assures adequate oxygenation (provided there is adequate tissue perfusion). Much higher levels of PaO_2 are often expected during anesthesia depending on the percentage of oxygen in the inspired gas. As a rule, the PaO_2 should be approximately 5 times the inspired oxygen concentration, so that when breathing 100% oxygen the arterial PaO_2 should approach 500 mmHg. An animal may be relatively hypoxemic in that its PaO_2 is less than would be expected for the particular inspired oxygen concentration. This can indicate concurrent hypoventilation (check the $PaCO_2$), ventilation-perfusion mismatching, a shunt, or diffusion impairment. Absolute hypoxemia with significant impairment of tissue oxygenation occurs at PaO_2 values < 60 mmHg. When PaO_2 falls to that level, measures should be taken to improve oxygenation immediately, as hypoxemia is poorly tolerated, such as maximizing the inspired oxygen concentration and improving ventilation.

W. End-tidal anesthetic concentration

An adjunct to monitoring anesthetic depth is monitoring the end-expiratory (end-tidal) inhalation agent concentration during the anesthetic procedure. As described with capnography, the end-expiratory concentration of an inhalation agent is assumed to be reflective of the arterial and brain concentrations of the agent being monitored. Typically, surgical anesthesia is achieved at 1.2–1.5 times the minimum alveolar concentration (MAC) of an inhaled anesthetic agent, and the MAC varies with the agent (Lobo et al., 2022). As an example, the average MAC of isoflurane in the cat was approximately 1.71% and sevoflurane was approximately 3.08% (Shaughnessy and Hofmeister, 2014). An end-tidal inhalation agent monitor will indicate if the alveolar concentration of gas is in the proper range and, in combination with observational signs of depth of anesthesia, will indicate if the animal is suitably anesthetized for a surgical procedure.

As with other parameters, using end-tidal agent concentration as the sole indicator of anesthetic depth can lead to erroneous conclusions and poor outcomes. The administration of other anesthetic drugs, especially opioids or alpha-2 agonists that have significant analgesic properties, will allow an animal to be adequately anesthetized at anesthetic concentrations much less than 1.5 times MAC. Hypothermia can also markedly decrease the MAC of inhalation agents, so relying on end-tidal concentration alone without also observing the animal may lead to inappropriately deep planes of anesthesia. It is important to recognize that the end-tidal gas concentration necessary to achieve surgical anesthesia is not the same thing as the concentration setting on the vaporizer. During the induction and equilibration phases of inhalation anesthesia, there can be a large difference between the vaporizer concentration and the end-tidal value (the vaporizer concentration being higher at the beginning of anesthesia). With time, the difference between these two concentrations narrows. Monitoring end-tidal agent concentrations can serve as a useful guide for when to decrease or increase the setting on the vaporizer, which is often necessary in a research setting to quantitatively establish the dose of drug delivered.

X. Electroencephalogram and bispectral index

To date, several different methods to describe and monitor the potency of anesthetic agents and patient anesthetic depth in animals have been described. The majority of these techniques merge the assessment of electroencephalography (EEG) data with other parameters to determine the degree of depression of the frontal cortex. The Bispectral Index (BIS) is an example of technology utilizing a predetermined algorithm of human EEG activity to provide the anesthetist with immediate feedback on the patient's CNS activity, and therefore anesthetic depth. Basically, a number between 0 and 100 is derived from EEG data collected from the patient during anesthesia. A typical BIS value of 40–60 is used to prevent intraoperative awareness in human anesthesia. The use of BIS technology has been reported recently with variable success in animals (cattle, dogs, chickens, and swine) (Deschk et al., 2015; Gallego et al., 2021; Jaber et al., 2015; Saenubol et al., 2020). However, as with similar modalities that assess the EEG, the implementation of BIS should be carefully considered because of the variable responses measured when using different classes of anesthetic agents, in addition to species-specific differences. Physical evaluation of anesthetic depth is still one of the best tools available (Haskins, 2015).

III. Special circumstances

A. Unique challenges of laboratory animals

Monitoring general anesthesia becomes more difficult when the patient size is reduced. The laboratory animal veterinarian is uniquely tasked with conducting anesthesia in a wide variety of species. Most of these species are small, such as rodents, and some are aquatic, such as zebrafish and amphibians. These challenges can make routine techniques used to monitor anesthesia (i.e., manual pulse, observations of respiratory effort, etc.) difficult. To compensate for this, the use of creative techniques and modified equipment is often necessary to be able to follow the status of these patients under anesthesia (Le et al., 2020; Smith et al., 2018). Other equipment, such as a BP-monitoring device, is often impractical. However, modifications can sometimes be made to existing equipment to accommodate the smaller species used in the laboratory setting (Pollock et al., 2020). Summary comments on anesthetic monitoring in the laboratory animal environment can be found in Table 10.2.

Further challenges facing the laboratory animal anesthetist are the necessity for physiologic stability for valid experimental data and accurate interpretation of research results. Anesthetics can have a profound effect on research results, and a well-documented anesthetic procedure is an important part of the experimental record. Data collected during anesthetic monitoring serves as the basis for the design of subsequent anesthetic procedures.

The need to minimize pain and distress is an important aspect of all veterinary anesthesia, but the regulatory environment adds an additional dimension in the research setting. An anesthetic protocol, approved by the Institutional Animal Care and Use Committee, is the first step toward this goal, but anesthetic monitoring and the provision of appropriate analgesics also play a role as tindicators of an animal's response to the procedure while under the influence of anesthetic drugs. Investigators are encouraged to seek the advice of trained professionals in laboratory animal medicine and anesthesiology, especially when developing new animal models or techniques.

The most successful anesthetic protocols, however, come with practice. To determine the best protocol for a

TABLE 10.2 Summary comments on anesthetic monitoring in the laboratory animal environment.

- Comprehensive and ongoing training program for *all* personnel conducting anesthesia
- Preanesthetic physical exam and ASA classification[a] as appropriate
- Create appropriate anesthetic plan
  - Include current ASA classification[a]
  - Consider research procedure
  - Consult previous anesthetic protocols/anesthetic records
- Minimum monitoring should include
  - Heart rate/rhythm and pulse pressure
  - Respiratory rate and pattern
  - CRT/mucous membrane color
  - Temperature
  - Blood loss
  - Anesthetic record
  - Consult AVCA suggested plan[b]
- Anesthetic depth
  - Use a combination of observations
  - Consider traditional methods
  - Consider BIS EEG monitoring
- Consider use of specialized monitors
  - NIBP and INBP
  - Pulse oximetry
  - Capnography
  - Peripheral nerve stimulator for NMB protocols
  - BIS

[a]*American Society of Anesthesiologists (2020).*
[b]*American College of Veterinary Anesthesiologists (2009).*

given research or surgical procedure, it is helpful to have anesthetic monitoring records of past procedures. Such records assist the anesthetist in anticipating problems that might be encountered in future procedures and evaluating the patient during the postprocedure period. In addition, good monitoring records are always necessary for demonstrating consistency in experimental protocols and for eliminating variability that may confound results.

IV. Summary and conclusions

Frequent evaluation of the physiologic status of an anesthetized animal leads to early recognition of homeostatic disturbances, facilitating timely and appropriate intervention to prevent anesthetic mishaps, and helping to provide a stable physiologic state consistent with the welfare of the patient and sound experimental data. An accurate interpretation of monitoring data begins with the knowledge of what is normal for the animal species, and this should always start with a preanesthetic evaluation. It is usually not feasible to monitor all possible parameters in every patient, especially in the smaller laboratory animal species, so the anesthetist must choose those parameters that are most likely to change in response to anesthesia and surgery and will have an impact on the well-being of the animal and on the research itself. The systems requiring at least some degree of monitoring in all patients include the cardiovascular, respiratory, and CNS. Therefore, the anesthetist must have a basic knowledge of the physiological effects of the anesthetic agents to be used, the procedures to be performed, and the experimental manipulations and data to be collected as part of the experimental protocol. When a change in a monitored parameter occurs, the anesthetist must accurately determine the cause of that change. Monitoring several parameters, with serial data collected, allows trends to be observed that enable the anesthetist to tailor the anesthetic protocol to the response of the animal. This is important because systems interact with each other to create a physiologic state, and because interventions will likely affect more than one system.

Acknowledgments

In preparation of this chapter for this third edition, the authors wish to acknowledge J.C. Smith and P.J. Danneman for their efforts in the preparation of Chapter 6 (Monitoring of Anesthesia) for the second edition of this text.

References

Adeyinka, A., Kondamudi, N.P., January 2022. Cyanosis. In: StatPearls [Internet]. StatPearls Publishing, Treasure Island (FL). Available from: https://www.ncbi.nlm.nih.gov/books/NBK482247/. (Accessed January 2022).

American College of Veterinary Anesthesiologists, 2009. Recommendations for Monitoring Anesthetized Veterinary Patients. https://acvaa.org/wp-content/uploads/2019/05/Small-Animal-Monitoring-Guidlines.pdf. (Accessed January 2022).

American Society of Anesthesiologists, 2020. Physical Status Classification in "Relative Value Guide". https://www.asahq.org/standards-and-guidelines/asa-physical-status-classification-system. (Accessed January 2022).

Antognini, J.F., Barter, L., Carstens, E., 2005. Movement as an index of anesthetic depth in humans and experimental animals. Comp. Med. 55 (5), 413–418.

Chan, E.D., Chan, M.M., Chan, M.M., June 2013. Pulse oximetry: understanding its basic principles facilitates appreciation of its limitations. Respir. Med. 107 (6), 789–799. https://doi.org/10.1016/j.rmed.2013.02.004. Epub 2013 Mar 13.

Comroe Jr., J.H., Botelho, S., 1947. The unreliability of cyanosis in the recognition of arterial anoxemia. Am. J. Med. Sci. 124 (1), 1–6.

Deschk, M., Wagatsuma, J.T., Araujo, M.A., Santos, G.G.F., Junior, S.S.R., Abimussi, C.J.X., Siqueira, C.E., Motta, J.C.L., Perri, S.H.V., Santos, P.S.P., 2015. Continuous infusion of propofol in calves: bispectral index and hemodynamic effects. Vet. Anaesth. Analg. 43 (3), 309–315.

Dorsch, J.A., Dorsch, S.E., 2008a. Monitoring devices. In: Understanding Anesthesia Equipment, fifth ed. Wolters Kluwer Health, Philadelphia, PA, pp. 685–858.

Dorsch, J.A., Dorsch, S.E., 2008b. Understanding Anesthesia Equipment, fifth ed. Wolters Kluwer Health, Philadelphia, PA, pp. 191–208.

Duke-Novakovski, T., 2017. Basics of monitoring equipment. Can. Vet. J. 58 (11), 1200–1208.

Gallego, M.L.V., Jurado, O.M., Hatt, J., 2021. Effects of isoflurane and sevoflurane alone and in combination with butorphanol or medetomidine on the bispectral index in chickens. BMC Vet. Res. 17 (1), 201.

Haskins, S.C., 2015. Monitoring anesthetized patients. In: Grimm, K.A., Lamont, L.A., Tranquilli, W.J., Greene, S.A., Robertson, S.A. (Eds.), Veterinary Anesthesia and Analgesia, fifth ed. Wiley Blackwell, New York, NY, pp. 86–113.

Jaber, S.M., Sullivan, S., Hankenson, F.C., Kilbaugh, T.J., Marguiles, S.S., 2015. Comparison of heart rate and blood pressure with toe pinch and bispectral index for monitoring the depth of anesthesia in piglets. J. Am. Assoc. Lab. Anim. Sci. 54 (5), 536–544.

Lafferty, K., Pollock, C., 2018. Capnometry in Exotic Animal Species. https://lafeber.com/vet/capnometry/. (Accessed February 2022).

Le, T., Zhang, J., Xia, X., Xu, X., Clark, I., Schmiess-Heine, L., Nguyen, A.H., Lau, M.P.H., Cao, H., 2020. Continuous electrocardiogram monitoring in zebrafish with prolonged mild anesthesia. Annu. Int. Conf. IEEE Eng. Med. Biol. Soc. 2020, 2610–2613.

Lobo, S.A., Ojeda, J., Dua, A., et al., 2022 Jan. Minimum alveolar concentration [Updated 2021 Sep 18]. In: StatPearls [Internet]. StatPearls Publishing, Treasure Island (FL).

MacLennan, D.H., Phillips, M.S., 1992. Malignant hyperthermia. Science 256 (5058), 789–794.

Magder, S., 2005. How to use central venous pressure measurements. Curr. Opin. Crit. Care 11 (3), 264–270.

Pollock, C., Nugent-Deal, J., O'Shea, R., 2020. Anesthetic Depth in Exotic Animals: Monitoring the Degree of Central Nervous System Depression. https://lafeber.com/vet/anesthetic-depth-in-exotic-animals-monitoring-the-degree-of-central-nervous-system-depression/. (Accessed January 2022).

Prisk, G.K., West, J.B., October 21, 2021. Non-invasive measurement of pulmonary gas exchange efficiency: the oxygen deficit. Front. Physiol. 12, 757857. https://doi.org/10.3389/fphys.2021.757857.

Rembert, M.S., Smith, J.A., Hosgood, G., 2004. A comparison of forced-air warming system to traditional thermal support for rodent microenvironments. Lab. Anim. 38 (1), 55–63.

Rocco, P.R.M., Zin, W.A., 2002. Respiratory effects of anesthesia. In: Gullo, A. (Ed.), Anaesthesia, Pain, Intensive Care and Emergency Medicine—A.P.I.C.E. Springer, Milano. https://doi.org/10.1007/978-88-470-2099-3_4.

Rodriguez Ziccardi, M., Khalid, N., 2021. Pulmonary Artery Catheterization. In: StatPearls [Internet]. StatPearls Publishing, Treasure Island (FL). Available from: https://www.ncbi.nlm.nih.gov/books/NBK482170/. (Accessed January 2022).

Rosenberg, H., Pollock, N., Schiemann, A., et al., 2015. Malignant hyperthermia: a review. Orphanet J. Rare Dis. 10, 93. https://doi.org/10.1186/s13023-015-0310-1.

Saenubol, P., Akatvipat, A., Pleumsamran, A., Chankrachang, S., 2020. Correlation between bispectral index value and modified Glasgow coma scale score in dogs with altered levels of consciousness. J. Vet. Emerg. Crit. Care 31 (1), 52–58.

Shafer, S.L., Stanski, D.R., 2008. Defining depth of anesthesia. Hanb. Exp. Pharmacol. 182, 409–423.

Shaughnessy, M.R., Hofmeister, E.H., January 2014. A systematic review of sevoflurane and isoflurane minimum alveolar concentration in domestic cats. Vet. Anaesth. Analg. 41 (1), 1–13. https://doi.org/10.1111/vaa.12083. Epub 2013 Sep. 10.

Skelding, A., Valverde, A., 2020. Non-invasive blood pressure measurement in animals: Part 1—Techniques for measurement and validation of non-invasive devices. La Revue Veterinaire Canadienne 61 (4), 368–374.

Skorupski, A.M., Zhang, J., Ferguson, D., Lawrence, F., Hankenson, F.C., 2017. Quantification of induced hypothermia from aseptic scrub applications during rodent surgery preparation. J. Am. Assoc. Lab. Anim. Sci. 56, 562–569.

Smith, B.D., Vail, K.J., Carroll, G.L., Taylor, M.C., Jeffery, N.D., Vemulapalli, T.H., Elliott, J.J., 2018. Comparison of etomidate, benzocaine, and MS222 anesthesia with and without subsequent flunixin meglumine analgesia in African clawed frogs (*Xenopus laevis*). J. Am. Assoc. Lab. Anim. Sci. 57 (2), 202–209.

Stypmann, J., 2007. Doppler ultrasound in mice. Echocardiography 24 (1), 97–112.

Santilli, R., Moïse, N.S., Pariaut, R., Perego, M., 2018. Electrocardiography of the dog and cat. In: Diagnosis of Arrhythmias, second ed. Edra S.p.A., Milano, Italia.

Wilde, E., Aubdool, A.A., Thakore, P., Baldissera Jr., L., Alawi, K.M., Keeble, J., Nandi, M., Brain, S.D., 2017. Tail-cuff technique and its influence on central blood pressure in the mouse. J. Am. Heart Assoc. 6, e005204.

Section IV

Periprocedural care

Chapter 11

General care: periprocedural management considerations for research animals

F. Claire Hankenson[1], K. Andrew Claude[2] and Vengai Mavangira[3]

[1]Laboratory Animal Medicine, School of Veterinary Medicine, University of Pennsylvania, Philadelphia, PA, United States; [2]Department of Clinical Science, Carlson College of Veterinary Medicine, Oregon State University, Corvallis, OR, United States; [3]Department of Veterinary Diagnostic and Production Animal Medicine, College of Veterinary Medicine, Iowa State University, Ames, IA, United States

Chapter outline

I. Introduction

Periprocedural management and postprocedural care are vital components of animal outcomes, regardless of whether they occur in general clinical practice, veterinary teaching hospitals, or animal research settings. As the complexity of translational animal models continues to evolve, considerations for skillful and specialized perioperative care measures are heightened. Periprocedural planning is crucial to ensure appropriate resources are committed to the project, including a dedicated animal environment, assigned personnel trained in animal research, with functional equipment and species-specific supplies at the ready. In addition, it is essential to ensure that appropriate anesthetic and analgesic drugs and therapeutics are in stock, in date, and formulated and/or diluted for the species of interest. Lastly, veterinary oversight and consultation in the days following the procedure are critical to assess recovery and address any unexpected clinical events.

The intentions of careful planning and preparation are to maximize positive outcomes for the animals and the animal care personnel involved. While institutions and sites may differ in which regulatory oversight groups and outside agencies participate in the review of their programs, the goal of this chapter is to provide insights into the care and support for a variety of species (as our animal patients) that are necessary for research, teaching, and production in both biomedical and agricultural realms. High-level discussions

Anesthesia and Analgesia in Laboratory Animals. https://doi.org/10.1016/B978-0-12-822215-7.00004-4

in this chapter will focus on care for laboratory mice and rats, larger nonrodent species (rabbits, cats, dogs, nonhuman primates) and agricultural animals. The topics herein are intended to be complimentary to other chapters in this text that provide more detailed guidance on pain assessments, anesthetics, and analgesics and on local and global aspects of regulatory oversight for animal research.

II. Oversight, planning, and organization

A. Veterinary consultation on the selected animal model

Prior to the initiation of any studies involving live animals, approval for all experimental protocols must be secured through application to the institutional animal care and use committee (IACUC) or its equivalent ethical review body if located outside of the United States. Inherent in the application is the need to justify the use of live animals and complete a search of the scientific literature to confirm that the proposed experiments are not duplicative with previously published work and to identify potential refinement, reduction, and replacement opportunities (Mihalko, 2013).

The consultative period required under present research regulations, standards, and the literature search required under the Animal Welfare Act (Title 9, USC, 1985 [AWA]) allows for key opportunities for veterinary team members to consult and clarify the benefits of perioperative planning with involved research personnel. Veterinary consultation can further assist with the determination of the preferred animal model in which the scientific hypothesis is best assessed. The search for alternatives to animal use can assist with the identification of nonanimal options to investigate biological questions. The requisite literature search facilitates a contemporary review of relevant scientific literature and helps to identify resources that may contribute to the design of novel experiments and the best choice of animal model.

The suitability of the selected animal model for the proposed project should be paramount in the overall justification of research work; this includes ethical consideration of issues surrounding the selected species and the benefit of the work to society versus potential harm or "cost" to the animals. Rodent models may be preferable due to their ability to undergo genetic manipulations directly relevant to a particular disease entity, while larger species may be useful for translational work that requires a similar scope of anatomy and physiology in which to evaluate human therapies. The final decision of which species is most appropriate for the research, teaching, or production interest will be the shared decision of the research team, clinical veterinary staff, animal facility personnel, internal administrators, and regulatory oversight bodies.

B. Procedural planning with PREPARE and ARRIVE guidance

Continued global emphasis about the importance of strategic experimental planning of animal experiments has been highlighted in the PREPARE guidance. The acronym "PREPARE" abbreviates the phrase "Planning Research and Experimental Procedures on Animals: Recommendations for Excellence" (Smith et al., 2018a). In this guidance, three overarching areas are emphasized for the research teams to highlight for maximal quality of animal study preparation: formulation of the planned experiments, dialogue (consultation) between scientists and the animal facility team, and quality control of various components of the studies. The authors of PREPARE contend that thorough planning will increase the likelihood of research success and serve to include apt consideration of the 3Rs (as coined by Russell and Burch, 1959).

As a compliment to PREPARE, aspects of reporting on experimental factors are highlighted in the ARRIVE 2.0 guidelines (Percie du Sert et al., 2020). The acronym "ARRIVE" stands for "Animal Research: Reporting of In Vivo Experiments." The ARRIVE "Essential 10" points directly to aspects of planning for animal research in the areas of "Experimental Research (Point 8)" and "Experimental Procedures (Point 9)." Specifically, the guidance encourages documenting all details about the species, strain (and substrain), sex, age, weight, health status, genotype, and any previous procedures conducted with the animals; in total, these specifics encompass the veterinary "history" of the selected animal patient.

The ARRIVE "Essential 10" are accompanied by the "Essential Set", which recommends the inclusion of more granular details of animal research that can impact overall well-being. For example, extrinsic factors, including housing and husbandry conditions, details of environmental enrichment, food and water types, cage mates, and socialization can have significant effects on data. In particular, the ARRIVE guidance prompts researchers to describe expected clinical signs, frequency of monitoring, interventions to be undertaken to reduce pain, distress, and suffering, details of any adverse outcomes and events, and descriptons of objective and humane endpoints established for the study.

1. *Consideration of species characteristics*

To plan, execute, and troubleshoot perioperative procedures, it is vital that personnel are trained and exhibit an understanding of anesthesia, clinical and behavioral signs of pain, and methods to provide supportive care for each species that may be evaluated.

Species-specific age and weight considerations for animal patients must be included in the procedural planning. During anesthetic induction, animals are considered anesthetized when they lose their righting reflex and no longer can ambulate or hold normal postures (McCarren et al., 2013). Further, one can extend the definition of general anesthesia in larger animal patients to the loss of the gag reflex and inability to swallow, thus allowing for airway intubation. For all species, the animal should *never* exhibit a response (i.e., withdrawal, increased respirations, awakening) to intentional stimulus, like a toe pinch or corneal reflex, prior to starting surgical and invasive procedures.

Typically, dedicated equipment is required for routinely checking pulse, blood pressure, oxygenation, and heart rate in laboratory rodents. It has been shown provision of supplemental oxygen, once gas anesthesia is discontinued in rodents, can signifiantly offset hypoxic states (Blevins et al., 2021). For larger species, like cats and dogs, between 47% and 60% of anesthesia-related mortality occurs during the postoperative period, most commonly within the first 3–4 hours, thus, heightened postanesthesia attention to monitoring these patients should be included in the research plan (Brodbelt, 2009; Brodbelt et al., 2008a,b). In certain animal patients, attention to body position during surgery or procedures is critical; for example, the administration of intraperitoneal fluids in rats placed in ventral recumbency for procedures may lead to respiratory distress due to compression of the limited lung field (Hankenson et al., 2021). The position of pregnant animals and ruminants can affect adequate tidal volume due to pressure on the diaphragm, whereas older (e.g., geriatric) animals may have inadequate gas exchange despite a relatively normal tidal volume and respiratory rate. In sum, older animals may be more prone to develop hypoxemia than younger animals (Moens, 2013).

It is recommended that all personnel working in research be versed in the specifics of the experimental protocol, the scientific literature related to the area of study, the animal species needed for the project, and the perceived intensity/invasiveness/impact of the procedures on the animals. Consideration of species-specific characteristics and unique clinical parameters (e.g., body temperature, blood pressure, body mass index, activity level, appetite, hydration) will better permit assessments of normal and abnormal parameters, balanced against the scientific objectives, by research and veterinary staff (Percie du Sert et al., 2020; Al Hussein et al., 2020). The emphasis on good planning to determine suitable severity classifications, appropriate monitoring and assessments and the expectation that staff are trained and competent is further endorsed by international organizations like FELASA, ECLAM, and ESLAV to abide by mandates outlined in Directive 2010/63/EU (Smith et al., 2018a, 2018b).

C. Equipment and animal environment

Most contemporary animal care programs have configured surgical and procedural space for use with research animals in much the same way that a veterinary teaching institution might approach the requirement. There may be single rooms that can be utilized for rodent surgery (in dedicated and uncluttered spaces; see Fig. 11.1) or multiple rooms for animal and surgeon preparation, surgery, and animal recovery, as expected for USDA-covered species (Institute of Laboratory Animal Resources, 2011).

Within surgical and procedural spaces, it is desirable for tables, monitors, and cages to be raised on casters to facilitate movement throughout the animal areas. Surfaces and mobile carts should be ample enough to accommodate stock supplies of instruments, surgical gloves, sterile instrument packs, critical care diagnostic equipment, and areas for refrigeration and/or incubation of key fluids and/or drugs,

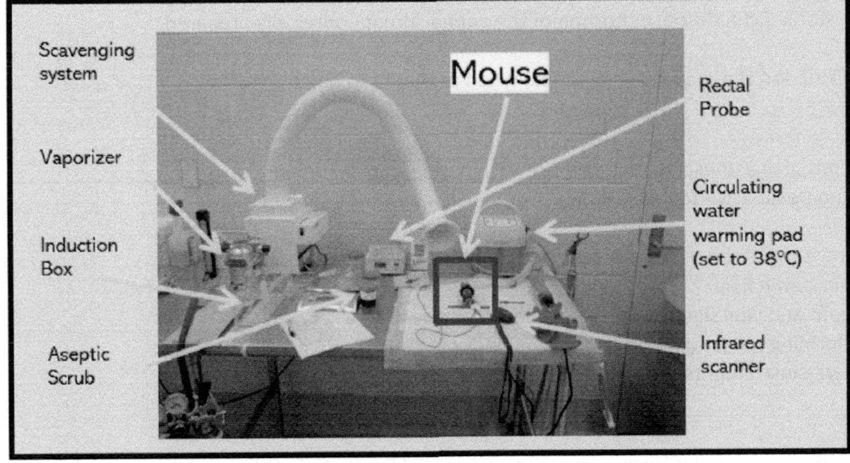

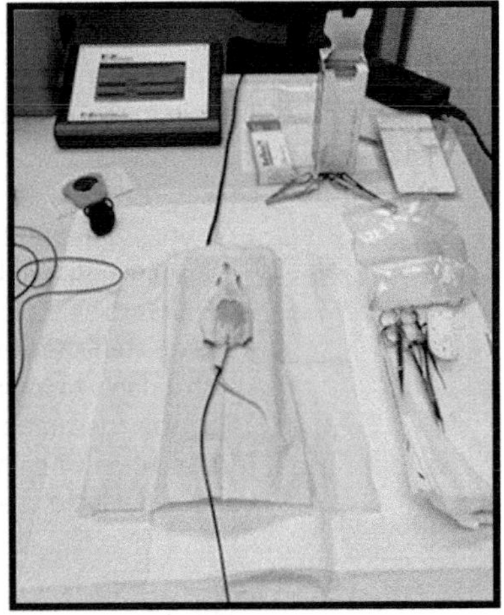

FIGURE 11.1 Rodent surgical areas with support equipment and heat supplementation. Note: mouse (on right) is in dorsal recumbency with body temperature monitoring using rectal thermometry. Thermometer is secured to tail using medical tape which assists with accuracy of data collection. *Images courtesy of FCH at Michigan State University.*

and specimens. Secure and locked safes for controlled substances should be near to procedure and surgical suites.

When working with animals, personal protective equipment (PPE) should be donned and worn throughout the procedure, including (at minimum) a clean laboratory coat and/or surgical scrubs, surgical mask, and sterile nitrile gloves (Adams and Pacharinsak, 2015). Floors, surfaces, and walls/ceilings should be constructed of materials that are easily able to be sanitized. Checklists (see Fig. 11.2) may be useful to remind the surgical team of the importance of maintaining sterile technique, that animals are to be appropriately supplemented with external heat sources, that animals are assessed regularly while under anesthesia (toe pinch, monitoring of vital signs, etc.), and that animals are appropriately monitored and positioned during recovery until return to righting reflex and consciousness.

For larger species, it is recommended that surgical tables are designed with a trough shape to better position and hold animals in dorsal recumbency. Further, these tables can tilt and adjust in height to meet the surgeon's comfort level. Metal stools, which can be easily sanitized, can be placed in procedural spaces for staff to use as needed for postural relief. Suction vacuum lines, oxygen tanks (or access to gas delivered from a central location), oxygen generators, pumps, and IV stands may all be necessary for large animal surgeries. If feasible, in large animal areas, the

Surgery Room/Area

- ☐ Clean, disinfect and dry working surfaces with appropriate agents before each surgery
- ☐ Provide adequate lighting throughout surgical area for visualizing surgical site and access
- ☐ Provide heat source (warm water recirculating blanket recommended at medium setting: 37°F)

Patient Preparation

- ☐ Prepare animal in an area separate from the surgical stage location
  - ☐ Remove hair from surgical site with clippers or minimal depilatory agent (timed for removal to avoid skin irritation)
  - ☐ Place non-medicated sterile ophthalmic ointment in patients' eyes and gently close lids together
- ☐ Administer pre-operative analgesics
- ☐ Transfer animal to the surgical stage/room/area
- ☐ Position animal using care not to overstretch limbs, bind them, or restrict circulation
- ☐ Perform surgical scrub using a skin disinfectant (then remove with ethanol wipe) or waterless alcohol-based scrub/rub that dries in place on skin
- ☐ Prepare warm saline or LRS-type fluids for prolonged or invasive procedures

Preparation of the Surgeon, Instruments, and Sterile Field

- ☐ Ensure appropriate instruments have been sterilized
- ☐ Don a clean laboratory coat and surgical mask; remove all jewelry from hands and wrists (rings, watches, etc.)
- ☐ Create a sterile area; cover the surgical site/animal with a sterile drape (transparent material is recommended)
- ☐ Anything touching the sterile field, drape, or portion of the animal already surgically prepared, must be sterile
- ☐ Scrub hands, then dry and don sterile gloves (non-latex) when prepared to begin surgery

Surgery and Intraoperative Monitoring

- ☐ Assure appropriate depth of anesthesia for animal prior to initiating surgical procedure
  - ☐ Animal should be nonresponsive to tactile stimuli, toe-pinch, etc. with a slowed rate of breathing
- ☐ Ensure sterile technique is maintained (can use cling wrap and foil coverings over knobs and instruments to maintain sterile field)
- ☐ Perform anesthetic depth and vital sign monitoring while under anesthesia
- ☐ Use caution when performing subsequent procedures on multiple animals; do not contaminate sterile field and use sterile instruments on each patient

Postoperative Care

- ☐ Monitor the animal continuously until it is conscious; then every 10-15 minutes until ambulatory
- ☐ House animals individually until fully ambulatory
- ☐ Do not return patient to housing area or cage until animal is in a normal ambulatory and conscious state
- ☐ Complete observations and record findings daily for 3 days (minimum) postoperatively

FIGURE 11.2 Sample Animal Surgery Checklist that highlights considerations for surgeon and patient prep, intraoperative monitoring, and postoperative care. *Courtesy of Campus Animal Resources, Michigan State University.*

availability of floor drains can more easily assist with cleaning, mopping, and disinfection of the area upon completion of procedures.

The procedural areas for agriculture species should address the complete recovery needs for the animals and the necessary means to monitor the development of post-procedural complications. Frequently, primary disease (induced or natural), pain, reduced feed intake (which can include presurgical fasting), and anesthesia type are associated with altered gastrointestinal motility in ruminants, therefore materials for stimulating appetite and returning to rumination should be available, as described in a later section of this chapter (Ness et al., 2017; Jasmin et al., 2011).

1. Considerations for rodent housing

a. Single versus social housing

It is preferable to isolate individual rodents during the immediate postprocedural period, particularly while recovering from anesthesia, to facilitate individual observations, enhance the quality of clinical assessments, and more easily provide intervention and treatment to specific animals. Some authors contend that individual housing will minimize chewing on sutures and skin staples by conspecifics and minimize the chance of self-injury due to disorientation in the immediate postprocedural course (Uchihashi et al., 2015). In contrast, solitary housing may contribute to distress and visceral sensitivities that can be overcome with a return to social housing (Larauche et al., 2010; Jirkof et al., 2012; Pham et al., 2010; Van Loo et al., 2007).

In addition, cages used for recovery should have a heat source available to a portion of the cage (e.g., placement of cages partly onto a warm water recirculating heat pad set to ~37°C; see Fig. 11.3) to allow the animal to reach body temperatures closer to the preferred thermoneutral zone for a smoother recovery (Adams and Pacharinsak, 2015; Hankenson et al., 2021). Animals may also benefit from prewarming, as well as postwarming efforts, potentially through means like forced warm air delivery or placement into small animal veterinary incubators prior to anesthetic induction (Zhang et al., 2017; Schuster and Pang, 2018; Rufiange et al., 2020; Hankenson et al., 2021).

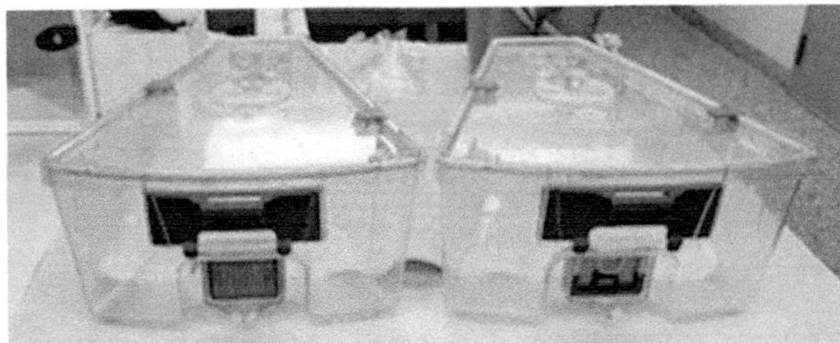

FIGURE 11.3 Rodent cages placed partially on warm-water reciculating blankets in preparation for postoperative recovery of animals. *Image courtesy of FCH at Michigan State University.*

It is critical to continue to assess animals during the postanesthetic recovery phase to monitor potential interference with the integrity and placement of skin closures. Rats are known to chew at incisional sites and can remove skin staples that may lead to dehiscence and significant self-injury. If rodents are attempting to remove stabilizing sutures or staples, it is recommended to reanesthetize the animals to disinfect and reinforce the skin closure, potentially with a suture at the incision line, placement of subcutaneous suture material, and/or application of tissue glue as an additional adhesive. Miniaturized e-collars can be purchased or fabricated to further dissuade self-injury; mini "jackets" and soft gauze bandaging can also be used to protect incision sites for healing (Brown, 2006a, 2006b). Topical anesthetics, like lidocaine and bupivacaine, can be injected at the incisional site to provide relief of discomfort and overcome the potential for self-injury secondary to breakthrough pain (Mihalko, 2013).

b. Bedding and enrichments

In the postprocedural period for rodents, bedding pieces may adhere to the incision line, leading to irritation; therefore, it is often recommended to recover rodents in static cages (removed from any ventilation rack) with padding, paper towels, or soft substrates on the cage bottom. Bedding (like corncob pieces) may be ingested by rodent patients, referred to as pica, and may result in a risk of choking or gastrointestinal obstruction (Clarke et al., 1997; Mihalko, 2013). An advantage of a paper towel, disposable underpad "blue diaper lining" (MedLine), or absorbent sheets on the cage bottom (Iso-PAD (Braintree Scientific, Braintree, MA)) is the ability to visually inspect for evidence of urine, blood, and any wound seepage. These substrates also provide sufficient foot traction to aid in ambulatory efforts of weakened (muscular) or impaired (peripheral nerve injury) animals.

Providing nesting material, opaque tubes for hiding, plastic huts for shelter and exercise, and other types of rodent cage enrichments will assist with assessments of species-typical behaviors, depending upon the observed level of interaction that animals have with manipulanda. The provision of pieces of paper substrates or cotton padding that can be retrieved and incorporated into an existing nest can be used as a measure of well-being in laboratory mice, referred to as the 'time to integrate nest' or TINT scale (Gaskill et al., 2013; Rock et al., 2014). TINT may be beneficial as a measure of postsurgical comfort because nest-consolidation and building behaviors can be suppressed if animals are experiencing pain or distress (Gallo et al., 2020). Nest-building behavior is not solely related to clinical health; some mouse strains are less prone to exhibit this behavior, and warmer ambient cage temperatures may reduce some of the thermoregulatory motivation for nest-building behavior. Therefore, TINT should be one of several considerations for return of normal mouse behaviors following surgery or related invasive or painful procedures.

Burrowing into bedding and other substrates by rats is an important species-specific behavior to facilitate in laboratory housing. Increasing evidence suggests that rats prefer to climb and burrow within their home environments (as opposed to the nest building described in mice). Therefore, one should consider encouraging these behaviors with the inclusion of elevated intracage "balcony" spaces and multi-tiered shelters within the home cage (Makowska and Weary, 2016). Additional bedding may be of benefit if its inclusion does not block airflow or watcr access for animals.

Following certain procedures, for example, placement of an indwelling catheter or chronic instrumentation of the animals, care should be taken to ensure that automatic watering devices can be reached and that implants do not get bumped or dislodged against wire-bar food holders or water bottle clasps. For animals with head implants, animals housed in metabolic caging, or other customized protocol-specific cage designs, advanced planning can address specialized cage needs. For example, a higher wire-bar lid can be customized by vendors, or if food is provided elsewhere in the cage, the wire-bar can be removed entirely. To creatively provide fluid, specialized water sources like fluid or gel packs can subsidize the animals' needs.

2. Considerations for housing of nonrodent larger species

A contemporary nonrodent, yet larger animal, post-procedural unit should be able to accommodate all the species housed in the facility, including rabbits, cats, and dogs, with considerations for the separation of species using visual, olfactory, auditory, and/or climatic barriers. This can be achieved using temporary or permanent walls, secondary enclosures, mobile dividers, or curtains. If possible, separate, dedicated recovery areas for individual animals (segregated by species) can provide a suitable environment during recovery. Individual recovery areas also encourage dedicated attention and postoperative nursing care; see Fig. 11.4 and 11.5 (Flecknell et al., 2007).

Polyvinyl-coated raised flooring has become the standard in primary and secondary enclosures for larger research animals. It is recommended that these species be kept in caging that permits easy access to intravenous (IV) ports, ready spot cleaning, and the ability for animal care staff to safely enter spaces and interact with these species to deliver treatments and conduct physical examinations. If recovery is to be conducted in transport cages prior to return to routine housing, consider door-mounted food and water receptacles that can be filled at the cage front and remain off the floor as animals may knock them over during return to righting reflex and recovery. Animals that have temporary Elizabethan collars, swivel systems for catheters, or mesh jackets to protect indwelling tubing or vascular access ports may benefit from the use of portable ball-valve bottles or J-feeders that remain off the floor surface.

Nonhuman primates (NHPs) should be socially housed whenever possible; however, following a specific surgery or procedure, reintroduction to a social pair or group should be done with heightened monitoring and oversight by veterinary staff. Even if NHPs are involved in studies that require surgical implants, food or water scheduling or restriction, use of tethers or jackets, and/or drug dosing, they can be safely socially housed without compromising the validity of these studies (Roberts and Platt, 2005). When NHPs must be singly housed based upon professional veterinary judgment, they may benefit from more space than is required for pair or group-housed primates, as well as the provision of additional enrichment, such as increased human interaction or periodic use of activity cages (Institute of Laboratory Animal Resources, 2011). The use of protected contact between compatible animals (for example, grooming bars) in these situations may be a means of improving their environment until such time as they can be returned to social housing (APV, 2019a).

3. Considerations for housing of large agricultural species

Housing requirements for agricultural species will depend on various factors, including, but not limited to, the type and age of the animal, the type of procedure (whether minimally invasive a major procedure within), and whether procedures are expected to interfere with return to normal behavioral and physiological routines for that animal.

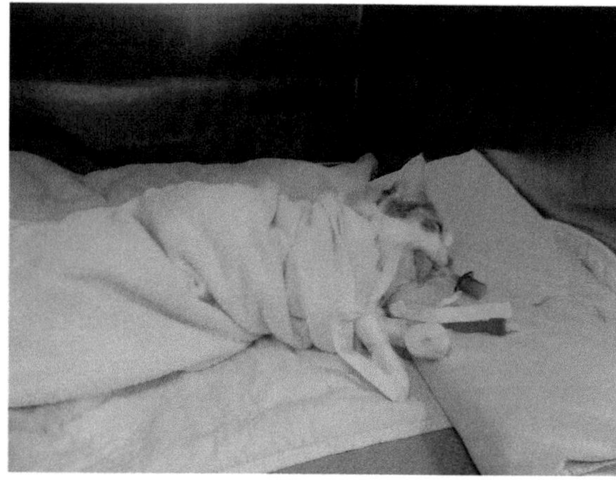

FIGURE 11.4 During recovery of felines, ensure animals are kept covered and warmed without obstructing the head. Animals should remain intubated until restoration of swallowing reflex. Cats can be readily extubated. *Image courtesy of KAC at Michigan State University.*

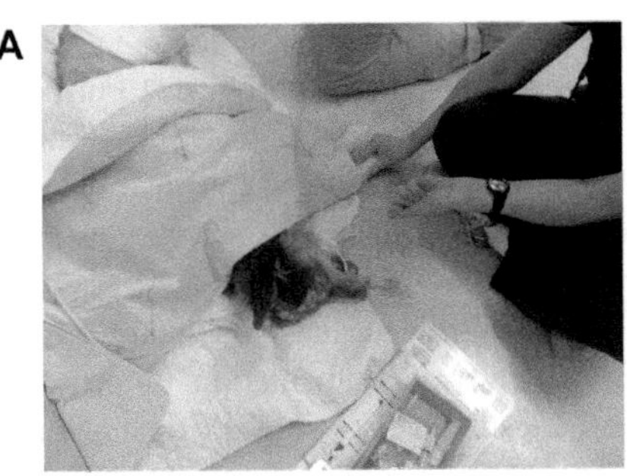
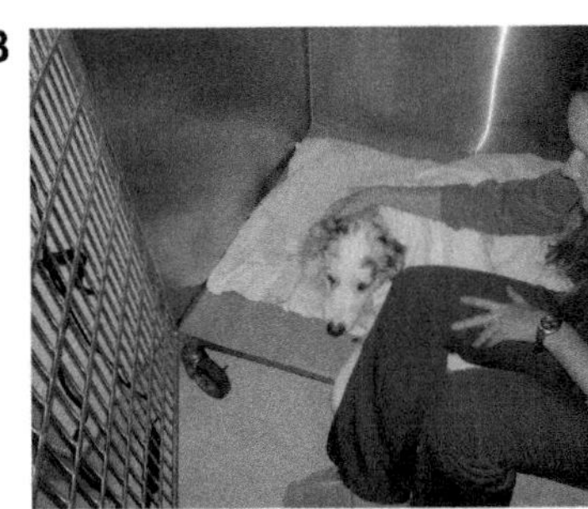

FIGURE 11.5 (A) During recovery of canines, ensure animals are kept covered and warmed without obstructing the head. Animals should remain intubated until restoration of swallowing reflex, after which time extubation can occur. (B) Veterinary personnel should remain with the animal as consciousness is gained to assess behavior and potential for delirium. Cats can be readily extubated. *Images courtesy of KAC at Michigan State University.*

Housing must meet the spacing requirements outlined in resources that include both the *Guide* (Institute of Laboratory Animal Resources, 2011) and the *Ag Guide* (American Dairy Science Association, American Society of Animal Science, Poultry Science Association., 2020).

a. Single versus social housing

In general, agricultural species are social animals and are accustomed to staying in groups (American Dairy Science Association, American Society of Animal Science, Poultry Science Association., 2020). When housed socially, the adequate stocking density of the field/pen/run must be followed to permit animals free access to food and water and room to express species-specific behaviors. Further, it is preferred to group animals from the same source (American Dairy Science Association, American Society of Animal Science, Poultry Science Association., 2020) to maintain biosecurity and limit the spread of pathogens. Commingling animals from different sources can result in fighting, as animals may seek to establish a social hierarchy. Where single housing may be preferred or necessary to meet research needs, measures should be taken to prevent the development of abnormal behaviors and stereotypies. With singly housed animals, appropriate accommodations should be made, including the use of enrichments, while maintaining visual and auditory interaction with conspecifics (Swanson et al., 2018).

b. Bedding

Bedding materials should provide comfortable surfaces to encourage lying-down behaviors. Cattle display decreased lying behavior on concrete, rubber, and wooden surfaces compared to dry bedded surfaces (Proudfoot, 2019). Various materials are available for use as supplementary substrates, including sawdust, straw, wood shavings, paper, hulls, composted and dried manure solids, and sand. The addition of these materials is critical to provide adequate footing support to prevent slip and fall injuries, minimize lameness and pressure-associated problems such as hock injuries, and minimize exposure to bedding-associated infections (Fig. 11.6). Historically, bacterial mammary infections in dairy cattle, including streptococcal species and coliforms are associated with straw, sawdust, and shavings (Hohmann et al., 2020). Regardless of the choice for bedding materials, monitoring the condition of the substrate may be more important because the quality of materials deteriorates with the accumulation of manure and moisture. Bedding depth should also be considered as an aspect of enrichment for optimization; studies have shown that lying behavior in cattle increases with greater bedding depth (Tucker et al., 2009).

Agricultural animals necessary for research and held in confinement can be acclimated to research surroundings to minimize stress and the potential for injuries, as well as improve the external validity of experimental results (Cox et al., 2019). Animals can be trained to utilize research handling facilities and be rewarded in the form of treats before experimental procedures begin (Cox et al., 2019). Research facilities should also seek to emulate the purpose for which the study is being performed. For example, agricultural species raised for production purposes should be in facilities that reflect their production settings.

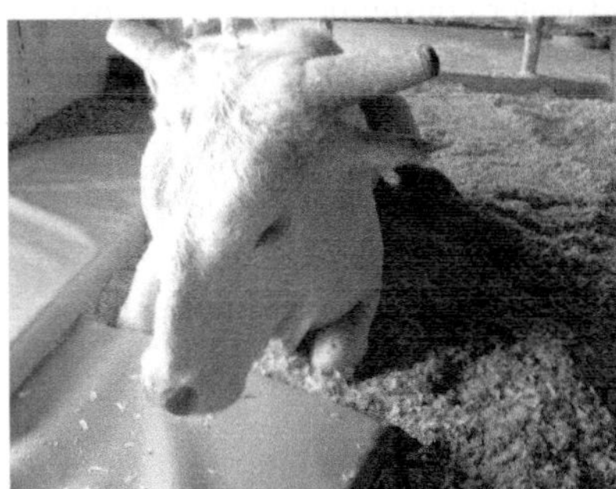
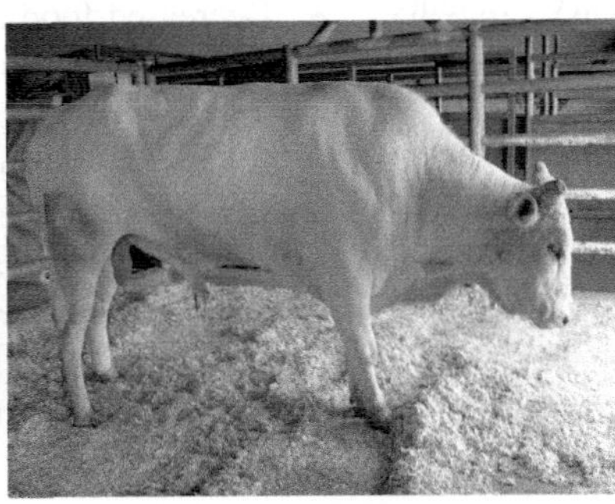

FIGURE 11.6 Bedded stalls are particularly important for postanesthetic recovery of cattle, prior to and after return to standing postures. *Images courtesy of VM at Michigan State University.*

D. Animal acclimation and baseline assessments

Animals destined for surgery or procedures should be identified well in advance to allow time (known as the conditioning phase) for staff to observe the animals prior to the procedure. This acclimation period allows for gentle handling of animals and introductions to the new environment, caging type, food and water receptacles, and nutritional supplements that are planned during the periprocedural period. During this time, baseline weight and an appreciation of normal posture and disposition (e.g., friendly, inquisitive, anxious, aggressive) can be obtained, and baseline hematologic, hemodynamic, and serum chemistries can be established.

Staff will learn the individual nuances of the animals under their care, which will make their observations and assessments more powerful. For rodents, gentle handling by hand and by tube transfer (Henderson et al., 2020) and by tickling and playful handling of adolescent rats (Cloutier et al., 2014; LaFollette et al., 2020) are continuing to grow in favor. These animal-human interactions are aimed to produce a positive social effect, which will facilitate the postprocedural manipulations that may be associated with dosing and treatment delivery.

Larger species are particularly responsive to human interaction and positive reinforcement with treats to assist with acclimation to new environments and completion of medical interventions (temperature collection, blood glucose monitoring, etc.). Cats, dogs, and to a limited degree, ferrets and rabbits tend to respond favorably to human contact, especially during stressful situations like post-anesthesia recovery. Postoperative nursing care can include brushing, combing, and petting the patient throughout the entire recovery phase. Human interaction can be incorporated readily into periods when vital parameters are being captured and can be important tools to aid in postoperative pain assessments (Flecknell, 2016). Depending on the nature of use, acclimation for agriculture animals in production studies depends on familiarizing them with the housing environment and daily routines. For agricultural animals in biomedical research settings, attempts should be made to maintain social groupings and address species-specific needs for thermal comfort, humidity levels, and husbandry practices (American Dairy Science Association, American Society of Animal Science, Poultry Science Association., 2020).

III. Medical recordkeeping and veterinary care

Monitoring animal wellness is the crux of postprocedural care. For this reason, medical record documentation and management are a mainstay for any animal care program. At any point in time, the IACUC can ask to review the medical records of the animals in the program. Further, outside regulatory oversight entities like the USDA, funding agencies, and AAALAC site visitors can also ask to review medical records for consistency and accuracy as part of overall program assessments.

The cornerstone of thorough veterinary medical records is documentation. Specifically, documentation of procedures, animal outcomes, anesthetic and analgesic dosing, and general subjective and objective observations of animals are expected in records. These records are essential for the oversight of the animal health by the veterinary team and are critical to recording welfare measures for research animals within an institution (Institute of Laboratory Animal Resources, 2011). Veterinarians are expected to be part of the professional team that establishes, reviews, and oversees medical and animal use records (Field et al., 2007; American College of Laboratory, 2020). Particularly, within any research animal program, appropriate compliance with federal and local laws, policies, and guidance related to work with animals is expected. Drugs that are delivered to animals periprocedurally must be appropriate for the species intended, documented in the medical record once administered, and of pharmaceutical grade, unless otherwise justified and approved by the IACUC.

The veterinary care program includes the timely review of all perioperative steps by a qualified veterinarian, which has been granted responsibility and authority by the institution for oversight. The American College of Laboratory Animal Medicine (ACLAM), which grants certifications to veterinary specialists that work in animal research programs, describes the inherent responsibilities of the veterinarian to include "overseeing and assessing the adequacy of surgical monitoring and providing recommendations concerning presurgical procedures, surgical techniques, the qualifications of approved personnel to perform surgery and the provision of peri-operative care" (American College of Laboratory Animal Medicine ACLAM, 2016).

1. Considerations for rodents

Potential signs associated with pain and distress in rodents can include the following (Hankenson, 2013; Turner et al., 2019):

- Decreased food and water consumption, weight loss
- Self-imposed isolation/hiding
- Rapid, open-mouth breathing
- Biting, aggression
- Increased/decreased movement, twitching, or trembling
- Unkempt appearance (rough, dull hair coat)
- Abnormal posture/positioning (hunched back, head-pressing)
- Dehydration, skin tenting, sunken eyes

When preparing documentation about the medical condition of the rodent patient, records should be sure to include identification of the animal (whether numerical or a physical description, with genotype (if available), vendor source, age, body weight, and sex). Details about the surgical procedure and date performed should be described.

These observations before, during and after surgery, at the conclusio of anesthesia, and typically well beyond the procedural phase itself (if the invasiveness of the procedure or the patient's status dictates) should be documented. Observations can be made by any personnel involved in the collaborative team of research and animal care and veterinary staff. Of note, entries in records should reflect the persons (often by the inclusion of personal initials) that complete the medical entries. Approved anesthetics and analgesics should be well-described within the IACUC protocol; however, the medical record should verify that the appropriate dosing route and frequency of dosing was accomplished and effectively mitigated painful behaviors and negative experiences of the animals. Staples and skin sutures should be removed within 7–10 days of placement, or within the period recommended by the IACUC. The inclusion of body condition scoring assessments is highly recommended as a measure of health in rodents (Ullman-Cullere and Foltz, 1999; Hickman and Swan, 2010). Lastly, postprocedural observations about behavior, appetite, appearance, and activity should be included in the record-keeping and initialed by the observer.

Medical records for rodents can be accomplished easily by creation of a card that fits into the cage card holder and contains all relevant information, itemized above (Fig. 11.7). With this type of rodent veterinary care record, one side can contain the objective information, while the other side can contain daily logs of written details or descriptors. Electronic databases can also manage rodent cases, as can contemporary regulatory technology programs

***POST OPERATIVE RECORD FORM:* Species** ______________

Principal Investigator________________ Protocol#____________
Person performing the procedure______________________________
Procedure___________________________ Date____________
Animal Identification______________________________________
Anesthetic /dose____
Analgesic /dose /route /frequency_____________________________
Day of Surgery/Postop care_________________________________
2nd Day/Postop care_______________________________________
3rd Day/Postop care_______________________________________
____
List any additional Procedure(s)____________________________
____
Staple/Suture: yes☐ no☐ Date removed:______________________
Contact Information____

FIGURE 11.7 Sample rodent medical record. The records may be kept on 3″ × 5″ cards maintained with the cage card in the cardholder. Medical cards may be removed from cage when observations are no longer needed. Alternatively, medical records may be maintained in a notebook placed in or near the animal room or in the laboratory. *Image courtesy of Campus Animal Resources at Michigan State University.*

that serve to partner IACUC, animal care, and environmental health data into a unified web-based resource.

Once the rodent patient is no longer under observation, the medical card can be removed from the cage and saved for future review by the clinical veterinary team, by personnel involved in postapproval monitoring, or by the research team for use in objective assessments and outcomes as part of the study data collection.

2. Considerations for nonrodent larger species

Larger animal species, like dogs and cats, typically have a more robust medical history and record-keeping expectations within the animal research environment. Medical records for larger species should be comprehensive and include all historical information about pathogen status, disease history, vaccination records, deworming protocols, daily checks, procedures, and anesthesia reports. The USDA requires a written program of veterinary care for dogs present at each research site. Details on this licensing rule (APHIS-2017-0062; https://www.aphis.usda.gov/aphis/ourfocus/animalwelfare/sa_regulated_businesses/new-licensing-rule/veterinary-care-for-dogs) clarify that veterinarians must conduct physical examinations no less than once annually on all canines at the premises and requires that:

- Medical records for each dog must be available at the time of inspection by the USDA.
- Medical records must include identification, records of routine husbandry, descriptions of any health-related issues, records of any tests and administration of vaccinations.
- Vaccinations for contagious and deadly diseases are administered.
- Dogs are sampled and treated for parasites and other pests.
- Preventive care plans ensure dogs have healthy haircuts, properly trimmed nails, and clean and healthy eyes, ears, skin, and teeth.

Anesthesia records are also critical as part of the comprehensive animal patient profile, whether through electronic and paper medical records. Ideally, anesthetic records should contain information regarding the individual animal patient's general health, plus all drugs, medications, fluids, and dosages administered, and chronological data representing the patient's vital parameters during anesthesia, adverse events, and postanesthetic monitoring (Kadry et al., 2012).

It is most common that larger research animals, particularly those that are covered by USDA oversight, have individual records. Medical records can be kept in a variety of formats and with varying arrangements; however, it is the authors' experience that certain standardized elements should be included in the medical record. For example, a listing of key points of contact (responsible personnel), IACUC protocol number, and space for master problem lists. Including relevant clinical blood work, test/assay results, and anesthesia records can help with visualizing trends and permit ease of health interpretations over time. Daily treatment and observation notes should be recorded so that in-depth findings and information can be interpreted (Haskins and Eisele, 1997).

Recognition of animal discomfort and pain, particularly in NHPs, is typically assessed through an evaluation of clinical presentation and behavior. With NHPs, because of personnel safety concerns, cage-side observation may be the only available assessment tool (APV, 2019b). Direct cage-side observations are relatively easy to perform and inexpensive because the animal is in clear view and can interact with the observer. The caveat to direct observations is that many animals mask signs of pain to human caregivers. Therefore, an extended observation period is often required to allow the animal to habituate to the observer and allow accurate assessment. Remote assessments may be acceptable with the appropriate installation of video monitoring equipment and access to recordings by personnel. The optimal assessments of a veterinary patient's pain will be accomplished by an observer who is not only knowledgeable about species- specific signs of pain but also familiar with the specific animal under consideration (APV, 2019b).

3. *Considerations for large animal agricultural species*

To facilitate the timely and accurate identification of postoperative complications and aberrant behavior in agricultural species that may be housed in rural barn settings, it is advised that a hybrid arrangement of animal facility personnel, research staff, and animal care professionals cooperate to identify clinical issues of concern. To facilitate the most rapid intervention and response should farm veterinary staff be located off-site, facility personnel can be trained on methods to triage supportive care to the herd or flock prior to the veterinarian's arrival. Standard operating procedures, for example, "Veterinary Care Guidelines" or a dedicated "Written Program of Veterinary Care," can help to guide nonveterinary personnel to initiate appropriate steps and treatments in advance of veterinary consultation. These types of guidance documents should clearly and specifically state the clinical signs of complications, provide a stepwise approach to diagnostic and therapeutic interventions, describe how to monitor responses to interventions, and highlight when to contact experienced personnel such as emergency veterinarians, principal investigators, or farm administrators to aid in the care of agriculture animals.

In production animal settings, group health records are appropriate for animals kept within a cohort, flock, or herd (American Dairy Science Association, American Society of Animal Science, Poultry Science Association., 2020). Animals with individual procedures require individual medical records with details adequate to monitor health status, recovery progress, and other outcomes of interest and production measures where applicable. Medical records for large agricultural species, and those species involved in translational biomedical research, should be in line with the expectations of ACLAM (Field et al., 2007; American College of Laboratory, 2020). Records must be readily accessible for review to form the basis for initiating, modifying, or ending interventions during postoperative care of large animal patients.

In agricultural settings, metallic 'tin back' flip charts or three-ring binders may be useful for protecting written records from moisture, dirt, and fecal contamination. Computerized record-keeping systems that are made for veterinary hospitals can also work for research animal settings, with the caveat that 'one size may not fit all' for the preferred electronic medical record approach.

IV. Interventions for care and well-being

A. Monitoring approaches

One of the most critical decisions to make during the periprocedural period is the appropriate frequency of observations of the patients to minimize distress and optimize evaluation and the potential need for intervention. Within the first few days following a procedure, the patient's status will dictate if more frequent and intensive assessments are necessary; therefore, staff must remain flexible and nimble to best support the animals under care. At a minimum, animals should be monitored continuously until they regain consciousness, and then every 10–15 minutes until alert, normothermic and ambulatory. Animals should not be returned to routine housing areas, nor placed with other animals until they are fully conscious.

Rodent species commonly assessed for 72 hours after the surgery or procedure. Invasiveness of the procedure or the patient's postoperative health status may warrant extended monitoring beyond 72 hours; this should be based upon consultation with veterinary staff. Medical records (as described previously) should document the observations and findings during this period. Removing visual barriers (the cage lid or opening cage/pen door) and observing from a distance may offer more information about attributes such as curiosity, gait, and neurologic status. For rodents, as mentioned previously, assessment of the home cage and nest-building activities may factor into overall health assessments. Objective considerations of 'where, what, and how' or WWHow, provide an additional tool for postoperative severity assessments in rodents (Tappe-Theodor et al., 2022).

For large, nonrodent species, the immediate postoperative period requires frequent monitoring and should include collection and documentation of respiratory and heart rates, mucus membrane color, capillary refill time, body temperature, level of consciousness, and intervention with analgesia. Postoperative monitoring should occur at least every 5–10 minutes during anesthetic recovery to check vital parameters, along with any other clinical findings and should be recorded within the anesthesia record (as part of the medical record). Once the animal has fully recovered, it is recommended that monitoring occur every 1–4 hours for the first 8–12 hours. Large-animal observations should include a minimum subjective data set of appetite (interest in food), thirst (interest in liquid), urination, defecation, overall behavior and attitude, and condition of hair or skin coat. Pain levels should also be assessed frequently following procedures. All species should be checked at least once per day after fully recovering from anesthesia to ensure that animals continue to recover and fare as predicted (Flecknell, 2016).

B. Postprocedural management

In brief, when animals are recovering from anesthesia and procedures, their environment should be warm and quiet with limited pedestrian traffic. The area should be appropriately lighted to enable observations by personnel and overall, the facilities should be clean, dry, and comfortable for the resting animal (Institute of Laboratory Animal Resources, 2011). Ideally, the postprocedural recovery area should offer temperature controls to maintain the spaces at warmer temperatures than housing areas to offset prolonged or spontaneous hypothermia in veterinary patients awakening from sedation. Common confounders to achieving thermoneutrality in research animals include the use of metallic transport cages and staging of larger animals in hallways or corridors that are not adequately warmed and may have significant cross-breezes from the proximity of personnel foot traffic.

In general, hypothermia is defined for rodents as a core body temperature that falls below 97°F (36°C). External warming devices such as thermogenic packs and sleeves for rodents (Caro et al., 2013; Beale et al., 2018), far-infrared warming devices, warm circulating water blankets, warm forced air devices, heat lamps, and incubators are all beneficial during the recovery phase. It is never advised to use commercial electric heating pads as they contain 'hot spots' that can lead to surface burns and endanger recumbent animals. Similarly, microwaveable heat sources may heat unevenly and cause injury. Hyperthermia, while occasionally reported during anesthesia, is uncommon in recovering animals unless there is a malfunction leading to excess heat supplementation; this may occur if heat lamps are placed too closely or focused for too long on animal patients. In horses, if hyperthermia is detected, supplemental oxygen, ventilation, and active cooling steps should be performed promptly to return the patient to normothermia (Mama et al., 2019).

Attention to sources of unanticipated noise and vibration within animal facilities warrants consideration for their potential adverse impacts on animal health. There are known areas of noise, like cage washers, loading docks, and large animal housing spaces; however, there are also sources of noise, like smoke detection devices, lighting systems, computer and equipment alarms, HVAC, and laminar flow hoods, that cumulatively can impact animals, and may or may not be at a frequency where certain animal species are affected (Reynolds et al., 2010; Turner et al., 2005). Noise exposure influences virtually every area of biomedical research, from the immune system to the development of tumors and heart disease, to typical circadian rhythms; noise and vibration are sources of stress and can lead to a cascade of stress responses in animals (Turner, 2020). Even at relatively low intensities, such noise can negatively impact research animals and humans alike; therefore, the recovery areas are best kept to low undisturbed sound volumes until animals can be returned to typical housing environments.

It is both an ethical and regulatory mandate to ensure that pain and distress are mitigated in animals, particularly when procedures are anticipated to cause more than momentary discomfort (Carbone, 2019). While there are numerous analgesics and dosing regimens for rodents, it is believed that current regimens may be insufficient in frequency and there may be pain experienced by rodents postoperatively (Waite et al., 2015), as demonstrated by adverse behaviors (Larson et al., 2019). Overall, multimodal analgesia is likely more effective for treating postsurgical pain than single-analgesic protocols; however, effects on appetite, activity,and body weight need to be considered during analgesic selection. Nesting consolidation and grooming transfer tests can be useful for refining the detection and treatment of postoperative pain in mice (Oliver et al., 2018).

Occasionally, the postprocedural period requires clinical interventions which may be a source of discomfort, such as wound debridement, bandage changes, or restraint to administer medications. In addition to pharmaceutical interventions, nontherapeutic postprocedural supportive care measures can be introduced, including softened bedding substrates for more comfortable postprocedural positioning, heat supplementation for prolonged recovery periods, and placement of feed and water sources in locations that are able to be accessed by animal without extending the neck up or down to reach bowls and lixits.

Effective pain management in larger nonrodent animals generally involves a balanced or multimodal strategy using several classes of pain-modifying medications. The rationale behind this approach is that it addresses targeting multiple sites in pain pathways, potentially allowing lower doses of each drug, and minimizing the potential for side effects associated with any single drug. The choice of medication should be based on anticipated pain levels and individual patient needs, particularly assessing species-specific issues like appropriate volume of agents, oprtional routes of delivery, and the potential for clinical side effetcts (Epstein et al., 2015; Gad et al., 2016; Turner et al., 2011a,b).

Regardless of the circumstances, patients recovering from anesthesia should continue to be monitored with special attention paid to heart rate, respiratory rate, body temperature, SpO2, and the ability to breathe and swallow effectively (Fig. 11.8); the research animal community can benefit from expectations for veterinary patient recovery as outlined by the American Animal Hospital Association (AAHA) (Grubb et al., 2020). In larger species, delayed recovery, dysphoria, and emergence of delirium can range from being minor issues to serious concerns. Postanesthesia dysphoria and emergence delirium present as clinically similar. Technically, dysphoria is a condition related to opioid intolerance and is typically managed by reversing the opioid effects. This is a critical decision because reversing the dysphoric effects of opioids also reverses their analgesia effects; therefore, it is best to rule out the emergence of delirium and/or breakthrough pain before reversing the opioid.

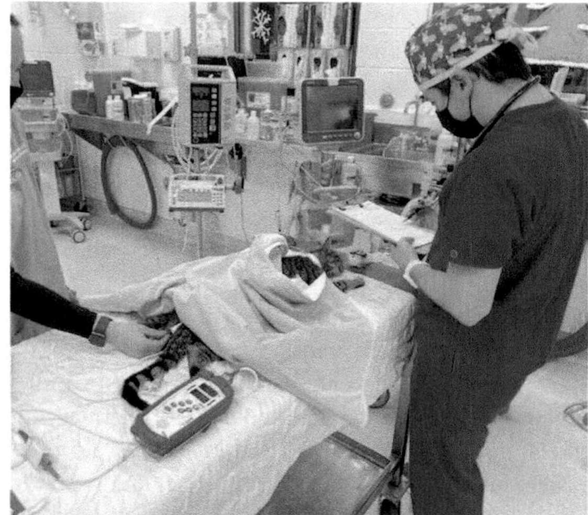

FIGURE 11.8 Postoperative monitoring of larger nonrodent species includes continuous assessments of temperature, pulse oximetry, blood pressure and heart rate, with attention to behavioral responses to drug interventions and supportive care. *Image courtesy of KAC at Michigan State University.*

Postoperative pain can be mitigated with additional opioid administration, whereas postoperative dysphoria tends to be aggravated with additional opioids. NHPs may exhibit additional behaviors like lip-biting and chewing that are indicative of pain and distress (Descovich et al., 2019). Emergence delirium (seen in cats and dogs) oftentimes can be managed using low doses of dexmedetomidine and/or acepromazine intravenously. The advantage of dexmedetomidine is that it provides both strong sedation and analgesic effects. In cases of severe delirium, alfaxalone and/or propofol IV may be necessary. Other sources of delayed recoveries and delirium in domestic species can be related to discomforts such as a full bladder, prolonged hunger, fear, loneliness, and inadequate padding. With small patients and/or neonatal animals, blood glucose should be monitored throughout the entire period of anesthesia to ensure normoglycemia until after the return to consciousness.

Rabbits have particularly special considerations regarding peri-operative anesthesia and analgesia. They have a higher risk of anesthesia-related morbidity and mortality (1.4%) compared to dogs and cats (0.17% and 0.24%, respectively) (Brodbelt, 2009). Rabbits are easily stressed, especially when handled and managed incorrectly. Anesthesia-related stress and pain can have adverse effects on rabbit gastrointestinal and cardiovascular function. It is important to minimize postoperative stress, manage and alleviate pain, and closely monitor feed intake and fecal output.

Laboratory personnel must be familiar with the unique husbandry and physiological needs of rabbits to mitigate potential life-threatening problems. Small rabbit species will be highly susceptible to the effects of hypothermia until they regain normal activity. Ideally, recovery for laboratory rabbits should not occur on sawdust, wood chips, or anything that could be inhaled or become lodged in their oral cavities (Flecknell, 2016). Once rabbits return to normal activity, they can be transferred to a cage containing substrates like hay and straw to provide warmth, an area of security, and an additional source of food. Subcutaneous warm fluid administration may be indicated, especially if the rabbits are not provided water prior to anesthesia or have reduced fluid intake.

Rabbits should be encouraged to eat as soon as possible after recovery to reduce the risk of postoperative digestive disturbances. Rabbits with decreased gut mobility can be treated with metoclopramide as a preanesthetic adjunct and/or postoperatively. Common signs of pain in rabbits include anorexia, aggression, altered breathing patterns, altered posture and/or gait, over- or under-grooming, chewing fur or self-mutilation, hiding, and decreased activity (Wenger, 2012). It is advisable to employ a standardized pain scoring system such as the Rabbit Grimace Scale to objectively assess levels of periprocedural pain

(Keating et al., 2012; Benato et al., 2021). Grimace scales are based on facial expressions in response to pain and are validated for a variety of species as an adjunct approach to pain assessment and scoring (Cohen and Beths, 2020).

The assessments described thus far rely on the ability of personnel to identify the behavioral, physiological, and physical indicators of pain. Aside from measurable and quantifiable physiological parameters, many of the assessments require expert training and may be affected by variability among observers. Pain assessment in agricultural animals can be challenging, particularly in stoic species. To an inexperienced observer, signs of pain may be difficult to detect in ruminants. Several objective and nonobjective methods can be used to judge if pain is present. In painful animals, a standard clinical evaluation may detect signs associated with pain including decreased movement, decreased interaction with other animals, limited feed intake, altered locomotion, flank watching, ear twitching, kicking, changes in posture, poor hair coat, changes in vital parameters including heart rate and respiratory rate, and teeth grinding (Hudson et al., 2008). In some cases, pain may only be detected when evoked, such as the grunting sounds that accompany a withers pinch test in cattle with cranial abdomen or caudal thoracic pain. Small ruminants and camelids similarly mask signs of pain (Smith et al., 2021). Horses in pain may display new and unusual behaviors with or without changes in physiological parameters, including alterations in heart rate, respiratory rate, blood pressure, and gut motility (Guedes, 2017). Grimace scaling in species like cattle, sheep, pigs and horses have been expolored and further research is needed to expand its applicability to diverse agricultural settings and procedures that may cause pain in agricultural animals (Cohen and Beths, 2020).

Provision of analgesics, reversal of anesthetic medications where applicable, nutritional support, and specific treatments for disease process are essential for maximizing well-being and expediting recovery postoperatively. In certain agricultural species or for field studies, regional blocks of analgesics may be preferable to and more efficiently administered than generalized anesthesia (Seddighi and Doherty, 2016).

Nonsteroidal antiinflammatory drugs (NSAIDs) and opioids are commonly used for analgesia. In some instances, gabapentin may be an option for chronic pain that is refractory to commonly used NSAIDs (Coetzee, 2013). The plan for analgesia will depend on the surgery and anticipated postoperative pain levels and must be designed in consultation with anesthesiologists and clinical veterinarians.

Altered gastrointestinal motility is a common occurrence postoperatively due to pain, complications of general anesthesia, reduced feed intake, and primary disease (Ness et al., 2017). Stimulation of GI motility may be necessary in the postprocedural period and prokinetic drugs may be helpful in ruminants. Prokinetic drugs include bethanechol, neostigmine, metoclopramide, and erythromycin, and their effects have been evaluated on the abomasum, small intestines, cecum, and the proximal ascending colon (Constable et al., 2012). Lidocaine has also been shown to promote GI motility through various effects, including reduction of circulating catecholamines, blockade of inhibitory reflexes, and decreasing inflammatory mediator production (Ness et al., 2017). Complete assessment for factors that contribute to altered GI motility, such as electrolyte imbalances like hypocalcemia, shock, inflammation, endotoxemia, and intestinal ischemia is critical. Addressing those factors, when present, will promote the effectiveness of motility modifiers.

In horses, given their size and strength, the chance for self-injury as they recover from the confusion of anesthesia is significant; this is true not only for the animals but also for the safety of the veterinary and research personnel involved in the patient's recovery. Therefore, ensuring there is appropriate support and oversight for this species is essential (see Fig. 11.9). Close postanesthetic monitoring is important to detect respiratory and gastrointestinal complications. The use of opioids and alpha-2 agonists may mask subtle abdominal discomfort postoperative. Similarly, the use of NSAIDs (e.g., flunixin meglumine) may mask abdominal pain; therefore, monitoring behavior and manure production are critical for the early identification of potentially significant gastrointestinal complications (Mama et al., 2019).

A 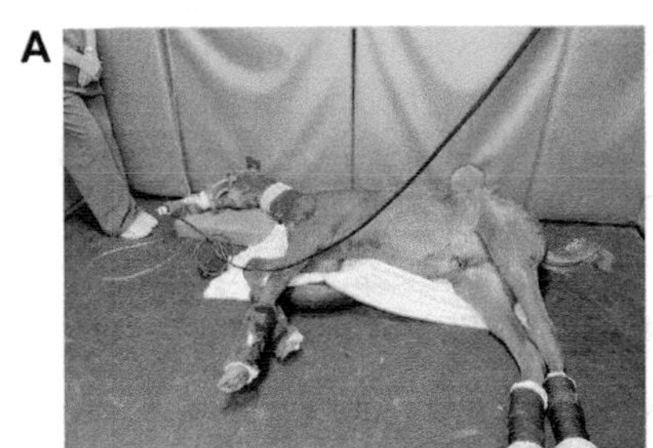

B 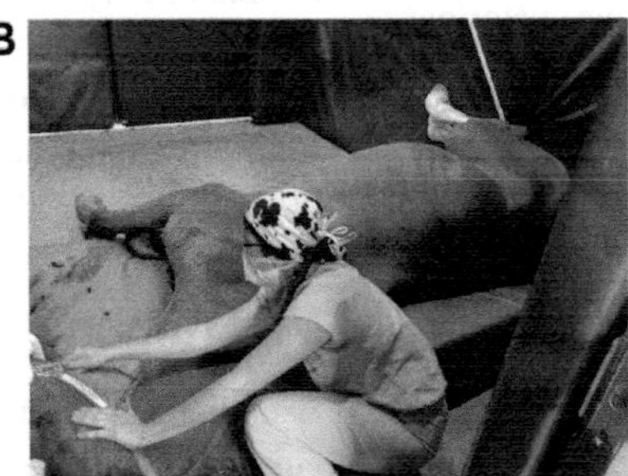

FIGURE 11.9 Equine recovery should include use of protective padding within the room and on the floor and surrounding the hoofs and lower limbs to protect animals from injury while coming out of anesthesia, for both foals (A) and adults (B). Supportive ropes will assist personnel in helping the animals to regain a standing posture. *Images courtesy of Michigan State University.*

C. Fluid therapy

The provision of adequate hydration and the restoration of normal tissue volume may be one of the most important interventions in the postprocedural period. This effort also supports normal renal and cardiac function as well as the distribution and elimination of necessary antibiotics, analgesics, and other experimental treatments. A variety of crystalloids and colloids, as well as improved filtration and administration systems for small-volume infusions are available for veterinary patient applications. Administration of fluids, including the selection of appropriate delivery routes, is a key consideration in small animal patients (Morton et al., 2001; Turner et al., 2011a; Turner et al., 2011b; Mazzaferro and Ford, 2012).

Aspects of critical care and fluid support for mice, rats, and guinea pigs are described in more detail elsewhere (Hankenson, 2013; Jensen, 2017). In general, to determine if a rodent is dehydrated, one should gently lift and pinch the skin over the back, just between the scapulae, and then observe the rate of return of the skin to its resting position. The slowness of return is correlated to various degrees of dehydration that can be offset with fluid supplementation (Hankenson, 2013). Any administered fluids should be from a sterile source to avoid the introduction of infectious agents to the patient; prophylactic fluids, like 0.9% NaCl or polystarch, given subcutaneously at a total volume of ~1.0 mL (mice) to ~2.0 mL (rats) can significantly improve survival rates in certain biomedical models (Smith et al., 1999).

Larger animals can also be assessed for fluid needs by using skin turgor (as described above for smaller rodents), as well as output and concentration of urine to estimate fluid loss (Mazzaferro and Ford, 2012). In ruminants, particularly younger calves, hydration status can be assessed using the means described above, in addition to eyeball recession scores; these estimates can then help to determine rehydration requirements (Roussel, 2014).

Fluid choice is going to be dictated by the type of procedure and other parameters specific to the project. Fluid rates should be established by veterinary staff and tailored to the patient's physiologic responses. Further specific recommendations regarding fluid choices are beyond the scope of this chapter and can be readily obtained from veterinary textbooks and online veterinary resources.

D. Nutritional support

Nutritional supplementation of high-quality, certified, and palatable feedstuffs is part of expected supportive care. Modifications of the laboratory rodent's own diet can be made with the addition of high-calorie, easily digested food items like Nutri-Cal or by soaking food pellets/biscuits in Ensure (Hankenson, 2013). An expansive selection of nutritional supplementation products is available for laboratory rodents and rabbits, including commercially available critical care supplements (Oxbow Animal Health ®). Food and fluid options can be provided on the cage floor in disposable trays/dishes or can be delivered by oral gavage for direct instillation into the stomach. Syringe feeding has been shown as a positive mechanism to deliver supportive nutritional care fluids to rodents (Turner et al., 2011a,b). Rodents can be supplemented with gel-based nutritional support, which can improve postoperative weight gain and assist with boosting calories, as well as hydration and pain management (Abelson et al., 2012; Hankenson, 2013; Taylor et al., 2016; Foley et al., 2019).

Large animals may also undergo periods of anorexia postoperatively, and opioids may further diminish appetite and food intake. Animals that are not eating after 5 days of optimal care should be considered candidates for supplemental fat, protein, and carbohydrates. AAHA provides recommendations to support anorexic patients by specific feeding techniques, including palatable and heated meals, high-fat diets, and agents like appetite stimulants, antiemetics, and prokinetics. If feeding techniques and medications do not improve total voluntary intake, feeding via enteral tubes (e.g., nasal, esophageal, or gastric) is strongly recommended over oral syringe feeding. Feeding protocols for nonrodent, larger species should promote the delivery of enteral nutrition over parenteral nutrition when assisted nutrition support is needed. Parenteral nutrition is reserved for select cases, generally in referral facilities with 24-hour care teams (Cline et al., 2021).

In ruminants, enteral feeding via stomach tubing or through the creation of a temporary rumen fistula may be appropriate to address inappetence postoperatively. In cattle unable to feed for various reasons, supportive care can be successfully delivered through temporary rumenotomy until animals recover (Chigerwe et al., 2005). As mentioned previously, sheep can be stimulated to restore ruminations via transfaunation from a clinically healthy conspecific. In addition, the provision of hay augments ruminations through the stimulatory effects on buccal receptors during chewing. Typically, healthy horses can tolerate food deprivation for up to 72 hours; however, postoperative animals likely will need nutritional support sooner because of an increased catabolic state. Specific details for enteral/parenteral nutritional support for horses are beyond the scope of this chapter and the readers are directed to additional resources (Carr, 2018).

V. Humane endpoint considerations

Establishing a humane study endpoint is critical to assuring animal well-being, by avoiding prolonged delay when the animal is not recovering or is moribund. Clinical and/or humane endpoints such as decreased appetite, significant weight loss, dehydration, altered hemogram values, and increased levels of pain should be clearly distinguished from experimental endpoints and described within an IACUC protocol. Research investigators should be advised that humane endpoints may precede experimental time points based on the condition and welfare of the animals. Ideally, endpoints should be identified that will provide the earliest relief possible to the animal; pilot studies may be utilized to identify and support the criteria for these experimental endpoints.

Scoring systems can be established to obtain objective criteria for the removal of animals from experimental studies (Hankenson, 2013; Nunamaker et al., 2013). Approaches from human medicine, described as frailty assessments, provide a global evaluation of the health of aged mice and rats. For example, prior to death from age-related disease, most mice develop marked reductions in body weight and temperature, thus providing signs (e.g., frailty scores) that close monitoring, intervention, or preemptive euthanasia may be necessary (Toth, 2018; Hankenson et al., 2013).

Humane endpoints may be physical, biochemical, behavioral, or a combination of these factors. Ideally, endpoints are study-specific and should be developed by the research team in collaboration with the veterinarian, animal care personnel, and behavioral staff. Whenever possible, surrogate endpoints, such as those developed using various imaging modalities or molecular biomarkers should be used to minimize animal pain and distress (APV, 2020). Endpoint criteria and facets of the anesthetic and analgesic regimen should be reported along with other methods in scientific manuscripts, as described in the PREPARE and ARRIVE guidelines (Smith et al., 2018a; Percie du Surt et al., 2020).

Regardless of species, timely preemptive euthanasia limits terminal suffering. Furthermore, interventional euthasia allows for antemortem collection of data and samples that would be lost if spontaneous death occurs. Veterinarians trained in laboratory animal medicine should use professional judgment to assess whether a proposed euthanasia method is aligned with the goals of the research and will yield valid data. When necessary, veterinarians should participate in the assessment and validation of euthanasia methods on a case-by-case basis (Shomer et al., 2020).

References

Abelson, K.S., Jacobsen, K.R., Sundbom, R., et al., 2012. Voluntary ingestion of nut paste for administration of buprenorphine in rats and mice. Lab. Anim. 46 (4), 349–351.

Adams, S., Pacharinsak, C., 2015. Mouse anesthesia and analgesia. Curr Protoc Mouse Biol 5 (1), 51–63.

American College of Laboratory Animal Medicine (ACLAM). Position Statement on adequate veterinary care. (2016). Subcommittee: Hankenson, F.C. (Chair), Laber, K.L, Eurell, L., Samer, J., Jackson, T., Maguire, S., Maurer, K., Scholz, J., Singer, L., Wood, J. Am. Assoc. Lab. Anim. Sci. 55 (6), 826–828.

American College of Laboratory Animal Medicine (ACLAM). Position on Medical Records Content and Scope. (2020). https://www.aclam.org/about/position-statements. (Accessed 3 January 2022)

American Dairy Science Association, American Society of Animal Science, Poultry Science Association., 2020. *Guide for the Care and Use of Agricultural Animals in Research and Teaching*, Fourth ed. Federation of Animal Science Societies, Champaign, IL https://poultryscience.org/files/galleries/AG_Guide_4th_Ed_2020.pdf. (Accessed 3 January 2023).

Al Hussein, H., Al Hussein, H., Sircuta, C., et al., 2020. Challenges in perioperative animal care for orthotopic implantation of tissue-engineered pulmonary valves in the ovine model. Tissue Eng. Regen. Med. 17 (6), 847–862.

Association of Primate Veterinarians (APV), 2019a. Socialization guidelines for nonhuman primates in biomedical research. J. Am. Assoc. Lab. Anim. Sci. 58 (6), 753–755.

Association of Primate Veterinarians (APV), 2019b. Guidelines for assessment of acute pain in nonhuman primates. J. Am. Assoc. Lab. Anim. Sci. 58 (6), 748–749.

Association of Primate Veterinarians (APV), 2020. Humane endpoint guidelines for nonhuman primates in biomedical research. J. Am. Assoc. Lab. Anim. Sci. 59 (1), 6–8.

Beale, C.N., Esmail, M.Y., Aguiar, A.M., et al., 2018. Use of air-activated thermal devices during recovery after surgery in mice. J. Am. Assoc. Lab. Anim. Sci. 57 (4), 392–400.

Benato, L., Murrell, J., Knowles, T.G., et al., 2021. Development of the Bristol Rabbit Pain Scale (BRPS): a multidimensional composite pain scale specific to rabbits (*Oryctolagus cuniculus*). PLoS One 16 (6), e0252417.

Blevins, C.E., Celeste, N.A., Marx, J.O., 2021. Effects of oxygen supplementation on injectable and inhalant anesthesia in C57BL/6 mice. J. Am. Assoc. Lab. Anim. Sci. 60 (3), 289–297.

Brodbelt, D.C., 2009. Perioperative mortality in small animal anaesthesia. Vet. J. 82 (2), 152–161.

Brodbelt, D.C., Blissitt, K.J., Hammond, R.A., Neath, P.J., et al., 2008a. The risk of death: the confidential enquiry into perioperative small animal fatalities. Vet. Anaesth. Analg. 35 (5), 365–373.

Brodbelt, D.C., Pfeiffer, D.U., Young, L.E., et al., 2008b. Results of the confidential enquiry into perioperative small animal fatalities regarding risk factors for anesthetic-related death in dogs. J. Am. Vet. Med. Assoc. 233 (7), 1096–1104.

Brown, C., 2006a. Restraint collars. Part I: Elizabethan collars and other types of restraint collars. Lab Anim (NY) 35, 23–25.

Brown, C., 2006b. Restraint collars. Part II: specific issues with restraint collars. Lab Anim (NY) 35, 25–27.

Carbone, L., 2019. Ethical and IACUC considerations regarding analgesia and pain management in laboratory rodents. Comp. Med. 69 (6), 443–450.

Caro, A.C., Hankenson, F.C., Marx, J.O., 2013. Comparison of thermoregulatory devices used during anesthesia of C57BL/6 mice and correlations between body temperature and physiologic parameters. J. Am. Assoc. Lab. Anim. Sci. 52 (5), 577–583.

Carr, E.A., 2018. Enteral/parenteral nutrition in foals and adult horses practical guidelines for the practitioner. Vet. Clin. N. Am. Equine Pract. 34 (1), 169–180.

Chigerwe, M., Tyler, J.W., Dawes, M.E., et al., 2005. Enteral feeding of 3 mature cows by rumenostomy. J. Vet. Intern. Med. 19 (5), 779–781.

Clarke, J.A., Myers, P.H., Goelz, M.F., et al., 1997. Pica behavior associated with buprenorphine administration in the rat. Lab. Anim. Sci. 47, 300–303.

Cline, M.G., Burns, K.M., Coe, J.B., et al., 2021. AAHA nutrition and weight management guidelines for dogs and cats. J. Am. Anim. Hosp. Assoc. 57 (4), 153–178.

Cloutier, S., Wahl, K., Baker, C., et al., 2014. The social buffering effect of playful handling on responses to repeated intraperitoneal injections in laboratory rats. J. Am. Assoc. Lab. Anim. Sci. 53 (2), 168–173.

Coetzee, J.F., 2013. A review of analgesic compounds used in food animals in the United States. Vet. Clin. N. Am. Food Anim. Pract. 29 (1), 11–28.

Cohen, S., Beths, T., 2020. Grimace scores: tools to support the identification of pain in mammals used in research. Animals (Basel) 10 (10), 1726.

Constable, P.D., Nouri, M., Sen, I., et al., 2012. Evidence-based use of prokinetic drugs for abomasal disorders in cattle. Vet. Clin. N. Am. Food Anim. Pract. 28 (1), 51–70.

Cox, R.J., Nol, P., Ellis, C.K., et al., 2019. Research with agricultural animals and wildlife. ILAR J. 60 (1), 66–73.

Descovich, K.A, Richmond, S.E, Leach, M.C, et al., 2019. Opportunities for refinement in neuroscience: Indicators of wellness and post-operative pain in laboratory macaques. ALTEX 36 (4), 535–554. https://doi.org/10.14573/altex.1811061. https://www.altex.org/index.php/altex/article/view/1204. (Accessed 3 January 2023).

Epstein, M., Rodan, I., Griffenhagen, G., et al., 2015. AAHA/AAFP pain management guidelines for dogs and cats. J. Am. Anim. Hosp. Assoc. 51 (2), 67–84.

Field, K., Bailey, M., Foresman, L.L., et al., 2007. Medical records for animals used in research, teaching, and testing: public statement from the American College of Laboratory Animal Medicine. ILAR J. 48 (1), 37–41.

Flecknell, P.A., 2016. *Laboratory Animal Anaesthesia*, Fourth ed. Flecknell P. Elsevier.

Flecknell, P.A., Richardson, C.A., Popovic, A., 2007. Chapter 30. Laboratory Animals. In: Tranquilli, W.J., Thurmon, J.C., Grimm, K.A. (Eds.), Lumb and Jones, Fourth ed. Blackwell Press.

Foley, P.L., Kendall, L.V., Turner, P.V., 2019. Clinical management of pain in rodents. Comp. Med. 69 (6), 468–489.

Gad, S.C., Spainhour, C.B., Shoemake, C., et al., 2016. Tolerable levels of nonclinical vehicles and formulations used in studies by multiple routes in multiple species with notes on methods to improve utility. Int. J. Toxicol. 35 (2), 95–178.

Gallo, M.S., Karas, A.Z., Pritchett-Corning, K., et al., 2020. Tell-tale TINT: does the time to incorporate into nest test evaluate post-surgical pain or welfare in mice? J. Am. Assoc. Lab. Anim. Sci. 59 (1), 37–45.

Gaskill, B.N., Karas, A.Z., Garner, J.P., et al., 2013. Nest building as an indicator of health and welfare in laboratory mice. J. Vis. Exp. (82), 51012.

Grubb, T., Sager, J., Gaynor, J.S., et al., 2020. AAHA anesthesia and monitoring guidelines for dogs and cats. J. Am. Anim. Hosp. Assoc. 56 (2), 59–82.

Guedes, A., 2017. Pain management in horses. Vet. Clin. N. Am. Equine Pract. 33 (1), 181–211.

Hankenson, F.C., 2013. *Critical Care Management for Laboratory Mice and Rats*. CRC Press Inc, Taylor and Francis Group.

Hankenson, F.C., Kim, J.J., Le, T.M., et al., 2021. Using waterless alcohol-based antiseptic for skin preparation and active thermal support in laboratory rats. J. Am. Assoc. Lab. Anim. Sci. 60 (3), 365–373.

Hankenson, F.C., Ruskoski, N., van Saun, M., et al., 2013. Weight loss and reduced body temperature determine humane endpoints in a mouse model of ocular herpesvirus infection. J. Am. Assoc. Lab. Anim. Sci. 52 (3), 277–285.

Haskins, S.C., Eisele, P.H., 1997. Postoperative support and intensive care. In: Kohn, D.F., Wixson, S.K., White, W.J., Benson, G.J. (Eds.), Anesthesia and Analgesia in Laboratory Animals. Academic Press, New York, pp. 381–382.

Henderson, L.J., Dani, B., Serrano, E.M.N., et al., 2020. Benefits of tunnel handling persist after repeated restraint, injection, and anaesthesia. Sci. Rep. 10, 14562.

Hickman, D.L., Swan, M., 2010. Use of a body condition score technique to assess health status in a rat model of polycystic kidney disease. J. Am. Assoc. Lab. Anim. Sci. 49, 155–159.

Hohmann, M.F., Wente, N., Zhang, Y., et al., 2020. Bacterial load of the teat apex skin and associated factors at herd level. Animals (Basel) 10 (9), 1647.

Hudson, C., Whay, H., Huxley, J., 2008. Recognition and management of pain in cattle. In Pract. 30 (3), 126–134.

Institute of Laboratory Animal Resources, 2011. *Guide for the Care and Use of Laboratory Animals*, Eighth ed. The National Academies Press, Washington, D.C. https://grants.nih.gov/grants/olaw/guide-for-the-care-and-use-of-laboratory-animals.pdf. (Accessed 3 January 2023)

Jasmin, B.H., Boston, R.C., Modesto, R.B., et al., 2011. Perioperative ruminal pH changes in domestic sheep (*Ovis aries*) housed in a biomedical research setting. J. Am. Assoc. Lab. Anim. Sci. 50 (1), 27–32.

Jensen, J., 2017. Chapter 6. Special Techniques and Species. In: *Handbook of Laboratory Animal Anesthesia and Pain Management Rodents*. CRC Press, Taylor & Francis Group.

Jirkof, P., Cesarovic, N., Rettich, A., et al., 2012. Individual housing of female mice: influence on postsurgical behaviour and recovery. Lab. Anim. 46 (4), 325–334.

Kadry, B., Feaster, W.W., Macario, A., et al., 2012. Anesthesia information management systems: past, present, and future of anesthesia records. Mt. Sinai J. Med. 79 (1), 154–165.

Keating, S.C.J., Thomas, A.A., Flecknell, P.A., et al., 2012. Evaluation of EMLA cream for preventing pain during tattooing of rabbits: changes in physiological, behavioural and facial expression responses. PLoS One 7 (9), e44437.

LaFollette, M.R., Cloutier, S., Brady, C.M., et al., 2020. Changing human behavior to improve animal welfare: a longitudinal investigation of training laboratory animal personnel about heterospecific play or "rat tickling". Animals (Basel) 10 (8), 1435.

Larauche, M., Gourcerol, G., Million, M., et al., 2010. Repeated psychological stress-induced alterations of visceral sensitivity and colonic motor functions in mice: influence of surgery and postoperative single housing on visceromotor responses. Stress 13 (4), 343–354.

Larson, C.M., Wilcox, G.L., Fairbanks, C.A., 2019. The study of pain in rats and mice. Comp. Med. 69 (6), 555–570.

Makowska, I.J., Weary, D.M., 2016. The importance of burrowing, climbing, and standing upright for laboratory rats. R. Soc. Open Sci. 3, 160136.

Mama, K.R., 2019. Chapter 22. Complications of inhalation anesthesia and their management. In: Auer, J.A., Stick, J.A. (Eds.), *Equine Surgery*, Fifth ed. W.B. Saunders, pp. 340–345.

Mazzaferro, E.M., Ford, R.B., 2012. Chapter 1. Emergency care. In: *Kirk and Bistner's Handbook of Veterinary Procedures and Emergency Treatment*, ninth ed. W.B. Saunders, Philadelphia.

McCarren, H., Moore, T., Kelz, B., 2013. Assessing changes in volatile anesthetic sensitivity of mice after local or systemic pharmacological intervention. J. Vis. Exp. 80, 1–8.

Mihalko, K.L., 2013. Care of rodent models used for preclinical evaluation of tissue-engineered/regenerative medicine product candidates. Methods Mol. Biol. 1001, 197–206.

Moens, Y., 2013. Mechanical ventilation and respiratory mechanics during equine anesthesia. Vet. Clin. N. Am. Equine Pract. 29 (1), 51–67.

Morton, D.B., Jennings, M., Buckwell, A., et al., 2001. Joint Working Group on Refinement. Refining procedures for the administration of substances. Report of the BVAAWF/FRAME/RSPCA/UFAW Joint Working Group on Refinement. British Veterinary Association Animal Welfare Foundation/Fund for the Replacement of Animals in Medical Experiments/Royal Society for the Prevention of Cruelty to Animals/Universities Federation for Animal Welfare. Lab. Anim 35 (1), 1–41.

Ness, S.L., Steiner, A., 2017. Chapter 7. Postoperative management. In: Fubini, S.L., Ducharme, N.G. (Eds.), *Farm Animal Surgery*, Second ed. W.B. Saunders.

Nunamaker, E.A., Artwohl, J.E., Anderson, R.J., et al., 2013. Endpoint refinement for total body irradiation of C57BL/6 mice. Comp. Med. 63 (1), 22–28.

Oliver, V.L., Thurston, S.E., Lofgren, J.L., 2018. Using cageside measures to evaluate analgesic efficacy in mice (*Mus musculus*) after surgery. J. Am. Assoc. Lab. Anim. Sci. 57 (2), 186–201.

Percie du Sert, N., Hurst, V., Ahluwalia, A., et al., 2020. The ARRIVE guidelines 2.0: updated guidelines for reporting animal research. PLoS Biol. 18 (7), e3000410.

Pham, T.M., Hagman, B., Codita, A., et al., 2010. Housing environment influences the need for pain relief during post-operative recovery in mice. Physiol. Behav. 99 (5), 663–668.

Proudfoot, K.L., 2019. Maternal behavior and design of the maternity pen. Vet. Clin. N. Am. Food Anim. Pract. 35 (1), 111–124.

Reynolds, R.P., Kinard, W.L., Degraff, J.J., et al., 2010. Noise in a laboratory animal facility from the human and mouse perspectives. J. Am. Assoc. Lab. Anim. Sci. 49 (5), 592–597.

Roberts, S.J., Platt, M.L., 2005. Effects of isosexual pair-housing on biomedical implants and study participation in male macaques. Laboratory animal facility from the human and mouse perspectives. J. Am. Assoc. Lab. Anim. Sci. 44 (5), 13–18.

Rock, M.L., Karas, A.Z., Rodriguez, K.B., et al., 2014. The time-to-integrate-to-nest test as an indicator of wellbeing in laboratory mice. J. Am. Assoc. Lab. Anim. Sci. 53 (1), 24–28.

Roussel, A.J., 2014. Fluid therapy in mature cattle. Vet. Clin. N. Am. Food. Anim. Pract. 30 (2), 429–439.

Rufiange, M., Leung, V.S., Simpson, K., et al., 2020. Prewarming followed by active warming is superior to passive warming in preventing hypothermia for short procedures in adult rats (*Rattus norvegicus*) under isoflurane anesthesia. J. Am. Assoc. Lab. Anim. Sci. 8;59 (4), 377–383.

Russell, W.M.S., Burch, R.L., 1959. The Principles of Humane Experimental Technique. Universities Federation for Animal Welfare, Wheathampstead.

Schuster, C.J., Pang, D.S.J., 2018. Forced-air pre-warming prevents peri-anaesthetic hypothermia and shortens recovery in adult rats. Lab. Anim. 52 (2), 142–151.

Seddighi, R., Doherty, T.J., 2016. Field sedation and anesthesia of ruminants. Vet. Clin. N. Am. Food Anim. Pract. 32 (3), 553–570.

Shomer, N.H., Allen-Worthington, K.H., Hickman, D.L., et al., 2020. Review of rodent euthanasia methods. J. Am. Assoc. Lab. Anim. Sci. 59 (3), 242–253.

Smith, D.E., Blumberg, J.B., Lipman, R.D., 1999. Improved survival rates in mice that received prophylactic fluids after carcinogen treatment. Contemp. Top. Lab. Anim. Sci. 38, 84–86.

Smith, A.J., Clutton, R.E., Lilley, E., et al., 2018a. PREPARE: guidelines for planning animal research and testing. Lab. Anim. 52 (2), 135–141.

Smith, D., Anderson, D., Degryse, A.D., et al., 2018b. Classification and reporting of severity experienced by animals used in scientific procedures: FELASA/ECLAM/ESLAV Working Group report. Lab. Anim. 52 (Suppl. 1), 5–57.

Smith, J.S., Schleining, J., Plummer, P., 2021. Pain management in small ruminants and camelids: applications and strategies. Vet. Clin. N. Am. Food Anim. Pract. 37 (1), 17–31.

Swanson, J.C., Chapin, L.T., Hankenson, F.C., 2018. Chapter 23. Agricultural animals. In: Weichbrod, R.H., Thompson, G.A., Norton, J.N. (Eds.), *Management of Animal Care and Use Programs in Research, Education, and Testing*, Second ed. CRC Press, Taylor & Francis Group, Boca Raton.

Tappe-Theodor, A., Pitzer, C., Lewejohann, L., et al., 2022. The "WWHow" concept for prospective categorization of post-operative severity assessment in mice and rats. Front. Vet. Sci. 15 (9), 841431.

Taylor, B.F., Ramirez, H.E., Battles, A.H., Andrutis, K.A., Neubert, J.K., 2016. Analgesic activity of tramadol and buprenorphine after voluntary ingestion by rats (*Rattus norvegicus*). J. Am. Assoc. Lab. Anim. Sci. 55 (1), 74–82.

Toth, L.A., 2018. Identifying and implementing endpoints for geriatric mice. Comp. Med. 68 (6), 439–451.

Tucker, C.B., Weary, D.M., von Keyserlingk, M.A., et al., 2009. Cow comfort in tie-stalls: increased depth of shavings or straw bedding increases lying time. J. Dairy Sci. 92 (6), 2684–2690.

Turner, J.G., 2020. Noise and vibration in the vivarium: recommendations for developing a measurement plan. J. Am. Assoc. Lab. Anim. Sci. 59 (6), 665–672.

Turner, J.G., Parrish, J.L., Hughs, L.F., et al., 2005. Hearing in laboratory animals: strain differences and nonauditory effects of noise. Comp. Med. 55 (1), 12–23.

Turner, P.V., Brabb, T., Pekow, C., et al., 2011a. Administration of substances to laboratory animals: routes of administration and factors to consider. J. Am. Assoc. Lab. Anim. Sci. 50 (5), 600–613.

Turner, P.V., Pekow, C., Vasbinder, M.A., et al., 2011b. Administration of substances to laboratory animals: equipment considerations, vehicle selection, and solute preparation. J. Am. Assoc. Lab. Anim. Sci. 50 (5), 614–627.

Turner, P.V., Pang, D.S., Lofgren, J.L., 2019. A review of pain assessment methods in laboratory rodents. Comp. Med. 69 (6), 451–467.

Uchihashi, M., Wilding, L.A., Nowland, M.H., 2015. Surgical correction of rectal prolapse in laboratory mice (*Mus musculus*). J. Am. Assoc. Lab. Anim. Sci. 54 (4), 433–438.

Ullman-Cullere, M.H., Foltz, C.J., 1999. Body condition scoring: a rapid and accurate method for assessing health status in mice. Lab. Anim. Sci. 49, 319–323.

Van Loo, P.L., Kuin, N., Sommer, R., Avsaroglu, H., et al., 2007. Impact of 'living apart together' on postoperative recovery of mice compared with social and individual housing. Lab. Anim. 41 (4), 441–455.

Waite, M.E., Tomkovich, A., Quinn, T.L., et al., 2015. Efficacy of common analgesics for postsurgical pain in rats. J. Am. Assoc. Lab. Anim. Sci. 54 (4), 420–425.

Wenger, S., 2012. Topics in medicine, and surgery; anesthesia and analgesia in rabbits and rodents. J. Exot. Pet Med. 21, 7–16.

Zhang, E.Q., Knight, C.G., Pang, D.S., 2017. Heating pad performance and efficacy of 2 durations of warming after isoflurane anesthesia of Sprague-Dawley rats (*Rattus norvegicus*). J. Am. Assoc. Lab. Anim. Sci. 56 (6), 786–791.

Chapter 12

Pain assessment in laboratory species

Alexandra L. Whittaker[1] and Chalette Brown[2]
[1]School of Animal and Veterinary Sciences, The University of Adelaide, Adelaide, SA, Australia; [2]Cerberus Sciences, Adelaide, SA, Australia

Chapter outline

I. Introduction

As humans, we are all aware of what pain means to us, and recognize that pain also occurs in nonhuman animals. However, pain is a complex biological process, and by analogy with humans, the pain experience in animals is likely to be uniquely individual. This renders it problematic to measure pain in animals with any kind of precision and challenges the assumption that we can generalize expected pain levels across all animals experiencing the same named procedure. This difficulty is further compounded when working with prey species since there is a prevalent viewpoint that these animals may mask pain to avoid predator attention (Stasiak et al., 2003). It has previously been suggested that there is little empirical data to back up this claim (Mogil, 2020), however recent studies have shown depression in behavioral pain indices in both mice (Miller and Leach, 2015) and guinea pigs (Oliver et al., 2017) when in the presence of an observer. An eloquent argument to explain the previous observation is that an assumption of pain masking may result from less strong human-rodent relationships, with the animals being somewhat fearful of humans (Carbone, 2020).

Recently, the International Association for the Study of Pain (IASP) revised the definition of pain to "an unpleasant sensory and emotional experience associated with or resembling that associated with, actual or potential tissue damage" (International Association for the Study of Pain (IASP), 2020). This definition aptly highlights the important components of the pain pathway, comprising sensory neuron activation and subsequent neurological transmission, with the final processing of the 'pain signal' in higher brain regions to create the emotional 'experience' of pain (Mota-Rojas et al., 2021). Some valuable guidance accompanies the new definition:

1. Pain is always a personal experience that is influenced to varying degrees by biological, psychological, and social factors.
2. Pain and nociception are different phenomena. Pain cannot be inferred solely from activity in sensory neurons.

Anesthesia and Analgesia in Laboratory Animals. https://doi.org/10.1016/B978-0-12-822215-7.00019-6

3. Through their life experiences, individuals learn the concept of pain.
4. A person's report of an experience as pain should be respected.
5. Although pain usually serves an adaptive role, it may have adverse effects on function and social and psychological well-being.
6. Verbal description is only one of several behaviors to express pain; inability to communicate does not negate the possibility that a human or a nonhuman animal experiences pain.

Pain research has typically focused at a biological level on sensory activation and neurological transmission using nociceptive tests. However, more recent theories have proposed that pain be viewed as part of a dynamic interaction between biological, psychological, and social factors unique to each individual: the so-called biopsychosocial model (Gatchel, 2004). In consideration of this model, there is now strong evidence that early life experiences, including pain, can impact later-life neural processing and may lead to hypersensitization or an exaggerated response to pain (Low and Fitzgerald, 2012; Walker et al., 2003) which may be of particular relevance to laboratory animals. In spite of the abundant evidence and widespread acceptance of the biopsychosocial model, it still remains unclear (and largely underinvestigated) as to what this model means for animal pain assessment and mitigation. At the current time, an overall attention to a general ethic of care to include frequent pain assessment, ideally using a range of assessment methods (Younger et al., 2009), with the provision of optimal analgesic treatment, and consideration of conditions that afford optimal well-being is perhaps the best that we can do.

The chapter begins with a brief overview of different types of pain since this influences assessment method choice and treatment selection. The term "pain" used throughout this chapter refers to the emotional experience of pain as opposed to nociception, even though it is acknowledged that the degree of conscious emotional state may vary between species (Prunier et al., 2013). A discussion on why pain prevention and assessment are important in laboratory animals follows. The remainder of the chapter discusses practicalities around pain assessment in laboratory animals, including the timing of pain assessment, assessment methods and challenges associated with using them, and the requirements for record keeping.

II. Types of pain

Pain can be variously described dependent on both its duration and source of origin. There is almost certainly an overlap between these definitions, and often a lack of clarity around the timing for the transition from one type to another.

Acute pain occurs at the time of surgery or injury and is regarded as adaptive since behavioral responses are usually made to avoid the pain source in the future. A subacute phase may subsequently develop to encourage protective behavior to promote healing (Bateson, 1991). Chronic pain is generally less well-defined in animals and refers to pain that persists beyond injury recovery (Whittaker and Howarth, 2014). However, there appears to be no established guidance as to what this duration may be in animals. In spite of this, chronic pain should be considered as a possibility when animals have cancer, musculoskeletal injuries, long-term illnesses, or head injuries. It should also be considered that acute painful insults may transition into chronic pain states, for example, when there is undertreatment of acute pain leading to hyperalgesia or when a nerve injury occurs leading to neuropathy (refer to Chapter 7 for further information).

An understanding of the source of the pain is also needed to determine assessment methods and appropriate treatment. Common classifications include nociceptive, neuropathic, mixed, and visceral (Melnikova, 2010). Laboratory animal models create all of these pain types, for example, arthritis models create a nociceptive insult, stroke and experimental autoimmune encephalomyelitis models can lead to neuropathic pain, tumor inoculation is a source of mixed pain, and visceral pain is created by intestinal disease models.

III. Why prevent pain?

Society, in our modern world, expects a high level of care and safeguarding of animal welfare for animals in research (National Research Council (US) Committee on Recognition and Alleviation of Pain in Laboratory Animals, 2009). Whilst there are differences across jurisdictions, laws protecting research animals generally ascribe sentience to nonhuman vertebrates, as well as their embryonic, fetal, or larval forms, and cephalopods (Mellor, 2019). As a result, these animals deserve our careful consideration of treatments, interventions, and pain relief as needed. Pain and emotional distress lead to suffering. Prevention of pain forms part of an animal welfare safeguard. Yet, in order to address pain, we need to be able to assess and prevent it to the greatest extent possible.

There are legal ramifications in place of not addressing pain. Moreover, from a research perspective, pain not related to the research intervention (e.g., intraspecific aggression leading to injuries), pain from veterinary treatment and husbandry procedures (e.g., physical identification measures, administering injections), and pain as a by-product of the research project (e.g., bone fractures) can all affect research outcomes (National Research Council (US) Committee on Recognition and Alleviation of Pain in Laboratory Animals, 2009). Separately, research on pain models or the use of painful stimuli in behavioral studies needs to be considered as these are pertinent to the study design, but the study design will need to include pain mitigation and be justifiable and defensible (National Research Council (US) Committee on Recognition and Alleviation of Pain in Laboratory Animals, 2009). Pain can also affect sleeping patterns, food and water consumption, weight, immune parameters, and cardiovascular parameters, among many other factors (for further reading, see Comparative Medicine—special edition, 69(6) 2019). Prevention of pain also allows quicker recovery postoperatively and aims to prevent sensitization to later painful insult, and the transition to chronic pain states.

IV. Pain assessment

A. Why assess pain?

The ultimate goal of pain assessment is to enable the employment of pain mitigation strategies through analgesic or anesthetic administration, physical interventions (such as joint immobilization), and addressing anxiety which may be associated or contributing to pain (National Research Council (US) Committee on Recognition and Alleviation of Pain in Laboratory Animals, 2009). For further information on the ethical, legal, and scientific rationale for preventing and assessing pain, see Chapters 1, 2, and 3.

Pain prediction and assessment in research studies allow humane endpoints to be implemented. Humane endpoints as defined by the NC3Rs (2021) are "clear, predictable, and irreversible criteria which substitute for more severe experimental outcomes such as advanced pathology or death." Humane endpoints can be arrived at by running pilot studies before commencing the research study (National Research Council (US) Committee on Recognition and Alleviation of Pain in Laboratory Animals, 2009), assessing similar studies in published literature, as well as recognizing that judgment will be required with each study often having its own unique endpoints.

The principles of the "Three Rs": replacement, reduction, and refinement (The Three R's or 3Rs) (Russell, 1959) allow the protection of animals in research by safeguarding their welfare, as well as minimizing their use. The definition of Refinement by the NC3Rs includes "methods which minimize animal suffering and improve welfare"(NC3Rs, 2020). Humane endpoints can also be considered as a form of refinement (National Research Council (US) Committee on Recognition and Alleviation of Pain in Laboratory Animals, 2009), as is improved analgesia. In the mid-2000s, it was thought that perhaps as low as 20% of painful studies in rodents include analgesia (Stokes et al., 2009). Even in nonrodent species where there may be greater consideration of the need for analgesia, rates of systemic analgesic administration were low, for example in experimental studies on rabbits rates of only 50% were seen in the mid-2000s (Coulter et al., 2009). A review of 400 scientific articles, using a range of species, between 2014 and 2015, as well as some before 2011, which involved invasive survival surgeries, showed 338 of those 400 articles mentioned the use of anesthesia and/or analgesia. 302 of the 400 articles did not mention analgesic use, nor express that analgesia was withheld (it is unclear whether this is due to a lack of reporting or a lack of discussion) (Carbone and Austin, 2016). In many regions of the world, there is a legal requirement to address and reduce pain in animals used for research. In a review of 684 surgical procedures from 506 experimental applications in Germany from 2010, 30% of surgeries did not have a proposed postoperative analgesia protocol (Herrmann and Flecknell, 2019).

Pain assessment and administration of appropriate analgesia assist in preventing those negative sequelae which impact research and animal welfare, as well as preventing wind-up and central nervous sensitization (Valverde and Gunkel, 2005) (refer to Chapters 4, 6, and 7).

B. Timing of pain assessment

1. Postprocedure

Reliable pain assessment should facilitate the use of analgesia. Preemptive analgesia is widely accepted as an ethical course of action and gold standard of practice. Once pain has been inflicted or is present, reliable pain assessment methods should be used in order to address the pain. There are some difficulties in assessing pain in laboratory species, and there is currently no gold standard for assessment of animal pain (Paul-Murphy et al., 2004). Human pain scales rely on verbal expressions of pain states. Since nonverbal humans and animals are not able to describe pain verbally (Paul-Murphy et al., 2004), pain assessment is always subjective. Reliable pain assessment can reduce the overuse of analgesics, and their accompanying side effects. For example, opioids may reduce gastrointestinal motility, lead to respiratory depression and variations in behavior (National Research Council (US) Committee on Recognition and Alleviation of Pain in Laboratory Animals, 2009; Valverde and Gunkel, 2005), and lead to body weight loss (Jirkof et al., 2020; Stasiak et al., 2003).

Pain assessment and management should be tailored to the species, strain, sex, age, type of procedure, and duration of the procedure (Whittaker and Howarth, 2014). Ideally, preemptive analgesia should be given to all animals undergoing surgical procedures. For both surgical and nonsurgical procedures, pain assessment should commence from soon after the procedure until a period of days following the procedure, when pain score has decreased. Additionally, pain should be assessed after analgesic administration, to ensure it is having the desired effect. Pain assessment should also be performed at time points where a waning of the known duration of action of the chosen analgesic occurs. The normal periods of activity and 24-hour pattern of behavior should be borne in mind for the pain assessments and decision making. Patterns of analgesic usage should follow this timespan with consideration for a gradual decrease in dose and volume of analgesic agents given, as well as use of other classes of agents, for example switching opioid agents to nonsteroidal antiinflammatory drugs as pain subsides in the days following the experimental intervention. "Cage-side" assessment, using animal or behavioral-based indices are ideal since they allow point of care intervention.

2. Chronic models

A brief summary on chronic pain in laboratory animals is provided here; please refer to Chapter 27 for greater detail. Chronic pain assessment tools have been less characterized compared to acute pain assessment tools (Whittaker and Howarth, 2014). In conducting chronic pain assessments, it is important to be aware of the possibility of pain and time of likely onset, for example, at a time when tumor size is significant, but pain assessment should still be conducted as part of routine monitoring. Often in chronic models, identification of pain behaviors is used in order to trigger interventions. There are few consistent and dependable indicators of chronic pain (Stasiak et al., 2003; Whittaker and Howarth, 2014). Chronic models involving pain, for example neoplasia studies, are common in biomedical research (Whittaker and Howarth, 2014), and development of reliable measures for chronic pain is imperative (Urban et al., 2011). It is important to note that in considering neoplastic pain, the delineation between acute versus chronic pain is not simplistic, as the pain experience follows the evolution of the disease state, and neoplastic damage to tissues (Caraceni and Shkodra, 2019).

C. Features of pain scales

Features of pain scales include their reliability, sensitivity, and validity (Rutherford, 2002). For example, when discussing a visual analog scale, when similar painful experiences are assessed, reassessed, and compared, reliability would infer that similar reproducible results are found. For example, within a painful state that does not change much during the assessment time point (Good et al., 2001). Sensitivity of a scale allows the identification of small changes in the perceived pain (Natelson et al., 1987). Validity of a scale indicates the ability of that scale to measure what is sought to be measured, as well as allowing the drawing of conclusions about the presence and grade of the parameter for the animal under investigation (Streiner et al., 2015). Content validity relates to whether the scale captures the measure of interest, whilst criterion validity is the comparison of a scale with an accepted standard. In human pain medicine, self-report is the "gold" standard. However, in nonverbal humans and animals criterion validity cannot be established. As a result, construct validity is often used to replace criterion validity (Turner et al., 2019). This relates the use of the scale to a known concept, for example, that the use of analgesics will reduce pain scores (Mogil and Crager, 2004). Practicality is important when it comes to the use of pain scales. Pain scales' criteria and indices should be easily understood by the users to aid applicability (Paul-Murphy et al., 2004). Ideally, pain scales will be generalizable, allow clinical decision-making, and guide intervention thresholds. Some pain scales are not generalizable and may have been developed for a discrete condition or evaluation after a particular intervention. There is some benefit in having a variety of pain scales available as they may control better for confounding variables; however using a smaller number of assessment tools may increase the ability to compare between research studies, for example (Paul-Murphy et al., 2004). A validated pain scale is well placed to provide accurate measurements. However, a further consideration in terms of validity relates to interobserver reliability. This means that two independent observers who complete the pain assessment at the same time should reach the same pain score (Stasiak et al., 2003). This is of particular concern in clinical laboratory animal medicine since a variety of staff are likely to be involved in pain assessment.

V. Pain assessment methods

As laboratory animal practitioners needing to assess animal pain there are two key questions. First, it is necessary to determine if the animal is in pain. Second, a determination of the level of pain is needed. This then guides the selection of appropriate interventions. Due to the complexity of pain perception, the experience is subjective and cannot be objectively measured. However, there are a number of tools which can be used to infer a painful state.

A physiological response, primarily mediated by the autonomic nervous system, accompanies activation of the pain pathways. This largely reflects the stress response and is not specific to pain (Middleton, 2003). Changes in behavior, posture and facial expression also occur in painful states and have varying specificity to pain itself (Jirkof et al., 2013; Whittaker and Howarth, 2014). The following will provide a brief overview of commonly used assessment methods, with an outline of the benefits and drawbacks associated with them. Table 12.1 summarizes common methods used for pain assessment in mammals.

A. Physiological markers

Physiological changes related to pain are generally a result of the stimulation of interrelated mechanisms. Pain acts as a

TABLE 12.1 List of general physiological and behavioral signs of pain in mammals.

Physiological indicators	Behavioral indicators
Hormone levels in blood/other tissues: Adrenal axis: cortisol/corticosterone Sympathetic axis: epinephrine/norepinephrine	Vocalizations: Number/duration Intensity Spectral characteristics
Inflammatory markers in blood e.g., haptoglobin, fibrinogen, IL-1	Postures: Abnormal lying Abnormal standing Abnormal sitting
Autonomic nervous system activation: Heart rate Respiratory rate Blood pressure Body temperature Heart rate variability	Behaviors: Licking, scratching, rubbing Avoidance/escape Tonic immobility Aggressiveness Isolation Loss of appetite Inactivity or excessive locomotion Sleep disturbance

Adapted from Prunier, et al. (2013). Copyright 2021, with permission from Elsevier.

stressor, leading to direct stimulation of the hypothalamic-pituitary-adrenal (HPA) and sympathetic axes. This leads to the production of hormones such as corticosterone (or cortisol dependent on species), adrenaline, and noradrenaline. Therefore, common physiological indicators of pain include products of the activation of HPA and sympathetic axes, and indicators of their downstream effects, such as elevations in heart rate, respiratory rate, or body temperature, and body weight changes. Tissue injury also causes immune system activation and the release of inflammatory mediators, such as interleukin-1. These substances can go on to cause additional activation of the HPA axis. Inflammation generates a range of other substances, such as haptoglobin and fibrinogen. Whilst these substances are not directly involved in pain mediation, since inflammation is a common cause of pain, they are commonly measured to infer a pain state (Prunier et al., 2013). However, some studies have suggested that these markers show minimal linkage with pain occurrence (see, e.g., Paull et al., 2009).

Physiological markers have the advantage of being objective and potentially indicating the intensity of pain response to guide treatment selection and dose. However, they need to be interpreted with caution since they are also influenced by stress and illness in the absence of pain. For example, restraint of animals commonly induces cortisol elevations. Furthermore, measures related to stimulation of the sympathetic axis are often highly sensitive, but also short-lived. Similarly, cortisol levels in plasma and saliva are also highly variable due to their rapid onset and decline in concentration (Wiechers et al., 2021; Wright-Williams et al., 2007). In spite of this sensitivity, these measures are often nonspecific, and it is almost impossible to tease apart the stress versus pain component (Prunier et al., 2013).

Use of physiological indicators is likely to be poorly suited to a clinical situation, and they may be better utilized as research tools. For example, a number of these markers require invasive sampling, such as the taking of a blood sample and subsequent laboratory analyses. Alternately, remote data acquisition techniques may be required to reduce the influence of human handling on the outcomes. This may involve specialized, expensive equipment. These sampling processes render the methods retrospective in nature precluding timely clinical intervention (Prunier et al., 2013). There are, however, a range of devices that are minimally invasive and might be acquired at a reasonable cost allowing real-time monitoring of physiological parameters such as heart rate, body temperature, and activity. For example, telemetry uses small implanted devices which allow automated and wireless transmission of physiological data to a receiver outside of the animals' cage (Niemeyer, 2016). These devices can range from requiring complex implantation surgery, such as the placing of electrodes in the brain (Niemeyer, 2016), to the use of minimally invasive radiofrequency identification microchips which can measure body temperature and activity (Redfern et al., 2017). Thermal imaging may also be an option to monitor activity and respiratory rate (Pereira et al., 2018) via noninvasive method.

The value of commonly used physiological indices is largely as determinants of acute pain based on their release being coincident with injury. Furthermore, chronic states tend to prolong cortisol secretion with the risk of creating a maladaptive response with compensatory down-regulation and blunting of cortisol responses (Hannibal and Bishop, 2014). There are, however, two possible exceptions to this arising from recent research. There is growing interest in the use of hair cortisol levels as an indicator for chronic stress (Burnard et al., 2017; Shi et al., 2021; Wiechers et al., 2021). Whilst the linkage between ongoing stress and cortisol levels in the hair is far from proven, and subject to multiple confounders, this method may become more promising following further research. Heart rate variability is under the control of the sympathetic and parasympathetic systems, and there is evidence from the human literature that decreased high-frequency variability occurs in chronic pain, as a result of decreased parasympathetic activation (Tracy et al., 2016). There has been a minimal investigation of this idea in the veterinary context, although one study provided evidence of its utility to detect mild-to-moderate pain in mice following laparotomy (Arras et al., 2007).

Akin to the parameters with an acute onset, these methods are nonspecific to pain.

B. Behavioral methods of pain assessment

Behavioral signs of pain are used in animals and nonverbal humans, as they are not able to express their experience of pain with verbal language (Paul-Murphy et al., 2004). These methods are widely applicable, minimally resource-intensive, and often allow assessment in real-time, allowing timely intervention (Wright-Williams et al., 2007). A range of methods based on spontaneous behavioral expression are available.

1. Animal-based indices and pain-specific behaviors

There has been a consideration for pain assessment and tool development across a range of laboratory species. Many behavioral changes have been considered, including, amongst others, behavioral signs of pain such as autotomy focused on the painful region, guarding behavior, grooming behavior, reduction in locomotion, reduction in appetite, lack of attention to environmental stimuli, and various vocalizations (Mogil and Crager, 2004). Many of these behaviors are species-specific, and thus recognition often requires some knowledge and experience of the species concerned.

In many research facilities, scoring systems to guide the need for intervention rely on an assessment of general clinical signs. Many of the signs considered and scoring methods are based on the seminal work by Morton and Griffiths in 1985 (Morton and Griffiths, 1985). This schema considered animal-based indices such as food/water intake, behavioral signs, and animal appearance, and system-based measures such as fecal volume and consistency, body weight, body temperature, and pallor. The criteria are usually developed into a scoring tool where an overall score can be assigned. These measures are often easy to observe and document objectively. However, simple assessment methods are likely to be fairly crude and fail to identify pain in its early stages (Turner et al., 2019). Furthermore, these methods are nonspecific to pain and more aptly considered as markers of pain or distress (Morton and Griffiths, 1985). Additionally, there is evidence that analgesic administration may actually increase some clinical scores (George et al., 2019), largely due to the common side effect of reducing food consumption (Cooper et al., 2009; Jablonski et al., 2001; Whittaker et al., 2016), although presumably simultaneously reducing pain as suggested in other studies (Oliver et al., 2017; Oliver et al., 2018).

In rodents, a suite of pain-specific behaviors has been identified, although much of the research was performed in models expected to induce visceral pain, such as laparotomy procedures (Affaitati et al., 2002; Roughan and Flecknell, 2001). These behaviors include fairly subtle, short-duration behaviors such as writhing, abdominal press and twitching, weight shifting and back arching (Affaitati et al., 2002; Dunbar et al., 2016). These appear to be highly specific to pain and correlations have been seen between behavioral pain scoring and peak corticosterone after a painful intervention in mice (Wright-Williams et al., 2007). However, they can often be missed due to the rapid movements of rodents, and the difficulties in visualizing animals in their home cage due to cage furniture. Methods to overcome this include removal of the animals from the home cage, and the use of video recording for retrospective analysis. However, this limits the practical application of these methods. Whilst it is generally assumed that a greater frequency of pain behaviors correlates with increased pain, and this may then guide the assessment of pain intensity, in reality, minimal observation time is likely to be available for this assessment. Furthermore, whilst the list of behaviors is well-developed for acute pain, these behaviors appear to be rare in models where chronic pain is to be expected (Roughan et al., 2004). Instead, there may be a different set of behaviors which are model-specific (Roughan et al., 2004), for example, lameness occurrence during osteosarcoma development (Husmann et al., 2015), or just a general increase in inactivity and reduction in maintenance behaviors such as grooming (Van Loo et al., 1997). This is an area where further research attention is needed.

2. Grimace scales

Recently, it has been proposed that evaluation of complex motor responses, such as facial and bodily expression could be an indicator of animal emotional experience (Ekman, 1992; Panksepp, 2005). Facial expressions have been the subject of significant study across species as potential indicators of both positive and negative emotional states (Whittaker and Marsh, 2019). There is also good evidence that facial expressions are associated with the emotional experience of pain, given that insular cortex lesions modulate expression and this region is involved in human pain perception (Langford et al., 2010). Criteria for assessment of facial expression have been standardized, resulting in the development of "grimace scales". Grimace scales utilize an assessment, and subsequent scoring of action units focused on the eyes, ears, and cheeks, which are assimilated to produce an overall score. These scales have now been developed for a range of lab species including; mice (Langford et al., 2010), rats (Sotocinal et al., 2011), rabbits (Keating et al., 2012), sheep (Häger et al., 2017), ferrets (Reijgwart et al., 2017), cats (Evangelista et al., 2019), pigs (Viscardi et al., 2017), and horses (Dalla Costa et al., 2014).

Grimace scales are now well characterized in rodents and are generally considered valid at identifying pain across a range of models commonly used in biomedical research, including those in oncology (Chartier et al., 2020; de Almeida et al., 2019, 2020), pain research (Akintola et al., 2019; Langford et al., 2010), infectious disease (Mai et al., 2018) and neurological conditions (Duffy et al., 2016; Hassler et al., 2019). They particularly seem to have validity for assessment of acute pain, although there is also limited evidence for their utility in assessment of chronic pain states such as those arising from cancer (de Almeida et al., 2019, 2020; Whittaker et al., 2021). However, they are less well-characterized in larger laboratory species and therefore currently employed less. Additionally, in spite of the significant number of validation studies performed in rodents, they are not widely used in clinical laboratory animal practice. This likely stems from the lack of validation of the scales using real-time methods (Mota-Rojas et al., 2020). These methods are needed to support animal welfare by allowing effective intervention, and documentation of pain status over time. They need to be able to be performed in a minimally resource-intensive fashion, and outcomes should not be modified by observer presence. Development of these cage-side methods, as well as the creation of training opportunities for researchers and ethics committees on the grimace scales, should be a priority for laboratory animal professionals. There are a number of excellent reviews on the use of grimace scales in veterinary species for readers interested in learning more (see e.g., Descovich et al., 2017; McLennan et al., 2019; Mogil et al., 2020; Whittaker et al., 2021).

3. Vocalizations

Assessment of vocalizations has been proposed as a measure of the emotional pain response in a range of species. The rate and acoustic structure (e.g., frequencies, amplitude, and duration) of vocalizations have been considered to be fairly predictive of change in emotional arousal across species, i.e., they are produced at faster rates with higher amplitude and frequency (Laurijs et al., 2021). Therefore, they offer the opportunity to determine the intensity of the pain response, although this has been minimally investigated in the scientific literature. Animals may vocalize spontaneously or on handling, but vocalization may not be specific to pain, and not all animals in pain will vocalize (Carstens and Moberg, 2000). For example, vocalization in dogs after surgery is more commonly a sign of anxiety than pain, and cats tend not to vocalize unless pain is extreme (Gassel et al., 2005). In ruminants, vocalization is uncommonly reported in the face of acute pain, and was absent in a study on heat branding by Lay et al., (1992), in spite of the treatment causing increases in cortisol, heart rate, and aversive behavior (Lay et al., 1992).

For rodents both audible, and perhaps more commonly, ultrasonic vocalizations have been used. Emitted frequencies of 22–28 kHz have been considered to arise as a result of stress or pain (Jourdan et al., 1995, 1998), whereas higher frequencies signal social affiliative interactions (Wöhr and Schwarting, 2013). They have also been shown to be modified after the acute painful challenge of vasectomy (Smith et al., 2020), and in chronic pain states such as arthritis (Calvino et al., 1996). However, their utility as a reliable pain assessment method has been called into question since it has been shown that this number is poorly correlated with other pain behavior signs in rat inflammatory, visceral, and neuropathic pain models in one study (Wallace et al., 2005), and were not found to be modified by analgesics in another (Jourdan et al., 2002). Moreover, there has been little discussion on how vocalization monitoring might be incorporated in a practical fashion into vivarium routines. Given that recording needs microphones, as well as other equipment and software programs for analysis this method is unlikely to be feasible for practical pain assessment. For a recent review on the linkage between rodent ultrasonic vocalizations and emotional states, see Simola and Granon (2019).

4. Alternate behavioral indicators

Locomotion is frequently modified if an animal is in pain. Modification may be in the form of reduced distance traveled or inability to perform specific behaviors, such as rearing. For example, rabbits were less active following surgery (Karas et al., 2007), and similar findings have been found in models of acute pain in mice (Flecknell and Liles, 1991). Running wheel activity may be a practical way of assessing this outcome in rodents (Cobos et al., 2012; Tubbs et al., 2011). Furthermore, there is evidence that this method may have application not just in models where the pain insult is directed toward the musculoskeletal system, for example after hepatectomy (Tubbs et al., 2011). However, given that rodents are highly motivated toward running wheel activities, it may be that this method is only sensitive to relatively severe pain (Whittaker and Howarth, 2014). Gait assessment is also valuable as an indication of pain in models where animals tend to shift weight toward the unaffected limb, for example, inflammatory or orthopedic disease conditions (Medhurst et al., 2002; Stevenson et al., 2011).

Alternatively, in some species, increases in activity may occur when pain is experienced. In farm animals, restlessness often manifests as frequent attempts to rise, with altered postures after surgical procedures. Pigs (Hay et al., 2003), lambs (Molony et al., 2002), and calves (Robertson et al., 1994) were observed to lie more on their sides with extended legs after castration than before. Abnormal ventral lying with legs being tucked under the body may also be observed, for instance in lambs and pigs after castration and tail docking (Hay et al., 2003; Molony et al., 1993, 2002).

These postural alterations appear to be a common manifestation of acute pain in younger animals (Eicher and Dailey, 2002). Moreover, other postural changes such as aspects of the head, back, and ear position have been evaluated as pain indicators, for example in cows (Gleerup et al., 2015), sheep (Silva et al., 2020), and pigs (Luna et al., 2020). These indicators are often incorporated into composite pain assessment scales (Steagall et al., 2021). A range of studies have also demonstrated that sociability and interactions with pen mates are reduced in painful conditions, with an associated increase in aggressive behaviors (see, e.g., Guesgen et al., 2013; Sutherland et al., 2012; Taylor et al., 2001). For further details on methods of pain assessment in farm animals, refer to the review of Steagall et al. (2021).

Sleep behavior may also be disturbedby decreased total sleep time, increased number of arousals, and increased time is taken to enter sleep (Andersen and Tufik, 2000; Schütz et al., 2003). Whilst sleep disturbance might be a useful indicator of chronic and severe pain, it is probably best regarded as a general indicator of pain and distress, rather than pain-specific.

There has been considerable attention in recent years on the performance of nonessential behaviors as an indicator of emotional state. These behaviors, which are usually highly motivated and nonessential, have been equated with well-being. As a result, they are often the first behaviors to be reduced in the face of pain or distress (Jirkof, 2014). These might include play, social affiliative behaviors, or species-specific behaviors. The latter category includes behaviors such as dust bathing, beak wiping, and preening in birds; body shaking and rubbing in cattle and pigs; as well as nest building and burrowing in rodents (Whittaker and Marsh, 2019). At least in rodents where nest building and burrowing have been reduced after interventions expected to induce pain and are corroborated using data from other pain assessment methods, there is good evidence to support the link with pain (Jirkof, 2014). Furthermore, analgesics can often reinstate these behaviors (Andrews et al., 2012; Arras et al., 2007). The behaviors are easily observed and encouraged through the provision of bedding or burrowing substrate. However, these behaviors have also been modified by the stress evoked by housing conditions, which hints at their nonspecificity for pain (Bangsgaard Bendtsen et al., 2012). They can also be highly variable between individuals and may have a ceiling effect, where all the substrate is used up so differences cannot be observed (Deacon, 2006).

A range of other methods for assessing affective states have been proposed. These may be nonspecific to pain, instead being general indicators of distress, or the corollary, that of well-being. These include apparatus-based behavioral tests such as judgment bias or conditioned place preference (CPP) testing. Since cognition is simpler to assess in animals than emotion, the judgment bias task is based on the recognized linkage between cognition and emotional state, i.e., decisions influence emotional state and vice versa (Jirkof et al., 2019). The tests require a training period where associations are learned based on a graded stimulus requiring some action (or inaction), which leads to attainment of a reward or punishment (or lesser reward). Once these associations are learned, a novel (ambiguous) stimulus of the same nature, and that lies in between the previous learned associations is introduced (Whittaker and Barker, 2020). The choice made allows prediction of whether the animal is in a positive or negative affective state. There has been little evaluation of the test in rodents where the pain is expected, as opposed to distress or anxiety (Jirkof et al., 2019). However, there is some limited evidence of utility. For example, chemotherapy-induced mucositis in rats altered judgment biasing (George et al., 2018). Furthermore, a number of studies in large animals have demonstrated the impact of pain on test outcomes; see e.g., Neave et al. (2013), and LeCorps et al. (2019) evaluating calves after disbudding. A further benefit of this test is that it allows the prediction of positive affective states which are often difficult to ascertain through other testing methods. The drawback is that training periods are often lengthy. Therefore at the current time, the method is not suitable for clinical pain assessment in research animals, especially when they are on short-duration studies. CPP testing has been adapted from studies evaluating drug psychoactive properties to being used for welfare determination. The animals are conditioned to one location, which is paired with a drug treatment, and receive a placebo in another location. When given the choice, animals in pain typically spend more time in the drug-paired location as it is assumed to be a positive experience (Roughan et al., 2014). Mice with bladder cancer developed a morphine preference in the CPP, indicating they were in pain (Roughan et al., 2014), although a later study could not confirm a pain association (Miller et al., 2016a,b). The benefit of this test is its potential to evaluate pain rather than nociception. However, the complex nature of the conditioning process renders it unsuitable for use as a routine welfare assessment tool.

A relatively simple newer behavioral test that may indicate pain is the grooming transfer test. This test relies on the propensity of mice to groom, and hence a fluorescent powder is applied to their coat. Latency to groom has been shown to increase following laparotomy surgery, with a subsequent decrease upon analgesic administration (Oliver et al., 2018).

VI. Challenges in assessment of pain

Analgesiometry has been the traditional method of measuring nociception and analgesic effectiveness by applying an uncomfortable stimulus to a body part and measuring the pain threshold exhibited. This is often by withdrawal away from the nociceptive stimulus (a motor response) (Stasiak et al., 2003). Analgesiometry inflicts the stimulus onto a control animal(s) and a treated animal(s) (diseased or intervention); however it does not measure the pain behaviors shown spontaneously by an animal and therefore may not truly reflect the emotional experience of pain (Whittaker and Howarth, 2014).

All species, both mammalian and nonmammalian, should have considerate practices in place, and assessment tools used to assess their pain. However, there are differences between species in how they respond to painful experiences (Paul-Murphy et al., 2004; Stasiak et al., 2003; Valverde and Gunkel, 2005). It is therefore important to have deep knowledge of species and their pain behaviors (Stasiak et al., 2003). For example, it has been proposed that prey species like rats, mice, and ruminants may hide signs of pain (Stasiak et al., 2003). Other species may have more subtlety to how they display signs of pain, for example, avian species (Stasiak et al., 2003). Horses may have more demonstrative behaviors when in pain, like kicking at the abdomen in colic episodes (Paul-Murphy et al., 2004). Guinea pigs may be quiet when in pain, instead of their usual flight (stampeding behavior) or vocalizations (Mayer, 2007). Training and experience may be of importance may also impact upon assessment with overlap in signs to the untrained eye, for example, rabbits showing teeth grinding behavior when experiencing abdominal pain, compared to rabbits showing relaxed "teeth purring" behavior when resting (Mayer, 2007). Table 12.2 presents proposed behavioral indicators of pain in common laboratory animals.

TABLE 12.2 List of general physiological and behavioral signs of pain in mammals.

Species	General behavior
Rat	Reduced activity; reduced appetite; reduced drinking; licks; guards limbs; self-mutilates; increased aggression and vocalization; aversion toward con-specifics
Mouse	As rat; increased vibrissa movement, hunched back
Guinea pig	Squeals, stampedes when handled; or quiet
Rabbit	Anxious; hides; squeals or cries; or aggressive; scratches/bites; reduced appetite; cannibalizes young; tonic immobility
Dog	Bites, scratches, guards; whimpers or howls; growls; quiet, submissive; or more aggressive to handling
Cat	Quiet; hisses or spits; hides; licks excessively; limps; guards limbs; stilted gait; reduced appetite; escape response to handling
Horse	Reluctant to be handled; decreased activity; disrupted feeding; restlessness or depression; reluctance to move; unusual limb position
Nonhuman primate	Screams or moans; reduced feeding and drinking; aggression

Adapted from Carstens and Moberg (2000).

For some species, pain scales are well-characterized, for example, the previously discussed acute postoperative pain scales in rats (Whittaker and Howarth, 2014) or the Mouse Grimace Scale (Langford et al., 2010). There are other pain scales and scoring systems in place, but they may not be fully validated. For example, few studies have evaluated nonfacial, behavioral pain indices in the mouse, but one by Wright-Williams et al. (2007) shows some overlap with the rat ethogram, with the addition of a few mouse-specific behaviors. Ideally, pain scales would be developed to consider characteristics inclusive of the environment animals were raised and kept in during the experiment, the current housing environment, and the animal's age or stage of development (Paul-Murphy et al., 2004) (Wright-Williams et al., 2007).

There are some practicalities which affect the assessment of pain behaviors in vivaria. Notwithstanding that staff needs training and experience in recognizing both normal and abnormal species behaviors (Mayer, 2007), their presence will also affect their ability to assess pain behavior (see e.g., Miller and Leach, 2015; Oliver et al., 2017). Handling animals may be inherently stressful and may alter the behavior observed. Fear and apprehension in an unfamiliar environment, for example being housed singly for an experiment, will also affect behavior and therefore behavior analysis (Wright-Williams et al., 2007). In addition, mice move very rapidly, which makes reliable pain assessment somewhat challenging (Wright-Williams et al., 2007). Due to these animals being fast-moving, cage-side live scoring on the Mouse Grimace Scale is often lower than those delivered by poststudy image analysis (Miller and Leach, 2015). Furthermore, animals may be hidden from view due to the housing setup, making assessment difficult. Rodents show burrowing habits (Mayer, 2007), which will affect the observer's ability to watch the animal without interrupting its normal behavior. Some behaviors are also found to be highly variable not just within individual laboratories or animals, but between laboratories (Jirkof et al., 2020). If handling is needed for assessment, consideration needs to be given to natural behavior expressions such as immobility when handled, which makes pain assessment difficult (Mayer, 2007). Animals may also habituate to humans over time, which may alter their display of pain behaviors.

Mice and rats are nocturnal species, therefore pain assessments which are made during the light phase are unlikely to give a full picture of pain in the animals observed. Mice may show greater pain behaviors in the first part of the dark phase (Whittaker and Howarth, 2014). Assessment of other factors is also dependent on the circadian rhythm; for example, around only 5% of food and water consumption occurs during the light phase in rats (Liles and Flecknell, 1993). Options to increase the efficacy of assessments include examination of the animals under red light or during the dark phase of the day using reverse lighting systems.

Measures may also have variable specificity, practicality, and have confounds (for example that of sedation, learning, or fear) that need to be borne in mind (Mogil and Crager, 2004). Pain assessments may be impacted by the anesthetics and analgesics used during the study and around the time of pain assessment. There are also strain differences in how mice or rats, for example, respond to anesthetics (e.g., isoflurane) and analgesics (e.g., buprenorphine) and the behaviors shown (Miller et al., 2015, 2016a,b). This may be especially relevant with opioid-based agents. For example, buprenorphine has been shown to change motor activity by causing increased hopping and walking in mice (Miller et al., 2015; Tubbs et al., 2011).

Disagreeable sensations are associated with nociceptive pain as well as other physical disorders (for example, hypoxia, vomiting, and thermal discomfort). Negative affective states like fear, distress, and isolation may also lead to disagreeable feelings (McMillan, 2003). Discerning between nociceptive physical pain and emotional components of pain is important yet objective scales to characterize emotional responses to pain are not well typified (Whittaker and Howarth, 2014). Furthermore, whilst pain can certainly contribute to stress, it is important to remember that pain assessment methods may inadvertently measure stress-related behaviors rather than the pain itself. These behaviors may therefore not be responsive or amenable to analgesics. When assessing pain, it is important that behaviors and responses categorized as pain responses are not confounded with other etiologies, which may include fear, anxiety, sickness behavior, or paresthesia (Mogil and Crager, 2004; Whittaker and Howarth, 2014).

Sickness behaviors are a common confounding factor in pain assessment. Sickness behaviors include nonspecific behavioral signs secondary to cytokine release from inflammation, infection, or stressors (Tizard, 2008; Vollmer-Conna, 2001). Common sickness behaviors include social withdrawal, an increase in resting, a reduction in explorative behavior, a reduction in self-care activities like grooming, anhedonia, impaired learning and recall, a decrease in consumption of food and water and somnolence, among others (Tizard, 2008; Bowen, 2013; Dantzer et al., 2008; Stella et al., 2011; Tizard, 2009). Sickness behavior often shows a typical pattern in the first 24 hours after cytokine release, followed by the second phase of depressed behavior and anhedonia (Bowen, 2013). Sickness behavior can be triggered by psychological stressors, for example, guinea pig pups separated from their mother in a novel environment exhibit sickness behaviors (Hennessy et al., 2014). Cats, privately owned or in vivaria, are sensitive to changes in their environment and show sickness behaviors in response to unfamiliar staff, a new cage environment, a change in the daily routine of feeding, or a lack of agency in their environment (Stella et al., 2011). In a traditional sickness model sense, it is thought that sickness behaviors may aid in recovery, and animals are motivated to participate in sickness behaviors when feeling unwell (Dantzer et al., 2008; Tizard, 2008; Vollmer-Conna, 2001), but from a pain assessment perspective, we need to aim to discern between true pain behaviors and pain-like behaviors seen in sickness behavior.

A. Automation of assessment

A challenge with many of the behavioral assessment methods described above is that they can be subjective, time-consuming, and occurring at times of day when animals are less active due to normal staffing patterns being during the daylight hours (Richardson, 2015). In addition, typical animal pens or cages may obscure animals preventing accurate observation. Behavioral automation has multiple advantages, including: allowing continuous recording, introducing objectivity due to the technology design, reducing the effects of observer presence, reducing human labor requirements, and minimizing stress on the animals due to a reduced need to handle and remove them from their home cage environment. There are a number of high-throughput automated home cage systems available for rodents which variously combine systems that detect floor movement, utilize infrared beams, automate video analysis, and monitor food/water consumption (Richardson, 2015; Grieco et al., 2021). There has also been considerable progress in developing automated facial pain expression systems using deep learning methods in animals (Andresen et al., 2020; Tuttle et al., 2018). These techniques are only likely to become more valid and commonplace in the coming years.

VII. Documentation and record-keeping

A nonstandardized approach to pain assessment is likely to result in wide variations in opinions between individuals caring for animals. Therefore, a pain assessment goal should be to use validated and objective methods where possible. In many cases, the use of a combination of methods will increase certainty in the assessment outcome.

Since a number of the measures discussed are often fairly subjective, the development of situation- and species-specific score sheets which may combine physiological and behavioral variables can add objectivity and encourage transparency in decision-making (Bugnon et al., 2016).

These score sheets may encourage a binary response, i.e., present, or determine the degree of variation of the criteria from the normal parameters see, e.g., (Morton and Griffiths, 1985) with a numerical score assigned. The former may be less sensitive to animal distress. Score sheets should make it clear at what point intervention is required based on the cumulative score, and what specific intervention should be made. In the case of grimace scales there has been a range of attempts to develop intervention thresholds such that attainment of scores above a certain level signal the need to provide rescue analgesia (Evangelista et al., 2019; McLennan et al., 2016; Oliver et al., 2014).

Consideration should also be given to whether there are any score sheet criteria which should have a higher weighting and therefore trigger an intervention point in their own right. Attention should be directed toward making use of the score sheet as efficient and easy as possible, through avoiding use of an excessive number of criteria or highly subjective parameters (Bugnon et al., 2016). It is recommended that piloting of new sheets be performed by those who will ultimately use it, and that investigators be trained in recognition of the parameters and on the method of scoring.

Given that there are a variety of documented confounders in pain assessment, such as observer presence, time of day and between animal variability, establishing a written record of scores can be valuable since it allows contrast of scores over time within the same animal, rather than utilizing an absolute score cut-off which may fail to accurately represent the animal's response to pain and the changing nature of this response. In this sense, a level of clinical discretion may need to be built into scoring systems and ethical approvals to encourage consideration of individual differences in response to pain.

VIII. Summary

There are clear ethical and legal obligations to reduce pain in animals undergoing research procedures. Reduction of pain also benefits scientific outcomes since physiological and behavioral responses to pain can confound data interpretation. Therefore, pain prevention in the first place and pain assessment to enable the employment of mitigation strategies are essential. Pain assessment can be achieved using physiological or behavioral indicators. The latter have greater utility for clinical pain assessment since they provide instantaneous data which is immediately actionable. Behavioral methods are also likely to be more specific to pain rather than general sickness behaviors, although there are few methods which are completely unique to the pain response. Pain assessment should be performed by individuals who are trained and experienced with the species in question, at a frequency that allows early recognition of pain and intervention, which may be tailored for the procedure performed and the individual. Common behavioral-based pain assessment methods use observation of clinical signs, pain-specific behaviors, and the grimace scales. Other methods such as the assessment of nonessential behavior performance and activity monitoring are available but are less well-validated and have reduced specificity for pain. Use of standardized score sheets introduces greater objectivity in scoring and increases transparency in decision-making.

References

Affaitati, G., Giamberardino, M., Lerza, R., Lapenna, D., Laurentis, S., Vecchiet, L., 2002. Effects of tramadol on behavioural indicators of colic pain in a rat model of ureteral calculosis. Fund. Clin. Pharmacol. 16, 23–30.

Akintola, T., Tricou, C., Raver, C., Castro, A., Colloca, L., Keller, A., 2019. Search of a rodent model of placebo analgesia in chronic orofacial neuropathic pain. Neurobiol. Pain 6, 100033.

Andersen, M., Tufik, S., 2000. Altered sleep and behavioral patterns of arthritic rats. Sleep Res. Online: SRO 3 (4), 161–167.

Andresen, N., Wöllhaf, M., Hohlbaum, K., Lewejohann, L., Hellwich, O., Thöne-Reineke, C., Belik, V., 2020. Towards a fully automated surveillance of well-being status in laboratory mice using deep learning: starting with facial expression analysis. PLoS One 15, e0228059.

Andrews, N., Legg, E., Lisak, D., Issop, Y., Richardson, D., Harper, S., Pheby, T., Huang, W., Burgess, G., Machin, I., 2012. Spontaneous burrowing behaviour in the rat is reduced by peripheral nerve injury or inflammation associated pain. Eur. J. Pain 16, 485–495.

Arras, M., Rettich, A., Cinelli, P., Kasermann, H.P., Burki, K., 2007. Assessment of post-laparotomy pain in laboratory mice by telemetric recording of heart rate and heart rate variability. BMC Vet. Res. 3, 1–10.

Bangsgaard Bendtsen, K.M., Krych, L., Sørensen, D.B., Pang, W., Nielsen, D.S., Josefsen, K., Hansen, L.H., Sørensen, S.J., Hansen, A.K., 2012. Gut microbiota composition is correlated to grid floor induced stress and behavior in the BALB/c mouse. PLoS One 7 (10), e46231.

Bateson, P., 1991. Assessment of pain in animals. Anim. Behav. 42, 827–839.

Bowen, J., 2013. Effects of sickness behaviour and pain on behaviour. Proc. AWWA Annu. Conf. D4.2.1–D4.2.3.

Bugnon, P., Heimann, M., Thallmair, M., 2016. What the literature tells us about score sheet design. Lab. Anim. 50, 414–417.

Burnard, C., Ralph, C., Hynd, P., Hocking Edwards, J., Tilbrook, A., 2017. Hair cortisol and its potential value as a physiological measure of stress response in human and non-human animals. Anim. Prod. Sci. 57, 401–414.

Calvino, B., Besson, J., Boehrer, A., Depaulis, A., 1996. Ultrasonic vocalization (2R 28 kHz) in a model of chronic pain, the arthritic rat: effects of analgesic drugs. Neuroreport 7, 581–584.

Caraceni, A., Shkodra, M., 2019. Cancer pain assessment and classification. Cancers 11.

Carbone, L., Austin, J., 2016. Pain and Laboratory animals: publication practices for better data reproducibility and better animal welfare. PLoS One 11 (5), 1–24.

Carbone, L., 2020. Do "prey species" hide their pain? Implications for ethical care and use of laboratory animals. J. Appl. Anim. Ethics Res. 2, 216–236.

Carstens, E., Moberg, G.P., 2000. Recognizing pain and distress in laboratory animals. ILAR J. 41, 62–71.

Chartier, L.C., Hebart, M.L., Howarth, G.S., Whittaker, A.L., Mashtoub, S., 2020. Affective state determination in a mouse model of colitis-associated colorectal cancer. PLoS One 15, e0228413.

Cobos, E.J., Ghasemlou, N., Araldi, D., Segal, D., Duong, K., Woolf, C.J., 2012. Inflammation-induced decrease in voluntary wheel running in mice: a nonreflexive test for evaluating inflammatory pain and analgesia. Pain 153, 876–884.

Cooper, C.S., Metcalf-Pate, K.A., Barat, C.E., Cook, J.A., Scorpio, D.G., 2009. Comparison of side effects between buprenorphine and meloxicam used postoperatively in Dutch belted rabbits (*Oryctolagus cuniculus*). J. Am. Assoc. Lab. Anim. Sci.: JAALAS 48, 279–285.

Coulter, C.A., Flecknell, P.A., Richardson, C.A., 2009. Reported analgesic administration to rabbits, pigs, sheep, dogs and non-human primates undergoing experimental surgical procedures. Lab. Anim. 43, 232–238.

Dalla Costa, E., Minero, M., Lebelt, D., Stucke, D., Canali, E., Leach, M.C., 2014. Development of the Horse Grimace Scale (HGS) as a pain assessment tool in horses undergoing routine castration. PLoS One 9, e92281.

Dantzer, R., O'connor, J.C., Freund, G.G., Johnson, R.W., Kelley, K.W., 2008. From inflammation to sickness and depression: when the immune system subjugates the brain. Nat. Rev. Neurosci. 9, 46–56.

de Almeida, A.S., Rigo, F.K., De Prá, S.D., Milioli, A.M., Dalenogare, D.P., Pereira, G.C., Ritter, C.D.S., Peres, D.S., Antoniazzi, C.T.D., Stein, C., Moresco, R.N., Oliveira, S.M., Trevisan, G., 2019. Characterization of cancer-induced nociception in a murine model of breast carcinoma. Cell. Mol. Neurobiol. 39, 605–617.

de Almeida, A.S., Rigo, F.K., De Prá, S.D., Milioli, A.M., Pereira, G.C., Lückemeyer, D.D., Antoniazzi, C.T., Kudsi, S.Q., Araújo, D., Oliveira, S.M., Ferreira, J., Trevisan, G., 2020. Role of transient receptor potential ankyrin 1 (TRPA1) on nociception caused by a murine model of breast carcinoma. Pharmacol. Res. 152, 104576.

Deacon, R.M.J., 2006. Burrowing in rodents: a sensitive method for detecting behavioral dysfunction. Nat. Protoc. 1, 118–121.

Descovich, K., Wathan, J., Leach, M.C., Buchanan-Smith, H.M., Flecknell, P., Farningham, D., Vick, S.-J., 2017. Facial expression: an under-utilised tool for the assessment of welfare in mammals. ALTEX 34 (3), 409–429.

Duffy, S.S., Perera, C.J., Makker, P.G., Lees, J.G., Carrive, P., Moalem-Taylor, G., 2016. Peripheral and central neuroinflammatory changes and pain behaviors in an animal model of multiple sclerosis. Front. Immunol. 7, 369.

Dunbar, M.L., David, E.M., Aline, M.R., Lofgren, J.L., 2016. Validation of a behavioral ethogram for assessing postoperative pain in Guinea pigs (*Cavia porcellus*). JAALAS: J. Am. Assoc. Lab. Anim. Sci. 55 (1), 29–34.

Eicher, S.D., Dailey, J.W., 2002. Indicators of acute pain and fly avoidance behaviors in holstein calves following tail-docking. J. Dairy Sci. 85, 2850–2858.

Ekman, P., 1992. Are there basic emotions? Psychol. Rev. 99 (3), 550–553. https://doi.org/10.1037/0033-295X.99.3.550.

Evangelista, M.C., Watanabe, R., Leung, V.S., Monteiro, B.P., O'Toole, E., Pang, D.S., Steagall, P.V., 2019. Facial expressions of pain in cats: the development and validation of a Feline Grimace Scale. Sci. Rep. 9, 1–11.

Flecknell, P., Liles, J., 1991. The effects of surgical procedures, halothane anaesthesia and nalbuphine on locomotor activity and food and water consumption in rats. Lab. Anim. 25, 50–60.

Gassel, A.D., Tobias, K.M., Egger, C.M., Rohrbach, B.W., 2005. Comparison of oral and subcutaneous administration of buprenorphine and meloxicam for preemptive analgesia in cats undergoing ovariohysterectomy. J. Am. Vet. Med. Assoc. 227, 1937–1944.

Gatchel, R.J., 2004. Comorbidity of chronic pain and mental health disorders: the biopsychosocial perspective. Am. Psychol. 59, 795–805.

George, R.P., Barker, T.H., Lymn, K.A., Bigatton, D.A., Howarth, G.S., Whittaker, A.L., 2018. A judgement bias test to assess affective state and potential therapeutics in a rat model of chemotherapy-induced mucositis. Sci. Rep. 8 (1), 1–9.

George, R.P., Howarth, G.S., Whittaker, A.L., 2019. Use of the rat grimace scale to evaluate visceral pain in a model of chemotherapy-induced mucositis. Animals 9, 678.

Gleerup, K.B., Andersen, P.H., Munksgaard, L., Forkman, B., 2015. Pain evaluation in dairy cattle. Appl. Anim. Behav. Sci. 171, 25–32.

Good, M., Stiller, C., Zauszniewski, J.A., Anderson, G.C., Stanton-Hicks, M., Grass, J.A., 2001. Sensation and distress of pain scales: reliability, validity, and sensitivity. J. Nurs. Meas. 9, 219–238.

Grieco, F., Bernstein, B.J., Biemans, B., Bikovski, L., Burnett, C.J., Cushman, J.D., van Dam, E.A., Fry, S.A., Richmond-Hacham, B., Homberg, J.R., Kas, M.J.H., Kessels, H.W., Koopmans, B., Krashes, M.J., Krishnan, V., Logan, S., Loos, M., McCann, K.E., Parduzi, Q., Pick, C.G., Prevot, T.D., Riedel, G., Robinson, L., Sadighi, M., Smit, A.B., Sonntag, W., Roelofs, R.F., Tegelenbosch, R.A.J., Noldus, L.P.J.J., 2021. Measuring behavior in the home cage: study design, applications, challenges, and perspectives. Front. Behav. Neurosci. 15, 735387.

Guesgen, M.J., Beausoleil, N.J., Stewart, M., 2013. Effects of early human handling on the pain sensitivity of young lambs. Vet. Anaesth. Analg. 40, 55–62.

Häger, C., Biernot, S., Buettner, M., Glage, S., Keubler, L., Held, N., Bleich, E., Otto, K., Müller, C., Decker, S., 2017. The Sheep Grimace Scale as an indicator of post-operative distress and pain in laboratory sheep. PLoS One 12, e0175839.

Hannibal, K.E., Bishop, M.D., 2014. Chronic stress, cortisol dysfunction, and pain: a psychoneuroendocrine rationale for stress management in pain rehabilitation. Phys. Ther. 94, 1816–1825.

Hassler, S.N., Ahmad, F.B., Burgos-Vega, C.C., Boitano, S., Vagner, J., Price, T.J., Dussor, G., 2019. Protease activated receptor 2 (PAR2) activation causes migraine-like pain behaviors in mice. Cephalalgia 39, 111–122.

Hay, M., Vulin, A., Génin, S., Sales, P., Prunier, A., 2003. Assessment of pain induced by castration in piglets: behavioral and physiological responses over the subsequent 5 days. Appl. Anim. Behav. Sci. 82, 201–218.

Hennessy, M.B., Deak, T., Schiml, P.A., 2014. Sociality and sickness: have cytokines evolved to serve social functions beyond times of pathogen exposure? Brain Behav. Immun. 37, 15–20.

Herrmann, K., Flecknell, P., 2019. Retrospective review of anesthetic and analgesic regimens used in animal research proposals. ALTEX 36 (1), 65–80.

Husmann, K., Arlt, M.J.E., Jirkof, P., Arras, M., Born, W., Fuchs, B., 2015. Primary tumour growth in an orthotopic osteosarcoma mouse model is not influenced by analgesic treatment with buprenorphine and meloxicam. Lab. Anim. 49 (4), 284–293.

International Association for the Study of Pain (IASP), 2020. IASP Announces Revised Definition of Pain. Available online: https://www.iasp-pain.org/PublicationsNews/NewsDetail.aspx?ItemNumber=10475#:~:text=Jul%2016%2C%202020&text=The%20definition%20is%3A%20%E2%80%9CAn%20unpleasant,pain%20for%20further%20valuable%20context. (Accessed 13 November 2020).

Jablonski, P., Howden, B.O., Baxter, K., 2001. Influence of buprenorphine analgesia on post-operative recovery in two strains of rats. Lab. Anim. 35, 213–222.

Jirkof, P., 2014. Burrowing and nest building behavior as indicators of well-being in mice. J. Neurosci. Methods 234, 139–146.

Jirkof, P., Abdelrahman, A., Bleich, A., Durst, M., Keubler, L., Potschka, H., Struve, B., Talbot, S.R., Vollmar, B., Zechner, D., Häger, C., 2020. A safe bet? Inter-laboratory variability in behaviour-based severity assessment. Lab. Anim. 54, 73–82.

Jirkof, P., Fleischmann, T., Cesarovic, N., Rettich, A., Vogel, J., Arras, M., 2013. Assessment of postsurgical distress and pain in laboratory mice by nest complexity scoring. Lab. Anim. 47, 153–161.

Jirkof, P., Rudeck, J., Lewejohann, L., 2019. Assessing affective state in laboratory rodents to promote animal welfare-what is the progress in applied refinement research? Animals 9 (12), 1026.

Jourdan, D., Ardid, D., Chapuy, E., Eschalier, A., Le Bars, D., 1995. Audible and ultrasonic vocalization elicited by single electrical nociceptive stimuli to the tail in the rat. Pain 63, 237–249.

Jourdan, D., Ardid, D., Chapuy, E., Le Bars, D., Eschalier, A., 1998. Effect of analgesics on audible and ultrasonic pain-induced vocalization in the rat. Life Sci. 63, 1761–1768.

Jourdan, D., Ardid, D., Eschalier, A., 2002. Analysis of ultrasonic vocalisation does not allow chronic pain to be evaluated in rats. Pain 95, 165–173.

Karas, A.Z., Weaver, L.A., Andrutis, K.A., Blaze, C.A., 2007. A model for clinical evaluation of perioperative analgesia in the rabbit. In: 6th World Congress on Alternatives and Animals in the Life Sciences, Tokyo, Japan.

Keating, S.C., Thomas, A.A., Flecknell, P.A., Leach, M.C., 2012. Evaluation of EMLA cream for preventing pain during tattooing of rabbits: changes in physiological, behavioural and facial expression responses. PLoS One 7 (9), e44437.

Langford, D.J., Bailey, A.L., Chanda, M.L., Clarke, S.E., Drummond, T.E., Echols, S., Glick, S., Ingrao, J., Klassen-Ross, T., LaCroix-Fralish, M.L., 2010. Coding of facial expressions of pain in the laboratory mouse. Nat. Methods 7, 447–449.

Laurijs, K.A., Briefer, E.F., Reimert, I., Webb, L.E., 2021. Vocalisations in farm animals: a step towards positive welfare assessment. Appl. Anim. Behav. Sci. 236, 105264.

Lay Jr., D., Friend, T., Bowers, C., Grissom, K., Jenkins, O., 1992. A comparative physiological and behavioral study of freeze and hot-iron branding using dairy cows. J. Anim. Sci. 70, 1121–1125.

Lecorps, B., Ludwig, B.R., von Keyserlingk, M.A., Weary, D.M., 2019. Pain-induced pessimism and anhedonia: evidence from a novel probability-based judgment bias test. Front. Behav. Neurosci. 13, 54.

Liles, J.H., Flecknell, P.A., 1993. The effects of surgical stimulus on the rat and the influence of analgesic treatment. Br. Vet. J. 149, 515–525.

Low, L., Fitzgerald, M., 2012. Acute pain and a motivational pathway in adult rats: influence of early life pain experience. PLoS One 7, e34316.

Luna, S.P., de Araújo, A.L., da Nóbrega Neto, P.I., Brondani, J.T., de Oliveira, F.A., Azerêdo, L.M., Telles, F.G., Trindade, P.H., 2020. Validation of the UNESP-Botucatu pig composite acute pain scale (UPAPS). PLoS One 15 (6), e0233552.

Mai, S.H., Sharma, N., Kwong, A.C., Dwivedi, D.J., Khan, M., Grin, P.M., Fox-Robichaud, A.E., Liaw, P.C., 2018. Body temperature and mouse scoring systems as surrogate markers of death in cecal ligation and puncture sepsis. Intensive Care Med. Exp. 6, 1–14.

Mayer, J., 2007. Use of behavior analysis to recognize pain in small mammals. Lab. Anim. 36, 43–48.

McLennan, K.M., Miller, A.L., Dalla Costa, E., Stucke, D., Corke, M.J., Broom, D.M., Leach, M.C., 2019. Conceptual and methodological issues relating to pain assessment in mammals: the development and utilisation of pain facial expression scales. Appl. Anim. Behav. Sci. 217, 1–15.

McLennan, K.M., Rebelo, C.J.B., Corke, M.J., Holmes, M.A., Leach, M.C., Constantino-Casas, F., 2016. Development of a facial expression scale using footrot and mastitis as models of pain in sheep. Appl. Anim. Behav. Sci. 176, 19–26.

McMillan, F.D., 2003. A world of hurts—is pain special? J. Am. Vet. Med. Assoc. 223, 183–186.

Medhurst, S.J., Walker, K., Bowes, M., Kidd, B.L., Glatt, M., Muller, M., Hattenberger, M., Vaxelaire, J., O'Reilly, T., Wotherspoon, G., Winter, J., Green, J., Urban, L., 2002. A rat model of bone cancer pain. Pain 96, 129–140.

Mellor, D.J., 2019. Welfare-aligned sentience: enhanced capacities to experience, interact, anticipate, choose and survive. Animals 9 (7), 440.

Melnikova, I., 2010. Pain market. Nat. Rev. Drug Discov. 9, 589–590.

Middleton, C., 2003. Understanding the physiological effects of unrelieved pain. Nurs. Times 99, 28–31.

Miller, A., Burson, H., Söling, A., Roughan, J., 2016a. Welfare assessment following heterotopic or orthotopic inoculation of bladder cancer in C57BL/6 mice. PLoS One 11 (7), e0158390.

Miller, A., Kitson, G., Skalkoyannis, B., Leach, M., 2015. The effect of isoflurane anaesthesia and buprenorphine on the mouse grimace scale and behaviour in CBA and DBA/2 mice. Appl. Anim. Behav. Sci. 172, 58–62.

Miller, A.L., Leach, M.C., 2015. The mouse grimace scale: a clinically useful tool? PLoS One 10, e0136000.

Miller, A.L., Golledge, H.D., Leach, M.C., 2016b. The influence of isoflurane anaesthesia on the rat grimace scale. PLoS One 17 (11), e0166652. https://doi.org/10.1371/journal.pone.0166652. PMID: 27855184; PMCID: PMC5114010.

Mogil, J., 2020. The measurement of pain in the laboratory rodent. In: Wood, J.N. (Ed.), The Oxford Handbook of the Neurobiology of Pain. Oxford University Press, New York, NY.

Mogil, J.S., Crager, S.E., 2004. What should we be measuring in behavioral studies of chronic pain in animals? Pain 112, 12–15.

Mogil, J.S., Pang, D.S., Dutra, G.G.S., Chambers, C.T., 2020. The development and use of facial grimace scales for pain measurement in animals. Neurosci. Biobehav. Rev. 116, 480–493.

Molony, V., Kent, J., Robertson, I., 1993. Behavioural responses of lambs of three ages in the first three hours after three methods of castration and tail docking. Res. Vet. Sci. 55, 236–245.

Molony, V., Kent, J.E., McKendrick, I.J., 2002. Validation of a method for assessment of an acute pain in lambs. Appl. Anim. Behav. Sci. 76, 215–238.

Morton, D.B., Griffiths, P.H., 1985. Guidelines on the recognition of pain, distress and discomfort in experimental animals and an hypothesis for assessment. Vet. Rec. 116, 431–436.

Mota-Rojas, D., Napolitano, F., Strappini, A., Orihuela, A., Ghezzi, M.D., Hernández-Ávalos, I., Mora-Medina, P., Whittaker, A.L., 2021. Pain at the slaughterhouse in ruminants with a focus on the neurobiology of sensitisation. Animals 11.

Mota-Rojas, D., Olmos-Hernández, A., Verduzco-Mendoza, A., Hernández, E., Martínez-Burnes, J., Whittaker, A.L., 2020. The utility of grimace scales for practical pain assessment in laboratory animals. Animals 10, 1838.

Natelson, B.H., Creighton, D., McCarty, R., Tapp, W.N., Pitman, D., Ottenweller, J.E., 1987. Adrenal hormonal indices of stress in laboratory rats. Physiol. Behav. 39, 117–125.

National Research Council (US) Committee on Recognition and Alleviation of Pain in Laboratory Animals, 2009. Recognition and Alleviation of Pain in Laboratory Animals. National Academy of Sciences, Washington, DC.

NC3Rs, 2020. 3Rs Advice for Project Licence Applicants: Refinement. Available online: https://nc3rs.org.uk/3rs-advice-project-licence-applicants-refinement. (Accessed 28 August 2021).

NC3Rs, 2021. Humane Endpoints. Available online: https://www.nc3rs.org.uk/humane-endpoints. (Accessed 28 August 2021).

Neave, H.W., Daros, R.R., Costa, J.H.C., von Keyserlingk, M.A.G., Weary, D.M., 2013. Pain and pessimism: dairy calves exhibit negative judgement bias following hot-iron disbudding. PLoS One 8 (12), e80556.

Niemeyer, J., 2016. Telemetry for small animal physiology. Lab. Anim. (Lond.) 45, 255–257.

Oliver, V., De Rantere, D., Ritchie, R., Chisholm, J., Hecker, K.G., Pang, D.S.J., 2014. Psychometric assessment of the rat grimace scale and development of an analgesic intervention score. PLoS One 9, e97882.

Oliver, V.L., Athavale, S., Simon, K.E., Kendall, L.V., Nemzek, J.A., Lofgren, J.L., 2017. Evaluation of pain assessment techniques and analgesia efficacy in a female Guinea pig (*Cavia porcellus*) model of surgical pain. JAALAS: J. Am. Assoc. Lab. Anim. Sci. 56 (4), 425–435.

Oliver, V.L., Thurston, S.E., Lofgren, J.L., 2018. Using cageside measures to evaluate analgesic efficacy in mice (*Mus musculus*) after surgery. JAALAS: J. Am. Assoc. Lab. Anim. Sci. 57 (2), 186–201.

Panksepp, J., 2005. Affective consciousness: core emotional feelings in animals and humans. Conscious. Cognit. 14, 30–80.

Paul-Murphy, J., Ludders, J.W., Robertson, S.A., Gaynor, J.S., Hellyer, P.W., Wong, P.L., 2004. The need for a cross-species approach to the study of pain in animals. J. Am. Vet. Med. Assoc. 224, 692–697.

Paull, D., Lee, C., Colditz, I., Fisher, A., 2009. Effects of a topical anaesthetic formulation and systemic carprofen, given singly or in combination, on the cortisol and behavioural responses of Merino lambs to castration. Aust. Vet. J. 87 6, 230–237.

Pereira, C.B., Kunczik, J., Zieglowski, L., et al., 2018. Remote welfare monitoring of rodents using thermal imaging. Sensors 18 (11). https://doi.org/10.3390/s18113653.

Prunier, A., Mounier, L., Le Neindre, P., Leterrier, C., Mormède, P., Paulmier, V., Prunet, P., Terlouw, C., Guatteo, R., 2013. Identifying and monitoring pain in farm animals: a review. Animal 7, 998–1010.

Redfern, W.S., Tse, K., Grant, C., Keerie, A., Simpson, D.J., et al., 2017. Automated recording of home cage activity and temperature of individual rats housed in social groups: the Rodent Big Brother project. PLoS One 12 (9), e0181068.

Reijgwart, M.L., Schoemaker, N.J., Pascuzzo, R., Leach, M.C., Stodel, M., de Nies, L., Hendriksen, C.F., Van Der Meer, M., Vinke, C.M., van Zeeland, Y.R., 2017. The composition and initial evaluation of a grimace scale in ferrets after surgical implantation of a telemetry probe. PLoS One 12, e0187986.

Richardson, C.A., 2015. The power of automated behavioural homecage technologies in characterizing disease progression in laboratory mice: a review. Appl. Anim. Behav. Sci. 163, 19–27.

Robertson, I., Kent, J., Molony, V., 1994. Effect of different methods of castration on behaviour and plasma cortisol in calves of three ages. Res. Vet. Sci. 56, 8–17.

Roughan, J.V., Coulter, C.A., Flecknell, P.A., Thomas, H.D., Sufka, K.J., 2014. The conditioned place preference test for assessing welfare consequences and potential refinements in a mouse bladder cancer model. PLoS One 9 (8), e103362.

Roughan, J.V., Flecknell, P.A., 2001. Behavioural effects of laparotomy and analgesic effects of ketoprofen and carprofen in rats. Pain 90, 65–74.

Roughan, J.V., Flecknell, P.A., Davies, B.R., 2004. Behavioural assessment of the effects of tumour growth in rats and the influence of the analgesics carprofen and meloxicam. Lab. Anim. 38, 286–296.

Russell, W.M.S., 1959. In: Russell, W.M.S., Burch, R.L. (Eds.), The Principles of Humane Experimental Technique. Methuen, London.

Rutherford, K.M., 2002. Assessing pain in animals. Anim. Welf. 11, 31–53.

Schütz, T.C.B., Andersen, M.L., Tufik, S., 2003. Sleep alterations in an experimental orofacial pain model in rats. Brain Res. 993, 164–171.

Shi, R., Dou, J., Liu, J., Sammad, A., Luo, H., Wang, Y., Guo, G., Wang, Y., 2021. Genetic parameters of hair cortisol as an indicator of chronic stress under different environments in Holstein cows. J. Dairy Sci. 104, 6985–6999.

Silva, N.E., Trindade, P.H., Oliveira, A.R., Taffarel, M.O., Moreira, M.A., Denadai, R., Rocha, P.B., Luna, S.P., 2020. Validation of the Unesp-Botucatu composite scale to assess acute postoperative abdominal pain in sheep (USAPS). PLoS One 15 (10), e0239622.

Simola, N., Granon, S., 2019. Ultrasonic vocalizations as a tool in studying emotional states in rodent models of social behavior and brain disease. Neuropharmacology 159, 107420.

Smith, B.J., Bruner, K.E.P., Hess, A.M., Kendall, L.V., 2020. Female urine-induced ultrasonic vocalizations in male C57BL/6J mice as a proxy indicator for postoperative pain. JAALAS: J. Am. Assoc. Lab. Anim. Sci. 59 (2), 204–211.

Sotocinal, S.G., Sorge, R.E., Zaloum, A., Tuttle, A.H., Martin, L.J., Wieskopf, J.S., Mapplebeck, J.C., Wei, P., Zhan, S., Zhang, S., McDougall, J.J., King, O.D., Mogil, J.S., 2011. The Rat Grimace Scale: a partially automated method for quantifying pain in the laboratory rat via facial expressions. Mol. Pain 7, 55.

Stasiak, K.L., Maul, D., French, E., Hellyer, P.W., Vandewoude, S., 2003. Species-specific assessment of pain in laboratory animals. JAALAS: J. Am. Assoc. Lab. Anim. Sci. 42, 13–20.

Steagall, P.V., Bustamante, H., Johnson, C.B., Turner, P.V., 2021. Pain management in farm animals: focus on cattle, sheep and pigs. Animals 11 (6), 1483.

Stella, J.L., Lord, L.K., Buffington, C.T., 2011. Sickness behaviors in response to unusual external events in healthy cats and cats with feline interstitial cystitis. J. Am. Vet. Med. Assoc. 238, 67–73.

Stevenson, G.W., Mercer, H., Cormier, J., Dunbar, C., Benoit, L., Adams, C., Jezierski, J., Luginbuhl, A., Bilsky, E.J., 2011. Monosodium iodoacetate-induced osteoarthritis produces pain-depressed wheel running in rats: implications for preclinical behavioral assessment of chronic pain. Pharmacol. Biochem. Behav. 98, 35–42.

Stokes, E.L., Flecknell, P.A., Richardson, C.A., 2009. Reported analgesic and anaesthetic administration to rodents undergoing experimental surgical procedures. Lab. Anim 43, 149–154.

Streiner, D.L., Norman, G.R., Cairney, J., 2015. Health Measurement Scales: A Practical Guide to Their Development and Use. Oxford University Press, USA.

Sutherland, M.A., Davis, B.L., Brooks, T.A., Coetzee, J.F., 2012. The physiological and behavioral response of pigs castrated with and without anesthesia or analgesia. J. Anim. Sci. 90 (7), 2211–2221.

Taylor, A.A., Weary, D.M., Lessard, M., Braithwaite, L., 2001. Behavioural responses of piglets to castration: the effect of piglet age. Appl. Anim. Behav. Sci. 73 (1), 35–43.

Tizard, I., 2008. Sickness behavior, its mechanisms and significance. Anim. Health Res. Rev. 9, 87–99.

Tizard, I., 2009. Veterinary Immunology an Introduction. Saunders Elsevier, St. Louis.

Tracy, L.M., Ioannou, L., Baker, K.S., Gibson, S.J., Georgiou-Karistianis, N., Giummarra, M.J., 2016. Meta-analytic evidence for decreased heart rate variability in chronic pain implicating parasympathetic nervous system dysregulation. Pain 157, 7–29.

Tubbs, J.T., Kissling, G.E., Travlos, G.S., Goulding, D.R., Clark, J.A., King-Herbert, A.P., Blankenship-Paris, T.L., 2011. Effects of buprenorphine, meloxicam, and flunixin meglumine as postoperative analgesia in mice. JAALAS: J. Am. Assoc. Lab. Anim. Sci. 50, 185–191.

Turner, P.V., Pang, D.S., Lofgren, J.L., 2019. A review of pain assessment methods in laboratory rodents. Comp. Med. 69, 451–467.

Tuttle, A.H., Molinaro, M.J., Jethwa, J.F., Sotocinal, S.G., Prieto, J.C., Styner, M.A., Mogil, J.S., Zylka, M.J., 2018. A deep neural network to assess spontaneous pain from mouse facial expressions. Mol. Pain 14, 1744806918763658.

Urban, R., Scherrer, G., Goulding, E.H., Tecott, L.H., Basbaum, A.I., 2011. Behavioral indices of ongoing pain are largely unchanged in male mice with tissue or nerve injury-induced mechanical hypersensitivity. Pain 152, 990–1000.

Valverde, A., Gunkel, C.I., 2005. Pain management in horses and farm animals. J. Vet. Emerg. Crit. Care 15, 295–307.

Van Loo, P., Everse, L., Bernsen, M., Baumans, V., Hellebrekers, L., Kruitwagen, C., Den Otter, W., 1997. Analgesics in mice used in cancer research: reduction of discomfort? Lab. Anim. 31, 318–325.

Viscardi, A.V., Hunniford, M., Lawlis, P., Leach, M., Turner, P.V., 2017. Development of a piglet grimace scale to evaluate piglet pain using facial expressions following castration and tail docking: a pilot study. Front. Vet. Sci. 4.

Vollmer-Conna, U., 2001. Acute sickness behaviour: an immune system-to-brain communication? Psychol. Med. 31, 761–767.

Walker, S.M., Meredith-Middleton, J., Cooke-Yarborough, C., Fitzgerald, M., 2003. Neonatal inflammation and primary afferent terminal plasticity in the rat dorsal horn. Pain 105, 185–195.

Wallace, V., Norbury, T., Rice, A., 2005. Ultrasound vocalisation by rodents does not correlate with behavioural measures of persistent pain. Eur. J. Pain 9, 445–452.

Whittaker, A., Marsh, L., 2019. The role of behavioural assessment in determining "positive" affective states in animals. Cab Rev.: Perspect. Agric., Vet. Sci., Nutr. Nat. Resour. 14.

Whittaker, A.L., Barker, T.H., 2020. A consideration of the role of biology and test design as confounding factors in judgement bias tests. Appl. Anim. Behav. Sci. 20, 105126.

Whittaker, A.L., Howarth, G.S., 2014. Use of spontaneous behaviour measures to assess pain in laboratory rats and mice: how are we progressing? Appl. Anim. Behav. Sci. 151, 1–12.

Whittaker, A.L., Liu, Y., Barker, T.H., 2021. Methods used and application of the mouse grimace scale in biomedical research 10 years on: a scoping review. Animals 11.

Whittaker, A.L., Lymn, K.A., Wallace, G.L., Howarth, G.S., 2016. Differential effectiveness of clinically-relevant analgesics in a rat model of chemotherapy-induced mucositis. PLoS One 11, e0158851.

Wiechers, D.-H., Brunner, S., Herbrandt, S., Kemper, N., Fels, M., 2021. Analysis of hair cortisol as an indicator of chronic stress in pigs in two different farrowing systems. Front. Vet. Sci. 8.

Wöhr, M., Schwarting, R.K., 2013. Affective communication in rodents: ultrasonic vocalizations as a tool for research on emotion and motivation. Cell Tissue Res. 354, 81–97.

Wright-Williams, S.L., Courade, J.-P., Richardson, C.A., Roughan, J.V., Flecknell, P.A., 2007. Effects of vasectomy surgery and meloxicam treatment on faecal corticosterone levels and behaviour in two strains of laboratory mouse. Pain 130, 108–118.

Younger, J., McCue, R., Mackey, S., 2009. Pain outcomes: a brief review of instruments and techniques. Curr. Pain Headache Rep. 13, 39–43.

Chapter 13

Basic considerations for pain management in laboratory animals

James O. Marx[1] and Mark A. Suckow[2]

[1]*Department of Pathobiology, School of Veterinary Medicine, University of Pennsylvania, Philadelphia, PA, United States;* [2]*Department of Biomedical Engineering, University of Kentucky, Lexington, KY, United States*

Chapter outline

I. Rationale for pain mitigation

The relationship between humans and animals is influenced not only by individual experience and observation but also by the larger perspective of society. With respect to pain and pain relief in animals, ethical, scientific, and regulatory aspects are all important factors that guide approaches when working with animals in research. In many ways, regulatory and guidance documents reflect the prevailing societal perspective and provide a framework for oversight to ensure humane care and use. As societal attitudes change, so may regulatory expectations (Kirkwood and Hubrecht, 2001). Additional detail and perspective are offered elsewhere in this book (see Chapters 1, 2, and 3 for details).

The control of pain in laboratory animals is complicated by many factors, not the least of which is the difficulty in detection of pain in these animals, which is addressed in Chapter 12. The prescription of analgesia can be based on either (1) the prediction that an animal will experience pain after a procedure or (2) the identification of pain in the animal. After the identification of the need for analgesia, there are several things to consider before prescribing an analgesic protocol, including the type of pain, duration of pain, and species-specific responses to drugs and therapies.

II. Considerations for prescription of analgesia

There are many factors for scientists and clinicians to consider when addressing analgesia in laboratory animals. The potential sources of pain for laboratory animals vary

Anesthesia and Analgesia in Laboratory Animals. https://doi.org/10.1016/B978-0-12-822215-7.00027-5

and may limit the treatment options available to the animal for analgesia. Potential causes of pain include painful, protocol-related events (surgery or induced disease), spontaneous injury or disease not associated with an experimental procedure or animal models of pain. In studies specifically examining pain, and in some experimental protocols, the use of analgesia may be either completely eliminated or at least greatly limited with scientific justification. Approving the scientific justification to withhold analgesics is one of the most challenging animal welfare issues confronting Institutional Animal Care and Use Committee (IACUCs).

The treatment of pain depends upon the identification of both the type of pain and its duration. Treating all pain as acute, somatic pain responsive to nonsteroidal antiinflammatories or opiates will lead to treatment failures and result in a compromise in both the quality of the scientific results and the animal's welfare. Therefore, a basic understanding of the different types of pain and effective analgesic usage for that type of pain is critical for animal welfare.

A. Somatic pain

Somatic pain is the most common type of pain in laboratory animal medicine and is associated with the peripheral tissues of the body, skin, bone, muscle, etc., and tends to be focal, easily localized, sharp pain. It can be induced by a myriad of causes, including incision, crush, bone injury, ischemia, chemical, or thermal injury, and the severity of the pain can be augmented by inflammation associated with the injury. In fact, in some pain categorization systems, inflammatory pain is considered to be a separate category of pain. Most traumatic nonprotocol-related injuries will result in somatic pain, in addition to postoperative surgical pain. There are many animal models of somatic pain including, for example, the plantar incision model, or irritant-based injections, and much of our understanding of analgesia in animals comes from animal models and injuries resulting in somatic pain (Abboud et al., 2021). Since somatic pain is frequently easily localized and the pain pathways are well characterized, there are many treatment options for somatic pain, making multimodal analgesia a viable option. This frequently takes the form of local analgesics, nonsteroidal antiinflammatory drugs (NSAIDs), opiates, and nonpharmacological pain control (Foley et al., 2019).

B. Visceral pain

Visceral pain is associated with the organs in the thorax, abdomen, and pelvis. It differs from somatic pain in that it is characterized as a dull diffuse pain which can be difficult to localize, can radiate to other parts of the body, and result in mild to intense pain (Cervero and Laird, 1999). The pain may be accompanied by symptoms such as nausea, vomiting, changes in vital signs, and emotional manifestations. The afferent neurons sensing visceral pain differ from somatic afferent neurons in that they are most sensitive to factors such as stretch, ischemia, pH, bacterial products, and immune mediators (Grundy et al., 2019). The identification of the cause of spontaneous visceral pain can be more challenging than in somatic pain, and, as with all plans to address pain, is critical to effective analgesia. Animal models of visceral pain typically include the induction of inflammation and traction/distension models of abdominal organs (Hockley et al., 2018; Johnson et al., 2020). Inflammatory bowel disease is frequently used as a model of visceral pain. Opioids form the backbone of treatment of visceral pain, but they have questionable efficacy and side effects that can complicate the cause of visceral pain due to potential constipation, sedation, and GI irritation, making visceral pain a therapeutic challenge (Camilleri and Boeckxstaens, 2017; Johnson and Greenwood-Van Meerveld, 2016).

C. Neuropathic pain

Neuropathic pain results from injury or inflammation to the peripheral or central nervous system and is considered maladaptive, in that the pain is disproportional to the amount of tissue damage and can continue on beyond the point of tissue damage (Grubb, 2010; Kaliyaperumal et al., 2020). Humans describe this pain as shooting or burning and can be associated with allodynia and hyperalgesia. Injury to the nervous tissues means that neuropathic pain may be associated with other types of pain. Many studies have shown that the efficacy of NSAIDs and opiates in treating neuropathic pain is limited, meaning that the identification of the presence of neuropathic pain in our patients is critical to its effective treatment. Several studies have reported that calcium channel blockers gabapentin and pregabalin and sodium channel blocker lidocaine have been shown to be effective at relieving neuropathic pain by decreasing the release of neurotransmitter from the damaged neurons (Grubb, 2010; Wiffen et al., 2017). In humans, tricyclic antidepressants also have shown potential in the treatment of neuropathic pain. Environmental enrichment in mice and rats has also proven to be beneficial at altering neuropathic pain, a fact which is very relevant in animal models of neuropathic pain (Stagg et al., 2011; Tai et al., 2021; Vachon et al., 2013). There are many surgical models of neuropathic pain, including chronic constriction injury to the sciatic nerve, sciatic nerve ligation, spinal nerve ligation, spared nerve injury, brachial plexus avulsion, sciatic nerve transaction, and sciatic nerve trisection, as well as animal models of diabetic neuropathy (Gao and Zheng, 2014; Jaggi et al., 2011).

D. Cancer pain

Cancer pain is less commonly confronted in laboratory animal medicine than the other forms of pain, as many animals in biomedical research are euthanized if a spontaneous tumor develops. In humans, the most common locations of cancer pain are in the bones, with tumor invasion of nervous tissue or hollow viscid being the second and third most common locations of cancer pain (Foley, 1999). The most common cancer models utilize subcutaneous tumors in rodents, and many of these models do not appear to elicit pain in the animal. That said, this pain needs to be addressed when animals with cancer are maintained under an IACUC-approved protocol or used as animal models of cancer (Brabb et al., 2014; Carbone, 2011; Turner et al., 2019). The pain from cancer comes from the invasion of the tumor into tissues or due to damage to peripheral neural plexi, in which case neuropathic signs may predominate. In both human and veterinary medicine, there are many treatment options for increasing levels of cancer pain, including the use of nutraceuticals, physical therapy, progressing to both NSAID and opiate pharmacological control, and ultimately neuroablative surgery (Looney, 2010; Pacharinsak and Beitz, 2008).

E. Acute and chronic pain

Pain has evolved to inform the organism of actual or potential tissue damage. When the pain persists beyond the resolution of the injury and healing, or the injury fails to heal (i.e., arthritis), then the pain becomes maladaptive and is considered chronic, becoming the problem in and of itself. Acute pain can be treated with a myriad of drugs and therapies; however, the treatment of chronic pain can require long-term administration of drugs, increasing the risk of drug side effects. Further, it is possible to assume an animal with chronic pain is acting normally "for that animal" when its behavior and activity are being altered persistently by chronic pain. It is then important to appreciate the role which chronic pain can have on research results, affecting the animal's behavior, immune function, and endocrine systems. The study of chronic pain presents an important challenge for researchers, IACUCs, and institutions due to the welfare of animals being subjected to long-term pain with no or limited use of analgesia. In addition to the government regulatory requirements, the Animal Research Advisory Committee of the NIH has produced guidance for IACUCs in the study of pain in the guidelines for pain and distress in laboratory animals: responsibilities, recognition, and intervention. Chronic pain is discussed in greater detail in Chapter 27.

F. Effects of stress on pain perception

Both psychological and physiological stress has been shown to impact the perception of pain in both humans and animals (Council, 2009). Considering that the definition of pain includes an unpleasant emotional experience to a potentially noxious stimulus [(International Association for the Study of Pain [IASP] Task Force on Taxonomy, 1994), Merskey H., Bogduk N., Part III: Pain terms, a Current List with Definitions and Notes on Usage Classification of Chronic Pain. IASP Task Force on Taxonomy. Second edition. Seattle (WA): IASP Press, 1994. pp. 209–214.] it is not surprising that the psychological state of the animal plays an important role in its perception and response to pain. The nature of the psychological stress is critical to determining how this effect manifests itself. Fear has been shown to induce a "stress-induced analgesia", with animals showing a decrease in responsiveness to noxious stimuli (Turner et al., 2019; Ferdousi and Finn, 2018). On the other hand, anxiety and other psychological and physiological stressors have been shown to induce increased pain responses in animals, a "stress-induced hyperalgesia." There is a myriad of animal models of stress which have been shown to result in increased pain responsiveness, including restraint, sleep deprivation, cold exposure, noise stress, and social defeat; and as would be expected, procedures to decrease the stress in research animals, including the use of environmental enrichment, socialization, gentle handling techniques, and familiarization to experimental procedures, have been shown to decrease the response to pain in animal models (Council, 2009; Neely et al., 2018). Failing to control stressors in animals either experiencing painful procedures or experiencing pain from a nonprotocol related injury will unnecessarily increase the pain experienced by experimental animals. The impact of psychological and physiological stress on pain in research animals means that the use of environmental enrichment and control of other potential stressors needs to be carefully controlled, in any animal potentially experiencing pain, but particularly in animal models studying pain, as it can create an uncontrolled variable potentially affecting the reproducibility of the experimental results.

III. Nonpharmacological treatments for pain

There are many factors to consider when selecting an analgesia plan, either for an animal on an experimental protocol or following a painful injury or disease. Ideally, the protocol will completely control the pain so the animal does not experience any pain, will be similar to the analgesics used by humans with the disease being modeled or conditioned, and will have no impact on any dependent variables being studied. Obviously, these goals are almost impossible to ever completely achieve, meaning careful consideration of scientific goals and animal welfare are critical to addressing with each animal use protocol reviewed or animal being treated for nonprotocol-related pain. Further compounding the difficulties addressing the use of analgesics in laboratory animal medicine are the need to use analgesics acceptable to journal reviewers/editorial boards and the restrictions on the use and availability of opiates in animals due to the human opioid epidemic.

With the concerns of the ongoing opioid epidemic, nonpharmacologic control of pain is becoming increasingly important. As discussed above, the control of both psychological and physiological stress is critical in minimizing the pain perceived by the animals. Further, while some techniques used in human medicine are not a viable option in veterinary medicine (relaxation therapy, guided imagery, audio-visual distraction, hypnosis, mindful meditation, etc.), there are many analgesic techniques which are either well established or are being developed in veterinary medicine. Most of these techniques currently focus on companion animals or equine medicine; however, some have been tested in other laboratory species and likely could be applied to these species. This section will focus on the use of these techniques for pain control.

A. Acupuncture and electroacupuncture

Traditional Chinese Medicine describes diseases as disturbances of the flow of energy (Qi) in the body and uses the stimulation of acupuncture points to correct these disturbances, bringing the two types of energy, the Yin and Yang, into proper balance. Research has demonstrated several physiological mechanisms for the analgesic activity of acupuncture, including the release of endogenous opioids, serotonin and norepinephrine, diffuse noxious inhibitory controls, and stimulation of the autonomic nervous system (Kawakita and Okada, 2014; Zhang et al., 2014). There are extensive publications and textbooks describing the use of acupuncture in dogs, cats, and horses and many ways of stimulating the acupuncture points, including traditional needles, moxibustion, injection, and laser stimulation of points (Dewey and Xie, 2021; Fry et al., 2014; Xie and Preast, 2007). There are few published articles describing the use of acupuncture in the most commonly used species in biomedical research (Magden, 2017). There are two reports using acupuncture for osteoarthritis in NHP and one showing that acupuncture was able to help provide effective analgesia in rabbits following ovariohysterectomy (Magden et al., 2013; Parmen et al., 2015). One limitation of acupuncture for many of our species is that anesthesia is proposed to decrease the efficacy of acupuncture due to the decrease in neural activity during the procedure. While we are able to train many of our animals to self-present a limb for procedures, the use of acupuncture for spontaneous painful procedures may well be limited by this.

B. Physical therapy/exercise induced analgesia

As with acupuncture, physical therapy is gaining popularity as a pain control strategy for chronic pain in dogs, cats, and horses (Kaneps, 2016; Millis and Ciuperca, 2015). And, as with acupuncture, the mechanisms of this analgesia are only beginning to come to light and are the result of several physiologic responses. Again, evidence supports the roles of endogenous opioids, cannabinoids, activation of descending inhibitory pathways, secretion of serotonin, increases in antiinflammatory cytokines, and peripheral changes in neural activity in the beneficial effects of these therapies (Chimenti et al., 2018; Lesnak and Sluka, 2020). Physical therapy has been reported to be beneficial in osteoarthritis in rhesus macaques and for the general well-being of aged chimpanzees (Neal Webb et al., 2020). While there is little published data about the use of physical therapy in common laboratory animal species, many veterinarians and animal physical therapists are developing protocols for a broad array of species. While this therapy certainly has the potential to aid animals, care must be taken to prevent inducing further injury and actually increasing pain with a loss of function in animals. Further, without control animals to compare these results with, it is impossible to assess the beneficial, or harmful, effects of the therapy.

C. Cryotherapy

Cryotherapy is the localized cooling of a potentially painful part of the body. Ultimately, the cooling effect can extend 2–4 cm into the tissues, resulting in a decrease in nociceptive nerve fiber stimulation and conduction, a decrease in local blood flow resulting in a decrease in edema and localized inflammation, and a decrease in reflex muscle contraction (Wright et al., 2020). Cryotherapy has been successfully used in dogs following orthopedic surgery, providing benefit for the first 24 hours after surgery (Drygas et al., 2011) and is also been suggested for animals following soft tissue surgery (Corti, 2014). An additional benefit of this is that it is an easy and inexpensive treatment that could be applied to many animals early in the postoperative period. As with physical therapy, care must be taken to ensure that excessive cold is not applied to the treated area, inducing tissue damage.

D. Laser therapy (photobiomodulation)

The absorption of light causing changes in cellular activity and processes is well documented in science (see photosynthesis/vitamin D production). A wealth of research has gone into how the absorption of light by cytochrome C and its effects on the mitochondria results in pain relief, a reduction in inflammation, and increased healing (Pryor and Millis, 2015). The use of therapeutic lasers in small animal practice has rapidly grown, with as many as 20% of small animal clinics reporting they own a laser for localized therapy. Lasers have been shown to be beneficial in the pain relief of dogs following orthopedic surgery, but again, little work has been done in commonly used research species (Looney et al., 2018).

E. Pheromones

Canine and feline pheromones have been used in small animal clinics because of their effects on minimizing stress for hospitalized animals. There is some data supporting these effects, particularly in cats (Vitale, 2018). The pheromones react with receptors in the vomeronasal organ, which then connect with the limbic system in the brain, producing their calming effects. Any therapy which can reliably reduce stress in animals will likely benefit in pain control of our patients. Again, little work has been done testing these strategies in most research species.

F. Neonatal procedures

There are several nonpharmacological analgesic techniques which have been shown to be beneficial in the pain control of neonatal children which could be beneficial to neonatal and young animals as well. The administration of sucrose before a painful procedure combined with nonnutritive suckling or warming has been shown to ease the pain response in neonatal children (Blass and Watt, 1999; Gray et al., 2015). Additionally, swaddling and facilitated tucking has been shown to decrease the pain response in neonatal children (Shiff et al., 2021). While these techniques may be beneficial to neonatal animals, none have been shown to work adequately on their own as the sole form of analgesia in children, and pharmacological control of pain is strongly recommended unless not using them is scientifically justified.

IV. Operational aspects of pain management

An essential aspect of ensuring adequate pain management is implementing practices that enable an institutional culture that is favorable toward animal wellbeing, that is, a culture of care. Toward this end, the focus should be placed on individual abilities and attitudes, as well as a broader engagement of these principles at the institutional level.

A. Personnel

1. Training

All personnel directly involved with animal care and use, or its oversight, should have a high level of appreciation for the importance of practices that minimize pain and distress to the animals. While the specifics of such training logically vary with the specific roles of individuals, it should never be assumed that personnel will fully learn neither in a classroom setting nor on the job; that is, that relevant aspects of pain management will be learned and mastered during the course of normal professional activity. Certainly, some knowledge can be gained and refined through direct experience, and personnel may bring a strong knowledge base with them from previous training; however, training should be easily available and encouraged for all.

The precise content of training will, of course, depend on the species being used, the types of experimental procedures to be performed, and the role of the individual. For example, the Institutional Official and members of the IACUC or Animal Welfare Board should understand the ethical and regulatory expectations with respect to pain management, as well as the potential impact of pain and distress on experimental outcomes. This would include a general understanding of the importance to consider nonanimal or alternative approaches for work that involves the potential for pain or distress to animals.

For research staff (including principal investigators, students, and technicians), veterinarians, and animal care personnel, appropriate training might include background information similar to that for the IACUC/Animal Welfare Board, including information on methods to mitigate pain and distress, both pharmacological and nonpharmacological. An essential part of such training includes specific information on pain recognition. Since clinical evidence of pain can vary greatly between species, personnel should clearly understand how to evaluate if an animal is in pain and what actions are to be taken if an animal is found to be in pain. All personnel should understand that, unless required as part of the approved experimental design and justified with a scientific rationale, animals found to be in pain should receive interventions intended to abrogate the pain and distress. Establishing and assessing the proficiency of personnel with specific procedures or interventions to mitigate pain and distress can be helpful. As part of this process, personnel who are not directly charged with implementing such interventions should be instructed with respect to the recognition of pain in animals and the mechanisms for reporting affected animals to others, such as veterinary staff, who are qualified and authorized to invoke appropriate measures.

2. Performance expectations

To some great extent, the success of training can be measured by its outcomes in terms of compliance. With respect to animal pain and distress, a hoped-for outcome is that no incidents of unexpected, unaddressed pain and distress are observed or reported. With many invasive procedures, however, and because animals may respond differently to pain mitigation efforts, it is unlikely that all evidence of pain and distress will be uniformly absent. In such cases, the measure of success can be placed on consistent reporting to the veterinary staff for further evaluation and intervention and the ability of the veterinary staff to work with the researchers to effectively relieve the pain and distress without affecting the experimental goals of the project.

It is certainly possible that some personnel will engage in their work without sufficient training or acumen. Such instances often require remediation through additional training, and perhaps more robust supervision. In the rare circumstance where blatant disregard for animals is determined to have occurred and resulted in unnecessary pain or distress, more significant sanctions might be justified. In contrast, the human-animal bond can provide a foundation for compassion and diligence with respect to ensuring the humane care and use (Bayne, 2002; Greenhough and Roe, 2019). Indeed, compassion is a feature that should be encouraged, and attention should be given to avoiding compassion fatigue among personnel (Dowling, 2018; LaFollette et al., 2020; Pavan et al., 2020; Randall et al., 2021).

B. Creating an ecosystem for cooperation

Though skills and knowledge are critical components to the effective management of pain and distress, establishing a broad, supportive institutional culture of care and responsibility that centers around expectations for minimizing the pain of animals will facilitate the consistent application of basic principles (Klein and Bayne, 2007). Such practices operate most effectively when there is trust and cooperation among those having a role in ensuring the proper care and use of animals. In this way, then, institutions should work to establish an ecosystem that engenders support and synergy between individuals, units, and roles.

1. Institutional oversight

The tone for proper care and use of animals in research and teaching should be widely understood, and it is best set at the level of institutional animal care and use oversight. Institutional position statements or policies embraced by, and communicated from the upper administrative levels, such as the Institutional Official, should definitively state a commitment to, and expectation for, practices that will reduce pain and distress experienced by animals to that which is unavoidable. That commitment should be widely disseminated, evident, and understood by all those participating in the institutional animal research enterprise. Oversight committees, such as the IACUC, should not only define expectations for the minimization of pain and distress but also ensure that personnel are adequately qualified and that training is available when needed (Rush and Dyson, 2000). The IACUC/Animal Review Board should be easily consulted for information and to answer questions. This can be done electronically by telephone, email, or websites; during open office hours; and by direct interaction with research and animal care personnel through regular meetings, such as those organized for continuing education and post approval monitoring.

It is essential that institutional administration and oversight committees harmonize expectations and that the administration support, and provide the needed resources for the oversight committee in its efforts. Failure to demonstrate commitment to animal care and use through the allocation of institutional resources is likely to result in a minimal positive impact or may even negatively impact welfare. Institutional recognition through awards or other acknowledgments can also be an effective means to reinforce the importance of innovation and efforts to promote humane animal care and use.

2. Veterinary and animal care staff

Those who provide hands-on daily and veterinary care to animals are often adept at recognizing subtle changes in behavior and appearance that may signal pain or distress and are often looked to as sources of expertise with regard to matters of animal pain and distress. In this regard, such personnel should have adequate training with respect to both pain recognition and alleviation; and they should be educated with respect to institutional policies and expectations. Importantly, those providing direct animal care should be provided a clear sense of support by the institution for their role in ensuring animal welfare. Because communication is essential, the veterinary and animal care staff should be available and approachable by research personnel to address concerns or questions that might arise. Additionally, such individuals should ensure that investigators and research staff have the needed resources for the management of animal pain and distress. For example, opportunities should be created to train and educate research personnel on matters related to pain and distress. Further, the veterinary staff may consider developing or recommending a formulary to provide specific information for the pharmacologic management of pain and distress (Hawk et al., 2005). It is important for all personnel at the institution to manifest a collaborative demeanor, though they should also feel empowered to intervene when animal welfare is at risk beyond the defined experimental parameters.

3. Investigators and research staff

It is important that all research personnel handling animals clearly understand the procedures to be followed to mitigate pain and distress to animals, the potential impact of pain and distress on experimental results, as well as the expectation to closely follow defined protocols. As part of this, the principal investigator should ensure that all such personnel clearly understand not only institutional expectations but also that the investigator is clearly committed to animal welfare. Further, research personnel should recognize who to contact (e.g., veterinary and animal care staff), and how to do so, in the event that animals experience unexpected pain or distress, and they should readily engage in this interaction.

4. Productive outcomes

The primary goal is, of course, to promulgate sound animal care in support of scientific excellence, which are undeniably linked. Instances of failure to adequately control animal pain and distress are one metric that can be used to assess success (or failure); however, it is also useful to examine the overall tenor of cooperation between animal care and veterinary staff with the investigators with respect to reducing pain and distress in animals. For example, the ready willingness of personnel to ask questions, seek training and advice, and communicate problems can all be taken as evidence of an ecosystem that promotes efforts to mitigate pain and distress.

References

Abboud, C., Duveau, A., Bouali-Benazzouz, R., Masse, K., Mattar, J., Brochoire, L., Fossat, P., Boue-Grabot, E., Hleihel, W., Landry, M., 2021. Animal models of pain: diversity and benefits. J. Neurosci. Methods 348, 108997.

Bayne, K., 2002. Development of the human-research animal bond and its impact on animal well-being. ILAR J. 43, 4–9.

Blass, E.M., Watt, L.B., 1999. Suckling- and sucrose-induced analgesia in human newborns. Pain 83, 611–623.

Brabb, T., Carbone, L., Snyder, J., Phillips, N., 2014. Institutional animal care and use committee considerations for animal models of peripheral neuropathy. ILAR J. 54, 329–337.

Camilleri, M., Boeckxstaens, G., 2017. Dietary and pharmacological treatment of abdominal pain in IBS. Gut 66, 966–974.

Carbone, L., 2011. Pain in laboratory animals: the ethical and regulatory imperatives. PLoS One 6, e21578.

Cervero, F., Laird, J.M., 1999. Visceral pain. Lancet 353, 2145–2148.

Chimenti, R.L., Frey-Law, L.A., Sluka, K.A., 2018. A mechanism-based approach to physical therapist management of pain. Phys. Ther. 98, 302–314.

Corti, L., 2014. Nonpharmaceutical approaches to pain management. Top. Companion Anim. Med. 29, 24–28.

Council, N.R., 2009. Recognition and Alleviation of Pain in Laboratory Animals. National Academies Press, Washington, DC.

Dewey, C.W., Xie, H., 2021. The scientific basis of acupuncture for veterinary pain management: a review based on relevant literature from the last two decades. Open Vet. J. 11, 203–209.

Dowling, T., 2018. Compassion does not fatigue! Can. Vet. J. = La revue veterinaire canadienne 59, 749–750.

Drygas, K.A., McClure, S.R., Goring, R.L., Pozzi, A., Robertson, S.A., Wang, C., 2011. Effect of cold compression therapy on postoperative pain, swelling, range of motion, and lameness after tibial plateau leveling osteotomy in dogs. J. Am. Vet. Med. Assoc. 238, 1284–1291.

Ferdousi, M., Finn, D.P., 2018. Stress-induced modulation of pain: role of the endogenous opioid system. Prog. Brain Res. 239, 121–177.

Foley, K.M., 1999. Advances in cancer pain. Arch. Neurol. 56, 413–417.

Foley, P.L., Kendall, L.V., Turner, P.V., 2019. Clinical management of pain in rodents. Comp. Med. 69, 468–489.

Fry, L.M., Neary, S.M., Sharrock, J., Rychel, J.K., 2014. Acupuncture for analgesia in veterinary medicine. Top. Companion Anim. Med. 29, 35–42.

Gao, F., Zheng, Z.M., 2014. Animal models of diabetic neuropathic pain. Exp. Clin. Endocrinol. Diabetes: Off. J. German Soc. Endocrinol. [and] German Diabetes Assoc. 122, 100–106.

Gray, L., Garza, E., Zageris, D., Heilman, K.J., Porges, S.W., 2015. Sucrose and warmth for analgesia in healthy newborns: an RCT. Pediatrics 135, e607–e614.

Greenhough, B., Roe, E., 2019. Attuning to laboratory animals and telling stories: learning animal geography research skills from animal technologists. Environ. Plann. Soc. Space 37, 367–384.

Grubb, T., 2010. Chronic neuropathic pain in veterinary patients. Top. Companion Anim. Med. 25, 45–52.

Grundy, L., Erickson, A., Brierley, S.M., 2019. Visceral pain. Annu. Rev. Physiol. 81, 261–284.

Hawk, C.T., Leary, S.L., Morris, T.H., 2005. Formulary for Laboratory Animals, third ed. ed. Wiley-Blackwell, Ames, IA.

Hockley, J.R.F., Smith, E.S.J., Bulmer, D.C., 2018. Human visceral nociception: findings from translational studies in human tissue. Am. J. Physiol. Gastrointest. Liver Physiol. 315, G464–G472.

Jaggi, A.S., Jain, V., Singh, N., 2011. Animal models of neuropathic pain. Fund. Clin. Pharmacol. 25, 1–28.

Johnson, A.C., Greenwood-Van Meerveld, B., 2016. The pharmacology of visceral pain. Adv. Pharmacol. 75, 273–301.

Johnson, A.C., Farmer, A.D., Ness, T.J., Greenwood-Van Meerveld, B., 2020. Critical evaluation of animal models of visceral pain for therapeutics development: a focus on irritable bowel syndrome. Neuro Gastroenterol. Motil.: Off. J. Eur. Gastrointest. Motil. Soc. 32, e13776.

Kaliyaperumal, S., Wilson, K., Aeffner, F., Dean Jr., C., 2020. Animal models of peripheral pain: biology review and application for drug discovery. Toxicol. Pathol. 48, 202–219.

Kaneps, A.J., 2016. Practical rehabilitation and physical therapy for the general equine practitioner. Vet. Clin. N. Am. Equine Pract. 32, 167–180.

Kawakita, K., Okada, K., 2014. Acupuncture therapy: mechanism of action, efficacy, and safety: a potential intervention for psychogenic disorders? Biopsychosoc. Med. 8, 4.

Kirkwood, J.K., Hubrecht, R., 2001. Animal consciousness, cognition and welfare. Anim. Welf. 10, S5–S17.

Klein, H.J., Bayne, K.A., 2007. Establishing a culture of care, conscience, and responsibility: addressing the improvement of scientific discovery and animal welfare through science-based performance standards. ILAR J. 48, 3–11.

LaFollette, M.R., Riley, M.C., Cloutier, S., Brady, C.M., O'Haire, M.E., Gaskill, B.N., 2020. Laboratory animal welfare meets human welfare: a cross-sectional study of professional quality of life, including compassion fatigue in laboratory animal personnel. Front. Vet. Sci. 7, 114.

Lesnak, J.B., Sluka, K.A., 2020. Mechanism of exercise-induced analgesia: what we can learn from physically active animals. Pain reports 5, e850.

Looney, A., 2010. Oncology pain in veterinary patients. Top. Companion Anim. Med. 25, 32–44.

Looney, A.L., Huntingford, J.L., Blaeser, L.L., Mann, S., 2018. A randomized blind placebo-controlled trial investigating the effects of photobiomodulation therapy (PBMT) on canine elbow osteoarthritis. Can. Vet. J. = La revue veterinaire canadienne 59, 959–966.

Magden, E.R., 2017. Spotlight on acupuncture in laboratory animal medicine. Vet. Med. 8, 53–58.

Magden, E.R., Haller, R.L., Thiele, E.J., Buchl, S.J., Lambeth, S.P., Schapiro, S.J., 2013. Acupuncture as an adjunct therapy for osteoarthritis in chimpanzees (*Pan troglodytes*). J. Am. Assoc. Lab. Anim. Sci.: JAALAS 52, 475–480.

Millis, D.L., Ciuperca, I.A., 2015. Evidence for canine rehabilitation and physical therapy. Vet. Clin. N. Am. Small Anim. Pract. 45, 1–27.

Neal Webb, S.J., Bridges, J.P., Thiele, E., Lambeth, S.P., Schapiro, S.J., 2020. The implementation and initial evaluation of a physical therapy program for captive chimpanzees (*Pan troglodytes*). Am. J. Primatol. 82, e23109.

Neely, C., Lane, C., Torres, J., Flinn, J., 2018. The effect of gentle handling on depressive-like behavior in adult male mice: considerations for human and rodent interactions in the laboratory. Behav. Neurol. 2018, 2976014.

Pacharinsak, C., Beitz, A., 2008. Animal models of cancer pain. Comp. Med. 58, 220–233.

Parmen, V., Pestean, C., Ober, C., Mircean, M., Oana, L., 2015. Paraclinical investigations of electroacupuncture analgesia in a rabbit ovariohysterectomy. J. Acupunct. Merid. Stud. 8, 44–47.

Pavan, A.D., O'Quin, J., Roberts, M.E., Freed, C.L., 2020. Using a staff survey to customize burnout and compassion fatigue mitigation recommendations in a lab animal facility. J. Am. Assoc. Lab. Anim. Sci.: JAALAS 59, 139–147.

Pryor, B., Millis, D.L., 2015. Therapeutic laser in veterinary medicine. Vet. Clin. N. Am. Small Anim. Pract. 45, 45–56.

Randall, M.S., Moody, C.M., Turner, P.V., 2021. Mental wellbeing in laboratory animal professionals: a cross-sectional study of compassion fatigue, contributing factors, and coping mechanisms. J. Am. Assoc. Lab. Anim. Sci.: JAALAS 60, 54–63.

Rush, H.G., Dyson, M., 2000. Personnel training. In: Silverman, J., Suckow, M.A., Murthy, S. (Eds.), The IACUC Handbook. CRC Press, Boca Raton.

Shiff, I., Bucsea, O., Pillai Riddell, R., 2021. Psychosocial and neurobiological vulnerabilities of the hospitalized preterm infant and relevant non-pharmacological pain mitigation strategies. Front. Pediatr. 9, 568755.

Stagg, N.J., Mata, H.P., Ibrahim, M.M., Henriksen, E.J., Porreca, F., Vanderah, T.W., Philip Malan Jr., T., 2011. Regular exercise reverses sensory hypersensitivity in a rat neuropathic pain model: role of endogenous opioids. Anesthesiology 114, 940–948.

Tai, W.L., Sun, L., Li, H., Gu, P., Joosten, E.A., Cheung, C.W., 2021. Additive effects of environmental enrichment and ketamine on neuropathic pain relief by reducing glutamatergic activation in spinal cord injury in rats. Front. Neurosci. 15, 635187.

Turner, P.V., Pang, D.S., Lofgren, J.L., 2019. A review of pain assessment methods in laboratory rodents. Comp. Med. 69, 451–467.

Vachon, P., Millecamps, M., Low, L., Thompsosn, S.J., Pailleux, F., Beaudry, F., Bushnell, C.M., Stone, L.S., 2013. Alleviation of chronic neuropathic pain by environmental enrichment in mice well after the establishment of chronic pain. Behav. Brain Funct. : BBF 9, 22.

Vitale, K.R., 2018. Tools for managing feline problem behaviors: pheromone therapy. J. Feline Med. Surg. 20, 1024–1032.

Wiffen, P.J., Derry, S., Bell, R.F., Rice, A.S., Tolle, T.R., Phillips, T., Moore, R.A., 2017. Gabapentin for chronic neuropathic pain in adults. Cochrane Database Syst. Rev. 6, CD007938.

Wright, B., Kronen, P.W., Lascelles, D., Monteiro, B., Murrell, J.C., Robertson, S., Steagall, P.V.M., Yamashita, K., 2020. Ice therapy: cool, current and complicated. J. Small Anim. Pract. 61, 267–271.

Xie, H., Preast, V., 2007. Xie's Veterinary Acupuncture. Blackwell Publishing, Ames, IA.

Zhang, R., Lao, L., Ren, K., Berman, B.M., 2014. Mechanisms of acupuncture-electroacupuncture on persistent pain. Anesthesiology 120, 482–503.

Section V

Practical considerations by species

Chapter 14

Anesthesia and analgesia in laboratory rodents

Paulin Jirkof[1] and Jennie Lofgren[2]
[1]*Office for Animal Welfare and 3Rs, University of Zurich, Zurich, Switzerland;* [2]*Animal Welfare Compliance, Novartis Institutes for Biomedical Research, Cambridge, MA, United States*

Chapter outline

Anesthesia and Analgesia in Laboratory Animals. https://doi.org/10.1016/B978-0-12-822215-7.00007-X

I. Introduction

Rodents, especially mice and rats, are by far the most common laboratory animal species and needed by virtually all fields of biomedical research. In the biomedical research environment, the administration of anesthesia and analgesia of rodents is routinely performed by scientists and members of the scientific team without the direct supervision of a veterinarian. Institutions provide advice and training to these scientists through their veterinary and training staff. For rodents, many national regulations allow anesthesia in locations remote from the central vivarium, such as the laboratory, where direct observation of the efficacy of anesthesia by laboratory animal veterinarians is not routine. Because of the indirect role of the veterinarian in anesthesia and the frequently remote location of rodent anesthesia, we have selected the most reliable, safest, and simplest methods of anesthesia and analgesia in this chapter. Other, seldom-used methods have been de-emphasized to focus the reader's attention on current best practice methods of laboratory animal anesthesia and analgesia. We have supplemented this selection with information about those additional anesthetics and analgesics that are used due to their special characteristics, such as minimal cardiovascular depression. Tables 14.3, 14.5, and 14.6 list the commonly used anesthetics, analgesics, and reversal agents, with their trade names and recommended dose ranges by species.

Assessment of discomfort and distress in animals can be difficult, particularly in prey species like rodents that tend naturally to hide overt signs of pain that could impact their vulnerability to predation and therefore their survival (Miller and Leach (2015a); Oliver et al., 2017; Pinho et al., 2020). Personnel may neglect to provide appropriate anesthesia or analgesia to rodents due to their inability to assess and recognize pain in animals, lack of knowledge about appropriate medications, and fear of untoward side effects (Peterson et al., 2017; Jirkof, 2017). Please, see Chapter 12 for an introduction to pain assessment in laboratory animals. See also Turner et al. for a review on rodent-specific pain signs (Turner et al., 2019).

Laboratory animal professionals are mandated by several national regulations (see Chapter 2) to select appropriate agents for use in various animal species that are compatible with sound scientific methods. More specifically, one must administer appropriate sedation, analgesia, or anesthesia to animals undergoing procedures that cause more than momentary or slight pain or distress. Sedative drugs induce a relaxed state, analgesics reduce or relieve pain without loss of consciousness, and anesthetics render the animal unconscious without loss of vital functions. The avoidance or minimization of discomfort, distress, and pain in laboratory animals is an ethical imperative for all individuals who work with these species in biomedical research. See Chapter 1 for a more in-depth discussion.

No matter which type of anesthetic is selected, it is important to provide appropriate and gentle restraint before and after the administration of anesthetics, sufficient analgesia during and after the procedure, and relaxation of muscle tone to the degree that procedures can be performed quickly and efficiently. Strain differences in rodents must be considered, and pilot studies should be undertaken when changing to a new anesthetic or analgesic regimen in research models (Flecknell, 1993a; Flecknell, 2015; Hurley and Adams (2008)).

Materials in this chapter have been derived in part from the chapter, "Anesthesia and Analgesia in Rodents" in the first and second editions of *Anesthesia and Analgesia in Laboratory Animals* (Wixson and Smiler, 1997; Gaertner et al., (2008)). Descriptions of historic anesthetics more commonly utilized in the past for specific research needs have been limited in this edition, and an increased emphasis has been placed on current state recommendations. For more information about these historic anesthetics, please refer to previous versions of this text/chapter.

II. Pre-procedural considerations

A. Planning

Every anesthetic affects an animal's physiology as well as its pain perception; therefore in some cases avoidance of anesthesia while maintaining high standards of animal welfare, such as through habituation and positive reinforcement, is preferable. When anesthetics must be used, the selection of an appropriate anesthetic regimen requires careful consideration of multiple factors to maximize effectiveness and minimize risks. Considerations of the animal's own characteristics, the intended procedure, research aims, and the practicality of available agents all contribute to the choice of analgesics and anesthetics utilized in each unique situation.

1. Health and safety

Any anesthetic choice involves consideration of the animal's needs, the agent's availability, the equipment required, and the impact on experimental aims and training. Inhalant anesthetics require the use of calibrated vaporizers and gas scavenging systems and appropriate training and monitoring to ensure staff safety. See Chapter 6 for more details on the safe and effective management of waste gases. Infusion methods may require an infusion pump for precise control. Recovery support may include a need for heated cages or chambers and supplemental oxygen. Personnel must be trained in procedures, such as injection techniques, must be familiar with the use of any equipment required for administration and monitoring, and should also be knowledgeable regarding potential adverse anesthetic effects and appropriate responses.

The number of animals to undergo a procedure on the same day may influence the choice of anesthetics, since rodent anesthesia for groups of rodents is often done in an assembly line fashion with individual animals proceeding sequentially through induction, surgery, and supervised recovery phases. The availability of resources such as a centralized surgery facility and staff with experience in rodent anesthesia may increase the options available for scientists by providing access to drugs, equipment, and personnel who can provide experienced, specialized support, and training opportunities. The expense of agents or equipment, technical challenges, and safety considerations may all affect whether a specific agent may be suitable in a given situation.

It is common for surgery to be performed on a number of rodents in the same session, but this practice requires some special considerations. There should be enough staff participating in the session to ensure that each animal is adequately observed and treated during induction and anesthesia, until full recovery from anesthesia. Regardless of the number of animals operated upon in a single session, it is important to provide individualized care to each one. Injectable anesthetics may be preferred since it is generally not necessary to adjust the dose once given, but this does not preclude the need to monitor the depth of anesthesia closely. Education of personnel and proper aseptic techniques are essential to avoid compromise of animal welfare.

The animal may need to be transported while under anesthesia or may be undergoing a procedure in a location that sets limitations on access and anesthetic equipment, such as magnetic resonance or other imaging studies, which are addressed elsewhere in this text (Chapter 29). Consideration for maintaining animal security, ability to monitor anesthesia and respond to changes in anesthetic depth (if under anesthesia during transport), and animal emergencies while en route, risk of allergen or biohazard exposure to personnel and passerby, and temperature control for the animals must be made to ensure animal and personnel safety during transport.

2. History and records

The anesthetic regimen must be compatible with the needs and restrictions of the procedure to be performed. Different agents have different durations of effect, so the anticipated length of the procedure must be a primary consideration. It is also essential that contingency plans be in place to ensure continued depth of anesthesia should the procedure last longer than expected. The choice of anesthetics may depend on whether or not the animal is intended to survive the procedure, and the degree of invasiveness of the proposed procedure needs to be anticipated. Scientific goals may require specific physiologic effects such as muscle relaxation or avoidance of cardiac or respiratory disturbances, and the anesthetic regimen must be adjusted to provide or avoid these effects (see also Chapter 3). The use of stereotaxic surgery or procedures on the eyes, nasal, or oral cavities may limit the anesthetic options.

Understanding the background health status of the rodents can be helpful for anticipating potential anesthetic complications, such as those induced by respiratory pathogens. Additionally, if anesthesia has been performed in the same model before carrying forward any lessons learned can be valuable.

Records of the date, time of induction, name of surgeon/anesthetist and their contact information, protocol number, procedure a performed, animal's identification, body weight, health status, name, dose, and route of anesthetics, analgesics, and any adjunct therapies administered should be created for each procedure (Lofgren et al., 2020). Additionally, recording of monitored physiologic variables, even if intermittent, as well as any notes regarding an individual animal's adverse events during the procedure or anesthesia, such as excessive blood loss, animals requiring additional anesthetics, fluids, or other interventions taken as a result, should be included. The time of recovery from anesthesia and any notes regarding any complications or difficulty experienced during this time is helpful to inform post-procedural monitoring and care. Postprocedural monitoring records should be tailored to the procedure performed and anticipated risks to the patient. Records should capture monitoring progress for each animal, with documented health and pain status and provision of analgesia and supportive care noted more intensively in the first 72 h after a procedure and then at least daily until animals are fully recovered, pain-free, and sutures or staples (where applicable) are removed. While legal requirements for maintaining rodent anesthesia or surgery records vary, it can be useful to maintain these records for a year to allow veterinary and IACUC staff the opportunity to assure compliance with approved protocols and practices, troubleshoot any future animal health or welfare issues and maintain an institutional "memory" for how well or poorly a given procedure and associated anesthetics and analgesics worked for various strains, sexes, or other specific conditions.

3. Patient evaluation

Many animal species' characteristics may influence the choice or route of administration of anesthetic agents. The small size of rodents imposes limitations on the volume of an agent that can be administered by a particular route. Table 14.1 lists the amounts of drugs that can be given by various routes in rodent species. Within a species, strain, sex, genotype, age, and other external factors can affect response to anesthetic or analgesic agents (e.g., Fagioli et al., 1990; Hurley and Adams, 2008; Jauchem and Frei, 1991; Mecklenburg et al., 2017; Pick et al., 1991; Sonner et al., 2000; see also Chapter 30). Genetically modified rodents may have unexpected variability in their response to anesthetics compared with background strains. Drug pharmacokinetics and pharmacodynamics may differ in obese or lean animals. Pregnant animals require special consideration depending on the stage of pregnancy, whether the agent under consideration crosses the placenta, and whether potential effects on the fetus will alter experimental data. While a primary consideration is that animals are anesthetized gently with as little physiological disturbance as possible, a second important consideration is that the anesthetic to be used should minimally affect research data. The health status of an individual animal also requires consideration. While it may be impractical to perform a complete physical exam on every rodent, a useful assessment can be made quite quickly and score sheets should be implemented whenever possible. Detection of any potential health issues should initiate a closer examination of the individual animal and reassessment of the anesthetic protocol, associated risks, the planned anesthetic dose, and whether this animal is a suitable subject for the proposed research.

a. Physical exam

Animals that have been recently shipped should be allowed several days to recover from the stress of transport. A minimum of 72 h acclimation is recommended for general studies, but for some types of research, such as evaluations of microbiota, 5 days are necessary to stabilize changes, with behavioral or physiology research 1–3 weeks may be necessary, and for breeding performance up to a month (Obernier and Baldwin, 2006; Hoorn et al., 2011; Arts et al., 2014; Montonye et al., 2018). During this time, they are acclimating to changes in their surroundings, which may include the cage environment, feed and water, light cycle, cage mates, noise levels, and handlers. Gentle handling with the provision of positive reinforcement in the form of a small, preferred treat for all rodents and, for rats "tickling" can also reduce stress before and during the study (Fridgeirsdottir et al., 2014; Cloutier et al., 2018; Leidinger et al., 2017).

As close as possible to the time of anesthesia, animals should receive at least a brief health assessment including elements that reflect cardiac and respiratory function, such as general level of activity and response to stimuli such as handling, mucous membrane color, and characterization of respiratory effort (Lofgren et al., 2020). For injectable anesthetics, it is highly desirable to measure the actual body weight of each animal rather than using a single dose for all

TABLE 14.1 Volumes and routes of administration by species and anatomical site.

Species	Oral (mL/kg)	Subcutaneous (mL/kg)[a]	Intraperitoneal (mL/kg)	Intramuscular (mL per injection site)	Intravenous (bolus, mL/kg)	(Infusion, mL/kg)[b]
Mouse	10 (total max 1 mL)	Scruff 10 (25 G)	10 (25–27 G)	Quadriceps or caudal thigh 0.05 (27 G) (IM not recommended)	Lateral tail vein 5 (26–28 G)	Max. 25
Rat	10 (total max 5 mL)	Scruff or back 10 (25 G)	10 (23–25 G)	Quadriceps or caudal thigh 0.1 (23–25 G)	Lateral tail vein 5 (25–27 G)	Max. 20
Gerbil	10 (total max 1 mL)	Scruff 5 (23 G)	10 (25 G)	Quadriceps or caudal thigh 0.1 (24 G)	Lateral tail vein 5 (25 G)	Max. 25
Hamster	10 (total max 1 mL)	Scruff 5 (23 –25 G)	10 (23–25 G)	Quadriceps or caudal thigh 0.1 (25 G)	Femoral or jugular vein 5 (25–27 G)	Max. 25
Guinea pig	10 (gavage not recommended)	Scruff or back 5 (23–25 G)	10 (23–25 G)	Quadriceps or caudal thigh 0.1 (25)	Ear vein or saphenous vein 5 (25–27 G)	Max. 20

G = gauge of needle to be used.
[a]*The injection volume depends on skin mobility and may have to be distributed over several injection sites.*
[b]*With infusions over 2 h, the maximum volume should be <10% of blood volume.*
Based on GV-SOLAS, Committee for Animal Welfare Officers, and TVT, Administration of substances to laboratory animals, March 2017.

animals in a group. Because of their small body size and the small volumes used for injection, it is relatively easy to inadvertently overdose or underdose an individual rodent. This is particularly important in cohorts of older animals, which may have more variation in weight than those at a younger age.

b. Labs

Preanesthetic blood work is not frequently required or performed prior to anesthesia in rodents, as most will be healthy. However, for animals that may be compromised due to their phenotype or induced model, such as diabetic, aged, etc., appropriate clinical labs may inform anesthetic and monitoring choices.

4. Fasting

Rodents do not require fasting or withholding of water prior to anesthesia. Rodents cannot vomit, therefore the risk of aspiration during induction or recovery is significantly reduced. Additionally, they have a high metabolic rate and can more easily become hypoglycemic and experience other metabolic or physiologic changes when fasting (Jensen et al., 2019). In some rodents, like guinea pigs and hamsters, cheek or pharyngeal pouches are used to store food, etc., and may need to be cleaned of debris after induction. Three hours of preanesthetic fasting has been shown to have no significant impact on induction time, total sleep time, or loss of toe pinch response in rats undergoing ketamine/xylazine anesthesia (Struck et al., 2011). If gastric emptying is required for the procedure for which anesthesia is being performed, 4–6 h results in the same gastric emptying as fasting rodents for 12–18 h, therefore the shorter time period should suffice without adding extra stress to the animals (Jensen et al., 2013). As rodents are nocturnal and consume as much as two-thirds of their food overnight, if fasting must occur, a fasting period of 5–6 h during the day is more comparable to humans and recommended as an alternative to overnight fasting (Jensen et al., 2013).

B. Chemical restraint versus anesthesia

The choice of anesthetic is largely informed by the goal of the anesthesia—to reduce movement and facilitate reducing stress and increasing compliance for a nonpainful procedure like imaging, dosing, or sample collection, or for an otherwise painful procedure such as surgery—and with due consideration to experimental aims. Some agents (e.g., ketamine, diazepam, acepromazine, or an α-2 agonist) can provide sedation suitable for nonpainful procedures when given at an appropriate dose and time. Deeper levels of sedation, and general anesthesia, require drug combinations to meet the goals of achieving loss of consciousness, immobility, and analgesia.

The objectives of chemical restraint are to inhibit purposeful movements by the animal that could cause injury or escape of the animal, as well as reduce the distress associated with restraint or minor procedures. As with anesthesia, efforts should be made to ensure the animal does not become hypothermic or suffer other untoward effects like driedout corneas. In laboratory rodents, brief inhalant anesthesia or ketamine/xylazine, alone or in combination are often used. For many, mainly larger species and for minor procedures heavy sedation alone may be sufficient. Some agents inappropriate for a surgical plane of anesthesia, such as alfaxalone or acepromazine and butorphanol, may work well for chemical restraint for non or minimally invasive procedures. Frequently, an opioid agonist is used in combination with another sedative drug from a different class. The degree and frequency of monitoring for animals under chemical restraint or sedation is less than for animals maintained under general anesthesia, but still requires consistent attention to provide needed corrections to maintain normal physiology and respond to emergencies. Where appropriate for the agent used, chemical restraint should be reversed once the restraint is no longer needed.

In some instances, additional drugs given before or during anesthesia may improve the quality of the anesthesia and/or recovery. The most commonly used premedications are sedatives and analgesics. Sedatives calm the animal, smooth anesthetic induction and recovery, and reduce the dose of anesthetic agent needed, but are seldom used prior to rodent anesthesia due to the additional stress of administering a second injection (and associated restraint). Systemic and/or local analgesics can profoundly reduce anesthetic requirements, thus minimizing the adverse effects of general anesthetics (e.g., isoflurane) by reducing the dose required, and contributing to preemptive and preventive analgesia, which persists into the recovery period (Karas, 2002; Penderis and Franklin, 2005). Other agents that may be used prior to or during anesthesia are anticholinergics, antibiotics, parenteral fluids, supplemental oxygen, and paralytic agents. These are discussed in greater detail in other sections of this chapter and in Chapter 5.

C. Need for analgesia

One of the great challenges of caring for rodents is their ability to hide evidence of pain in the presence of an observer (i.e., real-time, cage side), sometimes resulting in an assumption that they are not experiencing pain (Sorge et al., 2014; Miller and Leach, 2015a; Oliver et al., 2017; Whittaker et al., 2021; Chartier et al., 2020; Mogil et al., 2020). Additionally, if a model has been traditionally performed without analgesia, there is a concern that addition of analgesia will invalidate the model and historic data collected with it. However, growing bodies of literature are providing evidence that rodents do experience significant pain after procedures that are expected to cause pain in humans or other vertebrates and if unmitigated, pain can have significant impacts on not just animal welfare but research results as well. Models that do not incorporate analgesia when they should are likely to produce poor-quality data, negatively impacting their translatability and reproducibility. Therefore, for reasons of ethics, meeting regulatory requirements which dictate that which is expected to cause pain in humans should be assumed to also cause pain in laboratory animals, and for the scientific validity of the data being generated, analgesia must be provided unless strong veterinary or scientific justification can be made and is accepted and approved by the relevant authorities or ethical review bodies. For more information about the assessment of pain in rodents, please see Chapter 12 and Section 6.c below, as well as Chapter 3 about the relative impact of pain and analgesia on a variety of research models.

D. Balanced anesthesia

The concept of combining different anesthetic drugs is often referred to as balanced anesthesia. By combining an inhalant with another anesthetic, analgesic, or sedative, the overall safety and efficacy of the anesthetic protocol can be improved. For example, the dose-dependent cardiovascular and respiratory depressant effects of volatile agents can be reduced by the addition of sedatives or analgesics with fewer cardiorespiratory depressant effects (e.g., benzodiazepines and opioids). Their addition allows a lower dose of volatile agent to be given while achieving the same depth of anesthesia. Inhalant anesthesia can be supplemented with the administration of parenteral drugs (e.g., fentanyl-midazolam followed by sevoflurane) (Lipiski et al., 2017). Care must be taken during the selection of drug combinations, and doses should be reduced in order to minimize adverse effects. For instance, sevoflurane and isoflurane potentiate seizure and arrhythmia activity in rats given concurrent high doses of intravenous bupivacaine (Dwyer et al., 1994).

III. Anesthesia

A. Premedication

In some instances, additional drugs given before or during anesthesia may improve the quality of the anesthesia and/or recovery. The most commonly used premedications are sedatives and analgesics. Sedatives calm the animal, smooth anesthetic induction and recovery, and reduce the dose of anesthetic agent needed, for example, an injectable sedative followed by a transition to an inhalant anesthetic. Systemic and/or local analgesics may also reduce the anesthetic requirements and have a preemptive/preventative effect on pain perception, which persists into the recovery period (Karas, 2002; Penderis and Franklin, 2005). Other agents that may be used prior to or during anesthesia are anticholinergics, antibiotics, parenteral fluids, supplemental oxygen, and paralytic agents. These are discussed in greater detail in other sections of this Chapter 11 and in Chapter 5.

B. Induction

Table 14.2 displays some examples of induction agents and their common concentrations for rats and mice.

TABLE 14.2 Induction agents (examples).

Drug	Use	Dose mg/kg unless otherwise specified	Route	References
Rat				
Isoflurane (Forane)	I	5%	Inhaled	Smith et al. (2004) Vaillancourt et al. (1999), Wood et al. (2001), Flecknell (2015)
Propofol (Rapinovet)	I	10	IV, IP	Cantwell (2001), Flecknell (2015)
Sevoflurane	I	Up to 5%	Inhaled	
Mouse				
Isoflurane (Forane)	I Neonatal mice I	0.04 2%–4%	Inhaled	Szczensy et al. (2004) Drobac et al. (2004), Gotoh et al. (2004)
Propofol (Rapinovet)	I	26	IV, IP	Cantwell (2001), Flecknell (2015)
Sevoflurane	I	Up to 5%	Inhaled	

C. Pharmacological options

1. Inhalation anesthetics

Inhalant anesthetics provide a safe, reliable, reversible, and reproducible means of rendering rodents unconscious to perform surgeries and other intricate or potentially painful procedures. This section will provide a review of the use of inhalant anesthetics in mice and rats. For more information regarding the pharmacokinetics of anesthetic agents, please refer to Chapter 6.

a. Delivery systems

Inhalation anesthesia involves the delivery of a volatile compound or a high concentration of a gas to the rodent via the respiratory tract. An "anesthesia box," usually made of Plexiglas and attached to an inhalant agent vaporizer or gas line, and a scavenging system is commonly used for induction. Inhalant anesthesia of small rodents is generally maintained utilizing face masks or nose cones, applied either to a single animal or to a group of animals by use of a manifold connected to a vaporizer.

With improved training programs and equipment (Jou et al., 2000; Ordodi et al., 2005), endotracheal intubation has become a more common practice in mice and rats. Because anesthetic-induced respiratory depression is not uncommon, the anesthetist will often choose to mechanically ventilate the rodent patient. Due to the compliant pulmonary system of the rodent, it is possible to ventilate a rodent with a nosecone. Today, there are commercial nose cones designed for rodents, which closely fit the rodent snout and thus minimize the amount of waste gas exiting the cone around the patient–mask interface and facilitate ventilation. Close-fitting "masks" for small rodents can also be easily fashioned out of trimmed latex exam gloves fitted snugly over a mask adapter. Rodents are obligate nasal breathers; therefore, a nosecone is an ideal way to deliver inhalant anesthesia.

Endotracheal intubation of mice and rats is facilitated by equipment and techniques that have been refined and customized for these species. Depending on the species and technique, visualization of the laryngeal orifice may involve ventral transillumination of the oropharynx, use of a customized laryngoscope, or conventional pediatric equipment (several detailed descriptions of intubation techniques can be found in the literature; for example, Nelson et al., 2020, and Thomas et al., 2014). Intubation can be accomplished in dorsal recumbency or by using customized or commercially available inclined rodent boards. Similar to other rodent equipment refinements, many manufacturers of mechanical ventilators have specifically designed and calibrated models for use in small rodents.

At times, large numbers of rodents may need to be anesthetized in quick succession to allow for procedures of short duration to be performed humanely and efficiently. Commercially available manifolds requiring only one vaporizer and input of air/oxygen have become much more popular when attached via nose cones or masks to several rodents undergoing similar experimental surgical procedures.

Scavenging of anesthetic gases is essential to protect laboratory personnel working with animals. In a barrier setting, many rodent procedures are best performed within secondary enclosures such as a cage changing station or a biosafety cabinet (BSC). If this BSC is hard-ducted and exhausts to the outside (Class II, Type B2), then supplemental scavenging is not needed. Otherwise, the exhaust from the induction chamber must be attached either to a wall-mounted vacuum system or to commercial charcoal canisters that remove the anesthetic agents from expired and excess anesthetic mixture. Canisters must be routinely monitored to ensure they do not exceed their scavenging capacity. Prefabricated induction chambers should exhaust through a carbon filter, a calibrated vacuum system (hard ducted to the exhaust system), or into a fume hood, vacuum exhaust, or ducted BSC. Even if the induction chamber is attached to a scavenging system, opening the chamber to retrieve the anesthetized rodent releases the vaporized inhalant into the surrounding area. National standards for exposure to unscavenged anesthetics in humans should be followed as chronic exposure to volatile anesthetics in excess of these limits can have a serious impact on the health of staff (Deng et al., 2018). The institution's occupational health program should define the proper use of inhalant anesthetics by trained personnel.

b. Advantages and disadvantages of inhalation anesthesia in rodents

Over the years, inhalant anesthesia has proven to be safe and reliable in rodents. The most important advantages of inhalant anesthesia are the steep dose-response curve, predictable and rapid control of anesthetic depth and duration, their safety, and the minimal influence on research data (Flecknell, 2015; Navarro et al., 2021a). These factors directly relate to increased survival rates and optimal data acquisition from rodent models of biomedical research.

Anesthetic induction with inhalants often requires closer attention than with parenteral anesthetics. Induction doses (e.g., isoflurane 4%–5%) are usually significantly higher than maintenance doses (e.g., isoflurane 1%–3%), and prolonged exposure to these higher percentages may lead to mortality via cardiovascular and respiratory depression.

A drawback of inhalant anesthetics is the lack of analgesic properties (Miller et al., 2021). Perioperative analgesia, i.e., preemptive, during, and postsurgery, is therefore paramount.

The induction, delivery, and scavenging systems all add to the cost and technical training necessary to provide safe and reliable inhalation anesthesia.

Required training is not the only cost related to inhalant anesthesia—an even more direct expense is the equipment itself. Complete systems to anesthetize a number of rodents may cost several thousand dollars. Fortunately, these are start-up costs and inhalant anesthesia equipment will function well for years with regular servicing. Anesthetic vaporizers should be recalibrated at appropriate intervals (typically, annually) to ensure the correct dosage.

It is important to note that the significance of the advantages of inhalant anesthetic delivery (relative safety for the animal and ease of adjusting anesthetic depth) far outweighs the disadvantages. We advocate for the appropriate use of these agents.

c. Volatile inhalation agents

The blood:gas partition coefficient of any volatile anesthetic determines the rapidity of induction, how quickly the anesthetist can alter the depth of anesthesia, and how rapidly the animal recovers from anesthesia. The lower the blood:gas coefficient, the more rapidly the induction, adjustment, and recovery will occur. The newer agents (e.g., sevoflurane) have a lower blood:gas coefficient, and thus work slightly more rapidly than other agents (e.g., isoflurane) (Heavner, 2001). The minimum alveolar concentration (MAC) is a measure of volatile agent potency, and it allows different agents to be compared. It is defined as the agent concentration necessary to prevent gross, purposeful movement in 50% of an animal population exposed to a noxious stimulus (usually equivalent to a surgical stimulus) (Heavner, 1997). MAC is inversely proportional to the potency of the gas, i.e., anesthetics with a low MAC have a relatively high potency. MAC is typically described as the "effective dose" when 50% of the patients are "anesthetized," or the ED_{50}. The ED_{50} equaling 1 MAC generally represents "light" anesthesia. ED_{95} represents 1.2−1.4 MAC—when 95% of the patients are anesthetized. MAC 2.0 is considered very deep anesthesia and may be fatal (Rampil and King, 1996).

The primary effects of volatile and gas anesthetics are to produce loss of consciousness with associated muscle relaxation. Clinical and physiologic signs of adequate anesthetic depth in rodents include increases in arterial CO_2, reduced eyelid aperture, and absence of the withdrawal reflex, commonly the toe pinch, and no response to surgical incision (Steffey et al., 2003). The primary negative side effect seen with all volatile anesthetics is an agent-dependent depression of the cardiovascular system, resulting in decreased cardiac output, reduced contractility, decreased respiratory rate, and systemic hypotension (Rampil and King, 1996).

The pharmacology of inhalant anesthetics is detailed in Chapter 6.

Isoflurane Isoflurane is a preferred anesthetic for all rodents when appropriate equipment and scavenging are available and is the most commonly used inhalation anesthetic in rodents (Richardson and Flecknell, 2005). For procedures where only very short durations of anesthesia are required, isoflurane provides a rapid onset of induction and recovery (Flecknell, 2015). For these reasons, and its extremely limited metabolism (inhalant agents are largely removed unchanged via exhalation; see Chapter 6 for details), its use has increased over the last years (Stokes et al., 2009, Flecknell, 2015). Isoflurane causes moderate respiratory and cardiovascular system depression but maintains better cardiac function than for example the combination of ketamine and xylazine (Flecknell, 2015). Isoflurane is used far more often than other inhaled agents and has been shown to be very safe when used appropriately, even for long periods of anesthesia in both mice (Szczensy et al., 2004; Ewald et al., 2011) and rats (Wood et al., 2001).

In mice and rats, repeated exposure to isoflurane has been shown to be aversive (Moody and Weary, 2014). Thus, for studies requiring repeated isoflurane anesthesia, such as serial imaging over time, this increasing aversion should be considered when weighing the cumulative welfare impact of the study.

Isoflurane as well as sevoflurane are known to have neuroprotective effects on the brain, e.g., during ischemia or infarction, but may also cause neurotoxicity under certain conditions (Neag et al., 2020). At typical anesthetic levels, isoflurane significantly reduces serotonin levels in mice (Whittington and Virag, 2006) and increases the survivability of oxygen- and glucose-deprived hippocampal cells of the rat (Zhan et al., 2006). Isoflurane offers a protective effect on ischemic rat neuronal cells (Kawaguchi et al., 2004) and in a perinatal stroke model in rats (Zhao and Zuo, 2004). In rats, isoflurane improves spatial memory following general hypoxia (Bekker et al., 2006). Isoflurane was also found to cause reversible deficits in object recognition tests (Ding et al., 2016), impaired learning function in fear conditioning tests, and more anxiety-related behavior in the elevated plus maze in mice in the post-anesthetic period (Yonezaki et al., 2015).

Isoflurane may be the best inhalant anesthetic agent to be used in rodent models of human traumatic brain injury. While injured rats anesthetized with isoflurane developed a clinically relevant decrease in MAP, the intracranial pressure did not change (Goren et al., 2001). Not only do injured rats anesthetized with isoflurane have the best cognitive outcome and neuronal survival compared with other common anesthetics (Statler et al., 2006), anesthesia with isoflurane before and immediately after the traumatic brain injury showed no alterations in histopathology compared with control animals (Statler et al., 2006). See also Rowe et al. (2013) for a review.

The most used inhalation anesthetics have an impact in general and on parameters of interest in cardiovascular studies in specific. Relative to general impacts, isoflurane causes decreased systemic vascular resistance with hypotension (Evers et al., 2006). In a compensatory manner, the heart rate can slightly increase (Evers et al., 2006). While isoflurane acts as a bronchodilator, it can irritate and stimulate tracheal and bronchial reflexes and can trigger laryngospasm (Evers et al., 2006). The vasodilatory effect of isoflurane can result in a slightly increased cerebral blood flow with minor risk for increased intracranial pressure (Evers et al., 2006). Compared to pentobarbital, isoflurane produces less deleterious cardiac effects, demonstrated by a higher mean coronary blood flow in rats due to a larger ejection fraction and higher cardiac output (Iltis et al., 2005). In mice (CD-1, Swiss, and C57BL), cardiac output decreased by only 5% compared with awake, resting control mice (Janssen et al., 2004). Wistar rats anesthetized with 0.9% isoflurane have significantly reduced MAP and perfusion pressure of the brain as compared with rats anesthetized with propofol (Kahveci et al., 2001).

In regard to model-specific impacts, isoflurane has protective effects in models of ischemic cardiac disease. Mice anesthetized with isoflurane and subjected to coronary artery occlusion develop smaller infarct sizes (Tsutsumi et al., 2006b). In mice and rats, cardioprotective effects can last for 2 weeks following the anesthetic episode (Tsutsumi et al., 2006a; Wakeno-Takahashi et al., 2005). The mechanism of these cardioprotective effects may be a reduction of superoxide production and adherence of neutrophils (Hu et al., 2003).

Isoflurane has inconsistent effects in the pulmonary system and can have both protective and deleterious effects. At the cellular level, isoflurane causes a significant ciliary dysfunction of rat trachea epithelial cells at normal anesthetic doses (Matsuura et al., 2006). Anesthesia with isoflurane worsens the sequelae in patients with neurogenic pulmonary edema, a trait linked to the excessive release of endothelial growth factor from bronchial cells in rats (Kandatsu et al., 2005). Long-term exposure of rats to isoflurane inhibits the release of inflammatory cytokines by the pulmonary epithelium (Giraud et al., 2003). Isoflurane has protective effects on the vascular endothelium when rats are anesthetized before lipopolysaccharide (LPS) administration. LPS-induced vasodilation and the subsequent drop in MAP, increase in tumor necrosis factor-α (TNF-a), and direct vascular damage can all be attenuated by prior exposure of rats to isoflurane (Plachinta et al., 2003).

Isoflurane is only minimally metabolized by the liver; therefore, adverse hepatic effects are rare following short-to-moderate duration anesthesia. Rats can be anesthetized for short periods of time with isoflurane without any change in the activity of cytochrome P450 enzymes (Plate et al., 2005). Compared to the cardiovascular and nervous systems, the gastrointestinal system is generally spared of side effects of anesthesia with volatile agents. However, rats briefly anesthetized with isoflurane demonstrated a 50% reduction in gut motility for up to 2 h (Torjman et al., 2005). Another important consideration is the use of anesthesia for hematologic measurements. C3H/HeN mice have been shown to develop leukopenia, neutropenia, and thrombocytopenia within 48 h following only 30 min of isoflurane anesthesia (Jacobsen et al., 2004).

Isoflurane may be safely used in pregnant or neonatal rodents and can be recommended for embryo transfer (ET) procedures (Smith et al., 2004). Exposure of pregnant ICR mice to isoflurane in the first gestational week produces slight growth retardation in preterm fetuses (Haque et al., 2004). Caesarian-derived pups of pregnant rats administered 2.5% isoflurane have more physiologically normal levels of lactate, pO_2, and pCO_2 than those at higher doses of isoflurane (Vaillancourt et al., 1999). Isoflurane produces hypoglycemia and metabolic acidosis in neonatal mice. Mechanical ventilation greatly improves survivability in neonatal mice over spontaneous breathing when exposed to long anesthetic regimens (Loepke et al., 2006; Yu et al., 2020). Despite these physiologic effects, isoflurane is generally safe to use in neonatal mice (Drobac et al., 2004; Gotoh et al., 2004) and can be recommended for brief procedures such as tail biopsy for genotyping or toe clipping for identification.

The specific effects of isoflurane on DNA and gene expression are inconsistent. Although isoflurane has been shown to offer protection of the brain and heart following hypoxia to anoxia, normal anesthetic doses of isoflurane can produce oxidative DNA damage in lymphocytes, spleens, and bone marrow of rats as well as in brain, liver, and lung tissue (Kim et al., 2006). Conversely, in rat neuronal cultures, exposure to isoflurane upregulates protective genes and downregulates damaging genes (Huang and Zuo, 2005). Isoflurane has been shown to alter the expression of hundreds of genes in the rat brain, as detected by gene microarrays (Rampil et al., 2006).

Isoflurane and other volatile agents may have a hyperalgesic effect if the inhaled concentration becomes too low. In rats recovering from anesthesia, a concentration of 0.5 MAC is high enough to produce an antinociceptive effect, while 0.1–0.2 MAC produces hyperalgesia (Flood et al., 2002; Zhang et al., 2000). Therefore, it is of great importance to have completed all painful procedures prior to lowering the dose of isoflurane and beginning the recovery of the rodent. It is also recommended that perioperative analgesics be administered well before the patient begins recovering from isoflurane anesthesia, ideally before an invasive procedure begins (preemptive analgesia).

Sevoflurane Isoflurane might be more common, but both isoflurane and sevoflurane provide an equally effective anesthesia with acceptable and similar adverse effects. It shows very rapid induction, ease of maintenance, and rapid recovery of rodents (Cesarovic et al., 2010; Lipiski et al., 2017). Sevoflurane does have direct cardiodepressant effects, most notably on myocardial contractility, but this effect is similar to that of isoflurane and not severe (Park et al., 1996). Pretreatment with clinically relevant doses of sevoflurane is cardioprotective, similar to many other fluorinated anesthetics (Obal et al., 2001), and is most significant in animals pretreated 48 h before infarction (Lutz and Liu, 2006) and in septic animals (Serita et al., 2002). This protective effect further extends into the reperfusion phase in these models. Sevoflurane delivered during the first few minutes of reperfusion significantly reduces infarct size, but a longer duration of anesthesia did not further improve the protective effects (Obal et al., 2003).

At normal anesthetic doses, sevoflurane does not produce ciliary dysfunction in rat tracheal epithelial cells (Matsuura et al., 2006). In cases of neurogenic pulmonary edema, sevoflurane does not worsen and may improve the overall outcomes (Kandatsu et al., 2005). Furthermore, sevoflurane induces an epithelium-dependent bronchodilation (Park et al., 1998), which may improve both anesthetic and oxygen delivery to patients with pulmonary compromise.

Ischemia-induced cerebral apoptosis is reduced if rats are anesthetized with sevoflurane (Pape et al., 2006). General neuroprotection from preconditioning occurs whether sevoflurane is inhaled minutes to days before an ischemic event (Payne et al., 2005). When compared with isoflurane, the most widely used anesthetic in neurophysiology, sevoflurane offers similar rates of the rebuilding high-energy phosphate stores following cerebral ischemia in rats (Payne et al., 2005). Sevoflurane does not have the same neuroprotective effects in experimental spinal cord ischemia in rats (Zvara et al., 2006). Behaviorally, exposure to about 0.1 MAC of sevoflurane significantly enhances the memory of aversive stimuli in the rat (Alkire et al., 2005).

As seen in mice anesthetized with halothane, repeated anesthesia with sevoflurane has been shown to produce a peripheral leukopenia and lymphopenia that can persist for several days (Elena et al., 2003).

On a cellular level, sevoflurane inhibits oxytocin-induced contractions of the pregnant myometrium at normal anesthetic doses (Gultekin et al., 2006; Yazmakage et al., 2002). This effect, combined with other positive physiologic effects of sevoflurane, could be useful in improving the success rate of cesarean sections in rodents. Adolescent rats require a higher MAC of sevoflurane than do young adult rats (Kashimoto et al., 1997).

"Compound A" (fluoromethyl-2,2-difluoro-1-trifluoromethyl vinyl ether), a by-product of the interaction between sevoflurane and soda lime is nephrotoxic in rats. There is evidence that there may be species differences with regards to the renal metabolism of inhaled Compound A (Kharasch and Jubert, 1999), but it has not been shown to be neurotoxic in clinical situations (Konat et al., 2003). It is also a potent upregulator of genes involved in apoptosis, oxidative injury, the inflammatory response (Kharasch et al., 2006), and the cytochrome P450 system (Sheffels et al., 2004).

A deterrent to the use of sevoflurane over other inhalants is its higher cost.

Desflurane Desflurane is infrequently used in rodents because of its low boiling point (necessitating the use of a specialized electrically powered vaporizer) and high cost of use. It is also associated with cardiovascular stimulation during acute increases in concentration and is a significant contributor to climate change (more so than isoflurane). Its primary advantage is its lower solubility, which results in an extremely rapid recovery from anesthesia compared with, for example, isoflurane.

Methoxyflurane Methoxyflurane is the most soluble volatile agent in the blood and brain, and thus the most potent inhalant. It has an analgesic effect. Currently, methoxyflurane has limited availability in some countries, and its veterinary use is limited.

Enflurane Induction and recovery with enflurane are fast. It has a depressing effect on respiration and the cardiovascular system (Flecknell, 2015). The most recent use is experimental rather than clinical.

Halothane Halothane was historically utilized as an inhalant anesthetic but has been replaced by safer alternatives isoflurane and sevoflurane, and is no longer commercially available in pharmaceutical grade in the United States.

d. Nonvolatile inhalation agents

Nitrous oxide Nitrous oxide was among the first inhalant anesthetic gases used in a clinical setting in the early 19th century. It has many desirable characteristics, including low solubility in the blood, low toxicity, and minimal cardiopulmonary depression. However, since its anesthetic properties are insufficient for surgical anesthesia, it is most often used as a supplemental inhalant gas anesthetic. It is seldom used in rodents, and its clinical use in other species is increasingly limited.

Xenon Xenon's profound neuroprotective effects stem from its antagonism of the *N*-methyl-D-aspartic acid (NMDA) receptor (Watkins and Jane, 2006), which is implicated in neuronal damage (Wilhelm et al., 2002). Like many other gaseous anesthetics, xenon has cardioprotective (Weber et al., 2005) and neuroprotective (Petzelt et al., 2003) effects if animals are pretreated with the gas before an ischemic episode. In addition, xenon was shown to provide short-term neuroprotection when administered after an episode of hypoxia in neonatal rats (Dingley et al., 2006). When used for anesthesia in rats, xenon may potentiate gas emboli formation in procedures involving cardiopulmonary bypass, which can impair motor performance and cognition (Jungwirth et al., 2006).

The high cost of xenon gas has limited its use as an anesthetic in animal experiments.

In summary, volatile and other gas anesthetics can be extremely useful in rodent models. As with any other method of anesthesia, there may be undesirable side effects or potentially confounding variables; thus, a method must be chosen that protects the health and welfare of the animal while maintaining a minimal impact on the research.

2. *Injectable*

a. General considerations in the use of injectable anesthetics in rodents

Injectable anesthetics are commonly preferred over inhalant anesthetics, particularly for short-term anesthesia, because of ease of use. In cases when inhalant administration would physically interfere with the work being performed (e.g., surgery of the head, nasal, or oral cavities) or when inhalant equipment or staff trained in its use, is unavailable, injectables can be administered readily. Injectable anesthetics require only a needle, syringe, and the appropriate training to give a simple injection in a defined anatomic location (Flecknell, 1993b). Injectable agents also more easily allow several animals to be maintained under anesthesia at the same time. When using parenteral anesthetics, it is important to consider accurate dosing with correct multidrug use ratios, storage conditions, and feasibility of immediate use following reconstitution. It is critical to weigh each animal accurately prior to administration of a calculated dose of anesthesia to avoid over- or underdosing. Injectables in rodents are usually administered intraperitoneally (IP); however, in larger species (e.g., adult rats, guinea pigs), anesthetics may be administered intramuscularly (IM) or intravenously (IV). Both the volume administered, and the gauge of the needle used for administration should be considered, particularly for the IM route. Table 14.1 gives guidance for appropriate routes, volumes, and needle gauges for various rodent species.

When drugs are given by injection, the dosage cannot be reduced after induction. Therefore, drugs either at a low dose or with a wide safety margin should be used. Subcutaneous (SC) administration of anesthetics is not recommended because the induction of anesthesia is prolonged and variable in onset. Intravenous injections in rodents can be performed by more highly trained personnel. For most purposes, general anesthesia in rodents is preferred to local anesthetic techniques because it is believed to reduce stress to the animal and increase safety for personnel (Hall et al., 2001).

Many small mammals become distressed by handling, subsequently increasing the risk of injury and adverse physiologic effects that might lead to complications while under anesthesia. The risk of injury is considerably reduced by proper handling by trained personnel.

A multimodal approach is the most common method for administering anesthetics and analgesics in laboratory rodents. As the mechanism of action of these drugs varies, depending on target sites and receptors within the central and peripheral pain pathways, the overall doses of individual drugs used in combination can often be decreased to reduce the occurrence of side effects (Robertson, 2001). A considerable increase in the use of injectable anesthetic combinations compared to single-injected agents has been documented (Richardson and Flecknell, 2005). Injectable and inhalant agents must be used with caution and careful monitoring in neonatal rodents due to the significant differences between neonatal and adult physiology. Anesthesia for neonatal rodents is discussed briefly later in this chapter and in detail in Chapter 28.

b. Dissociative anesthetics

Ketamine Ketamine is a potent analgesic at low doses and has a short half-life in rodents of several minutes following IP injection (Navarro et al., 2021a). Compared to other injectable anesthetics, ketamine has the least depressant effects on heart rate and left ventricular function parameters (Pachon et al., 2015). For anesthesia, ketamine combinations, usually with xylazine, dexmedetomidine, or one of these agents plus acepromazine, are a preferred anesthetic when equipment for inhalant anesthesia is not available. Ketamine is a noncompetitive NMDA receptor antagonist that can prevent central sensitization and provide analgesia in the face of ischemic and somatic pain (Robertson, 2001). For more information on ketamine's analgesic properties, see Section E.4 in this chapter.

Anesthetic doses of ketamine produce a dissociative state and behavioral effects. It is not recommended as a sole anesthetic agent in rodents (Flecknell, 1987b). Ketamine does not lead to muscle relaxation, and tonic-clonic spasms of limb muscles may occur even in the absence of surgical or other stimulation. The absence of muscle relaxation makes ketamine a poor choice as the sole anesthetic for many surgical procedures, but particularly those that require considerable muscle relaxation, e.g., intraabdominal surgery. Although single doses are short-acting, they effectively produce sedation rather than a classic ketamine-induced dissociative state characterized by an abnormal, often exaggerated response to the local environment and stimuli. Ketamine can stimulate increased salivation and secretions can obstruct the airways, although laryngeal and pharyngeal reflexes are retained. Ketamine can induce a transient rise in arterial pressure, usually measured as hypertension in rodents. Ketamine, like most nonvolatile anesthetic agents, is broken down into metabolites in the liver prior to urinary excretion. Incremental additional doses of ketamine can be given to extend the period of anesthesia, but can cause severe respiratory depression, as anesthetic depth is hard to titrate with bolus injections (Flecknell, 1987b). Another disadvantage of ketamine is the occasional production of apneustic ventilation, a pattern characterized by a prolonged pause after inspiration. Ketamine suppresses respiration at high doses in mice; an effect typically not observed in other species due to the low doses used in combination with other agents (Navarro et al., 2021a).

Despite these disadvantages, when combined with other agents, ketamine remains the drug of choice for injectable anesthesia. Ketamine is used preferentially due to its (1) ease of IP administration; (2) relative safety among injectable agents; (3) ability to produce a cataleptic state characterized by CNS excitement rather than depression, along with analgesia, immobility, dissociation from the environment, and amnesia; and (4) complementary properties with adjuvant agents, allowing for a decrease in the amount of general anesthetic needed. To reduce adverse effects, a variety of other compounds, both injectables and inhalants, are typically administered along with ketamine (Hall et al., 2001b; Navarro et al., 2021a). Ketamine combinations are common first choices for injectable rodent anesthesia (Richardson and Flecknell, 2005; Flecknell, 2009; Flecknell, 2015).

Ketamine combined with A-2 agonists A-2 agonists are extremely useful in combination with ketamine because they smooth induction, can be used for chemical restraint and sedation at lower doses, or for general anesthesia at higher doses; additionally, the combination provides muscle relaxation that is absent if ketamine is given alone. These combinations should be administered IP or SC, as ketamine can cause muscle necrosis due to its low pH (Gaertner et al., 1987). SC injection may reduce the risk of injury and partial failure rates as compared to IP but may also lengthen the time to onset of anesthesia due to a decreased absorption rate (Miner et al., 1969; Turner et al., 2011).

Ketamine and xylazine. Ketamine/xylazine combinations are commonly used injectable combinations for anesthesia of mice, rats, hamsters, and guinea pigs (Branson, 2001; Gilroy and Varga, 1980; Green et al., 1981; Van Pelt, 1977). The availability of mobile apps to assist with ketamine/xylazine dosing calculations can be additive in further refining doses and reducing anesthetic-associated deaths (Jara et al., 2021). While some rodent studies report that ketamine/xylazine combinations produce a surgical anesthesia depth, others failed to inhibit motor responses following a noxious stimulus with the combination alone (reviewed by Navarro et al., 2021a). Therefore, ketamine/xylazine has been combined with other drugs like acepromazine, buprenorphine, carprofen, azaperone, and lidocaine (Buitrago et al., 2008; Gergye et al., 2020; Dholakia et al., 2017; Olson and Renchko, 1988; Navarro et al., 2021a) to safely achieve surgical anesthesia depth.

If careful monitoring is performed, the ketamine/xylazine combination can be used for long-term procedures, reducing mobility and allowing calm restraint while maintaining spontaneous ventilation. If the patient's pedal withdrawal reflex begins to return, redosing of either 50% of the initial ketamine dose or 25% of the initial ketamine/xylazine dose is recommended to extend the surgical plane of anesthesia in mice (Jaber et al., 2014). Ketamine/xylazine also has been effective in anesthetizing pregnant mice (Furukawa et al., 1998). Serial use of ketamine/xylazine in rats should be carefully considered. While heart rate and blood pressure were consistent when this combination was used to anesthetize rats six times over 3 weeks, rats were also more likely to fail to reach a surgical plane of anesthesia, had reduced sleep times, decreases in body weight, and developed necrosis at the injection site (Albrecht et al., 2014).

Adverse side effects of ketamine plus xylazine must also be considered. Body temperature in rodents may decrease by several degrees following the administration of ketamine/xylazine, and this decrease may be exacerbated by increased urination, defecation, and salivation (Wixson and Smiler, 1997; Wixson et al., 1987c). Profound reductions in rectal and core body temperatures have been noted in rats, demonstrated by a decrease of up to 4°C over 60 min of anesthesia (Wixson et al., 1987c). It has been documented that rats anesthetized with ketamine plus xylazine may develop a variety of corneal lesions, including keratoconjunctivitis sicca, focally severe and permanent band keratopathy of the cornea, but interestingly protected rats from retinal degeneration (Kufoy et al., 1989; Turner and Albassam, 2005; Koehn et al., 2015; Arango-Gonzalez et al., 2012). However, transient cataracts previously ascribed to xylazine have subsequently been determined to be from drying of the cornea (Calderone et al., 1986; Lee et al., 2020). Corneal opacities are lessened in severity in certain strains of rats that receive yohimbine for reversal of ketamine plus xylazine anesthesia (Turner and Albassam, 2005; Koehn et al., 2015). Muscle necrosis may occur following IM injections in small rodents; therefore, IP injections are recommended (Gaertner et al., 1987; Smiler et al., 1990). Additionally, ketamine/xylazine negatively impacts respiration, even at subtherapeutic doses (Massey and Richerson, 2017). SpO2 levels of mice anesthetized with these combinations can drop precipitously; therefore, supplemental oxygen can be especially valuable whenever these combinations are used (Burnside et al., 2013).

Ketamine combined with medetomidine or dexmedetomidine. Ketamine/medetomidine produces sedation and anesthesia (depending on dose) suitable for minor procedures in mice, such as retroorbital bleeding, but may not lead reliably to surgical anesthesia (Burnside et al., 2013). Female inbred and outbred mice appeared to be more resistant to the effects of this anesthetic combination than male mice (Cruz et al., 1998; Taylor et al., 2000). It can be reversed rapidly by atipamezole (Cruz et al., 1998; Taylor et al., 2000), but early reversal may lead to prolonged recovery times in rats (Wellington et al., 2013; Baker et al., 2011). One advantage of medetomidine-midazolam-fentanyl is that the same negative outcomes with serial ketamine/xylazine use did not develop with serial anesthesia of this cocktail (Albrecht et al., 2014). In rats, ketamine/medetomidine anesthesia can be prolonged with the addition of buprenorphine (Hedenqvist et al., 2000a). Though caution with this combination (ketamine/medetomidine/buprenorphine) in rats should be exercised as an increase in risk for respiratory failure resulting in mortality has been documented (Roughan et al., 1999). Less muscle and tissue inflammation has been observed when medetomidine is combined with ketamine (vs. ketamine alone) for IM injections (Sun et al., 2003) or IP injections (vs. ketamine/xylazine) in rats (Wellington et al., 2013). The addition of medetomidine to ketamine may cause hyperglycemia and polyuria, similar to that observed with xylazine. In rats, bradycardia, respiratory depression, and subsequent hypoxemia have been described (Wellington et al., 2013). In C57BL/6 male mice anesthetized with medetomidine/ketamine, a small percentage (3%) of mice developed obstructive uropathy due to seminal coagulum release, an adverse effect not observed with xylazine/ketamine anesthesia (Wells et al., 2009).

Medetomidine is not currently commercially available as it has been replaced by dexmedetomidine, its racemic isomer. Ketamine/dexmedetomidine was found comparable to medetomidine in mice and can be used with a 50% reduction in dose rate (Burnside et al., 2013). Recommended doses in rats are 75 mg/kg ketamine with 0.25−1 mg/kg dexmedetomidine (Wellington et al., 2013; Flecknell, 2015). In BALB/c mice, when dexmedetomidine (0.2 mg/kg) and tiletamine-zolazepam (40 mg/kg) were administered with the addition of butorphanol (3 mg/kg), the resulting sleep time was longer (143 min) and more reliable (24/24 mice) than when given without the butorphanol (Cagle et al., 2017e). As with ketamine/xylazine, if animals must be redosed to maintain the surgical plane of anesthesia, only ketamine should be redosed. While some literature has supported a concern that atipamezole and yohimbine may counteract the analgesic effectiveness of opiates, the reversal of ketamine-dexmedetomidine with atipamezole did not alter antinociceptive effects of preemptively administered butorphanol and buprenorphine in C57BL/6 mice (Iglesias et al., 1992; Izer et al., 2014). When administered multiple times over several weeks to BALB/c male mice, dexmedetomidine administration was associated with a high incidence (67%) of urethral plugs and obstruction, an effect that was independent of dose and administration of other anesthetics (Cagle et al., 2017).

Ketamine combined with promazine or acepromazine Promazine, combined with ketamine and aminopentamide hydrogen sulfate, has been documented to produce effective anesthesia in several species. The combination of drugs suppresses the protective reflexes such as coughing and swallowing during anesthesia, which otherwise remain under ketamine anesthesia alone (Mulder, 1978; Mulder and Johnson, 1978). Promazine alone provides CNS depression without marked motor function impairment. The combination is fairly potent, and minimal doses can provide sedative effects with minimal impact on cardiovascular or respiratory depression. Dosing of ketamine plus promazine in rodents is based on the volume of ketamine and allows 40−50 min of anesthesia after IM injection. Ketamine plus promazine is nonreversible, and hypothermia and hypotension may develop with longer durations of anesthesia.

The administration of ketamine with acepromazine provides only light anesthesia, which is not sufficient for surgical procedures (Flecknell, 1987b). Instead, the addition of xylazine to the ketamine/acepromazine mixture, given SC, has been shown to induce rapid and long-acting sedation and analgesia in rats and mice (Arras et al., 2001; Welberg et al., 2006; Navarro et al., 2021a).

Ketamine combined with benzodiazepines: diazepam and midazolam Diazepam is a benzodiazepine that provides sedation and good muscle relaxation and can potentiate the action of anesthetics and opioid analgesics (Flecknell, 1996). Classically, diazepam has been used as an anticonvulsant, and it can be antagonized in rodents by flumazenil (Metten et al., 2007). Midazolam has a shorter duration of action and can be administered IM as it is formulated as an aqueous solution.

The benzodiazepines are generally considered to cause few adverse cardiorespiratory effects. Minimal adverse cardiovascular effects are observed with ketamine/diazepam combinations, in particular minimal hypotension, especially when compared to ketamine/xylazine (Wixson et al., 1987b). Ketamine/midazolam were found to have no impact on learning and therefore were recommended for use in mouse studies where spatial and motor tasks are utilized (Valentim et al., 2013). Adverse respiratory effects are also minimal and may be limited to a slight decrease in respiratory rate and tidal volume. Ketamine/diazepam provides only light anesthesia (Flecknell, 1987b) with poor muscle relaxation, and a hyperacusis response in rats. When compared to other multimodal methods of anesthesia, higher mortality has been observed within 15 min of induction. Diazepam may also potentiate the heat loss observed with ketamine (Wixson et al., 1987c).

Ketamine combined with butyrophenones Butyrophenones are neuroleptic agents that include azaperone, droperidol, and haloperidol. Droperidol, when combined with an opioid (e.g., fentanyl), has not been documented to produce surgical anesthesia in rodents and neonates, but induces respiratory depression (Danneman and Mandrell, 1997). Azaperone is a sedative neuroleptic. When used alone, azaperone provides sedation in mice; however, in rats, it may induce tachypnea (Olson and Renchko, 1988). When combined with ketamine, azaperone produces a surgical plane of anesthesia in both mice and rats (Olson and Renchko, 1988).

Dissociative agent and muscle relaxant: telazol Telazol, a unique combination of dissociative agent (tiletamine hydrochloride) and muscle relaxant (zolazepam hydrochloride), is a nonnarcotic and nonbarbiturate combination. Telazol has characteristics similar to those of ketamine, including the maintenance of a number of reflexes under anesthesia. Corneal and pedal reflexes make it difficult for the anesthetist to assess the depth of anesthesia. Tiletamine is more potent, yet structurally similar to ketamine, with a longer duration of action. Zolazepam is a benzodiazepine derivative, licensed for use only with tiletamine. It has a rapid onset of action, but lacks analgesic properties (Ferrari et al., 2005) and is used to offset the cataleptic effects of tiletamine.

Telazol produces anesthesia in rats and can be combined with medetomidine, xylazine, or butorphanol to prolong the duration of effects (Ferrari et al., 2005; Silverman et al., 1983; Wilson et al., 1992). This anesthetic agent is not recommended for solitary use in mice or hamsters due to difficulties in inducing anesthesia and a very narrow margin of safety in these species (Silverman et al., 1983). When combined with 20 mg/kg xylazine, 80 mg/kg telazol produced surgical tolerance (pedal withdrawal) in mice but was outperformed by 100 mg/kg ketamine/20 mg/kg xylazine/3 mg/kg acepromazine (Arras et al., 2001). In rats, doses of 40–50 mg/kg Telazol resulted in fewer adverse cardiovascular effects as compared to ketamine/xylazine combinations or pentobarbital (Saha et al., 2007). It is important to note that, as with many agents, higher doses of telazol result in prolonged recovery times; therefore, laboratory animals should be monitored closely to ensure a safe recovery when using higher dosages. Due to its status as a schedule III-controlled substance, telazol procurement and usage require controlled substance registration, careful documentation, and secure storage.

c. Alfaxalone

Alfaxalone is a neuroactive steroid whose mechanism of action is as a GABA agonist. It was discontinued from the market due to high risks of anaphylaxis due to the solubilizing agent. However, reformulation has allowed it to reenter the market, where it is gaining traction in veterinary medicine to induce anesthesia, provide sedation, or, if used in combination with other drugs, achieve general anesthesia. When given alone, alfaxalone was not found to be appropriate for anything more than light sedation in both mice and rats with some mice developing behavioral hyperresponsiveness (Siriarchavatana et al., 2016; West et al., 2020). When combined with xylazine and administered IP, alfaxalone was appropriate for orthopedic surgery but resulted in high mortality when used for laparotomy, and mild adverse behavioral responses remained in some mice (Erickson et al., 2019; Siriarchavatana et al., 2016). Survival increased when the drugs were given to SC (Erickson et al., 2019). Significant sex and strain differences resulted in differing dosage recommendations: 80–120 mg/kg IP alfaxalone with 10 mg/kg IP xylazine for male mice and 40–80 mg/kg IP alfaxalone with 10 mg/kg IP xylazine for female mice (Erickson et al., 2019). Female rats administered 30 mg/kg alfaxalone with 0.05 mg/kg dexmedetomidine IP achieved surgical levels of anesthesia. As with the mice, significant sex differences were found with female rats experiencing longer periods of sedation than males, such that the authors did not have a recommended dose for male rats (West et al., 2020). When first induced with ketamine (80 mg/kg)/xylazine (8 mg/kg) SC, rats receiving a CRI of 10 mg/kg/hr IV alfaxalone maintained a surgical plane anesthesia (no pedal withdrawal reflex) for the duration of the CRI (Heng et al., 2020). No sex differences were identified in the CRI study.

d. α-2 agonists: xylazine, medetomidine, dexmedetomidine

As discussed in Chapter 4 and above, α-2 agonists xylazine, medetomidine, and dexmedetomidine are commonly used to supplement the primary anesthetic ketamine or ketamine plus acepromazine (Burnside et al., 2013; Flecknell, 2015). See the above section on ketamine for details. Another potential combination for reaching surgical plane anesthesia in C57BL/6 mice is xylazine combined with etomidate. However, the value of this combination was restricted to the C57BL/6 strain and not recommended for BALB/cJ or NU/J; thus, caution should be exercised regarding the general use of this anesthetic cocktail (Gergye et al., 2020). Although rarely used alone, α-2 agonists can produce sedation, analgesia, and muscle relaxation. The α-2 agonists may be used as a preanesthetic, which reduces the dosage of an inhalant primary anesthetic. While α-2 agonists have some analgesic properties and potentiate general anesthetics, they do not provide sufficient analgesia to be considered appropriate to minimize postoperative pain. See Section E.5. for more information about the analgesic properties of α-2 agonists.

A significant advantage of xylazine is its ability to be reversed by specific receptor antagonists, including atipamezole or yohimbine, and less commonly tolazoline, 4-aminopyridine, and idazoxan (Wixson and Smiler, 1997; Hsu et al., 1986; Lipman et al., 1987; Komulainen and Olson, 1991; Flecknell, 1996). In mice, atipamezole administration led to faster recovery of righting reflex compared to yohimbine (Janssen et al., 2017). Reversal leads to early termination of surgical anesthesia, which may reduce mortality and allow rapid return of the rodents to the home cage environment. Reversal agents also reverse bradycardia, bradypnea, and polyuria, but do not eliminate the hypothermic effects; thus, thermal support remains essential (Komulainen and Olson, 1991). Importantly, antagonist administration will also reverse the analgesic effects of α-2 agonists, so that analgesia should be provided by other means, as necessary.

The disadvantages of xylazine (and other α-2 agonists) include transient hyperglycemia, bradycardia, peripheral vasoconstriction, hypothermia, and diuresis; however, these effects are reduced in rodents compared to dogs because xylazine is most commonly administered by the IP route rather than the IV route. When administering xylazine, cardiac output decreases secondary to bradycardia (a response to peripheral vasoconstriction). Blood pressure is transiently increased due to vasoconstriction, followed by a return of blood pressure into the normal/low-normal range as vasoconstriction wanes. The effects on the pulmonary system are generally minimal when xylazine (or other drugs in the same class) are given alone, but respiratory depression can occur when combined with other drugs or in compromised animals. The α-2 agonists sensitize the myocardium to catecholamines and may elicit significant bradycardia and sinoatrial block. Xylazine should be avoided for studies of cardiac function due to its depressant effect on the heart, including reduced left ventricular ejection fraction and significant bradycardia (Pachon et al., 2015). It is also contraindicated in studies of muscle function due to a depressant effect on the contractility of skeletal muscle (Ingalls et al., 1996). Xylazine was initially thought to cause transient cataracts; however, subsequent studies suggest these effects may be due to the drying of the cornea (Calderone et al., 1986; Lee et al., 2020). Xylazine has also been documented to increase gastrointestinal transit time in mice (Hsu, 1982), cause severe hyperglycemia in mice (Windeløv et al., 2016), and induce diuresis via decreased release of antidiuretic hormone (Milanez et al., 2019). For further discussion of specific drug combinations, the reader should refer to Section IV.B.

Medetomidine is an α-2 agonist with 10 times greater specificity than xylazine and fewer notable side effects (Virtanen, 1989). Medetomidine alone can be used for deep sedation and analgesia with rapid reversal by its specific antagonist, atipamezole (Virtanen, 1989). Medetomidine has been used in combination with the opioids fentanyl (Hu et al., 1992) or sufentanil (Hedenqvist et al., 2000b) for reliable and reversible anesthesia in the rat. A main advantage to the use of these two combinations is their reversibility with nalbuphine or butorphanol, and atipamezole (Hahn et al., 2005; MacDonald et al. (1989)).

e. Barbiturate anesthetics

Along with the dissociatives described above, barbiturates constitute the other major group of injectable agents. Barbiturates act as CNS depressants and cause decreases in blood pressure, body temperature, renal filtration and function, and peripheral vasodilation (Wixson et al., 1987b). The liver is responsible for the metabolism of barbiturates, as for most nonvolatile anesthetic agents.

Barbiturates may have a narrow margin of safety (Flecknell, 1993b). Anesthetic duration may be impacted by environmental conditions, such as raw pine bedding, that cause induction of hepatic microsomal enzymes. Due to cumulative effects, barbiturates are not suitable for repeated administration (Flecknell, 1996). One can observe a dose-dependent cardiac and respiratory depression, with prolonged recovery times and a predisposition toward hypothermia. Depending on the strain, sex, and body composition of animals, barbiturates will often exhibit effects specific to each individual rodent (Flecknell, 1993a). Due to their status as controlled substances, the procurement and usage of barbiturates require controlled substance registration, careful documentation, and secure storage.

Pentobarbital Sodium pentobarbital, also commonly referred to as pentobarbital, or pentobarbitone, is known to have a narrow margin of safety in most animal species. It has been used historically because it provides a surgical plane of anesthesia following IV or IP administration but has been largely replaced by ketamine. Commercial solutions may contain propylene glycol, which can cause pain, tissue damage, and thrombophlebitis. For these reasons, the SC and intramuscular routes of injection are not recommended (Papich, 2016).

In laboratory rodents, pentobarbital provides no analgesic effect independent of the ability of barbiturates to induce unconsciousness (Brammer et al., 1993; Field et al., 1993). More importantly, the quality of anesthesia provided by pentobarbital is generally regarded as poor (Flecknell, 1996), and the assessment of pedal reflex is a poor indicator of anesthetic depth with this drug (Haberham et al., 1999).

Pentobarbital administration has been shown to be more reliable for rats than for mice and provides approximately 60–120 min of anesthesia (Wixson et al., 1987a). Higher doses (80 mg/kg IP) have been utilized for carotid catheterization in rats (Lawson et al., 2001). Mice and rats may experience initial hyperexcitability, including hyperalgesia, during the induction phase and upon recovery with this agent (Field et al., 1993; Wixson et al., 1987d). Significant cardiovascular depression has been noted in pregnant and nonpregnant mice (Furukawa et al., 1998). In contrast, little effect on heart rate has been noted in rats, as compared to anesthesia with other injectable agents (Sage et al., 1985; Wixson et al., 1987b). Hypotension and uncompensated respiratory acidosis have been documented in rats (Field et al., 1993). Sex differences in tolerance have been noted with this agent, in that male rats clear the drug more rapidly than do females (Zambricki and Dalecy, 2004). A low incidence of irreversible corneal lesions has been noted in rats anesthetized with pentobarbital (Turner and Albassam, 2005). Hypothermia is common and is most likely a result of decreased metabolism, vasodilation, and depression of thermoregulation. Respiratory depression can be increased if pentobarbital is administered with tranquilizers, benzodiazepines, opioids, α2 agonists, propofol, and inhalant anesthetic agents. A supplemental heat source and oxygen, as well as close monitoring, are therefore advised (Papich, 2016).

Pentobarbital can be combined with other anesthetic agents, in particular medetomidine and tiletamine/zolazepam (Telazol), for long-term anesthesia in rats (Ferrari et al., 2005). Rats that received pentobarbital 1 h after buprenorphine had longer sleep times and longer durations of surgical anesthesia when compared to ketamine/xylazine (Roughan et al., 1999).

Thiobarbital (inactin) Thiobarbital [5-ethyl-5-(1-methyl propyl)-2-thiobarbiturate] induces anesthesia of longer duration than pentobarbital. Pharmaceutical-grade thiobarbital is no longer commercially available in the United States but may be found in other parts of the world or provided, with approval of the institutional IACUC or other appropriate governing bodies, in nonpharmaceutical-grade formulations. Anesthesia for 3 h has been documented in rats. Nevertheless, several authors report a certain variability in effect (Flecknell, 2015; Vogler, 2006). Administration of additional anesthetic boluses, typically given by the IP route, may be necessary for anesthesia of longer duration. This agent is most useful when a long anesthetic period is needed; however, redosing (in rats) using higher than published doses may be needed to maintain the absence of pedal withdrawal reflexes (Brammer et al., 1993). Thiobarbital, like pentobarbital, has variable analgesic activity (Brammer et al., 1993; Flecknell, 1996) and may impact liver function (Nemeth et al., 1985).

f. Alkylphenol derivative: propofol

Propofol represents the alkylphenol class of anesthetics (Wixson and Smiler, 1997). This agent is administered strictly IV, resulting in a smooth induction of anesthesia and rapid recovery. The major advantage of propofol is the lack of residual effects following administration; recovery is rapid and complete. There are no known active metabolites of propofol, and 90% of the drug is excreted in the urine as water-soluble by-products. Recovery remains rapid when delivered by short-duration infusions or repeated boluses to maintain anesthesia. This quick recovery is important for rodents to minimize complications, including hypothermia, dehydration, and prolonged fasting that can accompany prolonged postsurgical recovery periods. Propofol is not suited as a sole anesthetic agent for invasive procedures as it is not analgesic (Alves et al., 2007).

In rats, mean blood pressures with propofol administration are very stable for up to 3 h, with excellent survival rates (Brammer et al., 1993). Premedication with other agents may be necessary to sedate rodents prior to IV cannulation for propofol infusion (Brammer et al., 1993; Cantwell, 2001). Target-controlled infusions (TCIs) may be used for IV administration but requires additional equipment and knowledge of pharmacokinetics (Hacker et al., 2005).

Drawbacks to the use of propofol include cardiopulmonary effects: hypotension results from direct myocardial depression and vasodilation, and bolus injections can result in hypoventilation and apnea (Hacker et al., 2005). These adverse effects warrant close monitoring. The injection of propofol has been documented to be painful in humans and dogs and may be painful in rodents, as evidenced by a hypertension observed on induction (Brammer et al., 1993; Jalota et al., 2011; Michou et al., 2012). In humans, pain associated with propofol injection was decreased by premedication with dexmedetomidine or pretreatment with lidocaine (Jalota et al., 2011; Lu et al., 2021). Propofol supports bacterial growth when it is not formulated with an antibacterial agent, so manufacturer guidelines should be followed regarding how long to keep open vials.

g. 2,2,2 tribromoethanol: former avertin

Anesthesia provided by TBE is relatively inexpensive with minimal cardiodepressive effects when compared to other agents. TBE is administered by IP and provides rapid induction and recovery, loss of reflex activity, and good muscle relaxation (Papaioannou and Fox, 1993; Silverman et al., 2003; Weiss and Zimmermann, 1999; Zeller et al., 1998).

Nevertheless, this anesthetic has been linked to animal welfare and health issues related to complications with the reconstituted solution (Buetow et al., 1999; Lieggi et al., 2005a, 2005b; Norris and Turner, 1983; Zeller et al., 1998; Weiss and Zimmermann, 1999). TBE is therefore replaced with inhalant anesthesia for routine procedures (Chu et al., 2006), and its use is recommended only for acute terminal studies when administered IP (Meyer and Fish, 2005). Additionally, TBE is only available in nonpharmaceutical grade formulations and therefore must receive specific consideration by the IACUC or appropriate ethical review body as to the strength of the scientific justification for its use versus pharmaceutical grade anesthetics that are safer for rodents.

h. Neuroleptanalgesic combinations

Commercially available preparations of neuroleptanalgesic consist of an opioid analgesic and a potent tranquilizer. A particular advantage to these agents is that the effects of the opioid may be reversed using a specific antagonist, like naloxone. This will also result in a complete reversal of analgesia produced by the opioid; therefore, buprenorphine can be administered to reverse the respiratory depressant effects of the opioid (i.e., fentanyl) and also provide analgesia into the postoperative period (Flecknell, 1987b). One should be cautious with repeated dosing, which can be detrimental to the animal due to the accumulation of the tranquilizing agent. Respiratory depression can result in hypercapnia and acidosis.

Fentanyl/fluanisone Fentanyl/fluanisone, or Hypnorm, is the most popular combination of neuroleptanalgesic. Hypnorm is administered IM or IP, yet repeated boluses may not provide additional analgesia (Brammer et al., 1993). Hypnorm is most commonly mixed with a benzodiazepine, like midazolam or diazepam, to provide excellent surgical anesthesia for short-term procedures (Flecknell, 1987b; Richardson and Flecknell, 2005). Fentanyl, midazolam, and medetomidine are another possible combination for use in mice, which can be antagonized with naloxone/flumazenil/atipamezole (Fleischmann et al., 2016). Tachycardia, hypotension, or hypothermia may be noted with these combinations; plans for giving receptor antagonists and appropriate perioperative care should be in place (Brammer et al., 1993; Flecknell and Mitchell, 1984; Fleischmann et al., 2016). A low incidence of irreversible corneal lesions has been noted in rats anesthetized with Hypnorm/midazolam (Turner and Albassam, 2005). Hyperglycemia has also been induced in fed (not fasted) rats when placed under Hypnorm anesthesia (Johansen et al., 1994).

D. TIVA

Total intravenous anesthesia, or continuous infusion of intravenous injectable anesthetic, has been used in rodents but may be more appropriate as a method for chemical restraint than for invasive procedures that could induce pain. For example, TIVA with propofol and remifentanil only resulted in a successful surgical plane of anesthesia in 9 of 17 Sprague Dawley rats; in comparison, all 19 rats anesthetized with inhaled isoflurane achieved surgical plane anesthesia (Gazzaz et al., 2018). When paired with inhalant anesthesia for induction followed by maintenance with IV propofol from a syringe pump and buprenorphine to alleviate postsurgical pain, surgical resection of primary mammary tumors was possible in mice (Dubowitz et al., 2021).

E. Anesthetic adjuvants

Adjuvant agents for anesthesia are agents that are combined with the primary anesthetic agent or agents to gain specific advantages. Such advantages include a reduction in the dose of the primary anesthetic (with an associated reduction in adverse effects), an increase in the duration of the surgical plane of anesthesia or muscle relaxation, an increase in the depth of anesthesia, perioperative analgesia, or a more rapid recovery from anesthesia. However, there are disadvantages to adding adjuvant agents to the anesthetic regimen. The addition of any drug beyond the primary anesthetic potentially complicates the course of anesthesia for the animal. Since an unanticipated adverse effect is possible with the administration of any drug, each drug added to the regimen increases the possibility of an adverse reaction. The addition of drugs that depress essential functions, such as the cardiovascular and respiratory systems, means that supplemental doses of the primary anesthetic(s) may need to be reduced. The discussion below focuses on the advantages and disadvantages of drugs commonly used as anesthetic adjuvants (see also Chapter 5).

Of general note, many of the adjuvant agents described below are administered by injection and may require manual restraint of rodents. It should be noted that some restraint techniques can have direct and deleterious effects on health and stress parameters. For example, severe bradycardia and arrhythmia can occur if mice are scrunched too tightly (Labitt et al., 2021). Therefore, it is recommended to carefully consider restraint techniques and to minimize impacts on the animal while administering these agents.

1. *Anticholinergics*

Anticholinergics, such as atropine, are seldom utilized in the anesthesia of rodents. Their primary uses in anesthesia

TABLE 14.3 Anesthetic agents.

Drug	Dose mg/kg unless otherwise specified	Route	References
Rat			
Alphaxolone-alphadolone (Saffan, Althesin)	6–9 25	IV	Flecknell (2015)
Isoflurane (Forane)	0.25–2.5	Inhaled	Smith et al. (2004) Vaillancourt et al. (1999), Wood et al. (2001), Flecknell (2015)
Isoflurane/morphine	2% I/5 M	Inhaled, IP	Smith et al. (2004)
Ketamine (Ketaset)/diazepam	40–75 K: 5 D	IP	Wixson et al. (1987a), Flecknell (2015)
Ketamine/medetomidine	60–75 K/0.4–0.5 M	IP	Hedenqvist et al. (2000a), Flecknell (2015)
Ketamine/xylazine	40–100 K/5–10 X	IM, IP	Hsu et al. (1986), Stringer and Seligmann (1996), Wixson et al. (1987a), Flecknell (2015)
Ketamine/xylazine/acepromazine	40–50 K/2.5–8.0 X/0.75–4.0 a	IM, IP	Lawson et al. (2001), Flecknell (2015)
Medetomidine/fentanyl	200–300 M/300 F	IP	Hu et al. (1992)
Medetomidine/sufentanil	150 M/40–50 S	SC	Hedenqvist et al. (2000b)
Sevoflurane (Ultane)	2%–4%	Inhaled	Pape et al. (2006), Payne et al. (2005), Flecknell (2015)
Sodium pentobarbital (Nembutal)	30–60	IP	Rao (1990), Wixson et al. (1987a–d)
Tiletamine/zolazepam (Telazol)	20–40	IP	Ferrari et al. (2005), Wilson et al. (1992), Flecknell (2015)
Mouse			
Alphaxolone-alphadolone (Saffan, Althesin)	10–15	IV	Flecknell (2015)
Fentanyl/fluanisone/diazepam	0.1–0.4 mL of a 1:10 dilution of Hypnorm: 5 D	IP	Green (1975), Flecknell (2015)
Fentanyl/fluanisone/midazolam	10 mL/kg (one part Hypnorm, two parts water for injection, one part M (5 mg/mL)	IP	Flecknell (2015)
Isoflurane (Forane)	0.08%–2.8% Neonatal mice: 0.25%–2.5%	Inhaled	Szczensy et al. (2004), Cesarovic et al. (2010) Drobac et al. (2004), Gotoh et al. (2004)
Ketamine (Ketaset)/diazepam	100 K: 5 D	IP	Flecknell (2015)
Ketamine/medetomidine	50–75 K/L-10 M	IP	Cruz et al. (1998), Flecknell (2015), Hahn et al. (2005), Hedenqvist et al. (2000a), Taylor et al. (2000)
Ketamine/xylazine	80–150 K/7.5–16 X	IP	Clifford (1984), Flecknell (2015), Furukawa et al. (1998), Hahn et al. (2005), Zeller et al. (1998)
Ketamine/xylazine/acepromazine	80–100 K/2.5–10 X/2.5–3 a	IM, IP	Flecknell (1996, 2016)
Sevoflurane (Ultane)	4.9%	Inhaled	Cesarovic et al. (2010)
Sodium pentobarbital (Nembutal)	30–90	IP	Flecknell (1993b), Gardner et al. (1995)
Thiobarbital [5-ethyl-5-(l-methylpropyl)-2-thiobarbiturate] (Inactin)	80	IP	Buelke-Sam et al. (1978)
Reversal agents (rodents)			
Flumazenil (Romazicon) reverses benzodiazepines	10 nmol	IP	Sarlis and Kaniaris (1991), Stackman and Walsh (1992)
Atipamezole (Antisedan) reverses alpha-2 agonists	0.5	SC	Hahn et al. (2005), Hedenqvist et al. (2000b), MacDonald et al. (1989)
Naloxone hydrochloride (Narcan) reverses opioids	20	IP	Gross (2001), Levine et al. (1988)

of larger species are for their parasympatholytic actions of decreased salivation, decreased secretions in the respiratory tract, and prevention of vagus inhibition of the heart (Thurmon et al., 1996a). The need for these actions is much reduced or absent in rodents, eliminating the routine need to use these drugs. However, inclusion of atropine and increased inspired oxygen, improved recovery from ovariectomy surgery in obese BALB/c females from 0% to 83%; though the authors did not separately assess the two refinements, so their relative contributions to increased survival are not evident (Mattheis et al., 2016). Similar utility has not been observed in rats, perhaps because the rat rapidly metabolizes atropine due to its hepatic atropine esterase (Thurmon et al., 1996a).

2. Phenothiazine tranquilizers

Phenothiazine tranquilizers such as acepromazine, chlorpromazine, and promazine are often used in combination with ketamine or in combination with ketamine plus xylazine in mice and rats. Phenothiazines act to depress the brain stem and connections to the cerebral cortex (Gross, 2001). The addition of these tranquilizers improves muscle relaxation and decreases the total dose needed of ketamine or ketamine plus xylazine. Phenothiazine tranquilizers also reduce ventricular arrhythmias and cardiac fibrillation, especially those that are induced by epinephrine (Grimm et al., 2015). Acepromazine and chlorpromazine are suitable for imaging of the pupil and photoresponse measurements (Eckley et al., 2020). Tranquilizers do not provide analgesia, as evidenced by increased vocalization in response to a formalin test in ketamine/xylazine/acepromazine-treated rats (Alemán-Laporte et al., 2020) and a lack of reduced pain or distress when acepromazine was used prior to CO2 euthanasia in mice (Valentine et al., 2012). However, especially in higher doses, phenothiazine tranquilizers depress cardiac and respiratory function. They cause a decrease in arterial blood pressure as a result depression of vasomotor reflexes and vasodilation. They also have peripheral vasodilatory actions and central hypothermic effects, which can contribute to decreased body temperature in rodents and other small animals (Thurmon et al., 1996a). In combination with ketamine, acepromazine produced significant, prolonged, and variable decreases in heart rate and other echocardiography changes (Rottman et al., 2003). Providing supplementary oxygen during anesthesia with ketamine/xylazine/acepromazine significantly reduces the risk of hypoxia and improves mouse survival (Blevins et al., 2021). Acepromazine, a potent neuroleptic agent with a high margin of safety, is the most widely used phenothiazine tranquilizer in rodents and should be the first choice among these agents because of its long history of safe use in rodents. The combination of ketamine/acepromazine is unlikely to provide a surgical plane of anesthesia at typical doses, but may be adequate to promote a smooth induction of anesthesia with inhalants, or to provide deep sedation/light anesthesia suitable for noninvasive procedures (Gardner et al., 1995), and can be paired with appropriate analgesics for more invasive procedures. Ketamine/xylazine/acepromazine anesthesia can be delivered via intraperitoneal continuous rate infusion (CRI) using a butterfly needle and syringe pump; a method that may reduce the risks associated with bolus dosing of these drugs (Erickson et al., 2016). Several publications have evaluated potential beyond use dates for combined ketamine/xylazine/acepromazine mixtures, which may be useful for clinicians and in vivo scientists (Taylor et al., 2009; Dodelet-Devillers et al., 2016). Chlorpromazine has been identified as having varied neurotoxicity on ICR, BALB/c, and C57/BL6 and CDF1 mice (Messiha, 1991), though no similar reports have documented this in rodents due to acepromazine.

3. Benzodiazepines: diazepam

Benzodiazepines such as diazepam and midazolam are sometimes used in combination with ketamine or as a preanesthetic adjuvant for inhalant anesthetics. In therapeutic doses, there are minimal respiratory and cardiac effects. Neither have analgesic effects and diazepam may even cause hyperalgesia, and therefore should be avoided for sedation in the postsurgical period (Flecknell, 2009). Midazolam is very similar to diazepam but has a shorter duration of action and is water soluble, making it easier to mix with other agents (Flecknell, 2009). Both diazepam and midazolam have muscle-relaxant and anticonvulsant activities and act on parts of the limbic system, the thalamus, and the hypothalamus to produce calming effects (Grimm et al., 2015). In combination, they can counteract muscle rigidity induced by ketamine. Because of their anticonvulsant activities, they are an anesthetic adjuvant of choice for models of head trauma but should be avoided if seizures are the subject of study. The muscle relaxant activity is centrally mediated at the spinal cord (Thurmon et al., 1996a). Diazepam enhances blockade induced by neuromuscular blocking agents and other centrally acting muscle relaxants (Dretchen et al., 1971). The effects of diazepam can be antagonized by utilizing flumazenil (Lemke et al., 1996).

4. The action and use of opioids in anesthesia

Opioids, such as fentanyl, morphine, and buprenorphine are added to anesthetic regimens because they provide substantial analgesia in addition to allowing reduction of the dose of the primary anesthetic. Opioids produce a greater level of analgesia than xylazine, at commonly used dosages. This analgesic effect is produced by interacting with opioid receptors that normally act as receptors for the naturally occurring endogenous opioids, endorphins, and enkephalins (Branson and Gross, 2001; Grimm et al., 2015). The pharmacology of opioids and other analgesics is covered in Chapter 7. Unlike xylazine and phenothiazine tranquilizers, therapeutic doses of opioids given by SC or IP injection cause minimal depression of cardiovascular function, with minimal depression of the cardiac rate, rhythm, and cardiac output; thus, they can be used where cardiovascular parameters are under study or where the animal enters the anesthetic period with prior cardiovascular compromise. Additional discussion regarding the actions of opioid drugs is provided in Section 7.

a. Morphine and methadone

The primary beneficial pharmacologic effect of morphine is analgesia. Morphine is MAC-sparing in rats in a dose-dependent manner (Abreu et al., 2012). The primary disadvantage of morphine is depression of respiration. The effects of morphine are species-specific, and morphine produces analgesia without CNS or respiratory depression in the hamster (Gross, 2001). In guinea pigs, rats, and mice, a low dose of morphine causes elevations in body temperature, while larger doses cause body cooling (Branson and Gross, 2001). Unwanted systemic side effects of morphine, like respiratory depression, can be decreased by intrathecal administration (Thomas et al., 2017). Morphine is not recommended for animals with head trauma due to its role in increasing intracranial pressure (via hypoventilation, respiratory acidosis, and cerebral vasodilation). Morphine may be used by SC or IM injection in the mouse, rat, and guinea pig as a preanesthetic or analgesic and will be effective within 15 min. At 10 mg/kg, methadone reduced sevoflurane MAC up to 100% (Abreu et al., 2012). Of note, the study used the tail clamp method of nociceptive stimulus and not true surgical stimulus, and therefore during a surgery some inhalant anesthesia would likely still be needed; additionally, this dose of methadone also caused apnea in some rats.

b. Buprenorphine and butorphanol

Buprenorphine hydrochloride is a partial agonist with a high affinity for the mu-opioid receptor but only partial activity (Branson and Gross, 2001). It is slow in onset and long in duration. It is primarily used for postoperative analgesia because of its long duration of action and minimal adverse side effects and is used more often than morphine (Gross, 2001). In its standard HCl formulation, buprenorphine's analgesic effects may only last 4–6 h depending on dose and species; it may be used for preemptive analgesia (Myers et al., 2021; Foley et al., 2019). Buprenorphine can also be provided via oral dosing in a food substrate like nut paste or in a sustained or extended-release formulation. The sustained-release formulations show promise for providing at least 12–24 h of analgesia, possibly more (Myers et al., 2021; Foley et al., 2019). Butorphanol, dosed at 5 mg/kg, reduced sevoflurane MAC by 30% in rats, indicating a ceiling effect had been reached and higher doses would not further increase MAC sparing. At 10 mg/kg of butorphanol, some rats developed apnea (Abreu et al., 2012). When combined with medetomidine and midazolam, butorphanol resulted in 45 min sleep time in C57BL/6 and BALB/c mice (Kirihara et al., 2013).

c. Fentanyl citrate

Fentanyl citrate, a phenylpiperidine derivative, is more lipid-soluble than morphine, acts rapidly, and is approximately 50–100 times more potent than morphine (Gross, 2001). Fentanyl provides analgesia and sedation with a relatively short duration of action of less than 30 min, but is also a respiratory depressant. Plasma levels of fentanyl can remain above therapeutic levels for 12 h of analgesia in mice when provided in a sustained-release formulation (Kendall et al., 2014). Fentanyl with midazolam can induce sedation and attenuate aversive behaviors during induction of inhalant anesthesia in mice (Cesarovic et al., 2012). Fentanyl is recommended in combination with fluanisone, diazepam, midazolam, and/or medetomidine for anesthesia; however, these combinations may not be appropriate for an invasive surgery (Flecknell and Mitchell, 1984; Green, 1975; Ter Horst et al., 2018; Fleischmann et al., 2016). Fentanyl is also used to relieve postoperative pain via a transdermal patch (Duragesic) in larger species. Administration via transdermal patch may circumvent the short duration of action via continuous administration. These methods have been used with some success in larger animals but are not reported for rodents. With fentanyl, analgesia may last for a shorter period of time than does respiratory depression, which may last for several hours after dosing (Thurmon et al., 1996b). Fentanyl has been reported to increase auditory-evoked potential (AEP) and electroencephalogram (EEG) magnitude during anesthesia (Antunes et al., 2003). Fentanyl can be reversed by the narcotic antagonists nalorphine and levallorphan (Fleischmann et al., 2016).

d. Naloxone, nalorphine, and levallorphan—opioid antagonists

Naloxone hydrochloride is a competitive nonselective opioid receptor antagonist and is primarily used to antagonize the effects of the potent mu opioids (hydromorphone, methadone, morphine, meperidine, and fentanyl). Because it lacks agonist properties, it does not produce analgesia or respiratory depression when used alone. Due to its relatively short half-life, the reversal effects of naloxone may wane/disappear before the respiratory depression effects of the opioid that is being reversed, so animals should be observed until fully recovered. Naloxone also reduces the duration of anesthesia and LD_{50} of pentobarbital in rats (Branson and Gross, 2001; Lumb and Jones, 1984). Nalorphine hydrochloride and levallorphan tartrate are synthetic mixed agonist (kappa receptor)-antagonists (mu receptor) agents only available as nonpharmaceutical grade in the US. They can be used to partially reverse opiates to maintain some analgesia while reversing sedative and respiratory depression of mu agonists (Thurmon et al., 1996b).

5. Cholinergic agents

Physostigmine and 4-aminopyridine are central cholinergic agents that have been shown to shorten the duration of action of ketamine, but these agents are not commonly used as antagonists following ketamine anesthesia in rodents.

6. Local anesthetics for anesthesia and analgesia

a. Injectable local anesthetics

Local anesthetics such as lidocaine, bupivacaine, and others, may be used to block nerve transmission of pain at the surgical site as local or regional anesthetics. In conjunction with other agents, their use allows a substantial reduction in the requirement of general anesthetics, which will reduce adverse effects and speed recovery. However, they are seldom used alone in rodents because, unlike general anesthetics, they do not eliminate stressful perceptions or give immobility during the procedure. The use of local anesthetics without general anesthesia is not recommended for experimental rodents due to humane concerns and the chances of bite injury to humans. When carefully used, local anesthetics administered intravenously can be a useful adjunct to anesthesia (Arevalo et al., 2004; Flecknell et al., 1990; Sintov and Shapiro, 2004; Foley et al., 2019). Local anesthetics can preempt the priming of pain perception mechanisms. Local anesthetics, especially long-acting local anesthetics such as bupivacaine, also provide some analgesic effect in the postoperative period. The primary disadvantage of effective use of local analgesics is that they take time to full effect after topical application, and their duration of action can be short (30–60 min for lidocaine, longer for bupivacaine). Starting the surgery or procedure prior to full effectiveness negates the positive effects of using these drugs.

The two most useful injectable anesthetics for local or regional anesthesia in rodents are lidocaine and bupivacaine. Lidocaine has a fast onset of action with a moderate duration of analgesia, is very stable in solution, and spreads through local tissues (Branson and Gross, 2001). It is also effective when applied to the surface of mucous membranes or the cornea. Lidocaine has been shown to cross the placenta and, in the liver of fetal guinea pigs, reaches levels higher than maternal hepatic levels (Finster et al., 1972). Bupivacaine has a slower onset than lidocaine, but a longer duration of action. Bupivacaine is also stable in solution and is approximately four times as potent as lidocaine on a percent volume basis. Analgesic duration is at least twice as long as lidocaine and has been reported to last as long as 12 h in larger species (Hassan et al., 1993; Hayes and Flecknell, 1999), but can be expected to last only 1–7 h in most rodents (Roughan and Flecknell, 2004; Foley et al., 2019). Bupivacaine can be used to successfully perform a brachial plexus block in rats (Zhang et al., 2019). Either morphine alone or bupivacaine plus buprenorphine have been shown to be effective agents for epidural anesthesia in the rat (Akerman, 1985; Morimoto et al., 2001; Thomas et al., 2017).

IV. Historic anesthetic regimens used for special purposes

The following anesthetics have been used historically for specific research purposes; often prolonged anesthesia which require minimal impacts on specific physiological parameters. All of these historic anesthetics have the potential for increased pain or distress for animals, particularly if invasive procedures are required, and several have health and safety concerns for both the animals and staff exposed to these agents. In most cases, pharmaceutical-grade alternative anesthetic regimens have replaced these agents and offer equivalent benefits to the research, as well as superior animal welfare and safety. For this reason, many institutions have banned the use of these historic anesthetics. If an institution still allows the use of these agents, the below anesthetics should only be used for terminal procedures in which all other pharmaceutical-grade anesthetics have been found to be incompatible with research aims. Pairing with appropriate adjunct anesthetics and analgesics is recommended, and all uses of these anesthetics must be carefully reviewed and approved by the facility veterinarian, IACUC, or appropriate ethical review body, as well as health and safety experts.

- **i.** Inactin (thiobutabarbital sodium salt hydrate), a barbiturate with sedative and hypnotic properties, is primarily used in rodents where a longer duration of anesthesia is needed and may be combined with ketamine for a deeper plane of anesthesia (Lorenz, 2002).
- **ii.** Alpha chloralose depresses the CNS to result in a loss of consciousness while increasing reflex activity (Thurmon et al., 1996b) and has minimal depression of respiratory and cardiac reflexes such as baroreceptors and chemoreceptor activities (Branson and Gross, 2001; Thurmon et al., 1996b; Becker et al., 2016). Fentanyl-

fluazinone-midazolam provides more stable conditions for physiologic studies (Jong et al., 2002).

iii. Ethyl carbamate (urethane) has been used for procedures of exceptionally long duration where preservation of autonomic reflexes is needed but may be inferior to fentanyl-fluanisone-midazolam combinations (Jong et al., 2002).

iv. Chloral hydrate was historically utilized as it preserves some cardiovascular parameters; however, its use in rodents has largely been discontinued by the availability of safer anesthetics that provide better analgesia, such as ketamine/xylazine (Rodrigues et al., 2006).

A. Steroid anesthetics

The neuroactive steroid anesthetics, alphaxolone, and alphadolone, were originally formulated as a combination for use in humans and animals. More recently, a commercial formulation was developed containing alfaxalone (previously "alphaxalone") that is licensed for use in cats and dogs, with use reported in a range of laboratory species (Erickson et al., 2019). Alfaxalone produces sedative and anesthetic effects with no analgesia and can induce adverse behaviors in rodents. Therefore, alfaxalone is usually combined with other agents, such as xylazine, dexmedetomidine, and/or ketamine, and with analgesics for any procedures that could induce pain (Nadeson and Goodchild, 2000; Siriarchavatana et al., 2016; Erickson et al., 2019; West et al., 2020). It can be recommended for intravenous administration to hamsters and both IV and IP in rats and mice (Siriarchavatana et al., 2016; Erickson et al., 2019; West et al., 2020; Ferrini et al., 2020). Alfaxalone can be given as a CRI with ketamine-xylazine in rats to achieve a prolonged surgical plane of anesthesia (Heng et al., 2020). Significant sex and strain differences have been found in dose responsiveness to alfaxalone in mice (Erickson et al., 2019). Alfaxalone may be useful where inhalation anesthesia is not an option because it can be given repeatedly or continuously to maintain anesthesia for long periods without the development of tolerance or cumulation (Green et al., 1978; Ferrini et al., 2020). The original alphaxolone -alphadolone formulation can cause seizures in mice, and the newer formulations of alfaxalone were associated with hyperresponsiveness and intense scratching in mice, indicating this anesthetic is not appropriate as a single agent in rodents (File and Simmonds, 1988; Siriarchavatana et al., 2016).

V. Use of neuromuscular blocking agents and antagonists

See Chapter 8 for detailed information about the use of neuromuscular blocking agents (such as atracurium) as adjuvants to anesthesia when animal movement must be avoided. If used, ensure respiratory support (controlled ventilation) is provided, and confirm the chosen drug regimen adequately maintains anesthesia and analgesia for the duration of the procedure. The use of neuromuscular blocking agents requires additional training and experience to ensure welfare is not compromised through inappropriate use of these drugs. The use of paralyzing agents requires specific written justification in the animal care and use protocol and close collaboration with the facility veterinarian.

A. Depolarizing neuromuscular blocking agents

Succinylcholine is a commonly used depolarizing agent for mice and rats, which has a rapid onset and a short duration of action, making it useful in short clinical procedures where immobility is needed. Partial paralysis of rats may be maintained with approximately 10–50 μg/(kg min) constant-rate IV infusions with or without an initial IV bolus of 1 mg/kg of succinylcholine (Mishra and Ramzan, 1992b; Rana and Ramzan, 1995).

B. Nondepolarizing neuromuscular blocking agents

Nondepolarizing neuromuscular blocking agents act as competitive antagonists to acetylcholine (ACh) at postsynaptic ACh receptors. Some of these agents are closely related to or derived from curare, a plant toxin from South America, and have more pronounced systemic effects due to histamine release. Nondepolarizing agents that have been used in rodents include atracurium and gallamine. Other agents, including vecuronium, pancuronium, and rocuronium, are steroid analogs that have less deleterious physiologic effects (Hildebrand, 1997).

Atracurium has a quick onset and a relatively short duration of action, thus making it a suitable nondepolarizing agent for short procedures. Under 1.25 MAC of isoflurane or sevoflurane anesthesia, atracurium produces 50% paralysis in rats using an initial bolus dose of 0.31–0.36 mg/kg with maintenance using 3.7–5.0 mg/(kg h) (Shin et al., 1992). Much higher doses are necessary to provide for complete paralysis in rats. Under fentanyl anesthesia (1.25 g/(kg h)), a bolus of atracurium 4 mg/kg followed by 15 mg/(kg h) CRI results in 95% twitch suppression (Bohrer et al., 1994). Cisatracurium outperformed pancuronium at effectively preserving vagal function and baroreflex under anesthesia in rats (Kandukuri et al., 2018).

Gallamine is a neuromuscular blocker with parasympatholytic actions. Approximately 50% paralysis can be achieved with 4 mg/kg bolus and 3 mg/(kg h) IV (Mishra and Ramzan, 1992a, 1992b). In guinea pigs, gallamine produces dose-dependent bronchoconstriction and thus should be used with caution (Del Monte et al., 1990).

Vecuronium may be administered to rats in numerous ways. With a dose of 0.3 mg/kg injected IV, the induction of paralysis is very rapid (18 s), but the duration of action is very short (90 s). If administered intratracheally or IM (doses of 1.5 and 2.25 mg/kg, respectively), the duration of action is approximately 8 min after induction. The onset of action with intratracheal instillation in rats is about 4.5 min, while the onset with IM injection is more than doubled (Sunaga et al., 2006). Infusion of a lower dose of vecuronium (0.14 mg/(kg h)) produces a stable 50% neuromuscular depression (Weinger et al., 1995). When anesthetized with 1.25 MAC isoflurane or sevoflurane anesthesia, vecuronium produces 50% paralysis in rats in a dose range of 0.15–0.19 mg/kg bolus and can be maintained at 2 mg/(kg h) (Shin et al., 1992). Higher bolus (1.5 mg/kg) and infusion doses (7.5 mg/(kg h)) are needed to produce near-complete paralysis in rats (Bohrer et al., 1994). Under deep fentanyl anesthesia, a 0.75 mg/kg bolus and a 2.5 mg/(kg h) CRI of pancuronium produce similar results (Bohrer et al., 1994). Rocuronium, another nondepolarizing agent in the curare family, when infused IV at 12–19 nmol/(kg min), gradually increases blockade and produces a steady-state 90% neuromuscular block after 30 min (Epemolu et al., 2003).

C. Neuromuscular blocker antagonists

Neostigmine and physostigmine are acetylcholinesterase (ACH) inhibitors, which act to increase the amount of ACh at the neuromuscular junction by interfering with the enzyme that degrades ACh. They effectively act to reverse the effects of nondepolarizing agents that rely on low levels of ACh to work effectively. Neostigmine (0.03 mg/kg IV) can reverse the neuromuscular blocking effects of pancuronium in rats (Henning et al., 1993).

These agents also have effects not directly associated with the antagonism of neuromuscular blockers. Neostigmine has been demonstrated to counteract the opioid-induced ileus common with morphine and other opioids and slightly increase gastrointestinal motility in rats (Erbil et al., 1998). Physostigmine (0.1 mg/kg IP) may act to antagonize the effects of ketamine in rats, as evidenced by approximately 10%–20% reduction in the anesthesia time produced by ketamine alone (75 or 100 mg/kg IP) (Kubota et al., 1999; Mimura et al., 1992), but it does not decrease the limited analgesia provided by ketamine (Mimura et al., 1990). Interestingly, higher doses of physostigmine (up to 0.6 mg/kg) are not as effective as 0.1 mg/kg at antagonizing ketamine (Mimura et al., 1990). In comparison, the ketamine-reversal characteristic of neostigmine increases with an increase in dosage between 100 µg/kg and 200 µg/kg. Neostigmine has also been shown to shorten the duration of anesthesia from pentobarbital when used in the dose range of 150–200 µg/kg (Leeuwin et al., 1984) (see also Table 14.4 for dosages and routes).

D. Anesthetic management and monitoring

1. Peri-anesthetic support

Because rodents have a high surface area to body mass ratio, it is extremely important to provide thermal support starting immediately after anesthetic induction and continuing throughout full recovery (Taylor, 2007; Wixson et al., 1987c). Body heat is lost rapidly through anesthetic-mediated depression of thermoregulation, and this loss is accelerated when the fur is clipped and liquid disinfectants are applied. Body heat is also lost if the anesthetized rodent is in contact with conductive surfaces such as metals. Intra and postoperative thermal support can be accomplished

TABLE 14.4 Neuromuscular blocking agents.

Drug	Dose mg/kg unless otherwise specified	Route	References
Rat			
Atracurium (Tracrium)/Fentanyl	15 mg/(kg h) a CRI/1.25 mg/(kg h) F	IV	Bohrer et al. (1994)
Atracurium/isoflurane	360 µg/kg A/1.25 MAC I	IV	Shin et al. (1992)
Atracurium/sevoflurane	311 µg/kg A/1.25 MAC S	IV	Shin et al. (1992)
Vecuronium/fentanyl	1.5 bolus/7.5 mg/(kg h) CRI	IV	Bohrer et al. (1994)
Vecuronium/isoflurane	0.15–0.19 bolus V then IV 5.0 mg/(kg h) V CRI/1.25 MAC I	IV	Shin et al. (1992)
Vecuronium/sevoflurane	0.15–0.19 bolus V then 2.0 mg/(kg h) CRI/1.25 MAC S	IV	Shin et al. (1992)
Mouse			
Tubocurarine	1	IV	Flecknell (2016)

through the use of a heated surgery platform, heating pad, heated chamber or cubicle, or an in-cage heat source such as a sealed container of warm water or nontoxic self-heating chemical warming packs, which can be left in the animal's cage overnight. Recently, there has been some success with applying a prewarming strategy; raising core body temperature before induction of anesthesia in order to delay the onset of hypothermia (Schuster and Pang, 2018; Rufiange et al., 2020). Even if normothermia is maintained during anesthesia, external heat support can be useful in promoting a faster recovery. Where heat pads are used, their performance should be confirmed periodically (Zhang et al., 2017). Small rodents become easily hypoxic under anesthesia; oxygen supplementation can therefore reduce mortality or prolonged recovery (Blevins et al., 2021).

2. *Anesthetic monitoring*

General guidance on monitoring of anesthesia can be found in Chapter 10, and peri-procedural care can be found in Chapter 11. As with all species, ensuring the depth of anesthesia is appropriate for minimizing pain and distress is paramount. Depth of anesthesia in rodents is typically assessed by response to a noxious stimulus like a toe or tail pinch in smaller rodents like mice or rats or pinching an ear in guinea pigs (Flecknell, 2009). Hindlimb withdrawal response is lost before the withdrawal response of the forelimbs as the depth of anesthesia increases. Loss of palpebral reflex and eye position are difficult and unreliable measures of anesthetic depth in rodents; in addition, ketamine can reduce palpebral reflexes even if the animal is still only lightly anesthetized (Flecknell, 2009). The color of mucous membranes can also be helpful, as the color will become lighter if perfusion is significantly decreased, again indicating the animal may be too deeply anesthetized. However, observing for changes in color is an insensitive indicator of perfusion and hypoxemia and should not be the sole method of monitoring in use. Respiratory rate and quality can be easily observed in rodents. If respiratory rate decreases and deep, infrequent breaths are taken the animal is likely too deeply anesthetized and anesthesia should be turned off temporarily, reduced (if inhalant), or partially reversed (if possible, with injectables used) to avoid cardiac arrest. If heart rate, oxygen saturation, and respiratory rate are being monitored, these parameters should remain stable as a painful procedure begins and can be monitored to indicate if additional analgesia is needed throughout the procedure. Pulse oximeters for rodents are commercially available and can be a valuable addition for monitoring anesthesia, particularly when a single individual is both monitoring anesthesia and performing the procedure (not advised and in some locations not allowed) or when the animal needs to be monitored from a distance such as during a prolonged imaging procedure. Pulse oximetry is considered a fail-safe monitor as, while hypoxemia may not be common, it is poorly tolerated and can rapidly lead to death. Body temperature should also be closely monitored, as rodents lose significant amounts of body heat in a matter of minutes (10–15), which can result in prolonged recovery from anesthesia. Some homeothermic heating devices not only help monitor body temperature via a rectal probe but also feedback into a heating pad to adjust the degree of heat provided to maintain the animal at an appropriate temperature. While a financial investment, the speed, and quality of rodent recovery from anesthesia make them more than worthwhile.

E. Common anesthetic emergencies

Pulmonary and cardiovascular failure leading to hypoventilation and hypotension are the most common anesthetic emergencies. Careful monitoring to catch emergencies as early as possible is essential to allow for appropriate interventions to be applied. If the animal is too deeply anesthetized, steps must first be taken to lighten the anesthetic depth. This is one of the greatest advantages of inhalant anesthetics as the vaporizer can be turned down, or even off, until anesthetic depth returns to an appropriate level. If injectable anesthesia is used, the appropriate antagonist may need to be given. 100% oxygen should be supplied, where possible, by facemask or even flow-by. If the animal has stopped breathing and is intubated, external ventilatory support can be very carefully provided, ensuring not to exceed a peak end-expiratory pressure of about 15–20 cm H_2O. If not intubated, the bulb syringe portion of a medicine dropper can be used by placing the open end over the nose of the rodent and squeezing in puffs of air. Intermittent compression of the chest wall can also be commenced by holding the animal's thorax between the forefinger and thumb and gently but rapidly compressing the chest wall. To stimulate respiration, doxapram can also be administered, but care should be taken to provide oxygen as it increases systemic oxygen consumption. If a cardiac arrest has occurred, the compressions at the area over the heart can be made at about 90 times a minute. Emergency resuscitation drugs can be administered: epinephrine at 1 μg/kg or 0.2 mL per 20 mg of a 1:10,000 solution if blood pressure is low; if ventricular tachycardia is confirmed, lidocaine at 2 mg/kg IV, followed by 5 mg/kg IV if no response or epinephrine at 30 μg per kg. If bradycardia occurs, atropine at 0.02 mg/kg can be used (all emergency drug dosages from Flecknell, 2009).

VI. Anesthesia for specific situations

Examples: See Section 7.d for specific situations for anesthesia and analgesia, as well as Chapter 28 Anesthesia and analgesia in the fetus and neonate; Chapter 29

Anesthetic considerations for in vivo imaging studies; Chapter 27 Management of chronic pain, and Chapter 3 Optimizing anesthesia and analgesia for specific research projects for related information.

Return to group housing: Most rodents are social species. Social housing and the provision of enrichment have been shown to decrease the amount of analgesia mice self-administer after surgery (Pham et al., 2010) and improve recovery (Jirkof et al., 2015). Social enrichment has also been shown to decrease chronic pain in rodents (Bushnell et al., 2015). If stably housed with conspecifics, rodents, once fully recovered from anesthesia, should be returned to their cage mates. Rodents can be recovered from anesthesia with cage mates if they can be continuously observed to ensure they do not injure one another while in various states of recovery.

VII. Post-procedural recovery and care

In addition to the selection of the anesthetic regimen, it is important to have a general plan in place that includes animal preparation and postanesthetic recovery. All animals should be observed during recovery until they are able to move around independently. This is especially important for group-housed rodents because each cage group maintains a dominance hierarchy, and partially awake rodents may serve as targets for aggression. Anesthesia is a stressful event, independent of any other procedures performed, and alleviating other stressors as much as possible will maximize the animal's overall well-being.

A. Recovery period

Animals should be assessed frequently for signs of pain or distress over the following 24–72 h and appropriate treatment given. In general, since rodents are prey species that may mask signs of distress, it is better to err on the side of providing analgesics for too long a time than too short. Animals may also require assistance meeting their nutritional and fluid needs. Contingency plans should be in place for the treatment or euthanasia of animals experiencing adverse effects from anesthesia or the procedure. See Chapter 11 for more details.

B. Supportive care

Returning rodents to a home cage with an already established nest or hiding spot to facilitate some affiliative pheromones, as well as supplying some easily accessible and highly palatable food can also assist with recovery. Studies in hamsters and guinea pigs have demonstrated that even immediately after surgery, rodents will very quickly consume a preferred treat, which can serve as a quick source of nutrition and reduce stress (Oliver et al., 2017; Edmunson et al., 2021). Supplemental heat under a portion of the primary enclosure should be provided while animals are recovering. In addition, supplying warmed SC fluids or even temporarily housing animals in static cages rather than IVCs can also improve thermal support during post-anesthesia and operative recovery (Szilagyi et al., 2018). The recovery space should be quiet, warm, and somewhat darkened to alleviate the stress of these prey species.

C. Pain assessment

For an overview of general approaches to pain assessments, see Chapter 12. For an overview of pain assessments in rodents, see Turner et al. (2019). Early and accurate recognition of unalleviated pain in rodents can be exceptionally challenging. Since rodents are prey species that live in large colonies, individuals exhibiting weakness may be targeted as prey by aggressive conspecifics or predators. Rodents may minimize pain-associated behaviors, such as facial grimaces in mice and rats or weight shifting in guinea pigs in the presence of a cage-side observer, limiting the utility of real-time assessments of pain that require the animal to actively display a behavior, posture, or expression during the observation (Sorge et al., 2014; Miller and Leach, 2015a; Oliver et al., 2017; Whittaker et al., 2021; Chartier et al., 2020). If cage-side pain assessments are used, blinding observers to reduce the risk of bias may be an important consideration (Nunamaker et al., 2018). Taken together, these measures may allow for delineation between animals that underwent a painful procedure and those that did not, but it can be difficult to accurately assess how well their pain has been alleviated using real-time cage-side methods (Leung et al., 2016). Another approach to pain assessment is to identify evidence that normal behavior is not being performed, such as decreased wheel running, burrowing, nesting, or grooming (Turner et al., 2019). The advantage of these approaches is that they do not require the animal to perform a specific behavior in the presence of the observer, but rather are evident via proxy indicators, such as a poorly formed nest, food pellets not displaced, nest pieces not consolidated to the primary nest, or a poorly groomed coat, that reflects what the animals were doing/or not doing when the observer was out of the room. While these measures can be influenced by nonpainful stimuli, they can be scored cage side while also being sensitive enough to detect not just the presence of unalleviated pain but also discriminate between gradations of pain, such as differences in analgesia effectiveness between analgesic regimens (Oliver et al., 2018; Gallo et al., 2020; Alexander et al., 2019). Some pain assessment methodologies, like grimace scales, nesting, and ambulatory behaviors, are modulated by inhalant and injectable anesthetics or opioid analgesics, hypothermia, or by the presence of conspecifics, like nesting scores, and these effects should be considered and parsed, where possible, from the presence of unalleviated pain (Miller and Leach, 2015a; Miller et al., 2015; Miller and Leach, 2016; Miller et al., 2016a; Klune et al., 2020; Gallo et al., 2020; Avsaroglu et al., 2008; Oliver et al., 2018; Nunamaker et al., 2018; Mogil et al., 2020). Where each pain assessment method has its strengths and weaknesses, the most effective approach to pain assessment in rodents is to triangulate for the presence of pain by utilizing a variety of methods, including assessments of the animal's environment, such as nest building and cage organization (Arras et al., 2007), as well as direct animal assessments such as signs of effective grooming, body posture, and facial action units. Taken together, these signs will help alert staff that animals require veterinary attention and can be helpful as a red flag that additional analgesia and monitoring are needed. Signs of pain in mice and rats are

Test	Stimulus	Method	Measurement
Tail-flick [8,69]	Radiant heat	Apply thermal radiation to tail	Reaction time of tail movement. Typically, does not exceed 2–10s
	Hot water immersion	Submerse tail in hot water	
Hot plate test [8,69]	Thermal heat, 50–55°C	Place animal on hot plate	Reaction time to paw licking and/or jumping. Baseline latency 5–10s
Paw withdrawal test [8,69]	Thermal and inflammatory	Carrageenin-induced inflammation followed by response to radiant heat	Reaction time to paw withdrawal from heat source
von Frey test [8,69]	Mechanical allodynia	Apply filaments to inflamed area that bend at calibrated pressure	Paw withdrawal associated with force of filament bending
Randall–Selitto test [8,69]	Mechanical allodynia	Application of a fixed element with linear increasing mechanical force in grams	Appearance of pain behavior such as paw withdrawal, struggling or vocalization
Formalin injection test [8,69]	Chemical	0.5–15% formalin injected into plantar surface of paw	Biphasic response: a) initial response within first few minutes is acute pain, b) secondary response at 20–30 min representing inflammatory pain. Analgesia often assessed using response to mechanical stimulus such as von Frey or Randall–Selitto
Complete Freund adjuvant test [8,69]	Inflammatory	Injection of CFA into hind paw	Response to thermal or mechanical stimuli
Neuropathic pain [8,69]	Thermal and mechanical	Ligation of the sciatic nerve. Often referred to as chronic constriction injury.	Response to thermal or mechanical stimuli
Writhing test [69]	Chemical	Intraperitoneal administration of acetic acid	Abdominal contractions, reduced motor activity, and incoordination
Facial Grimace Scale [65,130]	Various	Assess facial expression to noxious stimuli	Scoring based on orbital tightening, and position of nose, ears, cheeks and whiskers
Ultrasonic vocalization[8]	Various	Assess ultrasonic vocalizations—evoked or spontaneous	Emit ultrasonic vocalizations with acute pain
Nesting behavior [58,114]	Various	Assess nest building complexity	Animal in pain will be less inclined to build a nest or maintain them
		Time to integrate nest material (TINT)	
Burrowing behavior [57]	Various	Assess burrowing	Animal in pain will be less inclined to burrow
Ethograms [1,63,100,119]	Various	Observation of behavioral changes associated with pain	Animal in pain will demonstrate altered behaviors

FIGURE 14.1 Measures of pain and nociception in rodents.

listed in Fig. 14.1 and are also addressed in Chapter 12, which discusses strategies for assessing and minimizing pain in laboratory animals. The presence of preexisting pain increases the frequency and strength of some pain-associated behaviors, such as withdrawal response to the hot plate and tail-flick tests while reducing the frequency of other normal behaviors such as ambulation and feeding.

The impact of unrecognized and therefore unalleviated pain is first and foremost poor animal welfare, but also negatively impacts the resulting data, its reproducibility and translation. The effect of painful stimuli and the demonstration of pain-associated behaviors in mice are also influenced by rodent genotype (Liang et al., 2006) and sex (Mogil, 2020, 2021). The perception of pain in cage mates and neighboring mice may also influence the demonstration of pain behaviors in mice (Langford et al., 2006; Martin et al., 2015).

VIII. Analgesia

A. Approaches to analgesia in rodents

Improved pain management for rodents is an important goal in the use of experimental animals. In the past decade, as supported by numerous scientific publications on this topic, there has been an increased emphasis on minimizing pain in experimental rats and mice (see the special issue in Comparative Medicine, December 2019 devoted to the topic). Factors contributing to improved rodent pain management include the continued increased use of mice and rats in biomedical research, growing ethical consideration for rodents within the field and by the public, availability and uptake of validated rodent pain assessments, and enhanced understanding of the impact of unalleviated pain on rodent research models (Importance of Pain and Pain Management, *Comparative Medicine* 69(6), December 2019).

The analgesics most commonly used for rodents and other laboratory animal species are opioids and nonsteroidal antiinflammatory drugs (NSAIDs), as well as local anesthetics (to a lesser extent). The literature summarized in the below section and in Fig. 14.2, demonstrates that for minor procedures such as a vascular cannulization performed by skilled staff, an NSAID may be sufficient for treating pain in rodents, for more invasive procedures such as laparotomies, a multimodal combination of an NSAID plus buprenorphine is needed. Higher doses, closer to 20 mg/kg, may be needed to provide effective analgesia for both meloxicam and carprofen. While the provision of NSAIDs in drinking water or other oral formulations is desirable as animals can self-administer the analgesic, only carprofen was readily consumed in drinking water and resulted in significant, though incomplete, postoperative analgesia, improved by pairing with injectable buprenorphine (Ingrao et al., 2013; Oliver et al., 2018). There is more evidence to inform the likely duration of effective analgesia for the most commonly utilized analgesics: twice-daily dosing for the most commonly used NSAIDs, carprofen and meloxicam, and buprenorphine requiring three times a day or even more frequent dosing. Sustained-release formulations of buprenorphine are improving the duration of analgesia, and as FDA-approved options become commercially available, will facilitate increased access and use. The ultimate decision for selecting a drug must be based on the experimental model under study and the specific types of data to be collected, paired with postprocedural pain assessments to recognize when unalleviated pain remains and requires additional analgesics. In rodents, pain from typical surgical procedures, such as laparotomies and craniotomies, has been documented to be present for at least 2 days after surgery (Cho et al., 2019; Nunamaker et al., 2018; Oliver et al., 2017), therefore the analgesia plan for surgeries of equivalent invasiveness should at a minimum cover this period of time. Here we discuss pain in rodents and provide a discussion of analgesics that are useful in relieving pain in experimental rats and mice, emphasizing the effects of specific analgesics on major types of models. Recommended analgesics, doses, and routes are listed in Table 14.5. For a comprehensive list of drugs with doses, the reader is directed to the formularies by Flecknell (2015, 2018) and Foley et al. (2019); for the pharmacology of these drugs, see Chapter 7.

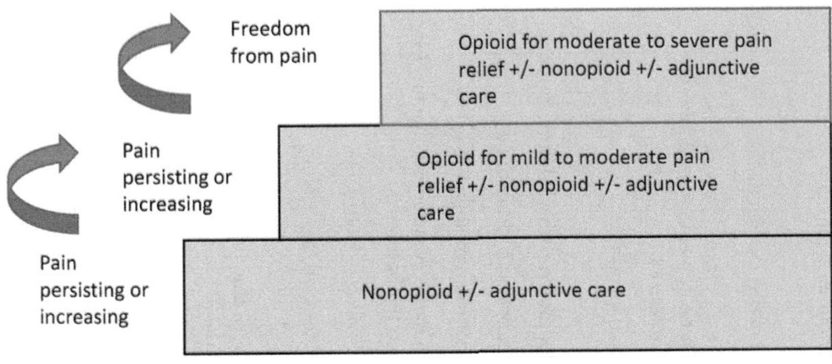

FIGURE 14.2 WHO's pain relief ladder for patient management. *Modified from https://www.who.int/cancer/palliative/painladder/en/.*

TABLE 14.5 Analgesic agents.

Drug	Use	Dose mg/kg unless otherwise specified	Route	References
Rat				
Acetaminophen (paracetamol, Tylenol)	AG	200–300	PO	Ince et al. (2015), Foley et al. (2019)
Aspirin	AG	100	PO	Jablonski and Howden (2002)
Bupivacaine (Marcaine)	LA	5	SC, local infiltration	GV-SOLAS (2020)
Buprenorphine (Buprenex)	AG	0.01–0.1 0.5	SC, IM PO	Foley et al. (2019), Hestehave et al. (2017)
Butorphanol (Torbugesic, Torbutrol, Stadol)	AG	1–2	SC	GV-SOLAS (2020), Flecknell (2015), Gades et al. (2000)
Carprofen (Rimadyl)	AG	2–5	SC	Foley et al. (2019)
Celecoxib (Celebrex)	AG	10–20	PO	Millecamps et al. (2005), Whiteside et al. (2004)
Dipyrone (Metamizole)	AG	100–250	SC, PO	Ince et al. (2015)
Dipyrone/morphine	AG	177–600 d/3.1–3.2 M	SC, IV	Hernandez-Delgadillo et al. (2002, 2003; Hernandez-Delgadillo and Cruz (2006)
Fentanyl (Sublimaze)	AG	0.01–1.0	SC, IV	Colpaert et al. (2001), Meert and Vermeirsch (2005), Stewart and Martin (2003a, 2003b), Ohtsuka et al. (2007)
Flunixin meglumine (Banamine, Flunazine)	AG	1–2,5	SC	GV-SOLAS (2020)
Gabapentin	AG	55 100	PO IP	Vollmer et al. (1986), Radulovic et al. (1995), Ma et al. (2011), McKeon et al., (2011), Zude et al. (2020)
Ibuprofen (Advil' Motrin, Nuprin)	AG	15–20	PO	Foley et al. (2019), GV-SOLAS (2020)
Ibuprofen/hydrocodone	AG	200 I/2.3 H	SC	Zelcer et al. (2005)
Ibuprofen/methadone	AG	200 I/1.7 M	SC	Zelcer et al. (2005)
Ibuprofen/oxycodone Inactin (ETMU): see thiobarbital	AG	200 I/0.5 O	SC	Zelcer et al. (2005)
Ketoprofen (Ketofen)	AG	2–5	SC	Foley et al. (2019)
Lidocaine (Xylocaine)	AG, LA	0.67–1.3 mg/(kg h) CRI	SC pump, SC local infiltration	Smith et al. (2002), GV-SOLAS (2020)
Lidocaine/prilocaine creme (EMLA Cream)	TA	Local application	Topical	Arevalo et al. (2004), Flecknell et al. (1990), Sintov and Shapiro (2004)
Meloxicam (Metacam)	AG	1–5	SC, IP, PO	Laird et al. (1997), Roughan and Flecknell (2003), Flecknell, (2015), Foley et al. (2019)
Meloxicam/tizanidine or clonidine	AG	0.5 M/0.25T	PO	Jain et al. (2002)
Metamizole	AG	100–250	SC, PO	Ince et al. (2015)
Methadone (Dolophine)	AG	0.5–3	SC	Erichsen et al. (2005)

Morphine (Duramorph)	AG	2.0–10 2.8	SC, IM SC local	Davis and Perkins (1993), Erichsen et al. (2005), Gades et al. (2000) Smith et al. (2003), Hestehave et al. (2019)
Naproxen/hydrocodone	AG	200 N/1.3 H	SC	Zelcer et al. (2005)
Ropivacaine	LA	2	SC local infiltration	Charlet et al. (2011)
Tramadol	AG	5–30	SC, IP	Taylor et al. (2016), Foley et al. (2019)
Mouse				
Acetaminophen (paracetamol, Tylenol)	AG	200	PO	Foley et al. (2019)
Bupivacaine (Marcaine)	LA	1–2 (max. 8)	SC, local infiltration	GV-SOLAS (2020)
Buprenorphine (Buprenex)	AG	0.05–0.1 1	SC PO	Foley et al. (2019), Jirkof et al. (2019)
Buprenorphine + carprofen	AG	0.1 B + 5 C	SC	Parker et al. (2011)
Butorphanol (Torbugesic, Torbutrol, Stadol)	AG	5	SC	Gades et al. (2000)
Carprofen (Rimadyl)	AG	2–20 10–25	SC PO	Matsumiya et al. (2012), Ingrao et al. (2013), Cho et al. (2019), Foley et al. (2019), GV-SOLAS (2020)
Diclofenac (Voltaren)	AG	8–28	IP, PO	Santos et al. (1998), Flecknell (2015)
Dipyrone (Metamizole)	AG	1.25 mg/mL drinking water	PO	Kumstel et al. (2020)
Flunixin meglumine (Banamine, Flunazine)	AG	4.0–11	IV, SC	Herrero and Headley (1996), Arras et al. (2007)
Ibuprofen (Advil' Motrin, Nuprin)	AG	30–40	PO	Foley et al. (2019)
Ketoprofen 2–5 SC	AG	2–5	SC	Foley et al. (2019)
Lidocaine (Xylocaine)	AG	2–4	SC local	GV-SOLAS (2020)
Lidocaine/bupivacaine	LA	10 L + 2–5 B	SC local	GV-SOLAS (2020)
Lidocaine/buprenorphine	AG	0.44 mM L/0.18 mM in DMSO	Topical	Kolesnikov et al. (2000)
Lidocaine/morphine	LA	0.85 mM L/1.7 mM in DMSO	Local	Kolesnikov et al. (2000)
Lidocaine/prilocaine creme (EMLA Cream)	TA	Local application	Topical	Arevalo et al. (2004), Flecknell et al. (1990), Sintov and Shapiro (2004)
Meloxicam (Metacam)	AG	2–10 10–20	SC, IP PO	Santos et al. (1998), Ingrao et al. (2013), Chen et al. (2016) Foley et al. (2019)
Morphine (Duramorph)	AG	10 6.1 mM in DMSO	SC Topical	Gades et al. (2000) Kolesnikov et al. (2000)
Ropivacaine	LA	1–2	SC local	GV-SOLAS (2020)
Tramadol (Zydol, Ultram)	AG	5–40	SC, IP, PO	Foley et al. (2019), Evangelista-Vaz et al. (2018a, 2018b), Jirkof et al. (2019)

AG, analgesic; I, induction agent; LA, local anesthetic; TA, topical anesthetic.

B. Timing of analgesia

1. Multimodal analgesia

In many models in rodents, multimodal analgesia has outperformed single-agent anesthesia, particularly for moderate to significantly invasive procedures. See the below sections on opioids and NSAIDs and Table 14.5 for specific recommendations.

2. Preventive analgesia

Preemptive analgesia, more recently referred to as preventive analgesia, or the provision of analgesic drugs in advance of the painful stimulus is well accepted for minimizing pain in humans and should be afforded to rodents as well (Foley et al., 2019; Dahl and Kehlet, 2011). While some conflicting evidence exists in the literature, the majority of reports align with what is well-known in human medicine, preventative analgesia can decrease the amount of postoperative analgesia required and can decrease secondary hyperalgesia (Dahl and Kehlet, 2011; Katz et al., 2011). Conversely, liposome-encapsulated hydromorphone provides preemptive analgesia for rats undergoing sciatic nerve resection (Smith et al., 2006), and bupivacaine local nerve blocks prevent subsequent hyperalgesia from thermal pain but fail to protect rats against hyperalgesia triggered by mechanical stimulation (Themistocleous et al., 2007). Preemptive buprenorphine given 30 min before surgery resulted in some protection from a postop decrease in food intake (Hayes and Flecknell, 1999), resulted in superior analgesia than when given at the time of anesthetic reversal administration (Izer et al., 2014), and preemptive pethidine prevented postovariohysterectomy hyperalgesia in rats (Lascelles et al., 1995).

At a minimum, analgesics should be provided in a way such that adequate plasma or local levels to minimize the anticipated pain are achieved by the time the animal will be conscious and able to experience both the physical and emotional components (suffering) incurred by a painful procedure. Therefore, it is critical to know the time expected for not only different analgesics, but also different routes of administration to achieve adequate concentrations to provide effective analgesia. Subcutaneously dosed analgesics may take 15–30 min and may be influenced by hypo or hyperthermia. Orally administered drugs, such as carprofen in drinking water can take 24 h before surgery to reach effective analgesic levels (Oliver et al., 2018). Not only preoperative but also immediate postoperative analgesic administration is important for adequate pain relief in postsurgical rodents. Intermediate doses of morphine (3 mg/kg) given parenterally 30 min before, and 30 min and 2 h after a simple abdominal surgery provide adequate pain relief over a 2-day period. Administration of this same dose later in the postsurgical period provides only transient relief (Gonzalez et al., 2000).

Presurgical administration of analgesics will reduce the amount of anesthesia needed during surgery. If analgesics with sedative effects are used preemptively, care should be taken to assure doses of anesthetics are adjusted to account for any synergistic effects on the depth of anesthesia and associated cardiovascular and respiratory effects. For example, when given preemptively, both the standard and sustained release formulations of buprenorphine reduced the concentration of isoflurane needed to achieve a surgical plane of anesthesia in mice (LaTourette et al., 2020). This is true for injectable anesthesia, as well; rats given buprenorphine at the beginning of a surgery require less propofol over the course of the surgery, resulting in a significantly reduced total anesthesia requirement and significantly improved recovery score (Penderis and Franklin, 2005). If using preemptive analgesics for the first time with a standard anesthetic regimen, careful monitoring should be used to titrate the amount of anesthetic required under new conditions, and a single animal should be anesthetized at a time to allow for the regimen to be optimized before a whole cohort of animals undergos anesthesia plus preemptive analgesia.

C. Pharmacologic options

1. Opioid analgesics

Opioids vary greatly in potency, duration of action, potential side effects, and negative interactions with other compounds. These factors and the expected level of post-procedural pain must be considered when choosing an appropriate opioid to administer to rodents (Gades et al., 2000; Genedani et al., 1999; Foley et al., 2019). Opioids act centrally to decrease pain perception and have anxiolytic properties, which may have the added effect of reducing the emotional, or suffering, component of the pain experience (Falcon et al., 2015). The most serious adverse effect of opioids is respiratory depression, which may occur depending on the agent, administration, and target receptor. Respiratory depression when the animal is under anesthesia is seen more in mu-and delta-agonists and less in kappa-agonists (Heavner, 1997). A common side effect of opioid analgesia is hypomotility of the gastrointestinal tract (Gawrisch and Cheng, 1990), ultimately leading to decreased food intake, which can prolong convalescence, and which may be of special concern in models involving gastrointestinal surgery. However, it is critical to note that unalleviated pain can induce equal degrees of decreased food intake and weight loss as buprenorphine in rodents but without the added benefit of comfort (Oliver et al., 2017, 2018). Therefore, this negative side effect of opioids should be balanced with the equivalent negative impacts of unalleviated pain. The development of dependence and tolerance is another important factor in determining the usefulness of the long-term administration of opioid analgesia (Roy et al., 2005).

Optimized opioid dosing of rodents is important, not only to prevent high-dose side effects such as respiratory depression but also to prevent hyperalgesic effects often seen in low-dose opioid administration (Crain and Shen, 2001). Many published rodent formularies offer very wide ranges of doses of opioids; therefore, investigators along with consulting laboratory animal veterinarians must evaluate individual animals to determine what agent and dose are appropriate for a particular species and protocol. These opioid regimens may need to be tested and customized for appropriate dose levels during model development.

Because of their potential for abuse and addiction, most opioids are controlled substances. Regulations delineated by federal or local agencies (e.g., Drug Enforcement Agency in the United States) will necessitate increased security in maintaining a stock of these drugs in animal facilities.

a. Morphine

Morphine is one of the classic opioids and is often used as a standard to measure comparative potency among opioid drugs. Morphine acts primarily at the mu-opioid receptor, as demonstrated by studies in mu-receptor knockout mice (Matthes et al., 1996). In vitro, morphine has been shown to bind to both delta and kappa receptors. Morphine interacts with other drugs, such as inhalant and injectable anesthetics and analgesics, to reduce the overall necessary dose of anesthetic or analgesic. Subanesthetic doses of ketamine not only potentiate the analgesic response of morphine but also may further reduce the activity level in rodents concurrently administered with both of these agents (Campos et al., 2006).

Regardless of route of administration, morphine has a relatively short duration of action, thus limiting its use in a laboratory animal setting where 24-h intensive care is not routinely provided. In rats and mice, 10 mg/kg of morphine provides analgesia adequate to relieve severe pain for only 2−3 h (Gades et al., 2000). A sustained-release formulation of morphine, provided by gavage, resulted in increased paw withdrawal latencies in rats for 11 h; however, the clinical effectiveness was not determined (Leach et al., 2010). Morphine can reduce remotely recorded and scored Rat Grimace Scale scores after laparotomy at 40 mg/kg SC (Sotocinal et al., 2011; Kawano et al., 2014). Morphine alone has been shown to be effective at alleviating pain due to bone cancer in mice, but more complete analgesia is achieved if morphine is administered concurrently with oral acetaminophen (Saito et al., 2005). In nerve injury models, morphine has been shown to be effective in alleviating pain in rats, contrary to the long-held belief that opioids in general are poor analgesics for neuropathic pain (Erichsen et al., 2005; Joshi et al., 2006). A commonly used dose range, 2−10 mg/kg, is useful to alleviate pain in rats with arthritis induced by complete Freund's adjuvant (CFA) (Davis and Perkins, 1993). Application of morphine in DMSO to the tails of mice produced local, dose-dependent analgesia with no uptake of the morphine by central receptors (Kolesnikov and Pasternak, 1999).

Although morphine administration in mice is not likely to produce inappetence due to ileus, gastrointestinal side effects can be noted in rats at doses as low as 10 mg/kg (Meert and Vermeirsch, 2005; Stevenson et al., 2006). Although rodents cannot vomit, opioid-induced nausea leading to pica behavior is possible and may be more severe with morphine than with other opioids, as is often observed in both humans and dogs (Ramsey et al., 2014). Small intestinal and cecal lumen bacterial counts are increased in morphine-treated rats with a 100% incidence of bacterial translocation through the intestinal wall (Erbil et al., 1998).

Encapsulation in a lipid-bilayer liposome greatly increases the intensity of analgesia and extends the duration of action of morphine (Smith et al., 2003) If encapsulated morphine is administered intrathecally, the onset of action is rapid, but analgesia is prolonged dramatically, up to 32 times longer duration than parenteral morphine (Kim et al., 1996). Intrathecal administration has been shown to be as efficacious as SC morphine or buprenorphine in rats (Thomas et al., 2017). Mice develop a tolerance to morphine after several days of repeated single doses (Tokuyama et al., 1998), although tolerance is not noted if the morphine is continuously administered for several days (Backonja et al., 1995). Therefore, morphine may not be an appropriate choice for the relief of chronic pain if a CRI is not practical or available. Parenteral dosing of morphine may also produce acute variations in circulating sex hormones in the rat (Ceccarelli et al., 2006).

b. Buprenorphine

Buprenorphine is a preferred analgesic to relieve moderate postsurgical pain in rodents. Buprenorphine is a partial mu-agonist and is much more potent than morphine, with a longer duration of action. In rats, it has a very wide safety margin, producing a low level of analgesia at low doses and much stronger analgesia at higher doses with little increase in side effects (Meert and De Kock, 1994; Meert and Vermeirsch, 2005). Buprenorphine is very useful to relieve moderate pain and is the most practical and clinically useful opioid analgesic for rodents (Roughan and Flecknell, 2002; Foley et al., 2019); particularly when given preemptively (Izer et al., 2014). Buprenorphine relieves many types of pain. It has been shown to increase the latency of thermal tests over a wide range of doses but is effective against inflammatory pain over a much narrower range. Buprenorphine is generally less effective against mechanically induced pain, but is effective at higher doses

(0.055 mg/kg IV and 0.129 mg/kg IP) in treating neuropathic pain (Christoph et al., 2005). In rat nerve injury models, buprenorphine in this same range reduces mechanical sensitivity without impacting postsurgical body weights (Stewart and Martin, 2003b). Buprenorphine (0.05 mg/kg s.c) was ineffective at allevaiting post-vasectomy pain in mice (Miller et al., 2016b). The duration of buprenorphine treatment and its dose have a significant effect on the maintenance of body weight in rats. Doses of 0.05 mg/kg versus 0.01 mg/kg appear to produce equivalent analgesia following laparotomy in Sprague–Dawley rats. Rats exhibit a dose-dependent response to the tail-flick test when buprenorphine is administered up to the maximal effective dose of 2.5 mg/kg. Doses exceeding 10 mg/kg SC (up to 80 mg/kg) reduce the pain, but to a lesser extent than lower doses (Meert and Vermeirsch, 2005). Repeated doses in the higher range reduce food intake, resulting in weight loss, a consequence not seen at the lower doses (Jablonski et al., 2001). If administered SC, 0.3 mg/kg is effective at eliminating low-intensity thermal pain in rats only 30 min postinjection but has limited efficacy for more intense pain over the same period. Higher doses have no additional analgesic effect on this short-time course (Abram et al., 1997). Over a longer time course, SC administration of 0.5 mg/kg in rats produces 6–8 h of analgesia, and 2.0 mg/kg in mice produces 3–5 h of analgesia (Gades et al., 2000). Therefore, while typically injectable buprenorphine is dosed at 12-hour intervals, pharmacokinetic profiles indicate it is likely only effective in rodents for 4–6 h and therefore should be dosed more frequently (Foley et al., 2019; Jirkof et al., 2015). When dosed with buprenorphine three times a day, postoperative male Wistar rats expressed more pica behavior, gnawing on petri dishes placed in their home cages, than when dosed twice a day; despite this, the rats dosed three times a day did not experience any differences in food consumption or body weight compared to the twice daily dosed rats (Schaap et al., 2012). Consumption of corn cob bedding was also observed in rats dosed twice-daily with 0.05–0.1 mg/kg standard buprenorphine, but significant impacts on overall health were not noted (Nunamaker et al., 2018).

Sustained- and extended-release formulations of buprenorphine are available through several means. An FDA-approved extended-release buprenorphine formulation for rodents is commercially available in the US and can be ordered with a researcher's license, i.e., does not require a veterinarian's prescription (Ethiqa, Fidelis, New Brunswick, NJ). A sustained-release buprenorphine formulation sold by a commercial compounding pharmacy, also commercially available in the US, requires a veterinary prescription (ZooPharm, Windsor, CO). Several bespoke formulations have been created at individual institutions using various stabilizers in suspension that can be of particular value in Europe and other parts of the world where the commercial formulations are not available (Liu et al., 2006; Traul et al., 2015; Jirkof, 2015; Schreiner et al., 2020; Guarnieri et al., 2018). The sustained and extended-release formulations indicated plasma levels believed to be therapeutic (1 ng/mL) were present in rodents over a wide range of durations, 12–72 h (Foley et al., 2011; Clark et al., 2014; Jirkof, 2015; Kendall et al., 2014; Traul et al., 2015; Navarro et al., 2021b; Levinson et al., 2021; Alamaw et al., 2022). In a tibial defect model in rats, sustained release buprenorphine (ZooPharm) resulted in rats being willing to perform significantly more vertical raises than those treated with the standard formulation of buprenorphine, but fewer vertical raises than the nonsurgical controls over the 3 days following surgery, indicating improved efficacy from the standard formulation but could still benefit from additional analgesia (Foley et al., 2011). In a rat plantar incisional model, twice-daily dosing of standard formulation buprenorphine (0.5 mg/kg) provided similar analgesia as sustained release buprenorphine (ZooPharm) at doses of 0.3–4.5 mg/kg for effective analgesia for incisional pain for 48–72 h; however, the highest dose (4.5 mg/kg) resulted in weight loss and sedation and was therefore not recommended (Chum et al., 2014). Effectiveness at preventing mechanical, but not thermal, hyperalgesia at a dose of 1.2 mg/kg (ZooPharm) was also found in a rat plantar incisional model, with some breakthrough pain on the 2nd day after surgery (Zude et al., 2020). A single dose of 0.5–1 mg/kg sustained-release buprenorphine (ZooPharm) effectively attenuated thermal hypersensitivity after skin incision in neonatal rat pups for at least 8 h after surgery (Blaney et al., 2021). In a mouse plantar incisional pain model, thermal and mechanical hypersensitivity were prevented with low (3.25 mg/kg) and high (6.5 mg/kg) doses of extended-release (Ethiqa) buprenorphine for at least 48 h, whereas sustained-release buprenorphine (ZooPharm) only attenuated mechanical, not thermal, hypersensitivity over that same time frame (Navarro et al., 2021b). Similarly, in a rat plantar incisional pain model comparing these same formulations, based on mechanimal hypersensitivity and plasma concentrations, the authors recommended a single SC dose of 0.65 mg/kg extended release buprenorphine (Ethiqa) to achieve 3 days of analgesia (Alamaw et al., 2022). One additional formulation of sustained-release buprenorphine FDA-approved for cats (Simbadol, Florham Park, NJ) has also been assessed in mice and rats and determined to not provide significant advantages over standard buprenorphine HCl formulations and perhaps does not outperform other extended or sustained-release formulations either (Kendall et al., 2021; Houston et al., 2021). Absorption of the sustained-release formulation may be limited in athymic nude rodents due to the deficient immune system being unable to dissolute the vehicle to absorb the buprenorphine (Page et al., 2019). Side effects of these prolonged-duration buprenorphine formulations can include body weight loss from decreased consumption, overgrooming, pica, and skin lesions at the site of injection (Allen and Johnson, 2018; Page et al., 2019; Levinson et al., 2021; Nunamaker et al., 2018).

When given alone, buprenorphine may not provide adequate analgesia for more invasive surgical procedures, such as laparotomy, but it can be combined effectively with other opioids or NSAIDs to provide even more effective analgesia (Oliver et al., 2017; Oliver et al., 2018; Foley et al., 2019). Buprenorphine was not effective when used alone in a rat bowel transplant model (Camprodon and Bowles, 2006), resulting in poor analgesia and high mortality. Other studies have shown that for specific surgeries, varying doses of parenteral buprenorphine in rats are not effective at reducing pain thresholds below vehicle/control levels (Kirsch et al., 2002) and may actually prolong recovery (Sharp et al., 2003). The analgesic effects of buprenorphine were not reduced when atipamezole was given to reverse injectable anesthetics in mice (Izer et al., 2014).

In rats, self-medication of buprenorphine (0.5 mg/kg in flavored gelatin) may provide pain relief adequate to maintain food and water intake, avoiding postsurgical weight loss (Flecknell et al., 1999b; Liles et al., 1998), and normal activity after surgery (Jablonski and Howden, 2002). Conflicting studies utilizing pain testing and scoring by Martin et al. have demonstrated that the pain threshold in rats is not increased with self-medicated oral dosages of buprenorphine. Instead, these reports advocate SC administration of 0.05 mg/kg as an effective dose to increase the pain threshold in rats (Martin et al., 2001; Thompson et al., 2004, 2006). Oral dosing, through medicated gels or in nut paste, can extend the duration of the analgesic effect of buprenorphine to 12−14 h and reduce the need for injections and peaks/troughs from periodic injectable delivery. However, ingestion, and therefore benefit from the drug can be variable, it requires the provision of the medicated substance well in advance of the painful stimuli to ensure adequate plasma levels are reached before pain begins, and the risk for diversion control must be considered (Goldkuhl et al., 2010; Hovard et al., 2015). Based on this balance of concerns, it is recommended that caution be exercised while administering buprenorphine by ingestion.

Administration of buprenorphine has been shown to result in pica (e.g., ingestion of bedding) and overgrooming to the point of self-injury in rats both with and without prior laparotomy (Clark et al., 1997; Allen and Johnson, 2018; Levinson et al., 2021). Buprenorphine-induced pica may reduce long-term growth (Jacobson, 2000). Pica has not been documented as a side effect of buprenorphine in mice. Parenteral dosing of buprenorphine may also produce acute variations in circulating sex hormones in the rat (Ceccarelli et al., 2006). Chronic administration of buprenorphine to rats (1.2 mg/kg twice daily for 14 days) produces analgesic tolerance (Gringauz et al., 2001).

c. Fentanyl

Fentanyl is a potent and relatively short-acting full mu-agonist. Due to this short duration, it is typically utilized to control postoperative pain as a continuous infusion or transdermally and, as such, is rarely used as postprocedural analgesia in rodents. Fentanyl is more commonly found as part of an anesthetic regimen for rodents or for analgesia in larger species, where fentanyl patches can be more practically and safely applied. Meert and Vermeirsch (Meert and Vermeirsch, 2005) determined that 0.16 mg/kg of fentanyl administered subcutaneously in rats has an onset of action within 15 min and produces analgesia for at least 2 h. Sustained release formulations have been assessed in mice and provided 12 h of plasma levels greater than what is presumed to be therapeutic (Kendall et al., 2014). In rat nerve injury models, fentanyl reduces mechanical sensitivity while allowing for the maintenance of body weight following surgery (Stewart and Martin, 2003b). Fentanyl is administered to rats and mice in a wide range of doses with 0.01−1.0 mg/kg IP having been reported to be effective (El Mouedden and Meert, 2005; Stewart and Martin, 2003a, 2003b). Chronically arthritic rats self-medicated with fentanyl in drinking water and altered their intake based on the pain they experienced, not due to the development of a progressive opioid dependence (Colpaert et al., 2001).

Fentanyl patches designed for transdermal delivery, which are used in a variety of larger animals, are not yet used in rodents due to practical considerations such as the size of the patient relative to the patch and the amount of fentanyl contained in patches originally designed for humans. Because the fentanyl gel matrix is released through the transmembrane at a titered rate, patches cannot be cut into pieces prior to use without risking a fatal analgesic overdose. Fentanyl may be applied topically to nonhaired skin in an aqueous cream base, and in this preparation, fentanyl improved wound healing, wound contracture, cellular proliferation, and angiogenesis in rats (Poonawala et al., 2005). A technique to extend the duration of effectiveness of fentanyl and to mimic the sustained release seen in transdermal delivery is to encapsulate the opioid in liposomes. Encapsulation greatly increases the intensity of analgesia and extends the duration of action of fentanyl (Thornton et al., 1998); however, producing encapsulated fentanyl in-house is an intricate process, and commercial availability is limited (Smith et al., 2003).

Fentanyl analogs, such as remifentanil, alfentanil, and sufentanil, are not currently or commonly used as analgesics in rodents due to the very short duration of analgesia and rapid development of analgesic tolerance (Kissin et al., 1996).

Parenteral dosing of fentanyl may produce acute variations in circulating sex hormones in the rat (Ceccarelli et al., 2006). In rodents, single boluses as well as short-term infusions of fentanyl and fentanyl analogs may result in prolonged hyperalgesia following the surgical procedure (Celerier et al., 2000, 2006). It is advised that complete analgesic coverage postoperatively should combine fentanyl (or its analogs) with other pain medications. In rats, the use of subanesthetic doses of ketamine alleviates this postoperative hyperalgesia state (Richebe et al., 2005). In rats, gastrointestinal side effects from fentanyl are less than those noted with other opioids and generally occur at doses higher than those necessary to produce analgesia (Meert and Vermeirsch, 2005).

d. Methadone, oxymorphone, and hydromorphone

Methadone, a μ selective opiate with additional analgesic properties via NMDA antagonist actions, is increasingly being utilized for larger species due to fewer opiate-associated nausea and vomiting and a wider range of licensing. Publications of its analgesic efficacy in rodents are limited, but where methadone is replacing oxymorphone in larger veterinary species, increased use in rodents may follow. When administered to mice with intraperitoneal Ehrlich carcinoma, methadone reduced mouse grimace scores only 40 min after administration and was outperformed by morphine (Rusch et al., 2021). In nerve injury models, methadone, a mu-agonist, has been shown to be effective in alleviating pain in rats (Erichsen et al., 2005), contrary to the long-held belief that opioids in general are poor analgesics for neuropathic pain (Kupers and Gybels, 1995). Methadone has been shown to produce additive analgesic effects when paired with other opioids (Bolan et al., 2002), an effect that may be due to its partial NMDA-antagonist activity (Ebert et al., 1995).

Oxymorphone has limited use because of its abbreviated analgesic duration. Chronically administered oxymorphone reduces pain-related behavioral changes such as altered grooming behavior, squinting eyes, activity, and agitation in rats subjected to a laparotomy (Gillingham et al., 2001). Oxymorphone was also demonstrated to effectively treat visceral pain in a gastrointestinal distension model (Briggs et al., 1995). Sustained-release oxymorphone in the form of liposome encapsulation has allowed for some use in mice (Thornton et al., 1998) and rats (Krugner-Higby et al., 2003; Smith et al., 2003); however, producing encapsulated oxymorphone in-house is an intricate process, and commercial availability is limited (Clark et al., 2004).

Commercially available extended-release hydromorphone capsules, delivered by gavage, resulted in 3 h of prolonged latency to withdrawal in Hargreaves tests in rats (Leach et al., 2010). However, where sustained-release buprenorphine provides longer-duration analgesia in rodents, current applications of the extended-release hydromorphone formulations are likely limited. Although not commercially available as a ready-to-use product, hydromorphone-impregnated rods may be relatively easily produced in the laboratory with some specialized equipment and skills and have been shown to provide some efficacy in rodents (Hasirci et al., 2003; Sendil et al., 2003).

e. Kappa receptor agonists: butorphanol, nalbuphine, and pentazocine

Butorphanol is a kappa-agonist and mu-antagonist more typically used for anesthetic purposes due to the short duration of action (1−2 h), and its utility is limited to minor pain (Gades et al., 2000). Even a compounded sustained-release formulation of butorphanol resulted in dramatic decreases in plasma concentrations 4 h after dosing in mice (Kendall et al., 2014). The unique opioid-receptor profile of this drug allows butorphanol to be administered to a patient that requires reversal of a mu-agonist, but avoids a complete reversal that otherwise might result in perceived pain. Butorphanol can reverse the effects of the mu receptor while providing short-term analgesia via the kappa receptor. Lower doses of butorphanol (0.4 mg/kg) and nalbuphine (2 mg/kg) than would otherwise be used for primary analgesia can be used in combination with atipamezole (1 mg/kg) to rapidly reverse the anesthetic and respiratory depression effects of fentanyl (0.3 mg/kg) and medetomidine (0.2−0.3 mg/kg) in rats (Hu et al., 1992) while still maintaining adequate analgesia. When butorphanol is administered preemptively with ketamine/medetomidine anesthesia in mice, analgesia is improved; however, respiratory support may be needed, particularly for male mice (Bauer et al., 2019). Like buprenorphine, the analgesic effects of butorphanol, were undiminished with the administration of atipamezole to reverse α-2 agonist anesthesia (Izer et al., 2014). Long-term administration of butorphanol may result in analgesic tolerance (Gringauz et al., 2001).

Nalbuphine is structurally similar to both naloxone and oxymorphone, and also has a kappa-agonism and mixed mu-agonism/-antagonism receptor profile. Similar to butorphanol, nalbuphine may be used to reverse the respiratory depression caused by mu-agonists, but still provide analgesia from the kappa-receptor activation (Loomis et al., 1989). Nalbuphine is a less effective analgesic than buprenorphine (Jeger et al., 2016), but causes minimal side effects and has a low potential for abuse. When administered with morphine to rats, nalbuphine eliminated the dependence and tolerance usually seen with chronically administered morphine (Jang et al., 2006; Lee et al., 1997). Unlike other opioids, it has minor effects on gastrointestinal motility and has been shown to promote food and water intake in postsurgical rats, as well as to increase activity

(Asai et al., 1998; Flecknell and Liles, 1991). Nalbuphine may offer some benefits over NSAIDs, such as not suppressing prostaglandins, and where it is not controlled, may be an opiate option when controlled substances are not possible and short-duration analgesia is needed, such as during dystocia (Narver, 2015). In mice, nalbuphine was more quickly absorbed when administered SC than IP, and its duration of action was 2 h, with a loss of detection in plasma after 12 h (Kick et al., 2017). In rats, its duration of action has also been shown to be 2 h, thus limiting its clinical usefulness to acute situations (Chen et al., 2002a). In vivo studies involving oil-based preparations of IM-administered nalbuphine have demonstrated that the duration of analgesia is extended to over 2 days (Liu et al., 2004; Wang et al., 2006).

Pentazocine is a kappa-agonist that may be administered for mild-to-moderate pain but is not often used due to the development of analgesic tolerance with chronic administration. Activation of the kappa receptor causes little, if any, respiratory depression, and its low addiction potential makes pentazocine a safe alternative to mu-agonists for mild-to-moderate pain-producing procedures. In rats, pentazocine increases the level of analgesia to heat-induced pain when coadministered with low doses of morphine (Hamura et al., 2000). Like other opioids, pentazocine markedly decreases gastric emptying time and gut transit time in rodents (Asai et al., 1998).

f. Miscellaneous opioids

Certain opioid drugs may be less commonly used in laboratory rodents primarily due to a lack of sufficient data about their scientific, pharmacologic, and clinical efficacy. A summary of these agents has been provided based on relevant literature.

Tramadol affects the CNS as an opioid agonist and acts as a serotonin reuptake inhibitor. Tramadol requires hepatic metabolism to produce the analgesic metabolites, resulting in marked variability in efficacy between species and individuals. At relatively low doses, an analgesic effect is not seen, but 20 or 40 mg/kg of tramadol increases the pain threshold in mice (Erhan et al., 2005). In rats, low doses such as 1.0 mg/kg are effective to increase the pain threshold in rats with experimentally induced arthritis (Kayser et al., 1991). As a single agent, tramadol is insufficient for treating postprocedural pain in mice and rats (Evangelista et al., 2018a, 2018b; McKeon et al., 2011; Wolfe et al., 2015; Rätsep et al., 2013). In a mouse osteotomy model, tramadol administered in drinking water provided a lower degree of analgesia, as evidenced by higher limping and flinching scores, than buprenorphine administered in the drinking water (Jirkof et al., 2019). However, as part of a multimodal analgesic approach, such as when combined with gabapentin, ketoprofen, or other opioids, improved analgesia efficacy in rodents is achieved (Foley et al., 2019; Romero et al., 2010; Miranda et al., 2012, 2018; Jirkof et al., 2018). Parenteral dosing of tramadol may produce acute variations in circulating sex hormones in the rat (Ceccarelli et al., 2006). In higher doses of tramadol, opioid-induced ileus is observed, but this reduced activity is overcome by concomitant use of clinically relevant doses of dipyrone, acetaminophen, or ibuprofen (Planas et al., 2003). Tramadol offers some benefits to particular models, like those studying bone and wound healing or immunological aspects of postoperative ileus, as it has minimal effects on the research outcomes (Huss et al., 2019; Hong et al., 2019). However, as mentioned above, tramadol should be paired with another analgesic to ensure the effective minimization of pain from invasive procedures.

Meperidine is a mu-agonist with some α-2 agonist properties (Takada et al., 2002). Meperidine is useful alone or in combination with other opioids to potentiate opioid analgesia. For example, when combined with paracetamol, meperidine resulted in increased latencies in a tail flick assay in mice (Kula et al., 2016). Meperidine can provide short-term relief from severe pain and has been shown to reduce the threshold for shivering (Paris et al., 2005). Meperidine has also been demonstrated to offer local anesthetic effects in doses greater than 1.0 mg/kg when injected perineurally (Hassan et al., 1989). While not commonly used in the United States, meperidine is more frequently used in Europe.

g. Opioid receptor antagonists

Naloxone is an opioid receptor antagonist that acts primarily on the mu receptor but also has some blocking activity of the kappa receptors (Kong et al., 1994; Tokuyama et al., 1998). At low doses, it can potentiate the analgesic effects of kappa-receptor agonists, such as pentazocine (Legros et al., 1984; Levine et al., 1988). Naloxone also reverses the analgesic effect of other agents that produce opioid-like analgesics, as well as the analgesic and euphoric effects of endogenous opioids.

Alvimopan is a peripherally acting opioid reversal agent (Greenwood-Van Meerveld et al., 2004). Opioid receptors involved with nociception are typically central (brain and spinal cord), but those involved with producing the side effect of ileus are found in the gut. Because the mu receptors associated with the reduction of gastrointestinal motility are peripheral and not central, peripherally acting reversal agents may be used to restore the normal physiology of the gastrointestinal tract with little impact on the analgesic effects of the opioid.

D. Nonsteroidal anti-inflammatory agents

1. Meloxicam and piroxicam

Meloxicam is a selective COX-2 inhibitor that reduces prostaglandin synthesis and therefore inflammation; it has fewer renal and gastric side effects than NSAIDs that inhibit both COX isoforms. Meloxicam is effective in both inflammatory and neurogenic pain but has limited analgesic abilities with visceral distension or thermal pain (Santos et al., 1998). Meloxicam often needs to be diluted to accurately dose rodents. When diluted 1:10 with sterile water and maintained in amber glass vials with rubber stoppers and stored in the dark at room temperature, meloxicam concentrations remained stable and free of bacterial contamination and endotoxin for 365 days (Kawano et al., 2019). When offered 20 mg/kg meloxicam in drinking water, C57BL6 mice would not drink it and therefore did not reach appreciable pK levels (Ingrao et al., 2013). Therefore, it is not recommended to provide meloxicam in drinking water to rodents. Based on pK data, the half-life of meloxicam administered via injection may be as short as 4 h in mice, and even SR formulations only achieved plasma levels believed to correlate with analgesia for approximately 12 h (Kendall et al., 2014). Therefore, at least twice-daily dosing of either standard or SR injectable formulations of meloxicam is needed. In postlaparotomy mice, meloxicam at doses of 5−20 mg/kg significantly reduced postsurgical inflammation; however, mice lost just as much weight as the saline controls and did not demonstrate any reductions in remotely recorded and scored Mouse Grimace Scale scores or improvements in remotely recorded and scored composite behavioral scores, indicating that while inflammation was decreased, the mice still experienced pain in the first 24 h after surgery (Roughan et al., 2016). In postpartial hepatectomy mice, 2 mg/kg meloxicam-treated mice had reduced wheel running in the first 24 h after surgery, but retained open-field activity at baseline levels, indicating possible evidence of anxiety or pain relief (Tubbs et al., 2011). After vascular cutdown and telemeter implantation in mice, preemptive 2 mg/kg meloxicam followed by 2 days of 1 mg/kg meloxicam, better preserved presurgical body weight and circadian rhythm of activity compared to mice treated with buprenorphine or tramadol (Rätsep et al., 2013). In postvasectomy mice, meloxicam at 5−10 mg/kg failed, but 20 mg/kg succeeded in significantly reducing remotely recorded and scored MGS, manually scored pain behavior scores, as well as preserved peak corticosterone levels that were not different from unoperated mice; of note, pain assessments were performed at 30 min after surgery, so the duration of effective analgesia was not determined (Miller et al., 2016b; Leach et al., 2012; Wright-Williams et al., 2007). In a rat incisional model, both the standard formulation of meloxicam and meloxicam SR failed to provide effective protection from postsurgical increases in nociception (von Frey and Hargreaves tests) compared to saline controls, and in one study, meloxicam was outperformed by both buprenorphine and buprenorphine SR (Seymour et al., 2016; Bennett et al., 2021). In postlaparotomy rats, 2 mg/kg meloxicam significantly reduced remotely recorded and scored composite behavior scores compared to saline-treated rats, but failed to significantly reduce remotely recorded and scored Rat Grimace Scale scores; in contrast 0.05 mg/kg buprenorphine more effectively reduced both composite behavior and RGS scores compared to saline-treated rats (Klune et al., 2019). In a rat laparotomy mode, 1−2 mg/kg meloxicam resulted in lower live/cage-side scored Rat Grimace Scale scores and cage-side observational scores than the saline-treated groups and RGS scores equivalent to the buprenorphine-treated groups, but the authors suggest multimodal approaches may have further improved analgesia efficacy (Nunamaker et al., 2018). Interestingly, remotely recorded and scored RGS performed by multiple blinded scorers and using randomized still images did not successfully distinguish between rats that underwent anesthesia only versus anesthesia plus surgery, and therefore, these scores were not used in the analysis. The authors suspect the ketamine/xylazine anesthesia may have masked remotely scored RGS changes; additionally, the cage-side/real-time RGS scores were performed by a single, nonblinded observer, which could have introduced bias (Nunamaker et al., 2018). Meloxicam raises the chronic hyperalgesia threshold in rats experiencing neuropathic pain (Takahashi et al., 2005). It reduces swelling in inflamed joints and diminishes pain-related behaviors in arthritic rats (Laird et al., 1997). Meloxicam may have offered some pain relief from bladder cancer in rats (Roughan et al., 2004). Meloxicam exhibits moderate synergistic effects with morphine (Pinardi et al., 2005), allowing a reduction in dose for both drugs and improving the safety margin. When meloxicam was dosed (0.2−2 mg/kg) in rats in combination with buprenorphine, in both surgical and carrageenan intraplantar injection models, there was no indication of enhanced analgesia compared to single-agent analgesic administration or increased dosing frequency of buprenorphine (Leung et al., 2016; Schaap et al., 2012). However, based on the above literature, which suggests meloxicam doses closer to 20 mg/kg may be required to provide effective pain relief for both mice and rats, the doses used in these multimodal studies may have been much too low; therefore, multimodal combinations with higher doses of meloxicam are worth exploring.

Meloxicam may be ulcerogenic in rats at doses of 1−3.2 mg/kg (Jain et al., 2002; Nunamaker et al., 2018), although this side effect is reduced by formulating the drug in polyethylene glycol for oral preparations (Vijaya Kumar and Mishra, 2006). Where meloxicam doses of 20 mg/kg may be necessary to confer adequate analgesia in mice, if the concentration is reduced to 1 mg/mL, skin ulceration in mice is minimized, and meloxicam can be dosed safely for six consecutive days and does not result in typical NSAID toxicities to the gastric or renal tissues (Sarfaty et al., 2019). Similarly, meloxicam dosed subcutaneously with 20 mg/kg daily in a 5 mg/mL concentration for 3 or 7 days did not result in any clinically significant changes in serum biochemistry profiles but did result in positive fecal occult blood and histologic evidence of gastritis on days 4 and 8, with complete recovery by day 15 (Kendall et al., 2022). Additionally, no skin ulcerations were observed. Gastric ulceration is also the primary drawback to piroxicam, which is more ulcerogenic than meloxicam (Engelhardt et al., 1995). There have been successful attempts to bypass this deficiency by formulating piroxicam in an orally absorbed preparation, which has been shown to have greater analgesic effects than a commercial tablet preparation (Attia et al., 2004). Both piroxicam and meloxicam may be administered in a topical gel, which produces therapeutic plasma levels while minimizing gastrointestinal side effects (Gupta et al., 2002). It is not recommended to provide meloxicam in drinking water to mice, as they will not readily consume it and therefore do not derive analgesic benefits from meloxicam provided in drinking water (Ingrao et al., 2013).

2. *Propionic acid derivatives: ibuprofen, carprofen, ketoprofen, ketorolac, and naproxen*

Carprofen, a COX-2 selective NSAID, is the most commonly used propionic acid derivative NSAID in rodents. Due to their small size, carprofen must often be diluted from 50 mg/mL to 0.5 or 1 mg/mL to allow for accurate dosing in rodents. Both aliquoted stock and diluted carprofen retain strength and sterility if kept refrigerated in sterile glass vials for 180 days or up to 60 days if kept in polypropylene conical tubes at room temperature (Xu et al., 2021). When mixed with a flavoring agent, carprofen should be stored in the refrigerator for a maximum of 21 days (Hawkins et al., 2006). While the frequently recommended dose of 5 mg/kg provides plasma levels thought to be analgesic for approximately 12 h, carprofen is frequently administered only once a day (Kendall et al., 2014). Sustained release carprofen resulted in a similar pK profile as standard carprofen, indicating both may require twice-daily dosing and no significant added benefit of using the SR formulation (Kendall et al., 2014). Efficacy studies for postoperative pain in mice indicate an even shorter period of efficacy, closer to 6 h in postoperative rats (Roughan and Flecknell, 2004). At standard doses, carprofen resulted in no or incomplete reductions in postsurgical decreases in nest building in mice, ambulation in mice or rats nor increases in postsurgical remotely recorded and scored Mouse Grimace Scale and visual assessment scores in mice or Rat Grimace Scale in rats (Jirkof et al., 2013; Matsumiya et al., 2012; Beninson et al., 2018; Adamson et al., 2010; Zegre Cannon et al., 2011; Waite et al., 2015). Compared to mice treated with 5 mg/kg carprofen, those treated with 50 mg/kg, carprofen had modestly improved nest complexity scores after sham ET surgery (Jirkof et al., 2013). In postlaparotomy mice, a reduction in remotely recorded and scored Mouse Grimace Scale was only observed at doses of 20–25 mg/kg and not in lower doses of 5–15 mg/kg (Matsumiya et al., 2012). Carprofen at 25 mg/kg, but not at 10 mg/kg significantly reduced remotely recorded and scored Mouse Grimace Scale scores after craniotomy compared to controls (Cho et al., 2019). When administered at 20 mg/kg subcutaneously daily for up to 7 days, no clinically significant changes in serum chemistry profiles, nor evidence of gastric ulceration were identified in mice (Kendall et al., 2022). Carprofen may have offered some pain relief from bladder cancer in rats (Roughan et al., 2004). Carprofen can be administered in drinking water to facilitate self-administration and is readily, if not preferably consumed by mice. However, even at the higher mg/kg doses consumed, analgesia efficacy was incomplete for typical postsurgical pain in mice, and in some cases resulted in very minor increases in BUN and creatinine, and in the majority of cases, the injectable route was determined to be more efficacious than the drinking water route (Ingrao et al., 2013; Oliver et al., 2018; Cho et al., 2019). In rats, oral administration of carprofen via self-administration may not be adequate for controlling pain associated with laparotomy when compared to similar SC doses (Flecknell et al., 1999a). Carprofen was not effective when used alone in a rat bowel transplant model (Camprodon and Bowles, 2006), nor was high-dose carprofen (15 mL/kg) effective in alleviating pain or elevating the pain threshold in rats subjected to acute muscle pain (Nielsen et al., 2004). Carprofen provided in a medicated food gel also failed to significantly attenuate postsurgical pain in rats (Seymour et al., 2016). While carprofen as a single agent, particularly at lower doses (5–10 mg/kg), has not demonstrated significant evidence of adequate analgesia for typical postsurgical pain in rodents, when provided as part of a multimodal regimen, analgesia efficacy is significantly increased. Carprofen coadministered with buprenorphine resulted in superior analgesia compared to either analgesic alone for postoperative mice and guinea pigs, and carprofen combined with tramadol provided superior analgesia compared to either analgesic alone for postoperative pain in rats (Oliver et al., 2017, 2018; Zegre Cannon et al., 2011; Ciuffreda et al., 2014). Carprofen and buprenorphine reduced postoperative depression, anorexia, and water intake (Liles and Flecknell, 1994), as well as other pain-related behaviors (Roughan and Flecknell, 2004), in postlaparotomy rats. This combination is effective for up to several hours over a wide range of doses in rats with laparotomies (Roughan and Flecknell, 2001, 2003). Carprofen administered with buprenorphine to provide multimodal analgesia had no positive or negative impacts on ET results in mice compared to when buprenorphine alone was used (Parker et al., 2011). Therefore, multimodal application of carprofen plus an opiate is preferred over carprofen alone for treating postlaparotomy (or equivalent invasiveness) pain in rodents.

Ibuprofen is sometimes provided to rodents in drinking water. It should be noted that pediatric ibuprofen suspensions are not very water-soluble and tend to settle out of solution (Foley et al., 2019). However, ibuprofen in drinking water was readily consumed and resulted in decreased pruritic behavior and improved healing of ulcerative dermatitis wounds in mice (Ezell et al., 2012). In both mouse and rat foot or joint inflammation models, while ibuprofen provided some evidence of increased locomotion, superior analgesia was provided by opioids and even other NSAIDs (Montilla-García et al., 2017; Cobos et al., 2012). Analgesic doses of ibuprofen, otherwise capable of pain relief in other models, did not significantly alleviate pain in capsaicin-induced neuropathic pain models (Joshi et al., 2006). In traumatic brain injury models, rats receiving ibuprofen postinjury developed significant learning dysfunction and cognitive deficits compared with injured rats not receiving ibuprofen (Browne et al., 2006). Rats trained to voluntarily consume an ibuprofen suspension had increased mobility compared to controls in the first 2 days after shoulder surgery; however, buprenorphine provided comparatively better analgesic coverage, indicating that for postoperative pain, ibuprofen might be best used as part of a multimodal analgesic approach (Caro et al., 2014). The combination of ibuprofen and hydrocodone or oxycodone provides better analgesia than these opioids or ibuprofen alone, as evidenced by the increased time to respond with the tail flick test. This synergistic effect was not seen when ibuprofen was combined with fentanyl or morphine; additional NSAIDs (ketorolac and aspirin) did not add to the effects of hydrocodone or oxycodone (Kolesnikov et al., 2003; Zelcer et al., 2005). In rats, when coadministered with caffeine, high-dose ibuprofen has an analgesic profile similar to that of morphine (Lopez et al., 2006), a level of analgesia that is not provided by ibuprofen alone.

Oral self-administration of ketoprofen to rats may not be adequate for controlling pain associated with laparotomy when compared to similar SC doses (Flecknell et al., 1999a). With less severe incisional pain, ketoprofen provides analgesia for up to 24 h at 10–20 mg/kg doses (Prado and Pontes, 2002). At 20 mg/kg, ketoprofen reduced remotely recorded and scored Mouse Grimace Scale scores in postlaparotomy mice (Matsumiya et al., 2012). At 25 mg/kg, if administered 15 min prior to surgery (preemptively), ketoprofen reduced remotely recorded and scored Rat Grimace Scale scores in postlaparotomy rats; the same dose of ketoprofen showed no effective analgesia when administered intraoperatively (Waite et al., 2015). Like ibuprofen, ketoprofen combined with caffeine produces analgesic efficacy in rats, which is two to three times that produced with ketoprofen alone (Diaz-Reval et al., 2001). Injectable ketoprofen dosed at 5–10 mg/kg, particularly when coupled with anesthesia, has resulted in significant gastrointestinal bleeding in rats; however, some interactions with rodent microbiota or pathogens may play a role in exacerbating this adverse effect (Shientag et al., 2012; Lamon et al., 2008).

Ketorolac tromethamine is less commonly used for treating clinical pain in rodents due to the risk of adverse effects such as gastric or renal toxicity; however, it can provide analgesia for properties of visceral, tonic, and inflammatory pain. Although it produces gastric lesions in high or prolonged doses (Padi et al., 2004), ketorolac does not interfere with platelet function. Ketorolac has analgesic effects comparable to strong opioids, yet its effectiveness in preventing pain from direct stimulation of nerves is questionable (Randolph and Peters, 1997). It has very rapid oral uptake (maximal plasma levels at approximately 20 min) and a half-life of 6 h (Granados-Soto and Flores-Murrieta, 1995). Ketorolac administered with the antibiotic gentamicin is contraindicated because both drugs have acute kidney effects and together have been shown to promote severe acute tubular necrosis over the course of 3 days (Jaquenod et al., 1998).

Naproxen is a long-acting COX inhibitor that has been seldom used in rodents because of the short duration of analgesia and the development of gastric ulceration (Whiteside et al., 2004). The use of this agent in rodents is not recommended.

3. *Salicylic acid acetate (aspirin)*

Aspirin, the oldest commercial NSAID that targets both COX-1 and COX-2, is an efficacious analgesic but has many side effects, including reduced hemostasis and increased incidence of gastric ulceration. Aspirin may reduce inflammation by reducing mast cell release of inflammatory mediators (Jiang et al., 2021). In rats undergoing laparotomies and organ transplants, oral administration of aspirin maintained a normal activity level (Jablonski and Howden, 2002). Aspirin and a glucose/aspirin combination both increased tail withdrawal latencies in tail flick and withdrawal tests as well as reduced carrageenan-induced paw swelling in mice (Jacob et al., 2013). Aspirin has been shown to be ineffective in restoring activity to control levels in CFA-induced arthritis models (Millecamps et al., 2005) and formalin-induced inflammatory pain models (Choi et al., 2001).

4. Acetaminophen

Acetaminophen reduces pyrexia and provides minor analgesia but is quite limited in reducing inflammation (Capetola et al., 1983). The analgesic effect of acetaminophen does not seem to be associated with the COX-1 or COX-2 pathways, as it produces very different analgesic profiles when compared with indomethacin, a well-known effector of the COX cascade. Thus, acetaminophen is an attractive option when looking to limit the impact to scientific goals requiring intact coagulation, prostaglandin synthesis, and inflammation (Abbott and Hellemans, 2000). Pediatric oral suspensions of acetaminophen are relatively insoluble in water, quickly settle out of suspension, and initial consumption can be reduced due to neophobia; therefore, the provision of these suspensions in water bottles is not a reliable method of delivery (Foley, 2014; Mickley et al., 2006). In addition, literature demonstrating effective analgesia of rodents by acetaminophen in drinking water is mixed and alternative analgesics or multimodal combinations have been shown to be more effective and reliable (Saito et al., 2005; Millecamps et al., 2005; Choi et al., 2001; Bauer et al., 2003; Mickley et al., 2006; Hayes et al., 2000; Miller et al., 2012; Montilla-García et al., 2017; Matsumiya et al., 2012; Romero et al., 2010; Stewart and Martin, 2003a; Shinozaki et al., 2015; Caro et al., 2014; Durst et al., 2021). Therefore, the provision of acetaminophen in drinking water alone is not a recommended means of pain relief in rodents.

5. Dipyrone

Dipyrone, also called Metamizol, inhibits prostaglandins and therefore inflammation, as well as the signaling of TRPA1, an ion channel present in a subpopulation of nociceptors. Dipyrone produces very good analgesia over a wide dosage range (150–600 mg/kg) and relieves inflammatory pain (Abbott and Bonder, 1997; Hernandez-Delgadillo et al., 2002), central pain (Beirith et al., 1998), thermal pain (Hernandez-Delgadillo and Cruz, 2006; Hernandez-Delgadillo et al., 2003), and visceral pain (Laird and Cervero, 1996; Laird et al., 1998). Dipyrone acts centrally in the brainstem (Tortorici and Vanegas, 1994; Tortorici et al., 1996) or spinal cord (Neugebauer et al., 1994), either alone or by activating the endogenous opioid pathways (Hernandez-Delgadillo and Cruz, 2006; Omisore et al., 2004). Despite this apparent mechanism of action, the effects of dipyrone may not be reversible by naloxone (Poveda et al., 2003; Taylor et al., 1998), nor does it produce opioid-induced ileus (Hernandez-Delgadillo et al., 2002). In postoperative mice, dipyrone improved gastrointestinal motility and reduced inflammation (Hong et al., 2019). When added to ketamine/medetomidine anesthesia in mice, dipyrone resulted in improved intraoperative analgesia (Bauer et al., 2019). Repeated doses of dipyrone eventually induce analgesic tolerance, a tolerance that is cross-reactive with morphine tolerance (Hernandez-Delgadillo and Cruz, 2004; Vanegas and Tortorici, 2002). When administered for four consecutive days, rats developed hyperalgesia, indicating that use should be limited to a shorter treatment course (Ruiz-Pérez et al., 2017).

Dipyrone use should be avoided for rodent epilepsy models, as intermediate-to-high doses (300–500 mg/kg) reduce limb extension and tonic-clonic plus limbic components of seizures induced by electroshock and sound (Doretto et al., 1998). The analgesic effect of dipyrone does not seem to be associated with the COX pathway (Abbott and Hellemans, 2000). It is suggested that the analgesic effect of dipyrone is not associated with its antiinflammatory effect (Beirith et al., 1998). Furthermore, dipyrone produces analgesia in adjuvant-induced arthritis models while not reducing inflammation, swelling, and edema (Tatsuo et al., 1994). Thus, dipyrone is a recommended analgesic for adjuvant-induced arthritis models and animal models involving coagulation, prostaglandin synthesis, and inflammation (Abbott and Hellemans, 2000).

6. Coxibs

Celecoxib and, to a lesser extent, parecoxib are two of the more commonly used highly specific COX-2 inhibitors used in rodents. In general, COX-2-specific agents impart less gastrointestinal effects and have better analgesic effects with inflammatory pain. In humans, coxibs are associated with an increased risk of cardiovascular side effects such as stroke and hypertension, and deletion of COX-2 in genetically modified mice similarly predisposes them to hypertension and thrombosis (Yu et al., 2012; Patrono, 2016).

Celecoxib alleviated pain-associated behavioral alterations following induced arthritis in rodents (Millecamps et al., 2005; Pomonis et al., 2005) and reduced swelling, chronic hyperalgesia, and joint pathology (Noguchi et al., 2005). Chronic administration effectively reduces the severity of endometriosis in mice, while not altering the estrous cycle (Efstathiou et al., 2005). When given for a long duration, celecoxib is effective in alleviating incisional pain (Whiteside et al., 2004). Preemptive administration of celecoxib, given prior to the painful stimulus, is highly effective (Veiga et al., 2004). Celecoxib at 20 mg/kg given 1 h prior to formalin paw injection significantly reduced licking and flinching, as well as protected against secondary hyperalgesia in mice (Zhao et al., 2017; Nishiyama, 2006) but had no local effects (Torres-Lopez et al., 2002). However, even when given up to 50 mg/kg orally, celecoxib did not provide effective analgesia in rats after knee surgery (Buvanendran et al., 2008). In rodents, celecoxib was ineffective at alleviating pain from bone cancer (Medhurst et al., 2002; Saito et al., 2005), thermal pain (Nishiyama, 2006; Veiga et al., 2004), and capsaicin-induced neuropathic pain (Joshi et al., 2006). When celecoxib is administered to rats with femoral fractures, there is increased fibrous repair but not a significantly increased time to healing (Brown et al., 2004). Unlike other NSAIDs, celecoxib does not cause gastric damage as it does not affect gastric prostaglandin E(2) synthesis (Wallace et al., 2000).

Parecoxib has more potent synergistic effects when combined with morphine than other COX-2 NSAIDs (Pinardi et al., 2005) and reduces the amount of opioids needed for adequate analgesia. This overall reduction in drug improves the safety margin of the analgesic regime and provides better analgesic coverage. Parecoxib provides relief from inflammatory pain, but it does not relieve visceral or tonic pain (Padi et al., 2004). Preemptive and postoperative treatment with parecoxib had no impact on bone healing in rats (Hjorthaug et al., 2019).

Firocoxib was assessed in a mouse plantar incisional model and found to reduce secondary hyperalgesia similarly to buprenorphine at both 10 and 20 mg/kg (Reddyjarugu et al., 2015). However, these same doses were assessed in a rat plantar incisional model and did not demonstrate any improvements in mechanical allodynia nor thermal hyperalgesia compared to saline-treated rats, indicating firocoxib, at least at these doses and for this type of pain, is not a good option for analgesia in rats (Bennett et al., 2021).

Robenacoxib is approved for analgesia in cats and holds promise due to its rapid central clearance and concentration at the local site of injury, also validated in rats, thereby reducing potential side effects from central exposure (King et al., 2009). While no significant impacts resulted on key model parameters, in a surgical mouse model of deep venous thrombosis, robenacoxib failed to provide evidence of effective analgesia; interestingly, the same results were found for a single dose of carprofen at 5 mg/kg (Beninson et al., 2018).

7. Miscellaneous NSAIDs

Flunixin meglumine, a nonselective COX inhibitor, though not frequently used in rodents, reduces inflammatory pain through the activation of spinal opioid receptors and is useful in inflammatory conditions (Herrero and Headley, 1996). Flunixin provides excellent antiinflammatory activity in rat nerve injury models and promotes greater weight gains than opioids. However, in a partial hepatectomy model, flunixin failed to provide adequate postoperative analgesia to mice (Tubbs et al., 2011). This agent has minimal antinociceptive properties and is less effective for providing analgesia following major surgery (Liles and Flecknell, 1994; Stewart and Martin, 2003b). Additionally, flunixin has been associated with renal tubular injury (Foley et al., 2019).

The primary mechanism of indomethacin is the blockade of prostaglandin synthesis due to nonselective COX-1/COX-2 inhibition. It may participate in the centrally located release of endogenous opioids (Suganuma et al., 1998). While indomethacin has been shown to be effective at alleviating bone cancer pain in mice (Saito et al., 2005), it prolongs bone fracture repair in rats (Brown et al., 2004). After surgical implantation of telemeters in mice, indomethacin-treated animals (preemptively with injectable indomethacin and the next day orally dosed via consumption of a food treat inoculated with indomethacin) had greater levels of lights on to lights off transition motor activity than mice treated with vehicle controls, indicating some degree of postoperative analgesia was conferred (Blaha and Leon, 2008). Interestingly, in rats, it has been shown to prevent the unusually rapid metastasis associated with untreated surgical pain (Page and Ben-Eliyahu, 2002). The use of indomethacin in pregnant rats should be avoided because it may cause significant neurologic and behavioral deficits in the pups as they mature (Benesova et al., 2001).

Mechanisms of analgesic and antiinflammatory actions of diclofenac are unclear; they may be through the inhibition of COX and possibly the lipooxygenase pathways (Scholer et al., 1986) or by activation of K^+ channels of afferent nerves (Ortiz et al., 2002). Diclofenac is primarily used for the relief of musculoskeletal or neurogenic pain (Santos et al., 1998). In inflammatory pain models, diclofenac has a very good analgesic effect when administered locally near the site of inflammation (Gupta et al., 2002; Jain et al., 2005; Torres-Lopez et al., 2002), but is less effective when administered systemically (Prado and Pontes, 2002). When given topically, diclofenac was found to be effective at reducing clinical signs associated with dry eye in mice (Kilic and Kulualp, 2016).

E. Other agents with analgesic action

1. Local and topical anesthetics

Administration of local anesthetics such as lidocaine has both analgesic and antiarrhythmic effects. Local anesthetics act locally on nerve endings or fibers, causing a temporary blockade of nerve impulse conduction, and recovery is spontaneous. Lidocaine has a very short duration of action of approximately 30 min, whereas bupivacaine may last around 60 min; though there are formulations that can extend this duration to 24–48 h (Foley et al., 2019). The duration of analgesia may be prolonged by the concurrent use of a vasoconstricting agent such as epinephrine (Branson and Gross, 2001). Caution should be used when using formulations with vasoconstricting properties in areas of the rodent where this could cause unintentional decreased blood flow, such as the tail and extremities, as this could result in ischemic injury. When 0.5 μg/kg dexmedetomidine was combined with lidocaine and injected into the plantar surface of the hind paw, local anesthesia was extended up to 35 min in rats, about the same period of time as when lidocaine was injected with epinephrine, but without some of the cardiovascular risks that can occur with epinephrine (Tsutsui and Sunada, 2017). Mice underwent a sham vasectomy or sham ET in male and female mice, respectively, and were treated with preemptive peri-incisional line blocks with a mix of 10 mg/kg lidocaine and 3 mg/kg bupivacaine, with or without also being provided 30 mg/mL paracetamol in the drinking water (Durst et al., 2021). Mice treated with local anesthetics only demonstrated no loss in body weight after surgery, the fewest increases in remotely recorded and scored Mouse Grimace Scale scores, with significant increases compared to baseline at 1 and 3 h postoperatively, indicating positive analgesic effects. Treatment with both paracetamol and local anesthetics did not outperform and in some cases underperformed in analgesia efficacy compared to the mice treated with local anesthetics only (Durst et al., 2021).

In a rat incisional model of pain, liposomal bupivacaine reduced thermal and mechanical nociception for up to 4 days (Kang et al., 2017). However, the commercial formulation of liposomal bupivacaine is only sold in large vials of 20 mLs which the manufacturers recommend be disposed of within 4 h of opening, resulting in a very high cost for use in rodents and limiting its clinical application. Lidocaine or bupivacaine may be combined with opioids and NSAIDs to fully relieve pain during the most painful period of 4–7 h postsurgery (Roughan and Flecknell, 2004). Continuously delivered lidocaine, via implantable osmotic pumps, at doses from 0.67 mg/kg/h to 1.3 mg/kg/h, provides analgesia to alleviate pain produced by a chronic constriction injury model of neuropathic pain and may even reverse the hyperalgesic peak if administered later at three postoperative days (Smith et al., 2002). Local anesthetics can also be used to decrease pain from IP injections of pentobarbital euthanasia in rats (Svendsen et al., 2007; Khoo et al., 2018).

Ammonium sulfate and bupivacaine are safe to use in neonatal rodents (Hertl et al., 1998). Analgesic effects are additive and may last for hours when a local anesthetic such as lidocaine or bupivacaine is combined with an opioid analgesic, such as morphine, levorphanol, or buprenorphine, delivered topically using DMSO (Hayes and Flecknell, 1999; Kolesnikov et al., 2000).

EMLA cream is a combination of lidocaine and prilocaine in equal amounts in an eutectic mixture. It is indicated for topical use to desensitize skin (usually before venipuncture or IV catheter placement); however, it can take up to an hour to provide a useful effect in humans, dogs, cats, pigs, and rabbits. It was less effective in rats and mice for venipuncture of the tail (Flecknell et al., 1990; David et al., 2014), tail biopsy (Dudley et al., 2016), and routine ear notching (Miller and Leach, 2015b; Burn et al., 2021), and therefore may have limited applications in rodents. Similarly, cetacaine (a topical benzocaine spray) was ineffective at reducing pain associated with tail biopsy in mice (Braden et al., 2015; Dudley et al., 2016). Mixed results of analgesia have been reported for immersion of the cut surface of the tail in bupivacaine for 30 s after biopsy in mice (Jones et al., 2012; Dudley et al., 2016). Analgesia may also be provided by immersing the tail in ice-cold 70% ethanol for 10 s prior to tail tip biopsy (Dudley et al., 2016). Topically applied lidocaine jelly did not significantly improve the recovery or welfare indices of mice with rectal prolapse (Mitchell et al., 2021).

2. *Gabapentin*

Several studies have demonstrated that while gabapentin, a GABA analogue, may provide some antinociception as a single agent when provided as part of a multimodal analgesic approach, gabapentin can be an effective additive to provide analgesia to rodents. Importantly, alone or in combination with other analgesics, gabapentin tends to underperform when compared to buprenorphine so should not be considered a preferential but additive analgesia strategy for postoperative pain in rodents. In STZ-induced diabetes model in mice, both gabapentin (efficacy seen as low as 9 mg/kg, assessed up to 100 mg/kg) and tramadol (up to 100 mg/kg) exerted antinociceptive effects as measured by tail flick, formalin, and hot plate tests, that were additive when provided together for multimodal analgesia (Miranda et al., 2018). In a plantar incisional model, rats treated with 10 mg/kg tramadol and 80 mg/kg gabapentin pre- and postoperatively had some relief from thermal hyperalgesia and normalized weight bearing. The postoperative analgesia provided by this combination was better than when tramadol was provided alone, but the combination underperformed compared to the analgesia provided by buprenorphine (McKeon et al., 2011). Rats that underwent shoulder surgery provided both tramadol at 10 mg/kg and gabapentin at 80 mg/kg preemptively and postoperatively achieved some improvements in ambulation, but to a much lower extent than rats treated with buprenorphine or ibuprofen (Caro et al., 2014). When carprofen (2 mg) and gabapentin (90 mg) were combined in an edible tablet (Rimadyl, Bio-Serv), consumption of the tablet decreased on the first day after plantar incision surgery, and these rats demonstrated mechanical hyperalgesia on that day, but reductions in mechanical hyperalgesia occurred on subsequent days 2 and 3 after surgery (Zude et al., 2020). Interestingly, when provided as a single agent (tablet with either carprofen or gabapentin), rats were protected from postsurgical increases in mechanical hyperalgesia, though not thermal hyperalgesia. Authors measured near complete consumption of the carprofen tab but much lower amounts of the gabapentin tabs, thus the gabapentin tablets may not be very palatable for rats (Zude et al., 2020). When gavaged, 50–100 mg/kg gabapentin significantly reduced mechanical hyperalgesia in a neuropathic pain model in rats synergistic when administered in a multimodal combination with donepezil and duloxetine (Hayashida and Eisenach, 2008). The multimodal combination of the anxiolytic trazodone (0.3 mg/kg) and gabapentin (3 mg/kg) administered to rats via injection in a neuropathic pain model of chronic constriction injury, outperformed each drug given alone in reducing mechanical hyperalgesia, preserving weight bearing, burrowing, and nest scores (Garrone et al., 2021). While the underlying mechanisms for this synergistic effect are not known, the authors hypothesize that it may be due to indirect inhibition of glutamate release, a primary excitatory neurotransmitter involved in central sensitization.

3. Synthetic cannabinoids

Synthetic cannabinoids are increasingly used to manage pain in human patient populations and have been shown to confer some analgesia in acute pain models in rodents, as well as in neuropathic, chronic inflammatory, and cancer pain rodent models (Tamba et al., 2020). Dosing routes vary from systemic to intrathecal and local. A comprehensive review of rodent studies evaluating the analgesic efficacy of various cannabinoids can be found in Soliman et al. (2021); overall, the meta-analysis of 374 rodent studies found selective CB1, CB2, nonselective cannabinoid receptor agonists, and PPAR-α agonists significantly reduced pain-associated behaviors in a variety of rodent models of inflammatory and neuropathic pain (Soliman et al., 2021). However, caution should be exercised before utilizing cannabinoids to treat clinical pain in rodents, as the International Association for the Study of Pain completed a comprehensive review of research on the effectiveness of cannabis for the treatment of pain and found a lack of sufficient evidence to support its use for this purpose, concluding more rigorous and robust research is needed (International Association for the Study of Pain, 2021).

4. Ketamine

Some studies indicate that the NMDA receptor antagonist ketamine improves analgesia when used in conjunction with other agents, especially opioids. In rats, ketamine used as part of the anesthetic combination or in the days following the painful procedure eliminates the hyperalgesia seen with the short-term use of fentanyl (Laulin et al., 2002). Similarly, when ketamine was added to the anesthesia protocol for a tibial defect model in mice, postoperative nociceptive measures were improved compared to mice that did not have ketamine added to their anesthetic protocol; additionally, ketamine-treated mice were more responsive to postoperative opioids (Minville et al., 2010). While none of the six NMDA receptor antagonists tested in a particular rat study were effective at improving tail-flick responses on their own, when combined with mu-opioids morphine and fentanyl, analgesia was enhanced (Redwine and Trujillo, 2003). Further research into the utility of NMDA antagonists has revealed a ketamine metabolite, hydroxynorketamine, was more effective than ketamine in reducing mechanical allodynia in three different chronic pain models in mice (Kroin et al., 2019).

5. α-2 agonists

In humans and rats, when administered intraoperatively, α-2 agonist dexmedetomidine improves pain management in the postoperative period (Yeo and Park, 2018; Bellon et al., 2016). However, the residual analgesia provided by α-2 agonists is insufficient unto itself to effectively alleviate postprocedural pain and therefore should not be relied upon for this purpose. These agents when combined with an opioid or NSAID, result in a synergistic effect, extending both the duration and potency of the total analgesic effect (Jain et al., 2002; McLaughlin and Dewey, 1994). Interestingly, when given at microdoses, much lower than those used for sedation or anesthetic purposes, analgesia can be conferred and may act via inhibition of TRPV1 receptors in the peripheral nervous system (Lee et al., 2020). In a rat model of carrageenan-induced nociception, 10 μM of dexmedetomidine injected locally into the hind paw significantly improved paw withdrawal thresholds in von Frey tests (Honda et al., 2015).

Clonidine is a centrally acting α-2 adrenergic agonist that provides short-acting analgesia in rodents alone and especially when coupled with an opioid (Hirst et al., 1984). Clonidine is not typically used to treat postprocedural pain in mice but may be of interest for very specific models. In a formalin model of visceral pain in mice, clonidine provides dose-dependent analgesia over a very wide dose range (0.001–0.1 mg/kg IP) for at least 1 h (Sabetkasaie et al., 2004). Clonidine given IP at doses greater than 0.02 mg/kg will alleviate hot plate nociception in rats (Sluka and Chandran, 2002). Significantly higher doses (2 mg/kg) have also been shown to provide mechanical analgesia in mice (Ozdogan et al., 2004; Sluka and Chandran, 2002). Clonidine (0.025 mg/kg) coadministered IP with low-dose morphine (0.5 mg/kg) produces a pronounced synergistic effect to alleviate inflammation pain. In contrast with morphine alone, tolerance does not develop with this combination (Gurtu et al., 1994). Administration of clonidine (0.1 and 1.0 mg/kg) seems to produce different effects in young, mature, and old mice during the active (dark) and inactive periods (Hirst et al., 1984).

6. *Cholinesterase inhibitors*

In addition to acting as neuromuscular blocking antagonists, neostigmine and physostigmine have significant analgesic properties when used in rodents. The exact mechanism of action for this analgesic effect is not known but may be through muscarinic and nicotinic receptors in the spinal cord; see Lauretti (2015) for a detailed review. Physostigmine at 50–200 μg/kg SC produces relief of mechanical and cold-based allodynia in rats, although it does not provide significant analgesia in hot plate tests (Poyhia et al., 1999). When neostigmine was provided with either diclofenac or celecoxib, antiinflammatory effects of the NSAIDs were enhanced, resulting in improved analgesia in rats across a variety of nonsurgical pain models; some liver and kidney values were negatively impacted, though histologically the organs remained within normal limits (Gowayed et al., 2021).

F. Nonpharmacologic options

1. *Acupuncture, nutrition, housing, conspecifics, etc.*

While opioids and NSAIDs are by far the most commonly used methods of alleviating pain in rodents, other "alternative" methods of analgesia that may not intuitively be associated with providing analgesia have recently been investigated. Alternatives with limited clinical documentation are not discussed here (see also Chapter 13 for more suggestions for nonpharmacological pain control.).

a. Diet and ingestion of sweets

In mice with bone cancer, soy-based diets reduced model-associated hyperalgesia (Zhao et al., 2004). The ingestion of sweet compounds produces low-level euphoria and analgesia. Nociception test latencies (e.g., tail flick) are increased in rats after the ingestion of sugar solutions, and this effect is reversed by administering opioid receptor antagonists. It is speculated that the sugar compounds not only trigger the release of endogenous opioids (Segato et al., 1997) but also act on serotonergic and noradrenergic receptors (Reboucas et al., 2005). Rats given a wide range of doses of aspartame, an artificial sweetener, exhibited an increased pain threshold (Sharma et al., 2005). There is a synergistic effect when aspartame is given along with various opioids and NSAIDs in rats and mice (Nikfar et al., 1997; Sharma et al., 2005). Rats have also been shown to regain body weight lost after surgery faster when provided a sugared cereal supplementation during the postoperative period (Welberg et al., 2006). Dipping oral gavage needles in sucralose was also found to decrease stress in mice during dosing (Hoggatt et al., 2010).

b. Acupuncture

Acupuncture has become more popular and accepted in veterinary medicine due to the increase in scientifically based studies investigating its mechanisms of action and documenting results. Many of these studies have been done using rodents. On an anatomic level, acupuncture analgesia seems to be regulated by the hypothalamus, while on a biochemical level an increase in arginine vasopressin seems to elicit an acupuncture-induced analgesic response in the rat hypothalamus (Yang et al., 2006). At the receptor level, naloxone often abolishes the clinical effects of acupuncture, though this may be frequency-specific for electroacupuncture (Huang et al., 2002), thus adding evidence to the notion of opioid receptor activation. Recent studies have shown that acupuncture triggers the upregulation of mu receptors in many areas of the rat brain, thus allowing for a greater effect of opioids (Zhu et al., 1995). Evidence suggests that the trigger for electroacupuncture-induced analgesia in mice is the release of brain endomorphins and other endogenous opioids (Huang et al., 2000), although some evidence exists that other mechanisms may also be involved. For example, electroacupuncture in a rat ankle sprain model increases stepping force equivalent to morphine analgesia (Koo et al., 2002), but this effect could not be reversed by naloxone. Electroacupuncture combined with low doses of indomethacin has a synergistic effect on the reduction of hyperalgesia (Zhang et al., 2004). In a rat plantar incision model, electroacupuncture reduced mechanical nociception as well as carprofen (Teixeira et al., 2012). In post-laparotomy rats, electroacupuncture improved postoperative ileus and improved remotely recorded and scored Rat Grimace Scale scores in the first 2 h after surgery (Murakami et al., 2019). Electroacupuncture in conscious, freely moving mice was demonstrated to reduce inflammation and nociception in a sickle cell disease model (Wang et al., 2016).

c. Dexamethasone

Dexamethasone provides significant relief from inflammation-based pain in chronic adjuvant-induced arthritis (Colpaert et al., 2001; Wilson et al., 2006). It also allows for a return of normal mobility in arthritic rats (Matson et al., 2007) and improves the clinical condition of aged, adrenalectomized arthritic rats (Yokoro et al., 2003). Dexamethasone does not provide analgesia in rodents with mechanical, neuropathic, and thermal pain (Veiga et al., 2004). While effective in increasing the threshold for pressure in endotoxin-induced hyperalgesia, dexamethasone was only marginally ineffective in alleviating the thermal pain associated with this model (Kanaan et al., 1997). Thus, the type of model will determine the potential usefulness of dexamethasone.

G. Specific situation analgesic recommendations

1. Analgesic use in immunologic, inflammation, and tumor studies

There is growing appreciation for the previously unmeasured impact of unalleviated pain on a variety of rodent models. Often, the concern first raised is whether analgesic use will introduce variability in the model, confounding research results. However, increasing literature is identifying the need to weigh the comparative impact of unalleviated pain and the use of analgesics in rodent models, sometimes even identifying that analgesia can correct for the variability introduced by pain and allow for possibly more translatable data. See Chapter 3 for an in-depth discussion of this topic. Additionally, the reader is referred to the following review articles for rodent-specific data relative to: Influence of Pain and Analgesia on Cancer Research Studies (Taylor, 2019), Defining and Managing Pain in Stroke and Traumatic Brain Injury Research (Larson et al., 2019), A Review of the Effects of Pain and Analgesia on Immune System Function and Inflammation: Relevance for Preclinical Studies (DeMarco and Nunamaker, 2019), Influence of Pain and Analgesia on Orthopedic and Wound-healing Models in Rats and Mice (Huss et al., 2019), The Influence of Pain and Analgesia in Rodent Models of Sepsis (Carpenter et al., 2019), and Interacting Influences of Sleep, Pain, and Analgesic Medications on Sleep Studies in Rodents (Toth, 2019).

2. Anesthesia and analgesia in neonatal mice and rats

It is now appreciated that neonatal animals, human and nonhuman, do experience pain and if left untreated, develop long-term changes affecting behavior and cognition. Therefore, it is imperative to adequately provide effective anesthesia and analgesia if invasive procedures are needed for neonatal rodents (Victoria and Murphy, 2016; Williams and Lascelles, 2020). The *Guidelines for the Care and Use of Mammals in Neuroscience and Behavioral Research* (ILAR, 2003) stipulate that for experiments involving late-term rodent fetuses after their removal from unanesthetized mothers (such as a dam euthanized by decapitation or cervical dislocation), guidelines for anesthesia and analgesia in neonates should be followed. Potentially painful experimental manipulations in neonatal rodents require the use of anesthesia or analgesia unless robust scientific justification is approved by the IACUC. The primary difficulty in using anesthesia or analgesia in the neonate is balancing its effectiveness and safety. Neonatal anesthesia and analgesia are covered in depth in Chapter 28, and the reader is referred to that chapter for more details. In general, the margin of safety for injectable anesthetics is narrowed in the neonate, and inhalation anesthesia is preferably recommended. Both isoflurane and sevoflurane maintained physiological parameters better than hypothermia in neonatal rat pups, and isoflurane was recommended as the anesthetic of choice for epilepsy research in neonatal rodents (Huss et al., 2016; Akman et al., 2018). Preemptive morphine or local nerve blocks in neonatal rats prevented behavioral and hormonal changes otherwise developed by adult rats if the pain was not minimized (Victoria et al., 2015; Walker et al., 2015).

H. Other rodents, including guinea pigs, hamsters, and gerbils

The rodent species discussed in this section are covered by the Animal Welfare Act and thus are required to receive appropriate relief to potentially painful or distressful procedures as described in the Act and in USDA Policy #11 (Code of Federal Regulations, 1997). As part of the Act and USDA Policy #12 (Code of Federal Regulations, 2000; Code of Federal Regulations, 2002), investigators must also perform a comprehensive literature search and consider any alternatives to potentially painful or distressful procedures performed on covered rodent species (Code of Federal Regulations, 2000). These alternatives may include refinements to the anesthetic and analgesic protocols used for these species.

Like mice and rats, these other rodents require special consideration when administering anesthetics and analgesics. Most small mammals are primary or obligate nasal breathers, and thus patency of the nares and nasopharynx is crucial whether using inhalant or injectable anesthesia (Heard, 2004). Even the large rodent species used commonly in biomedical research (e.g., *Marmota* or guinea pigs) are small enough to necessitate the use of nonrebreathing systems when using gas anesthesia (Lerche et al., 2000). There are few published reports describing the clinically relevant use of inhalant anesthetics in these other rodents.

1. Guinea pigs

Several anatomical aspects of the guinea pig (*Cavia porcellus*) are relevant to anesthesia for this species. Nearly the entire tongue of a guinea pig is both richly vascularized and tightly attached to the oropharynx; in addition, the epiglottis is behind the palatal ostium which makes it difficult to lower and visualize, making this one of the most difficult laboratory animal species to intubate (Karamichali et al., 2020; Johnson, 2010). Videoendoscopy can aid in the correct placement of endotracheal tubes in guinea pigs (Miranda et al., 2017). For guinea pigs, 380 ± 12 g, an 18 G intravenous catheter can be used for endotracheal intubation (Miranda et al., 2017). Guinea pigs can store food in the caudal oropharynx after eating, and therefore fasting is recommended for 2–3 h prior to anesthesia (Horn et al., 2013). In addition, a cotton swab should be used to sweep out food in the mouth after induction to reduce the risk of aspiration (author's experience and Horn et al., 2013). Atropine can reduce copious respiratory secretions and salivation while under anesthesia (Karamichali et al., 2020). The very large cecum can make drug calculations challenging, as the effective weight of the animal can be considerably less than the body mass with cecal contents. The pedal reflex is not always a reliable measure of anesthetic depth because guinea pigs make involuntary leg movements even while under a surgical plane of anesthesia (Harkness and Wagner, 1995). In the author's experience, careful and close monitoring is required when guinea pigs are under anesthesia, as they can very quickly alternate between too deep and too light. Thus, a separate veterinary anesthetist is recommended to monitor and adjust anesthetic administration and provide respiratory support as needed, rather than having the surgeon perform their own anesthetic monitoring. Like other rodents, guinea pigs rapidly lose body heat within 10–15 min of anesthesia. Heat support, such as with far-infrared active warming devices, can protect from anesthesia-associated hypothermia and should be applied as soon as possible (Zarndt et al., 2015).

a. Anesthetics

To safely achieve surgical plane anesthesia in guinea pigs, a combination of gas anesthetic for maintenance with injectable induction is recommended. Sevoflurane appears to be less irritating to their airways, so it is preferred to isoflurane when possible (Karamichali et al., 2020). Unlike other rodents, guinea pigs can breath-hold to such a considerable degree that an anesthetic chamber should not be used for induction (Karamichali et al., 2020). Breath-holding can result in a sudden deep breath of anesthetic gas followed by respiratory and/or cardiac arrest. The use of ketamine plus xylazine prior to inhalation anesthesia will avoid the induction of breath-holding by guinea pigs. For prolonged cardiorespiratory assessments in the guinea pig, combining low IV bolus doses of ketamine and xylazine hourly (14.6 and 3.7 mg/kg, respectively) with inhalants may be effective (Schwenke and Cragg, 2004). Guinea pig response to ketamine/xylazine is often both variable and insufficient to achieve a surgical plane of anesthesia; however, the combination is useful for inducing anesthesia prior to maintenance with an inhalant anesthetic (Quesenberry and Carpenter, 2012). The combination of 30 mg/kg ketamine and 5 mg/kg xylazine provides approximately 30–50 min of anesthesia and is preferred to other anesthetic options for noninvasive echocardiographic evaluations and blood collection from the vena cava but not surgical procedures (Schwenke and Cragg, 2004; Cetin et al., 2005; Dang et al., 2008). The combination of medetomidine-midazolam-fentanyl can be valuable in guinea pigs as a full reversal of anesthesia with atipamezole, flumazenil, and naloxone, respectively, which can reduce recovery time and the risk of hypothermia and hypoglycemia (Karamichali et al., 2020). Fentanyl (1.0 mg/kg IM) and diazepam (5 mg/kg IP) anesthesia have also been used for minor surgical procedures on guinea pigs without causing respiratory depression (Mertens and Muller-Deile, 1991). Telazol alone was ineffective for anesthesia in guinea pigs, but when telazol (60 mg/kg IP) was combined with xylazine (5 mg/kg IP) and butorphanol (0.1 mg/kg IM), prolonged anesthesia with minimal effects on physiologic parameters was achieved (Jacobson, 2001). In guinea pigs, IM injections are sometimes used for the administration of anesthetics. The maximum volume of injectable drugs into the semimembranosus muscle is 500 uL (Bencivenga et al., 2020).

Preoxygenation is of particular value if preexisting respiratory or cardiac disease is suspected. Respiratory support, preferably intubation, and placement of an intravenous catheter are recommended to ensure the ability to rapidly support the animal should they develop respiratory depression or dehydration.

b. Analgesics

Pain behaviors present after castration and laparotomy were subtle and performed infrequently, requiring manual scoring of videos, and included lying down with or without hind legs outstretched, weight shifting, abdominal contraction, back arching, twitching, and squinting; at the same time active behaviors significantly decreased (Chen et al., 2016; Dunbar et al., 2016; Oliver et al., 2017; Ellen et al., 2016). Pain assessment in guinea pigs is made challenging by significant suppression of pain behaviors in the presence of an observer (live score, cage side) versus remote scored from video, and therefore being able to remotely observe postprocedural guinea pigs by remote video (even by baby monitor) is valuable (Oliver et al., 2017). Attempts at establishing an easy on-demand cage-side indicator of postoperative pain like the time to integration of nest scores (TINT), such as measurements of latency to consuming a preferred food treat or hay, failed to identify unalleviated pain after castration or laparotomy in guinea pigs (Dunbar et al., 2016; Oliver et al., 2017). Where mouse and rat studies have identified evidence of pain for 48 h after major surgeries, guinea pigs were identified to express pain behaviors and mechanical hyperalgesia for 96 h after laparotomy and 24 h after castration (Oliver et al., 2017; Dunbar et al., 2016). Sustained-release (ZooPharm) buprenorphine at doses of 0.3–0.6 mg/kg resulted in plasma levels above 1 ng/mL for 48 h after injection (Zanetti et al., 2017). All guinea pigs lost approximately 10% of their body weight and had reduced fecal output during the 3 days after dosing, but they also experienced significantly reduced cortisol levels, indicating a reduction in stress. AST values were also elevated at these doses of sustained-release buprenorphine but remained within normal limits for the strain of guinea pig (Zanetti et al., 2017). In guinea pigs administered 0.3 mg/kg sustained-release buprenorphine (ZooPharm), a dosing regimen of 24–48 h is recommended versus every 8 h for the standard formulation of buprenorphine, based on the plasma values of the guinea pigs (Smith et al., 2016). An extended-release buprenorphine formulation (Animalgesic Laboratories, Millersville, MD, now reformulated and available as Ethiqa), administered at 0.48 mg/kg SC in guinea pigs resulted in plasma levels above 0.9 ng/mL from 8 to 96 h after dosing, suggesting this analgesic should be administered 8 h prior to surgery to ensure adequate plasma levels in the immediate postoperative period, or paired with a preemptive dose of standard buprenorphine formulation to provide analgesia while the extended-release formulation is absorbed. As with the sustained-release buprenorphine study, guinea pigs lost approximately 10% of their body weight with and without the addition of a laparotomy, indicating the extended-release buprenorphine prevented additional body weight loss associated with postsurgical pain and had behavioral evidence of analgesia, as well (Oliver et al., 2017). Carprofen (4 mg/kg SC every 24 h for 3 days) treated guinea pigs demonstrated more mechanical hypersensitivity and behaviors indicating unalleviated postlaparotomy pain compared to those treated with extended-release buprenorphine or those that received a multimodal combination of the two analgesics. Of the three analgesic regimens assessed, the multimodal combination resulted in the best analgesic coverage, though some unalleviated pain and hyperalgesia were present at 2 h postsurgery underscoring the need to dose the extended-release buprenorphine well before surgery to ensure adequate drug levels are reached prior to recovery from anesthesia (Oliver et al., 2017). Meloxicam (0.2 mg/kg SC) paired with an intratesticular lidocaine/bupivacaine block prior to castration in guinea pigs resulted in less weight loss 24 h after surgery than controls (Ellen et al., 2016). Meloxicam (0.5 mg/kg PO) and naproxen (5 mg/kg PO) produce significant analgesia in visceral pain tests in guinea pigs, while the addition of clonidine (0.25 mg/kg PO) improved analgesia even more so (Jain et al., 2002). Guinea pigs are sensitive to naproxen-induced gastric ulceration at high doses (80 mg/kg BID), a dose about five times greater than a known ulcerogenic dose in rats (Jain et al., 2002). The incidence of this gastric ulceration in guinea pigs occurs within a few days and decreases over a 3–21 day period as the cellular population of the stomach adapts to long-term administration of naproxen. Naproxen-induced ulceration is prevented by misoprostol, but not famotidine (Fitzpatrick et al., 1999). Indomethacin does not cause gastric ulceration in guinea pigs (Mariani and Bonanomi, 1978). Aspirin is ototoxic in guinea pigs at doses as low as 50 mg/kg (Crifo, 1975).

2. Hamsters

Hamsters have very large cheek pouches that can store food and even bedding or nesting material. Therefore, it is advisable to use a cotton swab to clean or use water to flush out, or to simply invert the cheek pouch after induction of anesthesia to reduce the risk of aspiration. As a general rule, because of the size and anatomical position of the testes, the careful and deliberate orientation of male hamsters receiving IP injections is vital to prevent accidental injection into the testes.

a. Anesthetics

A mixture of medetomidine (0.15 mg/kg), midazolam (2 mg/kg), and butorphanol (2.5 mg/kg) administered IM provided effective anesthesia in Syrian hamsters; atipamezole (0.15 mg/kg) successfully antagonized both anesthesia and associated alterations in glucose and insulin (Nakamura et al., 2017). Butorphanol (2.5 mg/kg) and midazolam (2 mg/kg) have been successfully used for transponder implantation, and ketamine (25 mg/kg) and midazolam (2 mg/kg) for intranasal administration of virus in a SARs-CoV-2 model (Osterrieder et al., 2020). As with other rodent species, inhalant anesthesia is reliable and easily titratable. Isoflurane has been used to facilitate blood collection in hamsters (Picazo et al., 2009), and intranasal inoculation for SARS-CoV-2 research (Francis et al., 2021).

In Syrian hamsters, a dose of 150 or 200 mg/kg ketamine with 10 mg/kg xylazine IP fairly consistently produces an adequate level of anesthesia for most procedures for 30–60 min (Curl and Peters, 1983; Payton et al., 1993; Flecknell, 2009). Ketamine (100 mg/kg) with medetomidine (0.25 mg/kg) given IP also appears to produce effective surgical anesthesia, which can be partially reversed with atipamezole (1 mg/kg) (Flecknell, 2009). Lower doses of ketamine are less reliable in this species. In Dzungarian hamsters (*Phodopus* spp.), ketamine 50–100 mg/kg and xylazine 5–10 mg/kg administered IP produce a satisfactory level of general anesthesia. Although ketamine is generally considered very safe in most species, twice this dose of ketamine in *Phodopus* hamsters (200 mg/kg) is fatal in about 50% of the recipients (Curl, 1988). In neonatal *Phodopus*, a lower dose of ketamine (40 mg/kg) and xylazine (4 mg/kg) administered IP produces a surgical plane of anesthesia within 3–4 min, which lasted for at least 30 min (Vella et al., 2004). Although ketamine and xylazine in combination appear to be very safe in hamsters, Gaertner et al. (1987) demonstrated that IM injections of 100–200 mg/kg ketamine with 10 mg/kg xylazine consistently produce moderate-to-severe muscle necrosis at the injection site. When possible, ketamine should be administered IP in hamsters. If IM injections are required, injection-related necrosis may be reduced by diluting the stock concentration.

Telazol 20 mg/kg and xylazine 10 mg/kg IP in hamsters were adequate for restraint, but necrotic muscle lesions may appear following IM injection. Higher doses of telazol (30 mg/kg) combined with 10 mg/kg xylazine IP produce a safe and reliable level of surgical anesthesia (Forsythe et al., 1992). Lower dosages of telazol in hamsters are suitable for less painful, noninvasive experimental manipulations (Hrapkiewicz et al., 1989). Hamsters may exhibit poor respiration following telazol administration (Silverman et al., 1983).

Though not available in the United States, fentanyl/fluanisone (Hypnorm) paired with midazolam or diazepam, administered IP, works well in hamsters and provides surgical anesthesia for 20–40 min, and can be partially reversed with nalbuphine or butorphanol (Flecknell, 2009).

Pentobarbital (50–90 mg/kg IP) produces profound respiratory perturbations and high mortality; with much safer options available, pentobarbital is not recommended for anesthesia for this species (Skornik and Brain, 1990).

b. Analgesics

Clinical signs of pain in hamsters include weight loss and prolonged periods of sleep, as well as behaviors including hunched posture with head down, reluctance to move, increased depression or aggression, incision grooming, back arch, fall/stagger, twitch, writhe, hind kick, dart, vocalize, and weight shift. While these behaviors were found to be quite specific for pain in Syrian hamsters, they were performed infrequently and even less so in the presence of an observer versus remote video (Edmunson et al., 2021). Pain behaviors were identified for 3 days postlaparotomy, thus analgesia should be provided throughout this period for procedures of equivalent invasiveness. A Syrian Hamster Grimace Scale was found to be quite specific for postsurgical pain but was only sensitive enough to accurately identify about 30% of the postsurgical hamsters. Of the facial action units scored, the orbital tightening was the most prominent pain-associated feature. While grimace scores were assigned from the video, the video was recorded with an observer in the room. Like mice, study data suggested hamsters may suppress pain faces in the presence of observers. Therefore, the grimace scale does not appear to be a reliable cage-side indicator for identifying postoperative pain in hamsters (Edmunson et al., 2021). Like guinea pigs, hamsters were just as rapid at taking treats after surgery as they were without any manipulations or after anesthesia alone, and thus latency to taking a preferred treat is also not a reliable indicator of unalleviated pain in either species (Edmunson et al., 2021).

High doses of morphine (80 mg/kg) produce sedation in hamsters, while lower doses (10 mg/kg) do not appear to have any behavioral effects, except a reduction in sexual response in females (Ostrowski et al., 1979). This diminished sexual activity is reversible by naloxone. Meloxicam is recommended at 0.5 mg/kg, PO or SC, at least once daily, and carprofen at 5 mg/kg, SC, at least once daily, though in mice twice-daily dosing and/or much higher doses (20 mg/kg) have been required to reach adequate efficacy. Buprenorphine is recommended at 0.5 mg/kg, SC every 8 h (Dutton, 2020).

3. Gerbils

Isoflurane and sevoflurane induction and maintenance work well in gerbils, and appear to have lower MAC required than is typically needed for mice and rats, about 1.6% isoflurane for maintance of anesthesia (Flecknell, 2009; Griffiths et al., 2010; de Segura et al., 2009; Moons et al., 2007). Ketamine (75 mg/kg) and medetomidine (0.5 mg/kg), given IP, provide at least 30 min of safe, repeatable anesthesia in Mongolian gerbils (*Meriones unguiculatus*) (Perez-Garcia et al., 2003). Ketamine (30 mg/kg), xylazine (6 mg/kg), and acepromazine (1 mg/kg) administered IP facilitated jugular venipuncture in fat-tailed gerbil (*Pachyuromys duprasi*) (Felt et al., 2009). Ketamine alone or in combination with only one of the following: xylazine, acepromazine, or diazepam, produced sedation but did not consistently provide deeper anesthesia appropriate for surgery in gerbils (Flecknell et al., 1983). However, ketamine (100 mg/kg) and xylazine (5 mg/kg) dosed IP were appropriate for EEG and ABR readings in gerbils (Jing et al., 2021); and fentanyl (0.03 mg/kg), midazolam (7.5 mg/kg), and medetomidine (0.15 mg/kg) dosed IP may be preferable for 18F-FDG-PET imaging as it has fewer effects on glucose than ketamine/xylazine in gerbils (Kessler et al., 2018). Hypnorm (fentanyl/fluanisone) dosed with diazepam, but not xylazine, provides both anesthesia and analgesia for minor surgical procedures and can be partially reversed with nalbuphine or butorphanol (Flecknell et al., 1983, 2009). Diazepam (5 mg/kg IP) or midazolam (5 mg/kg IP) can be used for sedation and immobilization but do not provide any analgesia (Flecknell, 2009). Alfaxalone resulted in severe respiratory depression in gerbils and is not recommended (Flecknell et al., 1983). Pentobarbital resulted in profound hypothermia and high mortality during relatively simple 60-minute surgical procedures in gerbils (Weinandy et al., 2005; Flecknell, 2009) and prolonged recovery times compared with ketamine (Lightfoote and Molinari, 1978). With much safer anesthetic options for this species, pentobarbital is not recommended for use in gerbils.

Carprofen (5 mg/kg SC) is described for treating postoperative pain in gerbils; however, analgesia efficacy was not assessed, and more frequent dosing (twice daily) and/or much higher doses (20 mg/kg) have recently been identified to provide effective analgesia in mice (Moons et al., 2007). Buprenorphine may be dosed at 0.1–0.2 mg/kg, SC every 8 h, and meloxicam at 0.5 mg/kg, PO or SC at least once per day (Dutton, 2020) (Table 14.6).

4. Other rodents: see Chapter 22 Other Mammals for additional rodents species

TABLE 14.6 Anesthesia and analgesia agents for other rodents.

Drug	Species	Use	Dose mg/kg unless otherwise specified	Route	References
Acetaminophen (paracetamol, Tylenol)	Hamster	AG	200	PO, IP	Neiger-Aeschbacher (2002)
Aspirin	Guinea pig	AG	87	PO	Flecknell (2015)
Atipamezole (Antisedan)	Rodents	R	0.1–1	IM, IP, SC, PO, IV	Flecknell (2015)
Buprenorphine (Buprenex)	Hamster, Guinea pig, Chinchilla	AG	0.05–0.1	SC, IP	Mueller (2018), Foley et al. (2019)
Butorphanol (Torbugesic, Torbutrol, Stadol)	Guinea pig	AG	1–2	SC	Flecknell (2015)
Carprofen (Rimadyl)	Hamster, Guinea pig, Chinchilla	AG	2–5	SC, IM	Foley et al. (2019), Neiger-Aeschbacher (2002), Oliver et al. (2017)
Diclofenac (Voltaren)	Guinea pig	AG	2.1	PO	Flecknell (2015)
Dipyrone (Metamizole)	Guinea pig, Chinchilla	AG	100–200	PO	GV-SOLAS (2020)
Flunixin meglumine (Banamine, Flunazine)	Hamster Guinea pig Chinchilla	AG	2.5 3–5 1–3	SC	Emmerich and Hein (2018) Fehr et al. (2014)
Isoflurane (Forane)	Guinea Pig	I A	5% induction, 1.5-2% maintenance	Inhaled	Ross et al. (2000)
Ibuprofen	Guinea pig	AG	10	PO	Foley et al. (2019)
Ketamine (Ketaset)/diazepam	Guinea pig	A	100 K/5 D	IM	Flecknell (2015)
Ketamine/medetomidine	Guinea pig	A	40 K/0.5 M	IP	Flecknell (2015)
Ketamine/xylazine	Guinea pig	A	40 K/5 X	IP	
Ketamine/xylazine/acepromazine (not approriate for surgery)	Gerbil	A	30 K/6 X /1A	IP	Felt et al. (2009)
Lidocaine/prilocaine creme (EMLA Cream)	Rodents	TA	Local application	Topical	Arevalo et al. (2004), Flecknell et al. (1990), Sintov and Shapiro (2004)
Meloxicam (Metacam)	Guinea pig	AG	0.1–0.3	SC, PO	Foley et al. (2019)
Morphine	Guinea pig	AG	2.5	SC, IM	Flecknell (2015)
Nalbuphine	Guinea pig	AG	1–2	IV, IP, IM	Flecknell (2015)

A, anesthetic; AG, analgesic; I, induction agent; LA, local anesthetic; NMB, neuromuscular blockade; PA, preanesthetic; R, reversal agent; SC-L, subcutaneous in liposomes; TA, topical anesthetic.

References

Abbott, F.V., Bonder, M., 1997. Options for management of acute pain in the rat. Vet. Rec. 140 (21), 553–557.

Abbott, F.V., Hellemans, K.G., 2000. Phenacetin, acetaminophen and dipyrone: analgesic and rewarding effects. Behav. Brain Res. 112 (1–2), 177–186.

Abram, S.E., Mampilly, G.A., Milosavljevic, D., 1997. Assessment of the potency and intrinsic activity of systemic versus intrathecal opioids in rats. Anesthesiology 87 (1), 127–134 (discussion 27A–29A).

Abreu, M., Aguado, D., Benito, J., Gómez de Segura, I.A., 2012. Reduction of the sevoflurane minimum alveolar concentration induced by methadone, tramadol, butorphanol and morphine in rats. Lab. Anim. 46 (3), 200–206.

Adamson, T.W., Kendall, L.V., Goss, S., Grayson, K., Touma, C., Palme, R., Chen, J.Q., Borowsky, A.D., 2010. Assessment of carprofen and buprenorphine on recovery of mice after surgical removal of the mammary fat pad. JAALAS 49 (5), 610–616.

Akerman, S.B., 1985. A methodological study of spinal (subarachnoid) anaesthesia in the rat and the mouse. Br. J. Anaesth. 57 (3), 329–332.

Akman, O., Raol, Y.H., Auvin, S., Cortez, M.A., Kubova, H., de Curtis, M., Ikeda, A., Dudek, F.E., Galanopoulou, A.S., 2018. Methodologic recommendations and possible interpretations of video-EEG recordings in immature rodents used as experimental controls: a TASK1-WG2 report of the ILAE/AES Joint Translational Task Force. Epilepsia Open 3 (4), 437–459.

Alamaw, E.D., Franco, B.D., Jampachaisri, K., Huss, M.K., Pacharinsak, C., 2022. Extended-release buprenorphine, an FDA indexed analgesic, attenuates mechanical hypersensitivity in rats (*Rattus norvegicus*). J. Am. Assoc. Lab. Anim. Sci. 61 (1), 81–88.

Albrecht, M., Henke, J., Tacke, S., Markert, M., Guth, B., 2014. Influence of repeated anaesthesia on physiological parameters in male Wistar rats: a telemetric study about isoflurane, ketamine-xylazine and a combination of medetomidine, midazolam and fentanyl. BMC Vet. Res. 10, 310.

Alemán-Laporte, J., Bandini, L.A., Garcia-Gomes, M.S., Zanatto, D.A., Fantoni, D.T., Amador Pereira, M.A., Navas-Suárez, P.E., Kirsten, T.B., Jimenez, R.R., Alvarado, G., Mori, C.C., 2020. Combination of ketamine and xylazine with opioids and acepromazine in rats: physiological changes and their analgesic effect analysed by ultrasonic vocalization. Lab. Anim. 54 (2), 171–182.

Alexander, K.S., Rodriguez, T.R., Sarfo, A.N., Patton, T.B., Miller, L.L., 2019. Effects of monoamine uptake inhibitors on pain-related depression of nesting in mice. Behav. Pharmacol. 30 (6), 463–470.

Alkire, M.T., Nathan, S.V., McReynolds, J.R., 2005. Memory enhancing effect of low-dose sevoflurane does not occur in basolateral amygdala-lesioned rats. Anesthesiology 103 (6), 1167–1173.

Allen, M., Johnson, R.A., 2018. Evaluation of self-injurious behavior, thermal sensitivity, food intake, fecal output, and pica after injection of three buprenorphine formulations in rats (*Rattus norvegicus*). Am. J. Vet. Res. 79, 697–703.

Alves, H.C., Valentin, A.M., Olsson, I.A., Antunes, L.M., 2007. Intraperitoneal propofol and propofol fentanyl, sufentanil and remifentanil combinations for mouse anaesthesia. Lab. Anim 41, 329–336.

Antunes, L.M., Roughan, J.V., Flecknell, P.A., 2003. Excitatory effects of fentanyl upon the rat electroencephalogram and auditory-evoked potential responses during anaesthesia. Eur. J. Anaesthesiol. 20 (10), 800–808.

Arango-Gonzalez, B., Schatz, A., Bolz, S., Eslava-Schmalbach, J., Willmann, G., Zhour, A., Zrenner, E., Fischer, M.D., Gekeler, F., 2012. Effects of combined ketamine/xylazine anesthesia on light induced retinal degeneration in rats. PLoS One 7 (4), e35687.

Arevalo, M.I., Escribano, E., Calpena, A., Domenech, J., Queralt, J., 2004. Rapid skin anesthesia using a new topical amethocaine formulation: a preclinical study. Anesth. Analg. 98 (5), 1407–1412.

Arras, M., Autenried, P., Rettich, A., Spaeni, D., Rulicke, T., 2001. Optimization of intraperitoneal injection anesthesia in mice: drugs, dosages, adverse effects, and anesthesia depth. Comp. Med. 51 (5), 443–456.

Arras, M., Rettich, A., Cinelli, P., Kasermann, H.P., Burki, K., 2007. Assessment of post-laparotomy pain in laboratory mice by telemetric recording of heart rate and heart rate variability. BMC Vet. Res. 3 (1), 1–10.

Arts, J.W., Kramer, K., Arndt, S.S., Ohl, F.S., 2014. Ex differences in physiological acclimatization after transfer in wistar rats. Animals (Basel) 30 (4), 693–711.

Asai, T., Mapleson, W.W., Power, I., 1998. Effects of nalbuphine, pentazocine and U50488H on gastric emptying and gastrointestinal transit in the rat. Br. J. Anaesth. 80 (6), 814–819.

Attia, M.A., El-Gibaly, I., Shaltout, S.E., Fetih, G.N., 2004. Transbuccal permeation, anti-inflammatory activity and clinical efficacy of piroxicam formulated in different gels. Int. J. Pharm. 276 (1–2), 11–28.

Avsaroglu, H., Sommer, R., Hellebrekers, L.J., van Zutphen, L.F., van Lith, HA.., 2008. The effects of buprenorphine on behaviour in the ACI and BN rat inbred strains. Lab. Anim. 42 (2), 171–184. In this issue.

Backonja, M.M., Miletic, G., Miletic, V., 1995. The effect of continuous morphine analgesia on chronic thermal hyperalgesia due to sciatic constriction injury in rats. Neurosci. Lett. 196 (1–2), 61–64.

Baker, N.J., Schofield, J.C., Caswell, M.D., McLellan, A.D., 2011. Effects of early atipamezole reversal of medetomidine–ketamine anesthesia in mice. J. Am. Assoc. Lab. Anim. Sci. 50, 916–920.

Bauer, D.J., Christenson, T.J., Clark, K.R., Powell, S.K., Swain, R.A., 2003. Acetaminophen as a postsurgical analgesic in rats: a practical solution to neophobia. Contemp. Top. Lab. Anim. Sci. 42 (2), 20–25.

Bauer, C., Schillinger, U., Brandl, J., Meyer-Lindenberg, A., Ott, A., Baumgartner, C., 2019. Comparison of pre-emptive butorphanol or metamizole with ketamine +medetomidine and s-ketamine + medetomidine anaesthesia in improving intraoperative analgesia in mice. Lab. Anim. 53 (5), 459–469.

Becker, K., Bergadano, A., Eberspacher, E., Haberstroh, J., Henke, J., Sager, M., Zahner, D., Arras, M., 2016. The use of alpha-chloralose in experiments with rodents and rabbits. In: From the Committee for Anaesthesia (GV-SOLAS) in Collaboration with Working Group 4 of the Veterinary Assocation for Animal Welfare. GV-SOLAS. http://www.gv-solas.de/fileadmin/user_upload/pdf_publikation/Anaest._Analgesie/Chloralose_Maerz_2016_e.pdf. (Accessed 7 January 2022).

Beirith, A., Santos, A.R., Rodrigues, A.L., Creczynski-Pasa, T.B., Calixto, J.B., 1998. Spinal and supraspinal antinociceptive action of dipyrone in formalin, capsaicin and glutamate tests. Study of the mechanism of action. Eur. J. Pharmacol. 345 (3), 233–245.

Bekker, A., Shah, R., Quatermain, D., Li, Y.S., Blanck, T., 2006. Isoflurane preserves spatial working memory in adult mice after moderate hypoxia. Anesth. Analg. 102 (4), 1134–1138.

Bellon, M., Le Bot, A., Michelet, D., Hilly, J., Maesani, M., Brasher, C., Dahmani, S., June 2016. Efficacy of intraoperative dexmedetomidine compared with placebo for postoperative pain management: a meta-analysis of published studies. Pain Ther. 5 (1), 63–80.

Bencivenga, M.A., Bowling, P.A., Fiallos, J.O., Gehling, A.M., Stafford, R.G., Long, S.Y., Fetterer, D.P., Bocan, T.M., Hofer, C.C., May 1, 2020. Investigation of various intramuscular volumes delivered to the semimembranosus muscle of cavia porcellus. J. Am. Assoc. Lab. Anim. Sci. 59 (3), 310–321.

Benesova, O., Tejkalova, H., Kristofikova, Z., Husek, P., Nedvidkova, J., Yamamotova, A., 2001. Brain maldevelopment and neurobehavioural deviations in adult rats treated neonatally with indomethacin. Eur. Neuropsychopharmacol. 11 (5), 367–373.

Beninson, J.A., Lofgren, J.L., Lester, P.A., Hileman, M.M., Berkowitz, D.J., Myers Jr., D.D., May 1, 2018. Analgesic efficacy and hematologic effects of robenacoxib in mice. J. Am. Assoc. Lab. Anim. Sci. 57 (3), 258–267.

Bennett, T.E., Pavek, T.J., Schwark, W.S., Singh, B., 2021. Comparison of nociceptive effects of buprenorphine, firocoxib, and meloxicam in a plantar incision model in sprague-dawley rats. JAALAS 60 (5), 539–548.

Blaha, M.D., Leon, L.R., 2008. Effects of indomethacin and buprenorphine analgesia on the postoperative recovery of mice. JAALAS 47 (4), 8–19.

Blaney, A., Jampachaisri, K., Huss, M.K., Pacharinsak, C., 2021. Sustained release buprenorphine effectively attenuates postoperative hypersensitivity in an incisional pain model in neonatal rats (*Rattus norvegicus*). PLoS One 16 (2), e0246213.

Blevins, C.E., Celeste, N.A., Marx, J.O., 2021. Effects of oxygen supplementation on injectable and inhalant anesthesia in C57BL/6 mice. J. Am. Assoc. Lab. Anim. Sci. 60 (3), 289–297.

Bohrer, H., Schmidt, H., Bach, A., Martin, E., Kohl, B., Bolsen, K., Goerz, G., 1994. Porphyrinogenic effects of atracurium, vecuronium, and pancuronium in a primed rat model. Lab. Anim. Sci. 44 (4), 326–330.

Bolan, E.A., Tallarida, R.J., Pasternak, G.W., 2002. Synergy between mu opioid ligands: evidence for functional interactions among mu opioid receptor subtypes. J. Pharmacol. Exp. Ther. 303 (2), 557–562.

Braden, G.C., Brice, A.K., Hankenson, F.C., May 2015. Adverse effects of vapocoolant and topical anesthesia for tail biopsy of preweanling mice. J. Am. Assoc. Lab. Anim. Sci. 54 (3), 291–298.

Brammer, A., West, C.D., Allen, S.L., 1993. A comparison of propofol with other injectable anaesthetics in a rat model for measuring cardiovascular parameters. Lab. Anim. 27 (3), 250–257.

Branson, K.R., 2001. Injectable anesthetics. In: Adams, H.R. (Ed.), Veterinary Pharmacology and Therapeutics, eighth ed. Iowa State University Press, Ames, IA, pp. 213–268.

Branson, K.R., Gross, M.E., 2001. Opioid agonists and antagonists. In: Adams, H.R. (Ed.), Veterinary Pharmacology and Therapeutics. Iowa State University Press, Ames, Iowa, pp. 268–298.

Briggs, S.L., Sawyer, D.C., Rech, R.H., Galligan, J.J., 1995. Oxymorphone-induced analgesia and colonic motility measured in colorectal distension. Pharmacol. Biochem. Behav. 52 (3), 561–563.

Brown, K.M., Saunders, M.M., Kirsch, T., Donahue, H.J., Reid, J.S., 2004. Effect of COX-2-specific inhibition on fracture-healing in the ratfemur. J. Bone Joint Surg. Am. 86-A (1), 116–123.

Browne, K.D., Iwata, A., Putt, M.E., Smith, D.H., 2006. Chronic ibuprofen administration worsens cognitive outcome following traumatic brain injury in rats. Exp. Neurol. 201 (2), 301–307.

Buelke-Sam, J., Holson, J.F., Bazare, J.J., Young, J.F., 1978. Comparative stability of physiological parameters during sustained anesthesia in rats. Lab. Anim. Sci. 28 (2), 157–162.

Buetow, B.S., Chen, L.I., Maggio-Price, L., Swisshelm, K., 1999. Peritonitis in nude mice in a xenograft study. Contemp. Top. Lab. Anim. Sci. 38 (6), 47–49.

Buitrago, S., Martin, T., Tetens-Woodring, J., et al., 2008. Safety and efficacy of various combinations of injectable anesthetics in BALB/c mice. JALAAS 47 (1), 11–17.

Burn, C.C., Mazlan, N.H.B., Chancellor, N., Wells, D.J., June 3, 2021. The pen is milder than the blade: identification marking mice using ink on the tail appears more humane than ear-punching even with local anaesthetic. Animals (Basel) 11 (6), 1664.

Burnside, W.M., Flecknell, P.A., Cameron, A.I., et al., 2013. A comparison of medetomidine and its active enantiomer dexmedetomidine when administered with ketamine in mice. BMC Vet. Res. 9, 48.

Bushnell, M.C., Case, L.K., Ceko, M., Cotton, V.A., Gracely, J.L., Low, L.A., Pitcher, M.H., Villemure, C., 2015. Effect of environment on the long-term consequences of chronic pain. Pain 156 (Suppl. 1), S42–S49.

Buvanendran, A., Kroin, J.S., Kari, M.R., Tuman, K.J., 2008. A new knee surgery model in rats to evaluate functional measures of postoperative pain. Anesth. Analg. 107 (1), 300–308.

Cagle, L.A., Franzi, L.M., Epstein, S.E., Kass, P.H., Last, J.A., Kenyon, N.J., 2017. Injectable anesthesia for mice: combined effects of dexmedetomidine, tiletamine-zolazepam, and butorphanol. Anesth. Res. Pract. 9161040.

Calderone, L., Grimes, P., Shalev, M., 1986. Acute reversible cataract induced by xylazine and by ketamine–xylazine anesthesia in rats and mice. Exp. Eye Res. 42 (4), 331–337.

Campos, A.R., Santos, F.A., Rao, V.S., 2006. Ketamine-induced potentiation of morphine analgesia in rat tail-flick test: role of opioid-, alpha2-adrenoceptors and ATP-sensitive potassium channels. Biol. Pharm. Bull. 29 (1), 86–89.

Camprodon, R.A., Bowles, M.J., 2006. Perioperative analgesia in experimental small bowel transplantation. Transplant. Proc. 38 (6), 1857–1858.

Cantwell, S.L., 2001. Ferret, rabbit, and rodent anesthesia. Vet. Clin. North Am. Exot. Anim. Pract. 4 (1), 169–191.

Capetola, R.J., Rosenthale, M.E., Dubinsky, B., McGuire, J.L., 1983. Peripheral antialgesics: a review. J. Clin. Pharmacol. 23 (11–12), 545–556.

Caro, A.C., Tucker, J.J., Yannascoli, S.M., Dunkman, A.A., Thomas, S.J., Soslowsky, L.J., 2014. Efficacy of various analgesics on shoulder function and rotator cuff tendon-to-bone healing in a rat (Rattus norvegicus) model. J. Am. Assoc. Lab. Anim. Sci. 53, 185–192.

Carpenter, K.C., Hakenjos, J.M., Fry, C.D., Nemzek, J.A., 2019. The influence of pain and analgesia in rodent models of sepsis. Comp. Med. 69 (6), 546–554.

Ceccarelli, I., De Padova, A.M., Fiorenzani, P., Massafra, C., Aloisi, A.M., 2006. Single opioid administration modifies gonadal steroids in both the CNS and plasma of male rats. Neuroscience 140 (3), 929–937.

Celerier, E., Gonzalez, J.R., Maldonado, R., Cabanero, D., Puig, M.M., 2006. Opioid-induced hyperalgesia in a murine model of postoperative pain: role of nitric oxide generated from the inducible nitric oxide synthase. Anesthesiology 104 (3), 546–555.

Celerier, E., Rivat, C., Jun, Y., Laulin, J.P., Larcher, A., Reynier, P., Simonnet, G., 2000. Long-lasting hyperalgesia induced by fentanyl in rats: preventive effect of ketamine. Anesthesiology 92 (2), 465–472.

Cetin, N., Cetin, E., Toker, M., 2005. Echocardiographic variables in healthy Guinea pigs anaesthetized with ketamine–xylazine. Lab. Anim. 39 (1), 100–106.

Cesarovic, N., Nicholls, F., Rettich, A., et al., 2010. Isoflurane and sevoflurane provide equally effective anaesthesia in laboratory mice. Lab. Anim 44 (4), 329–336.

Cesarovic, N., Jirkof, P., Rettich, A., Nicholls, F., Arras, M., 2012. Combining sevoflurane anesthesia with fentanyl-midazolam or s-ketamine in laboratory mice. J. Am. Assoc. Lab. Anim. Sci. 51 (2), 209–218.

Charlet, A., Rodeau, J.L., Poisbeau, P., 2011. Radiotelemetric and symptomatic evaluation of pain in the rat after laparotomy: long-term benefits of perioperative ropivacaine care. J. Pain 12, 246–256.

Chartier, L.C., Hebart, M.L., Howarth, G.S., Whittaker, A.L., Mashtoub, S., 2020. Affective state determination in a mouse model of colitis-associated colorectal cancer. PLoS One 15 (1), e0228413.

Chen, P.H., Boyd, K.L., Fickle, E.K., Locuson, C.W., 2016. Subcutaneous meloxicam suspension pharmacokinetics in mice and dose considerations for postoperative analgesia. J. Vet. Pharmacol. Ther. 39 (4), 356–362.

Chen, K.T., Hu, O.Y., Ho, S.T., Chen, Y.W., Wang, J.J., 2002a. The analgesic effect of nalbuphine and its long-acting prodrug, nalbuphine pivalate, in rats. Acta Anaesthesiol. Sin. 40 (4), 191–195.

Cho, C., Michailidis, V., Lecker, I., Collymore, C., Hanwell, D., Loka, M., Danesh, M., Pham, C., Urban, P., Bonin, R.P., Martin, L.J., 2019. Evaluating analgesic efficacy and administration route following craniotomy in mice using the grimace scale. Sci. Rep. 9 (1), 359.

Choi, S.S., Lee, J.K., Suh, H.W., 2001. Antinociceptive profiles of aspirin and acetaminophen in formalin, substance P and glutamate pain models. Brain Res. 921 (1–2), 233–239.

Christoph, T., Kogel, B., Schiene, K., Meen, M., De Vry, J., Friderichs, E., 2005. Broad analgesic profile of buprenorphine in rodent models of acute and chronic pain. Eur. J. Pharmacol. 507 (1–3), 87–98.

Chu, D.K., Jordan, M.C., Kim, J.K., Couto, M.A., Roos, K.P., 2006. Comparing isoflurane with tribromoethanol anesthesia for echocardiographic phenotyping of transgenic mice. J. Am. Assoc. Lab. Anim. Sci. 45 (4), 8–13.

Chum, H.H., Jampachairsri, K., McKeon, G.P., Yeomans, D.C., Pacharinsak, C., Felt, S.A., 2014. Antinociceptive effects of sustained-release buprenorphine in a model of incisional pain in rats (*Rattus norvegicus*). JAALAS 53 (2), 193–197.

Ciuffreda, M.C., Tolva, V., Casana, R., Gnecchi, M., Vanoli, E., Spazzolini, C., Roughan, J., Calvillo, L., 2014. Rat experimental model of myocardial ischemia/reperfusion injury: an ethical approach to set up the analgesic management of acute post-surgical pain. PLoS One 9 (4), e95913.

Clark, T.S., Clark, D.D., Hoyt Jr., R.F., 2014. Pharmacokinetic comparison of sustained- release and standard buprenorphine in mice. J. Am. Assoc. Lab. Anim. Sci. 53, 387–391.

Clark Jr., J.A., Myers, P.H., Goelz, M.F., Thigpen, J.E., Forsythe, D.B., 1997. Pica behavior associated with buprenorphine administration in the rat. Lab. Anim. Sci. 47 (3), 300–303.

Clark, M.D., Krugner-Higby, L., Smith, L.J., Heath, T.D., Clark, K.L., Olson, D., 2004. Evaluation of liposome-encapsulated oxymorphone hydrochloride in mice after splenectomy. Comp. Med. 54 (5), 558–563.

Clifford, D.H., 1984. Preanesthesia, anesthesia, analgesia and euthanasia. In: Fox, J.G., Cohen, B.J., Loew, F.M. (Eds.), Laboratory Animal Medicine. Academic Press, New York, pp. 527–562.

Cloutier, S., LaFollette, M.R., Gaskill, B.N., Panksepp, J., Newberry, R.C., 2018. Tickling, a technique for inducing positive affect when handling rats. JoVE (135), 57190.

Cobos, E.J., Araldi, D., Segal, D., Duong, K., Woolf, C.J., 2012. Inflammation-induced decrease in voluntary wheel running in mice: a nonreflexive test for evaluating inflammatory pain and analgesia. Pain 153 (4), 876–884.

Code of Federal Regulations, 1997. Title 9: Animals and Animal Products; Chap. 1 Animal and Plant Health Inspection Service, United States Department of Agriculture; Policy #11, Painful Procedures. Office of the Federal Register, Washington, DC.

Code of Federal Regulations, 2000. Title 9: Animals and Animal Products; Chap. 1 Animal and Plant Health Inspection Service, United States Department of Agriculture; Policy #12, Alternatives to Painful Procedures. Office of the Federal Register, Washington, DC.

Code of Federal Regulations, 2002. Title 9, Animals and Animal Products, Subchapter A, Part 1–3. Animal Welfare Act, Washintgon, D.C.

Colpaert, F.C., Tarayre, J.P., Alliaga, M., Bruins Slot, L.A., Attal, N., Koek, W., 2001. Opiate self-administration as a measure of chronic nociceptive pain in arthritic rats. Pain 91 (1–2), 33–45.

Crain, S.M., Shen, K.F., 2001. Acute thermal hyperalgesia elicited by low-dose morphine in normal mice is blocked by ultra-low-dose naltrexone, unmasking potent opioid analgesia. Brain Res. 888 (1), 75–82.

Crifo, S., 1975. Aspirin ototoxicity inthe Guinea pig. ORL 37 (1), 27–34.

Cruz, J.I., Loste, J.M., Burzaco, O.H., 1998. Observations on the use of medetomidine/ketamine and its reversal with atipamezole for chemical restraint in the mouse. Lab. Anim. 32 (1), 18–22.

Curl, J.L., 1988. Ketamine–xylazine anaesthesia in the Djungarian hamster (*Phodopus sungorus*). Lab. Anim. 22 (4), 309–312.

Curl, J.L., Peters, L.L., 1983. Ketamine hydrochloride and xylazine hydrochloride anaesthesiainthe golden hamster (*Mesocricetus auratus*). Lab. Anim. 17 (4), 290–293.

Dahl, J.B., Kehlet, H., 2011. Preventive analgesia. Curr. Opin. Anaesthesiol. 24 (3), 331–338.

Dang, V., Bao, S., Ault, A., Murray, C., McFarlane-Mills, J., Chiedi, C., Dillon, M., Todd, J.P., Detolla, L., Rao, S., November 2008. Efficacy and safety of five injectable anesthetic regimens for chronic blood collection from the anterior vena cava of Guinea pigs. J. Am. Assoc. Lab. Anim. Sci. 47 (6), 56–60.

Danneman, P.J., Mandrell, T.D., 1997. Evaluation of five agents/methods for anesthesia of neonatal rats. Lab. Anim. Sci. 47 (4), 386–395.

David, J.M., Duarte Vogel, S., Longo, K., Sanchez, D., Lawson, G., November 2014. The use of eutectic mixture of lidocaine and prilocaine in mice (Mus musculus) for tail vein injections. Vet. Anaesth. Analg. 41 (6), 654–659.

Davis, A., Perkins, M.N., 1993. The effect of capsaicin and conventional analgesics in two models of monoarthritis in the rat. Agents Actions 38 (Spec No), C10–C12.

DeMarco, G.J., Nunamaker, E.A., 2019. A review of the effects of pain and analgesia on immune system function and inflammation: relevance for preclinical studies. Comp. Med. 69 (6), 520–534.

Del Monte, M., Omini, C., Subissi, A., 1990. Mechanism of the potentiation of neurally-induced bronchoconstriction by gallamine in the guinea-pig. Br. J. Pharmacol. 99 (3), 582–586.

de Segura, I.A., de la Víbora, J.B., Criado, A., 2009. Determination of the minimum alveolar concentration for halothane, isoflurane and sevoflurane in the gerbil. Lab. Anim. 43 (3), 239–242.

Deng, H.B., Li, F.X., Cai, Y.H., et al., 2018. Waste anesthetic gas exposure and strategies for solution. J. Anesth. 32, 269–282.

Dholakia, U., Clark-Price, S., Keating, S., et al., 2017. Anesthetic effects and bodyweight changes associated with ketamine xylazine- lidocaine administered to CD-1 mice. PLoS One 12 (9), e0184911.

Diaz-Reval, M.I., Ventura-Martinez, R., Hernandez-Delgadillo, G.P., Dominguez-Ramirez, A.M., Lopez-Munoz, F.J., 2001. Effect of caffeine on antinociceptive action of ketoprofen in rats. Arch. Med. Res. 32 (1), 13–20.

Ding, F., Zheng, L., Liu, M., Chen, R., Leung, L.S., Luo, T., 2016. Ciproxifan, an H3 receptor antagonist, improves short-term recognition memory impaired by isoflurane anesthesia. J. Anesth. 30, 684–690.

Dingley, J., Tooley, J., Porter, H., Thoresen, M., 2006. Xenon provides short-termneuroprotection in neonatal rats when administered after hypoxia– ischemia. Stroke 37 (2), 501–506.

Dodelet-Devillers, A., Zullian, C., Vachon, P., Beaudry, F., 2016. Assessment of stability of ketamine-xylazine preparations with or without acepromazine using high performance liquid chromatography-mass spectrometry. Can. J. Vet. Res. 80 (1), 86–89.

Doretto, M.C., Garcia-Cairasco, N., Pimenta, N.J., Souza, D.A., Tatsuo, M.A., 1998. Dipyrone, a novel anticonvulsant agent? Insights from three experimental epilepsy models. Neuroreport 9 (10), 2415–2421.

Dretchen, K., Ghoneim, M.M., Long, J.P., 1971. The interaction of diazepam with myoneural blocking agents. Anesthesiology 34 (5), 463–468.

Drobac, E., Durand, E., Laudenbach, V., Mantz, J., Gallego, J., 2004. A simple method forshort-term controlled anesthesiainnewbornmice. Physiol. Behav. 82 (2–3), 279–283.

Dubowitz, J.A., Jost-Brinkmann, F., Ziegler, A.I., Gillis, R.D., Riedel, B., Sloan, E.K., 2021. An in vivo mouse model of total intravenous anesthesia during cancer resection surgery. J. Vis. Exp. (172).

Dudley, E.S., Johnson, R.A., French, D.C., Boivin, G.P., 2016. Effects of topical anesthetics on behavior, plasma corticosterone, and blood glucose levels after tail biopsy of C57BL/6NHSD mice (Mus musculus). J. Am. Assoc. Lab. Anim. Sci. 55 (4), 443–450.

Dunbar, M.L., David, E.M., Aline, M.R., Lofgren, J.L., 2016. Validation of a behavioral ethogram for assessing postoperative pain in Guinea Pigs (*Cavia porcellus*). J. Am. Assoc. Lab. Anim. Sci. 55 (1), 29–34.

Durst, M.S., Arras, M., Palme, R., et al., 2021. Lidocaine and bupivacaine as part of multimodal pain management in a C57BL/6J laparotomy mouse model. Sci. Rep. 11, 10918.

Dutton, M., 2020. Selected veterinary concerns of geriatric rats, mice, hamsters, and gerbils. Vet. Clin. North Am. Exot. Anim. Pract. 23 (3), 525–548.

Dwyer, R.C., Rampil, I.J., Eger II, E.I., Bennett, H.L., 1994. The electroencephalogram does not predict depth of isoflurane anesthesia. Anesthesiology 81 (2), 403–409.

Ebert, B., Andersen, S., Krogsgaard-Larsen, P., 1995. Ketobemi-done, methadone and pethidine are non-competitive *N*-methyl-d-aspartate (NMDA) antagonists in the rat cortex and spinal cord. Neurosci. Lett. 187 (3), 165–168.

Eckley, S.S., Villano, J.S., Kuo, N.S., Wong, K.Y., 2020. Acepromazine and chlorpromazine as pharmaceutical-grade alternatives to chlorprothixene for pupillary light reflex imaging in mice. J. Am. Assoc. Lab. Anim. Sci. 59 (2), 197–203.

Edmunson, A.M., Duke Boynton, F.D., Rendahl, A.K., Merley, A.L., Koewler, N.J., Dunbar, M.L., Sivula, C.P., 2021. Indicators of postoperative pain in Syrian hamsters (Mesocricetus auratus). Comp. Med. 71 (1), 76–85.

Efstathiou, J.A., Sampson, D.A., Levine, Z., Rohan, R.M., Zurakowski, D., Folkman, J., D'Amato, R.J., Rupnick, M.A., 2005. Nonsteroidal antiinflammatory drugs differentially suppress endometriosis in a murine model. Fertil. Steril. 83 (1), 171–181.

Elena, G., Amerio, N., Ferrero, P., Bay, M.L., Valenti, J., Colucci, D., Puig, N.R., 2003. Effects of repetitive sevoflurane anaesthesia on immnue response, select biochemical parameters and organ histology in mice. Lab. Anim. 37 (3), 193–203.

Ellen, Y., Flecknell, P., Leach, M., September 1, 2016. Evaluation of using Behavioural changes to assess post-operative pain in the Guinea pig (Cavia porcellus). PLoS One 11 (9), e0161941.

El Mouedden, M., Meert, T.F., 2005. Evaluation of pain-related behavior, bone destruction and effectiveness of fentanyl, sufentanil, and morphine in a murine model of cancer pain. Pharmacol. Biochem. Behav. 82 (1), 109–119.

Emmerich, I.E., Hein, J., 2018. Dosierungsvorschläge für Arzneimittel bei Kleinnagern, Kaninchen, Frettchen und Igeln, 2 edn. Dosivet, Thieme.

Engelhardt, G., Homma, D., Schlegel, K., Utzmann, R., Schnitzler, C., 1995. Anti-inflammatory, analgesic, antipyretic and related properties of meloxicam, a new non-steroidal anti-inflammatory agent with favourable gastrointestinal tolerance. Inflamm. Res. 44 (10), 423–433.

Epemolu, O., Bom, A., Hope, F., Mason, R., 2003. Reversal of neuromuscular blockade and simultaneous increase in plasma rocuronium concentration after the intravenous infusion of the novel reversal agent Org 25969. Anesthesiology 99 (3), 632–637.

Erbil, Y., Berber, E., Seven, R., Calis, A., Eminoglu, L., Kocak, M., Bilgic, L., 1998. The effect of intestinal transit time on bacterial translocation. Acta Chir. Belg. 98 (6), 245–249.

Erhan, E., Onal, A., Kocabas, S., Parlar, A., Yegul, I., Kosay, S., 2005. Ondansetron does not block tramadol-induced analgesia in mice. Methods Find. Exp. Clin. Pharmacol. 27 (9), 629–632.

Erichsen, H.K., Hao, J.X., Xu, X.J., Blackburn-Munro, G., 2005. Comparative actions of the opioid analgesics morphine, methadone and codeine in rat models of peripheral and central neuropathic pain. Pain 116 (3), 347–358.

Erickson, R.L., Blevins, C.E., Souza Dyer, C., Marx, J.O., 2019. Alfaxalone-xylazine anesthesia in laboratory mice (*Mus musculus*). J. Am. Assoc. Lab. Anim. Sci. 58 (1), 30–39.

Erickson, R.L., Terzi, M.C., Jaber, S.M., Hankenson, F.C., McKinstry-Wu, A., Kelz, M.B., Marx, J.O., 2016. Intraperitoneal continuous-rate infusion for the maintenance of anesthesia in laboratory mice (*Mus musculus*). JAALAS 55 (5), 548–557.

Evangelista-Vaz, R., Bergadano, A., Arras, M., Jirkof, P.D., 2018a. Analgesic efficacy of subcutaneous-oral dosage of tramadol after surgery in C57BL/6J mice. J. Am. Assoc. Lab. Anim. Sci. 57 (4), 368–375.

Evangelista Vaz, R., Draganov, D.I., Rapp, C., Avenel, F., Steiner, G., Arras, M., Bergadano, A., 2018b. Preliminary pharmacokinetics of tramadol hydrochloride after administration via different routes in male and female B6 mice. Vet. Anaesth. Analg. 45, 111–122.

Evers, A.S., et al., 2006. In: Brunton, L., Lazo, J., Parker, K. (Eds.), Goodman and Gilman's the Pharmacological Basis of Therapeutics. McGraw Hill, New York.

Ewald, A.J., Werb, Z., Egeblad, M., 2011. Monitoring of vital signs for long-term survival of mice under anesthesia. Cold Spring Harb. Protoc. (2).

Ezell, P.C., Papa, L., Lawson, G.W., 2012. Palatability and treatment efficacy of various ibuprofen formulations in C57BL/6 mice with ulcerative dermatitis. J. Am. Assoc. Lab. Anim. Sci. 51 (5), 609–615.

Fagioli, S., Consorti, D., Pavone, F., 1990. Age-related cholinergic drug effectsonanalgesiaintwo inbred strainsofmice. Brain Res. 510 (1), 150–153.

Falcon, E., Maier, K., Robinson, S.A., Hill-Smith, T.E., Lucki, I., 2015. Effects of buprenorphine on behavioral tests for antidepressant and anxiolytic drugs in mice. Psychopharmacology (Berl) 232 (5), 907–915.

Fehr, M., Sassenburg, L., Zwart, P., 2014. Krankheiten der Heimtiere, 8 edn. Schültersche Verlaggesellschaft.

Felt, S.A., Guirguis, F.I., Wasfy, M.O., Howard, J.S., Domingo, N.V., Hussein, H.I., January 2009. An effective venipuncture technique and normal serum biochemistry parameters of the captive fat-tailed jird (Pachyuromys duprasi). J. Am. Assoc. Lab. Anim. Sci. 48 (1), 57–60.

Ferrari, L., Turrini, G., Rostello, C., Guidi, A., Casartelli, A., Piaia, A., Sartori, M., 2005. Evaluation of two combinations of Domitor, Zoletil 100, and Euthatal to obtain long-term nonrecovery anesthesia in Sprague–Dawley rats. Comp. Med. 55 (3), 256–264.

Ferrini, E., Mecozzi, L., Corsi, L., Ragionieri, L., Donofrio, G., Stellari, F.F., 2020. Alfaxalone and dexmedetomidine as an alternative to gas anesthesia for micro-CT lung imaging in a bleomycin-induced pulmonary fibrosis murine model. Front. Vet. Sci. 8 (7).

Field, K.J., White, W.J., Lang, C.M., 1993. Anaesthetic effects of chloral hydrate, pentobarbitone and urethane in adult male rats. Lab. Anim. 27 (3), 258–269.

File, S.E., Simmonds, M.A., 1988. Myoclonic seizures in the mouse induced by alphaxalone and related steroid anaesthetics. J. Pharm. Pharmacol. 40 (1), 57–59.

Finster, M., Morishima, H.O., Boyes, R.N., Covino, B.G., 1972. The placental transfer of lidocaine and its uptake by fetal tissues. Anesthesiology 36 (2), 159–163.

Fitzpatrick, L.R., Sakurai, K., Le, T., 1999. Effect of naproxen on the hamster gastric antrum: ulceration, adaptation and efficacy of anti-ulcer drugs. Aliment. Pharmacol. Ther. 13 (11), 1553–1562.

Flecknell, P.A., 1987b. Laboratory mammal anesthesia. J. Assoc. Vet. Anesth. 14, 111–119.

Flecknell, P.A., 1993a. Anaesthesia of animals for biomedical research. Br. J. Anaesth. 71 (6), 885–894.

Flecknell, P.A., 1993b. Anesthesia and perioperative care. Methods Enzymol. 225, 16–33.

Flecknell, P.A., 1996. Laboratory Animal Anaesthesia: A Practical Introduction for Research Workers and Technicians. Academic Press, London.

Flecknell, P.A., 2009. Laboratory Animal Anesthesia, third ed. Academic Press, Elsevier, Ambsterdam, the Netherlands.

Flecknell, P.A., 2015. Laboratory Animal Anesthesia, fourth ed. Academic Press, Elsevier, Ambsterdam, the Netherlands.

Flecknell, P., 2018. Rodent analgesia: assessment and therapeutics. Vet. J. 232, 70–77.

Flecknell, P.A., John, M., Mitchell, M., Shurey, C., April 1983. Injectable anaesthetic techniques in 2 species of gerbil (Meriones libycus and Meriones unguiculatus). Lab. Anim. 17 (2), 118–122.

Flecknell, P.A., Liles, J.H., 1991. The effects of surgical procedures, halothane anaesthesia and nalbuphine on locomotor activity and food and water consumption in rats. Lab. Anim. 25 (1), 50–60.

Flecknell, P.A., Liles, J.H., Williamson, H.A., 1990. The use of lignocaine-prilocaine local anaesthetic cream for pain-free vene puncture in laboratory animals. Lab. Anim. 24 (2), 142–146.

Flecknell, P.A., Mitchell, M., 1984. Midazolam and fentanyl-fluanisone: assessment of anaesthetic effects in laboratory rodents and rabbits. Lab. Anim. 18 (2), 143–146.

Flecknell, P.A., Orr, H.E., Roughan, J.V., Stewart, R., 1999a. Comparison of the effects of oral or subcutaneous carprofen or ketoprofen in rats undergoing laparotomy. Vet. Rec. 144 (3), 65–67.

Flecknell, P.A., Roughan, J.V., Stewart, R., 1999b. Use of oral buprenorphine ('buprenorphine jello') for postoperative analgesia in rats—a clinical trial. Lab. Anim. 33 (2), 169–174.

Fleischmann, T., Jirkof, P., Henke, J., et al., 2016. Injection anaesthesia with fentanyl-midazolam-medetomidine in adult female mice: importance of antagonization and perioperative care. Lab. Anim. 50 (4), 264–274.

Flood, P., Sonner, J.M., Gong, D., Coates, K.M., 2002. Isoflurane hyperalgesia is modulated in nicotinic inhibition. Anesthesiology 97 (1), 192–198.

Foley, P.L., 2014. Current options for providing sustained analgesia to laboratory animals. Lab. Anim. 43, 364–371.

Foley, P.L., Haixiang, L., Crichlow, A.R., 2011. Evaluation of a sustained-release formulation of buprenorphine for analgesia in rats. J. Am. Assoc. Lab. Anim. Sci. 50 (2), 198–204.

Foley, P.L., Kendall, L.V., Turner, P.V., 2019. Clinical management of pain in rodents. Comp. Med. 69 (6), 468–489.

Forsythe, D.B., Payton, A.J., Dixon, D., Myers, P.H., Clark, J.A., Snipe, J.R., 1992. Evaluation of Telazol–xylazine as an anesthetic combination for use in Syrian hamsters. Lab. Anim. Sci. 42 (5), 497–502.

Francis, M.E., Goncin, U., Kroeker, A., Swan, C., Ralph, R., Lu, Y., Etzioni, A.L., Falzarano, D., Gerdts, V., Machtaler, S., Kindrachuk, J., Kelvin, A.A., 2021. SARS-CoV-2 infection in the Syrian hamster model causes inflammation as well as type I interferon dysregulation in both respiratory and non-respiratory tissues including the heart and kidney. PLoS Pathog. 17 (7), e1009705.

Fridgeirsdottir, G.A., Hillered, L., Clausen, F., 2014. Escalated handling of young C57BL/6 mice results in altered Morris water maze performance. Ups. J. Med. Sci. 119 (1), 1–9.

Furukawa, S., MacLennan, M.J., Keller, B.B., 1998. Hemodynamic response to anesthesia in pregnant and nonpregnant ICR mice. Lab. Anim. Sci. 48 (4), 357–363.

Gades, N.M., Danneman, P.J., Wixson, S.K., Tolley, E.A., 2000. The magnitude and duration of the analgesic effect of morphine, butorphanol, and buprenorphine in rats and mice. Contemp. Top. Lab. Anim. Sci. 39 (2), 8–13.

Gaertner, D.J., Boschert, K.R., Schoeb, T.R., 1987. Muscle necrosis in Syrian hamsters resulting from intramuscular injections of ketamine and xylazine. Lab. Anim. Sci. 37 (1), 80–83.

Gaertner, D., Hallman, T., Hankenson, C., Batchelder, M., 2008. Anesthesia and Analgesia for Laboratory Rodents. American College of Laboratory Animal Medicine, Anesthesia and Analgesia in Laboratory Animals, 2nd. Academic Press, pp. 239–297.

Gallo, M.S., Karas, A.Z., Pritchett-Corning, K., Garner Guy Mulder, J.P., Gaskill, B.N., 2020. Tell-tale TINT: does the time to incorporate into nest test evaluate postsurgical pain or welfare in mice? JAALAS 59 (1), 37–45.

Gardner, D.J., Davis, J.A., Weina, P.J., Theune, B., 1995. Comparison of tribromoethanol, ketamine/acetylpromazine, Telazol/xylazine, pentobarbi-tal, and methoxyflurane anesthesia in HSD:ICR mice. Lab. Anim. Sci. 45 (2), 199–204.

Garrone, B., di Matteo, A., Amato, A., Pistillo, L., Durando, L., Milanese, C., Di Giorgio, F.P., Tongiani, S., 2021. Synergistic interaction between trazodone and gabapentin in rodent models of neuropathic pain. PLoS One 16 (1), e0244649.

Gawrisch, E., Cheng, E.Y., 1990. Buprenorphine sedation of intensive care patients and ileus reversal. Crit. Care Med. 18 (9), 1034–1036.

Gazzaz, M., Saini, J., Pagliardini, S., Tsui, B., Jeffery, C., El-Hakim, H., 2018. Comparison of inhaled versus intravenous anesthesia for laryngoscopy and laryngeal electromyography in a rat model. J. Otolaryngol. Head Neck Surg. 47 (1), 64.

Genedani, S., Bernardi, M., Bertolini, A., 1999. Influence of antineoplastic drugs on morphine analgesia and on morphine tolerance. Eur. J. Pharmacol. 367 (1), 13–17.

Gergye, C., Zhao, Y., Moore, R., et al., 2020. A comparison of ketamine or etomidate combined with xylazine for intraperitoneal anesthesia in four mouse strains. JALAAS 59 (5), 519–530.

Gillingham, M.B., Clark, M.D., Dahly, E.M., Krugner-Higby, L.A., Ney, D.M., 2001. A comparison of two opioid analgesics for relief of visceral pain induced by intestinal resection in rats. Contemp. Top. Lab. Anim. Sci. 40 (1), 21–26.

Gilroy, B.A., Varga, J.S., 1980. Use of ketamine–diazepam and ketamine– xylazine combinations in Guinea pigs. Vet. Med. Small Anim. Clin. 75 (3), 508–509.

Giraud, O., Molliex, S., Rolland, C., Lecon-Malas, V., Desmonts, J.M., Aubier, M., Dehoux, M., 2003. Halogenated anesthetics reduce interleukin-1beta-induced cytokine secretion by rat alveolar type II cells in primary culture. Anesthesiology 98 (1), 74–81.

Goldkuhl, R., Jacobsen, K.R., Kalliokoski, O., Hau, J., Abelson, K.S.P., 2010. Plasma concentrations of corticosterone and buprenorphine in rats subjected to jugular vein catheterization. Lab. Anim. 44, 337–343.

Gonzalez, M.I., Field, M.J., Bramwell, S., McCleary, S., Singh, L., 2000. Ovariohysterectomy in the rat: a model of surgical pain for evaluation of pre-emptive analgesia? Pain 88 (1), 79–88.

Goren, S., Kahveci, N., Alkan, T., Goren, B., Korfali, E., 2001. The effects of sevoflurane and isoflurane on intracranial pressure and cerebral perfusion pressure after diffuse brain injury in rats. J. Neurosurg. Anesthesiol. 13 (2), 113–119.

Gotoh, H., Matsumoto, Y., Imamura, K., 2004. General anesthesia of infant mice by isoflurane inhalation for medium-duration surgery. Exp. Anim. 53 (1), 63–65.

Gowayed, M.A., Abdel-Bary, A., El-Tahan, R.A., May 1, 2021. The effective interplay of (non-) selective NSAIDs with neostigmine in animal models of analgesia and inflammation. BMC Pharmacol. Toxicol. 22 (1), 24.

Granados-Soto, V., Flores-Murrieta, F.J., 1995. Pharmacokinetics of oral ketorolac in the rat. Methods Find. Exp. Clin. Pharmacol. 17 (8), 535–538.

Green, C.J., 1975. Neuroleptanalgesic drug combinations in the anaesthetic management of small laboratory animals. Lab. Anim. 9 (3), 161–178.

Green, C.J., Halsey, M.J., Precious, S., Wardley-Smith, B., 1978. Alphaxolone–alphadolone anaesthesia in laboratory animals. Lab. Anim. 12 (2), 85–89.

Green, C.J., Knight, J., Precious, S., Simpkin, S., 1981. Ketamine alone and combined with diazepam or xylazine in laboratory animals: a 10 year experience. Lab. Anim. 15 (2), 163–170.

Greenwood-Van Meerveld, B., Gardner, C.J., Little, P.J., Hicks, G.A., Dehaven-Hudkins, D.L., 2004. Preclinical studies of opioids and opioid antagonists on gastrointestinal function. Neuro Gastroenterol. Motil. 16 (Suppl. 2), 46–53.

Griffiths, K.G., Alworth, L.C., Harvey, S.B., Michalski, M.L., May 2010. Using an intravenous catheter to carry out abdominal lavage in the gerbil. Lab. Anim. 39 (5), 143–148.

Grimm, K.A., Lamont, L.A., Tranquilli, W.J., Green, S.A., Robertson, S.A., 2015. Veterinary Anesthesia and Analgesia: The Fifth Edition of Lumb and Jones. Wiley Blackwell, Ames.

Gringauz, M., Rabinowitz, R., Stav, A., Korczyn, A.D., 2001. Tolerance to the analgesic effect of buprenorphine, butorphanol, nalbuphine, and cyclorphan, and cross-tolerance to morphine. J. Anesth. 15 (4), 204–209.

Gross, M.E., 2001. Tranquilizers, alpha-2-adrenergic agonists, and related agents. In: Adams, H.R. (Ed.), Veterinary Pharmacology and Therapeutics, eighth ed. Iowa State University Press, Ames, IA, pp. 299–343.

Guarnieri, M., Brayton, C., Tyler, B.M., 2018. A long-term study of a lipid-buprenorphine implant in rats. J. Vet. Med. 2616152.

Gultekin, H., Yildiz, K., Sezer, Z., Dogru, K., 2006. Comparing the relaxing effects of desflurane and sevoflurane on oxytocin-induced contractions of isolated myometrium in both pregnant and nonpregnant rats. Adv. Ther. 23 (1), 39–46.

Gupta, S.K., Bansal, P., Bhardwaj, R.K., Jaiswal, J., Velpandian, T., 2002. Comparison of analgesic and anti-inflammatory activity of meloxicam gel with diclofenac and piroxicam gels in animal models: pharmacokinetic parameters after topical application. Skin Pharmacol. Appl. Skin Physiol. 15 (2), 105–111.

Gurtu, S., Shukla, S., Mukerjee, D., 1994. Morphine, clonidine coadministration in subanalgesic doses: effective control of tonic pain. Neuroreport 5 (6), 715–717.

GV-SOLAS, 2020. Fachinformation Schmerztherapie bei Versuchstieren aus dem Ausschuss für Anästhesie der GV-SOLAS.

Haberham, Z.L., van den Brom, W.E., Venker-van Haagen, A.J., Baumans, V., de Groot, H.N., Hellebrekers, L.J., 1999. EEG evaluation of reflex testing as assessment of depth of pentobarbital anaesthesia in the rat. Lab. Anim. 33 (1), 47–57.

Hacker, S.O., White, C.E., Black, I.H., 2005. A comparison of target-controlled infusion versus volatile inhalant anesthesia for heart rate, respiratory rate, and recovery time in a rat model. Contemp. Top. Lab. Anim. Sci. 44 (5), 7–12.

Hahn, N., Eisen, R.J., Eisen, L., Lane, R.S., 2005. Ketamine– medetomidine anesthesia with atipamezole reversal: practical anesthesia for rodents under field conditions. Lab. Anim. 34 (2), 48–51.

Hall, L.W., Clarke, K.W., Trim, C.M., 2001. Anaesthesia of birds, laboratory animals and wild animals. In: Veterinary Anaesthesia. W.B. Saunders, London, England, pp. 463–478.

Hamura, H., Yoshida, M., Shimizu, K., Matsukura, T., Suzuki, H., Narita, M., Suzuki, T., 2000. Antinociceptive effect of the combination of pentazocine with morphine in the tail-immersion and scald-pain tests in rats. Jpn. J. Pharmacol. 83 (4), 286–292.

Haque, S.F., Izumi, S., Aikawa, H., Suzuki, T., Matsubayashi, H., Murano, T., Kika, G., Ikeda, M., Goya, K., Makino, T., 2004. Anesthesia and acoustic stress-induced intra-uterine growth retardation in mice. J. Reprod. Dev. 50 (2), 185–190.

Harkness, J.E., Wagner, J.E., 1995. The Biology and Medicine of Rabbits and Rodents. Williams & Wilkins, Baltimore.

Hasirci, V., Bonney, I., Goudas, L.C., Shuster, L., Carr, D.B., Wise, D.L., 2003. Antihyperalgesic effect of simultaneously released hydromorphone and bupivacaine from polymer fibers in the rat chronic constriction injury model. Life Sci. 73 (26), 3323–3337.

Hassan, H.G., Pilcher, C.W., Akerman, B., Renck, H., 1989. Antinociceptive effects of localized administration of opioids compared with lidocaine. Reg. Anesth. 14 (3), 138–144.

Hassan, H.G., Youssef, H., Renck, H., 1993. Duration of experimental nerve block by combinations of local anesthetic agents. Acta Anaesthesiol. Scand. 37 (1), 70–74.

Hawkins, M.G., Karriker, M.J., Wiebe, V., Taylor, I.T., Kass, P.H., September 15, 2006. Drug distribution and stability in extemporaneous preparations of meloxicam and carprofen after dilution and suspension at two storage temperatures. J. Am. Vet. Med. Assoc. 229 (6), 968–974.

Hayashida, K., Eisenach, J.C., November 19, 2008. Multiplicative interactions to enhance gabapentin to treat neuropathic pain. Eur. J. Pharmacol. 598 (1–3), 21–26.

Hayes, J.H., Flecknell, P.A., 1999. A comparison of pre- and post-surgical administration of bupivacaine or buprenorphine following laparotomy in the rat. Lab. Anim. 33 (1), 16–26.

Hayes, K.E., Raucci Jr., J.A., Gades, N.M., Toth, L.A., 2000. An evaluation of analgesic regimens for abdominal surgery in mice. Contemp. Top. Lab. Anim. Sci. 39 (6), 18–23.

Heard, D.J., 2004. Anesthesia, Analgesia, and Sedation of Small Mammals. Saunders, St. Louis, MO.

Heavner, J.E., 1997. Anesthesia and analgesia in laboratory animals: pharmacology of analgesics. In: Kohn, D.F., Wixson, S.K., White, W.J., Benson, G.J. (Eds.), American College of Laboratory Animal Medicine Series. Academic Press, San Diego.

Heavner, J.E., 2001. Anesthesia update: agents, definitions, and strategies. Comp. Med. 51 (6), 500–503.

Hedenqvist, P., Roughan, J.V., Flecknell, P.A., 2000a. Effects of repeated anaesthesia with ketamine/medetomidine and of pre-anaesthetic administration of buprenorphine in rats. Lab. Anim. 34 (2), 207–211.

Hedenqvist, P., Roughan, J.V., Flecknell, P.A., 2000b. Sufentanil and medetomidine anaesthesia in the rat and its reversal with atipamezole and butorphanol. Lab. Anim. 34 (3), 244–251.

Heng, K., Marx, J.O., Jampachairsi, K., Huss, M.K., Pacharinsak, C., 2020. Continuous rate infusion of alfaxalone during ketamine-xylazine anesthesia in rats. J. Am. Assoc. Lab. Anim. Sci. 59 (2), 170–175.

Henning, R.H., Nelemans, A., Houwertjes, M., Agoston, S., 1993. Reversal by suramin of neuromuscular block produced by pancuronium in the anaesthetized rat. Br. J. Pharmacol. 108 (3), 717–720.

Hernandez-Delgadillo, G.P., Cruz, S.L., 2004. Dipyrone potentiates morphine-induced antinociception in dipyrone-treated and morphine-tolerant rats. Eur. J. Pharmacol. 502 (1–2), 67–73.

Hernandez-Delgadillo, G.P., Cruz, S.L., 2006. Endogenous opioids are involved in morphine and dipyrone analgesic potentiation in the tail flick test in rats. Eur. J. Pharmacol. 546 (1–3), 54–59.

Hernandez-Delgadillo, G.P., Lopez-Munoz, F.J., Salazar, L.A., Cruz, S.L., 2003. Morphine and dipyrone co-administration delays tolerance development and potentiates antinociception. Eur. J. Pharmacol. 469 (1–3), 71–79.

Hernandez-Delgadillo, G.P., Ventura Martinez, R., Diaz Reval, M.I., Dominguez Ramirez, A.M., Lopez-Munoz, F.J., 2002. Metamizol potentiates morphine antinociception but not constipation after chronic treatment. Eur. J. Pharmacol. 441 (3), 177–183.

Herrero, J.F., Headley, P.M., 1996. Reversal by naloxone of the spinal antinociceptive actions of a systemically-administered NSAID. Br. J. Pharmacol. 118 (4), 968–972.

Hertl, M.C., Hagberg, P.K., Hunter, D.A., Mackinnon, S.E., Langer, J.C., 1998. Intrafascicular injection of ammonium sulfate and bupivacaine in peripheral nerves of neonatal and juvenile rats. Reg. Anesth. Pain Med. 23 (2), 152–158.

Hestehave, S., Abelson, K.S.P., Bronnum Pedersen, T., Munro, G., 2019. The analgesic efficacy of morphine varies with rat strain and experimental pain model: implications for target validation efforts in pain drug discovery. Eur. J. Pain 23 (3), 539–554.

Hestehave, S., Munro, G., Pedersen, T.B., Abelson, K.S.P., 2017. Antinociceptive effects of voluntarily ingested buprenorphine in the hot-plate test in laboratory rats. Lab. Anim. 51, 264–272.

Hildebrand, S.V., 1997. Paralytic Agents. Academic Press, San Diego.

Hirst, M., Kavaliers, M., Teskey, G.C., 1984. Age and day-night changes in clonidine-induced analgesia in mice. Can. J. Physiol. Pharmacol. 62 (9), 1102–1105.

Hjorthaug, G.A., Søreide, E., Nordsletten, L., Madsen, J.E., Reinholt, F.P., Niratisairak, S., Dimmen, S., November 2, 2019. Short-term perioperative parecoxib is not detrimental to shaft fracture healing in a rat model. Bone Joint Res. 8 (10), 472–480.

Hoggatt, A.F., Hoggatt, J., Honerlaw, M., Pelus, L.M., May 2010. A spoonful of sugar helps the medicine go down: a novel technique to improve oral gavage in mice. J. Am. Assoc. Lab. Anim. Sci. 49 (3), 329–334.

Honda, Y., Higuchi, H., Matsuoka, Y., Yabuki-Kawase, A., Ishii-Maruhama, M., Tomoyasu, Y., Maeda, S., Morimatsu, H., Miyawaki, T., October 5, 2015. The inhibitory effect of locally injected dexmedetomidine on carrageenan-induced nociception in rats. Eur. J. Pharmacol. 764, 215–219.

Hong, G.S., Stein, K., Lysson, M., Kalff, J., Wehner, S., December 2019. A comparative study about the immunomodulatory effects of tramadol and metamizole in a murine model of postoperative ileus. Lab. Anim. 53 (6), 610–618.

Hoorn, E.J., McCormick, J.A., Ellison, D.H., 2011. High tail-cuff blood pressure in mice 1 week after shipping: the need for longer acclimation. Am. J. Hypertens. 24 (5), 534–536.

Horn, C., Kimball, B., Wang, H., Kaus, J., Dienel, S., Nagy, A., Gathright, G., Yates, B., Andrews, P., 2013. Why can't rodents vomit? A comparative behavioral, anatomical, and physiological study. PLoS One 8, 101–171.

Houston, E.R., Tan, S.M., Thomas, S.M., Stasula, U.L., Burton, M.K., Knych, H.K., Kendall, L.V., 2021. Pharmacokinetics and efficacy of a long-lasting, highly concentrated buprenorphine solution in rats. J. Am. Assoc. Lab. Anim. Sci. 60 (6), 667−674.

Hovard, A., Teilmann, A., Hau, J., Abelson, K., 2015. The applicability of a gel delivery system for self-administration of buprenorphine to laboratory mice. Lab. Anim. 49, 40−45.

Hrapkiewicz, K.L., Stein, S., Smiler, K.L., 1989. A new anesthetic agent for use in the gerbil. Lab. Anim. Sci. 39 (4), 338−341.

Hsu, W.H., 1982. Xylazine-induced delay of small intestinal transit in mice. Eur. J. Pharmacol. 83 (1−2), 55−60.

Hsu, W.H., Bellin, S.I., Dellmann, H.D., Hanson, C.E., 1986. Xylazine−ketamine-induced anesthesia in rats and its antagonism by yohimbine. J. Am. Vet. Med. Assoc. 189 (9), 1040−1043.

Hu, C., Flecknell, P.A., Liles, J.H., 1992. Fentanyl and medetomidine anaesthesia in the rat and its reversal using atipamazole and either nalbuphine or butorphanol. Lab. Anim. 26 (1), 15−22.

Hu, G., Vasiliauskas, T., Salem, M.R., Rhone, D.P., Crystal, G.J., 2003. Neutrophils pretreated with volatile anesthetics lose ability to cause cardiac dysfunction. Anesthesiology 98 (3), 712−718.

Huang, C., Wang, Y., Chang, J.K., Han, J.S., 2000. Endomorphin and mu-opioid receptors in mouse brain mediate the analgesic effect induced by 2 Hz but not 100 Hz electroacupuncture stimulation. Neurosci. Lett. 294 (3), 159−162.

Huang, C., Wang, Y., Han, J.S., Wan, Y., 2002. Characteristics of electroacupuncture-induced analgesia in mice: variation with strain, frequency, intensity and opioid involvement. Brain Res. 945 (1), 20−25.

Huang, Y., Zuo, Z., 2005. Effects of isoflurane on oxygen-glucose deprivation-induced changes of gene expression profiling in glial-neuronal cocultures. Acta Anaesthesiol. Scand. 49 (10), 1544−1551.

Hurley, R.W., Adams, M.C.B., 2008. Sex, gender, and pain: an overview of a complex field. Anesth. Analg. 107 (1), 309−317.

Huss, M.K., Chum, H.H., Chang, A.G., Jampachairsi, K., Pacharinsak, C., 2016. The physiologic effects of isoflurane, sevoflurane, and hypothermia used for anesthesia in neonatal rats (Rattus norvegicus). JAALAS 55 (1), 83−88.

Huss, M.K., Felt, S.A., Pacharinsak, C., December 1, 2019. Influence of pain and analgesia on orthopedic and wound-healing models in rats and mice. Comp. Med. 69 (6), 535−545.

Iglesias, V., Alguacil, L.F., Alamo, C., Cuenca, E., 1992. Effects of yohimbine on morphine analgesia and physical dependence in the rat. Eur. J. Pharmacol. 211 (1), 35−38.

Iltis, I., Kober, F., Dalmasso, C., Lan, C., Cozzone, P.J., Bernard, M., 2005. In vivo assessment of myocardial blood flow in rat heart using magnetic resonance imaging: effect of anesthesia. J. Magn. Reson. Imaging 22 (2), 242−247.

International Association for the Study of Pain (IASP), July 2021. Cannabis and cannabinoid analgesia International association for the study of pain presidential task force on cannabis and cannabinoid analgesia position statement. Pain 162, S1−S2.

Ince, I., Aksoy, M., Ahiskalioglu, A., Comez, M., Dostbil, A., Celik, M., Yilmaz, I., Mammadov, R., Dogan, H., Boztok Ozgermen, B., Altuner, D., 2015. A comparative investigation of the analgesic effects of metamizole and paracetamol in rats. J. Invest. Surg. 28, 173−180.

Ingalls, C.P., Warren, G.L., Lowe, D.A., Boorstein, D.B., Armstrong, R.B., 1996. Differential effects of anesthetics on in vivo skeletal muscle contractile function in the mouse. J. Appl. Physiol. 80 (1), 332−340.

Ingrao, J.C., Johnson, R., Tor, E., Gu, Y., Litman, M., Turner, P.V., 2013. Aqueous stability and oral pharmacokinetics of meloxicam and carprofen in male C57BL/6 mice. J. Am. Assoc. Lab. Anim. Sci. 52 (5), 553−559.

Institute for Laboratory Animal Research (U.S.) (ILAR). Committee on Guidelines for the Use of Animals in Neuroscience and Behavioral Research and N. R. Council, 2003. Guidelines for the Care and Use of Mammals in Neuroscience and Behavioral Research. National Academy Press, Washington, DC.

Izer, J.M., Whitcomb, T.L., Wilson, R.P., 2014. Atipamezole reverses ketamine-dexmedetomidine anesthesia without altering the antinociceptive effects of butorphanol and buprenorphine in female C57BL/6J mice. JAALAS 53 (6), 675−683.

Jaber, S.M., Hankenson, F.C., Heng, K., McKinstry-Wu, A., Kelz, M.B., Marx, J.O., 2014. Dose regimens, variability, and complications associated with using repeat-bolus dosing to extend a surgical plane of anesthesia in laboratory mice. J. Am. Assoc. Lab. Anim. Sci. 53 (6), 684−691.

Jablonski, P., Howden, B.O., 2002. Oral buprenorphine and aspirin analgesia in rats undergoing liver transplantation. Lab. Anim. 36 (2), 134−143.

Jablonski, P., Howden, B.O., Baxter, K., 2001. Influence of buprenorphine analgesia on post-operative recovery in two strains of rats. Lab. Anim. 35 (3), 213−222.

Jacob, J.N., Badyal, D.K., Bala, S., March 2013. Evaluation of the in vivo anti-inflammatory and analgesic activity of a highly water-soluble aspirin conjugate. Basic Clin. Pharmacol. Toxicol. 112 (3), 171−174.

Jacobsen, K.O., Villa, V., Miner, V.L., Whitnall, M.H., 2004. Effects of anesthesia and vehicle injection on circulating blood elements in C3H/HeN male mice. Contemp. Top. Lab. Anim. Sci. 43 (5), 8−12.

Jacobson, C., 2000. Adverse effects on growth rates in rats caused by buprenorphine administration. Lab. Anim. 34 (2), 202−206.

Jacobson, C., 2001. A novel anaesthetic regimen for surgical procedures in Guinea pigs. Lab. Anim. 35 (3), 271−276.

Jain, N.K., Kulkarni, S.K., Singh, A., 2002. Modulation of NSAID-induced antinociceptive and anti-inflammatory effects by alpha2-adrenoceptor agonists with gastroprotective effects. Life Sci. 70 (24), 2857−2869.

Jain, S., Jain, N., Bhadra, D., Tiwary, A.K., Jain, N.K., 2005. Transdermal delivery of an analgesic agent using elastic liposomes: preparation, characterization and performance evaluation. Curr. Drug Deliv. 2 (3), 223−233.

Jalota, L., Kalira, V., George, E., Shi, Y.Y., Hornuss, C., Radke, O., Pace, N.L., Apfel, C.C., 2011. Perioperative Clinical Research Core. Prevention of pain on injection of propofol: systematic review and meta-analysis. BMJ. 342.

Jang, S., Kim, H., Kim, D., Jeong, M.W., Ma, T., Kim, S., Ho, I.K., Oh, S., 2006. Attenuation of morphine tolerance and withdrawal syndrome by coadministration of nalbuphine. Arch Pharm. Res. (Seoul) 29 (8), 677−684.

Janssen, C.F., Maiello, P., Wright Jr., M.J., Kracinovsky, K.B., Newsome, J.T., 2017. Comparison of atipamezole with yohimbine for antagonism of xylazine in mice anesthetized with ketamine and xylazine. JAALAS 56 (2), 142−147.

Janssen, B.J., DeCelle, T., Debets, J.J., Brouns, A.E., Callahan, M.F., Smith, T.L., 2004. Effects of anesthetics on systemic hemodynamics in mice. Am. J. Physiol. Heart Circ. Physiol. 287 (4), H1618−H1624.

Jara, C.P., Carraro, R.S., Zanesco, A., Andrade, B., Moreira, K., Nogueira, G., Souza, B.L., Prado, T.P., Póvoa, V., Velander, W., Velloso, L.A., Araújo, E.P., 2021. A smartphone app for individual xylazine/ketamine calculation decreased anesthesia-related mortality in mice. Front. Vet. Sci. 8, 651202.

Jaquenod, M., Ronnhedh, C., Cousins, M.J., Eckstein, R.P., Jordan, V., Mather, L.E., Power, I., 1998. Factors influencing ketorolac-associated perioperative renal dysfunction. Anesth. Analg. 86 (5), 1090−1097.

Jauchem, J.R., Frei, M.R., 1991. Cardiovascular changes in unanesthetized and ketamine-anesthetized Sprague−Dawley rats exposed to 2.8GHz radiofrequency radiation. Lab. Anim. Sci. 41 (1), 70−75.

Jeger, V., Hauffe, T., Nicholls-Vuille, F., Bettex, D., Rudiger, A., 2016. Analgesia in clinically relevant rodent models of sepsis. Lab. Anim. 50 (6), 418−426.

Jensen, T.L., Kiersgaard, M.K., Mikkelsen, L.F., Sørensen, D.B., 2019. Fasting of male mice - effects of time point of initiation and duration on clinical chemistry parameters and animal welfare. Lab. Anim. 53 (6), 587−597.

Jensen, T., Kiersgaard, M., Sørensen, D., Mikkelsen, L., 2013. Fasting of mice: a review. Lab. Anim 47 (4), 225−240.

Jiang, Y., Ye, F., Du, Y., Zong, Y., Tang, Z., July 2, 2021. P2X7R in mast cells is a potential target for salicylic acid and aspirin in treatment of inflammatory pain. J. Inflamm. Res. 14, 2913−2931.

Jing, Z., Pecka, M., Grothe, B., November 1, 2021. Ketamine-xylazine anesthesia depth affects auditory neuronal responses in the lateral superior olive complex of the gerbil. J. Neurophysiol. 126 (5), 1660−1669.

Jirkof, P., 2015. Effects of experimental housing conditions on recovery of laboratory mice. Lab. Anim. 44 (2), 65−70.

Jirkof, P., 2017. Side effects of pain and analgesia in animal experimentation. Lab. Anim. 46 (4), 123−128.

Jirkof, P., Arras, M., Cesarovic, N., 2018. Tramadol: paracetamol in drinking water for treatment of post-surgical pain in laboratory mice. Appl. Anim. Behav. Sci. 198, 95−100.

Jirkof, P., Durst, M., Klopfleisch, R., et al., 2019. Administration of Tramadol or Buprenorphine via the drinking water for post-operative analgesia in a mouse-osteotomy model. Sci. Rep. 9, 10749.

Jirkof, P., Fleischmann, T., Cesarovic, N., Rettich, A., Vogel, J., Arras, M., July 2013. Assessment of postsurgical distress and pain in laboratory mice by nest complexity scoring. Lab. Anim. 47 (3), 153−161.

Jirkof, P., Tourvieille, A., Cinelli, P., Arras, M., 2015. Buprenorphine for pain relief in mice: repeated injections vs sustained-release depot formulation. Lab. Anim. 49 (3), 177−187.

Johansen, O., Vaaler, S., Jorde, R., Reikeras, O., 1994. Increased plasma glucose levels after Hypnorm anaesthesia, but not after pentobarbital anaesthesia in rats. Lab. Anim. 28 (3), 244−248.

Johnson, D.H., 2010. Endoscopic intubation of exotic companion mammals. Vet. Clin. North Am. Exot. Anim. Pract. 13, 273−289.

Jones, C.P., Carver, S., Kendall, L.V., November 2012. Evaluation of common anesthetic and analgesic techniques for tail biopsy in mice. J. Am. Assoc. Lab Anim. Sci. 51 (6), 808−814.

Jong, W.M., Zuurbier, C.J., De Winter, R.J., Van Den Heuvel, D.A., Reitsma, P.H., Ten Cate, H., Ince, C., 2002. Fentanyl-fluanisone-midazolam combination results in more stable hemodynamics than does urethane alpha-chloralose and 2,2,2-tribromoethanol in mice. Contemp. Top. Lab. Anim. Sci. 41 (3), 28−32.

Joshi, S.K., Hernandez, G., Mikusa, J.P., Zhu, C.Z., Zhong, C., Salyers, A., Wismer, C.T., Chandran, P., Decker, M.W., Honore, P., 2006. Comparison of antinociceptive actions of standard analgesics in attenuating capsaicin and nerve-injury-induced mechanical hypersensitivity. Neuroscience 143 (2), 587−596.

Jou, I.M., Tsai, Y.T., Tsai, C.L., Wu, M.H., Chang, H.Y., Wang, N.S., 2000. Simplified rat intubation using a new oropharyngeal intubation wedge. J. Appl. Physiol. 89 (5), 1766−1770.

Jungwirth, B., Gordan, M.L., Biobner, M., Schmehl, W., Kochs, E.F., Mackensen, G.B., 2006. Xenon impairs neurocognitive and histologic outcome after cardiopulmonary bypass combined with cerebral air embolism in rats. Anesthesiology 104 (4), 770−776.

Kahveci, F.S., Kahveci, N., Alkan, T., Goren, B., Korfali, E., Ozluk, K., 2001. Propofol versus isoflurane anesthesia under hypothermic conditions; effects on intracranial pressure and local cerebral blood flow after diffuse traumatic brain injury in the rat. Surg. Neurol. 56 (3), 206−214.

Kanaan, S.A., Safieh-Garabedian, B., Haddad, J.J., Atweh, S.F., Abdelnoor, A.M., Jabbur, S.J., Saade, N.E., 1997. Effects of various analgesic and anti-inflammatory drugs on endotoxin-induced hyperalgesia in rats and mice. Pharmacology 54 (6), 285−297.

Kandatsu, N., Nan, Y.S., Feng, G.G., Nishiwaki, K., Hirokawa, M., Ishikawa, K., Komatsu, T., Yokochi, T., Shimada, Y., Ishikawa, N., 2005. Opposing effects of isoflurane and sevoflurane on neurogenic pulmonary edema development in an animal model. Anesthesiology 102 (6), 1182−1189.

Kandukuri, D.S., Phillips, J.K., Tahmindjis, M., Hildreth, C.M., 2018. Effect of anaesthetic and choice of neuromuscular blocker on vagal control of heart rate under laboratory animal experimental conditions. Lab. Anim. 52 (3), 280−291.

Kang, S.C., Jampachaisri, K., Seymour, T.L., Felt, S.A., Pacharinsak, C., 2017. Use of liposomal bupivacaine for postoperative analgesia in an incisional pain model in rats (Rattus norvegicus). J. Am. Assoc. Lab. Anim. Sci. 56 (1), 63−68.

Karas, A.Z., 2002. Postoperative analgesia in the laboratory mouse, *Mus musculus*. Lab. Anim. (NY) 31 (7), 49−52.

Kashimoto, S., Furuya, A., Nonaka, A., Oguchi, T., Koshimizu, M., Kumazawa, T., 1997. The minimum alveolar concentration of sevoflurane in rats. Eur. J. Anaesthesiol. 14 (4), 359−361.

Karamichali, P., Ftergioti, K., Kazakos, G., 2020. Perioperative management of rabbits and domestic rodents: part one—sedation and anaesthesia. Hell. J. Companion Anim. Med. 9 (1), 48−62.

Katz, J., Clarke, H., Seltzer, Z., 2011. Review article: preventive analgesia: quo vadimus? Anesth. Analg. 113 (5), 1242−1253.

Kawano, H.K., Simonek, G.D., Moffitt, A.D., Tahara, J.M., Brignolo, A.L., 2019. Sterility and stability of diluted meloxicam in compounded multi-dose vial after 365 days. JAALAS 58 (5), 594−596.

Kawano, T., Takahashi, T., Iwata, H., Morikawa, A., Imori, S., Waki, S., Tamura, T., Yamazaki, F., Eguchi, S., Kumagai, N., Yokoyama, M., 2014. Effects of ketoprofen for prevention of postoperative cognitive dysfunction in aged rats. J. Anesth. 28, 932−936.

Kawaguchi, M., Drummond, J.C., Cole, D.J., Kelly, P.J., Spurlock, M.P., Patel, P.M., 2004. Effect of isoflurane on neuronal apoptosis in rats subjected to focal cerebral ischemia. Anesth. Analg. 98 (3), 798−805.

Kayser, V., Besson, J.M., Guilbaud, G., 1991. Effects of the analgesic agent tramadol in normal and arthritic rats: comparison with the effects of different opioids, including tolerance and cross-tolerance to morphine. Eur. J. Pharmacol. 195 (1), 37–45.

Kendall, L.V., Bailey, A.L., Singh, B., McGee, W., 2022. Toxic effects of high-dose meloxicam and carprofen on female CD1 mice. J. Am. Assoc. Lab. Anim. Sci. 99 (99), 1–6.

Kendall, L.V., Hansen, R.J., Dorsey, K., Kang, S., Lunghofer, P.J., Gustafson, D.L., 2014. Pharmacokinetics of sustained-release analgesics in mice. J. Am. Assoc. Lab. Anim. Sci. 53 (5), 478–484.

Kendall, L.V., Singh, B., Bailey, A.L., Smith, B.J., Houston, E.R., Patil, K., Doane, C.J., 2021. Pharmacokinetics and efficacy of a long-lasting, highly concentrated buprenorphine solution in mice. J. Am. Assoc. Lab. Anim. Sci. 60 (1), 64–71.

Kessler, M., Mamach, M., Beutelmann, R., Bankstahl, J.P., Bengel, F.M., Klump, G.M., Berding, G., December 2018. Activation in the auditory pathway of the gerbil studied with 18F-FDG PET: effects of anesthesia. Brain Struct. Funct. 223 (9), 4293–4305.

Kharasch, E.D., Jubert, C., 1999. Compound A uptake and metabolism to mercapturic acids and 3,3,3-trifluoro-2-fluoromethoxypropanoic acid during low-flow sevoflurane anesthesia: biomarkers for exposure, risk assessment, and interspecies comparison. Anesthesiology 91 (5), 1267–1278.

Kharasch, E.D., Schroeder, J.L., Bammler, T., Beyer, R., Srinouanprachanh, S., 2006. Gene expression profiling of nephrotoxicity from the sevoflurane degradation product fluoromethyl-2,2-difluoro-1-(trifluoromethyl) vinyl ether ("compound A") in rats. Toxicol. Sci. 90 (2), 419–431.

Khoo, S.Y., Lay, B.P.P., Joya, J., McNally, G.P., April 2018. Local anaesthetic refinement of pentobarbital euthanasia reduces abdominal writhing without affecting immunohistochemical endpoints in rats. Lab. Anim. 52 (2), 152–162.

Kick, B.L., Shu, P., Wen, B., Sun, D., Taylor, D.K., 2017. Pharmacokinetic profiles of nalbuphine after intraperitoneal and subcutaneous administration to C57BL/6 mice. J. Am. Assoc. Lab. Anim. Sci. 56 (5), 534–538.

Kilic, S., Kulualp, K., April 2016. Efficacy of several therapeutic agents in a murine model of dry eye syndrome. Comp. Med. 66 (2), 112–118.

King, J.N., Dawson, J., Esser, R.E., Fujimoto, R., Kimble, E.F., Maniara, W., Marshall, P.J., O'Byrne, L., Quadros, E., Toutain, P.L., Lees, P., February 2009. Preclinical pharmacology of robenacoxib: a novel selective inhibitor of cyclooxygenase-2. J. Vet. Pharmacol. Ther. 32 (1), 1–17.

Kim, H., Oh, E., Im, H., Mun, J., Yang, M., Khim, J.Y., Lee, E., Lim, S.H., Kong, M.H., Lee, M., et al., 2006. Oxidative damages in the DNA, lipids, and proteins of rats exposed to isofluranes and alcohols. Toxicology 220 (2–3), 169–178.

Kim, T., Murdande, S., Gruber, A., Kim, S., 1996. Sustained-release morphine for epidural analgesia in rats. Anesthesiology 85 (2), 331–338.

Kirihara, Y., Takechi, M., Kurosaki, K., Kobayashi, Y., Kurosawa, T., 2013. Anesthetic effects of a mixture of medetomidine, midazolam and butorphanol in two strains of mice. Exp. Anim. 62 (3), 173–180.

Kirsch, J.H., Klaus, J.A., Blizzard, K.K., Hurn, P.D., Murphy, S.J., 2002. Pain evaluation and response to buprenorphine in rats subjected to sham middle cerebral artery occlusion. Contemp. Top. Lab. Anim. Sci. 41 (6), 9–14.

Kissin, I., Lee, S.S., Arthur, G.R., Bradley Jr., E.L., 1996. Time course characteristicsofacute tolerance developmenttocontinuously infused alfentanil in rats. Anesth. Analg. 83 (3), 600–605.

Klune, C.B., Larkin, A.E., Leung, V., Pang, D., 2019. Comparing the Rat Grimace Scale and a composite behaviour score in rats. PLoS One 14 (5), e0209467.

Klune, C.B., Robbins, H.N., Leung, V.S., Pang, D.S., 2020. Hypothermia during general anesthesia interferes with pain assessment in laboratory rats (Rattus norvegicus). J. Am. Assoc. Lab. Anim. Sci. 59 (6), 719–725.

Koehn, D., Meyer, K.J., Syed, N.A., Anderson, M.G., 2015. Ketamine/xylazine-induced corneal damage in mice. PLoS One 10 (7), e0132804.

Kolesnikov, Y., Pasternak, G.W., 1999. Topical opioids in mice: analgesia and reversal of tolerance by a topical *N*-methyl-d-aspartate antagonist. J. Pharmacol. Exp. Ther. 290 (1), 247–252.

Kolesnikov, Y.A., Chereshnev, I., Pasternak, G.W., 2000. Analgesic synergy between topical lidocaine and topical opioids. J. Pharmacol. Exp. Ther. 295 (2), 546–551.

Kolesnikov, Y.A., Wilson, R.S., Pasternak, G.W., 2003. The synergistic analgesic interactions between hydrocodone and ibuprofen. Anesth. Analg. 97 (6), 1721–1723.

Komulainen, A., Olson, M.E., 1991. Antagonism of ketamine–xylazine anesthesia in rats by administration of yohimbine, tolazoline, or 4-aminopyridine. Am. J. Vet. Res. 52 (4), 585–588.

Konat, G.W., Kofke, W.A., Miric, S., 2003. Toxicity of compound A to C6 rat glioma cells. Metab. Brain Dis. 18 (1), 11–15.

Kong, H., Raynor, K., Yano, H., Takeda, J., Bell, G.I., Reisine, T., 1994. Agonists and antagonists bind to different domains of the cloned kappa opioid receptor. Proc. Natl. Acad. Sci. USA 91 (17), 8042–8046.

Koo, S.T., Park, Y.I., Lim, K.S., Chung, K., Chung, J.M., 2002. Acupuncture analgesia in a new rat model of ankle sprain pain. Pain 99 (3), 423–431.

Kroin, J.S., Das, V., Moric, M., Buvanendran, A., January 2019. Efficacy of the ketamine metabolite (2R,6R)-hydroxynorketamine in mice models of pain. Reg. Anesth. Pain Med. 44 (1), 111–117.

Krugner-Higby, L., Smith, L., Clark, M., Heath, T.D., Dahly, E., Schiffman, B., Hubbard-VanStelle, S., Ney, D., Wendland, A., 2003. Liposome-encapsulated oxymorphone hydrochloride provides prolonged relief of postsurgical visceral pain in rats. Comp. Med. 53 (3), 270–279.

Kubota, T., Hirota, K., Anzawa, N., Yoshida, H., Kushikata, T., Matsuki, A., 1999. Physostigmine antagonizes ketamine-induced noradrenaline release from the medial prefrontal cortex in rats. Brain Res. 840 (1–2), 175–178.

Kufoy, E.A., Pakalnis, V.A., Parks, C.D., Wells, A., Yang, C.H., Fox, A., 1989. Keratoconjunctivitis sicca with associated secondary uveitis elicited in rats after systemic xylazine/ketamine anesthesia. Exp. Eye Res. 49 (5), 861–867.

Kula, A., Akkar, O.B., Gulturk, S., Cetin, M., Cetin, A., August 2016. Combination of paracetamol or ketamine with meperidine enhances antinociception. Hum. Exp. Toxicol. 35 (8), 887–892.

Kumstel, S., Vasudevan, P., Palme, R., Zhang, X., Wendt, E.H.U., David, R., Vollmar, B., Zechner, D., 2020. Benefits of non-invasive methods compared to telemetry for distress analysis in a murine model of pancreatic cancer. J. Adv. Res. 21, 35–47.

Kupers, R., Gybels, J., 1995. The consumption of fentanyl is increased in rats with nociceptive but not with neuropathic pain. Pain 60 (2), 137–141.

Labitt, R.N., Oxford, E.M., Davis, A.K., Butler, S.D., Daugherity, E.K.A., 2021. Validated smartphone-based electrocardiogram reveals severe bradyarrhythmias during immobilizing restraint in mice of both sexes and four strains. J. Am. Assoc. Lab. Anim. Sci. 60 (2), 201–212.

Laird, J.M., Cervero, F., 1996. Effects of metamizol on nociceptive responses to stimulation of the ureter and on ureter motility in anaesthetised rats. Inflamm. Res. 45 (3), 150–154.

Laird, J.M., Herrero, J.F., Garcia de la Rubia, P., Cervero, F., 1997. Analgesic activity of the novel COX-2 preferring NSAID, meloxicam in mono-arthritic rats: central and peripheral components. Inflamm. Res. 46 (6), 203–210.

Laird, J.M., Roza, C., Olivar, T., 1998. Antinociceptive activity of metamizol in rats with experimental ureteric calculosis: central and peripheral components. Inflamm. Res. 47 (10), 389–395.

Lamon, T.K., Browder, E.J., Sohrabji, F., Ihrig, M., July 2008. Adverse effects of incorporating ketoprofen into established rodent studies. J. Am. Assoc. Lab. Anim. Sci. 47 (4), 20–24.

Langford, D.J., Crager, S.E., Shehzad, Z., Smith, S.B., Sotocinal, S.G., Levenstadt, J.S., Chanda, M.L., Levitin, D.J., Mogil, J.S., 2006. Social modulation of pain as evidence for empathy in mice. Science 312 (5782), 1967–1970.

Larson, C.M., Wilcox, G.L., Fairbanks, C.A., 2019. Defining and managing pain in stroke and traumatic brain injury research. Comp. Med. 69 (6), 510–519.

Lascelles, B.D., Waterman, A.E., Cripps, P.J., Livingston, A., Henderson, G., 1995. Central sensitization as a result of surgical pain: investigation of the pre-emptive value of pethidine for ovariohys terectomy in the rat. Pain 62, 201–212.

LaTourette, P.C., David, E.M., Pacharinsak, C., Jampachaisri, K., Smith, J.C., Marx, J.O., 2020. Effects of standard and sustained-release buprenorphine on the minimum alveolar concentration of isoflurane in C57BL/6 mice. JAALAS 59 (3), 298–304.

Lauretti, G.R., 2015. The evolution of spinal/epidural neostigmine in clinical application: thoughts after two decades. Saudi J. Anaesth. 9 (1), 71–81.

Laulin, J.P., Maurette, P., Corcuff, J.B., Rivat, C., Chauvin, M., Simonnet, G., 2002. The role of ketamine in preventing fentanyl-induced hyperalgesia and subsequent acute morphine tolerance. Anesth. Analg. 94 (5), 1263–1269.

Lawson, D.M., Duke, J.L., Zammit, T.G., Collins, H.L., DiCarlo, S.E., 2001. Recovery from carotid artery catheterization performed under various anesthetics in male, Sprague–Dawley rats. Contemp. Top. Lab. Anim. Sci. 40 (4), 18–22.

Leach, M.C., Bailey, H.E., Dickinson, A.L., Roughan, J.V., Flecknell, P.A., 2010. A preliminary investigation into the practicality of use and duration of action of slow-release preparations of morphine and hydromorphone in laboratory rats. Lab. Anim. 44 (1), 59–65.

Leach, M.C., Klaus, K., Miller, A.L., Scotto di Perrotolo, M., Sotocinal, S.G., Flecknell, P.A., 2012. The assessment of post-vasectomy pain in mice using behaviour and the mouse grimace scale. PLoS One 7 (4), e35656.

Lee, B.M., Jang, Y., Park, G., Kim, K., Oh, S.H., Shin, T.J., Chung, G., 2020. Dexmedetomidine modulates transient receptor potential vanilloid subtype 1. Biochem. Biophys. Res. Commun. 522 (4), 832–837.

Lee, H., Kim, H.K., Shin, H.S., Han, S.J., Yoon, S., Seong, J.K., Seo, K.Y., 2020. Evaluation of factors related to Anaesthesia-induced Lens opacity in experimental mice. Lab. Anim. Res. 36, 1.

Lee, S.C., Wang, J.J., Ho, S.T., Tao, P.L., 1997. Nalbuphine coadministered with morphine prevents tolerance and dependence. Anesth. Analg. 84 (4), 810–815.

Leeuwin, R.S., van der Wal, J.K., Spanjer, W., 1984. Interactions of cholinesterase inhibitors and glucocorticoids with ketamine and pentobarbitone-induced general anaesthesia in the rat: possible effects on central cholinergic activity. Br. J. Pharmacol. 82 (2), 339–347.

Legros, J., Khalili-Varasteh, H., Margetts, G., 1984. Pharmacological study of pentazocine–naloxone combination: interest as a potentially non abusable oral form of pentazocine. Arch. Int. Pharmacodyn. Ther. 271 (1), 11–21.

Lemke, K.A., Tranquilli, W.J., Thurmon, J.C., Benson, G.J., Olson, W.A., 1996. Ability of flumazenil, butorphanol, and naloxone to reverse the anesthetic effects of oxymorphone–diazepam in dogs. J. Am. Vet. Med. Assoc. 209 (4), 776–779.

Lerche, P., Muir III, W.W., Bednarski, R.M., 2000. Nonrebreathing anesthetic systems in small animal practice. J. Am. Vet. Med. Assoc. 217 (4), 493–497.

Leung, V., Zhang, E., Pang, D.S., 2016. Real-time application of the Rat Grimace Scale as a welfare refinement in laboratory rats. Sci. Rep. 6, 31667.

Levine, J.D., Gordon, N.C., Taiwo, Y.O., Coderre, T.J., 1988. Potentiation of pentazocine analgesia by low-dose naloxone. J. Clin. Invest. 82 (5), 1574–1577.

Levinson, B.L., Leary, S.L., Bassett, B.J., Cook, C.J., Gorman, G.S., LU, C., 2021. Pharmacokinetic and histopathologic study of an extended-release, injectable formulation of buprenorphine in Sprague-Dawley rats. J. Am. Assoc. Lab. Anim. Sci. 60 (4), 462–469.

Liang, D.Y., Guo, T., Liao, G., Kingery, W.S., Peltz, G., Clark, J.D., 2006. Chronic pain and genetic background interact and influence opioid analgesia, tolerance, and physical dependence. Pain 121 (3), 232–240.

Lieggi, C.C., Artwohl, J.E., Leszczynski, J.K., Rodriguez, N.A., Fickbohm, B.L., Fortman, J.D., 2005a. Efficacy and safety of stored and newly prepared tribromoethanol in ICR mice. Contemp. Top. Lab. Anim. Sci. 44 (1), 17–22.

Lieggi, C.C., Fortman, J.D., Kleps, R.A., Sethi, V., Anderson, J.A., Brown, C.E., andArtwohl, J.E., 2005b. An evaluation of preparation methods and storage conditions of tribromoethanol. Contemp. Top. Lab. Anim. Sci. 44 (1), 11–16.

Leidinger, C., Herrmann, F., Thöne-Reineke, C., Baumgart, N., Baumgart, J., 2017. Introducing clicker training as a cognitive enrichment for laboratory mice. J. Vis. Exp. 121, e55415.

Lightfoote, W.E., Molinari, G.F., 1978. Comparison of ketamine and pentobarbital anesthesia in the Mongolian gerbil. Am. J. Vet. Res. 39 (6), 1061–1063.

Liles, J.H., Flecknell, P.A., 1994. A comparison of the effects of buprenorphine, carprofen and flunixin following laparotomy in rats. J. Vet. Pharmacol. Ther. 17 (4), 284–290.

Liles, J.H., Flecknell, P.A., Roughan, J., Cruz-Madorran, I., 1998. Influence of oral buprenorphine, oral naltrexone or morphine on the effects of laparotomy in the rat. Lab. Anim. 32 (2), 149–161.

Lipiski, M., Arras, M., Jirkof, P., et al., 2017. Premedication with fentanyl-midazolam improves sevoflurane anesthesia for surgical intervention in laboratory mice. Exp. Biol. Med. (Maywood) 242 (12), 1287–1298.

Lipman, N.S., Phillips, P.A., Newcomer, C.E., 1987. Reversal of ketamine/xylazine anesthesia in the rabbit with yohimbine. Lab. Anim. Sci. 37 (4), 474–477.

Liu, K.S., Hu, O.Y., Ho, S.T., Tzeng, J.I., Chen, Y.W., Wang, J.J., 2004. Antinociceptive effect of a novel long-acting nalbuphine preparation. Br. J. Anaesth. 92 (5), 712–715.

Liu, K.S., et al., 2006. Novel depots of buprenorphine have a long-acting effect for the management of physical dependence to morphine. J. Pharm. Pharmacol. 58, 337–344.

Loepke, A.W., McCann, J.C., Kurth, C.D., McAuliffe, J.J., 2006. The physiologic effects of isoflurane anesthesia in neonatal mice. Anesth. Analg. 102 (1), 75–80.

Lofgren, J.L.S., Foley, P.L., Golledge, H., 2020. Chapter 17. Anesthesia, analgesia, and euthanasia. In: Suckow, M.A., Hankenson, F.C., Wilson, R.P., Foley, P.L. (Eds.), The Laboratory Rat, third edition. Academic Press, Elsevier, Amsterdam, the Netherlands.

Loomis, C.W., Penning, J., Milne, B., 1989. A study of the analgesic interaction between intrathecal morphine and subcutaneous nalbuphine in the rat. Anesthesiology 71 (5), 704–710.

Lopez, J.R., Dominguez-Ramirez, A.M., Cook, H.J., Bravo, G., Diaz-Reval, M.I., Deciga-Campos, M., Lopez-Munoz, F.J., 2006. Enhancement of antinociception by co-administration of ibuprofen and caffeine in arthritic rats. Eur. J. Pharmacol. 544 (1–3), 31–38.

Lorenz, J.N., 2002. A practical guide to evaluating cardiovascular, renal, and pulmonary function in mice. Am. J. Physiol. Regul. Integr. Comp. Physiol. 282 (6), R1565–R1582.

Lu, Y., Gu, Y., Liu, L., Tang, X., Xia, Q., Xu, Z., 2021. Intravenous dexmedetomidine administration prior anesthesia induction with propofol at 4°C attenuates propofol injection pain: A double-blind, randomized, placebo-controlled trial. Front. Med. 8.

Lumb, W.V., Jones, E.W., 1984. Preanesthetic agents. In: Lumb & Jones' Veterinary Anesthesia, second ed. Lea & Febiger.

Lutz, M., Liu, H., 2006. Inhaled sevoflurane produces better delayed myocardial protection at 48 versus 24 hours after exposure. Anesth. Analg. 102 (4), 984–990.

Ma, L.L., Liu, W., Huang, Y.G., Yang, N., Zuo, P.P., 2011. Analgesic effect of gabapentin in a rat model for chronic constrictive injury. Chin. Med. J. (Engl). 124 (24), 4304–4309.

MacDonald, E., Haapalinna, A., Virtanen, R., Lammintausta, R., 1989. Effects of acute administration of medetomidine on the behaviour, temperature and turnover rates of brain biogenic amines in rodents and reversal of these effects by atipamezole. Acta. Vet. Scand. Suppl. 85, 77–81.

Mariani, L., Bonanomi, L., 1978. Resistance of the Guinea pig to indomethacin ulcerogenesis. Toxicol. Appl. Pharmacol. 45 (2), 637–639.

Martin, L.J., Hathaway, G., Isbester, K., Mirali, S., Acland, E.L., Niederstrasser, N., Slepian, P.M., Trost, Z., Bartz, J.A., Sapolsky, R.M., Sternberg, W.F., Levitin, D.J., Mogil, J.S., 2015. Reducing social stress elicits emotional contagion of pain in mouse and human strangers. Curr. Biol. 25 (3), 326–332.

Martin, L.B., Thompson, A.C., Martin, T., Kristal, M.B., 2001. Analgesic efficacy of orally administered buprenorphine in rats. Comp. Med. 51 (1), 43–48.

Massey, C.A., Richerson, G.B., 2017. Isoflurane, ketamine-xylazine, and urethane markedly alter breathing even at subtherapeutic doses. J. Neurophysiol. 118 (4), 2389–2401.

Matson, D.J., Broom, D.C., Carson, S.R., Baldassari, J., Kehne, J., Cortright, D.N., 2007. Inflammation-induced reduction of spontaneous activity by adjuvant: a novel model to study the effect of analgesics in rats. J. Pharmacol. Exp. Ther. 320 (1), 194–201.

Matsumiya, L.C., Sorge, R.E., Sotocinal, S.G., Tabaka, J.M., Wieskopf, J.S., Zaloum, A., King, O.D., Mogil, J.S., January 2012. Using the Mouse Grimace Scale to reevaluate the efficacy of postoperative analgesics in laboratory mice. J. Am. Assoc. Lab. Anim. Sci. 51 (1), 42–49.

Matsuura, S., Shirakami, G., Iida, H., Tanimoto, K., Fukuda, K., 2006. The effect of sevoflurane on ciliary motility in rat cultured tracheal epithelial cells; a comparison with isoflurane and halothane. Anesth. Analg. 102 (6), 1703–1708.

Mattheis, L., Jung, J.S., Hiebl, B., Garrels, W., Kielstein, H., Spielmann, J., 2016. Perioperative support reduces mortality of obese BALB/c mice after ovariectomy. Lab. Anim. (NY) 45 (7), 262–267.

Matthes, H.W., Maldonado, R., Simonin, F., Valverde, O., Slowe, S., Kitchen, I., Befort, K., Dierich, A., LeMeur, M., Dolle, P., 1996. Lossofmorphine-induced analgesia, reward effect and withdrawal symptoms in mice lacking the mu-opioid-receptor gene. Nature 383 (6603), 819–823.

McKeon, G.P., Pacharinsak, C., Long, C.T., Howard, A.M., Jampachaisri, K., Yeomans, D.C., Felt, S.A., March 2011. Analgesic effects of tramadol, tramadol-gabapentin, and buprenorphine in an incisional model of pain in rats (Rattus norvegicus). J. Am. Assoc. Lab. Anim. Sci. 50 (2), 192–197.

McLaughlin, C.R., Dewey, W.L., 1994. A comparison of the antinociceptive effects of opioid agonists in neonatal and adult rats in phasic and tonic nociceptive tests. Pharmacol. Biochem. Behav. 49 (4), 1017–1023.

Mecklenburg, J., et al., 2017. Effects of local and spinal administrations of mu-opioids on postoperative pain in aged vs adult mice. Pain Rep. 2, 1.

Medhurst, S.J., Walker, K., Bowes, M., Kidd, B.L., Glatt, M., Muller, M., Hattenberger, M., Vaxelaire, J., O'Reilly, T., Wotherspoon, G., et al., 2002. A rat model of bone cancer pain. Pain 96 (1–2), 129–140.

Meert, T.F., De Kock, M., 1994. Potentiation of the analgesic properties of fentanyl-like opioids with alpha 2-adrenoceptor agonists in rats. Anesthesiology 81 (3), 677–688.

Meert, T.F., andVermeirsch, H.A., 2005. Apreclinical comparison between different opioids: antinociceptive versus adverse effects. Pharmacol. Biochem. Behav. 80 (2), 309–326.

Mertens, J., Muller-Deile, J., 1991. The value of fentanyl/diazepam anesthesia for experimental operations and recordings of compound action potentials in the Guinea pig cochlea. Eur. Arch. Oto-Rhino-Laryngol. 248 (7), 402–405.

Messiha, F.S., 1991. Neurotoxicity of chlorpromazine and modulation by amantadine as a function of mouse strain. Neurotoxicology 12 (3), 571–581.

Metten, P., Buck, K.J., Merrill, C.M., Roberts, A.J., Yu, C.H., Crabbe, J.C., 2007. Use of a novel mouse genotype to model acute benzodiazepine withdrawal. Behav. Genet. 37 (1), 160–170.

Meyer, R.E., Fish, R.E., 2005. A review of tribromoethanol anesthesia for production of genetically engineered mice and rats. Lab. Anim. (NY) 34 (10), 47–52.

Michou, J.N., Leece, E.A., Brearley, J.C., 2012. Comparison of pain on injection during induction of anaesthesia with alfaxalone and two formulations of propofol in dogs. Vet. Anaesth. Analg. 39 (3), 275–281.

Mickley, G.A., Hoxha, Z., Biada, J.M., Kenmuir, C.L., Bacik, S.E., 2006. Acetaminophen self-administered in the drinking water increases the pain threshold of rats (*Rattus norvegicus*). J. Am. Assoc. Lab. Anim. Sci. 45 (5), 48–54.

Milanez, M., Cabral, A.M., Pires, J., Bergamaschi, C.T., Campos, R.R., Futuro Neto, H.A., Silva, N.F., 2019. Impairment of natriuresis and diuresis induced by intrarenal adrenoceptor mechanisms in an experimental model of cirrhosis in rats. Heliyon 5 (12), e03066.

Millecamps, M., Jourdan, D., Leger, S., Etienne, M., Eschalier, A., Ardid, D., 2005. Circadian pattern of spontaneous behavior in monarthritic rats: a novel global approach to evaluation of chronic pain and treatment effectiveness. Arthritis Rheum. 52 (11), 3470–3478.

Miller, A.L., Golledge, H.D., Leach, M.C., 2016a. The influence of isoflurane anaesthesia on the rat grimace scale. PLoS One 11 (11), e0166652.

Miller, A.L., Kitson, G.L., Skalkoyannis, B., Flecknell, P.A., Leach, M.C., 2016b. Using the mouse grimace scale and behaviour to assess pain in CBA mice following vasectomy. Appl. Anim. Behav. Sci. 181, 160–165.

Miller, A., Kitson, G., Skalkoyannis, B., Leach, M., 2015. The effect of isoflurane anaesthesia and buprenorphine on the mouse grimace scale and behaviour in CBA and DBA/2 mice. Appl. Anim. Behav. Sci. 172, 58–62.

Miller, A.L., Leach, M.C., 2015a. The mouse grimace scale: A clinically useful tool? PLoS One 10 (9), e0136000. In this issue.

Miller, A.L., Leach, M.C., 2015b. Using the mouse grimace scale to assess pain associated with routine ear notching and the effect of analgesia in laboratory mice. Lab. Anim. 49 (2), 117–120.

Miller, A.L., Leach, M.C., 2016. The effect of handling method on the mouse grimace scale in two strains of laboratory mice. Lab. Anim. 50 (4), 305–307.

Miller, A.L., Theodore, D., Widrich, J., January 2021. Inhalational anesthetic [Updated 2021 Sep 24]. In: StatPearls [Internet]. StatPearls Publishing, Treasure Island (FL).

Miller, A.L., Wright-Williams, S.L., Flecknell, P.A., Roughan, J.V., 2012. A comparison of abdominal and scrotal approach methods of vasectomy and the influence of analgesic treatment in laboratory mice. Lab. Anim. 46, 304–310.

Mimura, M., Namiki, A., Kishi, R., Ikeda, T., Miyake, H., 1990. Antagonistic effect of physostigmine on ketamine-induced anesthesia. Psychopharmacology (Berl.) 102 (3), 399–403.

Mimura, M., Namiki, A., Kishi, R., Ikeda, T., Miyake, H., Iwasaki, H., 1992. Central cholinergic action produces antagonism to ketamine anesthesia. Acta Anaesthesiol. Scand. 36 (5), 460–462.

Miner, N.A., Koehler, J., Greenway, L., 1969. Intraperitoneal injection of mice. Appl. Microbiol. 17, 250–251.

Minville, V., Fourcade, O., Girolami, J.P., Tack, I., 2010. Opioid-induced hyperalgesia in a mice model of orthopaedic pain: preventive effect of ketamine. Br. J. Anaesth. 104, 231–238.

Miranda, A., Pêgo, J.M., Correia-Pinto, J., April 2017. Animal facility videoendoscopic intubation station: tips and tricks from mice to rabbits. Lab. Anim. 51 (2), 204–207.

Miranda, H.F., Romero, M.A., Puig, M.M., 2012. Antinociceptive and anti-exudative synergism between dexketoprofen and tramadol in a model of inflammatory pain in mice. Fundam. Clin. Pharmacol. 26 (3), 373–382.

Miranda, H.F., Sierralta, F., Aranda, N., Poblete, P., Noriega, V., Prieto, J.C., December 2018. Synergism between gabapentin-tramadol in experimental diabetic neuropathic pain. Fundam. Clin. Pharmacol. 32 (6), 581–588.

Mishra, Y., Ramzan, I., 1992a. Influence of cimetidine on gallamine-induced neuromuscular paralysis in rats. Clin. Exp. Pharmacol. Physiol. 19 (12), 803–807.

Mishra, Y., Ramzan, I., 1992b. Interaction between succinylcholine and cimetidine in rats. Can. J. Anaesth. 39 (4), 370–374.

Mitchell, C.M., Salyards, G.W., Theriault, B.R., Langan, G.P., Luchins, K.R., November 1, 2021. Evaluation of pain and distress and therapeutic interventions for rectal prolapse in mice to reduce early study removal. J. Am. Assoc. Lab. Anim. Sci. 60 (6), 692–699.

Mogil, J.S., 2020. Qualitative sex differences in pain processing: emerging evidence of a biased literature. Nat. Rev. Neurosci. 21, 353–365.

Mogil, J.S., 2021. Sources of individual differences in pain. Annu. Rev. Neurosci. 44, 1–25.

Montonye, D.R., Ericsson, A.C., Busi, S.B., Lutz, C., Wardwell, K., Franklin, C.L., 2018. Acclimation and institutionalization of the mouse microbiota following transportation. Front. Microbiol. 9, 1085.

Mogil, J.S., Pang, D.S.J., Silva Dutra, G.G., Chambers, C.T., 2020. The development and use of facial grimace scales for pain measurement in animals. Neurosci. Bio. Behav. Rev. 116, 480–493.

Montilla-García, Á., Tejada, M.Á., Perazzoli, G., Entrena, J.M., Portillo-Salido, E., Fernández-Segura, E., Cañizares, F.J., Cobos, E.J., October 2017. Grip strength in mice with joint inflammation: a rheumatology function test sensitive to pain and analgesia. Neuropharmacology 125, 231–242.

Moody, C.M., Weary, D.M., 2014. Mouse aversion to isoflurane versus carbon dioxide gas. Appl. Anim. Behav. Sci. 158, 95–101.

Moons, C.P., Hermans, K., Remie, R., Duchateau, L., Odberg, F.O., 2007. Intraperitoneal versus subcutaneous telemetry devices in young Mongolian gerbils (Meriones unguiculatus). Lab. Anim. 41 (2), 262–269.

Morimoto, K., Nishimura, R., Matsunaga, S., Mochizuki, M., Sasaki, N., 2001. Epidural analgesia with a combination of bupivacaine and buprenorphine in rats. J. Vet. Med. A Physiol. Pathol. Clin. Med. 48 (5), 303–312.

Mueller, K., 2018. Schmerztherapie bei Kaninchen, Meerschweinchen, Chinchillas und Frettchen – ein Update. Der Prakt. Tierarzt 99.

Mulder, J.B., 1978. Anesthesia in the mouse using a combination of ketamine and promazine. Lab. Anim. Sci. 28 (1), 70–71.

Mulder, J.B., Johnson Jr., H.B., 1978. Ketamine and promazine for anesthesia in the rat. J. Am. Vet. Med. Assoc. 173 (9), 1252–1253.

Murakami, H., Li, S., Foreman, R., Yin, J., Hirai, T., Chen, J., 2019. Ameliorating effects of electroacupuncture on dysmotility, inflammation, and pain mediated via the autonomic mechanism in a rat model of postoperative ileus. J. Neurogastroenterol. Motil. 25 (2), 286–299.

Myers, P.H., Goulding, D.R., Wiltshire, R.A., McGee, C.A., Dickerson, A.B., Comins, M.M., Shi, M., Kissling, G.E., Lih, F.B., Deterding, L.J., Laber-Laird, K.E., Blankenship-Paris, T.L., 2021. Serum buprenorphine concentrations and behavioral activity in mice after a single subcutaneous injection of simbadol, buprenorphine SR-LAB, or standard buprenorphine. J. Am. Assoc. Lab. Anim. Sci. 60 (6), 661–666.

Nadeson, R., Goodchild, C.S., 2000. Antinociceptive properties of neu-rosteroids II. Experiments with Saffan and its components alphaxalone and alphadolone to reveal separation of anaesthetic and antinociceptive effects and the involvement of spinal cord GABA(A) receptors. Pain 88 (1), 31–39.

Nakamura, T., Karakida, N., Dantsuka, A., Ichii, O., Elewa, Y., Kon, Y., Nagasaki, K.I., Hattori, H., Yoshiyasu, T., 2017. Effects of a mixture of medetomidine, midazolam and butorphanol on anesthesia and blood biochemistry and the antagonizing action of atipamezole in hamsters. J. Vet. Med. Sci. 79 (7), 1230–1235.

Narver, H.L., 2015. Nalbuphine, a non-controlled opioid analgesic, and its potential use in research mice. Lab. Anim. (NY) 44 (3), 106–110.

Navarro, K.L., Huss, M., Smith, J.C., Sharp, P., Marx, J.O., Pacharinsak, C., 2021. Mouse anesthesia: The art and science. ILAR J. 62 (1–2), 238–273.

Navarro, K., Jampachaisri, K., Huss, M., Pacharinsak, C., 2021. Lipid bound extended release buprenorphine (high and low doses) and sustained release buprenorphine effectively attenuate post-operative hypersensitivity in an incisional pain model in mice (*Mus musculus*). Animal Model. Exp. Med. 4 (2), 129–137.

Neag, M.A., Mitre, A.O., Catinean, A., Mitre, C.I., 2020. An overview on the mechanisms of neuroprotection and neurotoxicity of isoflurane and sevoflurane in experimental studies. Brain Res. Bull. 165, 281–289.

Neiger-Aeschbacher, G., 2002. Anaesthesia and analgesia of small mammals. Part 2: intra- and postoperative care. Schweiz. Arch. Tierheilkd. 144, 597–604.

Nelson, A.M., Nolan, K.E., Davis, I.C., March 27, 2020. Repeated orotracheal intubation in mice. J. Vis. Exp. (157).

Nemeth, S., Viskupic, E., Murgas, K., 1985. Intravenous thiobarbital anaesthesia for determination of liver glycogen phosphorylase activity in rats subjected to various forms of stress. Endocrinol. Exp. 19 (2), 91–95.

Neugebauer, V., Schaible, H.G., He, X., Lucke, T., Gundling, P., Schmidt, R.F., 1994. Electrophysiological evidence for a spinal antinociceptive action of dipyrone. Agents Actions 41 (1–2), 62–70.

Nielsen, A.N., Mathiesen, C., Blackburn-Munro, G., 2004. Pharmacological characterisation of acid-induced muscle allodynia in rats. Eur. J. Pharmacol. 487 (1–3), 93–103.

Nikfar, S., Abdollahi, M., Etemad, F., Sharifzadeh, M., 1997. Effects of sweetening agents on morphine-induced analgesia in mice by formalin test. Gen. Pharmacol. 29 (4), 583–586.

Nishiyama, T., 2006. Analgesic effects of intrathecally administered celecoxib, a cyclooxygenase-2 inhibitor, in the tail flick test and the formalin test in rats. Acta Anaesthesiol. Scand. 50 (2), 228–233.

Noguchi, M., Kimoto, A., Kobayashi, S., Yoshino, T., Miyata, K., Sasamata, M., 2005. Effect of celecoxib, a cyclooxygenase-2 inhibitor, on the patho-physiology of adjuvant arthritis in rat. Eur. J. Pharmacol. 513 (3), 229–235.

Norris, M.L., Turner, W.D., 1983. An evaluation of tribromoethanol (TBE) asananaesthetic agentinthe Mongolian gerbil (*Meriones unguiculatus*). Lab. Anim. 17 (4), 324–329.

Nunamaker, E.A., Goldman, J.L., Adams, C.R., Fortman, J.D., 2018. Evaluation of analgesic efficacy of meloxicam and 2 formulations of buprenorphine after laparotomy in female Sprague-Dawley rats. JAALAS 57 (5), 498–507.

Obal, D., Preckel, B., Scharbatke, H., Mullenheim, J., Hoterkes, F., Thamer, V., Schlack, W., 2001. One MAC of sevoflurane provides protection against reperfusion injury in the rat heart in vivo. Br. J. Anaesth. 87 (6), 905–911.

Obal, D., Scharbatke, H., Barthel, H., Preckel, B., Mullenheim, J., Schlack, W., 2003. Cardioprotection against reperfusion injury is maximal with only two minutes of sevoflurane administration in rats. Can. J. Anaesth. 50 (9), 940–945.

Obernier, J.A., Baldwin, R.L., 2006. Establishing an appropriate period of acclimatization following transportation of laboratory animals. ILAR J. 47 (4), 364–369.

Ohtsuka, H., Fujita, K., Kobayashi, H., 2007. Pharmacokinetics of fentanyl in male and female rats after intravenous administration. Arzneimittelforschung 57 (5), 260–263.

Oliver, V.L., Athavale, S., Simon, K.E., Kendall, L.V., Nemzek, J.A., Lofgren, J.L., 2017. Evaluation of pain assessment techniques and analgesia efficacy in a female Guinea pig (Cavia porcellus) model of surgical pain. J. Am. Assoc. Lab. Anim. Sci. 56 (4), 425–435.

Oliver, V.L., Thurston, S.E., Lofgren, J.L., 2018. Using cageside measures to evaluate analgesic efficacy in mice (Mus musculus) after surgery. J. Am. Assoc. Lab. Anim. Sci. 57 (2), 186–201.

Olson, M.E., Renchko, P., 1988. Azaperone and azaperone-ketamine as a neuroleptic sedative and anesthetic in rats and mice. Lab. Anim. Sci. 38 (3), 299–304.

Omisore, N.O., Adewunmi, C.O., Iwalewa, E.O., Ngadjui, B.T., Watchueng, J., Abegaz, B.M., Ojewole, J.A., 2004. Antinociceptive and anti-inflammatory effects of *Dorstenia barteri* (Moraceae) leaf and twig extracts in mice. J. Ethnopharmacol. 95 (1), 7–12.

Ordodi, V.L., Mic, F.A., Mic, A.A., Sandesc, D., Paunescu, V., 2005. A simple device for intubation of rats. Lab. Anim. (NY) 34 (8), 37–39.

Ortiz, M.I., Torres-Lopez, J.E., Castaneda-Hernandez, G., Rosas, R., Vidal-Cantu, G.C., Granados-Soto, V., 2002. Pharmacological evidence for the activation of K(+) channels by diclofenac. Eur. J. Pharmacol. 438 (1–2), 85–91.

Osterrieder, N., Bertzbach, L.D., Dietert, K., Abdelgawad, A., Vladimirova, D., Kunec, D., Hoffmann, D., Beer, M., Gruber, A.D., Trimpert, J., 2020. Age-dependent progression of SARS-CoV-2 infection in Syrian hamsters. Viruses 12 (7), 779.

Ostrowski, N.L., Stapleton, J.M., Noble, R.G., Reid, L.D., 1979. Morphine and naloxone's effects on sexual behavior of the female golden hamster. Pharmacol. Biochem. Behav. 11 (6), 673–681.

Ozdogan, U.K., Lahdesmaki, J., Hakala, K., Scheinin, M., 2004. The involvement of alpha 2A-adrenoceptors in morphine analgesia, tolerance and withdrawal in mice. Eur. J. Pharmacol. 497 (2), 161–171.

Pachon, R.E., Scharf, B.A., Vatner, D.E., Vatner, S.F., 2015. Best anesthetics for assessing left ventricular systolic function by echocardiography in mice. Am. J. Physiol. Heart Circ. Physiol. *308* (12), H1525–H1529.

Page, C.D., Sarabia-Estrada, R., Hoffman, R.J., Lo, C.P., Gades, N.M., 2019. Lack of absorption of a sustained-release buprenorphine formulation administered subcutaneously to athymic nude rats. JAALAS 58 (5), 597–600.

Padi, S.S., Jain, N.K., Singh, S., Kulkarni, S.K., 2004. Pharmacological profile of parecoxib: a novel, potent injectable selective cyclooxygenase-2 inhibitor. Eur. J. Pharmacol. 491 (1), 69–76.

Page, G.G., Ben-Eliyahu, S., 2002. Indomethacin attenuates the immunosuppressive and tumor-promoting effects of surgery. J. Pain 3 (4), 301–308.

Papaioannou, V.E., Fox, J.G., 1993. Efficacy of tribromoethanol anesthesia in mice. Lab. Anim. Sci. 43 (2), 189–192.

Pape, M., Engelhard, K., Eberspacher, E., Hollweck, R., Kellerman, K., Zinter, S., Hutzler, P., Werner, C., 2006. The long term effect of sevoflurane on neuronal cell damage and expression of apoptotic factors after cerebral ischemia and reperfusion in rats. Anesth. Analg. 103 (1), 173–179.

Papich, M.G., 2016. Saunders Handbook of Veterinary Drugs Small and Large Animal, fourth ed. Saunders, Elsevier, Amsterdam, Netherlands.

Paris, A., Ohlendorf, C., Marquardt, M., Bein, B., Sonner, J.M., Scholz, J., Tonner, P.H., 2005. The effect of meperidine on thermoregula-tion in mice: involvement of alpha2-adrenoceptors. Anesth. Analg. 100 (1), 102–106.

Park, K.W., Dai, H.B., Lowenstein, E., Sellke, F.W., 1998. Epithelial dependence of the bronchodilatory effect of sevoflurane and desflurane in rat distal bronchi. Anesth. Analg. 86 (3), 646–651.

Park, W.K., Pancrazio, J.J., Suh, C.K., Lunch, C., 1996. Myocardial depressant effects of sevoflurane. Mechanical and electrophysiologic actions in vivo. Anesthesiology 84 (5), 1166–1176.

Parker, J.M., Austin, J., Wilkerson, J., Carbone, L., 2011. Effects of multimodal analgesia on the success of mouse embryo transfer surgery. JAALAS 50 (4), 466–470.

Patrono, C., 2016. Cardiovascular effects of cyclooxygenase-2 inhibitors: a mechanistic and clinical perspective. Br. J. Clin. Pharmacol. 82 (4), 957–964.

Payne, R.S., Akca, O., Roewer, N., Schurr, A., Kehl, F., 2005. Sevoflurane-induced preconditioning protects against cerebral ischemic neuronal damage in rats. Brain Res. 1034 (1–2), 147–152.

Payton, A.J., Forsythe, D.B., Dixon, D., Myers, P.H., Clark, J.A., Snipe, J.R., 1993. Evaluation of ketamine–xylazine in Syrian hamsters. Cornell Vet. 83 (2), 153–161.

Penderis, J., Franklin, R.J., 2005. Effects of pre- versus post-anaesthetic buprenorphine on propofol-anaesthetized rats. Vet. Anaesth. Analg. 32 (5), 256–260.

Perez-Garcia, C.C., Pena-Penabad, M., Cano-Rabano, M.J., Garcia-Rodriguez, M.B., Gallego-Morales, D., Rios-Granja, M.A., Diez-Prieto, I., 2003. A simple procedure to perform intravenous injections in the Mongolian gerbil (*Meriones unguiculatus*). Lab. Anim. 37 (1), 68–71.

Peterson, N.C., Nunamaker, E.A., Turner, P.V., 2017. To treat or not to treat: the effects of pain on experimental parameters. Comp. Med. 67 (6), 469–482.

Petzelt, C., Blom, P., Schmehl, W., Muller, J., Kox, W.J., 2003. Prevention of neurotoxicity in hypoxic cortical neurons by the noble gas xenon. Life Sci. 71 (17), 1909–1918.

Pham, T.M., Hagman, B., Codita, A., Van Loo, P.L., Strömmer, L., Baumans, V., 2010. Housing environment influences the need for pain relief during post-operative recovery in mice. Physiol. Behav. 99 (5), 663–668.

Picazo, M.G., Benito, P.J., García-Olmo, D.C., June 2009. Efficiency and safety of a technique for drawing blood from the hamster cranial vena cava. Lab. Anim. (NY) 38 (6), 211–216.

Pick, C.G., Cheng, J., Paul, D., Pasternak, G.W., 1991. Genetic influences in opioid analgesic sensitivity in mice. Brain Res. 566 (1–2), 295–298.

Pinho, R.H., Leach, M.C., Minto, B.W., Rocha, F.D.L., Luna, S.P.L., 2020. Postoperative pain behaviours in rabbits following orthopaedic surgery and effect of observer presence. PLoS One 15 (10), e0240605.

Pinardi, G., Prieto, J.C., Miranda, H.F., 2005. Analgesic synergism between intrathecal morphine and cyclooxygenase-2 inhibitors in mice. Pharmacol. Biochem. Behav. 82 (1), 120–124.

Plachinta, R.V., Hayes, J.K., Cerilli, L.A., Rich, G.F., 2003. Isoflurane pretreatment inhibits lipopolysaccharide-induced inflammation in rats. Anesthesiology 98 (1), 89–95.

Planas, E., Poveda, R., Sanchez, S., Romero, A., Puig, M.M., 2003. Nonsteroidal anti-inflammatory drugs antagonise the constipating effects of tramadol. Eur. J. Pharmacol. 482 (1–3), 223–226.

Plate, A.Y., Crankshaw, D.L., Gallaher, D.D., 2005. The effect of anesthesia by diethyl ether or isoflurane on activity of cytochrome P450 2E1 and P450 reductases in rat liver. Anesth. Analg. 101 (4), 1063–1064.

Pomonis, J.D., Boulet, J.M., Gottshall, S.L., Phillips, S., Sellers, R., Bunton, T., Walker, K., 2005. Development and pharmacological characterization of a rat model of osteoarthritis pain. Pain 114 (3), 339–346.

Poonawala, T., Levay-Young, B.K., Hebbel, R.P., Gupta, K., 2005. Opioids heal ischemic wounds in the rat. Wound Repair Regen. 13 (2), 165–174.

Poveda, R., Planas, E., Pol, O., Romero, A., Sanchez, S., Puig, M.M., 2003. Interaction between metamizol and tramadol in a model of acute visceral pain in rats. Eur. J. Pain. 7 (5), 439–448.

Poyhia, R., Xu, M., Kontinen, V.K., Paananen, S., Kalso, E., 1999. Systemic physostigmine shows antiallodynic effects in neuropathic rats. Anesth. Analg. 89 (2), 428–433.

Prado, W.A., Pontes, R.M., 2002. Presurgical ketoprofen, but not morphine, dipyrone, diclofenac or tenoxicam, preempts post-incisional mechanical allodynia in rats. Braz. J. Med. Biol. Res. 35 (1), 111–119.

Quesenberry, K., Carpenter, J., 2012. Ferrets, Rabbits, and Rodents, Clinical Medicine and Surgery, third ed. Elsevier, Missouri, pp. 429–451.

Radulovic, L.L., Turck, D., von Hodenberg, A., Vollmer, K.O., McNally, W.P., DeHart, P.D., Hanson, B.J., Bockbrader, H.N., Chang, T., 1995. Disposition of gabapentin (neurontin) in mice, rats, dogs, and monkeys. Drug Metab. Dispos. 23 (4), 441–448.

Rampil, I.J., King, B.S., 1996. Volatile anesthetics depress spinal motor neurons. Anesthesiology 85 (1), 129–134.

Rampil, I.J., Moller, D.H., Bell, A.H., 2006. Isoflurane modulates genomic expression in rat amygdala. Anesth. Analg. 102 (5), 1431–1438.

Ramsey, D., Fleck, T., Berg, T., Nederveld, S., DeLong, D., Tena, J.-K., Aleo, M., McCall, R., 2014. Cerenia prevents perioperative nausea and vomiting and improves recovery in dogs undergoing routine surgery. Int. J. Appl. Res. Vet. Med. 12, 228–237.

Rana, J., Ramzan, I., 1995. Neuromuscular blocking drug pharmacodynamics after chronic exposure to H2-antagonists. In Vivo 9 (2), 163–166.

Randolph, B.C., Peters, M.A., 1997. Analgesic effectiveness of ketorolac compared to meperidine in the rat formalin test. Anesth. Prog. 44 (1), 11–16.

Rao, S.B., 1990. Comparative study on the effects of pentobarbitone sodium, thiopentone sodium and ketamine–diazepam on body temperature in rats. Indian Vet. J. 67, 339–342.

Rätsep, M.T., Barrette, V.F., Winterborn, A., Adams, M.A., Croy, B.A., September 2013. Hemodynamic and behavioral differences after administration of meloxicam, buprenorphine, or tramadol as analgesics for telemeter implantation in mice. J. Am. Assoc. Lab. Anim. Sci. 52 (5), 560–566.

Reboucas, E.C., Segato, E.N., Kishi, R., Freitas, R.L., Savoldi, M., Morato, S., Coimbra, N.C., 2005. Effect of the blockade of mu1-

opioid and 5HT2A-serotonergic/alpha1-noradrenergic receptors on sweet-substance-induced analgesia. Psychopharmacology (Berl.) 179 (2), 349–355.

Reddyjarugu, B., Pavek, T., Southard, T., Barry, J., Singh, B., 2015. Analgesic efficacy of firocoxib, a selective inhibitor of cyclo-oxygenase 2, in a mouse model of incisional pain. JAALAS 54 (4), 405–410.

Redwine, K.E., Trujillo, K.A., 2003. Effects of NMDA receptor antagonists on acute mu-opioid analgesia in the rat. Pharmacol. Biochem. Behav. 76 (2), 361–372.

Richardson, C.A., Flecknell, P.A., 2005. Anaesthesia and post-operative analgesia following experimental surgery in laboratory rodents: are we making progress? Altern. Lab. Anim. 33 (2), 119–127.

Richebe, P., Rivat, C., Laulin, J.P., Maurette, P., Simonnet, G., 2005. Ketamine improves the management of exaggerated postoperative pain observed in perioperative fentanyl-treated rats. Anesthesiology 102 (2), 421–428.

Robertson, S.A., 2001. Analgesia and analgesic techniques. Vet. Clin. North Am. Exot. Anim. Pract. 4 (1), 1–18.

Rodrigues, S.F., de Oliveira, M.A., Martins, J.O., Sannomiya, P., de Cassia Tostes, R., Nigro, D., Carvalho, M.H., Fortes, Z.B., 2006. Differential effects of chloral hydrate- and ketamine/xylazine-induced anesthesia by the sc route. Life Sci. 79 (17), 1630–1637.

Romero, A., Miranda, H.F., Puig, M.M., 2010. Analysis of the opioid-opioid combinations according to the nociceptive stimulus in mice. Pharmacol. Res. 61 (6), 511–518.

Ross, M.C., Zoeffel, L.D., McMonagle, J.D., McDonough, J.H., 2000. Isoflurane anesthesia for guinea pigs (Cavia porcella) in a stereotaxic surgical apparatus. Contemp. Top. Lab. Anim. Sci. 39 (2), 43–46.

Rottman, J.N., Ni, G., Khoo, M., Wang, Z., Zhang, W., Anderson, M.E., Madu, E.C., 2003. Temporal changes in ventricular function assessed echocardiographically in conscious and anesthetized mice. J. Am. Soc. Echocardiogr. 16 (11), 1150–1157.

Roughan, J.V., Bertrand, H.G., Isles, H.M., 2016. Meloxicam prevents COX-2-mediated post-surgical inflammation but not pain following laparotomy in mice. Eur. J. Pain 20 (2), 231–240.

Roughan, J.V., Flecknell, P.A., 2001. Behavioural effects of laparotomy and analgesic effects of ketoprofen and carprofen in rats. Pain 90 (1–2), 65–74.

Roughan, J.V., Flecknell, P.A., 2002. Buprenorphine: a reappraisal of its antinociceptive effects and therapeutic use in alleviating post-operative pain in animals. Lab. Anim 36 (3), 322–343.

Roughan, J.V., Flecknell, P.A., 2003. Evaluation of a short duration behaviour-based post-operative pain scoring system in rats. Eur. J. Pain 7 (5), 397–406.

Roughan, J.V., Flecknell, P.A., 2004. Behaviour-based assessment of the duration of laparotomy-induced abdominal pain and the analgesic effects of carprofen and buprenorphine in rats. Behav. Pharmacol. 15 (7), 461–472.

Roughan, J.V., Flecknell, P.A., Davies, B.R., July 2004. Behavioural assessment of the effects of tumour growth in rats and the influence of the analgesics carprofen and meloxicam. Lab. Anim. 38 (3), 286–296.

Roughan, J.V., Ojeda, O.B., Flecknell, P.A., 1999. The influence of pre-anaesthetic administration of buprenorphine on the anaesthetic effects of ketamine/medetomidine and pentobarbitone in rats and the consequences of repeated anaesthesia. Lab. Anim. 33 (3), 234–242.

Rowe, R.K., Harrison, J.L., Thomas, T.C., Pauly, J.R., Adelson, P.D., Lifshitz, J., 2013. Using anesthetics and analgesics in experimental traumatic brain injury. Lab. Anim. 42 (8), 286–291.

Roy, S., Guo, X., Kelschenbach, J., Liu, Y., Loh, H.H., 2005. Invivo activation of a mutant mu-opioid receptor by naltrexone produces a potent analgesic effect but no tolerance: role of mu-receptor activation and delta-receptor blockade in morphine tolerance. J. Neurosci. 25 (12), 3229–3233.

Rufiange, M., Leung, V.S.Y., Simpson, K., Pang, D.S.J., 2020. Pre-warming before general anesthesia with isoflurane delays the onset of hypothermia in rats. PLoS One 15 (3), e0219722.

Ruiz-Pérez, D., Benito, J., Largo, C., Polo, G., Canfrán, S., Gómez de Segura, I.A., August 2017. Metamizole (dipyrone) effects on sevoflurane requirements and postoperative hyperalgesia in rats. Lab. Anim. 51 (4), 365–375.

Rusch, E., Bovi, M.F., Martinelli, E.C., Garcia-Gomes, M.S., Mori, C.M., Martins, D.S., Carregaro, A.B., 2021. Effects of three consecutive days of morphine or methadone administration on analgesia and open-field activity in mice with ehrlich carcinoma. JAALAS 60 (3), 349–356.

Sabetkasaie, M., Vala, S., Khansefid, N., Hosseini, A.R., Sadat Ladgevardi, M.A., 2004. Clonidine and guanfacine-induced antinociception in visceral pain: possible role of alpha 2/I2 binding sites. Eur. J. Pharmacol. 501 (1–3), 95–101.

Sage, M.D., West, E.J., Gavin, J.B., 1985. Cardiac performance of isolated beating hearts obtained from rats anesthetized by three different agents. Lab. Anim. Sci. 35 (2), 153–155.

Saha, D.C., Saha, A.C., Malik, G., Astiz, M.E., Rackow, E.C., 2007. Comparison of cardiovascular effects of tiletamine-zolazepam, pentobarbital, and ketamine-xylazine in male rats. J. Am. Assoc. Lab. Anim. Sci. 46 (2), 74–80.

Saito, O., Aoe, T., Yamamoto, T., 2005. Analgesic effects of nonsteroidal antiinflammatory drugs, acetaminophen, and morphine in a mouse model of bone cancer pain. J. Anesth. 19 (3), 218–224.

Santos, A.R., Vedana, E.M., andDe Freitas, G.A., 1998. Antinociceptive effect of meloxicam, in neurogenic and inflammatory nociceptive models in mice. Inflamm. Res. 47 (7), 302–307.

Sarlis, N.J., Kaniaris, P.K., 1991. Physostigmine is equipotent to flumazenil only in excessive doses, while naloxone is ineffective in reversing midazolam anesthesia. Middle East J. Anesthesiol. 11 (3), 271–288.

Sarfaty, A.E., Zeiss, C.J., Willis, A.D., Harris, J.M., Smith, P.C., November 1, 2019. Concentration-dependent toxicity after subcutaneous administration of meloxicam to C57BL/6N mice (Mus musculus). J. Am. Assoc. Lab. Anim. Sci. 58 (6), 802–809.

Schaap, M.W., Uilenreef, J.J., Mitsogiannis, M.D., van 't Klooster, J.G., Arndt, S.S., Hellebrekers, L.J., 2012. Optimizing the dosing interval of buprenorphine in a multimodal postoperative analgesic strategy in the rat: minimizing side-effects without affecting weight gain and food intake. Lab. Anim. 46 (4), 287–292.

Scholer, D.W., Ku, E.C., Boettcher, I., Schweizer, A., 1986. Pharmacology of diclofenac sodium. Am. J. Med. 80 (4B), 34–38.

Schreiner, V., Durst, M., Arras, M., Detampel, P., Jirkof, P., Huwyler, J., 2020. Design and in vivo evaluation of a microparticulate depot formulation of buprenorphine for veterinary use. Sci. Rep. 10 (1), 17295.

Schuster, C.J., Pang, D.S.J., 2018. Forced-air pre-warming prevents peri-anaesthetic hypothermia and shortens recovery in adult rats. Lab. Anim. 52 (2), 142–151.

Schwenke, D.O., Cragg, P.A., 2004. Comparison of the depressive effects of four anesthetic regimens on ventilatory and cardiovascular variables in the Guinea pig. Comp. Med. 54 (1), 77–85.

Segato, F.N., Castro-Souza, C., Segato, E.N., Morato, S., Coimbra, N.C., 1997. Sucrose ingestion causes opioid analgesia. Braz. J. Med. Biol. Res. 30 (8), 981–984.

Sendil, D., Bonney, I.M., Carr, D.B., Lipkowski, A.W., Wise, D.L., Hasirci, V., 2003. Antinociceptive effects of hydromorphone, bupivacaine and biphalin released from PLGA polymer after intrathecal implantation in rats. Biomaterials 24 (11), 1969–1976.

Serita, R., Morisaki, H., Ai, K., Morita, Y., Innami, Y., Satoh, T., Kosugi, S., Kotake, Y., Takeda, J., 2002. Sevoflurane preconditions stunned myocardium in septic but not healthy isolated rat hearts. Br. J. Anaesth. 89 (6), 896–903.

Seymour, T.L., Adams, S.C., Felt, S.A., Jampachaisri, K., Yeomans, D.C., Pacharinsak, C., 2016. Postoperative analgesia due to sustained-release buprenorphine, sustained-release meloxicam, and carprofen gel in a model of incisional pain in rats (Rattus norvegicus). JAALAS 55 (3), 300–305.

Sharma, S., Jain, N.K., Kulkarni, S.K., 2005. Possible analgesic and anti-inflammatory interactions of aspartame with opioids and NSAIDs. Indian J. Exp. Biol. 43 (6), 498–502.

Sharp, J., Zammit, T., Azar, T., Lawson, D., 2003. Recovery of male rats from major abdominal surgery after treatment with various analgesics. Contemp. Top. Lab. Anim. Sci. 42 (6), 22–27.

Sheffels, P., Schroeder, J.L., Altuntas, T.G., Liggitt, H.D., Kharasch, E.D., 2004. Role of cytochrome P4503A in cysteine S-conjugates sulfoxidation and the nephrotoxicity of the sevoflurane degradation product fluoromethyl-2,2-difluoro-1-(trifluoromethyl)vinyl ether (compoundA) in rats. Chem. Res. Toxicol. 17 (9), 1177–1189.

Shientag, L.J., Wheeler, S.M., Garlick, D.S., Maranda, L.S., November 2012. A therapeutic dose of ketoprofen causes acute gastrointestinal bleeding, erosions, and ulcers in rats. J. Am. Assoc. Lab. Anim. Sci. 51 (6), 832–841.

Shin, Y.S., Miller, R.D., Caldwell, J.E., Eger, E.I., 1992. The neuromuscular effects of sevoflurane and isoflurane alone and in combination with vecuronium or atracurium in the rat. J. Anesth. 6 (1), 1–8.

Shinozaki, T., Yamada, T., Nonaka, T., Yamamoto, T., 2015. Acetaminophen and non-steroidal anti-inflammatory drugs interact with morphine and tramadol analgesia for the treatment of neuropathic pain in rats. J. Anesth. 29, 386–395.

Silverman, J., Huhndorf, M., Balk, M., Slater, G., 1983. Evaluation of a combination of tiletamine and zolazepam as an anesthetic for laboratory rodents. Lab. Anim. Sci. 33 (5), 457–460.

Silverman, J., Schucker, A.E., Anestidou, L., Villarreal Acosta, Y., 2003. Anesthetics in GEM: does TBE make the grade? Lab. Anim. (NY) 32 (2), 19–21.

Sintov, A.C., Shapiro, L., 2004. New microemulsion vehicle facilitates percutaneous penetration in vitro and cutaneous drug bioavailability in vivo. J. Control. Release 95 (2), 173–183.

Siriarchavatana, P., Ayers, J.D., Kendall, L.V., 2016. Anesthetic activity of alfaxalone compared with ketamine in mice. J. Am. Assoc. Lab. Anim. Sci. 55 (4), 426–430.

Skornik, W.A., Brain, J.D., 1990. Breathing and lung mechanics in hamsters: effect of pentobarbital anesthesia. J. Appl. Physiol. 68 (6), 2536–2541.

Sluka, K.A., Chandran, P., 2002. Enhanced reduction in hyperalgesia by combined administration of clonidine and TENS. Pain 100 (1–2), 183–190.

Smiler, K.L., Stein, S., Hrapkiewicz, K.L., Hiben, J.R., 1990. Tissue response to intramuscular and intraperitoneal injections of ketamine and xylazine in rats. Lab. Anim. Sci. 40 (1), 60–64.

Smith, J.C., Corbin, T.J., McCabe, J.G., Bolon, B., 2004. Isoflurane with morphine is a suitable anaesthetic regimen for embryo transfer in the production of transgenic rats. Lab. Anim. 38 (1), 38–43.

Smith, L.J., Krugner-Higby, L., Clark, M., Wendland, A., Heath, T.D., 2003. A single dose of liposome-encapsulated oxymorphone or morphine provides long-term analgesia in an animal model of neuropathic pain. Comp. Med. 53 (3), 280–287.

Smith, L.J., Shih, A., Miletic, G., Miletic, V., 2002. Continual systemic infusion of lidocaine provides analgesia in an animal model of neuropathic pain. Pain 97 (3), 267–273.

Smith, L.J., Valenzuela, J.R., Krugner-Higby, L.A., Brown, C., Heath, T.D., 2006. A single dose of liposome-encapsulated hydromorphone provides extended analgesia in a rat model of neuropathic pain. Comp. Med. 56 (6), 487–492.

Smith, B.J., Wegenast, D.J., Hansen, R.J., Hess, A.M., Kendall, L.V., 2016. Pharmacokinetics and paw withdrawal pressure in female guinea pigs (Cavia porcellus) treated with sustained-release buprenorphine and buprenorphine hydrochloride. JAALAS 55 (6), 789–793.

Soliman, N., Haroutounian, S., Hohmann, A.G., Krane, E., Liao, J., Macleod, M., Segelcke, D., Sena, C., Thomas, J., Vollert, J., Wever, K., Alaverdyan, H., Barakat, A., Barthlow, T., Bozer, A.L.H., Davidson, A., Diaz-delCastillo, M., Dolgorukova, A., Ferdousi, M.I., Healy, C., Hong, S., Hopkins, M., James, A., Leake, H.B., Malewicz, N.M., Mansfield, M., Mardon, A.K., Mattimoe, D., McLoone, D.P., Noes-Holt, G., Pogatzki-Zahn, E.M., Power, E., Pradier, B., Romanos-Sirakis, E., Segelcke, A., Vinagre, R., Yanes, J.A., Zhang, J., Zhang, X.Y., Finn, D.P., Rice, A.S.C., 2021. Systematic review and meta-analysis of cannabinoids, cannabis-based medicines, and endocannabinoid system modulators tested for antinociceptive effects in animal models of injury-related or pathological persistent pain. Pain 162 (Suppl. 1), S26–S44.

Sonner, J.M., Gong, D., Eger, E.I., 2000. Naturally occurring variability in anesthetic potency among inbred mouse strains. Anesth. Analg. 91 (3), 720–726.

Sorge, R.E., Martin, L.J., Isbester, K.A., Sotocinal, S.G., Rosen, S., Tuttle, A.H., Wieskopf, J.S., Acland, E.L., Dokova, A., Kadoura, B., Leger, P., Mapplebeck, J.C., McPhail, M., Delaney, A., Wigerblad, G., Schumann, A.P., Quinn, T., Frasnelli, J., Svensson, C.I., Sternberg, W.F., Mogil, J.S., 2014. Olfactory exposure to males, including men, causes stress and related analgesia in rodents. Nat. Methods 11 (6), 629–632.

Sotocinal, S.G., Sorge, R.E., Zaloum, A., Tuttle, A.H., Martin, L.J., Wieskopf, J.S., Mapplebeck, J.C., Wei, P., Zhan, S., Zhang, S., McDougall, J.J., King, O.D., Mogil, J.S., 2011. The rat grimace scale: a partially automated method for quantifying pain in the laboratory rat via facial expressions. Mol. Pain 7, 55.

Stackman, R.W., Walsh, T.J., 1992. Chlordiazepoxide-induced working memory impairments: site specificity and reversal by flumazenil (RO15-1788). Behav. Neural. Biol. 57 (3), 233–243.

Statler, K.D., Alexander, H., Vagni, V., Dixon, C.E., Clark, R.S., Jenkins, L., Kochanek, P.M., 2006. Comparison of seven anesthetic agents on outcome after experimental traumatic brain injury in adult, male rats. J. Neurotrauma 23 (1), 97–108.

Steffey, M.A., Brosnan, R.J., Steffey, E.P., 2003. Assessment of halothane and sevoflurane anesthesia in spontaneously breathing rats. Am. J. Vet. Res. 64 (4), 470–474.

Stevenson, G.W., Bilsky, E.J., Negus, S.S., 2006. Targeting pain-suppressed behaviors in preclinical assays of pain and analgesia: effects of morphine on acetic acid-suppressed feeding in C57BL/6J mice. J. Pain 7 (6), 408–416.

Stewart, A.S.L., Martin, W.J., 2003a. Evaluation of postoperative analgesia in a rat model of incisional pain. Contemp. Top. Lab. Anim. Sci. 42 (1), 28–34.

Stewart, L.S., Martin, W.J., 2003b. Influence of postoperative analgesics on the development of neuropathic pain in rats. Comp. Med. 53 (1), 29–36.

Stokes, E.L., Flecknell, P.A., Richardson, C.A., 2009. Reported analgesic and anaesthetic administration to rodents undergoing experimental surgical procedures. Lab. Anim. 43, 149–154.

Stringer, S.K., Seligmann, B.E., 1996. Effects of two injectable anesthetic agents on coagulation assays in the rat. Lab. Anim. Sci. 46 (4), 430–433.

Struck, M.B., Andrutis, K.A., Ramirez, H.E., Battles, A.H., 2011. Effect of a short-term fast on ketamine-xylazine anesthesia in rats. J. Am. Assoc. Lab. Anim. Sci. 50 (3), 344–348.

Suganuma, T., Suzuki, T., Oshimi, M., Hanano, M., 1998. Change of beta-endorphin concentration in rat brain after administration of indomethacin or carrageenin. Biol. Pharm. Bull. 21 (7), 756–760.

Sun, F.J., Wright, D.E., Pinson, D.M., 2003. Comparison of ketamine versus combination of ketamine and medetomidine in injectable anesthetic protocols: chemical immobilization in macaques and tissue reaction in rats. Contemp. Top. Lab. Anim. Sci. 42 (4), 32–37.

Sunaga, H., Kaneko, M., Amaki, Y., 2006. The efficacy of intratracheal administration of vecuronium in rats, compared with intravenous and intramuscular administration. Anesth. Analg. 103 (3), 601–607.

Svendsen, O., Kok, L., Lauritzen, B., April 2007. Nociception after intraperitoneal injection of a sodium pentobarbitone formulation with and without lidocaine in rats quantified by expression of neuronal c-fos in the spinal cord—a preliminary study. Lab. Anim. 41 (2), 197–203.

Szczensy, G., Veihelmann, A., Massberg, S., Nolte, D., Massmer, K., 2004. Long-term anesthesia using inhalatory isoflurane in different strains of mice—the haemodynamic effects. Lab. Anim. 38 (1), 64–69.

Szilagyi, K., Zieger, M.A., Kacena, M.A., 2018. Improving post-operative outcomes in aged and diabetic obese mice. Lab. Anim. Sci. Prof. 6 (3), 65–67.

Takada, K., Clark, D.J., Davies, M.F., Tonner, P.H., Krause, T.K., Bertaccini, E., Maze, M., 2002. Meperidine exerts agonist activity at the alpha(2B)-adrenoceptor subtype. Anesthesiology 96 (6), 1420–1426.

Takahashi, M., Kawaguchi, M., Shimada, K., Nakashima, T., Furuya, H., 2005. Systemic meloxicam reduces tactile allodynia development after L5 single spinal nerve injury in rats. Reg. Anesth. Pain Med. 30 (4), 351–355.

Tamba, B.I., Stanciu, G.D., Urîtu, C.M., Rezus, E., Stefanescu, R., Mihai, C.T., Luca, A., Rusu-Zota, G., Leon-Constantin, M.M., Cojocaru, E., Gafton, B., Alexa-Stratulat, T., 2020. Challenges and Opportunities in preclinical research of synthetic cannabinoids for pain therapy. Medicina (Kaunas, Lithuania) 56 (1), 24.

Tatsuo, M.A., Carvalho, W.M., Silva, C.V., Miranda, A.E., Ferreira, S.H., Francischi, J.N., 1994. Analgesic and antiinflammatory effects of dipyrone in rat adjuvant arthritis model. Inflammation 18 (4), 399–405.

Taylor, D.K., 2019. Influence of pain and analgesia on cancer research studies. Comp. Med. 69 (6), 501–509.

Taylor, J., Mellstrom, B., Fernaud, I., Naranjo, J.R., 1998. Metamizol potentiates morphine effects on visceral pain and evoked c-Fos immunore-activity in spinal cord. Eur. J. Pharmacol. 351 (1), 39–47.

Taylor, B.J., Orr, S.A., Chapman, J.L., Fisher, D.E., 2009. Beyond-use dating of extemporaneously compounded ketamine, acepromazine, and xylazine: safety, stability, and efficacy over time. J. Am. Assoc. Lab. Anim. Sci. 48 (6), 718–726.

Taylor, R., Hayes, K.E., Toth, L.A., 2000. Evaluation of an anesthetic regimen for retroorbital blood collection from mice. Contemp. Top. Lab. Anim. Sci. 39 (2), 14–17.

Taylor, D.K., 2007. Study of two devices used to maintain normothermia in rats and mice during general anesthesia. JAALAS 46 (5), 37–41.

Ter Horst, E.N., Krijnen, P.A.J., Flecknell, P., Meyer, K.W., Kramer, K., van der Laan, A.M., Piek, J.J., Niessen, H.W.M., 2018. Sufentanil-medetomidine anaesthesia compared with fentanyl/fluanisone-midazolam is associated with fewer ventricular arrhythmias and death during experimental myocardial infarction in rats and limits infarct size following reperfusion. Lab. Anim. 52 (3), 271–279.

Themistocleous, A., Kamerman, P., Mitchell, D., 2007. Pre-emptive ring-block with bupivacaine prevents the development of thermal hyperalgesia, but not sustained mechanical hyperalgesia, in rat tails exposed to ultraviolet a light. J. Pain 8 (3), 208–214.

Taylor, B.F., Ramirez, H.E., Battles, A.H., Andrutis, K.A., Neubert, J.K., 2016. Analgesic activity of tramadol and buprenorphine after voluntary ingestion by rats (Rattus norvegicus). J. Am. Assoc. Lab. Anim. Sci. 55 (1), 74–82.

Teixeira, F.M., Castro, L.L., Ferreira, R.T., Pires, P.A., Vanderlinde, F.A., Medeiros, M.A., 2012. High-frequency electroacupuncture versus carprofen in an incisional pain model in rats. Braz. J. Med. Biol. Res. 45 (12), 1209–1214.

Thomas, A.A., Detilleux, J., Sandersen, C.F., Flecknell, P.A., 2017. Minimally invasive technique for intrathecal administration of morphine in rats: practicality and antinociceptive properties. Lab. Anim. 51 (5), 479–489.

Thomas, J.L., Dumouchel, J., Li, J., Magat, J., Balitzer, D., Bigby, T.D., 2014. Endotracheal intubation in mice via direct laryngoscopy using an otoscope. J. Vis. Exp. (86), 50269.

Thompson, A.C., DiPirro, J.M., Sylvester, A.R., Martin, L.B., Kristal, M.B., 2006. Lack of analgesic efficacy in female rats of the commonly recommended oral dose of buprenorphine. J. Am. Assoc. Lab. Anim. Sci. 45 (6), 13–16.

Thompson, A.C., Kristal, M.B., Sallaj, A., Acheson, A., Martin, L.B., Martin, T., 2004. Analgesic efficacy of orally administered buprenorphine in rats: methodologic considerations. Comp. Med. 54 (3), 293–300.

Thornton, S.R., Compton, D.R., Smith, F.L., 1998. Ontogeny of mu opioid agonist anti-nociception in postnatal rats. Brain Res. Dev. Brain Res. 105 (2), 269–276.

Thurmon, J.C., Tranquilli, W.J., Benson, G.J., 1996a. Preanesthetics and anesthetic adjuvants. In: Lumb & Jones'VeterinaryAnesthesia, third ed. Williams & Wilkins, pp. 183–209.

Thurmon, J.C., Tranquilli, W.J., Benson, G.J., 1996b. Injectable anesthetics. In: Lumb & Jones' Veterinary Anesthesia, third ed. Williams & Wilkins, pp. 210–240.

Toth, L.A., 2019. Interacting influences of sleep, pain, and analgesic medications on sleep studies in rodents. Comp. Med. 69 (6), 571–578.

Tokuyama, S., Inoue, M., Fuchigami, T., Ueda, H., 1998. Lack of tolerance in peripheral opioid analgesia in mice. Life Sci. 62 (17–18), 1677–1681.

Torjman, M.C., Joseph, J.I., Munsick, C., Morishita, M., Grunwald, Z., 2005. Effects of isoflurane on gastrointestinal motility after brief exposure in rats. Int. J. Pharm. 294 (1–2), 65–71.

Torres-Lopez, J.E., Ortiz, M.I., Castaneda-Hernandez, G., Alonso-Lopez, R., Asomoza-Espinosa, R., Granados-Soto, V., 2002. Comparison of the antinociceptive effect of celecoxib, diclofenac and resveratrol in the formalin test. Life Sci. 70 (14), 1669–1676.

Tortorici, V., Vanegas, H., 1994. Putative role of medullary off- and on-cells in the antinociception produced by dipyrone (metamizol) administered systemically or microinjected into PAG. Pain 57 (2), 197–205.

Tortorici, V., Vasquez, E., Vanegas, H., 1996. Naloxone partial reversal of the antinociception produced by dipyrone microinjected into the periaque-ductal grayofrats. Possible involvement of medullary off- and on-cells. Brain Res. 725 (1), 106–110.

Traul, K.A., Romero, J.B., Brayton, C., DeTolla, L., Forbes-McBean, N., Halquist, M.S., Karnes, H.T., Sarabia-Estrada, R., Tomlinson, M.J., Tyler, B.M., Ye, X., Zadnik, P., Guarnieri, M., 2015. Safety studies of post-surgical buprenorphine therapy for mice. Lab. Anim. 49 (2), 100–110.

Tsutsumi, Y.M., Patel, H.H., Huang, D., Roth, D.M., 2006a. Role of 12-lipoxygenase in volatile anesthetic-induced delayed preconditioning in mice. Am. J. Physiol. Heart Circ. Physiol. 291 (2), H979–H983.

Tsutsumi, Y.M., Patel, H.H., Lai, N.C., Takahashi, T., Head, B.P., Roth, D.M., 2006b. Isoflurane produces sustained cardiac protection after ischemia-reperfusion injury in mice. Anesthesiology 104 (3), 495–502.

Tsutsui, Y., Sunada, K., 2017. Dexmedetomidine increases the latency of thermal antinociception in rats. Anesth. Prog. 64 (4), 230–234.

Tubbs, J.T., Kissling, G.E., Travlos, G.S., Goulding, D.R., Clark, J.A., King-Herbert, A.P., Blankenship-Paris, T.L., 2011. Effects of buprenorphine, meloxicam, and flunixin meglumine as postoperative analgesia in mice. JAALAS 50 (2), 185–191.

Turner, P.V., Albassam, M.A., 2005. Susceptibility of ratstocorneal lesions after injectable anesthesia. Comp. Med. 55 (2), 175–182.

Turner, P.V., Brabb, T., Pekow, C., Vasbinder, M.A., 2011. Administration of substances to laboratory animals: routes of administration and factors to consider. J. Am. Assoc. Lab. Anim. Sci. 50 (5), 600–613.

Turner, P.V., Pang, D.S., Lofgren, J.L., December 1, 2019. A review of pain assessment methods in laboratory rodents. Comp. Med. 69 (6), 451–467.

Vaillancourt, C., Berger, N., Boksa, P., 1999. Effects of vaginal birth versus caesarean section birth with general anesthesia on blood gases and brain energy metabolism in neonatal rats. Exp. Neurol. 160 (1), 142–150.

Valentim, A.M., Olsson, I.A., Antunes, L.M., 2013. The anaesthetic combination of ketamine/midazolam does not alter the acquisition of spatial and motor tasks in adult mice. Lab. Anim. 47 (1), 19–25.

Valentine, H., Williams, W.O., Maurer, K.J., 2012. Sedation or inhalant anesthesia before euthanasia with CO2 does not reduce behavioral or physiologic signs of pain and stress in mice. JAALAS 51 (1), 50–57.

Vanegas, H., Tortorici, V., 2002. Opioidergic effects of nonopioid analgesics on the central nervous system. Cell. Mol. Neurobiol. 22 (5–6), 655–661.

Van Pelt, L.F., 1977. Ketamine and xylazine for surgical anesthesia in rats. J. Am. Vet. Med. Assoc. 171 (9), 842–844.

Veiga, A.P., Duarte, I.D., Avila, M.N., da Motta, P.G., Tatsuo, M.A., Francis-chi, J.N., 2004. Prevention by celecoxib of secondary hyperalgesia induced by formalin in rats. Life Sci. 75 (23), 2807–2817.

Vella, E.T., Evans, C.C., Williams, S., Wynne-Edwards, K.E., 2004. Neonatal anesthesia for studies of hamster parental behavior when infanticidal aggression is a possibility. Comp. Med. 54 (2), 202–208.

Victoria, N.C., Karom, M.C., Murphy, A.Z., 2015. Analgesia for early-life pain prevents deficits in adult anxiety and stress in rats. Dev. Neurosci. 37 (1), 1–13.

Victoria, N.C., Murphy, A.Z., 2016. Exposure to early life pain: long term consequences and contributing mechanisms. Curr. Opin. Behav. Sci. 7, 61–68.

Vijaya Kumar, S.G., Mishra, D.N., 2006. Analgesic, antiinflammatory, and ulcerogenic studies of meloxicam solid dispersion prepared with polyethylene glycol 6000. Methods Find. Exp. Clin. Pharmacol. 28 (7), 419–422.

Virtanen, R., 1989. Pharmacological profiles of medetomidine and its antagonist, atipamezole. Acta Vet. Scand. Suppl. 85, 29–37.

Vogler, G.A., 2006. Chapter 19 - anesthesia and analgesia. In: Suckow, M.A., Weisbroth, S.H., Franklin, C.L. (Eds.), The Laboratory Rat, second ed. Academic Press, Elsevier, Amsterdam, the Netherlands.

Vollmer, K.O., von Hodenberg, A., Kolle, E.U., 1986. Pharmacokinetics and metabolism of gabapentin in rat, dog and man. Arzneimittelforschung 36 (5), 830–839.

Waite, M.E., Tomkovich, A., Quinn, T.L., Schumann, A.P., Dewberry, L.S., Totsch, S.K., Sorge, R.E., 2015. Efficacy of common analgesics for postsurgical pain in rats. JAALAS 54 (4), 420–425.

Wakeno-Takahashi, M., Otani, H., Nakao, S., Imamura, H., Shingu, K., 2005. Isoflurane induces second window of preconditioning through upregulation of inducible nitric oxide synthase in rat heart. Am. J. Physiol. Heart Circ. Physiol. 289 (6), H2585–H2591.

Wallace, J.L., McKnight, W., Reuter, B.K., Vergnolle, N., September 2000. NSAID-induced gastric damage in rats: requirement for inhibition of both cyclooxygenase 1 and 2. Gastroenterology 119 (3), 706–714.

Walker, S.M., Fitzgerald, M., Hathway, G.J., June 2015. Surgical injury in the neonatal rat alters the adult pattern of descending modulation from the rostroventral medulla. Anesthesiology 122 (6), 1391–1400.

Wang, J.J., Sung, K.C., Hu, O.Y., Yeh, C.H., Fang, J.Y., 2006. Submicron lipid emulsion as a drug delivery system for nalbuphine and its prodrugs. J. Control. Release 115 (2), 140–149.

Wang, Y., Lei, J., Gupta, M., Peng, F., Lam, S., Jha, R., Raduenz, E., Beitz, A.J., Gupta, K., 2016. Electroacupuncture in conscious free-moving mice reduces pain by ameliorating peripheral and central nociceptive mechanisms. Sci. Rep. 6, 34493.

Watkins, J.C., Jane, D.E., 2006. The glutamate story. Br. J. Pharmacol. 147, S100–S108.

Weber, N.C., Toma, O., Wolter, J.I., Obal, D., Mullenheim, J., Preckel, B., Schlack, W., 2005. The noble gas xenon induces pharmacological preconditioning in the rat heart in vivo via induction of PKC-epsilon and p38 MAPK. Br. J. Pharmacol. 144 (1), 123–132.

Weinandy, R., Fritzsche, P., Weinert, D., Wenkel, R., Gattermann, R., 2005. Indicators for post-surgery recovery in Mongolian gerbils (*Meriones unguiculatus*). Lab. Anim. 39 (2), 200–208.

Weinger, M.B., Partridge, B.L., Henry, A.F., 1995. Dexmedetomidine does not modify the neuromuscular blocking action of vecuronium in the anaesthetized rat. Br. J. Anaesth. 74 (4), 455–457.

Weiss, J., Zimmermann, F., 1999. Tribromoethanol (Avertin) as an anaesthetic in mice. Lab. Anim. 33 (2), 192–193.

Welberg, L.A., Kinkead, B., Thrivikraman, K., Huerkamp, M.J., Nemeroff, C.B., Plotsky, P.M., 2006. Ketamine–xylazine–acepromazine anesthesia and postoperative recovery in rats. J. Am. Assoc. Lab. Anim. Sci. 45 (2), 13–20.

Wellington, D., Mikaelian, I., Singer, L., 2013. Comparison of ketamine-xylazine and ketamine-dexmedetomidine anesthesia and intraperitoneal tolerance in rats. J. Am. Assoc. Lab. Anim. Sci. 52 (4), 481–487.

Wells, S., Trower, C., Hough, T.A., Stewart, M., Cheeseman, M.T., 2009. Urethral obstruction by seminal coagulum is associated with medetomidine-ketamine anesthesia in male mice on C57BL/6J and mixed genetic backgrounds. JAALAS 48 (3), 296–299.

West, S.E., Lee, J.C., Johns, T.N., Nunamaker, E.A., 2020. Intraperitoneal alfaxalone and alfaxalone-dexmedetomidine anesthesia in sprague-dawley rats (*Rattus norvegicus*). JAALAS 59 (5), 531–538.

Whiteside, G.T., Harrison, J., Boulet, J., Mark, L., Pearson, M., Gottshall, S., Walker, K., 2004. Pharmacological characterisation of a rat model of incisional pain. Br. J. Pharmacol. 141 (1), 85–91.

Whittaker, A.L., Liu, Y., Barker, T.H., 2021. Methods used and application of the mouse grimace scale in biomedical research 10 Years on: a scoping review. Animals 11 (3), 673.

Whittington, R.A., Virag, L., 2006. Isoflurane decreases extracellular serotonin in the mouse hippocampus. Anesth. Analg. 103 (1), 92–98.

Wilhelm, S., Ma, D., Maze, M., Franks, N.P., 2002. Effects of xenon on in vitro and in vivo models of neuronal injury. Anesthesiology 96 (6), 1485–1491.

Williams, M.D., Lascelles, B., 2020. Early neonatal pain-A review of clinical and experimental implications on painful conditions later in life. Front. Pediatr. 8, 30.

Wilson, A.W., Medhurst, S.J., Dixon, C.I., Bontoft, N.C., Winyard, L.A., Brack-enborough, K.T., De Alba, J., Clarke, C.J., Gunthorpe, M.J., Hicks, G.A., et al., 2006. An animal model of chronic inflammatory pain: pharmacological and temporal differentiation from acute models. Eur. J. Pain 10 (6), 537–549.

Wilson, R.P., Zagon, I.S., Larach, D.R., Lang, C.M., 1992. Antinociceptive properties of tiletamine–zolazepam improved by addition of xylazine or butorphanol. Pharmacol. Biochem. Behav. 43 (4), 1129–1133.

Windeløv, J.A., Pedersen, J., Holst, J.J., 2016. Use of anesthesia dramatically alters the oral glucose tolerance and insulin secretion in C57Bl/6 mice. Physiol. Rep. 4 (11), e12824.

Wixson, S.K., Smiler, K.L., 1997. Anesthesia and analgesia in rodents. In: Kohn, D.F., Wixson, S.K., White, W.J., Benson, G.J. (Eds.), Anesthesia and Analgesia of Laboratory Animals. Academic Press, pp. 166–203.

Wixson, S.K., White, W.J., Hughes Jr., H.C., Lang, C.M., Marshall, W.K., 1987a. A comparison of pentobarbital, fentanyl–droperidol, ketamine–xylazine and ketamine–diazepam anesthesia in adult male rats. Lab. Anim. Sci. 37 (6), 726–730.

Wixson, S.K., White, W.J., Hughes Jr., H.C., Lang, C.M., Marshall, W.K., 1987b. The effects of pentobarbital, fentanyl–droperidol, ketamine–xylazine and ketamine–diazepam on arterial blood pH, blood gases, mean arterial blood pressure and heart rate in adult male rats. Lab. Anim. Sci. 37 (6), 736–742.

Wixson, S.K., White, W.J., Hughes Jr., H.C., Lang, C.M., Marshall, W.K., 1987c. The effects of pentobarbital, fentanyl–droperidol, ketamine–xylazine and ketamine–diazepam on core and surface body temperature regulation in adult male rats. Lab. Anim. Sci. 37 (6), 743–749.

Wixson, S.K., White, W.J., Hughes Jr., H.C., Marshall, W.K., Lang, C.M., 1987d. The effects of pentobarbital, fentanyl–droperidol, ketamine–xylazine and ketamine–diazepam on noxious stimulus perception in adult male rats. Lab. Anim. Sci. 37 (6), 731–735.

Wolfe, A.M., Kennedy, L.H., Na, J.J., Nemzek-Hamlin, J.A., July 2015. Efficacy of tramadol as a sole analgesic for postoperative pain in male and female mice. J. Am. Assoc. Lab. Anim. Sci. 54 (4), 411–419.

Wood, A.K., Klide, A.M., Pickup, S., Kundel, H.L., 2001. Prolonged general anesthesia in MR studies of rats. Acad. Radiol. 8 (11), 1136–1140.

Wright-Williams, S.L., Courade, J.P., Richardson, C.A., Roughan, J.V., Flecknell, P.A., 2007. Effects of vasectomy surgery and meloxicam treatment on faecal corticosterone levels and behaviour in two strains of laboratory mouse. Pain 130 (1–2), 108–118.

Xu, J.J., Renner, D.M., Lester, P.A., July 1, 2021. Strength and sterility of stock and diluted carprofen over time. J. Am. Assoc. Lab. Anim. Sci. 60 (4), 470–474.

Yazmakage, M., Tsujiguchi, N., Chen, X., Kamada, Y., Namiki, A., 2002. Sevoflurane inhibits contraction of uterine smooth muscle from pregnant rats similarly to halothane and isoflurane. Can. J. Anaesth. 49 (1), 62–66.

Yang, J., Liu, W.Y., Song, C.Y., Lin, B.C., 2006. Through central arginine vasopressin, not oxytocin and endogenous opiate peptides, glutamate sodium induces hypothalamic paraventricular nucleus enhancing acupuncture analgesia in the rat. Neurosci. Res. 54 (1), 49–56.

Yeo, J., Park, S., 2018. Effect of dexmedetomidine on the development of mechanical allodynia and central sensitization in chronic post-ischemia pain rats. J. Pain Res. 11, 3025–3030.

Yokoro, C.M., Tatsuo, M.A., Pereira, L.S., Alves, D.L., Francischi, J.N., 2003. Role of endogenous glucocorticoids in hyperalgesia and edema in old arthritic rats. Braz. J. Med. Biol. Res. 36 (1), 77–83.

Yonezaki, K., Uchimoto, K., Miyazaki, T., Asakura, A., Kobayashi, A., Takase, K., et al., 2015. Postanesthetic effects of isoflurane on behavioral phenotypes of adult male C57BL/6J mice. PLoS One 10 (3), e0122118.

Yu, Q., Li, J., Dai, C.L., Li, H., Iqbal, K., Liu, F., Gong, C.X., 2020. Anesthesia with sevoflurane or isoflurane induces severe hypoglycemia in neonatal mice. PLoS One 15 (4), e0231090.

Yu, Y., Ricciotti, E., Scalia, R., Tang, S.Y., Grant, G., Yu, Z., et al., 2012. Vascular COX-2 modulates blood pressure and thrombosis in mice. Sci. Transl. Med. 4, 132ra54.

Zambricki, E.A., Dalecy, L.G., 2004. Rat sex differences in anesthesia. Comp. Med. 54 (1), 49–53.

Zanetti, A.S., Putta, S.K., Casebolt, D.B., Louie, S.G., November 1, 2017. Pharmacokinetics and adverse effects of 3 sustained-release buprenorphine dosages in healthy guinea pigs (Cavia porcellus). J. Am. Assoc. Lab. Anim. Sci. 56 (6), 768–778.

Zarndt, B.S., Buchta, J.N., Garver, L.S., Davidson, S.A., Rowton, E.D., Despain, K.E., November 2015. Use of a far-infrared active warming device in Guinea pigs (Cavia porcellus). J. Am. Assoc. Lab. Anim. Sci. 54 (6), 779–782.

Zegre Cannon, C., Kissling, G.E., Goulding, D.R., King-Herbert, A.P., Blankenship-Paris, T., March 2011. Analgesic effects of tramadol, carprofen or multimodal analgesia in rats undergoing ventral laparotomy. Lab. Anim. (NY) 40 (3), 85–93.

Zelcer, S., Kolesnikov, Y., Kovalyshyn, I., Pasternak, D.A., Pasternak, G.W., 2005. Selective potentiation of opioid analgesia by nonsteroidal anti-inflammatory drugs. Brain Res. 1040 (1–2), 151–156.

Zeller, W., Meier, G., Burki, K., Panoussis, B., 1998. Adverse effects of tribromoethanol as used in the production of transgenic mice. Lab. Anim. 32 (4), 407–413.

Zhang, Y., Cui, B., Gong, C., Tang, Y., Zhou, J., He, Y., Liu, J., Yang, J., 2019. A rat model of nerve stimulator-guided brachial plexus blockade. Lab. Anim. 53 (2), 160–168.

Zhan, X., Fahlman, C.S., Bickler, P.E., 2006. Isoflurane neuroprotection in rat hippocampal slices decreases with aging: changes in intracellular Ca^{2+} regulation and *N*-methyl-d-asparate receptor-mediated Ca^{2+} influx. Anesthesiology 104 (5), 995–1003.

Zhang, E.Q., Knight, C.G., Pang, D.S., 2017. Heating pad performance and efficacy of 2 durations of warming after isoflurane anesthesia of sprague-dawley rats (*Rattus norvegicus*). J. Am. Assoc. Lab. Anim. Sci. 56 (6), 786–791.

Zhang, R.X., Lao, L., Wang, X., Ren, K., Berman, B.B., 2004. Electroacupuncture combined with indomethacin enhances antihyperalgesia in inflammatory rats. Pharmacol. Biochem. Behav. 78 (4), 793–797.

Zhang, Y., Eger, E.I., Dutton, R.C., Sonner, J.M., 2000. Inhaled anesthetics have hyperalgesic effects at 0.1 minimum alveolar anesthetic concentration. Anesth. Analg. 91 (2), 462–466.

Zhao, C., Wacnik, P.W., Tall, J.M., Johns, D.C., Wilcox, G.L., Meyer, R.A., Raja, S.N., 2004. Analgesic effects of a soy-containing diet in three murine bone cancer pain models. J. Pain 5 (2), 104–110.

Zhao, Y.Q., Wang, H.Y., Yin, J.B., Sun, Y., Wang, Y., Liang, J.C., Guo, X.J., Tang, K., Wang, Y.T., May 2017. The analgesic effects of celecoxib on the formalin-induced short- and long-term inflammatory pain. Pain Physician 20 (4), E575–E584.

Zhao, P., Zuo, Z., 2004. Isoflurane preconditioning induces neuroprotection that is inducible nitric oxide synthase-dependent in neonatal rats. Anesthesiology 101 (3), 695–703.

Zhu, C.B., Li, X.Y., Zhu, Y.H., Xu, S.F., 1995. Binding sites of mu receptor increased when acupuncture analgesia was enhanced by droperidol: an autoradiographic study. Zhongguo Yaoli Xuebao 16 (4), 311–314.

Zude, B.P., Jampachaisri, K., Pacharinsak, C., 2020. Use of flavored tablets of gabapentin and carprofen to attenuate postoperative hypersensitivity in an incisional pain model in rats (*Rattus norvegicus*). JAALAS 59 (2), 163–169.

Zvara, D.A., Bryant, A.J., Deal, D.D., DeMarco, M.P., Campos, K.M., Mansfield, C.M., Tytell, M., 2006. Anesthetic preconditioning with sevoflurane does not protect the spinal cord after an ischemic-reperfusion injury in the rat. Anesth. Analg. 102 (5), 1341–1347.

Further reading

Bickler, P.E., Fahlman, C.S., 2006. The inhaled anesthetic, isoflurane, enhances Ca2+-dependent survival signaling in cortical neurons and modulates MAP kinases, apoptosis proteins and transcription factors during hypoxia. Anesth. Analg. 103 (2), 419–429.

Brown, E.T., Umino, Y., Loi, T., Solessio, E., Barlow, R., 2005. Anesthesia can cause sustained hyperglycemia in C57/BL6J mice. Vis. Neurosci. 22 (5), 615–618.

Chen, N., Restivo, A., Reiss, C.S., 2002b. Selective inhibition of COX-2 is beneficial to mice infected intranasally with VSV. Prostaglandins. Other Lipid Mediat. 67 (2), 143–155.

D'Amato, F.R., 1998. Kin interaction enhances morphine analgesia in male mice. Behav. Pharmacol. 9 (4), 369–373.

Engelhard, K., Werner, C., Reeker, W., Lu, H., Mollenberg, O., Mielke, L., Kochs, E., 1999. Desflurane and isoflurane improve neurological outcome after incomplete cerebral ischaemia in rats. Br. J. Anaesth. 83 (3), 415–421.

Flecknell, P.A., 1984. The relief of pain in laboratory animals. Lab. Anim. 18 (2), 147–160.

Flecknell, P.A., 1987a. Laboratory Animal Anaesthesia. Academic Press, London, UK.

Haseneder, R., Kurz, J., Dodt, H.U., Kochs, E., Zieglgansberger, W., Scheller, M., Rammes, G., Hapfelmeier, G., 2004. Isoflurane reduces glutamatergic transmission in neurons in the spinal cord superficial dorsal horn: evidence for a presynaptic site of an analgesic action. Anesth. Analg. 98 (6), 1718–1723.

Miller, A.L., Leach, M.C., April 2015. Using the mouse grimace scale to assess pain associated with routine ear notching and the effect of analgesia in laboratory mice. Lab. Anim. 49 (2), 117–120.

Navarro, K., Jampachaisri, K., Huss, M., Pacharinsak, C., 2021b. Lipid bound extended release buprenorphine (high and low doses) and sustained release buprenorphine effectively attenuate post-operative hypersensitivity in an incisional pain model in mice (*Mus musculus*). ANEM 4 (2), 129–137.

Smith, M.A., French, A.M., 2002. Age-related differences in sensitivity to the antinociceptive effects of kappa opioids in adult male rats. Psychopharmacology (Berl.) 162 (3), 255–264.

Takahashi, K., Shigemori, S., Nosaka, S., Morikawa, S., Inubushi, T., 1997. The effects of halothane and isoflurane on the phosphoenergetic state of the liver during hemorrhagic shock in rats: an in vivo 31P nuclear magnetic resonance spectroscopic study. Anesth. Analg. 85 (2), 347–352.

Tanaka, T., Ogli, K., Komatsu, H., Nogaya, J., Yokono, S., 1993. Strain-differences of sensitivity to volatile anesthetics and their genetic character in mice. J. Anesth. 7 (1), 75–81.

Tsukamoto, A., Niino, N., Sakamoto, M., Ohtani, R., Inomata, T., 2018. The validity of anesthetic protocols for the surgical procedure of castration in rats. Exp. Anim. 67 (3), 329–336.

Vahl, T.P., Ulrich-Lai, Y.M., Ostrander, M.M., Dolgas, C.M., Elfers, E.E., Seeley, R.J., D'Alession, D.A., Herman, J.P., 2005. Comparative analysis of ACTH and corticosterone sampling methods in rats. Am. J. Physiol. Endocrinol. Metab. 289 (5), E823–E828.

Van Loveren, H., Gianotten, N., Hendriksen, C.F., Schuurman, H.J., Van der Laan, J.W., 1994. Assessment of immunotoxicity of buprenorphine. Lab. Anim. 28 (4), 355–363.

Vergari, A., Gunnella, B., Rodola, F., Frassanito, L., Musumeci, M., Palazzesi, S., Casalinuovo, I.A., 2004. A new method of orotracheal intubation in mice. Eur. Rev. Med. Pharmacol. Sci. 8 (3), 103–106.

Vergari, A., Polito, A., Musumeci, M., Palazzesi, S., Marano, G., 2003. Video-assisted orotracheal intubation in mice. Lab. Anim. 37 (3), 204–206.

Verma-Gandhu, M., Bercik, P., Motomura, Y., Verdu, E.F., Khan, W.I., Blenner-hassett, P.A., Wang, L., El-Sharkawy, R.T., Collins, S.M., 2006. CD4+ T-cell modulation of visceral nociception in mice. Gastroenterology 130 (6), 1721–1728.

Vickery, B., 1979. Prolongation of gestation in the rat and hamster by naproxen. Prostaglandins Med. 2 (5), 325–335.

Volker, D., Bate, M., Gentle, R., Garg, M., 2000. Oral buprenorphine is anti-inflammatory and modulates the pathogenesis of streptococcal cell wall polymer-induced arthritis in the Lew/SSN rat. Lab. Anim. 34 (4), 423–429.

Walker, J.S., 2003. Anti-inflammatory effects of opioids. Adv. Exp. Med. Biol. 521, 148–160.

Walker, J.S., Chandler, A.K., Wilson, J.L., Binder, W., Day, R.O., 1996. Effect of mu-opioids morphine and buprenorphine on the development of adjuvant arthritis in rats. Inflamm. Res. 45 (11), 557–563.

Ward, G.S., Johnsen, D.O., Roberts, C.R., 1974. The use of CI 744 as an anesthetic for laboratory animals. Lab. Anim. Sci. 24 (5), 732–742.

Weichbrod, R.H., Cisar, C.F., Miller, J.G., Simmonds, R.C., Alvares, A.P., Ueng, T.H., 1988. Effects of cage beddings on microsomal oxidative enzymes in rat liver. Lab. Anim. Sci. 38 (3), 296–298.

Weksler, B., Ng, B., Lenert, J., Burt, M., 1994. A simplified method for endotracheal intubation in the rat. J. Appl. Physiol. 76 (4), 1823–1825.

West, C.D., Green, C.J., 1987. The sedative effects of climazolam and climazolam with fentanyl-fluanisone in rats (*Rattus norvegicus*). Lab. Anim. 21 (2), 143–148.

West, J.P., Dykstra, L.A., Lysle, D.T., 1998. Differential tolerance to morphine's immunomodulatory effects following continuous administration. Drug Alcohol Depend. 53 (1), 31–38.

White, W.J., Field, K.J., 1987. Anesthesia and surgery of laboratory animals. Vet. Clin. North Am. Small Anim. Pract. 17 (5), 989–1017.

Wiesmann, F., Ruff, J., Hiller, K.H., Rommel, E., Haase, A., Neubauer, S., 2000. Developmental changes of cardiac function and mass assessed with MRI in neonatal, juvenile, and adult mice. Am. J. Physiol. Heart Circ. Physiol. 278 (2), H652–H657.

Williams, J.L., Baez, C., Hladky, K.J., Camacho, C.A., 2005. Effects of synthetic predator odor (TMT) on freezing, analgesia, stereotypy, and spatial memory. Psychol. Rec. 55 (1), 3–38.

Wilson, S.G., Smith, S.B., Chesler, E.J., Melton, K.A., Haas, J.J., Mitton, B., Strasburg, K., Hubert, L., Rodriguez-Zas, S.L., Mogil, J.S., 2003. The heritability of antinociception: common pharmacogenetic mediation of five neurochemically distinct analgesics. J. Pharmacol. Exp. Ther. 304 (2), 547–559.

Woolfolk, D.R., Holtzman, S.G., 1995. Rat strain differences in the potentiation of morphine-induced analgesia by stress. Pharmacol. Biochem. Behav. 51 (4), 699–703.

Yamasaki, A., Takahashi, T., Suzuki, T., Fujiwara, T., Hirakawa, M., Ohmori, E., Akagi, R., 2001. Differential effects of isoflurane and halothane on the induction of heat shock proteins. Biochem. Pharmacol. 62 (3), 375–382.

Yamasaki, K., Kuroe, K., Kamimura, R., 2003. A new method of inhalation anesthesia with nasopharyngeal insufflation in rat experiment. Exp. Anim. 52 (4), 349–351.

Yu, J., Ogawa, K., Tokinaga, Y., Iwahashi, S., Hatano, Y., 2004. The vascular relaxing effects of sevoflurane and isoflurane are more important in hypertensive than in normotensive rats. Can. J. Anaesth. 51 (10), 979–985.

Zagon, I.S., Tobias, S.W., Hytrek, S.D., McLaughlin, P.J., 1998. Opioid receptor blockade throughout prenatal life confers long-term insensitivity to morphine and alters mu opioid receptors. Pharmacol. Biochem. Behav. 59 (1), 201–207.

Zatzman, M.L., Thornhill, G.V., 1988. Effects of anesthetics on cardiovascular responses of the marmot *Marmota flaviventris*. Cryobiology 25 (3), 212–226.

Zhou, J.X., Luo, N.F., Liang, X.M., Liu, J., 2006. The efficacy and safety of intravenous emulsified isoflurane in rats. Anesth. Analg. 102 (1), 129–134.

Zuurbier, C.J., Emons, V.M., Ince, C., 2002. Hemodynamics of anesthetized ventilated mouse models: aspects of anesthetics, fluid support, and strain. Am. J. Physiol. Heart Circ. Physiol. 282 (6), H2099–H2105.

Chapter 15

Anesthesia and analgesia in rabbits

Patrick A. Lester[1,2], Tara L. Martin[1] and Daniel D. Myers[1,2]

[1]*Unit for Laboratory Animal Medicine, University of Michigan, Ann Arbor, MI, United States;* [2]*Conrad Jobst Vascular Research Laboratories, University of Michigan, Ann Arbor, MI, United States*

Chapter outline

I. Introduction

Rabbits are routinely utilized as research subjects for in vivo studies. Their popularity is a result of availability, cost, size, ease of handling, vascular access, and a variety of specific anatomical, physiological, and biochemical features. Their use requires the routine administration of pharmacologic agents for restraint, vascular access, surgery, and supportive care.

In this third edition, we have updated the previous chapter, in which we review the topic of anesthesia and analgesia as it pertains to the rabbit and current advancements in laboratory animal and veterinary anesthesia. Biomethodology, pre, intra, and postoperative considerations, and special anesthetic procedures will also be discussed. This chapter gives the reader a general overview of the subject; detailed information should be sought from the references provided. Since the science of anesthesia is constantly changing, the reader should also consult pertinent journals for "state-of-the-art" information. The tables in this chapter can be consulted for quick reference to the agents and doses used for sedation, tranquilization, anesthesia, and analgesia in rabbits.

Anesthesia and Analgesia in Laboratory Animals. https://doi.org/10.1016/B978-0-12-822215-7.00021-4

II. Preoperative considerations

A. Physical examination

The selection of the experimental subject is as important as the choice of the appropriate anesthetic agent. Rabbits may have underlying pathology due to unique phenotypes (e.g., cardiovascular pathology in the Watanabe Heritable Hyperlipidemic Rabbit or genetically modified rabbits with disease-specific phenotypes) that may increase their risk of anesthesia. Age, weight, and body condition score may also play a role during anesthesia. In addition, infectious disease processes (e.g., *Pasteurella multocida,* which has been linked historically to pneumonia in rabbits) or subclinical to clinical organ system dysfunction, including metabolic or electrolytic disturbances, can lead to anesthetic complications requiring additional management or preventative strategies. As a result, a thorough physical examination evaluating all organ systems, including temperature, should be performed prior to anesthesia or surgery. Thoracic radiography to identify latent pulmonary consolidation, interstitial edema, and abscesses is advisable in rabbits from colonies with enzootic or suspect pulmonary pathogens. Specialized studies may require additional preoperative diagnostics.

B. Labs and special diagnostics

Robust health surveillance and availability of *specific pathogen-free* (SPF) rabbits from numerous vendors have greatly diminished the incidence of *Pasteurella multocida* infections. As a result, the careful selection, purchase, and maintenance of SPF rabbits will greatly reduce the overall risks associated with using animals that are compromised by pathogens. In addition, multiple diagnostic commercial laboratories offer extensive PCR and serology-based diagnostic panels to perform individual or colony-based health surveillance. Recently immunodeficient transgenic rabbits have been created and maintained for research use (Song et al., 2017). Their unique housing requirements and susceptibility to novel pathogens such as *Pneumocystis oryctolagi* and other environmental commensals have created unique challenges in assessing anesthesia risks (Song et al., 2018, 2021). As a result, rabbits may appear clinically normal despite significant respiratory pathology, which can lead to ventilation-perfusion mismatching and gas exchange abnormalities during anesthesia. In addition to health screening, clinical chemistry panels and complete blood counts should be considered for older rabbits or those that may have underlying pathology due to their research model or phenotype. Animals with specialized anatomic, physiologic, or biochemical features may be required in studies utilizing anesthesia. These specialized characteristics may occur spontaneously or can be experimentally induced. Rabbits with these features should be evaluated preoperatively to anticipate special factors that may impact anesthesia. Clinical chemistry panels can be useful for assessing renal and hepatic function, which are necessary for drug metabolism and clearance. Electrolyte imbalances, anion gaps, or acid-base disturbances may also be detected, which, if undetected or corrected lead to cardiovascular compromise during anesthesia.

C. Fasting

As rabbits are not able to vomit, the requirement or benefit of preanesthetic fasting is not fully known at this time. Previous literature recommends that smaller rabbits <3 kg not be fasted for more than 12 h due to the risk of hypoglycemia and potential for metabolic acidosis (Bonath et al., 1982). Due to large cecum and coprophagy, presurgical fasting in rabbits may not be effective in reducing abdominal contents and may predispose to postsurgical ileus (Flecknell, 2015a).

D. Stabilization—acclimation

Breed selection is frequently mandated by the size of the desired subject, specific anatomical or physiological features, and availability. The New Zealand White and Dutch Belted rabbits remain the most frequently used breeds for research in the United States. These outbred stocks are maintained by a variety of vendors in closed colonies; genetic differences do exist in members of the same stock obtained from different vendors. The choice of sex may also be a consideration. In addition, multiple transgenic rabbit models developed via gene-targeted technology have been produced to address basic science and translational research and to foster drug development (Song et al., 2017; Xu et al., 2021). Sufficient time should be allotted when planning and scheduling experimental procedures to allow for stabilization following shipment and acclimation to a new environment. Stress from shipment and handling may result in increased levels of circulating catecholamines, which may adversely affect the anesthetic course. Ideally, rabbits should be quarantined for a minimum of 72 h, habituated to handling, and evaluated clinically before being subjected to anesthesia.

III. Anesthesia

A. Premedications

1. *Anticholinergics (parasympatholytics)*

Anticholinergic agents (e.g., atropine and glycopyrrolate) may produce pharmacologic effects such as mydriasis, prevention of bradycardia from the vagal reflex, tachycardia, reduced or thickened salivary and bronchial secretions, and reductions in gastrointestinal motility and urinary bladder/urethral tone. Due to the potential for thickened bronchial secretions, smaller rabbits when intubated should be carefully monitored for airway obstruction. Rabbits are unique in that they may demonstrate reduced effects from anticholinergics due to the presence of atropinesterase (AtrE), which degrades atropine into inactive products. The presence of AtrE is inherited and is found in varying frequencies (up to 50%) in the sera and/or tissues of some rabbits in a variety of breeds (Ecobichon and Comeau, 1974). AtrE may be present in the liver and the brain without being detectable in the sera (Margolis and Feigelson, 1963). At least three different phenotypes have been described with low, intermediate, and high levels of AtrE activity (Ecobichon and Comeau, 1974). Since the duration of action of atropine may be reduced when administered to rabbits, additional redosing as frequently as every 10–15 min may be required (Sedgwick, 1986). However, higher or more frequent dosing may lead to tachycardia and cardiac dysrhythmias. Glycopyrrolate, a quaternary ammonium with powerful antisialagogue activity and a more rapid onset than atropine, can be utilized in rabbits with AtrE. Glycopyrrolate was shown to be an effective anticholinergic agent in rabbits when administered at a dose of 0.1 mg/kg intramuscular (IM) (Olson et al., 1994). Glycopyrrolate produced a significantly elevated heart rate that lasted 60 min when administered alone to rabbits free of AtrE as determined by the in vivo screening test, while doses of atropine as high as 2 mg/kg did not. Both atropine and glycopyrrolate can be administered by the following routes of administration: subcutaneously, intramuscularly, intravenously, and intratracheally (emergency use). As anticholinergics can increase heart rate and thus myocardial oxygen demand, their use in cases of hypovolemic shock or preexisting tachycardia should be carefully evaluated.

2. Tranquilizers

Tranquilizers/sedatives are frequently used as a premedication for anesthesia or alone for noninvasive procedures such as phlebotomy. Their use may reduce the dose of primary anesthetics and counteract or offset the potential adverse effects of anesthetic agents to produce a balanced or multi-agent anesthetic approach.

a. Phenothiazines

Phenothiazine tranquilizers have been utilized alone or in combination with a variety of agents to induce a state of calmness or to reduce stress. Acepromazine has been commonly used in rabbits to provide sedation or as a surgical premedication when combined with an opioid analgesic (neuroleptanalgesia) (Lipman et al., 1990; Ludders et al., 1987). Peripheral vasodilation, a result of adrenoceptor α_1 blockade, and dose-dependent sedation make it extremely useful for phlebotomy, yet this potentially can augment hypotension during surgery. Acepromazine, when combined with diazepam, may result in reduced tear production (Ghaffari et al., 2009). It is generally used alone at doses of 0.25–0.75 mg/kg intravenous (IV) or IM and in combination with ketamine/xylazine at 1 mg/kg IM for blood collection (Ludders et al., 1987). Although the rabbit dose for acepromazine ranges from 0.75 to 10 mg/kg IM in the literature (Lipman et al., 1990; Ludders et al., 1987; Sedgwick, 1986), doses of 0.75–2 mg/kg are generally recommended and on the lower range when acepromazine is utilized in combination with other agents.

b. Benzodiazepines

The benzodiazepine tranquilizers (diazepam, midazolam, and zolazepam) have been used either alone or combined with opioids or dissociative agents to produce additional sedation, muscle relaxation, or general anesthesia (when combined with a dissociative anesthetic). Diazepam has been used at doses of 1–2 mg/kg IM or IV (Flecknell et al., 1983). Higher doses have been cited (5–10 mg/kg IM) in the literature (Green et al., 1981). When diazepam (5 mg/kg IM) is utilized with ketamine (30 mg/kg IM), the combination produces good sedation and muscle relaxation but insufficient analgesia to carry out surgical procedures (Green et al., 1981). Midazolam, which is more potent than diazepam and is water soluble (less irritating when administered parenterally and may be more compatible when mixed with other anesthetics such as ketamine), has been successfully utilized for sedation, as a premedication, and to provide sedation and muscle relaxation in combination with a dissociative anesthetic such as ketamine. In combination with ketamine and xylazine (30 mg/kg IM; 3 mg/kg IM), midazolam (0.2 mg/kg IM) provides an adequate plane of anesthesia for 30–45 min, as evaluated by reflexes and an EEG spectral response to a painful stimulus; however, cardiac depression was observed, and oxygen supplementation is recommended when using this combination (Dupras et al., 2001; Henke et al., 2005). Midazolam (1 mg/kg IM) has also been administered concurrently with fentanyl and medetomidine (0.02 mg/kg IM; 0.20 mg/kg IM); however, a surgical plane of anesthesia was not achieved in all rabbits, and the combination resulted in respiratory depression (Henke et al., 2005).

B. Analgesia

1. Opioids

Opioid analgesics mimic the response of endogenous opioid peptides such as endorphins and enkephalins to modulate inhibition of pain-modulating pathways within the brain and dorsal horn of the spinal cord. Their pharmacologic effects are due to G-protein-coupled receptor interactions, which share significant homology. Three primary opioid receptor types, mu, kappa, and delta, have been identified (Mansour et al., 1995), and research in opioid receptor knockout mice has demonstrated receptor-mediated antinociception (Gaveriaux-Ruff and Kieffer, 2002). Depending upon binding affinity, receptor selectivity, and intrinsic activity, opioids when bound to a G-protein-coupled opioid receptor activate second messenger pathways leading to hyperpolarization of neuronal cells with subsequent analgesia, sedation, and synergy with sedative anesthetics that modulate pain nociception via similar G-protein interactions (e.g., alpha-2 agonists). Opioids can be classified as agonists, partial agonists (agonist-antagonists), and antagonists. Full agonist agents such as morphine, fentanyl, or hydromorphone are best suited for treating moderate-to-severe pain with partial agonists such as butorphanol or buprenorphine used to provide analgesia for mild-to-moderate pain or where extra sedation is needed. Opioids with similar therapeutic analgesic or intrinsic activity (e.g., full agonists such as morphine or fentanyl) may differ in potency or dose and have different pharmacokinetic profiles regarding distribution, metabolism, clearance, and secretion. Due to higher clearance rates and the need for frequent administration to maintain analgesic plasma concentrations, long-acting analgesic opioid-based formulations, including those incorporating buprenorphine have been developed and evaluated for use in rabbits (Andrews et al., 2020).

The use of opioid drugs pre or intraoperatively may reduce or eliminate the need for postoperative analgesia. Experimental evidence in rodents, as well as clinical experience in humans and animals, indicates that opioids used preoperatively may block afferent impulses from arriving within the CNS, preventing sensitization to pain that may develop from CNS nociceptive stimulation (Melzack et al., 2001). Their administration has been shown to reduce postoperative pain and analgesic requirements (Melzack et al., 2001). Classically, narcotic analgesics have been employed alone for pre and intraoperative analgesia or with sedatives or tranquilizers (e.g., neuroleptanalgesia) for chemical restraint preoperatively. Buprenorphine is most commonly used for both preemptive and postoperative pain and in conjunction with sedative-hypnotic and dissociative agents (Andrews et al., 2020; Murphy et al., 2010; Shafford and Schadt, 2008). Administration of buprenorphine for analgesia has been reported to cause reduced gastrointestinal motility, food consumption, and reduced fecal output in rabbits, yet severe gastrointestinal clinical signs requiring additional treatment were not observed (Feldman et al., 2021; Martin-Flores et al., 2017). Gastrointestinal stasis or severe ileus may be due to multifactorial causes such as stress, surgery, pain, hydration status, diet, reduced fiber supplementation, and administration of pharmacologic agents, primarily anticholinergics and opioids (Bellini et al., 2018; Brandão et al., 2020; Cooper et al., 2009). As a result, the use of an opioid such as buprenorphine is not directly contraindicated and could impact animal welfare if withheld due to overt concerns of gastrointestinal stasis. In these efforts, the authors recommend considering judicious use of opioids as warranted and monitoring food consumption, fecal output, hydration status, and weight in addition to behavioral signs of pain with the provision of hay for fiber supplementation if opioids will be used. Butorphanol, an agonist-antagonist opioid with antagonist actions at the mu receptors and agonist actions at the kappa receptors, possesses minimal respiratory depressant effects and can be used for mild-to-moderate analgesia. When butorphanol is combined with alpha-2 agonists, benzodiazepines, or dissociative agents, it provides additional sedation and analgesia, thus making it a useful premedication for surgery. Due to its agonist-antagonist profile, it can be used as a partial reversal agent without completely reversing analgesia and sedation. The half-life of butorphanol in rabbits is estimated to be 1.64 h after IV administration and 3.16 h after SC administration (Portnoy and Hustead, 1992). As a result, frequent readministration is needed if used for postoperative analgesia. Fentanyl is a potent mu receptor agonist with a short duration of action and is best suited for use as a presurgical premedication or for delivery via constant rate infusion during surgery, especially in conjunction with other sedative-hypnotics such as propofol (Baumgartner et al., 2011, 2009) or alfaxalone (Arenillas and Gomez de Segura, 2018). Fentanyl can be administered transdermal via a fentanyl patch for postoperative pain. Current recommendations are to use one half of a 25 μg/h patch for 3-kg rabbit every 72 h. As the 25 μg/h patches cannot be incised to accommodate a 12.5 μg/h dose, the best practice is to cover 50% of the patch (side in contact with skin) with adhesive tape to prevent absorption or release of drug. Depending upon the cycle of hair growth, rapid hair regrowth could lead to reduced drug absorption. As a result, the use of a depilatory cream is recommended to provide a hairless surface for patch placement. However, depilatory creams can cause skin irritation and increased vascularity that may alter drug absorption. In those cases, the patch placement can be delayed up to 24 h later. Cleaning the skin with alcohol following shaving may mitigate some of the effects of hair regrowth and promote patch adherence in the interscapular area (Mirschberger et al., 2020). Weight and appetite should be carefully monitored in rabbits administered fentanyl patches (Foley et al., 2001, Table 15.1).

2. NSAIDS

Nonsteroidal antiinflammatory drugs (NSAIDs) produce antiinflammatory and analgesic effects via the inhibition of cyclooxygenase (COX), which catalyzes the production of

TABLE 15.1 Premedication and preoperative analgesia.

Drug	Rabbit	Route of administration
Phenothiazine		
Acepromazine	0.25–1	IM
Acepromazine: Butorphanol	0.5: 0.5	IM
Benzodiazepine		
Diazepam	0.5–5	IV, SQ, IM
Midazolam	0.25–2	IV, SQ, IM
Alpha$_2$-agonists		
Xylazine	1–5	IM
Medetomidine	0.1–0.5	SQ, IM
Dexmedetomidine	0.05–0.25	SQ, IM
Opioids		
Buprenorphine	0.01–0.05	IV, SQ, IM
Morphine	2–5	SQ, IM
Hydromorphone	0.05–0.1	SQ, IM
Butorphanol	0.1–0.8	SQ, IM
Anticholinergics		
Atropine	0.8–1	IV, IM
Glycopyrrolate	0.01–0.02 0.1 mg/kg	IV SQ, IM

All doses are mg/kg unless stated otherwise and ideally administered 15–30 min prior to anesthesia or surgery.
Adapted from Lester, P.A. et al., 2012. Anesthesia and Analgesia. In: Sukow, M.A., Stevens, K.A., Wilson, R.P. (Eds.), The Laboratory Rabbit, Guinea Pig, Hamster, and Other Rodents. Academic Press, pp. 33–56, Waltham, M.A., Flecknell, P.A., 2015. Laboratory Animal Aneasthesia, 4nd ed. Academic Press, London, UK.

prostaglandins, prostacyclins, and thromboxane A2 from arachidonic acid. There are two primary isoforms of COX, COX-1 and COX-2. COX-1 is a constitutive enzyme essential for maintaining physiologic functions such as a gastroprotective mucosal barrier and renal blood flow. The COX-2 enzyme is induced and responsible for producing inflammatory prostaglandin mediators associated with swelling, fever, and pain. COX-1 versus COX-2 selectivity may vary between the pharmacologic agent, species, and target tissue (Bergh and Budsberg, 2005). Due to their potential gastric-renal protective effects, COX-2 inhibitors are generally preferred over COX-1 NSAIDs. Examples of nonselective COX inhibitors include aspirin, ketoprofen, and ketorolac. Examples of drugs with COX-2-selective inhibition include carprofen, etodolac, meloxicam, and deracoxib. Few studies have been done investigating the use of these medications in rabbits, but clinical experience seems to suggest that the COX-2-selective inhibitors produce fewer side effects when administered to rabbits. For additional information, in-depth reviews of antiinflammatory drugs in veterinary medicine have been published (Monteiro and Steagall, 2019). Meloxicam loading dose of 1 mg/kg followed by 0.5 mg/kg given orally to rabbits was able to provide some degree of analgesia postovariohysterectomy, yet the authors indicated that a higher dose of meloxicam or coadministration of an opioid may be needed for optimal analgesia (Leach et al., 2009).

Meloxicam administered orally at 0.3 mg/kg or 1.5 mg/kg in conjunction with butorphanol 0.4 mg/kg IV, did not demonstrate additional reduction in isoflurane minimum alveolar concentration or isoflurane-sparing effects compared to the isoflurane-sparing effects of butorphanol (Turner et al., 2006). Carprofen (a racemic mixture), when delivered subcutaneously, demonstrated a mean bioavailability of greater than 90% for both enantiomers (Hawkins et al., 2008). In rabbits undergoing maxillofacial surgery and sinus augmentation, carprofen 5 mg/kg subcutaneously, when combined with buprenorphine did not demonstrate a reduction in postoperative facial expression scores (Hedenqvist et al., 2016). Moreover, carprofen and buprenorphine were used in combination with local anesthetics to provide optimized analgesia for stifle joint arthrotomy (Kluge et al., 2017). Based upon results from previous publications and clinical experience, the authors recommend that carprofen and other NSAIDs when used as a solo analgesic should be reserved for the treatment of mild-to-moderate pain. For procedures with anticipated moderate or greater potential for pain, carprofen should be utilized with a multi-modal analgesia approach or in conjunction with pharmacologic analgesic agents having different pharmacologic mechanisms of action, such as an opioid or local anesthetic.

3. Alpha-2 agonists

The α-2 adrenergic agonists (xylazine, dexmedetomidine, and medetomidine) can be employed alone as tranquilizers or in combination with other agents for anesthesia. The α-2 adrenergic agonists are a unique class of pharmacologic agents that possess sedative, analgesic, and muscle relaxation effects. The pharmacology and clinical utility of α-2 adrenoceptor agonists has been reviewed (Doherty, 1988; Maze and Tranquilli, 1991; Paddleford and Harvey, 1999; Valverde and Skelding, 2019; Virtanen, 1989). Dexmedetomidine (Dexdomitor) has primarily replaced medetomidine as medetomidine may no longer be commercially available in most countries. To convert previous literature doses using medetomidine to dexmedetomidine, the medetomidine dose should be reduced by 50%. Xylazine administered to rabbits at 3–9 mg/kg IV produces sedation, excellent muscle relaxation, and, at the high dose, analgesia; however, when used alone it is not sufficient to provide surgical anesthesia and is reported to cause hyperacusis (Green, 1975). Moderate depression of cardiopulmonary parameters is observed following IM administration at 5 mg/kg (Sanford and Colby, 1980). Xylazine has been used in combination with a variety of agents, including ketamine, ketamine/acepromazine, ketamine/buprenorphine, ketamine/butorphanol, ketamine/midazolam, midazolam/alfentanil, and tiletamine/zolazepam to induce and/or maintain surgical anesthesia (Borkowski et al., 1990; Difilippo et al., 2004; Dupras et al., 2001; Green, 1975; Henke et al., 2005; Lipman et al., 1990; Marini et al., 1993; Popilskis et al., 1991; Sanford and Colby, 1980; Sedgwick, 1986; Vachon et al., 1999). The α-2 antagonist yohimbine (0.2 mg/kg IV) was shown to effectively reverse the effects of anesthesia in ketamine/xylazine-anesthetized rabbits (Lipman et al., 1987), (Table 15.1).

Prior to its racemic enantiomer dexmedetomidine, medetomidine, was the most selective α-2 agonist available for use in veterinary medicine. Previous publications provide guidance regarding the use of medetomidine alone and in combination with opioids or various tranquilizers (Difilippo et al., 2004; Hedenqvist et al., 2014; Ko et al., 1992; Navarrete-Calvo et al., 2014; Santangelo et al., 2016). When coadministered with opioids, profound sedation and enhanced analgesia are common. In addition, bradycardia can be potentiated due to augmented vagal tone and G-protein receptor synergy with opioids and α-2 agonists such as xylazine and dexmedetomidine. To reduce or offset potential bradycardia, prior or concurrent administration of an anticholinergic agent can be performed. The pharmacokinetics of dexmedetomidine have been assessed in rabbits administered inhalant anesthesia demonstrating a terminal half-life of approximately 80 min (Bailey et al., 2017). The α-2 agonists, including xylazine, dexmedetomidine, and previously medetomidine, are widely used in conjunction with parenterally administered anesthetic induction agents, including common dissociative agents such as ketamine and tiletamine. Such combinations allow for enhanced sedative, analgesic, and muscle relaxation effects and will be discussed in later sections of this chapter. Regarding potential side effects, alpha-2 agonists can induce systemic vascular resistance in peripheral tissues, leading to reflex bradycardia followed by a centrally mediated decrease in cardiac output and subsequent hypotension. Moreover, xylazine has variable effects on the respiratory system, while medetomidine is associated with significant respiratory depression when used at higher doses or in conjunction with other tranquilizers, opioids, or anesthetics. As a result, oxygen should be supplemented via a facemask, nosecone, supraglottic airway device, or endotracheal tube. In addition, supportive equipment for manual or mechanical ventilation should be available to support respiratory function if needed.

4. Tramadol

Tramadol is a centrally acting synthetic analog of codeine with a weak affinity for opiate receptors that possesses selectivity for μ receptors (Dayer et al., 1994; Raffa et al., 1992). The M1 metabolite demonstrates up to 200 times higher affinity toward opioid receptors versus the parent compound, yet the affinity for both compounds is much weaker than full μ agonists such as morphine (Hennies et al., 1988). In addition to its affinity and intrinsic activity at opioid receptors, tramadol also inhibits norepinephrine and serotonin reuptake and can increase the concentrations of norepinephrine and serotonin within the central nervous system (Raffa et al., 1992). This atypical mechanism of action makes tramadol a unique analgesic as endogenous norepinephrine and serotonin are integrated into pain modulation, yet it can also increase the potential for serotonin-related side effects or serotonin syndrome. When tramadol was dosed orally at 11 mg/kg to New Zealand white rabbits, the mean half-life was determined to be 145.4 ± 81 min with no adverse effects detected (Souza et al., 2008). Moreover, the rabbit plasma concentrations within 6 h were less than therapeutic analgesic plasma concentrations for clinical doses administered to humans (Souza et al., 2008). Tramadol administered intravenously at 4.4 mg/kg over 1 min had minimal clinical effects upon the minimum alveolar concentration of isoflurane in New Zealand white rabbits, with wide ranges in plasma concentrations for both tramadol and its M1 metabolite that did not correlate with changes in minimum alveolar concentrations of isoflurane (Egger et al., 2009). Plasma levels that correlate with clinical analgesia or augment anesthetic agents in the rabbit are not known at this time. In addition, tramadol as a solo analgesic has not been found to provide clinically significant analgesia in rodents (Evangelista-Vaz et al., 2018; Wolfe et al., 2015), which may also apply to rabbits unless future research determines differently. As a result, tramadol should be used cautiously or avoided as a solo anesthetic agent in rabbits, and the dose may need to be extrapolated from clinical experience or data acquired from other species. In these efforts, the dosing interval should be reduced or modified in conjunction with pain assessment, and/or tramadol should be administered in conjunction with other analgesic agents (Souza and Cox, 2011).

5. *Local anesthetics*

Local or regional techniques may be used in combination with inhalant or injectable anesthetics to enhance analgesia for a multimodal analgesia approach. A full description of local anesthetics and regional anesthesia techniques is beyond the scope of this chapter, yet has been reviewed in recent publications regarding companion animals (Grubb and Lobprise, 2020a, 2020b). Such techniques can be extrapolated for use in rabbit anesthesia and surgery. The ability of local anesthetics to block nerve transmission via inhibition of sodium channels is dependent upon the size of the nerve, degree of myelination, and chemical properties of the local anesthetic (pKa, lipophilicity, and protein binding), with blockade of pain followed by temperature, pressure, conscious proprioception, and motor function. Lidocaine and bupivacaine can be used topically (e.g., creams, ointments, or gels for mucous membrane application), infiltrated subcutaneously at the site of surgery (Raillard et al., 2019), including delivery as a continuous infusion via an indwelling catheter, for peripheral or local nerve block (de Miguel Garcia et al., 2020; Kluge et al., 2017) (ultrasound sound guided or use of nerve stimulator to facilitate location of nerve branch) (Mencalha et al., 2016; Najman et al., 2015; Otero et al., 2012), or for epidural/spinal blockade (Antonczyk et al., 2019; Ong et al., 2020) generally in combination with a preservative-free opioid or alpha-2 agonist (Santos et al., 2021). Bupivacaine should be aspirated during infiltration to avoid administering intravenously as can be cardiotoxic at higher doses if administered in direct circulation. For spinal and epidural procedures, rabbits should receive prior sedation so that the potential for movement during administration and the risk of subsequent nerve damage is reduced.

a. Anesthetic or induction agents

For practical purposes, anesthetics used in the rabbit can be divided into the broad categories of injectable and inhalational agents. Injectable techniques have a long history of use in the rabbit. Ease of administration, predictability for short procedures, reasonable efficacy, and avoidance of the technical demands of administering inhalants are features that have popularized the use of these agents in the rabbit. At the same time, however, untoward physiologic effects, inability to control anesthetic depth, variable distribution, and clearance effects with redosing, and prolonged recovery attendant with their use have prompted the search for newer agents or novel combinations of agents. Many injectable agents and combinations produce physiologic respiratory depression or alterations in ventilation-perfusion sufficient to produce hypoxemia and should therefore be used with oxygen supplementation. The literature abounds with descriptions of the use of various injectables; some are of historical interest, others are of limited availability, and still, others have become valuable agents in the anesthetist's armamentarium.

b. Inhalants

The use of inhalants, while requiring special equipment and training, provides excellent reliability, efficacy for both short and long surgical procedures, and rapid adjustments to anesthetic depth, facilitating anesthetic induction and recovery. These features are especially important in rabbit anesthesia where many injectable combinations that are adequate for procedures involving superficial structures are inadequate for more invasive manipulations. Reduction in recovery time is an additional benefit of inhalant anesthesia. Isoflurane and sevoflurane are commonly used volatile inhalant anesthetics with low blood/gas solubility in both blood and body tissues, properties that allow for rapid dose-dependent changes in anesthetic depth with quick inductions and recovery. Both agents can cause dose-dependent vasodilation and reductions in cardiac output, leading to hypotension along with respiratory depression. An inhalant-specific calibrated vaporizer is needed to accurately and safely deliver isoflurane or sevoflurane, as each vaporizer must be calibrated to the specific vapor pressure of each anesthetic agent. In addition, desflurane, an inhalant with a very low blood/gas solubility ratio and thus associated with rapid recoveries, has been studied to provide inhalant anesthesia for rabbits, yet its use requires a specialized heated vaporizer and thus is not commonly used in the laboratory animal setting (Hedenqvist et al., 2001).

Once the rabbit is intubated, inhalants may be administered using various circuits, and rabbits may be ventilated or be allowed to breathe spontaneously. In these efforts, one may choose to administer a volume of fresh gas that is two to three times the minute respiratory volume of the animal (Flecknell, 2015b). Monitoring end-tidal carbon dioxide ($ETCO_2$) helps avoid hypercapnia and its attendant metabolic effects. The dosing of inhalant anesthesia or the inspired concentration required for sedation or surgical anesthesia is based upon each agent-specific minimum alveolar concentration (MAC), or the concentration that will inhibit gross purposeful movement in 50% of patients. MAC is a measure of potency, but not intrinsic efficacy or therapeutic effectiveness if dosed properly.

Sevoflurane is characterized by rapid induction and recovery, reduced odor aversiveness, and good acceptance by human patients where the agent is administered by using a face mask (Flecknell et al., 1999). Anesthesia maintenance with sevoflurane at 3.7% (1 MAC) has been described after buprenorphine premedication (0.05 mg/kg IV) and propofol induction (8 mg/kg IV) (Martin-Cancho et al., 2006). Sevoflurane administration to rabbits causes a dose-dependent reduction in mean arterial pressure by both a direct myocardial depressant effect and a decrease in systemic vascular resistance (Ma et al., 1998). In the clinical setting, sevoflurane maintenance after propofol induction is associated with rapid, smooth recovery (P.A. Flecknell and author's personal experience).

c. Dissociative-combinations

Ketamine is a water-soluble phencyclidine derivative that possesses anesthesia-analgesia activity due to its ability to block pain impulses to cortical-thalamic regions of the brain. It is typically administered in combination with other agents as it does not provide adequate muscle relaxation or analgesia for surgical anesthesia when used alone (Green et al., 1981). As a sole agent, ketamine should be restricted to minimally invasive procedures (e.g., subcutaneous implant, manipulation of tissues for vascular implant, or superficial wound repair). Ketamine is generally administered by IV or IM routes of injection in rabbits. Due to its low pH, pain and irritation can be observed with IM injection, leading to self-mutilation (Beyers et al., 1991; Vachon, 1999). Ketamine undergoes hepatic metabolism to norketamine with renal and biliary excretion of metabolites. Ketamine administered alone intravenously at 15 mg/kg or intramuscularly from 10 to 60 mg/kg provided inconsistent sedation with an onset of 10 min and an average duration of 30−60 min. The authors reported poor analgesia and response to noxious stimuli (Green et al., 1981). When combined with benzodiazepines such as diazepam or midazolam, additional muscle relaxation and sedation are reported, yet these combinations will not suffice for general surgery (Green et al., 1981). However, a ketamine (22 mg/kg) and alpha-2 agonist xylazine (3 mg/kg) combination administered intravenously achieved minor surgical anesthesia with a 2-min onset and an approximate 35-min duration (Green et al., 1981). These initial reports have resulted in numerous publications demonstrating the effective utility of a dissociative agent such as ketamine combined with a benzodiazepine for additional sedation and muscle relaxation or, more commonly, with an alpha-2 agonist such as xylazine, dexmedetomidine, or medetomidine (if commercially available) for additional analgesia. The dose of each agent and route of administration can be altered to enhance the degree and duration of sedation, muscle relaxation, and analgesia needed for examinations, minor procedures, or as premedications for surgical induction and inhalant anesthesia. When used as an induction agent, ketamine is commonly administered with diazepam or midazolam.

Ketamine is commonly combined with xylazine with the 35 mg/kg ketamine and 5 mg/kg xylazine dose appearing most frequently in literature. The combination at this dose provided mean withdrawal reflex loss durations of 46.5 (Hobbs et al., 1991), 32 (Marini et al., 1992), and 57 min (Lipman et al., 1990), respectively. Considerable variation in the response to ketamine/xylazine exists among rabbits (Marini et al., 1992; Peeters et al., 1988). Incremental doses of one-third of the original dose IM can be used to prolong anesthesia, yet in the authors' experience, this can lead to inconsistent anesthesia, and inhalant anesthesia is recommended for longer procedures. A myriad of physiologic effects occurs with intramuscularly administered ketamine and xylazine. Depression of respiratory rate ranging from 40% to 77% of preanesthetic baseline values has been reported (Hobbs et al., 1991; Lipman et al., 1990; Marini et al., 1992; Peeters et al., 1988; Popilskis et al., 1991; Sanford and Colby, 1980; Wyatt et al., 1989). Associated blood gas changes included hypoxemia (43%−50% reduction) and CO_2 retention (25%−50% increase) (Marini et al., 1992; Peeters et al., 1988; Popilskis et al., 1991; Wyatt et al., 1989). To offset such respiratory and ventilation variances, the authors recommend to provide supplemental oxygen via facemask, nosecone, supraglottic airway device, or endotracheal tube. Arterial blood pH either remained unchanged (Marini et al., 1992; Popilskis et al., 1991; Wyatt et al., 1989) or increased marginally due to metabolic alkalosis with partial respiratory compensation (Peeters et al., 1988). Cardiovascular changes were manifest as decreases in heart rate (from insignificant change to 35% reduction) and hypotension (20%−35% reduction). The maximal alterations produced by the ketamine and xylazine combination paralleled those seen when either drug was administered alone; ketamine preservation of heart rate was the only exception (Sanford and Colby, 1980).

Additional side effects include atropine-responsive salivation, apneustic breathing (prolonged pause following inspiration), and emergence delirium characterized by ataxia, increased motor activity, hyperreflexia, muscle rigidity, and agitation. Rough recoveries can be reduced by combining with a benzodiazepine, phenothiazine tranquilizer, opioid, or alpha-2 agonist. Ketamine has been reported to antagonize the NMDA receptor, a glutamate excitatory receptor associated with dorsal horn neuronal sensitization, hyperalgesia, allodynia, and the temporal summation (wind-up) that is often associated with chronic pain (Persson et al., 1995).

Ketamine has also been combined with the selective alpha-2 agonists medetomidine and, more recently, dexmedetomidine. Ketamine (15 mg/kg) and medetomidine (0.25 mg/kg) produced a smooth induction and can be used for minor surgical procedures up to 15–30 min in duration (Hedenqvist et al., 2001). A ketamine-medetomidine-butorphanol combination administered subcutaneously led to hypoxemia. As a result, supplemental oxygen is recommended, especially if an opioid such as butorphanol is also added to a ketamine and medetomidine combination (Hedenqvist et al., 2002). Ketamine (35 mg/kg), and xylazine (5 mg/kg), and buprenorphine (0.03 mg/kg) were compared to ketamine (35 mg/kg), and medetomidine (0.5 mg/kg), and buprenorphine (both administered IM), demonstrating no differences in heart rate, respiratory rate, or return to spontaneous breathing, yet a longer anesthetic period with the medetomidine group (Difilippo et al., 2004). Murphy et al. (2010) demonstrated that buprenorphine (0.03 mg/kg) administered subcutaneously as a premedication increased the duration of the anesthesia with few negative effects. Because of the variable health status and breed differences likely encountered in a diverse pet population, the authors recommended lower doses of medetomidine and ketamine administered subcutaneously, along with using isoflurane supplementation as needed as the regimen of choice. Ketamine (15 mg/kg) and medetomidine (0.25 mg/kg), or (0.5 mg/kg) were compared between subcutaneous and IM dosing. Both combinations produced reliable surgical anesthesia in combination with inhalant anesthesia as needed. The subcutaneous route of administration had a slower onset of action compared to the IM route, yet was better tolerated (Orr et al., 2005). In rabbits anesthetized with medetomidine (0.35 mg/kg) IV and ketamine (5 mg/kg) IV, atipamezole administered at doses equivalent to or twice that of medetomidine rapidly reversed medetomidine-associated depression of heart rate, mean arterial pressure, and respiratory rate. At a medetomidine equivalent dose, atipamezole reduced mean arousal time from 40.5 ± 15 min to 1.5 ± 1 min (Kim et al., 2004; Orr et al., 2005).

A continuous rate infusion of ketamine in combination with dexamethasone and in conjunction with topical lidocaine provided an adjustable plane of anesthesia with minimal respiratory effects for laryngotracheal surgery performed in rabbits (Sayce et al., 2020).

Telazol is a combination agent consisting of the dissociative agent, tiletamine, and the benzodiazepine, zolazepam. Administered alone, it does not provide sufficient analgesia for surgery but is useful for restraint and immobilization. The agent appears to be nephrotoxic in rabbits, as manifested by postrecovery azotemia and urinary casts (Brammer et al., 1991). The addition of xylazine (5 mg/kg IM) to telazol (15 mg/kg IM) produced surgical anesthesia lasting approximately 70 min (Popilskis et al., 1991). In contrast, Doerning et al. (1992) reported that as little as 7.5 mg/kg tiletamine was sufficient to produce mild nephrosis manifested as "scattered dilated tubules and occasional cellular casts. Azotemia did not occur at this dose. Ketamine and tiletamine-zolazepam are Schedule III controlled substances.

Acepromazine combined with ketamine and xylazine increased the duration of anesthesia (as measured by the absence of pedal reflex) when compared to ketamine and xylazine, but did so at the expense of moderate increases in the degree of hypotension and hypothermia. Reported doses include ketamine (35 mg/kg), xylazine (5 mg/kg), acepromazine (0.75 mg/kg), and ketamine (40 mg/kg), xylazine (3 mg/kg), and acepromazine (1 mg/kg) (Hobbs et al., 1991; Lipman et al., 1990; Ludders et al., 1987). The addition of butorphanol to ketamine and xylazine also increased the duration of reflex loss but with less physiologic alterations to heart rate, respiratory rate, blood pressure, and arterial blood gases than that accompanying the addition of acepromazine (Marini et al., 1992).

d. Sedative hypnotics

Sedative hypnotics such as propofol and alfaxalone are generally used as induction agents to support endotracheal intubation, or the insertion of supraglottic airway devices. Propofol is formulated as an oil-in-water emulsion and thus can support microbial growth. As a result, most commercial products are to be used as single-dose vials, yet there are commercially approved formulations labeled for 28-day storage periods once opened. Propofol and alfaxalone are associated with rapid onset of action with rapid metabolism and rapid clearance when administered intravenously. Alfaxalone is also labeled for IM administration. Neither propofol nor alfaxalone have direct analgesic properties, so their combination with an analgesic is recommended for a multimodal anesthesia approach.

6. *Propofol*

Propofol, an IV sedative-hypnotic agent, was first studied as an induction agent after medetomidine and atropine or medetomidine combined with midazolam and atropine premedication in rabbits. Rabbits were administered medetomidine (0.25 mg/kg IM) and atropine (0.5 mg/kg IM) or medetomidine (0.25 mg/kg IM), midazolam

(0.5 mg/kg IM), and atropine (0.5 mg/kg IM) 5 min prior to propofol (4 mg/kg IV for the former group; 2 mg/kg IV for the latter). Each premedication combination produced a loss of righting reflex, butpersistence of the pedal, ear pinch, palpebral, and corneal reflexes. Propofol administration caused further loss of palpebral, ear pinch, and corneal reflexes, but the pedal withdrawal reflex was preserved. The addition of midazolam prolonged the loss of the ear pinch reflex from a mean of 25–37 min. No changes were seen from the preanesthetic baseline in heart rate, respiratory rate, mean arterial pressure, or end-tidal CO_2 ($ETCO_2$). These combinations provided sufficient anesthesia to achieve ET intubation and may therefore be useful for induction or short-term anesthesia (Ko et al., 1992). Aeschbacher and Webb (1993) reported a 50% effective IV induction dose of 6.44 mg/kg. Additional studies evaluating propofol as a solo infusion agent over 8 h indicated hypotension and hypoxemia to be common sequela with supplemental oxygen recommended to improve anesthetic outcomes. Concordantly, Hellebrekers et al. (1997) reported that medetomidine premedication (0.35 mg/kg IM) followed by intravenously administered propofol (3 mg/kg) was sufficient to produce anesthesia of short duration (mean of 11 min) and depth adequate to ablate the ear pinch and pedal withdrawal reflexes. In addition to the primary IV route of administration, propofol (12.5 mg/kg) delivered via intraosseous tibial plateau administration may be used as a safe and reliable alternative method of administration in rabbits (Mazaheri-Khameneh et al., 2012).

7. Alfaxalone

Alfaxalone (Alfaxan - Jurox, Kansas City, MO) was recently reformulated and introduced into the veterinary market for use in multiple species, including rabbits. Alfaxalone is a noncumulative, short-acting neuroactive steroid that acts upon GABA receptors to produce sedative and anesthetic effects. The new formulation utilizes hydroxy-propyl β-cyclodextrin to improve solubility including IM and IV administration with minimal tissue irritation secondary to extravasation. The new formulation was evaluated for use as an IV induction agent in rabbits. Rabbits were premedicated with buprenorphine (0.03 mg/kg) and received alfaxalone intravenously over 60 s at 2 mg/kg or 3 mg/kg in rabbits. Postadministration apnea ($\sim$45 s; range = 10–120 s) was similar for both dosages, while cardiovascular parameters remained stable and within normal reported values (Grint et al., 2008). Intravenous alfaxalone (3 mg/kg) administration over 60 s results in rapid and smooth loss of unconsciousness with a mean duration of anesthesia or return of pedal withdrawal reflex of 8.9 min $\pm$ 1.9 min. In addition, there was a decrease in heart rate and respiratory rate, yet both indices remained within the normal values reported for rabbits (Gil et al., 2012). Marsh et al. (2009) evaluated the use of alfaxalone (5 mg/kg) IM in wild rabbits pretreated with medetomidine (0.25 mg/kg) subcutaneously providing a smooth induction and surgical plane of anesthesia in combination with supplemental isoflurane and oxygen. When utilized as an induction agent in rabbits presedated with fentanyl (0.0125 mg/kg) and droperidol (0.625 mg/kg) IM, alfaxalone IV administration up to 3 mg/kg was associated with apnea and hypoxemia in several rabbits, requiring supplemental oxygen and manual ventilation (Tutunaru et al., 2013). Alfaxalone (6 mg/kg) IM was evaluated as a sedative-induction agent when administered alone and in combination with either butorphanol (0.3 mg/kg), midazolam (1 mg/kg), dexmedetomidine (0.2 mg/kg), or butorphanol (0.3 mg/kg) and dexmedetomidine (0.2 mg/kg) and shown to provide effective and consistent sedation, including short-term anesthesia in rabbits (Bradley et al., 2019). Similar to previous studies, alfaxalone yielded smooth induction and recovery from sedation or anesthesia with the combination of alfaxalone, dexmedetomidine, and butorphanol, demonstrating utility for short, minor surgical procedures (e.g., subcutaneous implants, superficial wound repair, or soft tissue manipulation for vascular catheterization) (Bradley et al., 2019). Due to additive or synergistic effects when administered in conjunction with various sedative-analgesic premedications, the authors recommend pretreating rabbits with supplemental oxygen prior to induction with alfaxalone (either IV or IM) and having equipment to intubate or use a supraglottic airway device in conjunction with manual or positive pressure ventilation.

a. Barbiturate

Barbiturates such as pentobarbital are not commonly used to support anesthesia in rabbits due to their narrow therapeutic window and potential for cardiovascular compromise, as the dose at which surgical anesthesia occurs is extremely close to the dose at which apnea occurs. Anecdotally, success in the use of this agent requires considerable finesse, and its use should be scientifically aligned with the specific research model. As with other respiratory depressant anesthetic agents or combinations, supplemental oxygen and or assisted ventilation should be provided or available if needed. Dosages range from 25 to 60 mg/kg IV (Borkowski et al., 1990; Flecknell, 2018; Peeters et al., 1988). A typical schedule of administration is to inject some fraction of the calculated dose (generally one-third) over a specified time period, followed by a slow infusion of the remainder. Incremental dosages of 3–5 mg/kg IV can be used to prolong anesthesia. Continuous IV infusions of 7.5 and 20 mg/kg/h after an initial pentobarbital bolus of 50 mg/kg have also been reported (Todd et al., 1994).

b. Neuroleptanalgesic

Neuroleptanalgesic (opioid and tranquilizer) combinations containing fentanyl such as fentanyl/fluanisone (Hypnorm) have been reported for use in rabbits. Fentanyl/fluanisone is available in Europe. At the time of this publication, the fentanyl/droperidol combination (Innovar-Vet) is no longer commercially available or limited. Due to the opioid component and potential for vagal-induced bradycardia, atropine or glycopyrrolate should be considered as a premedication to avoid the bradycardia associated with the use of fentanyl or any of its congeners. Although fentanyl/fluanisone (Hypnorm) is available in Europe, it must be imported as an investigational drug in the United States. The commercial preparation contains 0.3 mg/mL fentanyl and 10 mg/mL fluanisone. At doses of 0.3–0.5 mL/kg, Hypnorm has been used for superficial surgeries and as a sedative prior to the administration of inhalational agents (Green, 1975). Respiratory depression, bradycardia, and poor muscle relaxation are characteristics of this agent. A constant-rate infusion technique has been described in which a 1:10 dilution of Hypnorm is administered intravenously at a rate of 1–3 mL/kg/h (Flecknell et al., 1983). While most reports support the advantages of the Hypnorm and benzodiazepine combinations, Peeters et al. (1998) reported that only three of six rabbits were adequately anesthetized with Hypnorm (0.5 mL/kg IM) and diazepam (2 mg/kg IM). It should be noted, however, that forelimb withdrawal was used as the criterion for anesthesia in that study instead of the more commonly used parameter of hind limb withdrawal. These responses are lost at different times in the rabbit. Another regimen using agents of the same three classes midazolam (1.0 mg/kg) IM combined with medetomidine (0.2 mg/kg IM) and fentanyl (0.02 mg/kg) IM was evaluated in cross-bred chinchilla rabbits (Henke et al., 2005). This combination produced surgical anesthesia in most rabbits (14 of 19), but was associated with apnea of short duration (30 s) in a third of animals and respiratory depression sufficient to produce mild-to-moderate hypercapnia.

c. Total intravenous anesthesia

Total intravenous anesthesia (TIVA) can be used as an alternative to inhalant anesthesia or more commonly in conjunction with inhalant anesthesia as part of a balanced anesthesia approach to minimize drug effects upon the cardiovascular and respiratory systems while maintaining surgical anesthesia. In-depth reviews of TIVA, including concepts relating to pharmacokinetics and context-sensitive half-time, have been published (Beths, 2017). Wyatt et al. evaluated a ketamine (1 mg/min) and xylazine (0.1 mg/min) intravenous infusion in New Zealand white rabbits which received ketamine (35 mg/kg) and xylazine (5 mg/kg) intramuscularly as a preanesthetic. Moderate hypotension and profound hypoxemia were initially noted after induction and both gradually improved with no significant change in respiratory rate with heart rate. Heart rate, respiratory rate, and rectal temperature remained stable throughout the study (Wyatt et al., 1989). Reichert et al. (2013) utilized an intravenous anesthesia approach for brachial plexus surgery in the rabbit. A sufentanil and midazolam continuous rate infusion was evaluated in New Zealand white rabbits premedicated with midazolam (0.1 mg/kg) subcutaneously. A mixture of sufentanil (2.5 mcg/mL) and midazolam (0.45 mg/mL) was used for induction at a rate of 0.3 mL/kg/h and adjusted for maintenance of anesthesia or suppression of pedal withdrawal reflex. Side effects included hypotension and respiratory depression, requiring mechanical ventilation (Hedenqvist et al., 2013). At this time, there is a paucity of published data regarding infusion rates and anesthetic total intravenous anesthetic protocols for use in rabbits. Additional research is needed to explore the use of various sedative-hypnotics in conjunction with opioid and tranquilizer premedication for their utility in TIVA (Table 15.2).

IV. Anesthetic circuits, monitoring and support

A. Inhalant anesthetic equipment

1. Induction via chambers and masks

Inhalational agents may be administered via chamber for induction or face mask for either induction or maintenance (Bateman et al., 2005; Betteridge, 1973; Flecknell et al., 1996, 1999; Hedenqvist et al., 2001; Kent, 1971).

However, rabbits are not as compliant with face mask or chamber induction, as induction via face mask may lead to significant adverse and physiologic effects and should be avoided unless the use of injectable premedication agents is restricted by the experimental protocol. Adverse effects include struggling severe apnea, hypercapnia, and hypoxemia when using desflurane, isoflurane, and sevoflurane (Bateman et al., 2005; Flecknell et al., 1996, 1999; Hedenqvist et al., 2001). Although sevoflurane has been reported to have reduced odor aversiveness in humans, struggling can occur with all inhalants when using a chamber induction or face mask method. Firm restraint is typically required during mask induction, which rabbits find particularly stressful (Gil et al., 2010; Keating et al., 2012). Induction chambers present a refinement over mask induction in that animals do not require manual restraint, but rabbits exhibit breath-holding and avoidance behavior during chamber induction, indicating that this method is still stressful to the animals (Flecknell et al., 1996). In addition, a large depot of WAG builds up within the chamber, potentially exposing personnel when the chamber

TABLE 15.2 Injectable anesthetic combination and constant rate infusions.

Drug or combination	Rabbit	Route of administration
Alfaxalone	2 (to effect)	IV (induction) divided doses
Fentanyl/fluanisone	0.2–0.5 mL/kg	IM
Ketamine	25–50	IM
Ketamine:Xylazine[a]	10–40:3–5	IM
Ketamine:Xylazine:Butorphanol	35:5:0.1	IM
Ketamine:Diazepam[a]	4–10:0.25–5 20–40:1–5	IV IM
Ketamine:Acepromazine[a]	25–50: 0.25–1	IM
Ketamine:Medetomidine[a]	15–25:0.25–0.5	SQ, IM
Ketamine:Dexmedetomidine[a]	15: 0.125	SQ, IM
Pentobarbital	30–45	IV
Propofol bolus (induction)	3–10 (to effect)	IV (induction) divided doses
Constant rate infusions (IV)		
Ketamine: Fentanyl	5–20 μg/kg/h: 0.3–0.4 mg/kg/h	IV
Propofol (surgical maintenance)	0.2–0.6 mg/kg/min	IV

All doses are mg/kg unless stated otherwise and administered immediately prior to anesthesia or surgery.
[a]*Only redose during surgery with ketamine component at 1/3 the original dose.*
Adapted from Lester, P.A. et al., 2012. Anesthesia and Analgesia. In: Sukow, M.A., Stevens, K.A., Wilson, R.P. (Eds.), The Laboratory Rabbit, Guinea Pig, Hamster, and Other Rodents. Academic Press, pp. 33–56, Waltham, M.A., Flecknell, P.A., 2015. Laboratory Animal Aneasthesia, 4nd ed. Academic Press, London, UK.

is opened. If chambers must be used, they should be well sealed and sized just large enough to allow the animal to comfortably sit in a natural position. While maintaining gas anesthesia by the mask is not fraught with the same issues as induction, the increased risk of operator exposure to WAG, the inability to administer controlled or assisted ventilation, the possibility of airway obstruction and the considerable dead space provided by the mask must all be considered (Bateman et al., 2005). Rabbits should be premedicated with sedatives if a mask or chamber induction is used. Modified cat restraint bags have been used to mask induce previously sedated animals (Lindquist, 1972).

2. Anesthetic circuits

Various circuits may be used to deliver inhalant anesthetics, and animals may be ventilated or allowed to breathe spontaneously. The Rees-modified T-piece and Bain circuits are traditionally considered most appropriate for animals within the weight range of most rabbits; Magill and circle circuits have also been used (Peeters et al., 1988; Nelson et al., 1990). Fresh gas flows for maintenance of spontaneously breathing animals are typically set to 1–3 L/min (Kent, 1971; Kumar et al., 1993; Peeters et al., 1988), or they may be set to a volume that is two to three times the animal's minute respiratory volume (Flecknell, 2015b). The following equation can be used to calculate minute volume, using an estimated tidal volume of 4–6 mL/kg (Nowland et al., 2015):

$$\text{Tidal Volume} \times \text{Respiratory rate} = \text{Minute Volume}$$

For example, a 2-kg rabbit breathing at 30 times/min would be expected to have a respiratory minute volume of 0.24–0.36 L. Note that rabbits have a relatively low tidal volume when compared to companion animals, and methods should be employed to avoid barotrauma such as pressure release valves; the oxygen flush valve should not be used when the patient is attached to the circuit (Reuter et al., 2005). Rebreathing is likely to occur for small veterinary patients if a fresh gas flow of 500 mL/min is used with a coaxial circuit, such as the Bain circuit. Monitoring ETCO2 helps avoid hypercapnia and its attendant metabolic effects, though some capnometers may be less accurate in rabbits due to the high flow rates used in rabbits and their low tidal volume (Duke-Novakovski et al., 2020).

3. Intubation or supraglottic airway devices

Endotracheal intubation is notably challenging in the rabbit. The anatomy of the rabbit's oropharynx makes the epiglottis and larynx difficult to visualize because of the large incisors, the long and narrow oral cavity, a thick tongue, and the limited mobility of the temporomandibular joint (Fig. 15.1). Laryngospasm is also induced easily (Wixson, 1994). The epiglottis is large, U-shaped, soft, and flexible. Just beyond the base of the epiglottis is a deep sagittal niche, bordered on both sagittal recesses by the hamuli epiglottici (Fig 15.2). This structure lifts the local epithelial layer and can be damaged easily by rough or incorrect ET intubation (Schuyt and Leene, 1978). The diameter of the aditus laryngicus is smaller than the diameter of the tracheal lumen and dictates the size of the ET tube (Fig. 15.3) (Schuyt et al., 1978). The vocal cords are situated extremely craniad and run obliquely in a dorsal-ventral direction (Schuyt and Leene, 1978). This means rabbits are easily injured during intubation, and prolonged or repeated attempts can cause hypoxemia during the perioperative period (Fusco et al., 2021; Reuter et al., 2005).

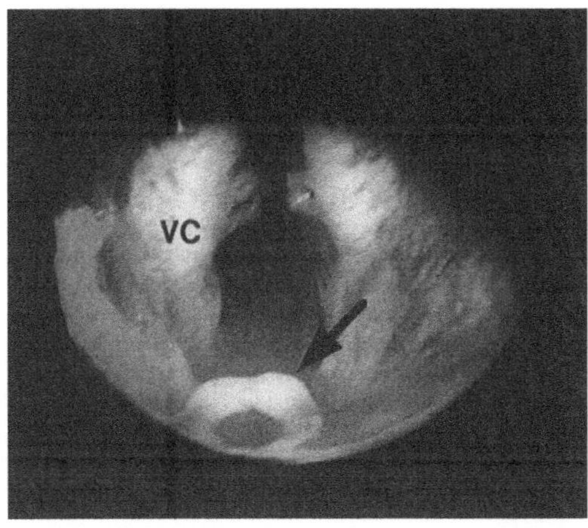

FIGURE 15.2 View of laryngeal structures in an anesthetized rabbit utilizing a 3.5 mm fiberoptic bronchoscope. The tip of the bronchoscope is depressing the epiglottis. The hamuli epiglotticiare visible (arrow) as are the vocal cords (VC).

There are numerous descriptions of techniques and devices which are useful in ET tube placement (Alexander and Clark, 1980; Bertolet and Hughes, 1980; N. L. Davis and Malinin, 1974; Fick and Schalm, 1987; Gografe et al., 2003; Kumar et al., 1993; Lindquist, 1972; Macrae and Guerreiro, 1989; Schuyt and Leene, 1978; Schuyt et al., 1978; Smith et al., 2004; Tran et al., 2001; Worthley et al., 2000). ET intubation can be performed with or without direct visualization of the larynx in the prone or supine position. For successful intubation, the mouth, larynx, and trachea must be brought into linear alignment (Fig. 15.4). Both upright (Alexander and Clark, 1980) and supine (Schuyt and Leene, 1978; Davis and Malinin, 1974) positions are described in the literature. Uncuffed (Cole or straight) or cuffed ET tubes (2.0–4.0 mm diameter) are used with or without an intubation stylet (Fig. 15.5). Intubation may be easier with cuffed tubes, likely because they are more rigid and less prone to bending on insertion (Lee et al., 2019; Smith et al., 2004). Wire-reinforced ET tubes should be used for procedures where kinking the tube is possible, such as stereotaxic surgery.

A pediatric laryngoscope (size 0–1 Wisconsin, size 0–1 Miller, neonatal, or size 1) may be used, depending on the size of the rabbit (Lindquist, 1972; Macrae and Guerreiro, 1989; Thompson et al., 2017). A handheld otoscope with a 5 mm ear speculum can be used to visualize the larynx and intubate small (~1.3 kg) rabbits (Weinstein et al., 2000). Video otoscopes can be used to more easily visualize the larynx, and at least one product is commercially marketed for this purpose (veterinary video otoscope system, VetOvation, Raleigh, NC). The larynx may be sprayed with a topical anesthetic (without epinephrine) and/or anesthetic lubricant applied to the tube to reduce

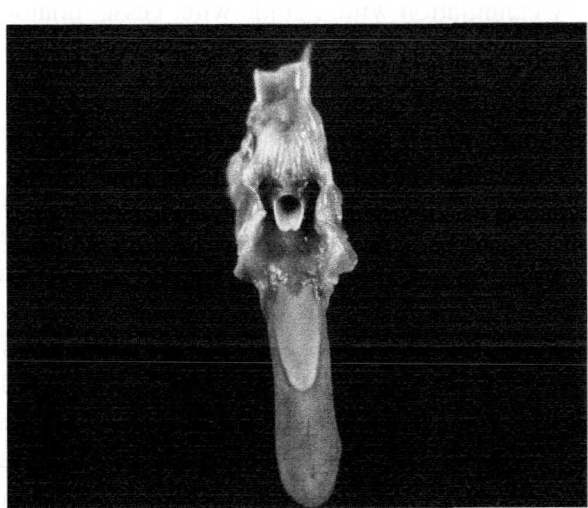

FIGURE 15.1 Dorsal view of the tongue, larynx, and proximal trachea from an adult New Zealand white rabbit. Note the long tongue and notched U-shaped epiglottis.

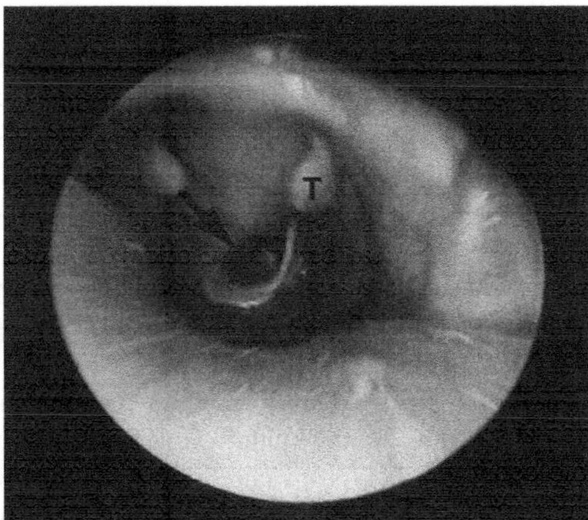

FIGURE 15.3 View of the oropharynx and larynx in an anesthetized rabbit utilizing a 3.5 mm fiberoptic bronchoscope. The laryngoscope blade is visible in the foreground. Note the tonsils (T) and the aditus laryngicus (arrow).

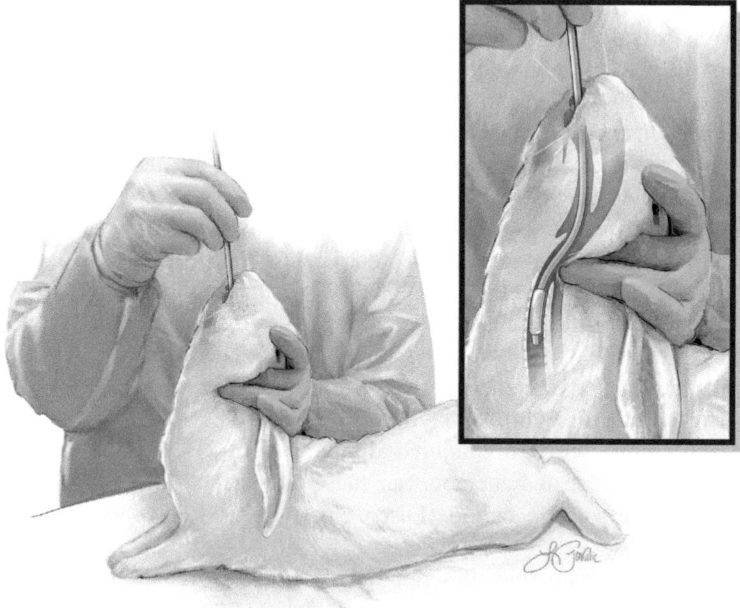

FIGURE 15.4 Endotracheal intubation of rabbit performed without direct visualization of the larynx. For successful intubation, the mouth, larynx, and trachea must be brought into linear alignment to permit passage of endotracheal tube.

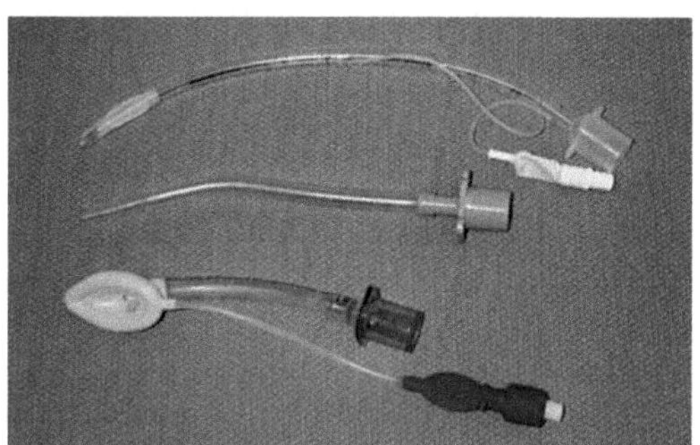

FIGURE 15.5 Devices used to deliver inhalational anesthetics to rabbits. From top to bottom: cuffed endotracheal tube (Murphy eye type), uncuffed endotracheal tube (Cole type), and laryngeal mask airway.

laryngeal irritability. Extreme caution should be used when spraying the larynx with any of the topical anesthetics, as overdosage is possible. Benzocaine-topical anesthetic spray has been shown to cause methemoglobinemia in rabbits following a second application, which may confound experimental results (Davis et al., 1993). Following visualization of the larynx, the tube is inserted gently on inspiration so that it passes through the aditus laryngicus when the vocal cords are abducted. If placement of the ET tube in the supraglottic region severely limits vision, the ET tube can be placed over a 0.97 mm flexible guidewire or a 5 or 6-Fr nylon IV or polypropylene urinary catheter (Gografe et al., 2003; Macrae and Guerreiro, 1989; Thompson et al., 2017; Weinstein et al., 2000). The guide wire or catheter can be advanced into the larynx under direct visualization before advancing the tube over the device. Thompson et al. (2017) have published step-by-step visual and video instructions to facilitate training in this process. Intubation can also be aided using a rigid 30 degree endoscope passed through a 4.5 mm ET tube (Tran et al., 2001). This method allows direct visualization as the tube is advanced. Similarly, (Worthley et al., 2000) used a 10 mm fiberoptic to visualize the larynx before passing an ET tube. Intubation has also been accomplished by inserting a 19 gauge, 20 cm catheter percutaneously through a guide needle into the trachea of an anesthetized rabbit, advancing the catheter retrograde through the larynx into the mouth, and finally, advancing the ET tube over the catheter, which serves as a guide (Bertolet and Hughes, 1980). Alternatively, a needle cricothyroidotomy can be performed, followed by cannulation with a guide wire, vessel dilator, and sheath introducer with side port extension (Irazuzta et al., 1997).

When intubation is performed blindly, the tube is placed in the supraglottic region and inserted into the larynx during inspiration, with the operator observing the respiratory pattern and rate or tube condensation or listening for breath sounds with or without a respiratory monitor to coordinate the advancement (Howard et al., 1990). Capnography can also be used to guide blind intubation, with mainstream capnography promoting faster intubation versus sidestream (Lee et al., 2019). Proper placement of the tube can be verified, as in other species, by palpation of the trachea and esophagus, listening for respiratory sounds, or observing air flow at the distal end of the tube by looking for displacement of plucked fur or condensation on a dental mirror.

ET tubes should be fixed in place with gauze or tape to avoid accidental extubation and should be routinely suctioned during procedures of modest or prolonged duration, as respiratory secretions may occlude the lumen. Tracheal mucosal injury may be a sequela to intubation in the rabbit (Grint et al., 2006; Nordin and Lindholm, 1977; Phaneuf et al., 2006). The pressure of the inflated cuff against the epithelium has been reported to interfere with blood flow and possibly cause necrosis (Nordin et al., 1977). Repeated intubation appears to be associated with a higher rate of injury when using both cuffed and uncuffed tubes (Phaneuf et al., 2006). Postintubation tracheal strictures have been described in rabbits 2–3 weeks after anesthesia (Grint et al., 2006). Although the definitive cause of the tracheal injury was unconfirmed, the location of the injury (adjacent to the tube's bevel) led the authors to speculate that the cause was either trauma or chemical injury from agents used to disinfect the ET tubes.

Because of the difficulties with intubation, alternatives to ET tube placement have been sought. Tracheostomies may be appropriate for nonsurvival surgical preparations requiring tracheal access. Administration of inhalational agents by mask has been described for both induction and/or maintenance of anesthesia, as previously discussed (Bateman et al., 2005; Betteridge, 1973; Flecknell et al., 1996, 1999; Hedenqvist et al., 2001; Kent, 1971). Laryngeal mask airway (LMA) devices are a type of supraglottic airway device (SGAD) developed for use in humans. Use in rabbits has been described in lieu of ET tube placement (Bateman et al., 2005; Smith et al., 2004). An LMA consists of an airway tube, a mask with an inflatable cuff, and a mask-inflation line (Fig. 15.5). The mask is designed to sit over and surround the larynx (Fig. 15.6). Smith et al. (2004) described placing an LMA with the rabbit in right lateral recumbency and the animal's head and neck tilted upward at a 90 degrees angle. The device is inserted with its aperture turned toward the tongue and its convex side against the left buccal wall blindly until it reaches the desired position. The device is then rotated 90 degrees counterclockwise so that the margins of the LMA's cuff cover the edges of the laryngeal aperture, and the cuff is inflated to reduce WAG escape and allow for positive pressure ventilation. LMAs are reportedly easier to place than ET tubes, but they have been associated with higher WAG emission, gastric tympany in ventilated animals, lingual cyanosis, and an incomplete airway seal (Bateman et al., 2005; Engbers et al., 2017). Imai et al. (2005) developed a device with features similar to an LMA, consisting of a spiral wire-containing tube, a mask designed to surround and seal the larynx, and an inflatable balloon designed to lie in the proximal esophagus. The device is inserted blindly, with the rabbit positioned in lateral recumbency with its neck in ventroflexion; the device allows for intermittent positive pressure ventilation (IPPV).

The V-gel (V-gel, Docsinnovent Ltd., Hemel Hempstead, UK) is a SGAD designed for use in rabbits (Fig 15.7). V-gels are cuffless with an extended, soft tip meant to sit in the esophagus, thus sealing the airway. However, imaging studies show that the tip does not always reach or remain within the esophagus, likely due to movement or improper placement of the V-gel (Engbers et al., 2017; Wenger et al., 2017). V-gel size is chosen based on the weight of the animal, and, when between sizes, the manufacturer recommends choosing the larger size, but Wenger et al. (2017) found that the recommended sizes may be too large to easily place in New Zealand white rabbits that weigh more than 5 kg. For placement, the V-gel is lubricated, and the animal is placed in sternal recumbency. The V-gel is inserted into the oropharynx and advanced until resistance is encountered or the device is within 1–2 cm of the fixation tabs (Engbers et al., 2017). V-gels are easier to place than human LMAs or ET

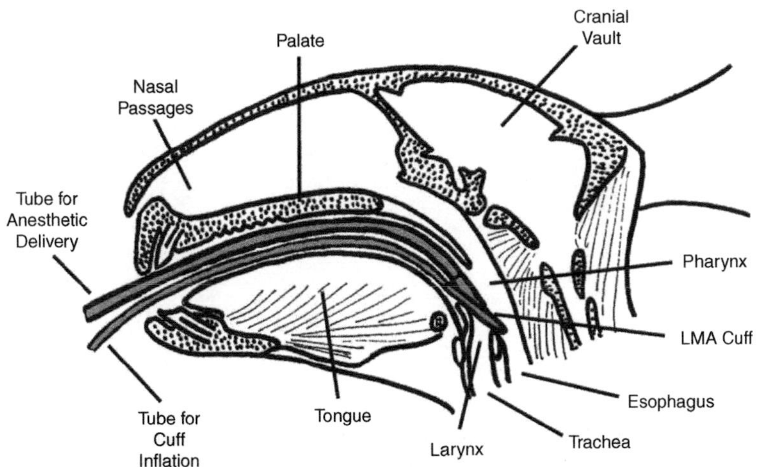

FIGURE 15.6 Diagram showing proper placement of a laryngeal mask airway with respect to the oropharyngeal cavity and upper airway of the rabbit.

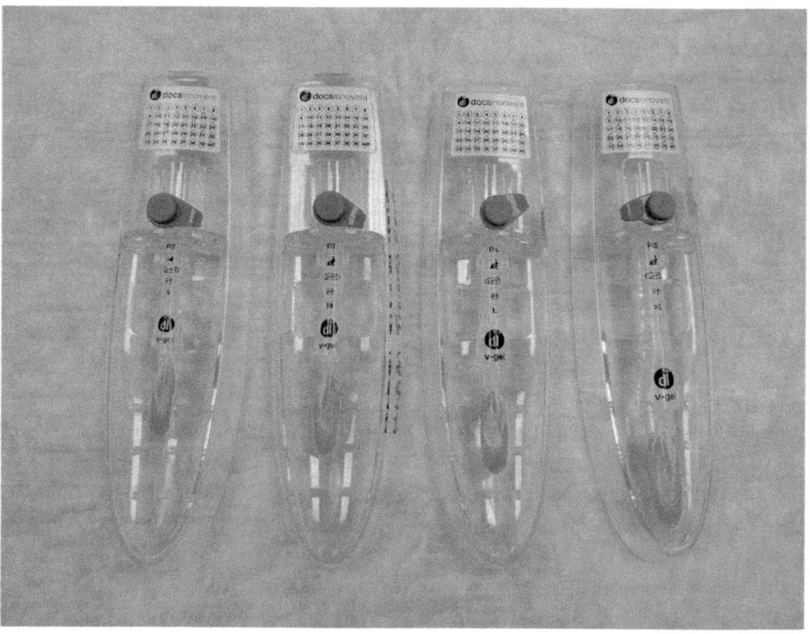

FIGURE 15.7 Photo demonstrating various sizes of supraglottic airway devices developed for use in rabbits.

tubes—even by inexperienced staff and may be associated with less sympathetic stimulation, fewer hemodynamic alterations, and fewer adverse effects (Comolli et al., 2020; Engbers et al., 2017; Raillard et al., 2019; Toman et al., 2015; Uzun et al., 2015; Wenger et al., 2017). However, placement may be more difficult in large rabbits (>5 kg) when using large-sized V-gels (Wenger et al., 2017) and V-gels may easily become displaced during long anesthetic events or if the patient is moved (Comolli et al., 2020). Capnography is highly recommended both to confirm appropriate placement and to ensure the V-gel remains in place for the entirety of the procedure because, in the authors experience, it is difficult to tell visually whether a V-gel has been displaced, and other methods of monitoring correct placement such as the development of a blue tint to the lips are likely associated with sequelae such as hypoxemia. Should the capnograph indicate obstruction, the V-gel can be slowly advanced or retracted to see if appropriate placement can be achieved. The manufacturer sells a specialized stand that can help prevent displacement (Fig. 15.8), though even with this in place, the V-gel should be detached from the anesthetic circuit prior to moving the animal and capnography should be used. A study by Engbers et al. (2017) indicated that V-gels were associated with less damage to the tracheal mucosa than blindly placed ET tubes. However, these and other authors also report a risk of hypercapnia when using V-gels, which may be addressed through IPPV (Comolli et al., 2020). Transient lingual cyanosis that resolves upon removal, laryngeal compression leading to airway obstruction, and gas leakage during mechanical ventilation have also been reported with V-gels (Wenger et al., 2017). The manufacturer of V-gels has recently released a new model that is softer and supposedly has an improved seal (V-gel ADVANCED, Docsinnovent Ltd., Hemel Hempstead, UK), but this device is intended for single use, and at the time of writing, no data has been published verifying these claims.

Fusco et al. developed two techniques for using the V-gel to guide ET tube placement (Fusco et al., 2021). These have the advantage of the easy placement associated with V-gels, the superior security and airway control associated with ET tubes, and the ability to continuously supplement oxygen during the intubation process. In the first method, which requires two people to perform, after correct V-gel placement is confirmed by capnography, a

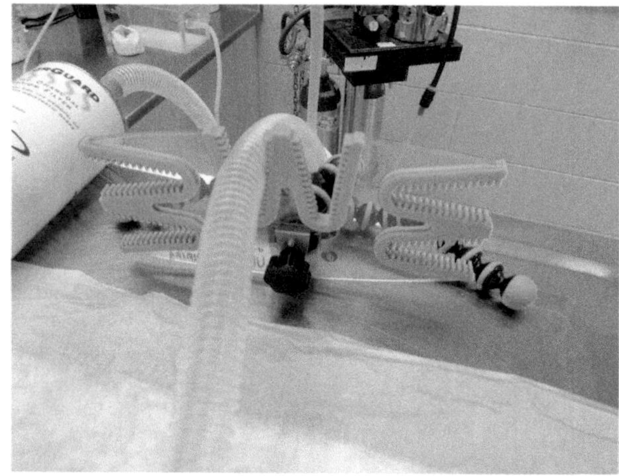

FIGURE 15.8 Specialized holding device or stand used in conjunction with a supraglottic airway device to prevent displacement during anesthesia.

polypropylene catheter is inserted through the V-gel lumen to act as a stylet. The V-gel is removed and a cuffed ET tube is threaded over the catheter and placed into the trachea, at which time the catheter is removed. In the second method, an uncuffed ET tube is inserted through the lumen of the V-gel prior to placement and both devices are inserted together and left in place for the duration of the anesthetic event. The authors were able to intubate rabbits in fewer attempts using this technique versus blind intubation, though the second method led to more leakage and contained more dead space than a V-gel alone.

4. Ventilators—general recommendations

A thorough review of mechanical ventilation is beyond the scope of this chapter. Mechanical ventilation has been reviewed for companion animal species, and many of the same principles can be applied to rabbit anesthesia (Hopper and Powell, 2013). In the author's experience, pressure control ventilators that allow for adjustments to minute ventilation, inspiratory pressure, and peak end-expiratory pressure in smaller animals to optimize oxygen hemoglobin saturation and maintain partial pressure of carbon dioxide a within normal physiologic range are recommended.

B. Anesthetic monitoring

The goal of monitoring should be to maintain normal cardiac function, respiratory function, and body temperature. Understanding the basic physiologic effects of the anesthetics used is paramount to correctly interpreting monitoring parameters. Reflexes or responses to surgical stimuli, body temperature, and the cardiopulmonary system should be thoroughly evaluated when monitoring animals under anesthesia.

Monitoring includes routine evaluation of anesthetic depth and physiologic functions and conditions, such as body temperature, cardiac and respiratory rates and patterns (Flegal et al., 2009a, 2009b, 2009c), and blood pressure (Fox et al., 2008), and should be appropriately documented. As breath holding and apnea can happen unexpectedly, close monitoring by a separate and dedicated anesthetist is recommended. ET CO2 can be monitored using a capnograph, which gives useful information about the patient's ventilatory status. Pulse oximeters can be used to monitor the hemoglobin oxygen saturation levels (SPO2), which correlates well with arterial oxygen levels (PaO2) but does not provide information on blood flow or tissue oxygenation. Arterial blood gas analysis can further improve a patient's monitoring by allowing evaluation of acid-base status, electrolytes, ventilation, and oxygenation if performed at protocol-specified intervals (Flegal et al., 2009b, 2009c).

The use of balanced anesthesia, including the addition of an intraoperative analgesic agent, can help minimize physiologic fluctuations during surgery. Maintenance of normal body temperature minimizes cardiovascular and respiratory disturbances caused by anesthetic agents (Dardai and Heavner, 1987; Fox et al., 2008) and is of particular importance in small animals, where the high ratio of surface area to body weight may easily lead to hypothermia. Fluid replacement may be a necessary component of intraoperative therapy depending on the duration and nature of the procedure.

1. Catheter placement and fluid support

Intravenous catheters may be placed at a variety of sites in the rabbit, including the cephalic, lateral saphenous, and marginal ear (caudal auricular) veins. The marginal ear vein is easy to access (Fig. 15.9) and it is relatively simple to restrain rabbits for catheterization of this vessel because no extension of the limbs is necessary. To catheterize the marginal ear vein, the rabbit should be restrained in sternal recumbency in a comfortable position. A cat restraint bag or towel may be used if necessary. Fur is first shaved or plucked from the ear, and the skin is aseptically prepared. Once dry, EMLA cream may be placed on the skin and the rabbit allowed to rest for approximately 20 min to reduce pain associated with catheterization (Keating et al., 2012). To place the catheter, the ear is gently extended, as shown in Fig. 15.10). A 23- to 25-gauge catheter may be inserted,

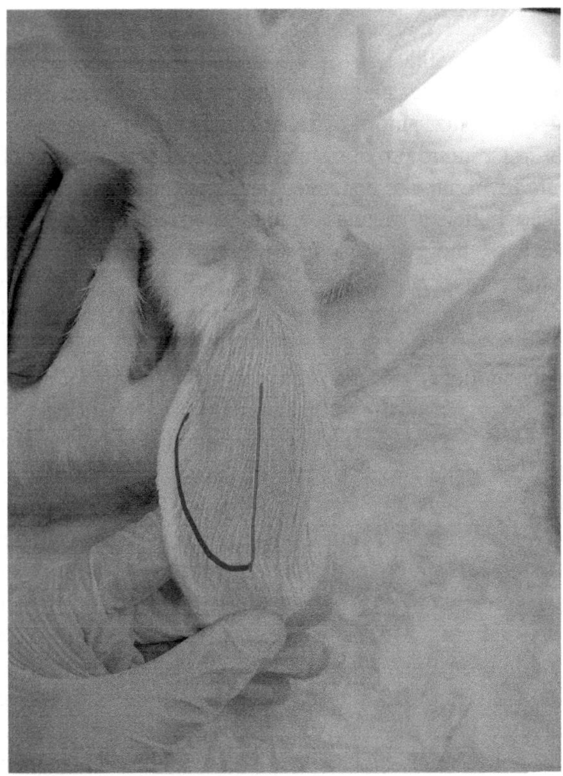

FIGURE 15.9 Photo demonstrating location of lateral marginal ear vein (purple) and central auricular artery (red).

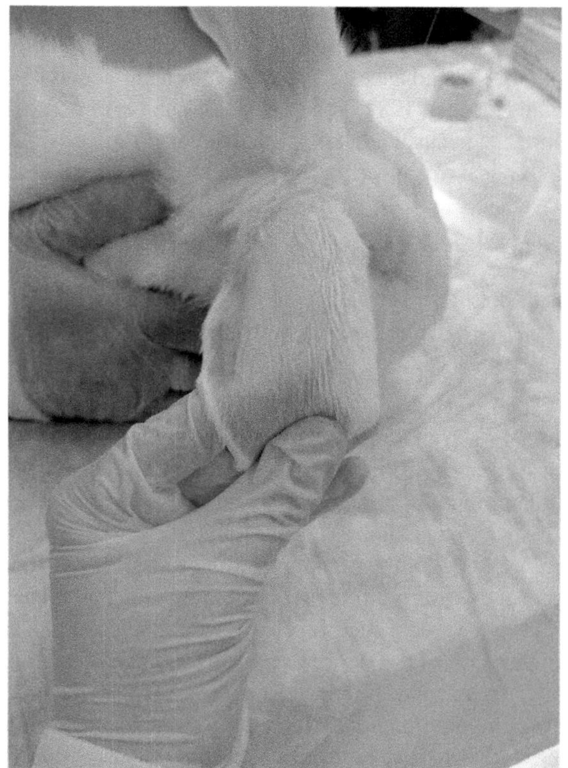

FIGURE 15.10 Photo demonstrating position of ear for catheterization of the lateral marginal ear vein. The ear is gently extended for placement of a catheter.

depending on the size of the animal (Pekow, 2012). To secure the catheter, the authors find it helpful to roll a stack of 4 × 4" gauze into a cylinder and place this into the ear prior to taping to provide stability. The catheter can then be secured with tape or bandage material as the user prefers. If using a butterfly catheter, the wings may be glued to the surface of the pinna (Pekow, 2012; Varga, 2014); this method is especially helpful when rapid access is necessary, such as in emergency situations. Care should be taken to appropriately maintain ear vein catheters, and noxious substances should not be injected via this route due to the risk of pinna necrosis. In the authors' experience, pinna necrosis following ear vein catheterization or blood collection is rare in New Zealand white rabbits, but this risk may be elevated in breeds with small ears (Brandão et al., 2020).

The cephalic vein in rabbits is often used for catheterization in pet rabbits. The area must be shaved carefully and many animals require sedation prior to catheter placement at this site (Brandão et al., 2020; Varga, 2014). When restraining for this procedure, the rabbit should be allowed to lie in a comfortable upright position. A 22- to 26-gauge catheter is inserted, depending on the size of the animal.

Rabbits are at high risk of hypotension during anesthesia (Hawkins and Pascoe, 2021). To treat or prevent hypotension, balanced electrolyte solutions may be administered at 10 mL/kg/h intraoperatively, though rabbits tolerate up to 50–70 mL/kg/day well in the absence of cardiac disease (Bennett, 2020; Brandão et al., 2020). Bolus doses of 10–20 mL/kg of crystalloid fluids may be administered to treat intraoperative hypotension (Hawkins and Pascoe, 2021). Colloid fluids may also be given as a 2–5 mL/kg bolus, as these are better retained within the vasculature, though there may be a risk of renal damage when using these products (Hawkins and Pascoe, 2021). For hypotension that is not resolved after decreasing the anesthetic dose and providing fluid therapy, positive inotropes such as norepinephrine may be necessary (Hawkins and Pascoe, 2021).

2. *Heat support or heated ventilator circuits*

Rabbits as well as other small mammals, due to their small body mass and high body surface-to-volume ratios, are highly susceptible to heat loss leading to hypothermia (Hawkins and Pascoe, 2021). Hypothermia is one of the most common causes of mortality during anesthesia in small mammals, along with respiratory compromise (Sikoski et al., 2007). All anesthetics affect thermoregulation, thus procedurally induced hypothermia has many untoward effects, including prolonged recovery times, altered hemostatic functions, and death (Shimokawa et al., 2003).

The use of external heating devices is necessary for the maintenance of normal body temperature in rabbits under general anesthesia. Specifically, forced-air warming devices and circulating warm-water blankets have been proven effective (Sikoski et al., 2007). Newer devices like the DarvallVet temperature-controlled breathing heated breathing circuits have been shown to protect against hypothermia, thus aiding in patient recovery (Website, 2021) (Figs. 15.11 and 15.12).

3. *Anesthetic depth and visual monitoring*

Traditional reflexes used in the monitoring of rabbit anesthesia include righting, palpebral, corneal, pedal withdrawal, and pinna reflexes. It is widely held that the pinna reflex (ear movement in response to a compressive force) is the most accurate measure of the depth of anesthesia, followed by the pedal withdrawal, corneal, and palpebral reflexes, in that order (Borkowski et al., 1990). The corneal reflex may be preserved until very deep levels of anesthesia are achieved. Care should be exercised, however, as the presence or absence of these reflexes may vary depending on the anesthetics used. Imai et al. determined that eyelid aperture increases with increasing anesthetic dose (0.8, 1.0, 1.5, and 2.0 MAC) for both isoflurane and halothane anesthesia in the rabbit (Imai et al., 1999). Muscle tone, jaw tone, vocalization, and gross purposeful movement in response to surgical stimulus are also indices of anesthetic depth.

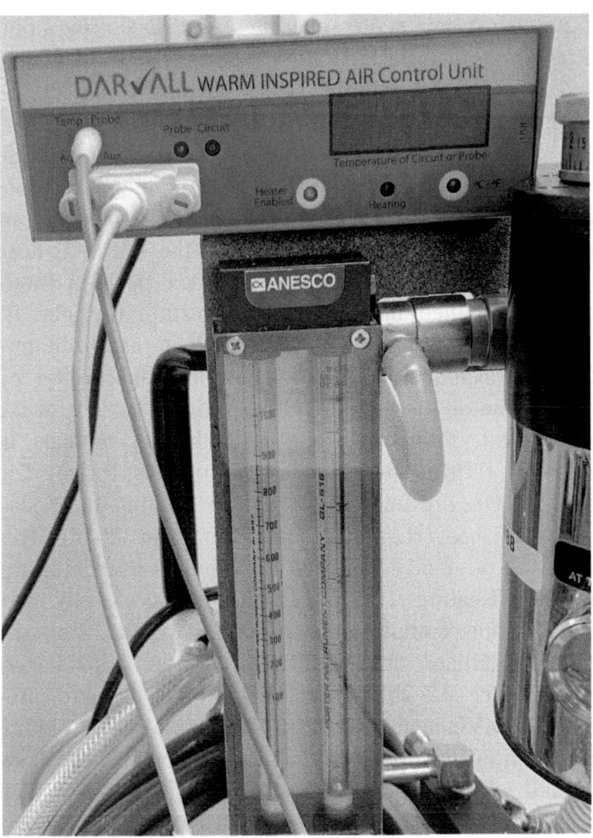

FIGURE 15.11 Photo demonstrating a temperature-controlled heated breathing circuit control system that can be used during anesthesia to prevent hypothermia.

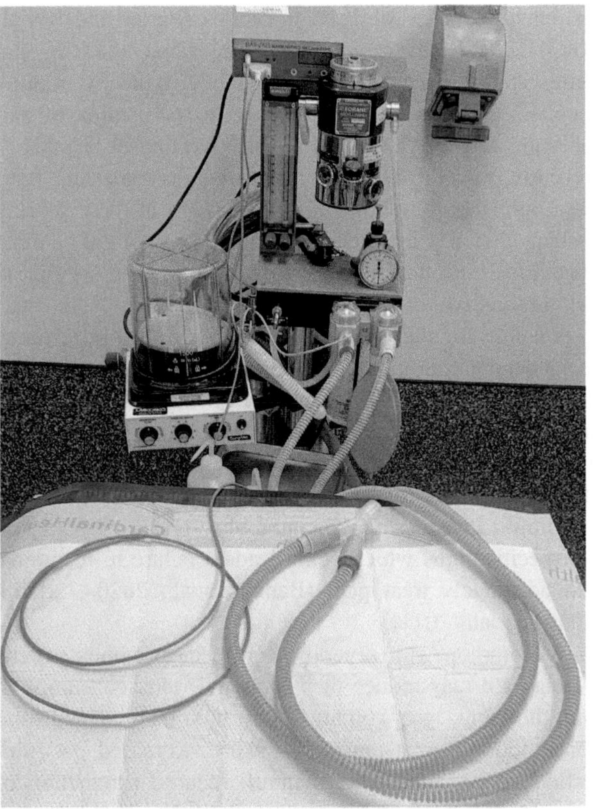

FIGURE 15.12 Photo demonstrating a temperature-controlled heated breathing circuit control system that can be used during anesthesia to prevent hypothermia.

4. *Anesthetic record keeping and regulations*

Documentation of patient monitoring is recommended throughout the anesthetic procedure at a minimum of every 15 min. The periodic evaluations of the patient's body temperature, pulse, respiration, blood pressure, and color of membranes pale or blue membranes, which are indicative of decreased blood volume, decreased perfusion, or respiratory distress) can effectively help you assess the status of your patient. Therefore, anesthetic record keeping also allows you to document and or go back and review to troubleshoot past anesthetic events for future corrective measures.

The Occupational Safety and Health Act requires employers to comply with hazard-specific safety and health standards and provide employees with a work environment free of hazards that can potentially cause death or serious physical harm (Occupational Safety & Health Administration [OSHA], 2022). OSHA has guidelines regarding anesthetic gases and workplace exposures, they are intended to assist employers with providing a hazard-free work environment. The National Institute for Occupational Safety and Health (NIOSH) currently recommends that no one be exposed at ceiling concentrations >2 ppm to any halogenated anesthetic (sampling period not to exceed 1 h). The American Conference of Governmental Industrial Hygienists (ACGIH) threshold limit value–time-weighted averages (TLV-TWA) for halothane and enflurane for a normal 8-h workday are 50 and 75 ppm, respectively. It is important to note that these are guidelines and not standards or regulations.

V. Postoperative analgesia

A. Pain assessment, monitoring, and record keeping

Effective pain control is essential to animal care—both for ethical reasons and because uncontrolled pain is a recognized experimental variable (Members et al., 2007). Pain cannot be effectively treated unless it is accurately recognized, which is difficult in rabbits because they tend to "freeze" or remain immobile when under stress (Paul-Murphy and Ramer, 1998; Leach et al., 2009). While tests relying on evoked stimuli such as thermal threshold testing have been validated in rabbits (Barter and Kwiatkowski, 2013), these are less useful when assessing patients at the cage-side because they typically require specialized equipment and training or acclimation of animals in a highly controlled setting (Keating et al., 2012). Recently, several behavior-based pain assessments have been published in rabbits. The foundation of these scoring systems is a clear understanding of normal animal behavior—both those typical to the species and specific to the individual patient under consideration. The staff responsible for daily animal care are a valuable resource for understanding individual behavior. Rabbits can also be filmed or observed and their normal behavior, growth rate, and food consumption recorded prior to initiating experiments. However, accurate behavior assessment can be challenging and many veterinary professionals report discomfort in assessing pain in rabbits, relying primarily on nonspecific signs which could lead to failure to recognize and adequately treat pain (Benato et al., 2020a, 2020b; Keown et al., 2011).

In common with several other species, rabbits experiencing pain may reduce their food and water consumption and, therefore, lose weight. Due to both this reduced food consumption and a tendency toward decreased gastrointestinal transit time when painful, reduced production of feces is also common (Benato et al., 2019). Fecal scoring systems have been developed to facilitate the visual assessment of fecal production in the cage pan (Weaver et al. 2010.) Failure to groom may result in the coat becoming ruffled and unkempt, because of the buildup of shed hair that would normally be removed by grooming. Other signs of pain in rabbits can include reduced activity, a hunched posture, increased hiding from caretakers (Pinho et al., 2020), isolation from cage-mates, and vocalizations such as screaming or squealing (Keating et al., 2012; Mayer, 2007). Subtle, inactive pain behaviors include twitching of the dorsal fur, sudden flinching or jerky movements without an obvious cause, wincing behavior, slow walking, slow postural adjustments, and abdominal pressing (Leach et al., 2009). The signs listed here are generalized and may not occur with every type of pain or in every individual, so scoring systems ought to be tailored to specific models or clinical conditions as necessary. For example, vocalization is associated with pain during ear tattooing (Keating et al., 2012), but does not typically occur following ovariohysterectomy or orchiectomy (Benato et al., 2021; Leach et al., 2009), indicating that vocalization may be a more useful indicator of sharp, acute pain than of postsurgical pain. Anesthetic and analgesic agents may confound behavioral assessment because some behaviors, such as an unkempt coat, reduced fecal output, or changes in activity level, may be associated with pain or with sedation. For example, grimace scores may be confounded by sedation.

Published pain scores may be used as a starting point for assessing pain in laboratory rabbits. The most widely used is the rabbit grimace scale (Keating et al., 2012). Similar to grimace scales in rodents and livestock, this scale assesses rabbit pain faces by scoring facial action units. Rabbits are assessed for orbital tightening (closure or squinting of the eye), cheek flattening (presence or absence of a sunken appearance to the cheeks), nose shape (U- vs. V-shaped nares), whisker position (horizontal vs. pulled back), and ear position (upright vs. pinned back). Representative images for use with this scale are available both in the original publication by Keating and on the website of the National Center for the replacement, refinement, and reduction of animals in research (https://www.nc3rs.org.uk/rabbit-grimace-scale (Fig. 15.13). Illustrations for use in training have also been published (Hampshire and Robertson, 2015). This scale was originally validated for rabbits undergoing ear tattooing (Keating et al., 2012), but has successfully been used for more complex models such as surgical calvarial defects (Raillard et al., 2019), catheter implantation (Andrews et al., 2020), and following orthopedic procedures (DiVincenti et al., 2016). This scale may require modification if working with breeds other than the New Zealand white—especially brachycephalic animals, such as many dwarf breeds, or those with lop ears.

The CANCRS composite pain scale for rabbits in a clinical environment relies on a combination of the rabbit grimace scale and on clinical parameters including heart rate percentage increase, respiratory rate and pattern, mental state, palpation, and vocalization (Banchi et al., 2020). If using this scale, clinical parameters alone should not be relied upon because doing so cannot differentiate between mild, moderate, or severe pain. The Bristol Rabbit Pain Scale is based on a 3-min observation of animals, which are scored for demeanor, locomotion, posture, ear position (with adjustments for lop ears), eye position (similar to orbital tightness in the rabbit grimace scale), and evidence of grooming (Benato et al., 2021). Both of these scales can be adapted to a variety of rabbit breeds, and they may provide more information about an animal's general health than the rabbit grimace scale alone.

When choosing pain assessments, the authors recommend adapting available scales for each particular model under consideration. More general markers of wellbeing such as weight, appetite, or fecal output may be affected by pain, but also by common anesthetics, postsurgical inappetence, or other causes of illness. Sedation caused by anesthetic or analgesic agents can confound behavioral analyses. A holistic approach is recommended, combining both more general assessments of well-being with measures specific to an individual model or disease process. For example, abdominal pressing can be assessed for animals undergoing abdominal surgery such as ovariohysterectomy

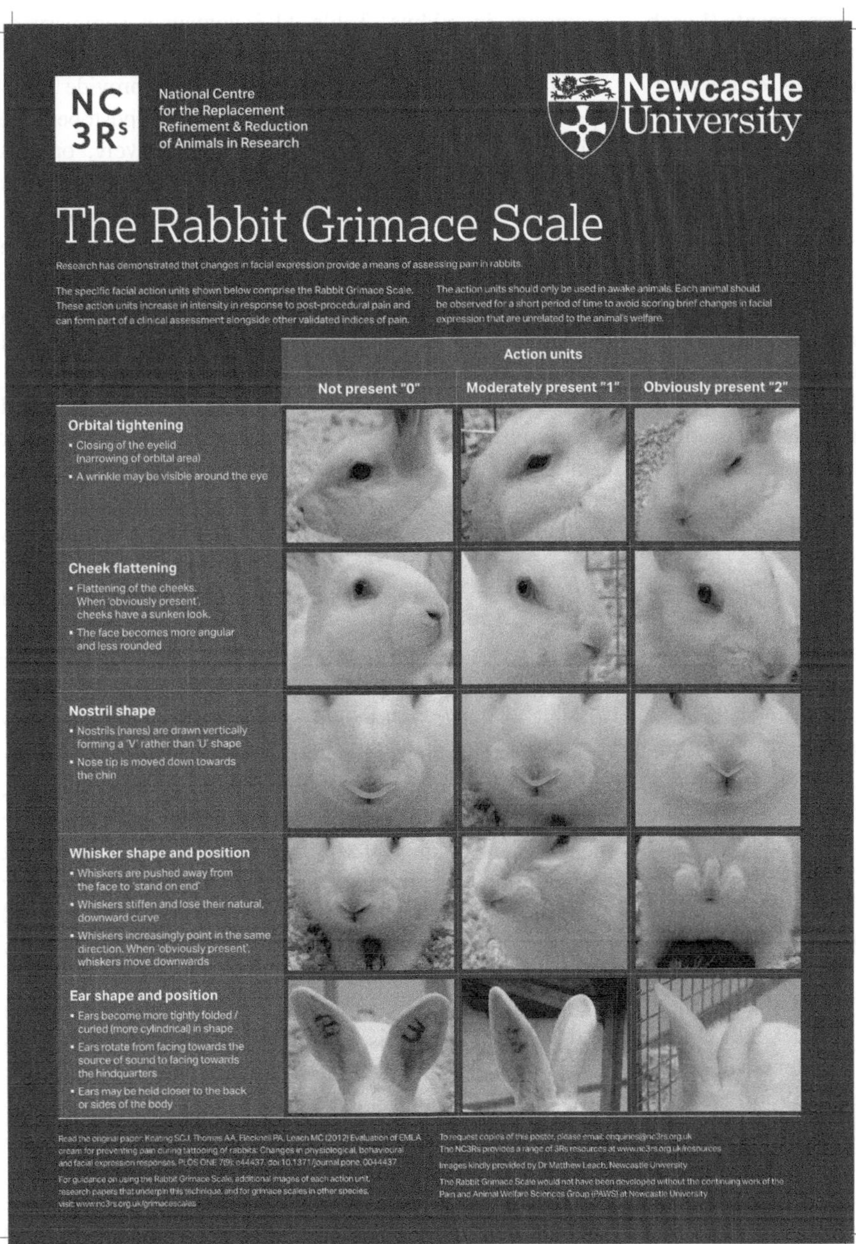

FIGURE 15.13 The Rabbit Grimace Scale can be used for assessing pain in New Zealand White laboratory rabbits.

(Leach et al., 2009). Animals undergoing orthopedic procedures may be more likely to show gait abnormalities or lameness (Pinho et al., 2020). Rabbits cannot express certain behaviors in standard laboratory caging due to size limitations (Coda et al., 2020; Weaver et al., 2010), so certain behaviors such as rearing and activity may be best assessed in pens or examination rooms. Published pain and clinical condition scores are available for a variety of models, including hepatectomy (Drude et al., 2016), sciatic nerve injury (Farinas et al., 2020), ovariohysterectomy (Leach et al., 2009), orthopedic procedures (Pinho et al., 2020), and bone defects (Raillard et al., 2019).

Because rabbits mask some pain behaviors in the presence of observers (Pinho et al., 2020), assessment may best be carried out using a video camera, or via an observation panel to view the animal in its cage or pen. Ideally, rabbits would be acclimated to this environment prior to any procedures, so that assessment is not confounded by fear. The authors of this chapter have had luck viewing animals in real-time using baby monitors, which are readily commercially available. If animals can only be assessed by a person physically present at cageside, a trusted caretaker with whom the animals are already comfortable may be the ideal choice. Rabbits are naturally less active in the morning, which may affect behavioral assessments (Leach et al., 2009). In addition, consideration should be given to the effects of analgesics, especially those that cause sedation, which may alter behavior and therefore confound pain assessment.

Regardless of assessment choice, records should be carefully kept. It is useful to design a pain assessment scoring sheet or template that can be rapidly completed at each postprocedural assessment. These records can then be reviewed, and refinements can be made as needed for future studies. Any time indications of pain are noted in an animal, this should be recorded, as should any rescue analgesics or nonpharmacologic methods of pain control applied to the animal. Animals requiring these interventions may need more frequent monitoring so that breakthrough pain can be treated quickly.

B. Selection of analgesics

A range of compounds are available to provide pain relief in the rabbit. However, the efficacy, pharmacodynamic, and pharmacokinetic profiles of few drugs have been established in this species. Some data can be gained through analgesiometric testing, where a noxious stimulus is applied until the rabbit makes a defined response such as a skin twitch. Changes in the response threshold after administration of an analgesic are used to determine the potency of the agent. A detailed description of analgesiometry methods in rabbits is beyond the scope of this chapter, but methods include application of thermal stimuli to the muzzle (Zhou et al., 1981), ear (McCallister et al., 1986; Piercey and Schroeder, 1980; Wynn et al., 1984), or skin (Barter and Kwiatkowski, 2013; Flecknell et al., 1990), electrical stimulation of the ears (Ayhan et al., 1983) or the tooth pulp (Mattila and Saarnivaara, 1968), and use of pressure on the hind limb (Lightowler and Smith, 1963).

When basing recommendations on data obtained using analgesiometry or other efficacy testing, it is important to appreciate that the severity of the painful stimuli used may vary considerably, and may also be qualitatively different from the pain experienced by a given animal, thus necessitating adjustment of doses. The potency of different analgesics assessed using analgesiometry correlates well with their potency in men, but the doses used to control clinical pain may vary considerably. Dose rates established using analgesiometry provide a safe starting point for clinical use of the agent. Surveys of veterinary professionals show that even experienced personnel express some uncertainty in designing rabbit analgesic plans (Benato et al., 2020a, 2020b; Keown et al., 2011). Still, where no data concerning particular analgesics are available for the rabbit, extrapolations may be made from data obtained in other species or based on clinical experience. Following are information and practical considerations for the most commonly used analgesics in rabbits. Table 11.3 contain a summary of recommended analgesic drugs, doses, and routes.

Opioid analgesics can be used both to provide intraoperative analgesia in rabbits and to provide postoperative pain relief. When given pre or intraoperatively, opioids may prolong anesthesia produced by other injectable agents (Gonzalez-Gil et al., 2015; Murphy et al., 2010). Side effects commonly associated with opioid analgesics in the rabbit include respiratory depression, increased gastrointestinal transit time, bradycardia, hypothermia, sedation, decreased arterial blood pressure, and increased arterial carbon dioxide (Benato et al., 2019).

The most commonly used opioid in rabbits is the partial mu agonist buprenorphine (Benato et al., 2019; Coulter et al., 2011). Typical recommendations are to administer buprenorphine at a range of 0.01–0.05 mg/kg every 6–12 h via the intramuscular, subcutaneous, or intravenous routes. However, buprenorphine has lower bioavailability and reaches lower peak serum concentrations when administered via the subcutaneous route (Askar et al., 2020), and so a best practice is to administer it via the IV or IM routes. If the SC route is used, initial doses should be administered IV or IM with SC reserved for maintaining serum concentrations. Regardless of route, onset of analgesia is delayed by 15–30 min following administration, which should be considered when developing an analgesic plan (Askar et al., 2020). For visceral pain, providing buprenorphine preemptively appears to be more effective than provision after the painful stimulus has occurred (Shafford and Schadt, 2008). Multiple studies have shown that buprenorphine alone may not provide adequate pain relief for procedures involving severe pain (DiVincenti et al., 2016; Hedenqvist et al., 2016)—in these cases, animals should be assessed frequently and multimodal analgesia should be considered.

Buprenorphine is available in sustained-release formulations. Pharmacokinetic studies of the compounded product Buprenorphine-SR (ZooPharm, Windsor, CO) show that, at a dose of 0.15 mg/kg, it takes approximately 15 h to reach presumed effective plasma concentrations, but that these concentrations are maintained for up to 77h following administration (Andrews et al., 2020). Buprenorphine-SR shows similar efficacy to buprenorphine-HCL in a tibial implant model (DiVincenti et al., 2016). Recently, an FDA indexed sustained-release buprenorphine has become available (Ethiqa XR, Fidelis Pharmaceuticals, North Brunswick, NJ), but at the time of writing, this preparation has not been tested in rabbits. High-concentration buprenorphine (Simbadol, Zoetis, Parsippany, NJ) is not recommended for use in rabbits because it can cause profound sedation and seizures when administered at the recommended dose for cats (0.24 mg/kg) (Andrews et al., 2020).

Buprenorphine generally has a low incidence of serious adverse effects in rabbits. Hypoxemia has been reported in rabbits anesthetized with combinations including buprenorphine but appears to be clinically insignificant unless animals have some form of respiratory compromise (Flecknell et al., 1989; Schroeder and Smith, 2011; Shafford and Schadt, 2008). Prolonged gastrointestinal transit time associated is discussed previously in this chapter. Gastrointestinal effects are not ameliorated by cisapride (Feldman et al., 2021) or methylnaltrexone (Martin-Flores et al., 2017), but may be partially relieved by providing easy access to water, such as providing a water bowl (Feldman et al., 2021). Because anorexia can also contribute to gastrointestinal stasis in rabbits, it is likely that the provision of palatable dietary supplements, including hay, could improve gut transit time following a painful procedure.

Following a 6–12 h lag time, transdermal fentanyl patches have been shown to yield presumed effective serum concentrations for up to 72 h after placement in rabbits (Foley et al., 2001; Mirschberger et al., 2020). However, to reach presumed effective serum concentrations, patches must be placed carefully and in the correct location as absorption can be affected by a variety of factors, including the temperature of the site, whether the skin is intact, and interindividual variation (Mirschberger et al., 2020). Patch dosing, application, and hair removal methods are discussed previously in this chapter. It is recommended that patches be placed in the interscapular area or on the outer surface of the pinna, though fentanyl concentrations will drop below effective levels by approximately 48h if placed on the ear (Mirschberger et al., 2020).

Non-steroidal antiinflammatory drugs (NSAIDs) are also commonly used in rabbits, but should be reserved for mild to moderate pain or used as part of a multimodal treatment plan as discussed previously in the chapter. Meloxicam may be given SC, IM, or orally. Oral absorption may be affected by food, so a best practice is to remove food for some period prior to oral dosing (Leach et al., 2009). Meloxicam appears safe for long-term dosing with little effect on gut microbiota (Cooper et al., 2009; Eshar and Weese, 2014). Pharmacokinetic data, is discussed previously in the chapter. An efficacy study of three doses, showed only the highest trialed (1 mg/kg loading dose followed by 0.5 mg/kg/day) provided any apparent analgesia following ovariohysterectomy (Leach et al., 2009).

Carprofen use is also reported, but less pharmacokinetic and efficacy data is available for this drug in rabbits (Hawkins et al., 2008). As discussed previously in the chapter, efficacy is questionable in rabbits, even when combined with buprenorphine (Hedenqvist et al., 2016). Carprofen does not affect antibody production in rabbits following administration of Complete Freund's Adjuvant (Fishback et al., 2016).

Local anesthetics may be associated with neurotoxicity in rabbits, so doses should be calculated carefully prior to infusion (Benato et al., 2019; Richard et al., 2012). "Splash blocks" at incision sites appear ineffective at controlling pain when used alone following major surgery (Cooper et al., 2009; DiVincenti et al., 2016). EMLA cream, a eutectic mixture of prilocaine and lidocaine, can be applied to the skin 20–30 min prior to a painful stimulus, such as tattoo application or catheterization, to effectively control pain (Keating et al., 2012). Lidocaine given as an IV infusion for 2 days following ovariohysterectomy appeared well-tolerated by rabbits and provided pain control with fewer gastrointestinal side effects than buprenorphine (Schnellbacher et al., 2017). Other uses of local anesthetics such as local, regional, and epidural anesthesia are discussed later in this chapter (Table 15.3).

1. Multimodal analgesia

Multimodal analgesia is advised as a best practice when possible. Using analgesics from multiple classes together provides numerous benefits, such as dose sparing, reduction in side effects caused by higher doses of individual drugs, and the ability to address multiple pain pathways at once. For example, following surgery, a local block can reduce incisional pain while an NSAID may help treat inflammatory pain. The most recent data in laboratory rabbits indicates that multimodal analgesia is uncommon (Coulter et al., 2011), but surveys of private practice veterinarians in the UK indicate that 70% of practitioners use multimodal analgesia (Benato et al., 2020b). It is possible that, as the benefits of multimodal analgesia have become more widely known, this effect is also occurring in laboratory rabbits, but more recent literature reviews or surveys are not currently available. In rabbits undergoing vascular cutdown, animals receiving both buprenorphine and meloxicam showed signs of improved pain control versus either drug alone (Goldschlager et al., 2013). Raillard et al. (2019) showed improved postoperative care in rabbits receiving multimodal analgesia following calvarial bone surgery, but many animals still required rescue buprenorphine, likely because this is an extensive and painful procedure.

2. Preventative analgesia

When possible, analgesics should be provided prior to a painful stimulus. For visceral pain, providing buprenorphine preemptively appears to be more effective than provision after the painful stimulus has occurred (Shafford and Schadt, 2008). Preemptive local anesthetics can prevent animals from perceiving pain from minor procedures such as tattoos or intravenous catheter placement (Keating et al., 2012).

C. Regional or spinal analgesia

Local or regional nerve blocks involve the infusion of a local anesthetic into the area surrounding a nerve, thus

TABLE 15.3 Analgesic agents.

Drug	Rabbit	Route of administration
Opioids		
Buprenorphine	0.01–0.05 q6-12h [a]	SQ, IM, IV[a]
Morphine	2–5 q4h	SQ
Hydromorphone	0.05–0.1	SQ, IM
Butorphanol	0.1–0.8 q4h	SQ
Oxymorphone	0.05–0.2 q8-12h	SQ, IM
Fentanyl patch	1/2 of a 25 μg/h patch	Topical
NSAIDs		
Carprofen	4 q24h	PO, SQ
Meloxicam	0.3 q24h	PO, SQ
Ketoprofen	1–2 q24h	PO, SQ
Local anesthetics		
Lidocaine	1–2 infiltrate	Topically, SQ
Bupivacaine	1–2 infiltrate	Topically, SQ

All doses are mg/kg unless stated otherwise.
[a]*Due to reduced plasma concentrations and bioavailability with subcutaneous administration, the intramuscular or intravenous route of administration is recommended as a loading dose or in circumstances where rapid analgesia is warranted. For chronic administration, a shorter dosing interval may be needed to optimize plasma concentrations and analgesia depending upon degree of pain.*
Adapted from Lester, P.A. et al., 2012. Anesthesia and Analgesia. In: Sukow, M.A., Stevens, K.A., Wilson, R.P. (Eds.), The Laboratory Rabbit, Guinea Pig, Hamster, and Other Rodents. Academic Press, pp. 33–56, Waltham, M.A., Flecknell, P.A., 2015. Laboratory Animal Aneasthesia, 4nd ed. Academic Press, London, UK.

preventing transmission of pain to the area served by that nerve. In the rabbit, they may be used in combination with inhalant or injectable anesthetics, as they are in other species (Lockhart et al., 1991; Madsen et al., 1993; Raman et al., 1989). Perhaps the most widely used examples of this technique in veterinary medicine are intratesticular blocks during castration and dental nerve blocks during tooth extraction surgery. Regional nerve blocks are commonly used to provide analgesia or anesthesia to other parts of the body, such as the limbs in larger species, such as livestock and dogs, and there are now numerous examples of the use of this technique in rabbits. Potential benefits include the ability to treat a localized painful area, thus avoiding potential systemic side effects that may be associated with other analgesic classes or delivery methods. Fonseca et al. (2015) describe the use of ultrasound to guide brachial plexus nerve blocks in rabbits undergoing forelimb surgery. Sensitivity was effectively blocked for approximately 319 min following infusion of ropivacaine and treated rabbits began eating soon after surgery. Kluge et al. (2017) present a method for blocking the sciatic and femoral nerves with a mixture of lidocaine and bupivacaine prior to stifle surgery. Rabbits given the local nerve block had a decreased need for opiates in the perioperative period. A long-acting, liposome-encapsulated form of bupivacaine (Nocita, Aratana Therapeutics Inc., Leawood, KS) has been approved for use in dogs. While no studies in rabbits using this product were found at the time of writing, safety and toxicity studies of a similar human preparation show that it is well tolerated by rabbits when given as a brachial plexus nerve block (Richard et al., 2012). Ultrasound-guided blockade of the lateral transversus abdominis plane (TAP block) is used to provide pain relief during abdominal surgery in dogs and cats; a recent publication using cadavers shows that this may also be feasible in rabbits (Di Bella et al., 2021).

Rabbits have been used to evaluate the pharmacology and toxicology of spinal anesthesia or analgesia (Adams et al., 1974; Crawford et al., 1993; Demirel et al., 2006; Dollo et al., 2004a, 2004a; Erdine et al., 1999; Hino et al., 2001; Hogan et al., 1998; Hughes et al., 1993; Jensen et al., 1992; Komoda et al., 2003; Langerman et al., 1990; Madsen et al., 1993; Malinovsky et al., 2002; Ugur et al., 2005; Vranken et al., 2006). Epidural or spinal anesthesia can act as an effective adjunct to other anesthetic methods, potentially sparing the use of inhalants or other classes of injectable anesthesia. Local anesthetics and opioids are most commonly administered via this route, and drugs of these classes can be safely combined for epidural injection in rabbits (Gusak et al., 2013). Typically, epidural injections are given at the lumbosacral junction. Inadvertent injection into the subarachnoid space can be avoided by using electrical stimulation to confirm appropriate placement in the epidural space (Otero et al., 2012). Subarachnoid injection can also be avoided by injecting at the level of the coccygeal spinal canal, but this risks inadvertent IV injection (Ong et al., 2020). Both epidural morphine and lidocaine have been shown to act as successful adjuncts for anesthesia during hind limb surgery (Antonczyk et al., 2019). In dogs, dexmedetomidine can prolong the analgesic effects of epidural lidocaine, but while this effect does appear to occur in rabbits, it was also associated with spinal cord lesions in a proportion of animals (Santos et al., 2021). Rabbits should be heavily sedated or anesthetized prior to administering spinal anesthesia to reduce the potential for movement during administration and subsequent nerve damage.

D. Supportive care and recovery period

Appropriate peri-procedural support is crucial to reducing pain and ensuring a safe recovery. This includes a variety of nonpharmaceutical interventions and preparatory steps. Many of the pain scales previously described in this chapter rely, in part, on assessing appetite and fecal output. In addition, buprenorphine can induce signs associated with gastrointestinal stasis in rabbits. Because of this, it is prudent to monitor weight, growth rate, appetite, and fecal output in rabbits prior to performing any painful procedures. This provides a baseline against which the recovery period can be judged.

The recovery area should be a calm, quiet environment. Cardiopulmonary function should continue to be monitored during recovery and into the postoperative period. Hypostatic pulmonary congestion should be avoided by altering the rabbit's position from left to right lateral recumbency every 15 min during anesthetic recovery. Thermal support should be provided because, like most small animals, rabbits have a high surface-area-to-volume ratio and therefore are especially prone to hypothermia, which can exacerbate pain and prolong anesthetic recovery periods. Rectal temperature should be monitored regularly during recovery. Thermal support consisting of circulating hot water blankets, hot water bottles, the Bair Hugger patient thermal warming system, hydrocollator packs, sodium acetate heat packs, microwavable heat packs, infant incubators, ICU cages, warming lamps, and/or blankets should be used to maintain body temperature. Where possible, animals in recovery should be provided with a thermal gradient within the environment so that they can self-regulate their temperature. Caution must be taken with sedated animals as they may not be able to remove themselves from hot surfaces effectively. Heat sources that reduce the risk of burns should be chosen.

Rabbits should be encouraged to eat and drink during the recovery period by providing them with water that is easy to access and palatable, nutritionally complete dietary supplements. Rabbits are prone to hypoglycemia because of high metabolic rates and, in neonates, limited fat reserves. They should be allowed access to a nutritious pelleted diet and hay as soon after surgery as is feasible. Anorexic animals can be given 5% dextrose solution SC, 50% dextrose orally, parenteral nutritional support through a stomach or nasoesophageal tube, or offered palatable supplements. Commercial products formulated to provide complete nutrition and high fiber for recovering animals are preferred. Fiber is especially important as it stimulates cecocolic motility and promotes peristalsis (Oglesbee, 2021). Examples include Oxbow Critical Care (Oxbow Animal Health Inc., Omaha, NE) or EmerAid for Herbivores (EmerAid Inc., Cornell, IL). Both supplements have formulations that can be provided by nasogastric tube, syringe, or given in a crock for self-feeding. Other supplements such as alfalfa cubes, dandelions, vegetables, or Nutrical per os may also be offered to stimulate appetite, but should not make up the bulk of the diet even in recovery. Persistent untreated anorexia causes fat mobilization and often leads to irreversible fatal hepatic lipidosis. The oral administration of probiotics such as Lactobacillus culture or a slurry of feces or cecal contents from healthy rabbits has been promulgated to return the gastrointestinal flora to normal following gastrointestinal surgery or the administration of flora-altering antibiotics (Gillett et al., 1983). To further minimize the risk of ileus after abdominal surgery, motility modifiers such as metoclopramide or ranitidine may be administered. Cisapride has been recommended previously, but recent work by Feldman et al. (2021) shows no effect on gastrointestinal transit time in rabbits. Dosage recommendations for metoclopramide are 0.2–0.5 mg/kg PO or SC, one to three times daily (Paul-Murphy and Ramer, 1998), and for ranitidine 2–5 mg/kg PO, twice daily (Kounenis et al., 1992). If ileus does develop, rabbits should be provided with fluid therapy to rehydrate the gut contents and analgesic drugs, as this condition is known to be painful (Oglesbee, 2021). The maintenance fluid requirement of the rabbit is reported as 100 mL/kg/day (Suckow and Schroeder, 2010). Fluids can be administered subcutaneously, intravenously, or intraperitoneally; water for oral intake should always be easily available. Treatment for ileus should continue until the rabbit is comfortable and passing normal feces, generally for 3–5 days (Oglesbee, 2021). Though not developed for this purpose, previously described fecal scoring systems may be useful when assessing these animals (Weaver et al. 2010).

Rabbits recovering from anesthesia may be lightly wrapped in a blanket or towel (burrito style) with the legs flexed against the body to prevent thrashing and damage to the spinal column. Dimming the lights and/or providing a darkened cage (e.g., by hanging a towel across the doorway) can also reduce stress in recovering animals.

Antibiotics may be necessary following select surgical procedures. They should not be used indiscriminately or as a substitute for aseptic technique. Clostridial enterotoxemia has been associated with the administration of a wide variety of antibiotics (Carman and Evans, 1984). Surgical sites should be evaluated daily for dehiscence, infection, and fluid accumulation. Nonabsorbable suture materials or staples should be removed as soon as wound healing permits to avoid their serving as a nidus of infection.

Finally, animals should be monitored consistently for signs of pain throughout the recovery period. Rabbits find handling stressful, so, if possible, restraint should be minimized and, where required, performed by experienced personnel who can accomplish goals efficiently. Postoperative rabbits with accessible sutures may be fitted with an Elizabethan collar ("e-collar") or cervical collar for the first postoperative week to prevent inadvertent suture removal. In most cases, problems can be avoided by the use of a subcuticular closure together with the use of a buried knot (Mehler, 2006). Supportive or protective care should be tailored to the study. For example, long plastic e-collars may be more effective than "bubble" e-collars at preventing animals from reaching incisions on the hindfoot. On the other hand, longer e-collars can make accessing feeders, water sources, and cecotropes more difficult and can prevent animals from accessing hiding spaces or shelves.

E. Nonpharmacologic (enrichment, acupuncture, nutrition, housing, conspecifics)

Nonpharmacologic pain control is a catch-all term that applies to a variety of measures, ranging from comfort care to alternative medicine modalities. To identify potential areas for intervention, it is helpful to consider the lived experience of the animal and to mentally walk through all aspects of an animal's typical day. For example, quiet environments with species-appropriate light cycles can promote rest and recovery. Therefore, it may be ideal to place postoperative animals at the end of a quiet hallway instead of in a busy room where people frequently enter and exit. Animals should be kept at an appropriate temperature and ideally, can be provided with the ability to thermoregulate, such as the provision of a temperature gradient within the cage or a nest box filled with nesting material that rabbits can enter or exit at will. Painful rabbits tend to spend more time at the back of their cages, away from humans. Nest boxes can also facilitate this natural instinct to hide. Soft resting areas with good traction give animals a comfortable space in which to recover and prevent injuries from slipping on cage floors. If an e-collar must be provided, ensure that animals can easily access all portions of the cage and can readily reach food and water.

Special consideration should be given to environmental enrichment in the postprocedural period. While enrichment is an important component of an animal care program, it cannot mitigate the stress of surgery alone (Coda et al., 2020). Enrichment should be assessed for safety and for its potential to act as an experimental confound. For example, it may be best to avoid enrichment that can become caught on external implants. Rabbits have a high preference for destructible enrichment (Hedenqvist et al., 2020; Thurston et al., 2018)—paperboard placed on the cage floor gives traction, insulation from cold floor surfaces, and an opportunity for chewing and shredding. Other destructible enrichment items include paper bags or cardboard tubes stuffed with hay—these can help prevent boredom and destructive behavior. As discussed previously in this chapter, meloxicam absorption may be reduced if animals have recently eaten, so the provision of food treats should be avoided just prior to dosing. Food treats may be provided to encourage rabbits to eat, but care should be taken to provide nutritionally complete supplements when possible. In the authors' experience, some rabbits will preferentially eat calorie-dense or sweet treats to the exclusion of their food or hay. In these cases, animals can gradually be provided with fewer treats and more of a complete diet over a period of days, with careful monitoring to ensure the animal continues to eat and produce feces.

Rabbits are a social species and should be socially housed whenever possible (Thurston et al., 2018). It is beyond the scope of this chapter to provide detailed instructions on rabbit social housing and maintenance, but rabbits in stable pairs or groups should be maintained with their conspecifics if possible. Successful maintenance of groups or pairs has been demonstrated following radius defect and femoral angioplasty procedures (Bartley and Johnson, 2019; Hedenqvist et al., 2020). Rabbits engage in more active behaviors when housed in larger pens with conspecifics (Coda et al., 2020; Hedenqvist et al., 2020). Because pain-associated behavior changes could disrupt social hierarchies, rabbits should be monitored carefully and, if needed, can be provided with additional destructible enrichment prior to separating the pair, as, in the authors' experience, increased destructible enrichment can promote the maintenance of pairs. To prevent animals from overgrooming their cagemates' incisions, commercially made jackets or modified human infant pants may be used (Bartley and Johnson, 2019). This method also allows rabbits to engage in grooming and coprophagy, both of which are prevented by e-collars.

Finally, a variety of nonpharmacologic pain control methods have been described in small animals, such as warm or cold compresses, low-level laser therapy, and acupuncture (Benato et al., 2019). However, few studies are available to validate these techniques in rabbits. If used, animals should be acclimated prior to the application of the painful stimulus, as many of these procedures require restraint. Rabbits have been used as an experimental model for acupuncture studies, but few of these describe analgesic benefits in the rabbits themselves. The application of acupuncture or electroacupuncture may be attempted to augment analgesia or improve gastrointestinal motility (Niu et al., 2007; Shi et al., 2020).

References

Adams, H.J., Mastri, A.R., Eicholzer, A.W., Kilpatrick, G., 1974. Morphologic effects of intrathecal etidocaine and tetracaine on the rabbit spinal cord. Anesth. Analg. 53 (6), 904–908. https://doi.org/10.1213/00000539-197453060-00018.

Aeschbacher, G., Webb, A.I., 1993. Propofol in rabbits. 2. Long-term anesthesia. Lab. Anim. Sci. 43 (4), 328–335. Retrieved from. https://www.ncbi.nlm.nih.gov/pubmed/8231090.

Alexander, D.J., Clark, G.C., 1980. A simple method of oral endotracheal intubation in rabbits (*Oryctolagus cuniculus*). Lab. Anim. Sci. 30 (5), 871–873. Retrieved from. https://www.ncbi.nlm.nih.gov/pubmed/7431872.

Andrews, D.D., Fajt, V.R., Baker, K.C., Blair, R.V., Jones, S.H., Dobek, G.L., 2020. A comparison of buprenorphine, sustained release buprenorphine, and high concentration buprenorphine in male New Zealand white rabbits. J. Am. Assoc. Lab. Anim. Sci. 59 (5), 546–556. https://doi.org/10.30802/AALAS-JAALAS-19-000132.

Antonczyk, A., Liszka, B., Skrzypczak, P., Kielbowicz, Z., 2019. Comparison of analgesia provided by lidocaine or morphine delivered epidurally in rabbits undergoing hindlimb orthopedic surgery. Pol. J. Vet. Sci. 22 (1), 31–35. https://doi.org/10.24425/pjvs.2018.125604.

Arenillas, M., Gomez de Segura, I.A., 2018. Anaesthetic effects of alfaxalone administered intraperitoneally alone or combined with dexmedetomidine and fentanyl in the rat. Lab. Anim. 52 (6), 588–598. https://doi.org/10.1177/0023677218764214.

Askar, R., Fredriksson, E., Manell, E., Hedeland, M., Bondesson, U., Bate, S., Hedenqvist, P., 2020. Bioavailability of subcutaneous and intramuscular administrated buprenorphine in New Zealand White rabbits. BMC Vet. Res. 16 (1), 436. https://doi.org/10.1186/s12917-020-02618-7.

Ayhan, I.H., Turker, R.K., Melli, M., 1983. A new method for the rapid measurement of analgesic activity in rabbits. Arch. Int. Pharmacodyn. Ther. 262 (2), 215–220. Retrieved from. https://www.ncbi.nlm.nih.gov/pubmed/6135398.

Bailey, R.S., Barter, L.S., Pypendop, B.H., 2017. Pharmacokinetics of dexmedetomidine in isoflurane-anesthetized New Zealand White rabbits. Vet. Anaesth. Analg. 44 (4), 876–882. https://doi.org/10.1016/j.vaa.2017.01.003.

Banchi, P., Quaranta, G., Ricci, A., Mauthe von Degerfeld, M., 2020. Reliability and construct validity of a composite pain scale for rabbit (CANCRS) in a clinical environment. PLoS One 15 (4), e0221377. https://doi.org/10.1371/journal.pone.0221377.

Barter, L.S., Kwiatkowski, A., 2013. Thermal threshold testing for evaluation of analgesics in New Zealand white rabbits. J. Am. Assoc. Lab. Anim. Sci. 52 (1), 44–47. Retrieved from. https://www.ncbi.nlm.nih.gov/pubmed/23562032.

Bartley, K.A., Johnson, C.H., 2019. Human infant pants for postoperative protection during social housing of New Zealand white rabbits (*Oryctolagus cuniculus*). J. Am. Assoc. Lab. Anim. Sci. 58 (4), 510–516. https://doi.org/10.30802/AALAS-JAALAS-18-000116.

Bateman, L., Ludders, J.W., Gleed, R.D., Erb, H.N., 2005. Comparison between facemask and laryngeal mask airway in rabbits during isoflurane anesthesia. Vet. Anaesth. Analg. 32 (5), 280–288. https://doi.org/10.1111/j.1467-2995.2005.00169.x.

Baumgartner, C., Koenighaus, H., Ebner, J., Henke, J., Schuster, T., Erhardt, W., 2011. Comparison of dipyrone/propofol versus fentanyl/propofol anaesthesia during surgery in rabbits. Lab. Anim. 45 (1), 38–44. https://doi.org/10.1258/la.2010.010091.

Baumgartner, C.M., Koenighaus, H., Ebner, J.K., Henke, J., Schuster, T., Erhardt, W.D., 2009. Cardiovascular effects of fentanyl and propofol on hemodynamic function in rabbits. Am. J. Vet. Res. 70 (3), 409–417. https://doi.org/10.2460/ajvr.70.3.409.

Bellini, L., Veladiano, I.A., Schrank, M., Candaten, M., Mollo, A., 2018. Prospective clinical study to evaluate an oscillometric blood pressure monitor in pet rabbits. BMC Vet. Res. 14 (1), 52. https://doi.org/10.1186/s12917-018-1369-4.

Benato, L., Murrell, J., Blackwell, E., Saunders, R., Rooney, N., 2020a. Pain and analgesia in pet rabbits: a survey of the attitude of veterinary nurses. J. Small Anim. Pract. 61 (9), 576–581. https://doi.org/10.1111/jsap.13186.

Benato, L., Murrell, J., Knowles, T.G., Rooney, N.J., 2021. Development of the Bristol Rabbit Pain Scale (BRPS): a multidimensional composite pain scale specific to rabbits (*Oryctolagus cuniculus*). PLoS One 16 (6), e0252417. https://doi.org/10.1371/journal.pone.0252417.

Benato, L., Murrell, J.C., Blackwell, E.J., Saunders, R., Rooney, N., 2020b. Analgesia in pet rabbits: a survey study on how pain is assessed and ameliorated by veterinary surgeons. Vet. Rec. 186 (18), 603. https://doi.org/10.1136/vr.105071.

Benato, L., Rooney, N.J., Murrell, J.C., 2019. Pain and analgesia in pet rabbits within the veterinary environment: a review. Vet. Anaesth. Analg. 46 (2), 151–162. https://doi.org/10.1016/j.vaa.2018.10.007.

Bennett, R.A., 2020. 30 - general principles of surgical techniques. In: Quesenberry, K.E., Orcutt, C.J., Mans, C., Carpenter, J.W. (Eds.), Ferrets, Rabbits, and Rodents, fourth ed. W.B. Saunders, Philadelphia, pp. 426–431.

Bergh, M.S., Budsberg, S.C., 2005. The coxib NSAIDs: potential clinical and pharmacologic importance in veterinary medicine. J. Vet. Intern. Med. 19 (5), 633–643. https://doi.org/10.1892/0891-6640(2005)19[633:tcnpca]2.0.co;2.

Bertolet, R.D., Hughes, H.C., 1980. Endotracheal intubation: an easy way to establish a patent airway in rabbits. Lab. Anim. Sci. 30 (2 Pt 1), 227–230. Retrieved from. https://www.ncbi.nlm.nih.gov/pubmed/7052377.

Beths, T., 2017. TIVA/TCI in veterinary practice. In: Absalom, A.R. (Ed.), Total Intravenous Anesthesia and Target Controlled Infusions. Springer, Cham, Switzerland, pp. 589–618.

Betteridge, K.J., 1973. A simple and inexpensive apparatus for halothane anaesthesia in rabbits and other small animals. Vet. Rec. 93 (14), 398–399. https://doi.org/10.1136/vr.93.14.398.

Beyers, T.M., Richardson, J.A., Prince, M.D., 1991. Axonal degeneration and self-mutilation as a complication of the intramuscular use of ketamine and xylazine in rabbits. Lab. Anim. Sci. 41 (5), 519–520. Retrieved from. https://www.ncbi.nlm.nih.gov/pubmed/1666163.

Bonath, K., Nolte, I., Schniewind, A., Sandmann, H., Failing, K., 1982. [Food deprivation as preparation for anesthesia and aftercare—effect of fasting on the acid-base status and glucose concentration in the blood of rabbits of different body weight]. Berl. Münchener Tierärztliche Wochenschr. 95 (7), 126–130. Retrieved from. https://www.ncbi.nlm.nih.gov/pubmed/7092793.

Borkowski, G.L., Danneman, P.J., Russell, G.B., Lang, C.M., 1990. An evaluation of three intravenous anesthetic regimens in New Zealand rabbits. Lab. Anim. Sci. 40 (3), 270–276. Retrieved from. https://www.ncbi.nlm.nih.gov/pubmed/2162982.

Bradley, M.P., Doerning, C.M., Nowland, M.H., Lester, P.A., 2019. Intramuscular administration of alfaxalone alone and in combination for sedation and anesthesia of rabbits (*Oryctolagus cuniculus*). J. Am. Assoc. Lab. Anim. Sci. 58 (2), 216–222. https://doi.org/10.30802/AALAS-JAALAS-18-000078.

Brammer, D.W., Doerning, B.J., Chrisp, C.E., Rush, H.G., 1991. Anesthetic and nephrotoxic effects of Telazol in New Zealand white rabbits. Lab. Anim. Sci. 41 (5), 432–435. Retrieved from. https://www.ncbi.nlm.nih.gov/pubmed/1666143.

Brandão, J., Graham, J., Quesenberry, K.E., 2020. 12—basic approach to veterinary care of rabbits. In: Quesenberry, K.E., Orcutt, C.J., Mans, C., Carpenter, J.W. (Eds.), Ferrets, Rabbits, and Rodents, fourth ed. W.B. Saunders, Philadelphia, pp. 150–161.

Carman, R.J., Evans, R.H., 1984. Experimental and spontaneous clostridial enteropathies of laboratory and free living lagomorphs. Lab. Anim. Sci. 34 (5), 443–452. Retrieved from. https://www.ncbi.nlm.nih.gov/pubmed/6096630.

Coda, K.A., Fortman, J.D., Garcia, K.D., 2020. Behavioral effects of cage size and environmental enrichment in New Zealand white rabbits. J. Am. Assoc. Lab. Anim. Sci. https://doi.org/10.30802/AALAS-JAALAS-19-000136.

Comolli, J., Schnellbacher, R., Beaufrere, H., Blas-Machado, U., Quandt, J., Mayer, J., Divers, S.J., 2020. Comparison of endoscopic endotracheal intubation and the v-gel supraglottic airway device for spontaneously ventilating New Zealand white rabbits undergoing ovariohysterectomy. Vet. Rec. https://doi.org/10.1136/vr.105746.

Cooper, C.S., Metcalf-Pate, K.A., Barat, C.E., Cook, J.A., Scorpio, D.G., 2009. Comparison of side effects between buprenorphine and meloxicam used postoperatively in Dutch belted rabbits (*Oryctolagus cuniculus*). J. Am. Assoc. Lab. Anim. Sci. 48 (3), 279–285. Retrieved from. https://www.ncbi.nlm.nih.gov/pubmed/19476717.

Coulter, C.A., Flecknell, P.A., Leach, M.C., Richardson, C.A., 2011. Reported analgesic administration to rabbits undergoing experimental surgical procedures. BMC Vet. Res. 7, 12. https://doi.org/10.1186/1746-6148-7-12.

Crawford, M.E., Jensen, F.M., Toftdahl, D.B., Madsen, J.B., 1993. Direct spinal effect of intrathecal and extradural midazolam on visceral noxious stimulation in rabbits. Br. J. Anaesth. 70 (6), 642–646. https://doi.org/10.1093/bja/70.6.642.

Dardai, E., Heavner, J.E., 1987. Respiratory and cardiovascular effects of halothane, isoflurane and enflurane delivered via a Jackson-Rees breathing system in temperature controlled and uncontrolled rats. Methods Find Exp. Clin. Pharmacol. 9 (11), 717–720. Retrieved from. https://www.ncbi.nlm.nih.gov/pubmed/3448450.

Davis, J.A., Greenfield, R.E., Brewer, T.G., 1993. Benzocaine-induced methemoglobinemia attributed to topical application of the anesthetic in several laboratory animal species. Am. J. Vet. Res. 54 (8), 1322–1326. Retrieved from. https://www.ncbi.nlm.nih.gov/pubmed/8214904.

Davis, N.L., Malinin, T.I., 1974. Rabbit intubation and halothane anesthesia. Lab. Anim. Sci. 24 (4), 617–621. Retrieved from. https://www.ncbi.nlm.nih.gov/pubmed/4369102.

Dayer, P., Collart, L., Desmeules, J., 1994. The pharmacology of tramadol. Drugs 47 (Suppl. 1), 3–7. https://doi.org/10.2165/00003495-199400471-00003.

de Miguel Garcia, C., Doss, G., Travis, M.L., Hetzel, S., Ferreira, T.H., 2020. Efficacy of greater auricular and auriculotemporal nerve blocks performed in rabbits. Vet. Anaesth. Analg. 47 (4), 567–573. https://doi.org/10.1016/j.vaa.2020.02.005.

Demirel, E., Ugur, H.C., Dolgun, H., Kahilogullari, G., Sargon, M.E., Egemen, N., Kecik, Y., 2006. The neurotoxic effects of intrathecal midazolam and neostigmine in rabbits. Anaesth. Intensive Care 34 (2), 218–223. https://doi.org/10.1177/0310057X0603400204.

Di Bella, C., Pennasilico, L., Staffieri, F., Serino, F., Palumbo Piccionello, A., 2021. Ultrasound-guided lateral transversus abdominis plane (TAP) block in rabbits: a cadaveric study. Animals 11 (7). https://doi.org/10.3390/ani11071953.

Difilippo, S.M., Norberg, P.J., Suson, U.D., Savino, A.M., Reim, D.A., 2004. A comparison of xylazine and medetomidine in an anesthetic combination in New Zealand White Rabbits. Contemp. Top. Lab. Anim. Sci. 43 (1), 32–34. Retrieved from. https://www.ncbi.nlm.nih.gov/pubmed/14984287.

DiVincenti Jr., L., Meirelles, L.A., Westcott, R.A., 2016. Safety and clinical effectiveness of a compounded sustained-release formulation of buprenorphine for postoperative analgesia in New Zealand White rabbits. J. Am. Vet. Med. Assoc. 248 (7), 795–801. https://doi.org/10.2460/javma.248.7.795.

Doerning, B.J., Brammer, D.W., Chrisp, C.E., Rush, H.G., 1992. Nephrotoxicity of tiletamine in New Zealand white rabbits. Lab. Anim. Sci. 42 (3), 267–269. Retrieved from. https://www.ncbi.nlm.nih.gov/pubmed/1320157.

Doherty, T.J., 1988. Physiologic effects of alpha 2-adrenergic receptors. J. Am. Vet. Med. Assoc. 192 (11), 1612–1614. Retrieved from. https://www.ncbi.nlm.nih.gov/pubmed/2900824.

Dollo, G., Le Corre, P., Chevanne, F., Le Verge, R., 2004a. Bupivacaine containing dry emulsion can prolong epidural anesthetic effects in rabbits. Eur. J. Pharmaceut. Sci. 22 (1), 63–70. https://doi.org/10.1016/j.ejps.2004.02.008.

Dollo, G., Malinovsky, J.M., Peron, A., Chevanne, F., Pinaud, M., Le Verge, R., Le Corre, P., 2004b. Prolongation of epidural bupivacaine effects with hyaluronic acid in rabbits. Int. J. Pharm. 272 (1–2), 109–119. https://doi.org/10.1016/j.ijpharm.2003.12.002.

Drude, N., Pawlowsky, K., Tanaka, H., Fukushima, K., Kogel, B., Tolba, R.H., 2016. Severity assessment in rabbits after partial hepatectomy: Part II. Lab. Anim. 50 (6), 468–475. https://doi.org/10.1177/0023677216677949.

Duke-Novakovski, T., Fujiyama, M., Beazley, S.G., 2020. Comparison of mainstream (Capnostat 5) and two low-flow sidestream capnometers (VM-2500-S and Capnostream) in spontaneously breathing rabbits anesthetized with a Bain coaxial breathing system. Vet. Anaesth. Analg. 47 (4), 537–546. https://doi.org/10.1016/j.vaa.2020.02.006.

Dupras, J., Vachon, P., Cuvelliez, S., Blais, D., 2001. [Anesthesia of the New Zealand rabbit using the the combination of tiletamine-zolazepam and ketamine-midazolam with or without xylazine]. Can. Vet. J. 42 (6), 455–460. Retrieved from. https://www.ncbi.nlm.nih.gov/pubmed/11424577.

Ecobichon, D.J., Comeau, A.M., 1974. Genetic polymorphism of plasma carboxylesterases in the rabbit: correlation with pharmacologic and toxicologic effects. Toxicol. Appl. Pharmacol. 27 (1), 28–40. https://doi.org/10.1016/0041-008x(74)90171-9.

Egger, C.M., Souza, M.J., Greenacre, C.B., Cox, S.K., Rohrbach, B.W., 2009. Effect of intravenous administration of tramadol hydrochloride on the minimum alveolar concentration of isoflurane in rabbits. Am. J. Vet. Res. 70 (8), 945–949. https://doi.org/10.2460/ajvr.70.8.945.

Engbers, S., Larkin, A., Rousset, N., Prebble, M., Jonnalagadda, M., Knight, C.G., Pang, D.S.J., 2017. Comparison of a supraglottic airway device (v-gel((R))) with blind orotracheal intubation in rabbits. Front. Vet. Sci. 4, 49. https://doi.org/10.3389/fvets.2017.00049.

Erdine, S., Yucel, A., Ozyalcin, S., Ozyuvaci, E., Talu, G.K., Ahiskali, B., Savci, N., 1999. Neurotoxicity of midazolam in the rabbit. Pain 80 (1–2), 419–423. https://doi.org/10.1016/s0304-3959(98)00240-1.

Eshar, D., Weese, J.S., 2014. Molecular analysis of the microbiota in hard feces from healthy rabbits (*Oryctolagus cuniculus*) medicated with long term oral meloxicam. BMC Vet. Res. 10, 62. https://doi.org/10.1186/1746-6148-10-62.

Evangelista-Vaz, R., Bergadano, A., Arras, M., Jirkof, P.D., 2018. Analgesic efficacy of subcutaneous-oral dosage of tramadol after surgery in C57BL/6J mice. J. Am. Assoc. Lab. Anim. Sci. 57 (4), 368–375. https://doi.org/10.30802/AALAS-JAALAS-17-000118.

Farinas, A.F., Stephanides, M., Kassis, S., Keller, P., Colazo, J.M., Thayer, W.P., 2020. Sciatic nerve injury model in rabbits: what to expect. Lab. Anim. 54 (6), 559–567. https://doi.org/10.1177/0023677219898481.

Feldman, E.R., Singh, B., Mishkin, N.G., Lachenauer, E.R., Martin-Flores, M., Daugherity, E.K., 2021. Effects of cisapride, buprenorphine, and their combination on gastrointestinal transit in New Zealand white rabbits. J. Am. Assoc. Lab. Anim. Sci. 60 (2), 221–228. https://doi.org/10.30802/AALAS-JAALAS-20-000064.

Fick, T.E., Schalm, S.W., 1987. A simple technique for endotracheal intubation in rabbits. Lab. Anim. 21 (3), 265–266. https://doi.org/10.1258/002367787781268837.

Fishback, J.E., Stronsky, S.M., Green, C.A., Bean, K.D., Froude, J.W., 2016. Antibody production in rabbits administered Freund's complete adjuvant and carprofen concurrently. Lab. Anim. 45 (2), 63–66. https://doi.org/10.1038/laban.937.

Flecknell, P., 2018. Analgesics in small mammals. Vet. Clin. North Am. Exot. Anim. Pract. 21 (1), 83–103. https://doi.org/10.1016/j.cvex.2017.08.003.

Flecknell, P.A., 2015a. Anaesthesia of common laboratory species: special considerations. In: Laboratory Animal Anesthesia, 4th. Elsevier, pp. 193–256.

Flecknell, P.A., 2015b. Basic principles of anaesthesia. In: Laboratory Animal Anesthesia, 4th. Elsevier, pp. 1–75.

Flecknell, P.A., Cruz, I.J., Liles, J.H., Whelan, G., 1996. Induction of anaesthesia with halothane and isoflurane in the rabbit: a comparison of the use of a face-mask or an anaesthetic chamber. Lab. Anim. 30 (1), 67–74. https://doi.org/10.1258/002367796780744910.

Flecknell, P.A., John, M., Mitchell, M., Shurey, C., Simpkin, S., 1983. Neuroleptanalgesia in the rabbit. Lab. Anim. 17 (2), 104–109. https://doi.org/10.1258/002367783780959420.

Flecknell, P.A., Liles, J.H., Williamson, H.A., 1990. The use of lignocaine-prilocaine local anaesthetic cream for pain-free venepuncture in laboratory animals. Lab. Anim. 24 (2), 142–146. https://doi.org/10.1258/002367790780890121.

Flecknell, P.A., Liles, J.H., Wootton, R., 1989. Reversal of fentanyl/fluanisone neuroleptanalgesia in the rabbit using mixed agonist/antagonist opioids. Lab. Anim. 23 (2), 147–155. https://doi.org/10.1258/002367789780863655.

Flecknell, P.A., Roughan, J.V., Hedenqvist, P., 1999. Induction of anaesthesia with sevoflurane and isoflurane in the rabbit. Lab. Anim. 33 (1), 41–46. https://doi.org/10.1258/002367799780578516.

Flegal, M.C., Fox, L.K., Kuhlman, S.M., 2009a. Principles of anesthesia monitoring and electrocardiogram. J. Invest. Surg. 22 (4), 316–317. https://doi.org/10.1080/08941930903042086.

Flegal, M.C., Fox, L.K., Kuhlman, S.M., 2009b. Principles of anesthesia monitoring—arterial blood pressure. J. Invest. Surg. 22 (2), 154–155. https://doi.org/10.1080/08941930902813537.

Flegal, M.C., Fox, L.K., Kuhlman, S.M., 2009c. Principles of anesthesia monitoring—respiration. J. Invest. Surg. 22 (1), 76. https://doi.org/10.1080/08941930802708167.

Foley, P.L., Henderson, A.L., Bissonette, E.A., Wimer, G.R., Feldman, S.H., 2001. Evaluation of fentanyl transdermal patches in rabbits: blood concentrations and physiologic response. Comp. Med. 51 (3), 239–244. Retrieved from. https://www.ncbi.nlm.nih.gov/pubmed/11924779.

Fonseca, C., Server, A., Esteves, M., Barastegui, D., Rosal, M., Fontecha, C.G., Soldado, F., 2015. An ultrasound-guided technique for axillary brachial plexus nerve block in rabbits. Lab. Anim. 44 (5), 179–184. https://doi.org/10.1038/laban.732.

Fox, L.K., Flegal, M.C., Kuhlman, S.M., 2008. Principles of anesthesia monitoring—body temperature. J. Invest. Surg. 21 (6), 373–374. https://doi.org/10.1080/08941930802411937.

Fusco, A., Douglas, H., Barba, A., Hopster, K., Stefanovski, D., Sinder, B., Schaer, T.P., 2021. V-Gel((R)) guided endotracheal intubation in rabbits. Front. Vet. Sci. 8, 684624. https://doi.org/10.3389/fvets.2021.684624.

Gaveriaux-Ruff, C., Kieffer, B.L., 2002. Opioid receptor genes inactivated in mice: the highlights. Neuropeptides 36 (2–3), 62–71. https://doi.org/10.1054/npep.2002.0900.

Ghaffari, M.S., Moghaddassi, A.P., Bokaie, S., 2009. Effects of intramuscular acepromazine and diazepam on tear production in rabbits. Vet. Rec. 164 (5), 147–148. https://doi.org/10.1136/vr.164.5.147.

Gil, A.G., Silvan, G., Villa, A., Illera, J.C., 2012. Heart and respiratory rates and adrenal response to propofol or alfaxalone in rabbits. Vet. Rec. 170 (17), 444. https://doi.org/10.1136/vr.100573.

Gil, A.G., Silvan, G., Villa, A., Millan, P., Martinez-Fernandez, L., Illera, J.C., 2010. Serum biochemical response to inhalant anesthetics in New Zealand white rabbits. J. Am. Assoc. Lab. Anim. Sci. 49 (1), 52–56. Retrieved from. https://www.ncbi.nlm.nih.gov/pubmed/20122317.

Gillett, N.A., Brooks, D.L., Tillman, P.C., 1983. Medical and surgical management of gastric obstruction from a hairball in the rabbit. J. Am. Vet. Med. Assoc. 183 (11), 1176–1178. Retrieved from. https://www.ncbi.nlm.nih.gov/pubmed/6643229.

Gografe, S.I., Wilson, J.S., Johnson, B.L., Rushing, G., Bowser, A., Parker, J.L., Cornelius, C.E., 2003. Successful management of long-term general anesthesia in rabbits used as an animal model of human disease. Contemp. Top. Lab. Anim. Sci. 42 (2), 16–19. Retrieved from. https://www.ncbi.nlm.nih.gov/pubmed/19757619.

Goldschlager, G.B., Gillespie, V.L., Palme, R., Baxter, M.G., 2013. Effects of multimodal analgesia with LowDose buprenorphine and meloxicam on fecal glucocorticoid metabolites after surgery in New Zealand white rabbits (*Oryctolagus cuniculus*). J. Am. Assoc. Lab. Anim. Sci. 52 (5), 571–576. Retrieved from. https://www.ncbi.nlm.nih.gov/pubmed/24041213.

Gonzalez-Gil, A., Villa, A., Millan, P., Martinez-Fernandez, L., Illera, J.C., 2015. Effects of dexmedetomidine and ketamine-dexmedetomidine with and without buprenorphine on corticoadrenal function in rabbits. J. Am. Assoc. Lab. Anim. Sci. 54 (3), 299–303. Retrieved from. https://www.ncbi.nlm.nih.gov/pubmed/26045456.

Green, C.J., 1975. Neuroleptanalgesic drug combinations in the anaesthetic management of small laboratory animals. Lab. Anim. 9 (3), 161–178. https://doi.org/10.1258/002367775780994574.

Green, C.J., Knight, J., Precious, S., Simpkin, S., 1981. Ketamine alone and combined with diazepam or xylazine in laboratory animals: a 10 year experience. Lab. Anim. 15 (2), 163–170. https://doi.org/10.1258/002367781780959107.

Grint, N.J., Sayers, I.R., Cecchi, R., Harley, R., Day, M.J., 2006. Post-anaesthetic tracheal strictures in three rabbits. Lab. Anim. 40 (3), 301–308. https://doi.org/10.1258/002367706777611415.

Grint, N.J., Smith, H.E., Senior, J.M., 2008. Clinical evaluation of alfaxalone in cyclodextrin for the induction of anaesthesia in rabbits. Vet. Rec. 163 (13), 395–396. https://doi.org/10.1136/vr.163.13.395.

Grubb, T., Lobprise, H., 2020a. Local and regional anaesthesia in dogs and cats: descriptions of specific local and regional techniques (Part 2). Vet. Med. Sci. 6 (2), 218–234. https://doi.org/10.1002/vms3.218.

Grubb, T., Lobprise, H., 2020b. Local and regional anaesthesia in dogs and cats: overview of concepts and drugs (Part 1). Vet. Med. Sci. 6 (2), 209–217. https://doi.org/10.1002/vms3.219.

Gusak, V., Turkovic, V., Nesek-Adam, V., Lerotic, I., Popovic, M., Brajenovic, N., Vnuk, D., 2013. Lidocaine serum concentration after epidural administration in combination with morphine and fentanyl in rabbit—a preliminary study. Res. Vet. Sci. 94 (3), 651–655. https://doi.org/10.1016/j.rvsc.2012.10.001.

Hampshire, V., Robertson, S., 2015. Using the facial grimace scale to evaluate rabbit wellness in post-procedural monitoring. Lab. Anim. 44 (7), 259–260. https://doi.org/10.1038/laban.806.

Hawkins, M.G., Pascoe, P.J., 2021. 37—anesthesia, analgesia, and sedation of small mammals. In: Quesenberry, K.E., Orcutt, C.J., Mans, C., Carpenter, J.W. (Eds.), Ferrets, Rabbits, and Rodents, fourth ed. W.B. Saunders, Philadelphia, pp. 536–558.

Hawkins, M.G., Taylor, I.T., Craigmill, A.L., Tell, L.A., 2008. Enantioselective pharmacokinetics of racemic carprofen in New Zealand white rabbits. J. Vet. Pharmacol. Therapeut. 31 (5), 423–430. https://doi.org/10.1111/j.1365-2885.2008.00975.x.

Hedenqvist, P., Edner, A., Fahlman, A., Jensen-Waern, M., 2013. Continuous intravenous anaesthesia with sufentanil and midazolam in medetomidine premedicated New Zealand White rabbits. BMC Vet. Res. 9, 21. https://doi.org/10.1186/1746-6148-9-21.

Hedenqvist, P., Edner, A., Jensen-Waern, M., 2014. Anaesthesia in medetomidine premedicated New Zealand White rabbits: a comparison between intravenous sufentanil-midazolam and isoflurane anaesthesia for orthopaedic surgery. Lab. Anim. 48 (2), 155–163. https://doi.org/10.1177/0023677213516311.

Hedenqvist, P., Orr, H.E., Roughan, J.V., Antunes, L.M., Flecknell, P.A., 2002. Anaesthesia with ketamine/medetomidine in the rabbit: influence of route of administration and the effect of combination with butorphanol. Vet. Anaesth. Analg. 29 (1), 14–19. https://doi.org/10.1046/j.1467-2987.2001.00058.x.

Hedenqvist, P., Roughan, J., Orr, H., Antunes, L.M., 2001a. Assessment of ketamine/medetomidine anaesthesia in the New Zealand White rabbit. Vet. Anaesth. Analg. 28 (1), 18–25. https://doi.org/10.1046/j.1467-2995.2001.00019.x.

Hedenqvist, P., Roughan, J.V., Antunes, L., Orr, H., Flecknell, P.A., 2001b. Induction of anaesthesia with desflurane and isoflurane in the rabbit. Lab. Anim. 35 (2), 172–179. https://doi.org/10.1258/0023677011911561.

Hedenqvist, P., Trbakovic, A., Mellgren, T., Ohman-Magi, C., Hammarstrom Johansson, P., Manell, E., Thor, A., 2020. The effect of housing environment on bone healing in a critical radius defect in New Zealand White rabbits. PLoS One 15 (5), e0233530. https://doi.org/10.1371/journal.pone.0233530.

Hedenqvist, P., Trbakovic, A., Thor, A., Ley, C., Ekman, S., Jensen-Waern, M., 2016. Carprofen neither reduces postoperative facial expression scores in rabbits treated with buprenorphine nor alters long term bone formation after maxillary sinus grafting. Res. Vet. Sci. 107, 123–131. https://doi.org/10.1016/j.rvsc.2016.05.010.

Hellebrekers, L.J., de Boer, E.J., van Zuylen, M.A., Vosmeer, H., 1997. A comparison between medetomidine-ketamine and medetomidine-propofol anaesthesia in rabbits. Lab. Anim. 31 (1), 58–69. https://doi.org/10.1258/002367797780600215.

Henke, J., Astner, S., Brill, T., Eissner, B., Busch, R., Erhardt, W., 2005. Comparative study of three intramuscular anaesthetic combinations (medetomidine/ketamine, medetomidine/fentanyl/midazolam and xylazine/ketamine) in rabbits. Vet. Anaesth. Analg. 32 (5), 261–270. https://doi.org/10.1111/j.1467-2995.2005.00242.x.

Hennies, H.H., Friderichs, E., Schneider, J., 1988. Receptor binding, analgesic and antitussive potency of tramadol and other selected opioids. Arzneimittel-forschung 38 (7), 877–880. Retrieved from. https://www.ncbi.nlm.nih.gov/pubmed/2849950.

Hino, Y., Inoue, H., Kudo, K., Nishida, N., Ikeda, N., 2001. Distribution of tetracaine and its metabolite in rabbits after high versus normal spinal anesthesia. Forensic Sci. Int. 124 (2–3), 130–136. https://doi.org/10.1016/s0379-0738(01)00585-0.

Hobbs, B.A., Rolhall, T.G., Sprenkel, T.L., Anthony, K.L., 1991. Comparison of several combinations for anesthesia in rabbits. Am. J. Vet. Res. 52 (5), 669–674. Retrieved from. https://www.ncbi.nlm.nih.gov/pubmed/1854090.

Hogan, Q.H., Amuzu, J., Clifford, P.S., Bosnjak, Z.J., Kampine, J.P., 1998. Hypoxia causes apnea during epidural anesthesia in rabbits. Anesthesiology 88 (3), 761–767. https://doi.org/10.1097/00000542-199803000-00028.

Hopper, K., Powell, L.L., 2013. Basics of mechanical ventilation for dogs and cats. Vet. Clin. North Am. Small Anim. Pract. 43 (4), 955–969. https://doi.org/10.1016/j.cvsm.2013.03.009.

Howard, P.J., Wittry, J.P., Blum, J.R., 1990. Use of an audible respiratory monitor to aid endotracheal intubation of the rabbit [abstract P22]. Lab. Anim. Sci. 40, 562–563.

Hughes, P.J., Doherty, M.M., Charman, W.N., 1993. A rabbit model for the evaluation of epidurally administered local anaesthetic agents. Anaesth. Intensive Care 21 (3), 298–303. https://doi.org/10.1177/0310057X9302100307.

Imai, A., Eisele, P.H., Steffey, E.P., 2005. A new airway device for small laboratory animals. Lab. Anim. 39 (1), 111–115. https://doi.org/10.1258/0023677052886484.

Imai, A., Steffey, E.P., Ilkiw, J.E., Farver, T.B., 1999. Comparison of clinical signs and hemodynamic variables used to monitor rabbits during halothane- and isoflurane-induced anesthesia. Am. J. Vet. Res. 60 (10), 1189–1195. Retrieved from. https://www.ncbi.nlm.nih.gov/pubmed/10791928.

Irazuzta, J., Hopkins, J., Gunnoe, P., Brittain, E., 1997. Simple method of multipurpose airway access through percutaneous tracheostomy in rabbits (*Oryctolagus cuniculus*). Lab. Anim. Sci. 47 (4), 411–413. Retrieved from. https://www.ncbi.nlm.nih.gov/pubmed/9306316.

Jensen, F.M., Dahl, J.B., Frigast, C., 1992. Direct spinal effect of intrathecal acetaminophen on visceral noxious stimulation in rabbits. Acta Anaesthesiol. Scand. 36 (8), 837–841. https://doi.org/10.1111/j.1399-6576.1992.tb03574.x.

Keating, S.C., Thomas, A.A., Flecknell, P.A., Leach, M.C., 2012. Evaluation of EMLA cream for preventing pain during tattooing of rabbits: changes in physiological, behavioural and facial expression responses. PLoS One 7 (9), e44437. https://doi.org/10.1371/journal.pone.0044437.

Kent, G.M., 1971. General anesthesia in rabbits using methoxyflurane, nitrous oxide, and oxygen. Lab. Anim. Sci. 21 (2), 256–257. Retrieved from. https://www.ncbi.nlm.nih.gov/pubmed/4325702.

Keown, A.J., Farnworth, M.J., Adams, N.J., 2011. Attitudes towards perception and management of pain in rabbits and Guinea pigs by a sample of veterinarians in New Zealand. N. Z. Vet. J. 59 (6), 305–310. https://doi.org/10.1080/00480169.2011.609477.

Kim, M.S., Jeong, S.M., Park, J.H., Nam, T.C., Seo, K.M., 2004. Reversal of medetomidine-ketamine combination anesthesia in rabbits by atipamezole. Exp. Anim. 53 (5), 423–428. https://doi.org/10.1538/expanim.53.423.

Kluge, K., Larenza Menzies, M.P., Kloeppel, H., Pearce, S.G., Bettschart-Wolfensberger, R., Kutter, A.P., 2017. Femoral and sciatic nerve blockades and incision site infiltration in rabbits undergoing stifle joint arthrotomy. Lab. Anim. 51 (1), 54–64. https://doi.org/10.1177/0023677215622734.

Ko, J.C., Thurmon, J.C., Tranquilli, W.J., Benson, G.J., Olson, W.A., 1992. A comparison of medetomidine-propofol and medetomidine-midazolam-propofol anesthesia in rabbits. Lab. Anim. Sci. 42 (5), 503–507. Retrieved from. https://www.ncbi.nlm.nih.gov/pubmed/1460852.

Komoda, Y., Nosaka, S., Takenoshita, M., 2003. Enhancement of lidocaine-induced epidural anesthesia by deoxyaconitine in the rabbit. J. Anesth. 17 (4), 241–245. https://doi.org/10.1007/s00540-003-0184-6.

Kounenis, G., Koutsoviti-Papadopoulou, M., Elezoglou, A., Voutsas, A., 1992. Comparative study of the H2-receptor antagonists cimetidine, ranitidine, famotidine and nizatidine on the rabbit stomach fundus and sigmoid colon. J. Pharmacobio-Dyn 15 (10), 561–565. https://doi.org/10.1248/bpb1978.15.561.

Kumar, R.A., Boyer, M.I., Bowen, C.V., 1993. A reliable method of anesthesia for extensive surgery in small rabbits. Lab. Anim. Sci. 43 (3), 265–266. Retrieved from. https://www.ncbi.nlm.nih.gov/pubmed/8355492.

Langerman, L., Chaimsky, G., Golomb, E., Tverskoy, M., Kook, A.I., Benita, S., 1990. A rabbit model for evaluation of spinal anesthesia: chronic cannulation of the subarachnoid space. Anesth. Analg. 71 (5), 529–535. https://doi.org/10.1213/00000539-199011000-00013.

Leach, M.C., Allweiler, S., Richardson, C., Roughan, J.V., Narbe, R., Flecknell, P.A., 2009. Behavioural effects of ovariohysterectomy and oral administration of meloxicam in laboratory housed rabbits. Res. Vet. Sci. 87 (2), 336–347. https://doi.org/10.1016/j.rvsc.2009.02.001.

Lee, L.Y., Lee, D., Ryu, H., Han, J.H., Ko, J., Tyler, J.W., 2019. Capnography-guided endotracheal intubation as an alternative to existing intubation methods in rabbits. J. Am. Assoc. Lab. Anim. Sci. 58 (2), 240–245. https://doi.org/10.30802/AALAS-JAALAS-17-000150.

Lightowler, J.E., Smith, A.E., 1963. Beta-(N-Pyrrolidyl)-Butyroanilid (Ws 10): its subacute toxicity, influence on morphine analgesia in the rat and morphine analgesia and respiratory depression in the rabbit. Arch. Int. Pharmacodyn. Ther. 144, 97–111. Retrieved from. https://www.ncbi.nlm.nih.gov/pubmed/14043657.

Lindquist, P.A., 1972. Induction of methoxyflurane anesthesia in the rabbit after ketamine hydrochloride and endotracheal intubation. Lab. Anim. Sci. 22 (6), 898–899. Retrieved from. https://www.ncbi.nlm.nih.gov/pubmed/4345312.

Lipman, N.S., Marini, R.P., Erdman, S.E., 1990. A comparison of ketamine/xylazine and ketamine/xylazine/acepromazine anesthesia in the rabbit. Lab. Anim. Sci. 40 (4), 395–398. Retrieved from. https://www.ncbi.nlm.nih.gov/pubmed/2166867.

Lipman, N.S., Phillips, P.A., Newcomer, C.E., 1987. Reversal of ketamine/xylazine anesthesia in the rabbit with yohimbine. Lab. Anim. Sci. 37 (4), 474–477. Retrieved from. https://www.ncbi.nlm.nih.gov/pubmed/3669601.

Lockhart, S.H., Cohen, Y., Yasuda, N., Freire, B., Taheri, S., Litt, L., Eger 2nd, E.I., 1991. Cerebral uptake and elimination of desflurane, isoflurane, and halothane from rabbit brain: an in vivo NMR study. Anesthesiology 74 (3), 575–580. https://doi.org/10.1097/00000542-199103000-00028.

Ludders, J.W., Thomas, C.B., Sharp, P., Sedgwick, C.J., 1987. An anesthetic technique for repeated collection of blood from New Zealand white rabbits. Lab. Anim. Sci. 37 (6), 803–805. Retrieved from. https://www.ncbi.nlm.nih.gov/pubmed/3437762.

Ma, D., Sapsed-Byrne, S.M., Chakrabarti, M.K., Whitwam, J.G., 1998. Effect of sevoflurane on spontaneous sympathetic activity and baroreflexes in rabbits. Br. J. Anaesth. 80 (1), 68–72. https://doi.org/10.1093/bja/80.1.68.

Macrae, D.J., Guerreiro, D., 1989. A simple laryngoscopic technique for the endotracheal intubation of rabbits. Lab. Anim. 23 (1), 59–61. https://doi.org/10.1258/002367789780886993.

Madsen, J.B., Jensen, F.M., Faber, T., Bille-Hansen, V., 1993. Chronic catheterization of the epidural space in rabbits: a model for behavioural and histopathological studies. Examination of meptazinol neurotoxicity. Acta Anaesthesiol. Scand. 37 (3), 307–313. https://doi.org/10.1111/j.1399-6576.1993.tb03720.x.

Malinovsky, J.M., Charles, F., Baudrimont, M., Pereon, Y., Le Corre, P., Pinaud, M., Benhamou, D., 2002. Intrathecal ropivacaine in rabbits: pharmacodynamic and neurotoxicologic study. Anesthesiology 97 (2), 429–435. https://doi.org/10.1097/00000542-200208000-00021.

Mansour, A., Fox, C.A., Akil, H., Watson, S.J., 1995. Opioid-receptor mRNA expression in the rat CNS: anatomical and functional implications. Trends Neurosci. 18 (1), 22–29. https://doi.org/10.1016/0166-2236(95)93946-u.

Margolis, F., Feigelson, P., 1963. Purification and characterization of a genetically determined rabbit serum esterase. J. Biol. Chem. 238, 2620–2627. Retrieved from. https://www.ncbi.nlm.nih.gov/pubmed/14063282.

Marini, R.P., Avison, D.L., Corning, B.F., Lipman, N.S., 1992. Ketamine/xylazine/butorphanol: a new anesthetic combination for rabbits. Lab. Anim. Sci. 42 (1), 57–62. Retrieved from. https://www.ncbi.nlm.nih.gov/pubmed/1316511.

Marini, R.P., Hurley, R.J., Avison, D.L., Lipman, N.S., 1993. An evaluation of three neuroleptanalgesic combinations in rabbits. Lab. Anim. Sci. 43 (4), 338–345. Retrieved from. https://www.ncbi.nlm.nih.gov/pubmed/7901451.

Marsh, M.K., McLeod, S.R., Hansen, A., Maloney, S.K., 2009. Induction of anaesthesia in wild rabbits using a new alfaxalone formulation. Vet. Rec. 164 (4), 122–123. https://doi.org/10.1136/vr.164.4.122.

Martin-Cancho, M.F., Lima, J.R., Luis, L., Crisostomo, V., Carrasco-Jimenez, M.S., Uson-Gargallo, J., 2006. Relationship of bispectral index values, haemodynamic changes and recovery times during sevoflurane or propofol anaesthesia in rabbits. Lab. Anim. 40 (1), 28–42. https://doi.org/10.1258/002367706775404462.

Martin-Flores, M., Singh, B., Walsh, C.A., Brooks, E.P., Taylor, L., Mitchell, L.M., 2017. Effects of buprenorphine, methylnaltrexone, and their combination on gastrointestinal transit in healthy New Zealand white rabbits. J. Am. Assoc. Lab. Anim. Sci. 56 (2), 155–159. Retrieved from. https://www.ncbi.nlm.nih.gov/pubmed/28315644.

Mattila, M.J., Saarnivaara, L., 1968. Modification by antihistaminic drugs of the morphine analgesia in rabbits. Ann. Med. Exp. Biol. Fenn. 46 (1), 72–77. Retrieved from. https://www.ncbi.nlm.nih.gov/pubmed/4387283.

Mayer, J., 2007. Use of behavior analysis to recognize pain in small mammals. Lab. Anim. 36 (6), 43–48. https://doi.org/10.1038/laban0607-43.

Mazaheri-Khameneh, R., Sarrafzadeh-Rezaei, F., Asri-Rezaei, S., Dalir-Naghadeh, B., 2012. Evaluation of clinical and paraclinical effects of intraosseous vs intravenous administration of propofol on general anesthesia in rabbits. Vet. Res. Forum 3 (2), 103–109. Retrieved from. https://www.ncbi.nlm.nih.gov/pubmed/25653755.

Maze, M., Tranquilli, W., 1991. Alpha-2 adrenoceptor agonists: defining the role in clinical anesthesia. Anesthesiology 74 (3), 581–605. Retrieved from. https://www.ncbi.nlm.nih.gov/pubmed/1672060.

McCallister, L.W., Lipton, J.M., Giesecke Jr., A.H., Clark, W.G., 1986. The rabbit ear-withdrawal test: a new analgesiometric procedure. Pharmacol. Biochem. Behav. 25 (2), 481–482. https://doi.org/10.1016/0091-3057(86)90027-4.

Mehler, S.J., 2006. Common surgical procedures. In: Flecknell, A.M.A.P.A. (Ed.), BSAVA Manual of Rabbit Medicine and Surgery. British Small Animal Veterinary Association, Gloucester, UK, pp. 166–168.

Melzack, R., Coderre, T.J., Katz, J., Vaccarino, A.L., 2001. Central neuroplasticity and pathological pain. Ann. N. Y. Acad. Sci. 933, 157–174. https://doi.org/10.1111/j.1749-6632.2001.tb05822.x.

Members, A.T.F., Kohn, D.F., Martin, T.E., Foley, P.L., Morris, T.H., Swindle, M.M., Wixson, S.K., 2007. Public statement: guidelines for the assessment and management of pain in rodents and rabbits. J. Am. Assoc. Lab. Anim. Sci. 46 (2), 97–108. Retrieved from. https://www.ncbi.nlm.nih.gov/pubmed/17427317.

Mencalha, R., Sousa, C.A., Costa, O., Abidu-Figueiredo, M., 2016. Ultrasound and gross anatomy of the brachial plexus and major nerves of the forelimb. An anesthetic approach using the domestic rabbit (Oyctolagus cuniculus) as an experimental modell. Acta Cir. Bras. 31 (4), 218–226. https://doi.org/10.1590/S0102-865020160040000001.

Mirschberger, V., von Deimling, C., Heider, A., Spadavecchia, C., Rohrbach, H., Zeiter, S., 2020. Fentanyl plasma concentrations after application of a transdermal patch in three different locations to refine postoperative pain management in rabbits. Animals 10 (10). https://doi.org/10.3390/ani10101778.

Monteiro, B., Steagall, P.V., 2019. Antiinflammatory drugs. Vet. Clin. North Am. Small Anim. Pract. 49 (6), 993–1011. https://doi.org/10.1016/j.cvsm.2019.07.009.

Murphy, K.L., Roughan, J.V., Baxter, M.G., Flecknell, P.A., 2010. Anaesthesia with a combination of ketamine and medetomidine in the rabbit: effect of premedication with buprenorphine. Vet. Anaesth. Analg. 37 (3), 222–229. https://doi.org/10.1111/j.1467-2995.2009.00525.x.

Najman, I.E., Ferreira, J.Z., Abimussi, C.J., Floriano, B.P., Meneghetti, T.M., Oliva, V.N., do Nascimento Jr., P., 2015. Ultrasound-assisted periconal ocular blockade in rabbits. Vet. Anaesth. Analg. 42 (4), 433–441. https://doi.org/10.1111/vaa.12237.

Navarrete-Calvo, R., Gomez-Villamandos, R.J., Morgaz, J., Manuel Dominguez, J., Fernandez-Sarmiento, A., Munoz-Rascon, P., Del Mar Granados, M., 2014. Cardiorespiratory, anaesthetic and recovery effects of morphine combined with medetomidine and alfaxalone in rabbits. Vet. Rec. 174 (4), 95. https://doi.org/10.1136/vr.101293.

Nelson, J.M., Krummel, T.M., Haynes, J.H., Flood, L.C., Sauer, L., Flake, A.W., Harrison, M.R., 1990. Operative techniques in the fetal rabbit. J. Invest. Surg. 3, 393–398. https://doi.org/10.3109/08941939009140366.

Niu, W.X., He, G.D., Liu, H., Qin, X.Y., 2007. Effects and probable mechanisms of electroacupuncture at the Zusanli point on upper gastrointestinal motility in rabbits. J. Gastroenterol. Hepatol. 22 (10), 1683–1689. https://doi.org/10.1111/j.1440-1746.2007.05049.x.

Nordin, U., Lindholm, C.E., 1977. The vessels of the rabbit trachea and ischemia caused by cuff pressure. Arch. Oto-Rhino-Laryngol. 215 (1), 11–24. https://doi.org/10.1007/BF00463187.

Nordin, U., Lindholm, C.E., Wolgast, M., 1977. Blood flow in the rabbit tracheal mucosa under normal conditions and under the influence of tracheal intubation. Acta Anaesthesiol. Scand. 21 (2), 81–94. https://doi.org/10.1111/j.1399-6576.1977.tb01198.x.

Nowland, B.B., Garcia, A., Rush, H.G., 2015. Biology and diseases of rabbits. In: JG, F. (Ed.), Laboratory Animal Medicine, third ed. Elsevier, Cambridge, MA, pp. 411–461.

Occupational Safety & Health Administration, (OSHA), 2022. Regulations (Standards-29 CFR 1910). https://www.osha.gov.

Oglesbee, B.L., 2021. Gastrointestinal diseases of rabbits. In: Quesenberry, C.J.O.K.E., Mans, C., Carpenter, J.W. (Eds.), Ferrets, Rabbits, and Rodents: Clinical Medicine and Surgery, fourth ed., pp. 174–187.

Olson, M.E., Vizzutti, D., Morck, D.W., Cox, A.K., 1994. The parasympatholytic effects of atropine sulfate and glycopyrrolate in rats and rabbits. Can. J. Vet. Res. 58 (4), 254–258. Retrieved from. https://www.ncbi.nlm.nih.gov/pubmed/7889456.

Ong, B.H.E., Hidaka, Y., Kaneko, Y., Yamamoto, S., Mizutani, S., Sekiguchi, S., Naganobu, K., 2020. Effects of a single-bolus bupivacaine injection into the coccygeal spinal canal of rabbits. J. Vet. Med. Sci. 82 (2), 197–203. https://doi.org/10.1292/jvms.19-0555.

Orr, H.E., Roughan, J.V., Flecknell, P.A., 2005. Assessment of ketamine and medetomidine anaesthesia in the domestic rabbit. Vet. Anaesth. Analg. 32 (5), 271–279. https://doi.org/10.1111/j.1467-2995.2005.00211.x.

Otero, P.E., Portela, D.A., Brinkyer, J.A., Tarragona, L., Zaccagnini, A.S., Fuensalida, S.E., Ceballos, M.R., 2012. Use of electrical stimulation to monitor lumbosacral epidural and intrathecal needle placement in rabbits. Am. J. Vet. Res. 73 (8), 1137–1141. https://doi.org/10.2460/ajvr.73.8.1137.

Paddleford, R.R., Harvey, R.C., 1999. Alpha 2 agonists and antagonists. Vet. Clin. North Am. Small Anim. Pract. 29 (3), 737–745. https://doi.org/10.1016/s0195-5616(99)50058-2.

Paul-Murphy, J., Ramer, J.C., 1998. Urgent care of the pet rabbit. Vet. Clin. North Am. Exot. Anim. Pract. 1 (1), 127–152. https://doi.org/10.1016/s1094-9194(17)30158-5. vi-vii.

Peeters, M.E., Gil, D., Teske, E., Eyzenbach, V., vd Brom, W.E., Lumeij, J.T., de Vries, H.W., 1988. Four methods for general anaesthesia in the rabbit: a comparative study. Lab. Anim. 22 (4), 355–360. https://doi.org/10.1258/002367788780746197.

Pekow, C.A., 2012. Basic experimental methods in the rabbit. In: Suckow, K.A.S.M.A., Wilson, R.P. (Eds.), The Laboratory Rabbit, Guinea Pig, Hamster, and Other Rodents. Elsevier, Waltham, MA, pp. 243–258.

Persson, J., Axelsson, G., Hallin, R.G., Gustafsson, L.L., 1995. Beneficial effects of ketamine in a chronic pain state with allodynia, possibly due to central sensitization. Pain 60 (2), 217–222. https://doi.org/10.1016/0304-3959(94)00139-6.

Phaneuf, L.R., Barker, S., Groleau, M.A., Turner, P.V., 2006. Tracheal injury after endotracheal intubation and anesthesia in rabbits. J. Am. Assoc. Lab. Anim. Sci. 45 (6), 67–72. Retrieved from. https://www.ncbi.nlm.nih.gov/pubmed/17089996.

Piercey, M.F., Schroeder, L.A., 1980. A quantitative analgesic assay in the rabbit based on the response to tooth pulp stimulation. Arch. Int. Pharmacodyn. Ther. 248 (2), 294–304. Retrieved from. https://www.ncbi.nlm.nih.gov/pubmed/7224712.

Pinho, R.H., Leach, M.C., Minto, B.W., Rocha, F.D.L., Luna, S.P.L., 2020. Postoperative pain behaviours in rabbits following orthopaedic surgery and effect of observer presence. PLoS One 15 (10), e0240605. https://doi.org/10.1371/journal.pone.0240605.

Popilskis, S.J., Oz, M.C., Gorman, P., Florestal, A., Kohn, D.F., 1991. Comparison of xylazine with tiletamine-zolazepam (Telazol) and xylazine-ketamine anesthesia in rabbits. Lab. Anim. Sci. 41 (1), 51–53. Retrieved from. https://www.ncbi.nlm.nih.gov/pubmed/1849587.

Portnoy, L.G., Hustead, D.R., 1992. Pharmacokinetics of butorphanol tartrate in rabbits. Am. J. Vet. Res. 53 (4), 541–543. Retrieved from. https://www.ncbi.nlm.nih.gov/pubmed/1586025.

Raffa, R.B., Friderichs, E., Reimann, W., Shank, R.P., Codd, E.E., Vaught, J.L., 1992. Opioid and nonopioid components independently contribute to the mechanism of action of tramadol, an 'atypical' opioid analgesic. J. Pharmacol. Exp. Therapeut. 260 (1), 275–285. Retrieved from. https://www.ncbi.nlm.nih.gov/pubmed/1309873.

Raillard, M., Detotto, C., Grepper, S., Beslac, O., Fujioka-Kobayashi, M., Schaller, B., Saulacic, N., 2019. Anaesthetic and perioperative management of 14 male New Zealand white rabbits for calvarial bone surgery. Animals 9 (11). https://doi.org/10.3390/ani9110896.

Raman, J., Montano, S.R., Lord, R.S., 1989. Assisted local anaesthesia in rabbits. Microsurgery 10 (1), 75–76. https://doi.org/10.1002/micr.1920100113.

Reichert, P., Rutowski, R., Kielbowicz, Z., Kuryszko, J., Kielbowicz, M., 2013. General intravenous anesthesia for brachial plexus surgery in the rabbit. Pol. J. Vet. Sci. 16 (4), 755–756. https://doi.org/10.2478/pjvs-2013-0108.

Reuter, J.D., Fowles, K.J., Terwilliger, G.A., Booth, C.J., 2005. Iatrogenic tension pneumothorax in a rabbit (*Oryctolagus cuniculus*). Contemp. Top. Lab. Anim. Sci. 44 (4), 22–25. Retrieved from. https://www.ncbi.nlm.nih.gov/pubmed/16050663.

Richard, B.M., Newton, P., Ott, L.R., Haan, D., Brubaker, A.N., Cole, P.I., Nelson, K.G., 2012. The safety of EXPAREL (R) (bupivacaine liposome injectable suspension) administered by peripheral nerve block in rabbits and dogs. J. Drug Deliv. 2012, 962101. https://doi.org/10.1155/2012/962101.

Sanford, T.D., Colby, E.D., 1980. Effect of xylazine and ketamine on blood pressure, heart rate and respiratory rate in rabbits. Lab. Anim. Sci. 30 (3), 519–523. Retrieved from. https://www.ncbi.nlm.nih.gov/pubmed/7431851.

Santangelo, B., Micieli, F., Mozzillo, T., Reynaud, F., Marino, F., Auletta, L., Vesce, G., 2016. Transnasal administration of a combination of dexmedetomidine, midazolam and butorphanol produces deep sedation in New Zealand White rabbits. Vet. Anaesth. Analg. 43 (2), 209–214. https://doi.org/10.1111/vaa.12278.

Santos, M.A., Lucera, T.M., Horr, M., Santana, I.N., Mattos-Junior, E., 2021. Comparative study on epidural administration of dexmedetomidine, dexmedetomidine-lidocaine or lidocaine in conscious rabbits. Lab. Anim. 55 (4), 341–349. https://doi.org/10.1177/0023677221993156.

Sayce, L.J., Powell, M.E., Kimball, E.E., Chen, P., Gartling, G.J., Rousseau, B., 2020. Continuous rate infusion of ketamine hydrochloride and dexmedetomidine for maintenance of anesthesia during laryngotracheal surgery in New Zealand white rabbits (*Oryctolagus cuniculus*). J. Am. Assoc. Lab. Anim. Sci. 59 (2), 176–185. https://doi.org/10.30802/AALAS-JAALAS-19-000076.

Schnellbacher, R.W., Divers, S.J., Comolli, J.R., Beaufrere, H., Maglaras, C.H., Andrade, N., Quandt, J.E., 2017. Effects of intravenous administration of lidocaine and buprenorphine on gastrointestinal tract motility and signs of pain in New Zealand White rabbits after ovariohysterectomy. Am. J. Vet. Res. 78 (12), 1359–1371. https://doi.org/10.2460/ajvr.78.12.1359.

Schroeder, C.A., Smith, L.J., 2011. Respiratory rates and arterial blood-gas tensions in healthy rabbits given buprenorphine, butorphanol, midazolam, or their combinations. J. Am. Assoc. Lab. Anim. Sci. 50 (2), 205–211. Retrieved from. https://www.ncbi.nlm.nih.gov/pubmed/21439214.

Schuyt, H.C., Leene, W., 1978. An improved method in rabbit intubation and thymectomy. Eur. Surg. Res. 10 (5), 362–372. https://doi.org/10.1159/000128027.

Schuyt, H.C., Meeder, P., Leene, W., 1978. A bit to immobilize the endotracheal tube in the intubated rabbit. Lab. Anim. Sci. 28 (4), 470–471. Retrieved from. https://www.ncbi.nlm.nih.gov/pubmed/703255.

Sedgwick, C.J., 1986. Anesthesia for rabbits. Vet. Clin. North Am. Food Anim. Pract. 2 (3), 731–736. https://doi.org/10.1016/s0749-0720(15)31214-7.

Shafford, H.L., Schadt, J.C., 2008. Effect of buprenorphine on the cardiovascular and respiratory response to visceral pain in conscious rabbits. Vet. Anaesth. Analg. 35 (4), 333–340. https://doi.org/10.1111/j.1467-2995.2007.00384.x.

Shi, X., Yu, W., Wang, T., Battulga, O., Wang, C., Shu, Q., Guo, C., 2020. Electroacupuncture alleviates cartilage degradation: improvement in cartilage biomechanics via pain relief and potentiation of muscle function in a rabbit model of knee osteoarthritis. Biomed. Pharmacother. 123, 109724. https://doi.org/10.1016/j.biopha.2019.109724.

Shimokawa, M., Kitaguchi, K., Kawaguchi, M., Sakamoto, T., Kakimoto, M., Furuya, H., 2003. The influence of induced hypothermia for hemostatic function on temperature-adjusted measurements in rabbits. Anesth. Analg. 96 (4), 1209–1213. https://doi.org/10.1213/01.ANE.0000050767.86196.AF.

Sikoski, P., Young, R.W., Lockard, M., 2007. Comparison of heating devices for maintaining body temperature in anesthetized laboratory rabbits (*Oryctolagus cuniculus*). J. Am. Assoc. Lab. Anim. Sci. 46 (3),

61–63. Retrieved from. https://www.ncbi.nlm.nih.gov/pubmed/17487956.

Smith, J.C., Robertson, L.D., Auhll, A., March, T.J., Derring, C., Bolon, B., 2004. Endotracheal tubes versus laryngeal mask airways in rabbit inhalation anesthesia: ease of use and waste gas emissions. Contemp. Top. Lab. Anim. Sci. 43 (4), 22–25. Retrieved from. https://www.ncbi.nlm.nih.gov/pubmed/15264765.

Song, J., Hoenerhoff, M., Yang, D., Yang, Y., Deng, C., Wen, L., Xu, J., 2021. Development of the nude rabbit model. Stem Cell Rep. 16 (3), 656–665. https://doi.org/10.1016/j.stemcr.2021.01.010.

Song, J., Wang, G., Hoenerhoff, M.J., Ruan, J., Yang, D., Zhang, J., Xu, J., 2018. Bacterial and Pneumocystis infections in the lungs of gene-knockout rabbits with severe combined immunodeficiency. Front. Immunol. 9, 429. https://doi.org/10.3389/fimmu.2018.00429.

Song, J., Yang, D., Ruan, J., Zhang, J., Chen, Y.E., Xu, J., 2017. Production of immunodeficient rabbits by multiplex embryo transfer and multiplex gene targeting. Sci. Rep. 7 (1), 12202. https://doi.org/10.1038/s41598-017-12201-0.

Souza, M.J., Cox, S.K., 2011. Tramadol use in zoologic medicine. Vet. Clin. North Am. Exot. Anim. Pract. 14 (1), 117–130. https://doi.org/10.1016/j.cvex.2010.09.005.

Souza, M.J., Greenacre, C.B., Cox, S.K., 2008. Pharmacokinetics of orally administered tramadol in domestic rabbits (*Oryctolagus cuniculus*). Am. J. Vet. Res. 69 (8), 979–982. https://doi.org/10.2460/ajvr.69.8.979.

Suckow, M.A., Schroeder, V., 2010. The Laboratory Rabbit, second ed. CRC Press/Taylor & Francis, Boca Raton, FL.

Thompson, K.L., Meier, T.R., Scholz, J.A., 2017. Endotracheal intubation of rabbits using a polypropylene guide catheter. JoVE 129. https://doi.org/10.3791/56369.

Thurston, S., Burlingame, L., Lester, P.A., Lofgren, J., 2018. Methods of pairing and pair maintenance of New Zealand white rabbits (Oryctolagus cuniculus) via behavioral ethogram, monitoring, and interventions. JoVE 133. https://doi.org/10.3791/57267.

Todd, M.M., Wu, B., Warner, D.S., Maktabi, M., 1994. The dose-related effects of nitric oxide synthase inhibition on cerebral blood flow during isoflurane and pentobarbital anesthesia. Anesthesiology 80 (5), 1128–1136. https://doi.org/10.1097/00000542-199405000-00022.

Toman, H., Erbas, M., Sahin, H., Kiraz, H.A., Uzun, M., Ovali, M.A., 2015. Comparison of the effects of various airway devices on hemodynamic response and QTc interval in rabbits under general anesthesia. J. Clin. Monit. Comput. 29 (6), 727–732. https://doi.org/10.1007/s10877-015-9659-x.

Tran, H.S., Puc, M.M., Tran, J.L., Del Rossi, A.J., Hewitt, C.W., 2001. A method of endoscopic endotracheal intubation in rabbits. Lab. Anim. 35 (3), 249–252. https://doi.org/10.1258/0023677011911705.

Turner, P.V., Kerr, C.L., Healy, A.J., Taylor, W.M., 2006. Effect of meloxicam and butorphanol on minimum alveolar concentration of isoflurane in rabbits. Am. J. Vet. Res. 67 (5), 770–774. https://doi.org/10.2460/ajvr.67.5.770.

Tutunaru, A.C., Sonea, A., Drion, P., Serteyn, D., Sandersen, C., 2013. Anaesthetic induction with alfaxalone may produce hypoxemia in rabbits premedicated with fentanyl/droperidol. Vet. Anaesth. Analg. 40 (6), 657–659. https://doi.org/10.1111/vaa.12071.

Ugur, B., Basaloglu, K., Yurtseven, T., Ates, U., Aydin, O.N., Ozenc, D., Gurel, A., 2005. Neurotoxicity with single dose intrathecal midazolam administration. Eur. J. Anaesthesiol. 22 (12), 907–912. https://doi.org/10.1017/S0265021505001547.

Uzun, M., Kiraz, H.A., Ovali, M.A., Sahin, H., Erbas, M., Toman, H., 2015. The investigation of airway management capacity of v-gel and cobra-PLA in anaesthetised rabbits. Acta Cir. Bras. 30 (1), 80–86. https://doi.org/10.1590/S0102-86502015001000011.

Vachon, P., 1999. Self-mutilation in rabbits following intramuscular ketamine-xylazine-acepromazine injections. Can. Vet. J. 40 (8), 581–582. Retrieved from. https://www.ncbi.nlm.nih.gov/pubmed/12001340.

Vachon, P., Dupras, J., Prout, R., Blais, D., 1999. EEG recordings in anesthetized rabbits: comparison of ketamine-midazolam and Telazol with or without xylazine. Contemp. Top. Lab. Anim. Sci. 38 (3), 57–61. Retrieved from. https://www.ncbi.nlm.nih.gov/pubmed/12086426.

Valverde, A., Skelding, A.M., 2019. Alternatives to opioid analgesia in small animal anesthesia: alpha-2 agonists. Vet. Clin. North Am. Small Anim. Pract. 49 (6), 1013–1027. https://doi.org/10.1016/j.cvsm.2019.07.010.

Varga, M., 2014. Rabbit basic science. In: Textbook of Rabbit Medicine, second ed.

Virtanen, R., 1989. Pharmacological profiles of medetomidine and its antagonist, atipamezole. Acta Vet. Scand. Suppl. 85, 29–37. Retrieved from. https://www.ncbi.nlm.nih.gov/pubmed/2571275.

Vranken, J.H., Troost, D., de Haan, P., Pennings, F.A., van der Vegt, M.H., Dijkgraaf, M.G., Hollmann, M.W., 2006. Severe toxic damage to the rabbit spinal cord after intrathecal administration of preservative-free S(+)-ketamine. Anesthesiology 105 (4), 813–818. https://doi.org/10.1097/00000542-200610000-00028.

Weaver, L.A., Blaze, C.A., Linder, D.E., Andrutis, K.A., Karas, A.Z., 2010. A model for clinical evaluation of perioperative analgesia in rabbits (*Oryctolagus cuniculus*). J. Am. Assoc. Lab. Anim. Sci. 49 (6), 845–851. Retrieved from. https://www.ncbi.nlm.nih.gov/pubmed/21205451.

Website, 2021. Retrieved from. https://darvallvet.com/heated-products/. (Accessed 13 September 2021).

Weinstein, C.H., Fujimoto, J.L., Wishner, R.E., Newton, P.O., 2000. Anesthesia of six-week-old New Zealand White rabbits for thoracotomy. Contemp. Top. Lab. Anim. Sci. 39 (3), 19–22. Retrieved from. https://www.ncbi.nlm.nih.gov/pubmed/11178320.

Wenger, S., Mullhaupt, D., Ohlerth, S., Prasse, S., Klein, K., da Silva Valente, B., Mosing, M., 2017. Experimental evaluation of four airway devices in anaesthetized New Zealand White rabbits. Vet. Anaesth. Analg. 44 (3), 529–537. https://doi.org/10.1016/j.vaa.2016.05.009.

Wixson, S.K, 1994. Anesthesia and analgesics. In: Manning, P.J., Ringler, D.H., Newcomer, C.E. (Eds.), The Biology of the Laboratory Rabbit. Academic Press Inc, Orlando, Fl, pp. 87–109.

Wolfe, A.M., Kennedy, L.H., Na, J.J., Nemzek-Hamlin, J.A., 2015. Efficacy of tramadol as a sole analgesic for postoperative pain in male and female mice. J. Am. Assoc. Lab. Anim. Sci. 54 (4), 411–419. Retrieved from. https://www.ncbi.nlm.nih.gov/pubmed/26224442.

Worthley, S.G., Roque, M., Helft, G., Soundararajan, K., Siddiqui, M., Reis, E.D., 2000. Rapid oral endotracheal intubation with a fibre-optic scope in rabbits: a simple and reliable technique. Lab. Anim. 34 (2), 199–201. https://doi.org/10.1258/002367700780457554.

Wyatt, J.D., Scott, R.A., Richardson, M.E., 1989. The effects of prolonged ketamine-xylazine intravenous infusion on arterial blood pH, blood gases, mean arterial blood pressure, heart and respiratory rates, rectal temperature and reflexes in the rabbit. Lab. Anim. Sci. 39 (5),

411–416. Retrieved from. https://www.ncbi.nlm.nih.gov/pubmed/2530398.

Wynn, R.L., El'Baghdady, Y.M., Ford, R.D., Thut, P.D., Rudo, F.G., 1984. A rabbit tooth-pulp assay to determine ED50 values and duration of action of analgesics. J. Pharmacol. Methods 11 (2), 109–117. https://doi.org/10.1016/0160-5402(84)90020-2.

Xu, J., Zhang, J., Yang, D., Song, J., Pallas, B., Zhang, C., Chen, Y.E., 2021. Gene editing in rabbits: unique opportunities for translational biomedical research. Front. Genet. 12, 642444. https://doi.org/10.3389/fgene.2021.642444.

Zhou, Z.F., Du, M.Y., Wu, W.Y., Jiang, Y., Han, J.S., 1981. Effect of intracerebral microinjection of naloxone on acupuncture- and morphine-analgesia in the rabbit. Sci. Sin. 24 (8), 1166–1178. Retrieved from. https://www.ncbi.nlm.nih.gov/pubmed/6272389.

Chapter 16

Anesthesia, restraint and analgesia in laboratory fishes

Almut Köhler[1], Karin Finger-Baier[2] and Luis Antunes[3,a]

[1]Safety and Environment, Karlsruhe Institute of Technology (KIT), Eggenstein-Leopoldshafen, Germany; [2]Max Planck Institute of Neurobiology (Now: Max Planck Institute for Biological Intelligence, Martinsried), Planegg, Germany; [3]School of Agrarian and Veterinary Sciences (ECAV), Department of Veterinary Sciences; Centre for the Research and Technology of Agro-Environmental and Biological Sciences (CITAB) UTAD, Vila Real, Portugal

Chapter outline

I. Introduction

Fish have gained increasing popularity as research models, resulting in constantly growing numbers of animals used to answer multiple scientific questions. In many countries, they already are counted as the second most used animal group after mice as a species. Basic research is mostly performed on relatively small fish species that can be housed and handled in a laboratory environment. Zebrafish dominate biomedical research. Medaka is mostly used in genomic studies. Cavefish help to understand the regulation of diurnal rhythms and metabolism. Cichlids are widely used to gain insight into the neuronal foundation of behavior. For toxicological and ecological studies, other species like fathead minnows, as well as zebrafish and medaka, are commonly used. Species like carp, tilapia, trout, salmon, sea bream, sea bass, and croaker are used for research regarding breeding, and growth trials with different nutrients and diets. Since these are commercially important species, also epizootic diseases and vaccine studies are of interest.

In research, fish are subjected to stressful conditions such as handling, transport, tagging, sampling, and invasive

[a] Supported by National Funds by FCT - Portuguese Foundation for Science and Technology, under the project UIDB/04033/2020.

procedures. Anesthesia is used daily in experimental procedures, such as when fish undergo painful procedures or have to be immobilized. This is crucial to the fish welfare as these vertebrates are capable of nociception and pain perception (Sneddon, 2009, 2019). The use of an inadequate anesthetic protocol can compromise not only the welfare of fish but also the reliability and reproducibility of the research results. Thus, the development of a suitable anesthetic regime for each fish species used in research is of high importance.

Anesthesia is normally defined as a reversible state produced by an external agent resulting in a loss of sensation through the depression of the central nervous system (CNS). Anesthetics may act locally or generally, depending on their application. General anesthesia suppresses CNS activity and results in unconsciousness and total lack of sensation; this may be followed by different levels of analgesia and muscle relaxation. Anesthesia and sedation are usually divided into several stages (see Table 16.1) that reflect the anesthetic depth. The administration of anesthetic agents by immersion, equivalent to inhalation anesthesia in mammals, is the most common anesthetic technique in fish due to its practicability (quick and easy). But there is a caveat: although the concentration of the anesthetic solution can be exactly determined, for most (if not all) compounds it remains unclear, what the internal dosage is and at what time it will be reached through immersion. It is also unclear whether immersion-applied painkillers act through skin receptors (locally) or centrally (by absorption through the gills). Nevertheless, in small fish, the administration of anesthesia by other routes, such as intramuscular (IM) or intraperitoneal (IP) injection, is unfeasible in a large-scale operation, and immersion has been selected as the routine technique.

Anesthesia in fish should only be done in healthy animals, acclimatized to the conditions of the vivarium. This issue and others related to preparation for anesthesia are developed in Section B (Planning). The selection of the anesthetics to use in fish is a complex decision. For example, regarding the induction of anesthesia, i.e., the period from anesthesia administration to loss of fish equilibrium and unconsciousness, the least aversive and quickest agent should be selected to reduce stress. However, not always the least aversive agent is the speediest one, and a compromise may have to be adopted between the stress caused and the time the fish is subjected to this stress. Maintenance of anesthesia is the period when anesthesia is kept at the desired level to conduct the procedure. Whenever a surgical plane of anesthesia needs to be induced and maintained, drugs with a narrow safety margin should be avoided. The best anesthetics must preserve the fish physiological variables within safety limits. One should consider that immersion, in contrast to injection, results in constant diffusion of anesthetic agents into the fish tissue, thus deepening the anesthesia over time. This may significantly depress cardiovascular and respiratory parameters with serious implications on the course and recovery from anesthesia. Drugs that reduce respiratory and heart rates cause high mortality under long-term exposure and sedation. The best drugs used in fish anesthesia should allow a quick and full recovery with fishes showing normal behaviors, such as normal swimming patterns in the water column and positive responses to food in a short period after anesthesia.

II. Preprocedural considerations

A. Planning and safety recommendations

Many anesthetics used for fish can cause harm to humans, either due to their chemical nature or improper usage. Some compounds have been shown to have irritating or even toxic qualities, which could have far-reaching health implications. Prior to establishing anesthetic protocols, MSDS (material safety data sheets) need to be consulted and the least hazardous compounds should be considered. If a hazardous, anesthetic substance (e.g., retinotoxic MS-222, neuropsychological active 2-phenoxyethanol) cannot be avoided due to species or procedure requirements, precautions have to be implemented to eliminate or at least minimize the risk to the human handler.

B. Health and fish evaluation

Although anesthesia is regarded as a method of refinement to avoid burden for the animals in form of pain and suffering, all forms of anesthesia are nevertheless stressful and challenging mostly for the respiratory, cardiovascular, and endocrine systems. The usual anesthetic compounds and techniques used cause increased adrenaline and cortisol levels that can lead to changes in homeostasis. Thus, a major point before anesthesia is to determine the health status of the fish. Fish with clinical symptoms of illness should not be used for research unless this is the focus of the study. Common indicators for the disease are an altered opercular beat rate (in− or decreased) and behavioral changes in the swimming pattern, like isolation from the shoal (in shoaling species like zebrafish) or swimming only close to the bottom or at the water surface or inlets. Additionally, rubbing against the tank walls or enrichment objects, loss of scales, changes in the color of the body pigmentation, misshapen or ragged fins, wounds, ulcers, or tumors are a sign of impaired well-being of the animal.

If possible, only animals with known health status reports should be used. However, this is not possible with several species and studies, with animals received from some aquacultures, and especially when wild animals are used. Under these circumstances, newly arrived animals

TABLE 16.1 Anesthetic agents.

Drug(s)	Species	Dose (immersion)	Comments
MS-222	Zebrafish (*Danio rerio*)	100–150 mg/L	75–200 mg/L immersion doses are reported
	Goldfish (*Carassius auratus*)	200–500 mg/L	
	Platyfish (*Xiphophorus maculatus*)	40 mg/L	
	Rainbow trout (*Oncorhynchus mykiss*)	40–100 mg/L	
	Hybrid tilapias	200 mg/L	
2-phenoxyethanol	Goldfish (*Carassius auratus*)	0.3–0.5 mL/L	
	Nile tilapia (*Oreochromis niloticus*)	0.5–2 mL/L	
	Rainbow trout (*Oncorhynchus mykiss*)	0.2 mL/L	
	Gilthead sea bream (*Sparus aurata*)	0.3–0.45 mL/L	
	Sea bass (*Dicentrarchus labrax*)	0.3–0.45 mL/L	
Clove oil	Zebrafish (*Danio rerio*)	60–140 mg/L	The response times to achieve loss of equilibrium and surgical anesthesia tended to plateau at concentrations higher than 60 mg/L
	Marine medaka (*Oryzias dancena*)	50–175 mg/L	Anesthesia induction time decreased as both anesthetic doses and water temperature increased
	Rainbow trout (*Oncorhynchus mykiss*)	20–140 mg/L	
	Nile tilapia (*Oreochromis niloticus*)	100–300 mg/L	
Metomidate	Zebrafish (*Danio rerio*)	2–10 mg/L	The time to recovery increase for the highest doses. Difficulty to achieve surgical anesthetic plane.
	Platyfish (*Xiphophorus maculatus*)	2 mg/L	
	Atlantic salmon (*Salmo salar*)	3–5 mg/L	
Etomidate	Zebrafish (*Danio rerio*)	2–8 mg/L	The time to recovery and mortality increase for the highest doses.
	Platyfish (*Xiphophorus maculatus*)	2–24 mg/L	
Propofol	Goldfish (*Carassius auratus*)	5–10 mg/L	
	Rainbow trout (*Oncorhynchus mykiss*)	10 mg/L	
	Nile tilapia (*Oreochromis niloticus*)	2.5–12.5 mg/L	
Lidocaine	Zebrafish (*Danio rerio*)	300–325 mg/L	
	Marine medaka (*Oryzias dancena*)	300–800 mg/L	Anesthesia induction time decreased as both anesthetic doses and water temperature increased. Smaller fish took less time than larger fish to recover from anesthesia
Combinations			
Propofol/Lidocaine	Zebrafish (*Danio rerio*)	2.5 mg/L + 50 mg/L	
Isoflurane/MS-222	Zebrafish (Danio rerio)	60–80 mg/L +60–80 mg/L	

Table 16.1 is adapted and based on data available at Martins et al. (2016) and Martins et al. (2019).

may need to be quarantined prior to establish their health status and to give them time for an acclimatization period in the procedure rooms prior to anesthesia. The quarantine period is very important for transported animals. Recently arrived animals may show different levels of stress and pathologies. These conditions may be induced by personnel handling the fish when carrying out the duty of transportation, being a direct effect of capturing and handling of fish before and during transportation, crowding of fish in the transport container, the temperature of the transporting water, and the various changing water parameters that may affect the water quality (e.g., oxygen saturation, pH, and TAN (total ammonia nitrogen) levels). Duration depends on origin and information about the introduced animal. For zebrafish, a suite of diagnostic testing services to proactively monitor the health of zebrafish colonies have been developed by different laboratories. These include whole fish health monitoring, histopathology, and infectious disease PCR testing to help maintain the colonies health. Microbiology testing (bioburden and identification) on water system samples and feed can be performed to ensure that unwanted agents are not introduced. Detailed recommendations for health monitoring and reporting for zebrafish research facilities can be found in Collymore et al. (2016) and Mocho et al. (2022a,b).

Before starting the anesthetic process, one should make sure that the set-up is complete and preparations for emergency cases are taken. In many cases, fish are immersed in a solution of the anesthetic compound in holding water (water originating from the aquatic system) to induce anesthesia. Since the uptake of chemicals is easy in fish due to the thin skin barrier, the anesthetic solution should be prepared with care, and especially the pH and temperature should be checked before transferring any fish to the anesthetic bath. It is of great benefit to use the normal holding water to set up the anesthetic solution since this avoids adaptational stress for the fish. This will ensure that water parameters are within acceptable range and the water also is at the same temperature as the fish are acclimatized to. Also, the recovery water tanks or aquariums (separate tanks with fresh holding water) should be prepared beforehand to facilitate both the recovery process (see also Section V) as well as a quick response to emergencies. Note that oxygenated holding water should be used during induction, maintenance, and anesthesia recovery to avoid hypoxia. To avoid emergencies, fish should be anesthetized in small batches (maximal 3–4 at a time) and remain no longer than 10 minutes in the anesthetic solution. Some anesthetic solutions need to be buffered before use (MS-222) or firstly prepared in stock solution in an organic solvent, such as ethanol or acetone (Benzocaine), in order to be used as well-tolerated immersion anesthetics with no effects on animal welfare. Although previous studies have shown that the use of ethanol (Readman et al., 2017) as a carrier solvent does not create an aversive response in itself, the solvent implication on the fish welfare and experimental results must be controlled if presolving in an organic solvent (e.g., ethanol, acetone, DMSO) is required. Given the relatively small differences between concentrations that are apparently safe and those that are clearly toxic (Maes et al., 2012), studies requiring anesthetics and compounds demanding any solvents and carriers require adequate control groups.

C. History and records

Before applying anesthesia to the animal, usually the already summarized burden of the animal should be considered and possible consequences for the process should be drawn. While this might be possible in bigger species where single animals can be marked by transponders permanently, there is limitation to smaller lab species like zebrafish or medaka where identification is not used on a regular basis. During the procedure, an experimental log should be used to record details about temperature, dosage, duration until the desired anesthetic plane is reached and time to recovery.

D. Fasting

Mostly, the fish remain in their social groups until anesthesia and are not singled out in advance. Individual feeding is not common. While in a laboratory environment it is possible to avoid feeding in defined time windows before the procedure, this is hardly possible when wild species are used that constantly find food in their natural environment. In the lab, fish should not be fed prior to anesthesia to not stress the metabolism as well as to avoid regurgitation of feed during hypnosis. Regurgitated food may reduce water quality and become lodged in the gills. To facilitate the fasting, anesthesia at the beginning of the working day is helpful, so that the companion fish are not stressed by being held off food. This will result in fasting periods of approx. 12–14 hours prior to anesthesia if feeding is stopped the night before. If automated feeding is used, the feeding regimen has to be adjusted so that those tanks are skipped during feeding. An additional benefit of fasting is the reduced production of feces, leading to less contamination of the anesthetic solution or the recovery bath.

III. Restraint

The simple handling of fish can cause a relevant physiological stress response in these animals. Thus, chemical restraint can increase fish safety by minimizing handling trauma and integument damage during longer and more rigid handling procedures. Nevertheless, the application of chemical restraining methods also affects animals through biochemical reactions and aversive behavior. Therefore, one should carefully consider the stressful effect on the fish in comparison with the benefit of the project by replacing a burden with another one to avoid unnecessary and unethical treatment. One has to differentiate between physical and chemical restraint.

Physical restraint, e.g., for imaging, is possible by embedding larval and juvenile fish in either low-melting agarose or methylcellulose. Anesthesia might be employed in addition to eliminate motion artifacts during high-resolution imaging, though compounds like MS-222 cannot be used for calcium imaging due to their means of action, blocking sodium action potentials.

Neuromuscular blocking agents (NMBAs) or similarly acting agents can be an effective modality to address physical restraints that arise daily in the laboratory. However, these drugs are often used to optimize anesthesia when proper unconsciousness is required to avoid animals' awareness during paralysis. Prior to use, some techniques described in the literature must be discussed and approved by your local animal welfare body. For example, for high-resolution calcium imaging, instead of tricaine anesthesia, fish can be injected with α-bungarotoxin, a neurotoxin contained in the venom of the Taiwanese many-banded krait, which produces paralysis of striated muscles by blocking cholinergic receptors in the neuromuscular junction. In zebrafish larvae, the intraspinal injection of α-bungarotoxin (Tesmer et al., 2022) will eliminate tail movements while still allowing heart contractions, gill movement, and neuronal activity. Prior to the intraspinal injection, fish should be anesthetized.

Electro anesthesia is widely used as an anesthetic method for wildlife monitoring of fish stocks in rivers or lakes (Reid et al., 2019; Hudson et al., 2011). Electric current is usually coming from a large battery or a portable generator. In some cases, stationary batteries/generators at the waterfront can be used. The cathode is placed in the water, and the anode is a net with a metal frame. The fish within the electric field between the poles are electro-anesthetized and usually orient themselves toward the anode (anodotaxis). For anesthesia mostly, smooth DC is used since pulse DC can lead to epileptic form insults. Depending on the current and length of the impulse the deepness of the anesthesia can be controlled. The effectiveness of the method depends greatly on the water quality (conductivity, pH), fish size (bigger fish respond better than smaller ones), and fish species (mostly the specific habitat: fish that are found in the mud are more difficult to reach). This method requires the use of dangerous electrical currents, 3000−15,000 W, 600−750 V. Therefore, it should only be performed with specialist certified equipment and conducted by trained/certified personnel.

Carbon dioxide is widely used for animal euthanasia. In fish, carbon dioxide is used mainly for the immobilization of salmon or carp, because it is safe, relatively cheap, and easy to apply by bubbling CO_2 in the water. Since it has no analgesic effect and its safety margin is low, it should be considered unsuitable for surgical procedures. It lowers the blood pH and can cause several side effects due to changes in enzyme activity affecting the experimental analysis. Nevertheless, changes are of short duration mostly (Bernier and Randall, 1998; Pirhonen and Schreck, 2003; Fish, 1943). Other studies showed that hyperoxygenation does not reduce primary stress responses after 30 and 90 minutes of CO_2 exposure in Arctic char (*Salvelinus alpinus* L.; Sandblom et al., 2013) and CO_2 narcosis induces violent aversive behavioral escape reactions that will negatively affect fish welfare (Gräns et al., 2016), although this technique elicited less pronounced physiological stress responses compared with dry electrical stunning.

Gradual cooling has been shown to be useful for sedation, immobilization for nonpainful procedures, and short-term procedures, such as IP injections (Collymore et al., 2014). Although this technique has been used in fish as a sedative and anesthetic, this method is highly questionable since it does not completely block nerve conduction and fish may be able to feel pain, making gradual cooling unsuitable for surgical procedures and unsuitable for fish acclimated to cold waters, thus it is not discussed in this review. Some of the most common anesthetic agents used in fish are briefly described below.

Besides minimizing stress responses and movement, the use of anesthetics is also crucial during invasive or surgical procedures. Teleost fish not only possess nociceptors but are also capable of experiencing pain. The literature regarding the use of anesthetics on fish is still scarce, and due to the high variability of fish species (size, natural habitat, behavior, and physiology), one must be careful when choosing the type, dose, and length of exposure of anesthetic or sedative drugs.

The use of anesthetic and analgesic methods is required to reduce stress and eliminate the pain perception thus applying relevant drugs being a matter of course for scientific and ethical reasons. Nevertheless, the use of chemicals should be analyzed with care before use. All drugs have side effects affecting the experimental outcome. The application as a bath as it is commonly performed, results in the fish being immersed in the drug with the whole-body surface. Most fish do have receptors in the skin reacting to chemical substances. This differs greatly from the situation in mammals, where substances are often applied by injection and bypass the active perception of the drug effect by body receptors. For many inhalants like CO_2 or anesthetic gases, it has been shown that they are aversive in conscious mammals. Studies show that fish present aversive behavior to most drugs that are usually applied, although to different degrees. Different restraint options need to be evaluated, and a decision between physical and chemical handling techniques has to be made based on animal welfare and scientific arguments.

IV. Analgesia, anesthesia and balanced anesthesia

Analgesia refers to the relief of pain, but since animals do not express pain in the same way humans do, this can be sometimes difficult to evaluate (Short, 1998). Arguments in favor of considering fish sentient animals can be of anatomical, physiological, behavioral, and pharmacological nature (Brown, 2015). The presence of nociceptors in fish indicates the occurrence of nociception, observed by motor responses of fish to noxious stimuli. Behavioral task performance showed rainbow trout seeking the analgesic agent when exposed to painful stimuli and learning to avoid a potentially noxious stimulus, indicating pain perception (Sneddon et al., 2003). Fish can also prioritize motivational drivers when in the presence of a noxious stimulus, indicating a central processing of pain. Other behavioral and physiological changes such as the reduction in swimming and food intake, the increase in gill ventilation rate, and the rubbing of the area affected by painful agents are also indicators of pain perception in fish like koi carp (Harms et al., 2005). These changes can be significantly reduced with the administration of an analgesic like morphine (Sneddon, 2003). Opioids, nonsteroidal antiinflammatory drugs (NSAIDs), and local anesthetics are three types of analgesic drugs that have been studied as potential analgesic agents in fish (see Section E).

Both opioids and NSAIDs have adverse side effects. However, analgesic agents can also provide better analgesia when combining different classes (multimodal therapy), which allows for the reduction of each analgesic dose, and thus causes less side effects. This approach is called balanced analgesia. The use of combined analgesics in fish shall improve analgesia and reduce side effects, being, therefore, an issue worthy to study.

A similar approach is called balanced anesthesia, wherein two or more drugs potentiate each other to produce the desired anesthesia effects, while reducing the risk of side effects, such as respiratory depression, hemodynamic instability, and mortality. This is possible when these drugs induce a synergetic and complementary effect, resulting in rapid full anesthesia with decreased doses and safer analgesia and anesthesia. Maintenance and recovery of anesthesia should also be more controlled and predictable. Unfortunately, there are not many studies of new anesthetic protocols to be used in fish by studying the quality of anesthesia and recovery induced by different concentrations of agents used alone and in combination (Chatigny et al., 2018). One example of balanced anesthesia in zebrafish is the use of propofol, a short-acting hypnotic agent, allowing a smooth anesthesia induction and a quick recovery with little cumulative effects but no analgesia properties, with lidocaine, a sodium-channel blocker with a large margin of safety in some species, with analgesia properties and poor hypnotic effects (Valentim et al., 2016). Anesthetic protocols of fish usually refer to one single agent, whereas protocols of human and veterinary medicine cover combinations of several drugs, each contributing to the effects needed in the anesthesia.

A. Anesthesia

The anesthetic agent should provide adequate immobilization and analgesia for the duration of the procedure and have a wide safety margin. An anesthetic agent that is easy to administer, and water-soluble, harmless to the environment and operator is preferred. Especially in smaller fish species, immersion anesthetics are preferred since handling and injection sites otherwise are limited. Immersion anesthesia is considered being physiologically and mechanistically comparable to inhalation anesthesia in mammals. The ideal anesthetic agent should have a rapid induction and recovery time with the least possible stress and side effects. Table 16.2 shows published options for anesthetic agents for different fish species, recommended doses, and comments. Anesthesia trials with small numbers of fish, i.e., pilot studies, must be performed to determine the optimal dosage and exposure time prior to the establishment of protocols and adjust the correct agents and doses to the anesthetic stage and type of procedure.

1. MS-222

Tricaine methane sulfonate, or MS-222, is the most used anesthetic in fish (Collymore et al., 2014; Sneddon, 2012; Ross and Ross, 2008; Readman et al., 2017), and its major mechanism of action is through the inhibition of sodium entrance into the cell. MS-222 is classified as a local anesthetic, but in an anesthetic bath, it induces general anesthesia as it is absorbed through the gills and partly through the skin of the fish (scaleless fish). The MS-222 solution needs to be buffered with sodium bicarbonate or TRIS to pH ~7.0 to prevent the pH of water from decreasing (Spears et al., 2014; Carter et al., 2011; Christiansen and Stoskopf, 2013). For storage, light-protective measures need to be taken as MS-222 is degraded by light (Katz et al., 2020; Carter et al., 2011). It is considered safe in fish, although, as other anesthetics, MS-222 can have secondary effects such as hypoxemia, hypercapnia, hypoglycemia, increased levels of lactic acid, erythrocyte swelling, elevated hematocrit, and changes in blood electrolytes, hormones, cholesterol, urea, and interrenal ascorbic acid, among others as shown in rainbow trout for example (Iwama et al., 1989). MS-222, in common with

TABLE 16.2 Anesthesia stages in fish.

Stage of anesthesia	Description	Physiological and behavioral signs	Clinical interest
0	Normal	Total equilibrium. Normal muscle tone. Normal reaction to visual and tactile stimuli. Normal respiratory rate.	
I	Light sedation	Slight loss of reaction to visual and tactile stimuli.	Can reduce stress and physical trauma during transport
II	Deep sedation	Slight decrease in muscle tone. No reaction to visual and light tactile stimuli. Small decrease in respiratory rate.	Appropriate stage for close visual observation and for minimal manipulation, weighing and measuring.
III	Light narcosis/ excitement phase	Partial loss of equilibrium/Weak responses to postural changes. Decrease in muscle tone. Increased reaction to visual and tactile stimuli. Respiratory rate increased and/or irregular.	Higher risk of physical injury or escape/jump from container or aquarium
IV	Deep narcosis	Total loss of equilibrium/Lack of responses to postural changes. No reaction to minor visual and tactile stimuli. Respiratory rate decreasing to almost normal.	Good plane for external sampling and blood sampling. Avoid painful procedures/analgesia may not be present. Suitable for imaging techniques
V	Light anesthesia	Complete loss of muscle tone. No reaction to painful stimuli. Decrease in respiratory rate. Decrease in heart rate.	Minor surgical procedures: fin biopsies and gill biopsies
VI	Surgical anesthesia	Absence of reaction to massive stimulation. Respiratory rate very low. Slow heart rate.	Major surgical procedures
VII	Medullary collapse/ overdose	Flaccid muscle tone. Apnea—absence of respiratory rate, which can be followed in several minutes by cardiac arrest if anesthesia depth is not decreased. Eventual death.	Appropriate for euthanasia

several other anesthetics has been shown to be aversive in zebrafish (Readman et al., 2013; Wong et al., 2014). MS-222 can cause mucous membrane irritation in humans (Carter et al., 2011), and there is a report of one episode of MS-222-related retinotoxicity (Davis et al., 2008), thus care should be taken during the handling of this substance (Bernstein et al., 1997). It is dissipated from the muscle tissue of carp within a few days (Qin et al., 2017). Currently, MS-222 is the only FDA-approved anesthetic available for aquatic organisms what has to be considered if food fish should be anesthetized that may end up in the food chain later. Withdrawal time is 21 days.

2. *Benzocaine*

Benzocaine is a white, odorless, and tasteless local anesthetic that is chemically similar to MS-222, but contrary to MS-222, it is almost insoluble in water (Ross and Ross, 2008). Due to its high lipophilicity, benzocaine requires a previous preparation of a stock solution in an organic solvent, such as ethanol or acetone, in order to be used as an immersion anesthetic. Benzocaine presents low toxicity to fish, since it does not have a negative impact on growth (Sørum and Damsgård, 2004) or reproductive capacity, although its safety margin may decrease at higher temperatures. Benzocaine is well tolerated by some fish species like the fathead minnow, carp, and rainbow trout (Readman et al., 2017), but similar to the results with MS-222, it can cause avoidance behaviors in others like zebrafish (Readman et al., 2013; Wong et al., 2014). Benzocaine and tricaine are commonly reported as the most effective anesthetics, with benzocaine being more economically affordable than MS-222 for use in large-scale procedures (Bolasina et al., 2017) but having a quite narrow safety margin (Gilderhus, 1990).

3. Clove oil compounds

Clove oil is extracted from the plant *Syzygium aromaticum*, and its major constituent, eugenol, is used as an immersion anesthetic in many species like a guppy, red pacu, or salmon (Bolasina et al., 2017; Sladky et al., 2001; Iversen et al., 2009). This oil needs to be mixed with ethanol to be used in an anesthetic bath as it is insoluble in water. Eugenol has been used as a local anesthetic, topical anesthetic, and analgesic in humans. It has rapid induction times and provides consistent anesthesia compared to other anesthetics, although it may have longer recovery times and increased mortality due to ventilatory failure when higher doses are used. It is efficient at a range of temperatures, easily available, relatively inexpensive, and generally regarded as safe for the user. As with other fish anesthetics, clove oil has been reported to change some physiological parameters such as reduced cardiovascular activity and prolonged cardiovascular recovery, lower feed intake after anesthesia, low net ion imbalances, and reduced stress response in some species like steelhead or rainbow trout, largemouth bass, and channel catfish (Cooke et al., 2004; Pirhonen and Schreck, 2003; Small, 2003; Wagner et al., 2003; Barata et al., 2016). Isoeugenol is another constituent of clove oil, and the active ingredient in Aqui-S, which is soluble in water. A similar product is called Aqui-S 20E, which has 10% of eugenol. Both products are candidates for a decreased withdrawal time sedative; however, in the transport of high stock densities, Aqui-S increased total ammonia, probably due to the increase in protein metabolism (Cupp et al., 2017; Becker et al., 2012). Although both eugenol and isoeugenol isolated are considered safe, clove oil solution should be avoided, since one of the compounds present, methyl eugenol, is a suspected carcinogenic, and the over-the-counter version of clove oil as a natural essence highly depends on environmental influences, requiring constant adaptation of protocols depending on the use of different batches.

4. Metomidate and etomidate

Metomidate and etomidate are both imidazole-based nonbarbiturate hypnotic drugs that act through the activation and modulation of the inhibitory gamma-aminobutyric acid type A (GABAA) receptors (Fish et al., 2008). They are used as immersion anesthetics in fish (Sneddon, 2012; Ross and Ross, 2008; Readman et al., 2017; Stoskopf and Posner, 2008) and produce a rapid anesthetic induction and recovery, although special care should be taken as they do not induce analgesia and surgical anesthetic stages. Also, these drugs suppress cortisol production (Witeska et al., 2017), and consequently the cortisol stress response, which should be considered, and their use is weighted in fish for research. In fact, etomidate prevented a delayed immunosuppressive effect of stress, and it has been recommended to use when long-term stress prevention is required. Although both agents have the same mechanism of action, they are different compounds, which implies some differences in their effects. While etomidate has minimal effects on respiratory function or the cardiovascular system, metomidate can induce respiratory depression and reduced circulation. The metomidate hydrochloride is commercially available under the name Aquacalm for sedation and anesthesia of ornamental finfish, but not for use in fish intended for human or animal consumption, and it is relatively expensive. Metomidate may enhance pigmentation in some species, probably due to an increase in melanocyte-stimulating hormone synthesis, and muscular tremors and involuntary movements may occur under metomidate anesthesia (Stoskopf, 2015).

5. 2-phenoxyethanol

2-phenoxyethanol is a colorless or straw-colored oily liquid with slight solubility in water, but soluble in ethanol, and is used as an immersion anesthetic (Adel et al., 2016; Zahl et al., 2012). This agent has bactericidal and fungicidal properties (Burka et al., 1997) and has been used as a topical anesthetic. This agent can provide deep stages of anesthesia and is relatively inexpensive, nevertheless, it has no other great advantages over other drugs. The use of 2-phenoxyethanol can elicit several side effects, such as decreased respiratory and heart rate, reduced blood pressure and blood oxygenation, alterations of blood parameters, and elevated plasma levels of adrenaline, glucose and cortisol as shown in bighead carp (Akbary et al., 2016). In addition, sustained and prolonged exposure to 2-phenoxyethanol can cause a neuropsychological syndrome in handlers. Although its mechanism of action is still unknown, this agent inhibited the NMDA receptor, which has been related to an analgesic effect (Grasshoff et al., 2006). However, the analgesia induced by phenoxyethanol may be incomplete (Burka et al., 1997). Nevertheless, it seems to be suitable to induce the light sedation needed for transportation of Persian sturgeons (*Acipenser persicus*) juveniles, being important for aquaculture and restocking purposes (Adel et al., 2016).

6. Lidocaine

Lidocaine hydrochloride inhibits the propagation of action potentials by blocking sodium channels and is used as a local anesthetic and analgesic. This drug is used as an immersion anesthetic in fish and produces a quick anesthetic induction and recovery (Sneddon, 2012; Ross and Ross, 2008). Furthermore, it is relatively inexpensive and safe for the handler.

7. Propofol

Propofol is a GABA A receptor agonist and a sedative-hypnotic anesthetic drug that can be injected or used as an immersion anesthetic, e.g., in rainbow trout or sturgeons (Prieto et al., 2017; Adel et al., 2016). Propofol induces an anesthetic state quickly and provides a rapid and complete recovery being described as a useful, safe, and effective depressant drug in a number of fish species like the Nile Tilapia (Valença-Silva et al., 2014). It has also been used for fish transportation, maintaining the ionic and respiratory homeostasis in goldfish (Gholipourkanani and Ahadizadeh, 2013), and preventing peroxidative damage in catfish (Gressler et al., 2016). Studies in humans indicate that propofol may provide inconsistent and temporary analgesia during general anesthesia by suppression of the CNS, but it is not considered an analgesic (Fassoulaki, 2011).

8. *New anesthetics—essential oils*

New drugs have been tested to reduce the side effects associated with anesthetics, as well as legal restraints or budgetary concerns. Essential oils (EOs), like menthol, and their constituents are the main tested sedative and anesthetic drugs for fish as a natural alternative to the commonly used synthetic drugs. More information regarding essential oils used in fish anesthesia may be found in Martins et al. (2019). However, experience with these compounds is still based on single cases, and it will be difficult to transpose to laboratory animal sciences due to large batch variations resulting from environmental or manufacturing differences.

Reported dose rates, as shown in Table 16.1, depend on the required anesthetic stage and type of procedure. There are substantial variations between fish species in response to anesthetic agents, as well as large individual differences within each species. Variations may be the result of pharmacokinetic differences, usually described as what the body does to the drug, and pharmacodynamic differences, usually described as what the drug does to the body. Both pharmacokinetic and pharmacodynamic differences in fish may be influenced by biological factors such as age, sex, life stage, body weight, growth rate, body composition, physiological condition, and health status, as well as environmental factors such as water temperature, salinity, pH, and oxygen level. Variations between doses reported in the table reflect the above reported reasons (Zahl et al., 2012).

B. Anesthesia monitoring

In fish, anesthesia effects may vary depending on the administration route, pH, temperature, salinity, oxygenation, nitrogenous compounds, and other water conditions. Furthermore, anesthesia depth and recovery depend on its duration, anesthetic concentration, animals' body weight and metabolism, gill surface, fish health status, strain, age, and the different particularities of each fish species (Ross and Ross, 2008; Nordgreen et al., 2014; Murray, 2002; Pereira, 2016). Proper training and supervision of fish anesthesia are essential to avoid complications that can lead to death. Not only anesthesia should be carefully monitored but also complete fish recovery. Depth of anesthesia or anesthesia stages in fish (Table 16.2) can be assessed by ataxia, loss of righting reflex, and response to stimuli (squeezing the base of the tail). The respiratory rate can be monitored by observing the movement of the operculum. Heart rate can be monitored by using a Doppler or/and electrocardiograph (using the pectoral and anal fins). The gills should be pink to light red. Pale gills are suggestive of hypoxemia, hypotension, or anemia (Neiffer and Stamper, 2009).

C. Common anesthetic emergencies

The most common emergency occurring during anesthesia in fish is cardiac or respiratory arrest (Coyle, 2004). Since typical monitoring known from mammals, like measuring the oxygen saturation in the blood as an early alarm parameter, is not possible in fish, methods to warn of the danger of cardiac or respiratory arrest are more difficult to follow. In contrast to mammals also the heart muscle tissue can contain a relatively high amount of glycogen and is highly capable of anaerobic energy mobilization (Gallego-Colon et al., 2016; Gamperl, 2017; Rodnick and Gesser, 2017; Short and Driedzic, 2018), making the heartbeat in fish independent from respiration to a certain degree. As poikilothermal animals, the whole metabolism can be reduced to very low levels, resulting in very faint movement of the operculum since oxygen consumption is low at that stage. When performing surgeries or procedures outside of the water a trick to identify ongoing breathing is to put small drops of water on the gills that should bubble when the fish respirates. Since the depth of the narcosis depends on the duration of the bath and the concentration of the solution (and the temperature of the water), a fast transfer of the fish to the recovery bath (normal holding water) is an important precaution to avoid the death of the animal. If respiration stops, the concentration of the anesthetic should be decreased or the fish placed in the recovery bath. Recovery is achieved by placing the fish in anesthetic-free aerated water, ensuring normograde water flow over the gills; a pump and tubing can facilitate this if strong spontaneous respiration is not present. This utilizes the buccal flow-heart rate reflex whereby water flow through the buccal cavity accelerates heart rate and normalizes hypoventilation-related bradycardia. Recovery is typically within 5–10 minutes. Reversal agents for injectables such as α2-agonists are available. The use of respiratory and cardiovascular emergency drugs is not well studied.

Doxapram 5 mg/kg IV or intracelomic for respiratory depression and epinephrine (1:1000) 0.2–0.5 mL IM, IC, IV, or intracelomic for cardiac arrest have been proposed (Schroeder et al., 2021; Goodman; Neiffer and Stamper, 2009). Doxapram may be used to stimulate respiration postanesthesia or to treat respiratory depression/failure, and epinephrine may be used to increase vascular smooth muscle contraction and heart rate. Nevertheless, for reducing fatalities it is always more advisable to avoid anesthetic emergencies requiring the use of those drugs. The constant monitoring of anesthesia depth prevents these situations that endanger the lives of animals.

As a safety measure to avoid anesthetic emergencies, a light sedation before full anesthesia (2-step anesthesia) can help to reduce cardiovascular responses and avoidance behavior, resulting in a decreased stress response of the fish.

D. Anesthesia for specific situations

For prolonged or repeated procedures, intubation-based administration seems to be the preferred choice, as it has a significantly lower mortality rate compared to extended or repetitive immersion baths, although Wynd et al. (2017) report a dynamic anesthesia flow system for long-term imaging of adult zebrafish with improved survival rates. A detailed protocol for intubation-based anesthesia in zebrafish was published by Xu et al. (2015). Out-of-water procedures, and ideally in-water procedures lasting longer than several minutes, should involve additional gill ventilation. This can be achieved via orally placed rubber tubing delivering normograde flow (i.e., from mouth to tail direction) of anesthetic-laden water over the gills at an approximate rate of 1–3 L/kg/min. A recirculation anesthetic delivery system is frequently used to perform surgical procedures in fish (Schroeder et al., 2021).

E. Analgesia

In larger fish species, some drugs have shown efficacy in terms of perioperative analgesia when administered intramuscularly or at the site of tissue damage. However, this is impractical in very small species (<1 g) and when large numbers need to be treated. Immersion is a commonly used route of administering anesthesia in fish and maybe a less invasive alternative to administering analgesia. Water-soluble analgesic drugs, like buffered acetylsalicylic acid (ASA), butorphanol tartrate, and lidocaine have been investigated to provide pre and post-surgery (tail fin clip) pain relief through addition to the tank water (Schroeder and Sneddon, 2017).

1. Pharmacologic options

There is a general agreement that analgesic additions to anesthetic protocols constitute a refinement (Sneddon, 2012; Chatigny et al., 2018), with usable options already published (Table 16.3). This table lists examples of potentially efficacious compounds from different pharmaceutical groups, for example, lidocaine, morphine, and nonsteroidal antiinflammatory drugs. Some analgesic drugs were previously described as anesthetic agents, namely tricaine, benzocaine, or lidocaine which are inducing loss of consciousness as well as local anesthetic functions by blocking sodium channels and inactivating local nociceptors. Nonsteroidal antiinflammatory drugs (NSAIDs) like acetylsalicylic acid (Aspirin), carprofen, or ketoprofen, and opioids like morphine, tramadol, or butorphanol do not result in loss of consciousness and should only be used for analgesic effects or in addition to anesthetic substances to reduce pain during surgical interventions.

a. Lidocaine

Lidocaine, a local anesthetic, is probably the most used and investigated analgesic in fish. This drug was already introduced in Section 6. Lidocaine has a large safety margin in some species, with good analgesia properties (Valentim et al., 2016). Low-dose lidocaine immersion can be recommended to aid perioperative analgesia, and provide a valuable refinement for reducing the impact of invasive procedures in zebrafish, and improve welfare. In rainbow trout (*Oncorhynchus mykiss*), lidocaine showed better results to ameliorate possible pain-related responses compared to an opioid, buprenorphine, and the NSAID, carprofen. Lidocaine reduced all of the pain indicators measured, with the most effective dose being 1 mg per fish (Mettam et al., 2011). Administration of 5 mg/L lidocaine in zebrafish at 5 days postfertilization prevented the behavioral changes induced by acetic acid (Lopez-Luna et al., 2017).

b. Opioids

Opioid analgesic drugs exert their effects through the activation of mu-, delta-, and kappa-opioid receptors (Raffa, 2014), thus inhibiting and modulating pain signals (Pergolizzi et al., 2017).

Morphine is a pure mu-opioid receptor agonist with a great hypoalgesia effect and frequently is used in veterinary medicine (Sneddon, 2003, 2009; Robertson and Taylor, 2004). Since pure mu-agonist opioids cause addiction in humans, the use of these opioids is strictly regulated (Schedule II controlled substance), which may limit their access and use (Center for Substance Abuse Treatment, 2004). Morphine in goldfish (*Carassius auratus*) may provide analgesia since it decreased MS-222 anesthetic needs in minimum anesthetic concentration (MAC) studies (Ward et al., 2012). Comparative analgesic efficacy of morphine and butorphanol have been tested in koi (*Cyprinus carpio*) undergoing surgery. Butorphanol and morphine appeared to have an analgesic effect, but morphine administration caused fewer deleterious adverse effects (Baker et al., 2013).

TABLE 16.3 Analgesia agents.

Drug(s)	Species	Dose (route of administration)	Comments
Local anesthetics			
Lidocaine	Atlantic salmon (*Salmo salar*) Rainbow trout (*Oncorhynchus mykiss*)	2 mg (0.1 mL/site of 2% solution) (Local infiltration)	Used at the sites of incisions
	Zebrafish (*Danio rerio*)	0.1–2 mg/kg (IM) and 2–5 mg/L Immersion	Very efficient at 1 mg/kg IM and pre and postsurgical immersion for tail fin clipping.
Opioids			
Butorphanol	Goldfish (*Carassius auratus*)	0.1 mg/kg (IM)	
	Koi carp (*Cyprinus carpio*)	0.4–10 mg/kg (IM)	Low dose—Attenuation of behavioral changes after surgery. High dose—induced temporary buoyancy problems. Decreased respiratory rate. Food consumption returned to baseline values within 3 hours after treatment. Efficient as an analgesic.
Morphine	Goldfish (*Carassius auratus*)	2–50 mg/kg (IP and IM)	Probably efficient at all doses
	Koi carp (*Cyprinus carpio*)	5 mg/kg (IM)	
	Winter flounder (*Pseudopleuronectes americanus*)	40 mg/kg (IP)	Effect 50 minutes after injection
	Rainbow trout (*Oncorhynchus mykiss*)	5–50 mg/kg (IM)	No side effects observed. Very efficient at 5 mg/kg.
Tramadol	Koi carp (*Cyprinus carpio*)	10, 30, 50, 80 and 100 nmol/g (IM)	The analgesic effect was dose-dependent. The higher the dose, the more quickly it acted.
NSAIDs			
Ketoprofen	Goldfish (*Carassius auratus*)	0.5, 1 and 2 mg/kg (IM)	Probably efficient at all doses.
Carprofen	Rainbow trout (*Oncorhynchus mykiss*)	1, 2.5 and 5 mg/kg (IM)	Depressed activity. Reduced time to feed using 2.5 and 5 mg/kg. Increased ventilation.
Acetyl-salicylic acid	Zebrafish (Danio rerio)	1 and 2.5 mg/L (immersion)	Ameliorated activity and ventilation

IM, intramuscular injection; *IP*, intraperitoneal injection.
Adapted and based on data from Sneddon (2012) and Martins et al. (2019).

Butorphanol is a kappa-opioid receptor agonist and a mu-antagonist, which limits its analgesic properties and efficacy. Buprenorphine is a partial mu-opioid receptor agonist, and its analgesic effect results from the combination of both opioid and nonopioid mechanisms of action. In addition, buprenorphine has a lower addiction potential compared to mu-agonists, and is one of the most used opioids in veterinary medicine. Both, buprenorphine (Schedule III) as well as butorphanol (Schedule IV) are controlled substances. In the rainbow trout (*Oncorhynchus mykiss*), buprenorphine had limited impact on the fish's response to painful stimulus (Gräns et al., 2014; Mettam et al., 2011). Administration of 48 mg/L morphine in zebrafish at 5 days postfertilization prevented the behavioral changes induced by acetic acid (Lopez-Luna et al., 2017).

Tramadol is a central analgesic and acts both as a mu-opioid receptor agonist (Duthie, 1998), although with weak affinity, and as an inhibitor of monoamine neurotransmitter reuptake, achieving its analgesic effects through the synergy of these mechanisms of action. Tramadol also is a Schedule IV controlled substance. Tramadol showed a beneficial effect in carp in a dose-dependent manner (Chervova and Lapshin, 2000), where its administration increased the nociceptive threshold in response to an electric shock.

In rainbow trout (*Oncorhynchus mykiss*), buprenorphine significantly decreased both ventilation and heart rates, and the effects were most pronounced at 4–7 days after anesthesia (Gräns et al., 2014). The routine uses of opioids in fish need to be carefully evaluated. In zebrafish, the use of tramadol results in increased oxygen consumption (Zhuo et al., 2016). Reductions in ventilation and heart rates are not caused by an analgesic effect of the drug, but may instead reflect a general sedative effect. This resembles what has previously been demonstrated in mammals, although the duration of the drug effect is considerably longer in this ectothermic animal. Thus, before using opioids for postoperative analgesic treatment in fish, these potentially adverse effects need further characterization.

c. Nonsteroidal antiinflammatory drugs

NSAIDs act through the inhibition of cyclooxygenase (COX) enzymes 1 and 2, which are responsible for the production of prostaglandins that are significantly increased in inflamed tissue and contribute to the development of signs of inflammation and pain (Papich, 2000). While COX-1 is constitutively produced to maintain homeostasis, COX-2 is mainly up-regulated in response to a noxious insult. Since COX-1's primary role is to protect the stomach and intestines and contribute to blood clotting, using drugs that inhibit it can lead to adverse side effects. Drugs that selectively inhibit COX-2, result in control of pain and inflammation with reduced side effects. NSAIDs are used in veterinary medicine, providing good and long-lasting analgesia (Jin and Chung, 2001). NSAIDs are also not subjected to the restrictions that opioids have (Dahl and Kehlet, 1991).

ASA, also known as aspirin, is used to reduce pain, fever, or inflammation. At least two different types of cyclooxygenases, COX-1 and COX-2, are acted on by ASA. It irreversibly inhibits COX-1 and modifies the enzymatic activity of COX-2. Administration of 2.5 mg/L aspirin in zebrafish at 5 days postfertilization prevented the behavioral changes induced by acetic acid (Lopez-Luna et al., 2017).

Ketoprofen is an NSAID with high selectivity for COX-1, but the elevated inhibitory effect over prostaglandin production may lead to gastrointestinal ulceration and nephrotoxicity (Pelligand et al., 2014). Ketoprofen in goldfish (*Carassius auratus*) may provide analgesia since it decreased MS-222 anesthetic needs in MAC studies (Ward et al., 2012).

Carprofen is an NSAID able to provide a good postoperative analgesia for up to 24 hours while having reduced side effects due to its limited COX-1 inhibition. Its specificity for COX-2 varies from species to species (Lascelles et al., 1995). In the rainbow trout (*Oncorhynchus mykiss*), carprofen ameliorated effects of noxious stimulation on time to resume feeding, but activity was reduced more than by noxious treatment alone (Mettam et al., 2011).

2. Refinement and preventive analgesia

Animals are premedicated to minimize stress resulting in hyperalgesia (Jennings et al., 2014), reduce the doses of induction and maintenance drugs, optimize conditions for a smooth induction and recovery, and provide preemptive analgesia. Lidocaine hydrochloride may be used to improve zebrafish fin clipping analgesia (Deakin et al., 2019). However, in fish, there are not many more viable published protocols with analgesics and anesthetics used as premedication. In addition, side effects, including effects on experimental results, of true analgesic compounds are either not well or not at all studied. It is generally accepted that stress increases the sensitivity to pain. Stress can be caused by inadequate housing conditions, e.g., wrong water parameters, social isolation, crowding, or rapid change of environmental conditions. Handling by unexperienced personnel can also lead to stress. Housing conditions should be adjusted to minimize stress, and fish should only be handled by staff trained in the specific handling technique required. Stress reduction may be considered a preanesthesia requirement.

3. Analgesia recommendations for specific situations

Several studies could show that a range of drugs with analgesic properties (ASA, lidocaine, flunixin, and morphine) can normalize behavior in fin-clipped fish, though one should note that the amount of fin clipped in these studies exceeded >20% of the tail fin, so this might not be applicable to fin-clipping for genotyping, where usually only the tail tip is clipped. Schroeder et al. (2021) published a detailed peri-operative analgesia protocol for zebrafish fin clipping. Lidocaine hydrochloride 2–5 mg/L may be added to the holding tanks preop and to the recovery tanks until the next water change (i.e., 48 hours) to improve analgesia.

As skin lesions can be painful, analgesic treatment should be considered. For group-housed fishes, this usually requires the removal of the affected fish from the group by netting. However, the chasing and netting might increase stress levels and pain to such an extent, that it might outweigh the benefit of the analgesic treatment. Many analgesic substances are administered by IM or IP injection (Table 16.3). Fish should be under general anesthesia to facilitate handling and to prevent pain at the injection site prior to these application procedures.

V. Postprocedural recovery and care

A. Recovery period and return to group housing

Compared to other species, postoperative care in fish is often compromised: analgesia, pain, and some adverse effects are more difficult to control and supplementary netting experiences should be avoided. Great care should be taken during the recovery stage to minimize stress and prevent mortality. If an animal fails to recover, increasing the flow of anesthetic-free water over the gills will often accelerate and normalize the heartbeat. Moving the fish backwards and forwards in the recovery bath or gently passing water over the gills with a hose will increase gill blood flow and eliminate the drug more rapidly.

For the recovery period, anesthetized fish should be kept isolated from untreated fish. Reactions are still slowed down and the fish have problems to keep their balance, thus not using the whole water column for swimming. This changed behavior can trigger other fish to become aggressive toward the recovering fish. This is of main importance in territorial species. In most cases fish recover very quickly and as soon as they show normal swimming behavior, they can be regrouped with their companions. In smaller species, for most surgical procedures, no sutures are required. To our knowledge, there isn't any report yet that suture material is attacked by companion fish in the same tank so that the individuals do not have to be kept isolated (Coyle, 2004).

B. Supportive care

Fishes are susceptible to diseases caused by a large number of infectious agents, including viruses, bacteria, true fungi, fungal-like microorganisms, other protists, and metazoans. The main problem during recovery is pathogens in the normal water, mainly bacterial or fungal infections, opportunist of the skin lesions caused by desiccation of the mucus layer when fish need to be kept outside of the water during a procedure. Thus, the constant moistening of the skin during anesthesia while the fish is removed from the water is of great importance. This can be reached by covering the animal in wet tissues around the surgical area. Fish can be placed in low-melting agarose or wet sponges when proper positioning is required. In bigger species, "custom-made" constructs creating a constant flow above the body have been applied (Harms, 2005).

In case of a bacterial or fungal infection, the fish should be isolated again to reduce the pathogen load in the system. If available, fish can be treated with antibiotics or antifungal drugs upon the advice of a veterinarian. However, external treatments are challenging. Preventative care with regular water changes, filtering, and UV treatments, is essential to maintain ideal aquarium chemistry. Undesirable environmental conditions, including poor water quality, overcrowding, and/or stress by incompatible conditions, create conditions that can lead to destructive outbreaks. Flukes are often present in aquariums but remain harmless under ideal conditions. Avoiding stressful conditions is a key to prevention, but once an outbreak occurs, prompt treatment is critical.

VI. Pain and welfare assessment

In addition to the importance of a good anesthetic protocol to ensure fish welfare during experimental procedures, animals should also be monitored for distress, discomfort, and pain during all the experimental protocol maintenance and recovery. Fish have demonstrated to react consistently to noxious chemical stimuli and present reliable phenotypes of stress, fear, and anxiety. Thus, the use of analgesic drugs in fish during and after painful experimental procedures should be considered, especially due to the fact that not all anesthetic agents available for fish have proved to have adequate analgesic properties (Zahl et al., 2012; Martins et al., 2019). The information concerning the use of analgesics in fish is extremely scarce (Table 16.3). In this context it is essential to assess pain and distress continuously to rapidly detect animal welfare changes. Welfare assessment may be based on physical appearance and behavioral observations (Table 16.4).

There have also been reports that physiological parameters may change due to pain and distress. These include increased blood pressure (Stasiak et al., 2003), elevated cortisol levels (Sloman et al., 2019) as well as altered blood biochemistry, e.g., plasma glucose, creatine kinase, potassium, and total protein, among others (Harms et al., 2005). As blood sampling is a final procedure in small fish, using these parameters to assess pain is limited to larger fish. These observations may be compiled to develop specific score sheets to evaluate pain and distress in laboratory fish. Researchers in Germany have designed an evaluation sheet for the assessment of the health and welfare risks of genetically altered teleost fish (Bert et al., 2016). Furthermore, by scoring clinical signs and their severity in a list, a health record is created over time. The score sheet can contain the number of animals affected as well as the severity of the observed changes. These data can be the basis for decisions on euthanasia. Score sheets for zebrafish can be downloaded at https://www.humane-endpoints.info/en/zebravis-v1/scoringslijsten.

TABLE 16.4 Fish welfare assessment parameters.

Behavioral abnormalities	Physical abnormalities
Fish breathing at surface or near water inlet	Color change (darkening)/loss of pigment
Rapid breathing/opercula movements	Weight loss/emaciation (low body to head ratio)
Sluggish movement/lethargy	Exophthalmia/pop-eyes
Flashing/rubbing on tank surface (itching)	Distended abdomen/heart edemas
Circling/twirling, spinning (itching)	Skeletal deformity (scoliosis, lordosis)
Loss of equilibrium	Mass/swelling
Aggression	Hemorrhage/redness
Shoal is swimming together very closely	Gas bubbles
Shoal "freezes" (fear behavior)	Protruding scales
Excited swimming	Fin erosion or lesion
Escape behavior	Skin ulceration or lesion
Hiding	Tumors
Isolation from shoal	Scabby mucus
Pendulum movement (floating position)	Bent body axis
Fins close to body	No production of eggs
Reduced/missing food consumption	Missing opercula/fins

References

Adel, M., Sadegh, A.B., Yeganeh, S., Movafagh, A.N., Saoud, I.P., 2016. Anesthetic efficacy of clove oil, propofol, 2-phenoxyethanol, and ketamine hydrochloride on Persian sturgeon, Acipenser persicus, juveniles. J. World Aquacult. Soc. 47 (6), 812–819. https://doi.org/10.1111/jwas.12286.

Akbary, P., Pirbeigi, A., Jahanbakhshi, A., 2016. Analysis of primary and secondary stress responses in bighead carp (Hypophthalmichthys nobilis) by anesthetization with 2-phenoxyethanol. Int. J. Environ. Sci. Technol. 13 (4), 1009–1016. https://doi.org/10.1007/s13762-015-0923-x.

Baker, T.R., Baker, B.B., Johnson, S.M., Sladky, K.K., 2013. Comparative analgesic efficacy of morphine sulfate and butorphanol tartrate in koi (*Cyprinus carpio*) undergoing unilateral gonadectomy. J. Am. Vet. Med. Assoc. 243 (6), 882–890. https://doi.org/10.2460/javma.243.6.882.

Barata, M., Soares, F., Aragão, C., Almeida, A.C., Pousão-Ferreira, P., Ribeiro, L., 2016. Efficiency of 2-phenoxyethanol and clove oil for reducing handling stress in reared meagre, Argyrosomus regius (Pisces: Sciaenidae). J. World Aquacult. Soc. 47 (1), 82–92. https://doi.org/10.1111/jwas.12245.

Becker, A.G., Parodi, T.V., Heldwein, C.G., Zeppenfeld, C.C., Heinzmann, B.M., Baldisserotto, B., 2012. Transportation of silver catfish, *Rhamdia quelen*, in water with eugenol and the essential oil of Lippia alba. Fish Physiol. Biochem. 38 (3), 789–796. https://doi.org/10.1007/s10695-011-9562-4.

Bernier, N.J., Randall, D.J., 1998. Carbon dioxide anaesthesia in rainbow trout: effects of hypercapnic level and stress on induction and recovery from anaesthetic treatment. J. Fish. Biol. 52 (3), 621–637. https://doi.org/10.1111/j.1095-8649.1998.tb02022.x.

Bernstein, P.S., Digre, K.B., Creel, D.J., 1997. Retinal toxicity associated with occupational exposure to the fish anesthetic MS-222. Am. J. Ophthalmol. 124 (6), 843–844. https://doi.org/10.1016/s0002-9394(14)71705-2.

Bert, B., Chmielewska, J., Bergmann, S., Busch, M., Driever, W., Finger-Baier, K., Hößler, J., Köhler, A., Leich, N., Misgeld, T., Nöldner, T., Reiher, A., Schartl, M., Seebach-Sproedt, A., Thumberger, T., Schönfelder, G., Grune, B., 2016. Considerations for a European animal welfare standard to evaluate adverse phenotypes in teleost fish. EMBO J. 35 (11), 1151–1154. https://doi.org/10.15252/embj.201694448.

Bolasina, S.N., de Azevedo, A., Petry, A.C., 2017. Comparative efficacy of benzocaine, tricaine methanesulfonate and eugenol as anesthetic agents in the guppy Poecilia vivipara. Aquacult. Rep. 6, 56–60. https://doi.org/10.1016/j.aqrep.2017.04.002.

Brown, C., 2015. Fish intelligence, sentience and ethics. Anim. Cognit. 18 (1), 1–17. https://doi.org/10.1007/s10071-014-0761-0.

Burka, J.F., Hammell, K.L., Horsberg, T.E., Johnson, G.R., Rainnie, D.J., Speare, D.J., 1997. Drugs in salmonid aquaculture–a review. J. Vet. Pharmacol. Therapeut. 20 (5), 333–349. https://doi.org/10.1046/j.1365-2885.1997.00094.x.

Carter, K.M., Woodley, C.M., Brown, R.S., 2011. A review of tricaine methanesulfonate for anesthesia of fish. Rev. Fish Biol. Fish. 21 (1), 51–59. https://doi.org/10.1007/s11160-010-9188-0.

Center for Substance Abuse Treatment, 2004. Clinical Guidelines for the Use of Buprenorphine in the Treatment of Opioid Addiction. Rockville (MD).

Chatigny, F., Creighton, C.M., Stevens, E.D., 2018. Updated review of fish analgesia. J. Am. Assoc. Lab. Anim. Sci. JAALAS 57 (1), 5–12. PMCID PMC5875091.

Chervova, L.S., Lapshin, D.N., 2000. Opioid modulation of pain threshold in fish. Dokl. Biol. Sci. Proc. Acad. Sci. USSR Biol. Sci. Sect. 375, 590–591. https://doi.org/10.1023/a:1026681519613.

Christiansen, E.F., Stoskopf, M.K., 2013. pH dynamics of tricaine methanesulfonate (MS-222) in fresh and artificial seawater. N. Am. J. Aquacult. 75 (3), 356–360. https://doi.org/10.1080/15222055.2013.783519.

Collymore, C., Crim, M.J., Lieggi, C., 2016. Recommendations for health monitoring and reporting for zebrafish research facilities. Zebrafish 13 (Suppl. 1), S138–S148. https://doi.org/10.1089/zeb.2015.1210.

Collymore, C., Tolwani, A., Lieggi, C., Rasmussen, S., 2014. Efficacy and safety of 5 anesthetics in adult zebrafish (*Danio rerio*). J. Am. Assoc. Lab. Anim. Sci. JAALAS 53 (2), 198–203. PMCID PMC3966278.

Cooke, S.J., Suski, C.D., Ostrand, K.G., Tufts, B.L., Wahl, D.H., 2004. Behavioral and physiological assessment of low concentrations of clove oil anaesthetic for handling and transporting largemouth bass (*Micropterus salmoides*). Aquaculture 239 (1–4), 509–529. https://doi.org/10.1016/j.aquaculture.2004.06.028.

Coyle, S.D., 2004. Anesthetics in aquaculture. With assistance of FAO of the UN: southern regional aquaculture center. Available online at: http://www.aces.edu/dept/fisheries/aquaculture/documents/5864154-3900fs.pdf.

Cupp, A.R., Schreier, T.M., Schleis, S.M., 2017. Live transport of yellow Perch and Nile Tilapia in AQUI-S 20E (10% eugenol) at high loading densities. N. Am. J. Aquacult. 79 (2), 176–182. https://doi.org/10.1080/15222055.2017.1281853.

Dahl, J.B., Kehlet, H., 1991. Non-steroidal anti-inflammatory drugs: rationale for use in severe postoperative pain. Br. J. Anaesth. 66 (6), 703–712. https://doi.org/10.1093/bja/66.6.703.

Davis, M.W., Stephenson, J., Noga, E.J., 2008. The effect of tricaine on use of the fluorescein test for detecting skin and corneal ulcers in fish. J. Aquat. Anim. Health 20 (2), 86–95. https://doi.org/10.1577/H07-023.1.

Deakin, A.G., Buckley, J., AlZu'bi, H.S., Cossins, A.R., Spencer, J.W., Al'Nuaimy, W., Young, I.S., Thomson, J.S., Sneddon, L.U., 2019. Automated monitoring of behaviour in zebrafish after invasive procedures. Sci. Rep. 9 (1), 9042. https://doi.org/10.1038/s41598-019-45464-w.

Duthie, D.J., 1998. Remifentanil and tramadol. Br. J. Anaesth. 81 (1), 51–57. https://doi.org/10.1093/bja/81.1.51.

Fassoulaki, A., 2011. Is propofol an analgesic? Eur. J. Anaesthesiol. 28 (7), 481–482. https://doi.org/10.1097/EJA.0b013e32834584a5.

Fish, F.F., 1943. The anaesthesia of fish by high carbon-dioxide concentrations. Trans. Am. Fish. Soc. 72 (1), 25–29. https://doi.org/10.1577/1548-8659(1942)72[25:TAOFBH]2.0.CO;2.

Fish, R.E., Danneman, P., Brown, M., Karas, A. (Eds.), 2008. Anesthesia and Analgesia in Laboratory Animals, 2. ed. Elsevier (American College of Laboratory Animal Medicine series), Amsterdam.

Gallego-Colon, E., Villalba, M., Tonkin, J., Cruz, F., Bernal, J.A., Jimenez-Borregureo, L.J., Schneider, M.D., Lara-Pezzi, E., Rosenthal, N., 2016. Intravenous delivery of adeno-associated virus 9-encoded IGF-1Ea propeptide improves post-infarct cardiac remodelling. NPJ Regen. Med. 1, 16001. https://doi.org/10.1038/npjregenmed.2016.1.

Kurt, G.A. (Ed.), 2017. The Cardiovascular System. Morphology, Control and Function. Elsevier Science, San Diego (Issn Ser, v.Volume 36A). Available online at: https://ebookcentral.proquest.com/lib/kxp/detail.action?docID=4982227.

Gholipourkanani, H., Ahadizadeh, S., 2013. Use of propofol as an anesthetic and its efficacy on some hematological values of ornamental fish *Carassius auratus*. SpringerPlus 2 (1), 76. https://doi.org/10.1186/2193-1801-2-76.

Gilderhus, P.A., 1990. Benzocaine as a fish anesthetic: efficacy and safety for spawning-phase salmon. Progress. Fish Cult. 52 (3), 189–191. https://doi.org/10.1577/1548-8640(1990)052<0189:BAAFAE>2.3.CO;2.

Goodman, G., Guidelines for anaesthesia and analgesia of fish. Available online at: https://norecopa.no/media/6360/guidelines-for-anaesthesia-and-analgesia-of-fish.pdf, checked on 2/1/2022.

Gräns, A., Niklasson, L., Sandblom, E., Sundell, K., Algers, B., Berg, C., Lundh, T., Axelsson, M., Sundh, H., Kiessling, A., 2016. Stunning fish with CO2 or electricity: contradictory results on behavioural and physiological stress responses. Anim. Int. J. Anim. Biosci. 10 (2), 294–301. https://doi.org/10.1017/S1751731115000750.

Gräns, A., Sandblom, E., Kiessling, A., Axelsson, M., 2014. Post-surgical analgesia in rainbow trout: is reduced cardioventilatory activity a sign of improved animal welfare or the adverse effects of an opioid drug? PLoS One 9 (4), e95283. https://doi.org/10.1371/journal.pone.0095283.

Grasshoff, C., Drexler, B., Rudolph, U., Antkowiak, B., 2006. Anaesthetic drugs: linking molecular actions to clinical effects. Curr. Pharmaceut. Des. 12 (28), 3665–3679. https://doi.org/10.2174/138161206778522038.

Gressler, L.T., Baldisserotto, B., Hundertmark Saccol, E.M., Jonas Sutili, F., Loebens, L., Pavanato, M.A., et al., 2016. Histological and Antioxidant Responses in *Rhamdia quelen* Sedated with Propofol. With Assistance of FAO of the UN. John Wiley & Sons, Ltd (Aquaculture research, vol. 47).

Harms, C.A., 2005. Surgery in fish research: common procedures and postoperative care. Lab. Anim. 34 (1), 28–34. https://doi.org/10.1038/laban0105-28.

Harms, C.A., Lewbart, G.A., Swanson, C.R., Kishimori, J.M., Boylan, S.M., 2005. Behavioral and clinical pathology changes in koi carp (*Cyprinus carpio*) subjected to anesthesia and surgery with and without intra-operative analgesics. Comp. Med. 55 (3), 221–226. PMCID 16089168.

Hudson, J.M., Johnson, J.R., Kynard, B., 2011. A portable electronarcosis system for anesthetizing salmonids and other fish. N. Am. J. Fish. Manag. 31 (2), 335–339. https://doi.org/10.1080/02755947.2011.578524.

Iversen, M., Eliassen, R.A., Finstad, B., 2009. Potential benefit of clove oil sedation on animal welfare during salmon smolt, *Salmo salar* L. transport and transfer to sea. Aquacult. Res. 40 (2), 233–241. https://doi.org/10.1111/j.1365-2109.2008.02091.x.

Iwama, G.K., McGeer, J.C., Pawluk, M.P., 1989. The effects of five fish anaesthetics on acid–base balance, hematocrit, blood gases, cortisol, and adrenaline in rainbow trout. Can. J. Zool. 67 (8), 2065–2073. https://doi.org/10.1139/z89-294.

Jennings, E.M., Okine, B.N., Roche, M., Finn, D.P., 2014. Stress-induced hyperalgesia. Prog. Neurobiol. 121, 1–18. https://doi.org/10.1016/j.pneurobio.2014.06.003.

Jin, F., Chung, F., 2001. Multimodal analgesia for postoperative pain control. J. Clin. Anesth. 13 (7), 524–539. https://doi.org/10.1016/s0952-8180(01)00320-8.

Katz, E.M., Chu, D.K., Casey, K.M., Jampachaisri, K., Felt, S.A., Pacharinsak, C., 2020. The stability and efficacy of tricaine methanesulfonate (MS222) solution after long-term storage. J. Am. Assoc. Lab. Anim. Sci. JAALAS. https://doi.org/10.30802/AALAS-JAALAS-19-000067.

Lascelles, B.D., Cripps, P., Mirchandani, S., Waterman, A.E., 1995. Carprofen as an analgesic for postoperative pain in cats: dose titration and assessment of efficacy in comparison to pethidine hydrochloride. J. Small Anim. Pract. 36 (12), 535–541. https://doi.org/10.1111/j.1748-5827.1995.tb02805.x.

Lopez-Luna, J., Al-Jubouri, Q., Al-Nuaimy, W., Sneddon, L.U., 2017. Reduction in activity by noxious chemical stimulation is ameliorated by immersion in analgesic drugs in zebrafish. J. Exp. Biol. 220 (Pt 8), 1451–1458. https://doi.org/10.1242/jeb.146969.

Maes, J., Verlooy, L., Buenafe, O.E., de Witte, P.A.M., Esguerra, C.V., Crawford, A.D., 2012. Evaluation of 14 organic solvents and carriers for screening applications in zebrafish embryos and larvae. PLoS One 7 (10), e43850. https://doi.org/10.1371/journal.pone.0043850.

Martins, T., Valentim, A., Pereira, N., Antunes, L.M., 2019. Anaesthetics and analgesics used in adult fish for research: a review. Lab. Anim. 53 (4), 325–341. https://doi.org/10.1177/0023677218815199.

Martins, T., Valentim, A.M., Pereira, N., Antunes, L.M., 2016. Anaesthesia and analgesia in laboratory adult zebrafish: a question of refinement. Lab. Anim. 50 (6), 476–488. https://doi.org/10.1177/0023677216670686.

Mettam, J.J., Oulton, L.J., McCrohan, C.R., Sneddon, L.U., 2011. The efficacy of three types of analgesic drugs in reducing pain in the rainbow trout, *Oncorhynchus mykiss*. Appl. Anim. Behav. Sci. 133 (3–4), 265–274. https://doi.org/10.1016/j.applanim.2011.06.009.

Mocho, J.P., Collymore, C., Farmer, S.C., Leguay, E., Murray, K.N., Pereira, N., et al., 2022a. FELASA-AALAS recommendations for monitoring and reporting of laboratory fish diseases and health status, with an emphasis on Zebrafish (*Danio rerio*). Comp. Med. 72 (3), 127–148. https://doi.org/10.30802/AALAS-CM-22-000034.

Mocho, J.P., Collymore, C., Farmer, S.C., Leguay, E., Murray, K.N., Pereira, N., et al., 2022b. FELASA-AALAS recommendations for biosecurity in an aquatic facility, including prevention of Zoonosis, introduction of new fish colonies, and quarantine. Comp. Med. 72 (3), 149–168. https://doi.org/10.30802/AALAS-CM-22-000042.

Murray, M.J., 2002. Fish surgery. Seminars Avian Exot. Pet Med. 11 (4), 246–257. https://doi.org/10.1053/saep.2002.126571.

Neiffer, D.L., Stamper, M.A., 2009. Fish sedation, analgesia, anesthesia, and euthanasia: considerations, methods, and types of drugs. ILAR J. 50 (4), 343–360. https://doi.org/10.1093/ilar.50.4.343.

Nordgreen, J., Tahamtani, F.M., Janczak, A.M., Horsberg, T.E., 2014. Behavioural effects of the commonly used fish anaesthetic tricaine methanesulfonate (MS-222) on zebrafish (*Danio rerio*) and its relevance for the acetic acid pain test. PLoS One 9 (3), e92116. https://doi.org/10.1371/journal.pone.0092116.

Papich, M.G., 2000. Pharmacologic considerations for opiate analgesic and nonsteroidal anti-inflammatory drugs. Vet. Clin. Small Anim. Pract. 30 (4), 815–837. https://doi.org/10.1016/s0195-5616(08)70009-3.

Pelligand, L., King, J.N., Hormazabal, V., Toutain, P.L., Elliott, J., Lees, P., 2014. Differential pharmacokinetics and pharmacokinetic/pharmacodynamic modelling of robenacoxib and ketoprofen in a feline model of inflammation. J. Vet. Pharmacol. Therapeut. 37 (4), 354–366. https://doi.org/10.1111/jvp.12107.

Pereira, N., 2016. Introduction to anaesthesia and surgery in fish. In: D'Almeida Bernardo, F. (Ed.), Maria Castilho Monteiro de Oliveira, Joana Espírito Santo Robalo, Practical Notions on Fish Health and Production. Bentham Science Publishers, pp. 127–182.

Pergolizzi, J.V., LeQuang, J.A., Berger, G.K., Raffa, R.B., 2017. The basic pharmacology of opioids informs the opioid discourse about misuse and Abuse: a review. Pain Ther. 6 (1), 1–16. https://doi.org/10.1007/s40122-017-0068-3.

Pirhonen, J., Schreck, C.B., 2003. Effects of anaesthesia with MS-222, clove oil and CO2 on feed intake and plasma cortisol in steelhead trout (*Oncorhynchus mykiss*). Aquaculture 220 (1–4), 507–514. https://doi.org/10.1016/S0044-8486(02)00624-5.

Prieto, G.F., Urzua, N.F., Mancini, M.A., Tonini, M.P., Messina, J., Salas, S., Errecalde, C.A., 2017. Anaesthetic effect of propofol on rainbow trout (*Oncorhynchus mykiss*) in two different concentrations. Iran. J. Vet. Surg. 12 (1), 18–24. https://doi.org/10.22034/ivsa.2017.51290.

Qin, Y., Zhang, J., Zhang, Y., Li, F., Li, Y., Han, Y., Zou, N., Pan, C., 2017. The effects of oxygenation aeration treatment on dissipation behaviors of tricaine mesylate in carp (*Cyprinus carpio*) muscle and water. Food Control 77, 50–56. https://doi.org/10.1016/j.foodcont.2017.01.027.

Raffa, R.B., 2014. On subclasses of opioid analgesics. Curr. Med. Res. Opin. 30 (12), 2579–2584. https://doi.org/10.1185/03007995.2014.952717.

Readman, G.D., Owen, S.F., Knowles, T.G., Murrell, J.C., 2017. Species specific anaesthetics for fish anaesthesia and euthanasia. Sci. Rep. 7 (1), 7102. https://doi.org/10.1038/s41598-017-06917-2.

Readman, G.D., Owen, S.F., Murrell, J.C., Knowles, T.G., 2013. Do fish perceive anaesthetics as aversive? PLoS One 8 (9), e73773. https://doi.org/10.1371/journal.pone.0073773.

Reid, C.H., Vandergoot, C.S., Midwood, J.D., Stevens, E.D., Bowker, J., Cooke, S.J., 2019. On the electroimmobilization of fishes for research and practice: opportunities, challenges, and research needs. Fisheries 44 (12), 576–585. https://doi.org/10.1002/fsh.10307.

Robertson, S.A., Taylor, P.M., 2004. Pain management in cats–past, present and future. Part 2. Treatment of pain–clinical pharmacology. J. Feline Med. Surg. 6 (5), 321–333. https://doi.org/10.1016/j.jfms.2003.10.002.

Rodnick, K., Gesser, H., 2017. Cardiac energy metabolism. Chapter 6. In: Kurt Gamperl, A. (Ed.), The Cardiovascular System. Morphology, Control and Function. Elsevier Science (Issn Ser, v.Volume 36A, San Diego, pp. 317–367.

Ross, L.G., Ross, B., 2008. Anaesthetic and Sedative Techniques for Aquatic Animals. Blackwell Publishing Ltd, Oxford, UK.

Sandblom, E., Seth, H., Sundh, H., Sundell, K., Axelsson, M., Kiessling, A., 2013. Stress responses in Arctic char (*Salvelinus alpinus* L.) during hyperoxic carbon dioxide immobilization relevant to aquaculture. Aquaculture 414–415, 254–259. https://doi.org/10.1016/j.aquaculture.2013.07.047.

Schroeder, P., Lloyd, R., McKimm, R., Metselaar, M., Navarro, J., O'Farrell, M., Readman, G.D., Speilberg, L., Mocho, J.-P., 2021. Anaesthesia of laboratory, aquaculture and ornamental fish: proceedings of the first LASA-FVS symposium. Lab. Anim. 55 (4), 317–328. https://doi.org/10.1177/0023677221998403.

Schroeder, P.G., Sneddon, L.U., 2017. Exploring the efficacy of immersion analgesics in zebrafish using an integrative approach. Appl. Anim. Behav. Sci. 187, 93–102. https://doi.org/10.1016/j.applanim.2016.12.003.

Short, C.E., 1998. Fundamentals of pain perception in animals. Appl. Anim. Behav. Sci. 59 (1–3), 125–133. https://doi.org/10.1016/S0168-1591(98)00127-0.

Short, C.E., Driedzic, W.R., 2018. Species-specific low plasma glucose in fish is associated with relatively high tissue glucose content and is inversely correlated with cardiac glycogen content. J. Comp. Physiol. B Biochem. Syst. Environ. Physiol. 188 (5), 809–819. https://doi.org/10.1007/s00360-018-1172-3.

Sladky, K.K., Swanson, C.R., Stoskopf, M.K., Loomis, M.R., Lewbart, G.A., 2001. Comparative efficacy of tricaine methanesulfonate and clove oil for use as anesthetics in red pacu (Piaractus brachypomus). Am. J. Vet. Res. 62 (3), 337–342. https://doi.org/10.2460/ajvr.2001.62.337.

Sloman, K.A., Bouyoucos, I.A., Brooks, E.J., Sneddon, L.U., 2019. Ethical considerations in fish research. J. Fish. Biol. 94 (4), 556–577. https://doi.org/10.1111/jfb.13946.

Small, B.C., 2003. Anesthetic efficacy of metomidate and comparison of plasma cortisol responses to tricaine methanesulfonate, quinaldine and clove oil anesthetized channel catfish *Ictalurus punctatus*. Aquaculture 218, 177–185.

Sneddon, L.U., 2003. The evidence for pain in fish: the use of morphine as an analgesic. Appl. Anim. Behav. Sci. 83 (2), 153–162. https://doi.org/10.1016/S0168-1591(03)00113-8.

Sneddon, L.U., 2009. Pain perception in fish: indicators and endpoints. ILAR J. 50 (4), 338–342. https://doi.org/10.1093/ilar.50.4.338.

Sneddon, L.U., 2012. Clinical anesthesia and analgesia in fish. J. Exot. Pet Med. 21 (1), 32–43. https://doi.org/10.1053/j.jepm.2011.11.009.

Sneddon, L.U., 2019. Evolution of nociception and pain: evidence from fish models. Philos. Trans. R. Soc. Lond. Ser. B Biol. Sci. 374 (1785), 20190290. https://doi.org/10.1098/rstb.2019.0290.

Sneddon, L.U., Braithwaite, V.A., Gentle, M.J., 2003. Novel object test: examining nociception and fear in the rainbow trout. J. Pain 4 (8), 431–440. https://doi.org/10.1067/s1526-5900(03)00717-x.

Sørum, U., Damsgård, B., 2004. Effects of anaesthetisation and vaccination on feed intake and growth in Atlantic salmon (*Salmo salar* L.). Aquaculture 232 (1–4), 333–341. https://doi.org/10.1016/S0044-8486(03)00529-5.

Spears, J., Kamunde, C., Stevens, E.D., 2014. Effect of TRIS and bicarbonate as buffers on anesthetic efficacy of tricaine methane sulfonate in Zebrafish (*Danio rerio*). Zebrafish 11 (6), 590–596. https://doi.org/10.1089/zeb.2014.0975.

Stasiak, K.L., Maul, D., French, E., Hellyer, P.W., VandeWoude, S., 2003. Species-specific assessment of pain in laboratory animals. Contemp. Top. Lab. Anim. Sci. 42 (4), 13–20. https://doi.org/10.1016/S0044-8486(02)00302-2.

Stoskopf, M.K., 2015. Biology and management of laboratory fishes. In: Fox, J.G., Anderson, L.C., Otto, G., Pritchett-Corning, K.R., Whary, M.T. (Eds.), Laboratory Animal Medicine. Elsevier, pp. 1063–1086.

Stoskopf, M.K., Posner, L.P., 2008. Anesthesia and restraint of laboratory fishes. In: Fish, R.E., Danneman, P., Brown, M., Karas, A. (Eds.), Anesthesia and Analgesia in Laboratory Animals. 2. Elsevier (American College of Laboratory Animal Medicine series), Amsterdam, pp. 519–534.

Tesmer, A.L., Fields, N.P., Robles, E., 2022. Input from torus longitudinalis drives binocularity and spatial summation in zebrafish optic tectum. BMC Biol. 20 (1), 24. https://doi.org/10.1186/s12915-021-01222-x.

Valença-Silva, G., Braz, M.G., Barreto, R.E., Salvadori, D.M.F., Volpato, G.L., 2014. Low dose of the anesthetic propofol does not induce genotoxic or mutagenic effects in Nile Tilapia. Trans. Am. Fish. Soc. 143 (2), 414–419. https://doi.org/10.1080/00028487.2013.856814.

Valentim, A.M., Félix, L.M., Carvalho, L., Diniz, E., Antunes, L.M., 2016. A new anaesthetic protocol for adult zebrafish (*Danio rerio*): propofol combined with lidocaine. PLoS One 11 (1), e0147747. https://doi.org/10.1371/journal.pone.0147747.

Wagner, G.N., Singer, T.D., Scott McKinley, R., 2003. The ability of clove oil and MS-222 to minimize handling stress in rainbow trout (*Oncorhynchus mykiss* Walbaum). Aquacult. Res. 34 (13), 1139–1146. https://doi.org/10.1046/j.1365-2109.2003.00916.x.

Ward, J.L., McCartney, S.P., Chinnadurai, S.K., Posner, L.P., 2012. Development of a minimum-anesthetic-concentration depression model to study the effects of various analgesics in goldfish (*Carassius auratus*). J. Zoo Wildl. Med. Off. Publ. Am. Assoc. Zoo Vet. 43 (2), 214–222. https://doi.org/10.1638/2010-0088.1.

Witeska, M., Teodorczuk, B., Lugowska, K., 2017. Hematological effects of etomidate and tricaine in common carp. Turk. J. Vet. Anim. Sci. 41, 93–98. https://doi.org/10.3906/vet-1603-30.

Wong, D., von Keyserlingk, M.A.G., Richards, J.G., Weary, D.M., 2014. Conditioned place avoidance of zebrafish (*Danio rerio*) to three chemicals used for euthanasia and anaesthesia. PLoS One 9 (2), e88030. https://doi.org/10.1371/journal.pone.0088030.

Wynd, B.M., Watson, C.J., Patil, K., Sanders, G.E., Kwon, R.Y., 2017. A dynamic anesthesia system for long-term imaging in adult zebrafish. Zebrafish 14 (1), 1–7. https://doi.org/10.1089/zeb.2016.1289.

Xu, C., Volkery, S., Siekmann, A.F., 2015. Intubation-based anesthesia for long-term time-lapse imaging of adult zebrafish. Nat. Protoc. 10 (12), 2064–2073. https://doi.org/10.1038/nprot.2015.130.

Zahl, I.H., Samuelsen, O., Kiessling, A., 2012. Anaesthesia of farmed fish: implications for welfare. Fish Physiol. Biochem. 38 (1), 201–218. https://doi.org/10.1007/s10695-011-9565-1.

Zhuo, H., Jin, H., Peng, H., Huang, H., 2016. Distribution, pharmacokinetics and primary metabolism model of tramadol in zebrafish. Mol. Med. Rep. 14 (6), 5644–5652. https://doi.org/10.3892/mmr.2016.5956.

Chapter 17

Anesthesia and analgesia in laboratory pigs

Thea Fleischmann[1], **R. Eddie Clutton**[2], **Henning Andreas Haga**[3], **Hugo van Oostrom**[4] **and Miriam Weisskopf**[1]

[1]*Center of Surgical Research, University Hospital Zurich, University of Zurich, Zurich, Switzerland;* [2]*Large Animal Research and Imaging Facility, The Roslin Institute, The University of Edinburgh, Roslin, United Kingdom;* [3]*Anaesthesia Unit, Faculty of Veterinary Medicine, Norwegian University of Life Sciences, Ås, Norway;* [4]*IVC/Evidensia, Utrecht, the Netherlands*

Chapter outline

Anesthesia and Analgesia in Laboratory Animals. https://doi.org/10.1016/B978-0-12-822215-7.00031-7

I. Introduction

A. Pigs in biomedical research

Pigs are commonly used in biomedical research, which is explained by both the clear physiological similarities between pigs and humans, and the creation of minipigs. Due to their significantly smaller size, the running costs of studies using minipigs are lower than studies using conventionally sized pigs. Taken together, pigs represent an affordable alternative to rodents with closer matching physio-pathological features to humans, which has led to an increase in the use of pigs in research.

Pigs are used in various studies, including cardiovascular, skin burns and wound healing, organ transplantation, drug or device safety, and studies for training surgeons. For a comprehensive review of the use of pigs in (biomedical) research see Gutierrez et al. (2015).

B. Specific anatomy and physiology of pigs relevant to anesthesia

Pigs are intelligent, inquisitive, stubborn, and easily stressed. While apparently friendly-looking, large, adult pigs can be fierce and dangerous. These combined features can complicate anesthesia in pigs. However, an understanding of pig behavior, combined with an appreciation of species-specific physiological and pharmacological characteristics is the basis of high-quality anesthetic management—as it is in other species. Depending on age and breed, the size of pigs can vary considerably, with body masses ranging from 1 to more than 100 kg. The size of the pig will determine the specifics of protocols, equipment, and other resources needed for safe and effective anesthetic management.

The inquisitive and intelligent nature of pigs can be used to train them for many procedures, and render handling easier, safer, and less stressful for the animal and handler. Training may even preclude the need for sedation and/or general anesthesia altogether. For more details on training pigs for procedures, see Section II of this chapter. Pigs have a stocky build and extensive subcutaneous fat deposits. This, combined with their behavior, may complicate venous access in the conscious animal. Generally, intravenous cannulation is only possible after adequate sedation has been achieved. For more details on IV catheter placement see Section V of this chapter.

Large subcutaneous fat deposits mean that attempted intramuscular injections are often made into adipose tissue. In the pelvic limb and lateral neck muscles just caudal to the ear, fat deposits are limited, and intramuscular injection easier to achieve. The cervical location is preferred over the pelvic limb, as it is easier to reach and the risk of accidently injecting into the sciatic nerve is avoided. For more details on intramuscular injections, see Section V of this chapter.

Pigs have a long snout and oral cavity, their epiglottis is often 'trapped' above the soft palate, the larynx is sensitive and the glottic airway follows a somewhat sigmoid course. Furthermore, their trachea is small in relation to the body mass. These factors can make endotracheal intubation in pigs challenging; however, with the correct technique, it is a feasible and recommended procedure. For more details on endotracheal intubation, see Section V of this chapter. Despite their subcutaneous fat deposits, their sparse bristle coat means that pigs readily develop hypothermia during anesthesia. Every effort should be made to keep the animal warm. In addition, due to the lack of a protective coat, the skin of pigs is easily damaged. Therefore, adequate padding and gentle manipulation and positioning of anesthetized pigs should be practiced.

This chapter aims to provide a comprehensive overview of these approaches, techniques, and protocols to aid research groups in achieving better anesthetic care for their research animals and consequently generating better research results.

For specific anesthesia-related questions not covered by this book, scientists are encouraged to consult specialists in Veterinary Anesthesia and Analgesia or Laboratory Animal Medicine.

II. Preprocedural considerations and planning

A. Health and safety

Animal risks: The risks of working with commercial pigs have been summarized (NCSV, 1995), with 20 specific occupational hazards identified by pig veterinarians (Hafer et al., 1996). The most common physical injuries result from lifting or moving pigs and accidents occurring during postmortem examination. Lung and skin injuries associated with exposure to formalin and disinfectants appear to be more common than the zoonotic agents they (presumably) are meant to control, e.g., Erysipelas, Staphylococcus, Streptococcus, Salmonella, and Klebsiella. However, these conditions, along with ecto- and endoparasites and mycoses, are probably less common in laboratory herds. Hearing damage is common amongst commercial pig veterinarians, which is unsurprising: screaming is a porcine defense mechanism and in reaching 110 dB (Weeks et al., 2009) is injurious to human hearing (Health USDoHHSNIo, 2010). High noise levels in housed pigs cause adrenocortical and sympathetic nervous system changes, which may lead to behavioral anomalies and growth retardation (Otten et al., 2004). They should be minimized in the laboratory by pig selection (laboratory-bred versus commercially sourced), effective training of personnel *and* pigs, and the judicious use of pharmacological rather than physical restraint methods.

B. Animal sourcing

The types of laboratory pig required (and its sourcing) are dictated by study requirements and cost. Laboratory suppliers or research institutes may breed "wild-type" or genetically modified animals modeling specific diseases. These and pigs reared on commercial farms will vary in genotype, disease and health status, production welfare standards, availability, and cost. Some biological features, i.e., genotype, growth rate, the onset of sexual maturity, adult size, and temperament, may be prioritized for experimental reasons. Some of these and other characteristics, e.g., pharmacogenomics, physiology, anatomy, and body composition, may affect anesthetic management. Information on physiological, biological, and hematological data exists for common breeds at different ages and sexes (Swindle, 2007) and should be consulted when concerns arise.

Size: The relatively slow growth rates and low body masses of mature adults make miniature laboratory pigs popular for chronic studies, or the initial testing of expensive reagents. Compared to larger commercial pigs favored for cost reasons in acute studies, or when human size relevance is important, the small size of minipigs means that using anesthetic equipment designed for pediatric humans, rather than adults (or pigs weighing 55 kg or more) may be advisable. This applies to equipment for tracheal intubation, venous access, anesthetic breathing systems, and monitoring sensors, e.g., for pulse oximetry or spirometry. In theory, smaller animals are more prone to hypothermia than larger pigs, so thermoregulatory measures must be applied more meticulously.

Breed: In addition to absolute size, ethological, anatomical, and physiological differences between different breeds may alter their responses to anesthetics. In general, laboratory-bred minipigs are docile, which may account for greater sensitivity to sedative drug combinations. Commercial pigs which are well-handled are likely to be similarly sensitive. Breed-related physiological differences may exist and affect study generalizability and responses to anesthetics, although age and body mass are confounding factors. Significant hemodynamic differences were found in 4-month-old Hanford, Yucatan miniature, and micropig during the same anesthetic (Smith et al., 1990). In contrast, no significant differences were found between Gottingen, Yucatan, and commercial pigs weighing 25 kg (Benharkate et al., 1993).

Genotype: Genetically modified pigs may have overt phenotypes presenting clear anesthetic challenges, e.g., glucose homeostasis in the diabetic GIPR^{dn} transgenic pig (Wolf et al., 2014). Whilst there appears to be little information on the subject, it seems possible that some marginally harmful phenotypes may only become apparent when affected animals are anesthetized and undergo biologically challenging procedures.

Age: Pre- and postnatal piglets are used to model neonatal human conditions (Svendsen and Koch, 2013) and present considerable anesthetic challenges. Literature describing anesthesia for piglet castration exists but is of little relevance to piglets used, for example, in studies of neonatal cerebral hypoxia. Defining the effects of age on response to anesthetics is difficult because age and body mass are closely related. However, neither age nor mass influenced the response of commercially bred pigs to intravenous anesthesia beyond 15 weeks of age or 57 kg body mass (Reed et al., 2015).

Sex: Sex is an important selection factor in reproductive or some experimental surgical studies. Otherwise, females have been excluded from basic and clinical research in anesthesia and other areas to avoid the variation in data produced by breeding, pregnancy, and hormonal changes (Mawhinney et al., 2013). However, males and female humans are physiologically distinct in their responses to various anesthetic agents so this exclusion represents considerable bias. Sex differences in sensitivity to anesthetics have been demonstrated repeatedly in mice (Hohlbaum et al., 2017) and rats (Zambricki and Dalecy, 2004), but there is no consistent pattern. The effect of sex on the sensitivity of pigs to anesthetics appears not to have been studied.

Health status: Pigs requiring anesthesia for experimental procedures will usually be healthy, as central nervous, cardiopulmonary, renal, or hepatic pathology will affect the response to anesthesia and increase morbidity and mortality. In chronic studies involving immunosuppressants and/or stressful procedures, freedom from specified pathogens may require that pigs be sourced from accredited specific pathogen-free herds. The propensity of certain genetic lines to develop malignant hyperthermia (MH) on exposure to volatile anesthetics, the related porcine stress syndrome during transport, or pale soft exudative pork (PSEP) postmortem must also be considered. The incidence of the "classical" phenotype appears to be waning although new forms have been identified (Nonneman et al., 2012) and a single case has been described in a Gottingen minipig (McInnes and McKeag, 2016). While animals may be screened by in-vitro caffeine-induced contracture or polymerase chain reaction tests, an examination of herd records for death during transit and carcass condemnation PSEP may be less expensive and adequately predictive.

Comprehensive recommendations on the health and welfare management of pigs bred on commercial farms, their transport to the facility, quarantine and acclimatization has been produced by the Federation of European Laboratory Animal Science Associations (FELASA) (Berset et al., 2021).

C. Transportation

Transportation stress results from noise, temperature extremes, crowding, pollutants, and infectious agents and may cause stress-induced cardiovascular, endocrine, immune, and reproductive changes (Seidler et al., 2001; Zucker and Kruger, 1998; Obernier and Baldwin, 2006). Using recently transported animals in experiments before their physiological status normalizes can have major confounding effects on research data (Obernier and Baldwin, 2006). While primary stress indices, e.g., catecholamines and glucocorticoids, normally return to physiological concentrations within 24 hours, immune and endocrine changes may take up to 7 days to normalize (Obernier and Baldwin, 2006). Upon arrival at the research facility, animals of unknown health status should be kept separately until their health status has been established (Kaiser et al., 2006).

D. Acclimatization

As transportation stress is likely to adversely affect research data, pigs should be acclimatized at the research facility for at least 7 days before experiments begin (Smith and Swindle, 2006). Acclimatization is also advisable when groups of pigs enrolled in chronic studies are transferred to laboratories from elsewhere. Acclimatization allows animals to (i) settle after transportation; (ii) become familiar with the new environment, diet, and personnel; (iii) be habituated and/or trained; (iv) undergo daily health checks; (v) be observed for behavior, food, and water intake and to be weighed (which facilitates the evaluation of post-procedural weight loss and other recovery complications). Acclimatization also allows the collection and analysis of baseline blood, urine, and other samples to facilitate the later interpretation of treatment effects. Acclimatization should last until these objectives are met and there is confidence that the study begins with each animal being biologically comparable, and at similarly low levels of stress. Acclimatization is also advisable (and for similar reasons) before short-term and/or acute studies.

Acclimatization may be less valuable when single pigs are required for terminal studies in which stress variables are unimportant, e.g., when exploratory surgical techniques are being developed, or when biosensors are being implanted and calibrated. Under these circumstances, a case may be made for anesthetizing singly-transported animals as soon as they reach the facility. This avoids problems with prolonged solitary housing—which may be as stressful as transport itself, or deciding the fate of any traveling "companion", which is superfluous to study requirements. This option should only be considered when animals are obtained from trusted farms with high herd health status and reliable health records, which are within brief traveling times from the facility, and when the scientific outcomes of the experiment are unaltered by transit stress.

E. Habituation and training

Training laboratory animals to participate in potentially stressful experimental procedures is seen as a major experimental refinement as it simultaneously improves animal welfare and data quality (Bailey, 2018). Training can be used to facilitate anesthesia, e.g., preoperative blood sampling, physical examination, accepting mask inductions, or replacing it entirely (thus avoiding the confounding effects of sedatives and anesthetics). Habituation techniques, which aim to decrease nonreinforced responses to stimuli by exposing the pig to repeated or prolonged stimulus exposure, have been used to replace anesthetics in chronic skin testing studies (Chilcott et al., 2001). Preprocedural habituation can also be used to improve an animal's postprocedural tolerance of surgical dressings, harnesses, being slung, and surgical implants. Positive reinforcement techniques, e.g., clicker training, have been used to promote voluntary participation of laboratory pigs in drug dosing, injections, clinical examinations, blood sampling, and repeated radiography (Herskin et al., 2021) (Fig. 17.1). Clicker training is rapidly effective in minipigs (Jonholt et al., 2021), and methods to accelerate its efficacy in farm-sourced laboratory pigs have been described (Thomsen and Kousholt, 2021). This is useful because animal training is time-consuming and increases study costs.

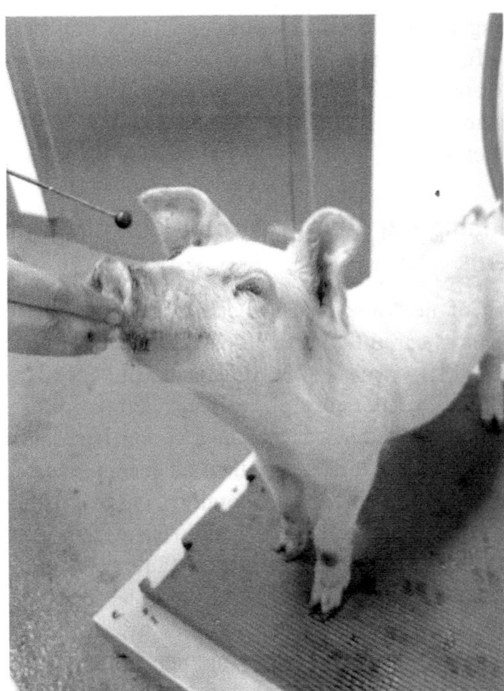

FIGURE 17.1 Pig being trained to follow target stick.

F. Preanesthetic examination

Pigs to be anesthetized are examined to: (i) indicate their suitability to undergo anesthesia and the proposed procedure by identifying and quantifying abnormalities that increase risk; (ii) determine whether preoperative preparation is required; and (iii) provide a datum against which the success of recovery may be gauged. Preanesthetic examination involves a perusal of the animal's records and a physical examination. If concerns are identified, more complex examinations may be required, but the animal should not be anesthetized for study until treatment—if indicated—is convincingly effective.

Individual health records may be available from suppliers or established during acclimatization. Of principle interest is the absence of health concerns and the presence of evidence that food intake and growth trajectories are normal.

Animals scheduled for anesthesia must be examined daily during acclimatization, or on the farm and immediately before transport if pigs are to be anesthetized on arrival. A physical (and hematological) examination is more difficult in pigs compared to other species and unless conducted sympathetically, is of less clinical value. Breed-related docility coupled with habituation to people, handling, nonaversive restraint, and physical examination will allow the collection of more meaningful information than possible when unhandled anxious animals are examined (or blood sampled) while physically restrained. The examination commonly begins with observation of the undisturbed animal amongst its undisturbed pen-mates to determine its: body and skin condition; spontaneous movement (if awake) and interactions with other pigs (including vocalization); respiratory pattern and rate; and ear, snout, and teat color. A note is taken of the presence or absence of gross lesions, e.g., skin erosions or hernias; ocular, nasal, and aural discharge; mouth breathing, coughing, or sneezing; or fecal staining of the perineum. The pen is then entered and the animal's response is noted. The bedding is checked for fecal consistency. Depending on the animal's reaction thus far, attempts may be made to usher the pig into a weighing crate where body weight is recorded, the rectal temperature is taken, and auscultation of the heart and lungs on the left and right sides is attempted.

When studies require preoperative hematological or biochemical values, then samples unaffected by stress at collection are best obtained from a heparinized venous cannula placed in the early stages of acclimatization. Habituating pigs to restraint in slings for blood sampling is widely advocated.

Technological advances in monitoring the health of commercially housed pigs remotely, e.g., using imagery and computer vision for the early detection of respiratory disease (Jorquera-Chavez et al., 2021) or ear-tag-based sensors to detect motion, vocalization, and temperature (Pandey et al., 2021), have considerable potential for assessing the study suitability of laboratory pigs in the near future.

G. Preoperative preparation

Preoperative preparation normally aims to resolve problems that increase anesthetic and procedural risk. However, low physical risk status is usually a prerequisite for the experimental use of laboratory pigs and so this measure is seldom necessary. Preoperative preparation also aims to ensure that all procedural requirements are available and functioning; this is facilitated by using available laboratory SOPs, consulting widely available recommendations for checking anesthetic equipment, and ensuring all items on the anesthetic plan are available in sufficient amounts. A further goal of preoperative preparation is to identify likely procedural problems and take steps to manage them should they arise. For example, preoperative blood collection is recommended before studies associated with critical hemorrhage, e.g., liver transplantation, or when extracorporeal support equipment requires priming with blood.

Blood typing and collection in pigs: Porcine blood group immunology is complex (Smith et al., 2006), and so studies requiring large volumes of blood avoid the risk of transfusion reactions (and the costs of cross-matching) by using autologous blood. This is a well-established approach, as the management of major intraoperative bleeding using traditional or experimental autotransfusion methods has been extensively studied in pigs (Solem et al., 1986). Autotransfusion also avoids the problems associated with autologous blood collection, which requires animal restraint for the collection of a finite blood volume. Porcine erythrocytes stored under standard human conditions are transfusable for up to 13 days after collection (Azevedo et al., 2009).

H. Food and water restriction

Preoperative food (and bedding) and water deprivation in pigs is said to prevent emesis, gastrointestinal gas accumulation, reduced venous return, gut wall edema, and cardiovascular failure, although evidence for this is scant. Arbitrary recommendations are potentially harmful because food and water restrictions cause adverse behavioral, biochemical, endocrine, hematologic, microbiological, thermoregulatory, and ulcerative gastric changes in pigs (Bradbury and Clutton, 2016a). Furthermore, there is little consensus and some confusion on the appropriate times: although stomach emptying in pigs requires only a few hours (Swindle, 2007), minimal recommended food restriction periods begin at 6 hours (Bradbury and Clutton, 2016a). Allowing ad libitum access to fresh water whilst removing edible bedding and food for 6–8 hours before anesthesia is recommended before most procedures. However, some gastro-intestinal studies may require a clean, empty motile intestine, in which case a combination of rectal enemata and a high-carbohydrate liquid diet as the sole energy source for 36–48 hours has proven acceptable, harmless, and effective (Gregson et al., 2021).

I. Preemptive analgesia

The merits of preemptive analgesia (PEA)—which aims to prevent the altered processing of nociceptive input that amplifies postoperative pain—are more demonstrable in animals (Woolf, 1983) than humans (Kissin, 2000) and in commercial pigs, preemptive meloxicam has benefits in both piglet castration (Keita et al., 2010) and farrowing (Mainau et al., 2012). This supports the practice of administering analgesics to pigs before noxious experimental procedures are begun. In practical terms, PEA involves incorporating opioid analgesics, ketamine, and alpha2-agonist drugs in preanesthetic medication, whereby the drugs' sedative effects augment those of other anxiolytics, e.g., benzodiazepines and/or butyrophenones, whilst simultaneously initiating a polymodal analgesic technique. The preemptive use of nonsteroidal antiinflammatory (NSAID) drugs should also be considered before operations involving extensive tissue destruction and inflammation. While PEA is intended to reduce postoperative pain (which is of greatest benefit in recovery procedures) its potential to reduce anesthetic doses also justifies its use in terminal experiments.

J. Planning the use of neuromuscular blocking agents

The use of neuromuscular blocking agents (NMBAs) in pigs requires careful consideration because the welfare effects of NMBAs misuse are dire, and while NMBAs are widely used in laboratory pigs, their incompetent use during noxious procedures is not uncommon (Bradbury and Clutton, 2016b). If the use of NMBAs is contemplated and experimentally justified in laboratory pigs, it is recommended that an experienced veterinary anesthesiologist, i.e., a Diplomate of the American (or European) College of Veterinary Anesthesia and Analgesia, be consulted or recruited. Maintaining anesthesia with a volatile agent is recommended because the measurement of end-tidal concentrations is straightforward and facilitates attempts to ensure the animal is anesthetized. Along with the ability to adequately ventilate the lungs of paralyzed animals, ensuring adequate anesthesia and analgesia is a minimum imperative when NMBAs are used. Both imperatives, but particularly the latter, should ideally be left to experienced personnel.

K. Repeated anesthesia

The interval permitted between repeated anesthetics, when required, is usually set by the Institutional Animal Care and Use Committee (IACUC) in resolving the opposing needs to maximize data collection while optimizing animal welfare. Such intervals will be arbitrary if they do not consider: (i) the drugs being given; (ii) the standard of anesthetic management provided; (iii) the procedure(s) for which the anesthetics are required; and; (iv) the duration of the repeated procedure. The intervals between which animals may be reanaesthetized without adverse effects are minimized when short-acting drugs with non cummulative properties are used for brief, innocuous procedures during which adverse physiological effects, such as hypotension and hypothermia, are prevented. Repeated anesthesia in pigs does not appear to cause adverse effects (Reed et al., 2015).

L. Documentation

Anesthesia-related documents, including the anesthetic record, may be required for legal, scientific, regulatory, accounting, and reporting reasons, and will be important in study planning, prosecution, and completion. An anesthetic plan providing the details of the intended anesthetic assists in preparatory discussions and assures a standardized anesthetic when several anesthesiologists participate in the same study. It also facilitates the completion of ARRIVE-compliant reports on the study's conclusion (Kilkenny et al., 2010).

Personnel training records and associated licenses are required in some countries before individuals can perform specified procedures on animals, including the administration of anesthetics. These should be examined to ensure legal compliance when extraordinary techniques, e.g., the use of NMBAs, are planned.

Individual animal records detailing breed, date of birth, health status, medical and experimental history, current medications, food and water intake, body weight and general health observations should be reviewed before recovery experiments and considered baseline information against which recovery can be gauged.

Anesthetic records are used to record animal details and pertinent information from the six major anesthetic periods, i.e., preoperative examination, preoperative preparation, preanesthetic medication, induction, maintenance, and recovery. Vital physiological information recorded at fixed, usually 5-minute intervals serves to focus the anesthetist's attention on those variables and their trajectories, and is an aid to good anesthetic management rather than the primary source of project data (Devitt et al., 1999).

Recovery records cover the periods from the discontinuation of anesthesia to the restoration of vital activity, and from the withdrawal of physiological support to the resumption of normal behaviors. These records must indicate the type (continuous vs. periodic) and extent of post-operative surveillance, the criteria triggering support measure withdrawal, e.g., O_2 delivery, and when certain end-points are reached. Recovery documents incorporating procedure-specific pain scoring systems are desirable when severe pain is likely and should include a clear indication for when rescue analgesia or euthanasia are required. The restoration (or otherwise) of ingestive, drinking, eliminative, grooming, and kinetic behaviors during recovery should be recorded and compared with the health record, as this will assist decisions over the animal's discharge from the recovery pen and reintroduction to pen-mates.

General recommendations for the objective recognition and assessment of pain in animals as well as systems for recording these, i.e., score sheets, have been formulated (Hawkins et al., 2011).

III. Sedation

A. Physical restraint

Pigs often forcefully object to being physically restrained and vocalize loudly. Depending upon the strength of the handler, pigs up to a certain size may be caught by a pelvic limb and lifted off the floor by supporting the ventral part of the body. A small piglet may be restrained on the handler's lap; however, this becomes difficult with increasing weight. If the pig is released into a small enclosure, for instance a cage-trolley, the pigs may be observed, a superficial clinical examination performed, and injections given intramuscularly. Even better access to the pig is achieved if the pig is placed in a hammock. These are commercially available from several providers, or can easily be manufactured. Most pigs will, after a little while, calm down in a hammock, and allow minor procedures to be performed (Fig. 17.2). If large pigs need to be forcefully restrained, a snout snare around the upper jaw can be used. The pig will commonly move backward after being caught by the snare. The result will be an immobilized but stressed animal.

B. Stress free injection methods

It is difficult to perform an intravenous injection in conscious pigs. Their skin, being adherent to the underlying tissue, makes a subcutaneous injection similarly difficult. Therefore, the intramuscular administration of preanesthetic medication is the most practical route. When extension tubing is used between the needle (a 0.8×40 mm needle is normally suitable) and syringe, injections can be made remotely from the pig (reducing its anxiety) while reducing the risk that movement will cause needle displacement (Fig. 17.3). Slow injections avoid the cannula being pushed out and also limit the pain of the injection. The muscles at the lateral side of the neck are commonly used and are associated with less avoidance behavior (Clutton et al., 1998).

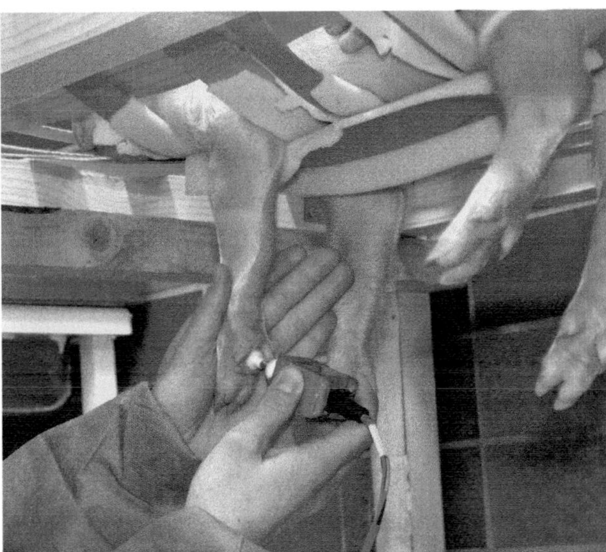

FIGURE 17.2 Pig in hammock for performance of minor procedures.

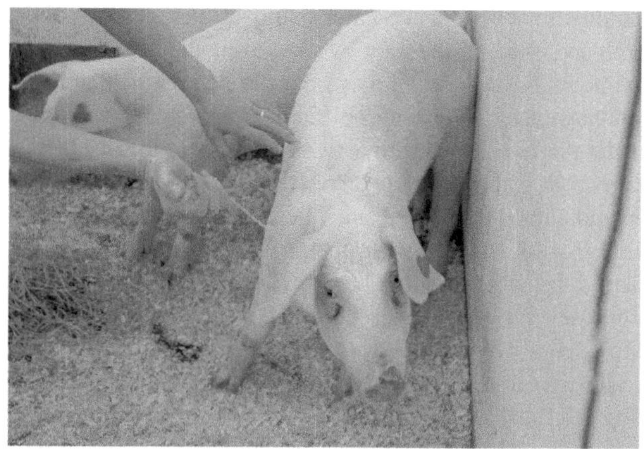

FIGURE 17.3 Pig being injected intramuscularly with extension tubing.

C. Agents

Sedative drugs are commonly used to facilitate the handling of pigs, or as part of preanesthetic medication. Drugs from several pharmacological classes are available, and the effects (both desirable and adverse) of numerous resulting combinations have been described. Examples of sedative agents are listed in Table 17.1.

1. Alpha2-agonists

Pigs appear to be less sensitive to alpha2-agonists than other mammals. Xylazine has limited efficacy as a sedative in pigs and high doses cause severe cardiovascular depression (Gomez de Segura et al., 1997). Medetomidine and dexmedetomidine induce dose-dependent sedation in pigs. There is an increasing sedative effect of medetomidine with increasing body weight (Ranheim and Haga, 2013). Medetomidine can lower plasma insulin concentrations and cause hyperglycemia (Nishimura et al., 1994), and if administered as a bolus there will be short-lasting hypertension, decreased cardiac output, and a longer-lasting bradycardia (Tendillo et al., 1996). The effects of medetomidine can be antagonized by atipamezole using 2–4 times higher dose than the medetomidine dose (Nishimura et al., 1992).

2. Phenothiazines

The sedative effect of acepromazine alone will be inadequate for most procedures (Nishimura et al., 1993a), and there are potential side effects such as hypotension and hypothermia. However, acepromazine may be usefully combined with other agents.

3. Butyrophenones

Azaperone has commonly been used as a sedative in commercial pig farming, to decrease fighting between pigs, for sedation, and as a premedication. Azaperone or droperidol can be used to achieve light to moderate sedation. The onset time is approximately 15 minutes after intramuscular administration and depending upon the dose used, the effect will last for several hours. Thermoregulation will be inhibited, and vasodilatation and hypotension can be expected (Nishimura et al., 1993a; Bustamante and Valverde, 1997; Clarke, 1969). Specific attention to monitoring and supporting body temperature and blood pressure is indicated.

TABLE 17.1 Examples of sedative agents.

Drug(s)	Dose (mg/kg)	Route of administration	Duration of action	Comments
Medetomidine	0.02–0.10	IV, IM	90–150 minutes	Minimal to deep sedation
Medetomidine Midazolam	0.02–0.08 0.2–0.6	IV, IM IV, IM	90–150 minutes	Moderate to deep sedation
Medetomidine Butorphanol	0.02–0.08 0.1–0.2	IV, IM IV, IM	90–150 minutes	Minimal to deep sedation
Azaperone	1–8	IM	120–600 minutes	Minimal to moderate sedation
Droperidol	0.1–0.4	IM	90–180 minutes	Minimal to moderate sedation
Midazolam	0.2–1.0	IV, IM	30–90 minutes	Minimal to moderate sedation
Ketamine Medetomidine Midazolam	5–10 20–60 0.4–0.8	IM IM IM	40–80 minutes	Deep sedation
Alfaxalone	4–6	IM		Moderate to deep sedation
Alfaxalone Midazolam	4 0.4	IM IM		Deep sedation

4. *Benzodiazepines*

Benzodiazepines can be used by themselves to induce light to moderate sedation and muscle relaxation, with little effect upon cardiac output (CO) (Smith et al., 1991). Both respiratory rate and tidal volume are reported to decrease (Klein and Reinhold, 2001), without significant influence upon arterial oxygen tension (Smith et al., 1991). Midazolam is water soluble and has a more predictable absorption after intramuscular administration compared to diazepam. The sedative effect of midazolam administered intramuscularly has an onset time of approximately 5 minutes and is, dose-dependent, lasting for up to an hour (Nishimura et al., 1993a; Bustamante and Valverde, 1997). Benzodiazepines are also useful as adjuncts to other drugs, either for sedation or for direct intramuscular induction of anesthesia. When combined with low-dose medetomidine a profound sedative effect is achieved (Nishimura et al., 1993b).

5. *Opioids*

Opioids are poor sedatives in pigs when administered as sole agents and can—dependent upon the dose—also result in excitation (Pavlovsky et al., 2021). If combined with other drugs opioids may enhance sedation. It has been demonstrated that butorphanol may enhance sedation with medetomidine (Sakaguchi et al., 1992), furthermore butorphanol is a common agent used in drug combinations for direct intramuscular induction of anesthesia.

D. Monitoring

Dependent upon the level of sedation the pig will have a more or less reduced ability for self-preservation. In addition, sedative drugs will have undesired physiological effects which can negatively affect the well-being of the animal. Thus, while being sedated the animal needs to be monitored, the level of monitoring needs to be adapted to the depth of sedation as well as the likelihood of negative effects. As a minimum, visual monitoring is needed until self-preservation is restored. Decreased ability for thermoregulation necessitates regular monitoring of body temperature, hypothermia being the most common problem, whereas hyperthermia may also ensue. The risk of hypoventilation or upper airway obstruction can be evaluated by monitoring respiratory movements of the thorax, respiratory sounds, and evaluating gas flow from the nostrils. Pulse-oximetry can be a valuable addition to manual monitoring.

E. Support

While being sedated, dry, well-tempered, and soft bedding is needed. If hypothermia is likely to occur, isolating material like a blanket or bubble wrap can be used. If warming mats are used, care must be taken not to overheat the surface of the animal since thermal burn is a well-known complication. Corneal injury is also possible if a heat source is applied too close to the eyes. If the animal hypoventilates, increasing the fraction of inspired oxygen by a loose-fitting mask or nostril prongs can be valuable. If a mask is used, the flow of gas needs to be high enough to prevent rebreathing of expired gas. If nasal prongs are used, rebreathing is not the same problem; however, obstruction of the nostrils needs to be avoided and the oxygen flow regulated to a level where it does not annoy the pig. If the oxygen is not humidified, excessive flow for some time may also dry out the nasal mucosa.

IV. General anesthesia

A. Preanesthetic evaluation

A good preanesthetic evaluation before starting the actual anesthetic procedure is paramount. Section II of this chapter discusses the importance of preprocedural considerations and planning. Next to these aspects, a history should be taken and a physical examination of the animal should be performed. For the history, animal caretakers can be asked whether the animal is behaving normally, whether the animal is fasting, and whether food and water intake have otherwise been normal. Thorough physical examination of pigs can at times be challenging; however, when observing the animal in its pen, a good impression of general demeanor, respiratory rate and type, and color of the skin can be obtained. With a calm approach, the ears or other extremities of the animal can be gently touched to get an impression of their temperature, and auscultation of the chest and measurement of rectal temperature can be performed. To facilitate the physical examination, small treats can be used to make the animal more cooperative. Based on the outcomes of the preanesthetic evaluation, it can be decided whether to proceed with the procedure or not and whether or not changes to the anesthetic protocol should be made.

B. Preanesthetic medication

1. *Aims*

The first aim of preanesthetic medication is to make the animal calm and cooperative. This is achieved by administering a sedative drug; see Section III of this Chapter. A second aim is to start analgesia when a painful procedure is planned, e.g., by including opioids in the premedication for a surgical procedure. A third aim is to counteract potential side effects of other anesthetic drugs that are used during the procedure, e.g., administering atropine to avoid opioid-induced bradycardia. A fourth aim is to be able to reduce the dose of the induction or maintenance agent used, e.g., less propofol or isoflurane is needed when sedatives and analgesics have been administered in the preanesthetic medication. The fifth and final aim is to plan ahead for a calm and comfortable recovery, i.e., when a sedative drug and adequate analgesia are provided, recoveries are usually smoother.

2. Routes of administration

Preanesthetic medication can be administered via different routes, e.g., orally, intranasally, oro-transmucosally, subcutaneously, intramuscularly, and intravenously. In pigs, the most reliable routes seem to be the intramuscular and intravenous route. As placement of an IV catheter is difficult in unsedated pigs, preanesthetic medication is usually given by intramuscular injection.

3. Agents

Sedative agents that can be used for pigs are described in Section IIIC of this chapter. Analgesic agents that can be included in preanesthetic medication are addressed in Sections VIII and IX.

Next to sedatives and analgesics, atropine or glycopyrrolate are sometimes added to preanesthetic medication. These are so-called antimuscarinic drugs and are usually administered to avoid bradycardia induced by opioids or vagal reflexes, e.g., the oculocardiac reflex during ocular surgery. Older texts describe administering antimuscarinic drugs as an antisialagogue, but this practice is nowadays considered obsolete. Preanesthetic medication greatly determines the quality of the rest of the anesthetic procedure and should therefore be carefully considered.

C. Induction

Induction of anesthesia involves administering anesthetic drugs, i.e., the induction agent(s), until the animal reaches a level of unconsciousness. Whether an animal has reached unconsciousness is arbitrary, but generally, it means the palpebral reflex of the animal is absent, the jaw tone is slack, and the animal will show little to no reaction to endotracheal intubation.

1. Methods for induction

General anesthesia can be induced in different ways. Intramuscular injections with a sufficient dose of induction agents will result in general anesthesia. However, this route is somewhat unpredictable in terms of the time of onset, and it is not possible to titrate the dose of the induction agent carefully to effect. Administering the induction agents intravenously overcomes these shortcomings. Another alternative of inducing general anesthesia is the so-called mask induction with a volatile anesthetic (Fig. 17.4). With this method, a tight-fitting mask connected to an anesthetic breathing system, is placed over the muzzle of the animal. After letting the animal breathe some oxygen, the vaporizer of the volatile anesthetic agent, e.g., isoflurane, can be activated and the percentage of volatile increased in a stepwise fashion until the animal has reached a state of general anesthesia. When general anesthesia is achieved, the vaporizer setting can be reduced or maintained at the set level, depending on the required depth of anesthesia. This latter method can be experienced as stressful by the animal as the pig needs to be physically restrained. Furthermore, personnel exposure levels to the volatile agent are high (Sare et al., 2011). However, particularly in piglets, mask-induction in a hammock with sevoflurane can be a good alternative to induction with injectable drugs.

As inducing general anesthesia causes significant changes to the animal's physiology, monitoring of at least respiratory rate and pattern and the peripheral pulse should be performed very regularly. Administration of any induction agent, especially via the intravenous route, can lead to apnea. Therefore, animals should be preoxygenated before starting induction, and adequate equipment and enough personnel should be ready to intubate the trachea of the animal so that the respiration can be taken over without unnecessary delay.

2. Agents

An overview of induction agents is provided in Table 17.2.

a. Ketamine

Ketamine is a so-called dissociative agent and exerts its effect by antagonism of the N-methyl-D-aspartate (NMDA) receptor. It leads to a form of general anesthesia where

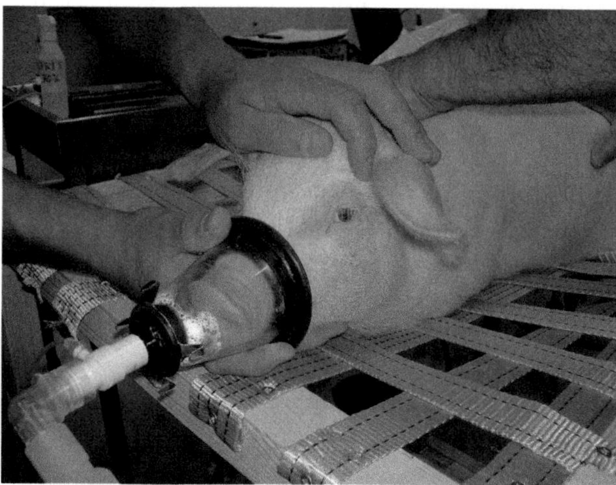

FIGURE 17.4 Pig in hammock; mask induction with volatile anesthetic.

TABLE 17.2 Overview of induction agents.

Drug(s)	Dose	Route of administration	Duration of action	Effects
Propofol	1–8 mg/kg depending on preanesthetic medication Dosed to effect	IV	15–20 minutes	Sedation, general anesthesia, vasodilation, decreased blood pressure, respiratory depression
Alfaxalone	0.5–6 mg/kg depending on preanesthetic medication Dosed to effect	IV, IM	15–20 minutes	Sedation, general anesthesia, vasodilation, decreased blood pressure, potentially increased heart rate, respiratory depression
Ketamine Usually in combination with alpha2-agonists	1–5 mg/kg depending on preanesthetic medication	IV, IM	15–20 minutes	Sedation, general anesthesia, analgesia, increased heart rate, increased blood pressure
Isoflurane/sevoflurane/desflurane	1%–4% 2%–6% 6%–15% depending on preanesthetic medication	Alveolar	Minutes	General anesthesia, vasodilation, decreased blood pressure, respiratory depression

some reflexes of the lower brain centers, e.g., swallowing, can remain present.

Ketamine is a versatile drug. It can be used as an analgesic and sedative, but also as an induction agent. It can be administered both intramuscularly and intravenously. Intramuscular administration of ketamine can be painful and often elicits an aversive reaction. Especially in animals that undergo sequential anesthetic procedures in a study, this can lead to learned avoidance behavior. Intramuscular injections are therefore best made in a calm and gentle fashion while the animal enjoys a treat. Ketamine provides analgesia and has no muscle relaxant properties, but might in fact induce muscle rigidity/spasm. Therefore it is usually combined with a drug that has muscle relaxant properties, e.g., a benzodiazepine (Linkenhoker et al., 2010), an alpha2-agonist (Sakaguchi et al., 1996; Santos et al., 2016), or propofol (Martinez-Taboada and Leece, 2014).

The cardiovascular side effects of ketamine are rather unique. The primary effect of ketamine is cardiovascular depression. However, through the release of endogenous catecholamines, heart rate, myocardial contractility, and blood pressure may increase. This leads to higher myocardial oxygen consumption (Patschke et al., 1975). These phenomena can be of importance in cardiovascular research. Ketamine is metabolized by the liver and excreted through the kidneys.

b. Propofol

Propofol is a hypnotic agent that exerts its effect via the GABA receptor. It should be administered intravenously. In low doses, it can be used as a sedative; higher doses will result in general anesthesia. Propofol does not provide analgesia but has good muscle relaxant properties. It can be easily titrated to effect and usually has a smooth recovery profile. Propofol induces vasodilation, resulting in a potential drop in blood pressure during induction of anesthesia. It is metabolized by the liver and extrahepatic pathways, i.e., the kidneys and small intestine (Sahinovic et al., 2018).

c. Alfaxalone

Alfaxalone is a so-called neuro-active steroid anesthetic. Like propofol, it exerts its anesthetic effects via the GABA receptor. It can be administered via both the intramuscular and intravenous route. In low doses, it can be used as a sedative, higher doses will result in general anesthesia (Bigby et al., 2017; Duval et al., 2018). Alfaxalone does not provide analgesia, but it has good muscle relaxant properties. It can be easily titrated to effect, and recoveries are generally smooth. Like propofol, alfaxalone produces vasodilation, which is often followed by an increase in heart rate (Rodriguez et al., 2012). Alfaxalone is metabolized by the liver.

d. Volatile anesthetics

All volatile anesthetics can induce general anesthesia. In modern laboratory animal anesthesia, isoflurane and sevoflurane are used most frequently. Volatile anesthetics are delivered through an anesthetic machine with an appropriate breathing system. For pigs, the most suitable and economical breathing system will be the circle system. Volatile anesthetics are delivered via the patient's airway. Induction with volatile anesthetics is usually stressful, partly because the animals resent the pungent smell and the airway irritation that may occur, partly because at subanesthetic levels they cause central nervous system (CNS) excitation (Becker et al., 2012). Volatile anesthetics do not provide analgesia but have excellent muscle relaxant properties. They induce dose-dependent vasodilation and myocardial depression, which can lead to significant hypotension. Volatile anesthetics are partly metabolized by the liver; however, this is insignificant to recovery, which occurs through exhaling the agent.

D. Maintenance of general anesthesia

1. General options

General anesthesia can be maintained in several different ways. Each way has its advantages and disadvantages and the option that best fits the study objectives, laboratory resources, personal experience, and preferences should be chosen.

The different ways to maintain general anesthesia in a pig include total intravenous anesthesia (TIVA), partial intravenous anesthesia (PIVA), and inhalational anesthesia. Although these ways differ, they all have at least one thing in common. The common denominator is the care for the anesthetized animal. What is pivotal for every general anesthetic is that the animal is kept warm, is provided with extra oxygen and that respiration and circulation are maintained. These aspects are discussed in more detail in Section VI of this chapter. Some maintenance agents and agents used for balanced anesthesia are listed in Table 17.3.

2. Total intravenous anesthesia

When using TIVA, general anesthesia is maintained by administering anesthetic drugs via the intravenous route. The three induction agents described above, propofol, alfaxalone, and ketamine, are also suitable to maintain general anesthesia. It is strongly advised to place an intravenous catheter, to ensure safe intravenous access. The maintenance agent of choice can be given as repeated boluses or as a continuous rate infusion (CRI). Next to the maintenance agent, CRIs of other anesthetics such as opioids (e.g., fentanyl) and/or alpha2-agonists (e.g., (dex-) medetomidine) should be given to provide additional analgesia and sedation and reduce the dose of maintenance agent needed. This will also reduce the dose-dependent side effects of the maintenance agent used and will give an overall more balanced anesthetic plane; hence, this approach is often referred to as 'balanced anesthesia'.

3. Inhalational anesthesia

During inhalational anesthesia, general anesthesia is maintained by an inhalant (volatile) agent. In modern

TABLE 17.3 Maintenance agents and agents used for balanced anesthesia.

Drug(s)	Dose	Route of administration	Effects
Propofol	10–20 mg/kg/hour depending on preanesthetic medication	IV	Sedation/general anesthesia, vasodilation, decreased blood pressure, respiratory depression
Alfaxalone	7–20 mg/kg/hour depending on preanesthetic medication	IV	Sedation/general anesthesia, vasodilation, decreased blood pressure, potentially increased heart rate, respiratory depression
Ketamine	1–5 mg/kg/hour depending on preanesthetic medication	IV	Sedation/general anesthesia, analgesia, increased heart rate, increased blood pressure
Isoflurane/sevo-flurane/ desflurane	1%–3% 2%–4% 6%–15% depending on preanesthetic medication	Alveolar	General anesthesia, vasodilation, decreased blood pressure, respiratory depression
Fentanyl	5–40 mcg/kg/hour depending on procedure and other medications administered	IV	Analgesia, bradycardia, respiratory depression
Remifentanil	0.2–0.8 mcg/kg/minute depending on procedure and other medications administered	IV	Analgesia, bradycardia, respiratory depression
Sufentanil	0.5–4 mcg/kg/hour depending on procedure and other medications administered	IV	Analgesia, bradycardia, respiratory depression
Dex-/ Medetomidine	1–5 mcg/kg/hour depending on procedure and other medications administered	IV	Analgesia, bradycardia, hypertension

laboratory animal anesthesia, isoflurane or sevoflurane are used most frequently. Desflurane is also a suitable agent, but the price and specific vaporizer needed may be a limiting factor (Varkey and Welliver, 2013). Inhalational anesthesia requires an anesthetic machine and a breathing circuit, and, ideally, the trachea of the animal is intubated with an endotracheal tube.

4. *Partial intravenous anesthesia*

PIVA is a combination of TIVA and inhalational anesthesia. General anesthesia is usually maintained with a volatile anesthetic agent, supplemented with intravenous CRIs of other anesthetics such as opioids (e.g., fentanyl), alpha2-agonists (e.g., (dex-)medetomidine), and ketamine to provide additional analgesia and sedation and reduce the dose of volatile agent needed. This will reduce the dose-dependent side effects of the volatile agent, creating a "balanced anesthesia" (Duval et al., 2018).

5. *Local anesthesia*

Local anesthetics are invaluable for balanced anesthesia. They can be used for so-called loco-regional techniques. These techniques inactivate the nerve(s) supplying a specified body area, resulting in complete numbness thereof. Incorporating a loco-regional technique greatly reduces the need of other analgesic, sedative, and general anesthetic agents to maintain the animal comfortable during an invasive procedure. The dose reductions will reduce the dose-dependent side effects and result in an anesthesia where it is easier to maintain the animal's normal physiology. In addition, loco-regional techniques result in excellent analgesia and prevent sensitization, reducing the amount of peri-procedural analgesia needed (Rivat et al., 2013).

V. Animal preparation

A. Presurgical preparation

The choice of anesthesia and analgesia should be made carefully and based on the pig's age, breed, disease status and the operation to be performed. It is important to choose a combination of drugs that minimally interferes with the systems being studied. If the research is intended to be used in human surgery, a drug regimen similar to those used in humans should be used (Souba and Wilmore, 2001). Induction of anesthesia is generally done in the animal's pen. To avoid vagal reflexes during endotracheal intubation antimuscarinic drugs can be administered simultaneously with the sedative-hypnotic agents intramuscularly (Chum and Pacharinsak, 2012). For drug combinations and dosages, please refer to Sections III and IV. Intramuscular injection is commonly performed in the neck just behind the base of the ear or less commonly in the major muscles of the thigh (Houpert et al., 1993). Safe intramuscular injection can be performed by using food (e.g., Yogurt) as a distraction and stress reliever (Kaiser et al., 2006). The needle can additionally be connected to an extension line, which will allow the pig to move freely while the drug is being injected. Smaller pigs can be restrainted in a humane restraint sling (Panepinto et al., 1983) or if trained can be picked up for injection (Ellegaard et al., 2010). Most of the common injectable tranquilizers and anesthetic agents can also be safely administered via the subcutaneous route and the induction time is similar to the intramuscular route (Swindle and Smith, 2013). Following anesthetic induction in the housing room, the animal is transported to the preparation room, where it is preoxygenated over a face-mask with 100% oxygen for 5–10 minutes. An ophthalmic ointment is applied to both eyes to avoid drying of corneal epithelium during the surgical procedure. An intravenous catheter (22G-18G) for anesthetic delivery and fluid substitution is placed in a readily accessible superficial vein. The most common sites are thereby the lateral auricular vein (Phillips et al., 2012), the cephalic vein, the lateral saphenous vein, or the coccygeal vein (Moon and Smith, 1996) (venipuncture sites are listed from the most common to the least common). If deeper veins, such as the jugular vein or the femoral vein need to be accessed, they should be cannulated under ultrasound guidance (Izer et al., 2017) (Pinkernelle et al., 2009) or following surgical exposure (Ettrup et al., 2011). A peripheral arterial catheter is placed for invasive blood pressure measurements. The coccygeal artery and the auricular artery (Bass et al., 2009) are easily accessible superficial arteries, deeper arterial vessels such as the carotid arteries or femoral arteries should again be cannulated under ultrasound guidance or following surgical exposure. A urinary catheter is then sterilely placed transurethral (female animals) (Li et al., 2017; Musk et al., 2015) or by cystotomy (male animals) (Holliman et al., 1982). Transurethral placement of a urinary catheter is best performed with the animal in the supine position. If a nonself-retaining vaginal speculum is used, an assisting person is needed to hold the lubricated speculum open, while the second person guides the Foley catheter with the help of a light source under vision into the urethral opening. The flow of urine is indicative of proper catheter placement. Based on experience, common catheter sizes used for farm pigs (25–100 kg) are 8–12 Charrière. Cystotomy can be performed via traditionally open celiotomy or laparoscopically (Zhang et al., 2014).

The surgical area is clipped and washed with antiseptic soap to eliminate gross dirt. The skin is then thoroughly rinsed and dried. Further disinfection of the surgical site will be done by the surgeon prior to cut down. Most surgical interventions will require endotracheal intubation to protect the airway, prevent aspiration of saliva, blood, and foreign materials, as well as to maintain positive pressure ventilation. For details on endotracheal intubation, please refer to part B of this section. Throughout the preparation of the animal thermal support should be provided and body temperature monitored rectally, pharyngeally, or esophageally (Musk et al., 2016), as hypothermia is a common complication of general anesthesia and occurs due to altered thermoregulatory control and evaporative and conductive heat loss.

B. Intubation

For endotracheal intubation, the pig can either be placed in a dorsal or sternal position (Swindle, 2007; Theisen et al., 2009). When intubating in the sternal position, an assisting person is needed to hold open the upper and lower jaws. Endotracheal intubation in pigs can be challenging due to a variety of anatomical features (Chum and Pacharinsak, 2012; Lumb et al., 2007; Smith et al., 1997; Dyce et al., 2009). The tongue of pigs is rather thick, and the oropharyngeal space is long and narrow. The elongated soft palate thereby hides the epiglottis and needs to be dislodged dorsally to get a clear vision of the tracheal opening. This is best achieved by performing a careful scooping motion with the endotracheal tube from the right piriform recess to the left along the soft palate (Ruemmler et al., 2020). After application of a topical anesthetic on the larynx (e.g., lidocaine), a long-bladed laryngoscope with a light source (19.5 cm (in smaller pigs up to 50 kg) −36 cm length (in larger pigs)) is used to gently depress the epiglottis in order to get a clear vision of the vocal cords and the tracheal opening (Fig. 17.5). The tip of a cuffed endotracheal tube (7−11 mm outer diameter, depending on the pig size, 30−56 cm in length) is passed through the cricoid cartilage and then rotated through an angle of 180 degrees while advancing. Using an intubation stylet with a ¼ curvature can facilitate tube guidance through the pharyngeal opening. Alternatively, curved endotracheal tubes made from PVC can be used. However, too much pressure during endotracheal intubation has to be avoided to not injure the vocal cords, which are caudoventrally located. PVC tubes thereby exert up to 10 times higher forces and pressures when compared to silicon or armored tubes (Joo et al., 2002) and can even cause laryngeal perforation (Steinbacher et al., 2012). Repeated attempts should be avoided, as pigs are prone to laryngospasm. Endotracheal intubation with the help of a flexible videoendoscope as national guidelines recommend in the condition of an anticipated difficult airway in patients has been shown feasible in pigs (Ruemmler et al., 2020; Apfelbaum et al., 2013).

The use of a laryngeal mask has shown to be successful in ensuring patent airways and adequate oxygenation (Wemyss-Holden et al., 1999) (Fig. 17.6). Care must be taken to use a model with an adequate seal or to place a gastric tube in pigs ventilated over a laryngeal mask, as gastric insufflation and regurgitation were previously described (Patil et al., 1997; Goldmann et al., 2005). A further alternative is the laryngeal tube, which has been used in human patients in Europe since the early 2000. The laryngeal tube is a supraglottic ventilatory device consisting of an airway tube and two low-pressure balloons forming an airtight seal with a decreased risk of gastro-esophageal regurgitation (Asai and Shingu, 2005). Successful application of the laryngeal tube has been described in pigs; however, special care has to be taken not to damage the balloons of the tube when coming into contact with the pig's sharp teeth (Birkholz et al., 2008). Surgical or percutaneous tracheostomies can be performed in cases of severe laryngeal swelling or persistent spasm (Guerra et al., 2012; Murphy et al., 2011). Complications can be bleeding and airway infections.

A double-lumen endobronchial tube can be used in thoracic surgical procedures such as lung separation, as it allows for isolated one-lung ventilation. However, due to interspecies differences in bronchial anatomy between pigs and humans, double-lumen endobronchial tubes designed

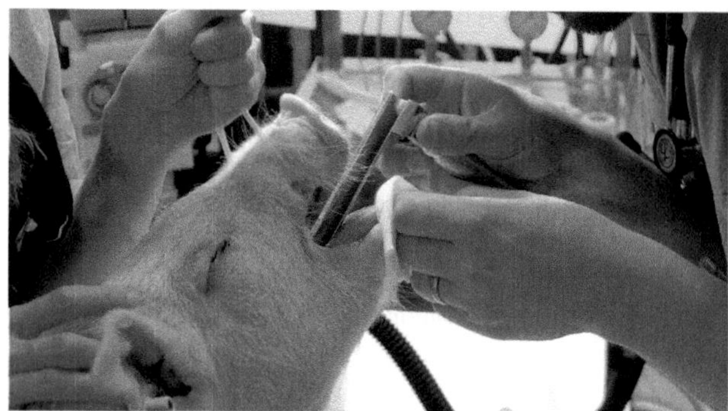

FIGURE 17.5 A long-bladed laryngoscope with a light source allows clear vision of the vocal cords and the tracheal opening.

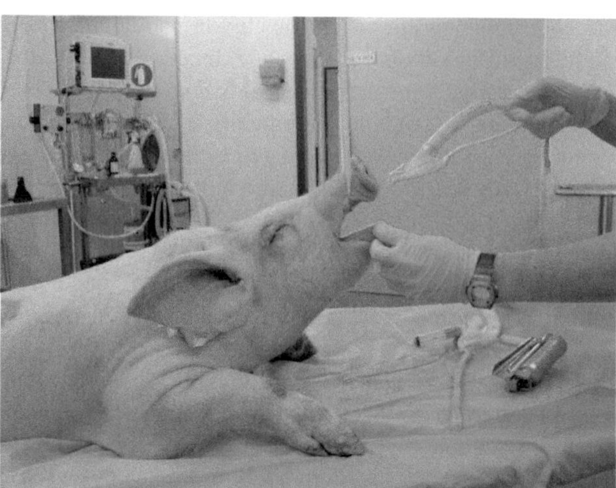

FIGURE 17.6 Introduction of a laryngeal mask in sternal recumbency.

for use in humans are not suitable for use in pigs and need to be adapted in design (Lesser et al., 2020).

VI. Anesthetic monitoring and support

Ensuring an appropriate depth of anesthesia as well as intact cardiovascular, respiratory, and metabolic function are imperative for animals undergoing invasive procedures. Due to the pig's size, instruments and tools developed for monitoring human patients during anesthesia can complement the standard veterinary anesthetic and monitoring equipment.

A. Central nervous system

General anesthesia is meant to induce a state of unconsciousness, a condition that is difficult to characterize and verify. In pigs, anesthetic depth is often determined by assessing the palpebral reflex, jaw tone, the occurrence of spontaneous movements, and response to noxious stimuli, such as mechanically clamping the coronary band of the medial or lateral dewclaw using forceps (Rydén et al., 2021). Additionally, changes in hemodynamic and respiratory variables in the absence of neuromuscular blockade can be used to determine sufficient suppression of nociceptive stimuli-induced sympathetic response (Kamiya et al., 2021). Mechanical ventilation and mechanical circulatory support systems (e.g., heart-lung machines, extracorporeal membrane oxygenation (ECMO) devices) hamper the interpretation of acute hemodynamic changes and respiration inflicted by insufficient anesthetic plane. It might therefore be desirable to include a more direct measure of central nervous system (CNS) function when establishing anesthetic depth. The electroencephalogram (EEG) reflects the general degree of cortical electrical activity and is thought to provide a clinically effective measure of the depth of cerebral depression under anesthesia. However, unprocessed EEG shows several limitations as a monitoring tool for anesthesia, especially due to its sensitivity to electrical interferences from the operating theatre. Several processing techniques have been implemented to overcome this problem and to provide a quantitative parameter reflecting the information of the EEG (Silva and Antunes, 2012). One of those quantitative parameters, the bispectral index (BIS)—derived from the EEG—is increasingly used to measure the depth of sedation, anesthesia, and awareness in pigs (Haga et al., 1999; Jaber et al., 2015). While there appears to be an agreeance that BIS decreases with increasing anesthetic doses in pigs its correlation to clinical scales of anesthetic depth remains limited (Martín-Cancho et al., 2003; Haga et al., 1999). Factors that appear to play a role in the limited usefulness of BIS as an objective monitor of anesthetic depth in pigs, are the algorithm, which is currently only based on data collected in humans, and the placement of the electrodes, which is more difficult in pigs due to the skin being thicker and furrier (Silva and Antunes, 2012).

B. Respiratory system

Respiratory depression by anesthetics, analgesics, surgical positioning, and the surgical intervention itself (thoracotomy, sternotomy) often requires mechanical ventilation to maintain adequate ventilation in pigs. Ventilation is readily adjusted to maintain a steady end-tidal carbon dioxide ($etCO_2$) of 35–45 mmHg, which is commonly achieved with a respiratory frequency of 16–25 breaths per minute and a tidal volume of 5.9–14.5 mL/kg bodyweight per breath (Hannon et al., 1990). $EtCO_2$ is measured with a mainstream or sidestream capnograph and should always be interpreted in conjunction with partial pressure of carbon dioxide in the arterial blood gas ($PaCO_2$). Normal $PaCO_2$-$EtCO_2$ difference is approximately 2–5 mmHg in pigs (Isbell et al., 2012). This gradient is a function of pulmonary dead space and CO. A ventilation-perfusion mismatch, described as a venous admixture or an increase in pulmonary dead space, will cause an increase in the $PaCO_2$-$EtCO_2$ gradient. The underlying causes range from changes in regional (pulmonary embolisms) or global pulmonary perfusion (pulmonary hypertension, cardiac failure, and hypovolemic shock) to changes in ventilation (high positive end expiratory pressure (PEEP), high inspiratory oxygen fraction) to atelectasis caused by body positioning as it is described in larger animals (Nyman et al., 1990).

A ventilation-perfusion mismatch will eventually cause an inadequacy in blood oxygenation and hypoxia. To determine arterial blood oxygenation, namely the amount of oxygen-carrying hemoglobin in the blood, a pulse oximeter is attached to either the tongue, the labial angle, or the snout (Thomas and Lerche, 2016). Partial pressure of oxygen (PaO_2) in the blood is determined by arterial blood gas analysis. PaO_2 is directly dependent on the inspiratory oxygen fraction and reflects a balance between arterial blood flow and tissue oxygen consumption (Ortiz-Prado et al., 2019).

C. Cardiovascular system

Anecdotally, the ventricular fibrillation (VF) threshold in pigs is markedly lower than in humans. One plausible reason is the Purkinje system, which is located transmurally in pigs and subendocardially in humans (Glomset and Glomset, 1940). With pigs being more prone to VF and other cardiac arrhythmias during cardiac interventions, thorough cardiovascular monitoring during anesthesia is essential. Clinical monitoring consists of regular auscultation of the heart, palpation of the pulse pressure, and assessment of mucous membrane color and the capillary filling time. As the pig is extensively used in cardiovascular research, a great variety of monitoring tools were adapted from human use and are regularly used in pig anesthesia. The pig should minimally be equipped with an arterial catheter for invasive blood pressure measurements, a central venous pressure line, and a standard three-limb electrocardiogram (ECG). Additional instrumentalization may consist of a Swan-Ganz thermodilution catheter or a pressure-volume (PV) catheter for cardiac output (CO) measurements.

Physiologic arterial blood pressure values in pigs are systolic 112−139 mmHg, mean 86−123 mmHg, and diastolic 72−98 mmHg (Hannon et al., 1990). The gold standard for blood pressure measurement is an invasive blood pressure technique via an arterial cannula (Kittleson and Olivier, 1983). Sites for arterial catheterization in pigs are described under Section VA. Auricular blood pressure measurements compare well to measurements in larger vessels such as the femoral artery, which in return correlates well with carotid blood pressure measurement (Bass et al., 2009; Aksakal et al., 2012). Non-invasive blood pressure measurement by a cuff placed circumferentially around the pelvic or thoracic extremities generally underestimates the true arterial pressure (Reed et al., 2018).

Heart rate and the ratio of diastole to systole of conventional and miniature pigs with the same body weight (30−50 kg) appear to be comparable (Bohn and Henner, 1968). ECG recordings are commonly obtained with the three standard limb leads. For detailed ECG analysis in pigs, please refer to further literature (Dukes and Szabuniewicz, 1969).

A Swan-Ganz thermodilution catheter can be placed through the jugular vein in the pulmonary artery to monitor mean pulmonary pressure, CO, and pulmonary capillary wedge pressure. Normal CO in pigs is 5−10 L/minute with a stroke volume of 65−81 mL (Jivegård et al., 1990). Pulse index continuous cardiac output, PV loop catheters, and transesophageal echocardiography are further methods to determine CO in pigs (Litton and Morgan, 2012; Ellenbroek et al., 2016; Weidemann et al., 2002).

D. Metabolism

A comprehensive metabolic panel describes a blood test to assess liver function, kidney function, and nutrient levels. Measurements include glucose, calcium, sodium, potassium, bicarbonate, chloride, blood urea nitrogen (BUN), creatinine, albumin, total protein, alkaline phosphatase, alanine aminotransferase, aspartate aminotransferase, and bilirubin. Glucose, calcium, sodium, potassium, bicarbonate, chloride, BUN, and creatinine should be part of the routine monitoring in pigs under anesthesia. Further analyzes can be performed depending on the duration and nature of the intervention.

Anesthetic and sedative agents such as alpha2-agonists (Daş et al., 2016), propofol (Manell et al., 2017), and volatile agents (Laber-Laird et al., 1992) are known to affect carbohydrate metabolism by decreasing insulin secretion during anesthesia in pigs, leading to hyperglycemia. Blood glucose levels appear not to be affected by NMDA-receptor antagonists such as ketamine and tiletamine (Manell et al., 2017). In case of prolonged anesthesia (>18 hours) blood glucose frequently and continuously decreases. To avoid glucose levels <2.0 mmol/L, 4.3% dextrose, and 0.18% saline solutions can be infused at 5−15 mL/kg/hour (Clutton et al., 2013).

Normal total blood calcium levels in pigs are 3.5−5.8 mg/dL, depending on the age and growth status of the animal (Gay et al., 2000). Approximately half of the total calcium is protein-bound and metabolically inactive. Ionized active calcium plays an important role in cardiac inotropy and vasomotor tone (Erdmann and Reuschel-Janetschek, 1991). The level of ionized calcium is thereby mainly dependent on the plasma concentration of albumin and the blood pH (Constable et al., 2019). The state of heparinization must be considered when interpreting calcium levels on a blood gas analyzer, as artifactual hypocalcemia may be seen in heparinized blood samples (Jonna et al., 1998). True ionized hypocalcemia appears to occur postresuscitation from VF in pigs, leading to refractory hypotension (Lindqwister et al., 2020).

Sodium, potassium, bicarbonate, and chloride are commonly balanced by the infusion of an isotonic crystalloid fluid replacement to maintain volume and electrolyte homeostasis during the course of anesthesia. A blood gas analyzer routinely analyzes their levels. Hypo- or Hyperkalemia are both common anesthetic emergencies in pigs (please see Section VII on common anesthetic emergencies).

E. Renal system

Urinary flow rate and glomerular filtration rate in pigs are comparable to humans (1−3 mL/kg/hour) (Dhondt et al., 2020). Release of antidiuretic hormone and consequently a reduction in urinary output is a natural response to perioperative stressors (e.g., hypoxia) and anesthesia itself (agents, cardio-vascular effects) (Forsling et al., 1980; Burchardi and Kaczmarczyk, 1994). The patency and positioning of the urinary catheter should always be verified before initiating treatment for oliguria or anuria. Furthermore, normovolemia and normotension have to be confirmed before administering diuretic agents. Perioperative acute kidney injury (AKI) is a possibly reversible syndrome associated with major surgeries in pigs in particular cardiac surgeries with cardiopulmonary bypass (Goebel et al., 2010). Serum creatinine and BUN have typically been used to diagnose AKI. However, as both factors are also dependent on nonrenal factors and their increase may lag several days behind, novel biomarkers for AKI have been suggested (Edelstein, 2008).

F. Integument

Special care must be taken when placing the pig on a heating mat with insulated heating elements, or when using containers filled with warm water or microwaveable heating bags for active warming during anesthesia, as they carry a relatively high potential for causing skin burns (Lumb et al., 2007). Bair huggers, for example, are commonly used across all species (including pigs) to provide thermal support but prevent burns. Periodic position change is recommended (if feasible) during prolonged anesthesia, as muscle and nerve damage (Clutton et al., 2013) and pressure sores on the skin may occur due to hypoperfusion of the affected body area.

G. Locomotor system

The occurrence of spontaneous movements and responses to noxious stimuli, such as mechanically clamping the coronary band of the medial or lateral dewclaw using forceps, are important indicators for anesthetic depth (Rydén et al., 2021). If the use of NMBAs is legally and ethically approved and indicated, the administration should occur once noxious stimulation demonstrably fails to elicit motor responses. Neuromuscular function after the administration of NMBAs can be monitored using an acceleromyograph, which determines the intensity of neuromuscular blockage by the train-of-four stimulation (Bellini and De Benedictis, 2018). In prolonged recovery procedures, physiotherapy, i.e., muscle massage and joint manipulation may relieve postoperative limb discomfort that discourages normal activity (Fig. 17.7).

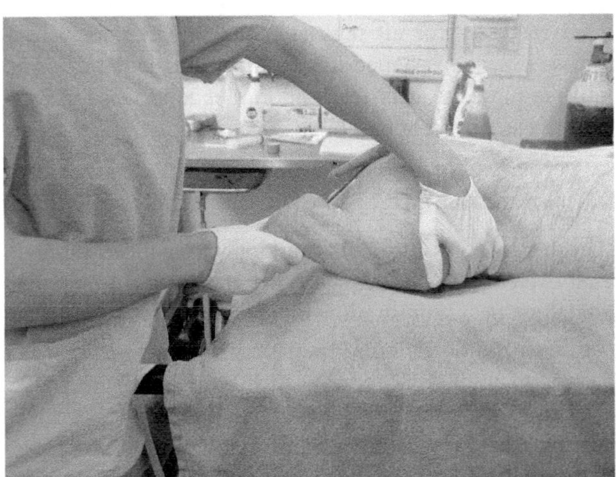

FIGURE 17.7 Physiotherapy during prolonged recovery procedure.

Intra-anesthetic shivering is a phenomenon that has been attributed to numerous other causes than cold-induced thermoregulation (De Witte and Sessler, 2002). In pigs, an association with artificial ventilation and shivering under normothermic conditions has been made. Inspiration of cold or room temperature air appears to induce respiratory shivering, possibly due to temperature receptors in the walls of the trachea, bronchi, or bronchioles with afferent fibers in the vagus, capable of initiating shivering (Cort and McCance, 1953).

H. Hemodynamic support

The primary hemodynamic parameters are blood pressure and heart rate; advanced hemodynamic parameters include CO and vascular resistance. Taken as a whole, all parameters are a function of preload, afterload, and cardiac contractility. Based on the underlying cause of hemodynamic instability, hemodynamic support is initiated (please refer to Section VIIA, hemodynamic instability).

I. Temperature support

Hypothermia is common under general anesthesia and is dependent on the duration of preanesthetic time, duration of anesthetic time, body condition, invasiveness of the surgery, and body positioning. External heat can be supplied in a variety of ways from simply increasing the ambient temperature, to heating blankets and circulating water mattresses, to forced-air and conductive fabrics (Dent et al., 2016). Accidental iatrogenic hyperthermia has to be avoided when applying external heat (Lumb et al., 2007). In case of accidental iatrogenic hyperthermia, the heating source should be removed and the animal cooled if necessary.

J. Urine output

Normovolemia and normotension have to be confirmed before administering diuretic agents to pigs. There are five classes of diuretics: thiazides and thiazide-like diuretics; loop diuretics; carbonic anhydrase inhibitors; potassium-sparing diuretics; and osmotic diuretics. Effects on renal clearance and electrolyte excretion vary markedly and should be considered in the choice of the proper diuretic agent (Gyrd-Hansen, 1969).

VII. Common anesthetic emergencies

A. Hemodynamic instability

The hemodynamic parameters commonly being monitored are blood pressure and heart rate. CO and vascular resistance are less commonly monitored. Based upon the underlying cause for hemodynamic instability, hemodynamic support is initiated. To maintain perfusion of vital organs, hypotension should be avoided. Dependent upon the anesthetic protocol, hypotension may be more or less common when anesthetizing pigs. Butyrophenone or phenothiazine premedication may cause hypotension through vasodilatation, and volatile agents possibly cause more hypotension than intravenous agents in pigs. If analgesia is provided through the effective use of local anesthetic techniques, less systemic anesthetic and analgesic drugs are needed, which can lessen the problem with hypotension. Anesthetic drugs potentially cause hypotension by inducing vasodilatation, and thus a relative hypovolemia, in which case boluses of a balanced crystalloid solution at a rate of 10–20 mL/kg over 10 minutes may ameliorate the problem. If the hypotension is rather caused by an increased vagal tone causing bradycardia, and by that reducing CO resulting in hypotension, antimuscarinic drugs can be used, either atropine at 20–50 μg/kg or glycopyrrolate at 4–10 μg/kg. If low CO is caused by a reduced cardiac contractility, an CRI of dobutamine at 1–5 μg/kg/minute can be initiated. If a reduced vascular resistance is suspected and boluses of crystalloids either do not increase the blood pressure sufficiently or are undesirable for any reason, norepinephrine as a CRI at 0.6–2.0 μg/kg/minute or phenylephrine as a bolus at 2–5 μg/kg or a CRI at 0.5–13 μg/kg/minute are possible treatments. Severe hemorrhage will, by reducing venous return, decrease cardiac output, which again leads to hypotension and increases heart rate through a baroreceptor response. Hemorrhage naturally will cause hypovolemia and thus decrease cardiac output. The preferred treatment is volume replacement, either by crystalloid or colloid fluids to effect.

B. Hypothermia/hyperthermia

Hypothermia will depress the immune response, inhibit hemostasis, depress drug metabolism, increase oxygen demand in recovery, and is likely unpleasant when recovering. When general anesthesia is induced, the differentiation between a peripheral and central heat compartment is lost and the thermoregulatory center is depressed. If the peripheral temperature was low prior to induction, the body temperature will drop. This temperature drop can be attenuated or avoided by prewarming the pig either by insulation or providing external heat prior to inducing anesthesia. During anesthesia, the compensatory responses are obtunded. To avoid further heat loss, the pig should be placed on an insulating surface, the body covered by insulating blankets or bubble wrap, and if possible, excessive use of water for washing or disinfecting should be avoided, the surgery time kept to a minimum, and fluids used for flushing should be body tempered. However, pigs may also become hyperthermic during anesthesia, in which case external cooling may be necessary to avoid an increase in the temperature. If unchecked, increasing body temperature may be lethal.

1. Malignant hyperthermia

MH is a syndrome caused by a recessive autosomal gene in the locus for the ryanodine receptor. The frequency of the gene differs between pig populations. In pigs, the syndrome is also called porcine stress syndrome. General anesthesia can trigger an episode of MH; volatile agents, halothane more than the others, and succinylcholine have specifically been recognized as triggers. Excessive calcium efflux from the sarcoplasmic reticulum will cause muscle rigidity, increase oxygen consumption and carbon dioxide production, a rapid increase in body temperature, blood lactate and blood potassium levels, and myoglobinuria. The gene coding for the syndrome has been isolated, and there are commercially available tests for the presence of this gene, so the best solution is to avoid obtaining pigs from a herd where the gene is present. If MH occurs during anesthesia, and the animal is still valuable as a research animal, the treatment consists of removal of the triggering agent, ventilation with 100% oxygen, aggressive cooling, dantrolene 2.5 mg/kg intravenously, monitoring electrolytes, and treating hyperkalemia if present.

C. Hypoglycemia

Young pigs originally bred for meat production are commonly used as research animals, and likely both due to the age of these animals as well as their high metabolic rate, hypoglycemia may occur during general anesthesia. In addition, they may have been fasted prior to the procedure. When being anesthetized, early clinical signs of hypoglycemia are difficult to detect, however, severe hypoglycemia is detrimental to the central nervous function. Blood glucose level can be easily monitored by a hand-held glucometer and hypoglycemia can be treated to effect if it occurs. Alternatively, an infusion of glucose may be provided routinely for all pigs at 50–100 mg/kg/hour. If a glucose infusion is started it is best to continue the infusion until the pig eats again to avoid that endogen insulin production causes a rebound hypoglycemia.

D. Hyperkalemia

The plasma potassium concentration is regulated through renal excretion and cellular uptake. Factors disturbing this regulation or administration of too much potassium can lead to hyperkalemia. This may happen, for instance, because of uroperitoneum, transfusion of old blood, iatrogenic administration of potassium, or acidosis. Hyperkalemia will disturb the de- and repolarization of the myocardium. If plasma potassium concentration gradually increases, the common pattern of changes being observed is first bradycardia, a peaked T-wave and broadened QRS complex prior to atrial standstill and ventricular escape rhythm, and in the end, asystole. Several other cardiac arrhythmias may also be observed. In case of severe hyperkalemia, progression toward fatal arrhythmias can be counteracted by administering 4.6–9.3 mg/kg of calcium intravenously, translating to 0.5–1.0 mL/kg of calcium gluconate at 100 mg/mL. An intravenous crystalloid infusion will dilute the plasma potassium concentration and infusion of glucose, optionally in addition with insulin, will shift potassium intracellularly. If hypercapnia is present, increasing ventilation to normalize arterial CO_2 and thus increase pH will facilitate the transport of potassium into the cell. If there is severe metabolic acidosis, administering $NaHCO_3$ will also increase pH and reduce the plasma potassium concentration.

E. Shivering

Shivering is a well-known problem in anesthetized pigs, to such a level that it can disturb the procedure being performed (Bradbury and Clutton, 2016b). Hypothermia may cause shivering, but shivering is also observed in normothermic animals using different anesthetic protocols. Fentanyl infusion has shown to elicit intraoperative shivering (Haga et al., 2018; Ringer et al., 2016). Anecdotal evidence indicates that the use of azaperone as a part of the anesthetic protocol can reduce the problem (Personal communication, Stijn Scuavliege, 2021).

F. Cardiac arrhythmia

Cardiac arrhythmias may arise during anesthesia for a variety of reasons. They may be a sign of another underlying problem, for instance hyperkalemia, in which case the cause of the problem needs to be identified and treated if possible. In pigs, nociception may induce both a rise and a drop in heart rate. The major problem arising will be if the arrhythmia causes a clinically relevant depression in cardiac output. In tachycardia, this happens because the time in diastole is decreased to a level where there is insufficient time for ventricular filling. The most likely causes of sinus tachycardia are either nociception or hypovolemia, which can be caused by hemorrhage without sufficient intravenous volume replacement. If tachycardia occurs, it is important to differentiate between these two causes because management will be very different. The vasovagal response is seen as severe bradycardia and vasodilation, which can occur because of intense, nociceptive stimulation. If occurring, the stimulation should be stopped, and an antimuscarinic drug administered to counteract the bradycardia prior to improving analgesic treatment. Opioids and alpha2-agonists are drugs that commonly induce bradycardia; however, some studies indicate that this is not universally observed when administered as an infusion in pigs (Haga et al., 2018). Tachycardia as a response to hypovolemia after hemorrhage may also be less pronounced than expected (Lervik et al., 2021).

G. Unexpected emergence from anesthesia

It is crucial to avoid unexpected emergence during the maintenance phase of anesthesia. The administration of the anesthetic drugs as well as the state of the pig needs to be continuously monitored. Equipment used for intravenous administration can fail, venous access can be lost, or syringes may need to be refilled. If volatile anesthesia is used, again the equipment can fail, or the endotracheal tube can dislodge. So, the anesthetist needs an additional plan for how to maintain anesthesia should the primary method fail. If emergence occurs, increasing a volatile agent will take too long time to have the desired effect, so a rapid-acting intravenous anesthetic agent must be readily available for administration. This becomes even more important if a neuromuscular blocking agent (NMBA) is used. In this case, the animal can regain awareness without being able to move. If an NMBA is used preferably anesthesia should be maintained by a volatile agent and the end-tidal concentration of the agent be measured to ascertain that the animal remains unconscious.

VIII. Postprocedural recovery and care

A. Recovery period

The postoperative recovery period is best supervised by veterinarians or specialized personnel.

Any installed monitoring devices during surgery should be continued as long as possible, depending on the performed intervention. Postoperative monitoring should at least include pulse rate and quality, body temperature, and respiration every 15 minutes until successful extubation and/or return of full consciousness. Additionally, after major procedures, blood pressure, cardiac parameters, urinary output, respiratory parameters (in case of intubation), drainage of indwelling tubes, etc., should be monitored as long as needed or as long as tolerated by the pig (Swindle and Smith, 2015). Intensive care monitoring and postoperative treatment should, however, always be adapted to the particular study protocol.

Once the intervention has been completed and all vital parameters are stable, the animal should be transported to an individual compartment in the stable and further monitored. The stable should not contain any straw or bedding due to the risk of suffocation in still not fully awake animals, but can be lined with blankets or a soft mat. Placing the animal in sternal recumbency supports respiration and facilitates physical examination. Heat support can be accomplished with heating lamps positioned above the animal or with warm water blankets. Extubation should only be performed after a strong swallowing reflex is present. Facilities and equipment should be available at hand to deal with complications during recovery. Suction should be available to clear airway passages of excessive secretions. In the event of laryngospasm or airway obstruction, intubation supplies, including a laryngoscope, need to be readily accessible (Fish et al., 2008).

B. Housing and enrichment

Whenever possible, pigs in the laboratory should be housed in small groups, as this is typical for the species and improves their well-being. Once a social order is established, it will be maintained as long as the group remains together (Smith and Swindle, 2006). Communal nesting, playing, or foraging/rooting usually is a sign of bonding and a stable group hierarchy. After interventions, the animals should, whenever possible, be returned to their companions once they have fully recovered from anesthesia. If individual housing is necessary, visual, olfactory, and auditory contact with other pigs should be ensured to prevent stress, and social deprivation and to support recovery (Smith and Swindle, 2006). Maintaining pigs as long as possible with familiar companions both before and after surgery helps to minimize stress and antisocial behavior.

Pigs are highly intelligent animals, which like to play, root, and explore their habitat. Thus, pigs kept in the laboratory require environmental enrichment to satisfy their natural needs and to prevent boredom and the emergence of antisocial and undesirable behavior. Straw, wood shavings, or other types of bedding encourage rooting and foraging and help the animals to control their microenvironment. Balls, toys on the ground or hanging from chains, or a nylon brush or broom head attached to the stable wall can be used as additional enrichment (Smith and Swindle, 2006). Additionally, some treats can also be hidden in toys or strewn in the bedding to occupy the animals further (Casey et al., 2007).

The environment can also be enriched by providing novel objects for investigation (such as cardboard boxes, mirrors, strips of rubber, and paper bags, etc.), by regular, positive interaction with care personnel (e.g., veterinarians, caretakers, researchers), or by playing music or radio in the background (Murison et al., 2009).

C. Supportive care

Supportive care includes medical or other means of helping the animal to recover quickly. Medical care includes the administration of analgesics, medical treatment, heat support, supplemental oxygen, or continued body-warm fluid administration during the immediate postoperative recovery phase. Eating can be encouraged by offering titbits, e.g., pellets mashed with warm water or mashed banana. Visual and olfactory contact with companions reassures pigs, but the presence of trusted personnel can also calm the animal and facilitate handling and postoperative medication, or examinations. Spending some time with the animals on a daily basis during the acclimatization phase is important, especially for chronic, long-term experiments, to build trust and to ensure calm and gentle handling of the animals during the study phase. In addition, well-acclimatized pigs are more likely to exhibit pain-related behavioral changes more overtly than pigs that are fearful of personnel. To achieve this, pigs should be accustomed to regular handling, body petting etc., by at least two persons before the beginning of the experiment or intervention (Nicholls et al., 2012).

D. Pain assessment; pain scoring and pain management

Pain assessment in pigs can be challenging, as pigs are prey animals and naturally try to hide any pain or discomfort. Pain or nociception may be assessed through objective or subjective methods. A wide range of behavioral indicators can be used in the assessment of pain in pigs, in addition to physiological and clinical measures as potential biomarkers of pain. Behavioral changes can include the appearance of pain-related behaviors (e.g., escape behavior, vocalization), a variation in normal behavior (e.g., disturbed resting behavior), or changes in body posture or pain grimace (Ison et al., 2016; Vullo et al., 2020; Viscardi et al., 2017).

Physiological measurements include cardiovascular and respiratory parameters, temperature, urination, and defecation; however, any changes can also alter due to other factors and have a low sensitivity for a clear assessment of pain. The same applies to other parameters such as cortisol or neuroendocrine changes (e.g., substance P) (Ison et al., 2016). Thus, behavioral changes are typically more helpful to assess discomfort or pain in pigs and can include the observation of basic needs such as water consumption or appetite; attitude, social behavior, or body posture; or further species-specific behaviors like rooting and nesting. The advantages of subjective, behavior-based methods in the assessment of pain are that they are not invasive, usually do not require equipment or restraint, and may be assessed by remote observation (Luna et al., 2020).

Pain assessment is essential to identify and quantify pain and to determine the need for and the effectiveness of analgesic treatment in animals. Most veterinarians and researchers are nowadays focusing on posture changes, variations in normal behavior, or pain-triggered behavior to detect signs of pain as well as subtle changes in well-being or signs of discomfort.

1. Pain scoring

Ideally, a scoring system is used for pain assessment, where some parameters can be clearly stated (e.g., by numerical values for heart rate, temperature, etc.), but other parameters need to be described in more detail (e.g., observation of behavior, response to the observer, etc.) to provide an overall picture of the animal's condition. The frequency of pain assessment and scoring strongly depends on the severity of the intervention, but should be maintained throughout the recovery phase or—in chronic studies—until the end of the experimental period.

2. Pain management

A good pain management combines a tailored analgesic regime with valid and reliable pain assessment methods to verify the efficacy of analgesic treatment and adjust it as necessary in each animal.

For further information, please refer to Chapters 7, 12, and 13.

IX. Analgesia

A. Approach to analgesia

In case an experiment or surgery will likely result in more than slight pain or distress, the use of appropriate analgesia (local, regional, or systemic) needs to be considered to avoid or minimize such pain or distress. The potential of analgesics to interfere with study objectives should be considered, and agents should be chosen that are not expected to alter the research outcome (CoRaAoP, 2009).

Timing of analgesia administration (preemptive, preventive), but also the route and adequate administration interval, and the composition of analgesics is important to cover the intra- as well as the postoperative phase (Rosero and Joshi, 2014).

Pain is a complex and multifactorial phenomenon, and combining analgesics of different classes that act at different target sites may provide better pain relief than using a single drug or technique. The drugs can be administered via the same or by different routes (Rosero and Joshi, 2014). Based on the understanding of the pathophysiology of pain development as well as the mechanisms of action of analgesics, a multimodal approach should always be tailored to the needs of each individual patient and to the experiment. All analgesic concepts aim at minimizing pain perception and at preventing the "wind up phenomenon" and central sensitization in the spinal cord or in the periphery after surgery.

B. Pharmacologic options

Currently available analgesics for postoperative pain management in pigs include opioids, local anesthetics (local, regional, or spinal anesthesia), nonsteroidal antiinflammatory drugs, and analgesic adjuncts such as steroids, ketamine, alpha2-agonists, and anxiolytics (Rosero and Joshi, 2014). Examples of analgesic agents are provided in Table 17.4.

1. Opioids

Opioids are effective for the treatment of moderate to severe pain and can be used as CRIs during or after surgery to provide adequate intra- and postinterventional pain relief. Fentanyl, sufentanil, or remifentanil are the most commonly used opioids during invasive surgeries in pigs. Depending on the type of intervention and postoperative care management, they can also be continued as low-dose intravenous infusions in the recovery phase. Most opioids have a relatively short-half life, limiting their use in the postprocedural recovery phase. Agents with half-lives of less than 4 hours include fentanyl, remifentanil, sufentanil, meperidine, oxymorphone, or morphine. However, morphine used as an epidural analgesic is effective for abdominal surgeries (Swindle and Smith, 2015). Buprenorphine has been extensively used in laboratory and companion animals and has proven to be a strong analgesic with a duration of action of at least 6–8 hours (Roughan and Flecknell, 2002), with little side effects in pigs (Swindle, 2009) It can be considered one of the primary opioid analgesics in pigs in research. Sustained-release formulations are now available on the market, as well as buprenorphine dermal patches.

2. NSAIDs

Non steroidal antiinflammatory drugs (NSAIDs) are analgesics with additional antipyretic, and antiinflammatory properties, hence, they are used for the treatment of pain, fever, and inflammatory processes. The effects are based on the inhibition of prostaglandin synthesis through the inhibition of cyclooxygenase enzymes. They typically have a high oral bioavailability and a long duration of action without causing sedation. Side effects typically include prevention of platelet aggregation, renal function changes, altered cartilage mechanism, and gastric ulceration (Junot et al., 2008). However, most side effects are usually related to long-term medication rather than to short-term use for postoperative analgesia (Swindle and Smith, 2015). Opioid administration should be preferred during and immediately after painful procedures, as their sedative and analgesic effects help to provide a smooth recovery. NSAIDs can either be combined with opioids and local anesthetics for the provision of multimodal analgesia or can be used as a single agent, depending on the type of intervention and the anticipated degree of pain. They have proven to be extremely valuable in the treatment of extensive inflammation or soft tissue trauma (Ranheim and Haga, 2013).

TABLE 17.4 Example of analgesic agents.

Drug(s)	Dose (mg/kg)	Route of administration	Duration of action	Comments
Opioids				
Buprenorphine	0.01–0.05	SC, IM, IV	6–8 hours	
Buprenorphine SR	0.12–0.24 (0.18 mg/kg)	SC	Up to 10 days	Sustained release
Buprenorphine TP	Patch 30, 35, 70 μg/hour	Transcutan	Up to 72 hours	Transdermal patch; application min. 12 hours before the intervention; highly variable
Butorphanol	0.2	SC, IM, IV	2–4 hours	
Fentanyl	CRI postop: 3–10 μg/kg/hour	IV	CRI	Continuous rate infusion
Fentanyl TP	Patch 50, 75, 100 μg/kg/hour	Transcutan	Up to 72 hours	Transdermal patch; application min. 12 hours before the intervention; highly variable
Fentanyl SR	1.3 mg/kg	Topical	Up to 7 days	Sustained release
Methadone	0.3	IV, IM	4 hours	
Morphine	0.2	IV, IM	4 hours	Apply slowly IV
Morphine	0.1	Epidural		
Pethidine	2	IM, IV	2 hours	Max. 1 g/animal
Piritramide	0.1–0.5	SC, IV	2–3 hours	
Local anesthetics				
Bupivacaine	1–2	SC (tissue infiltration, splash, epidural)	4–6 hours	Do not apply IV
Lidocaine	2–4	SC (tissue infiltration, splash, epidural)	30–60 minutes	
Ropivacaine	1–2	SC (tissue infiltration, splash, epidural)	4–6 hours	
NSAIDs				
Carprofen	2–4	SC, PO, IV	12–24 hours	
Flunixin-meglumine	2.2	IM	12–24 hours	Single dose recommended; 2nd dose possible
Ketoprofen	3	IM, PO	12–24 hours	
Ketorolac	1	IM, PO	12–24 hours	
Meloxicam	0.4	IM, PO, IV	24 hours	
Phenylbutazone	10	PO	12 hours	
Miscellaneous drugs				
Metamizole	20–50	IV, IM, PO	4–6 hours	Do not apply IV
Ketamine	0.6 mg/kg/hour	IV	CRI	As adjuvant therapy only; dose must be adjusted depending on substance combination

Ketoprofen, meloxicam, flunixin, and carprofen may even have some opioid-receptor activity (Swindle and Smith, 2015) and can—depending on the intervention—also be used as sole analgesic agents. Ketoprofen can be used to treat chronic pain, and carprofen is effective for soft tissue and orthopedic pain. All NSAIDs can be administered via various routes, e.g., parenteral or, per os as tablets or added to the food (i.e., in yogurt or mashed food). Sustained-release formulations of some NSAIDs are available on the market (Dunbar et al., 2019), but they have not yet been evaluated in pigs.

3. Ketamine, alpha2-agonists

Ketamine is an NMDA-receptor antagonist that is extremely effective in preventing central sensitization and "wind up" of the CNS. However, ketamine and alpha2-agonists are not effective analgesics when used alone in pigs. Their use is only recommended in anesthetic protocols in combination with other substances to ameliorate side effects and to strengthen anesthesia and analgesia.

4. Anxiolytics

Minor tranquilizers such as diazepam or midazolam induce sedation, anxiolysis, and muscle relaxation, but little or no analgesia. However, they can be administered postoperational to prolong sedation and provide a smoother recovery phase.

5. Local/regional anesthesia

Local or regional anesthesia is the temporary and reversible loss of sensation in a defined area of the body without loss of consciousness, achieved by local, regional, or spinal anesthesia. Most surgical procedures in research are performed under general anesthesia, and local/regional anesthesia may be used as part of a multimodal analgesia protocol to intercept pain transmission from the surgical site to the CNS. Local anesthetics work by blocking sodium channels and impulse conduction in nerve fibers, thereby interrupting neural transmission and reducing central sensitization. Examples of agents include lidocaine, bupivacaine, or ropivacaine, which are typically used for local tissue infiltration, regional nerve blocks (e.g., intercostal nerve block for lateral thoracotomy), or epidural anesthesia (Royal et al., 2013). When administered before surgery, the required amount of general anesthesia and opioids can be reduced, and by administering a longer-acting drug, local analgesia can even be maintained during the immediate recovery period (Lumb et al., 2007). Lidocaine has a fast onset and duration of action of 60−120 minutes, bupivacaine and ropivacaine have an intermediated onset of action, but provide analgesia for approximately 180−480 minutes (Lumb et al., 2007). Epidural analgesia is recommended for abdominal surgeries and can also be achieved with morphine instead of local anesthetics. Transdermal anesthetic patches or creams, containing lidocaine and/or prilocaine, can be used to prevent mild pain or distress caused by repeated injections or prior to the induction of injection anesthesia to minimize the stress for the animal. Lidocaine can also be used as an intraoperative CRI to prevent cardiac arrhythmias (Cobo et al., 2020), but it also provides excellent pain relief during surgery. A liposomal bupivacaine formulation has been shown to be a useful therapeutic option for prolonged alleviation of postsurgical pain (up to 72 hours) following soft tissue and orthopedic surgeries (Bergese et al., 2012), but its use has not yet been reported in animals.

C. Route of application

1. Injection, parenteral application

There are several options for the postoperative administration of analgesics. The most reliable option is by the parenteral injection technique. Intravenous injection is the safest and most efficient route for substance administration, but requires the placement of an indwelling catheter or vascular access port for multiple and/or repeated substance administration (Klein et al., 2019; Chuang et al., 2005). Most commonly, the jugular vein is used for long-term vascular access. Intramuscular or subcutaneous injections are usually well tolerated in well-handled and thoroughly acclimatized pigs for a short period of time, but are not appropriate when repeated injections over several days are required, as this may cause increased stress to the animals. In addition, periods of inadequate analgesia may occur with all injection methods if plasma concentrations fall below the effective level.

2. Osmotic pumps

Surgically implanted osmotic pumps and pellets can be used for prolonged and continuous administration of an analgesic. However, the costs and rather long minimum duration of use (7 days) make them impractical for routine postoperative analgesia.

3. Sustained-release formulations

Another option to overcome these problems are sustained-release formulations. A sustained-release buprenorphine formulation showed effective plasma levels in minipigs for more than 10 days (Thiede et al., 2014), and pharmacological and clinical efficacy for up to 7 days after surgery could be demonstrated after a single, topical application of a fentanyl solution in pigs (Goutchtat et al., 2021).

4. Transdermal patches

Transdermal patches have been used for many years in medical and veterinary practice for the transcutaneous administration of analgesics. Transdermal patches containing fentanyl or buprenorphine are also available for pigs. However, studies with fentanyl transdermal patches show a wide variability in terms of efficacy in pigs, and results are often contradictory (Royal et al., 2013; Harvey-Clark et al., 2000; Osorio Lujan et al., 2017; Wilkinson et al., 2001; Malavasi et al., 2006). One study demonstrated effective plasma levels for up to 72 hours with buprenorphine transdermal patches (Kittleson and Olivier, 1983), but another study failed to demonstrate stable plasma levels even with higher dosages (Osorio Lujan et al., 2017). Titration of the correct dosage can be difficult, and the patches need to be secured on the skin in such a way that they cannot be ingested or lose contact with the skin. Other factors which can influence the rate of absorption include breed, age, and size of the pig, as well as location of the patch, body temperature, or type of procedure. Hence, under or overdosing may occur (Swindle and Smith, 2015; Foley, 2014). Furthermore, most studies have been performed in miniature pigs, and different dosages may be required for farm breeds.

5. In-dwelling catheters

Local anesthetics (e.g., bupivacaine) or opiates can also be administered via in-dwelling catheters (e.g., "soaker" catheter) for additional pain relief on the surgical site.

6. Self-medication

Oral "self"-medication is another stress free option for administering analgesics, as the animals take the medication voluntarily. Most NSAIDs are available as palatable chewable tablets, capsules, or liquids and are readily consumed when mixed into yogurt or other treats. Oral administration of opioids is not ideal due to their lower bioavailability and metabolic first-pass effects. The general disadvantages of oral medication are the variability of gastrointestinal absorption and the difficulty in determining exactly which dose the animal has ingested. Nevertheless, oral administration in pigs is a viable, animal-friendly option if the uptake of the drug is monitored (Foley, 2014).

D. Prolonged postoperative analgesia

In case of major surgeries, prolonged pain relief after surgery is usually required. NSAIDs are generally longer lasting per se and often only need to be administered every 12 hours or once per day (Swindle, 2009). However, after major interventions, opioids are advisable due to their strong analgesic effect to cover the first days after surgery. Besides parenteral methods, fentanyl or buprenorphine transdermal patches or sustained-release formulations could be used. Both techniques can provide continuous, long-lasting analgesia, thus improving animal welfare by sustained analgesic effect and reduced handling (Roughan and Flecknell, 2002; Junot et al., 2008). Further, longer-lasting local anesthetics (e.g., bupivacaine) can be administered via in-dwelling catheters for additional pain relief at the surgical site.

Regardless of which route of administration or formulation is used, a pain assessment should be performed regularly and in case an animal is found to be under or overdosed, the analgesic regimen needs to be adjusted accordingly.

References

Aksakal, D., Hückstädt, T., Richter, S., Klitscher, D., Wowra, T., de Laffolie, J., et al., 2012. Comparison of femoral and carotid blood pressure during laparoscopy in piglets. J. Pediatr. Surg. 47 (9), 1688–1693.

Apfelbaum, J.L., Hagberg, C.A., Caplan, R.A., Blitt, C.D., Connis, R.T., Nickinovich, D.G., et al., 2013. Practice guidelines for management of the difficult airway: an updated report by the American Society of Anesthesiologists Task Force on Management of the Difficult Airway. Anesthesiology 118 (2), 251–270.

Asai, T., Shingu, K., 2005. The laryngeal tube. Br. J. Anaesth. 95 (6), 729–736.

Azevedo, L.C.P., Biagini, S., Costa, P.A., Rosário, A.L., Schettino, S.P., Wendel, S., et al., 2009. Feasibility of stored red blood cell transfusion in pigs. Crit. Care 13 (3), P2.

Bailey, J., 2018. Does the stress of laboratory life and experimentation on animals adversely affect research data? A critical review. Atla Altern. Lab. Anim. 46 (5), 291–305.

Bass, L.M.E., Yu, D.-Y., Cullen, L.K., 2009. Comparison of femoral and auricular arterial blood pressure monitoring in pigs. Vet. Anaesth. Analg. 36 (5), 457–463.

Becker, K., Eder, M., Ranft, A., von Meyer, L., Zieglgansberger, W., Kochs, E., et al., 2012. Low dose isoflurane exerts opposing effects on neuronal network excitability in neocortex and hippocampus. PLoS ONE 7 (6), e39346.

Bellini, L., De Benedictis, G.M., 2018. Neuromuscular blockade of atracurium in permissive hypercapnic versus normocapnic swine undergoing laparoscopy. PLoS ONE 13 (7), e0200439.

Benharkate, M., Zanini, V., Blanc, R., Boucheix, O., Coyez, F., Genevois, J.P., et al., 1993. Hemodynamic parameters of anesthetized pigs: a comparative study of farm piglets and Gottingen and Yucatan miniature swine. Lab. Anim. Sci. 43 (1), 68–72.

Bergese, S.D., Ramamoorthy, S., Patou, G., Bramlett, K., Gorfine, S.R., Candiotti, K.A., 2012. Efficacy profile of liposome bupivacaine, a novel formulation of bupivacaine for postsurgical analgesia. J. Pain Res. 5, 107–116.

Berset, C.M., Caristo, M.E., Ferrara, F., Hardy, P., Oropeza-Moe, M., Waters, R., et al., 2021. Federation of European Laboratory Animal Science Associations recommendations of best practices for the health management of ruminants and pigs used for scientific and educational purposes. Lab. Anim. 55 (2), 117–128.

Bigby, S.E., Carter, J.E., Bauquier, S., Beths, T., 2017. The use of alfaxalone for premedication, induction and maintenance of anaesthesia in pigs: a pilot study. Vet. Anaesth. Analg. 44 (4), 905–909.

Birkholz, T., Irouschek, A., Kessler, P., Blunk, J.A., Labahn, D., Schmidt, J., 2008. Feasibility of the laryngeal tube airway for artificial ventilation in pigs and comparison with the laryngeal mask airway. Lab Anim. (NY) 37 (8), 371–379.

Bohn, F., Henner, S., 1968. Electrocardiographic studies in miniature swine. Zeitschrift fur die gesamte experimentelle Medizin einschliesslich experimentelle Chirurgie 145 (4), 356–358.

Bradbury, A.G., Clutton, R.E., 2016a. Review of practices reported for preoperative food and water restriction of laboratory pigs (*Sus scrofa*). J. Am. Assoc. Lab. Anim. Sci. 55 (1), 35–40.

Bradbury, A.G., Clutton, R.E., 2016b. Are neuromuscular blocking agents being misused in laboratory pigs? Br. J. Anaesth. 116 (4), 476–485.

Burchardi, H., Kaczmarczyk, G., 1994. The effect of anaesthesia on renal function. Eur. J. Anaesthesiol. 11 (3), 163–168.

Bustamante, R., Valverde, A., 1997. Determination of a sedative dose and influence of droperidol and midazolam on cardiovascular function in pigs. Can. J. Vet. Res. 61 (4), 246–250.

Casey, B., Abney, D., Skoumbordis, E., 2007. A playroom as novel swine enrichment. Lab. Anim. 36 (3), 32–34.

Chilcott, R.P., Stubbs, B., Ashley, Z., 2001. Habituating pigs for in-pen, non-invasive biophysical skin analysis. Lab. Anim. 35 (3), 230–235.

Chuang, M., Orvieto, M., Laven, B., Gerber, G., Wardrip, C., Ritch, C., et al., 2005. Comparison of external catheters with subcutaneous vascular access ports for chronic vascular access in a porcine model. Contemp. Top. Lab. Anim. Sci. 44 (2), 24–27.

Chum, H., Pacharinsak, C., 2012. Endotracheal intubation in swine. Lab. Anim. 41 (11), 309–311.

Clarke, K.W., 1969. Effect of azaperone on the blood pressure and pulmonary ventilation in pigs. Vet. Rec. 85 (23), 649–651.

Clutton, R.E., Bracken, J., Ritchie, M., 1998. Effect of muscle injection site and drug temperature on pre-anaesthetic sedation in pigs. Vet. Rec. 142 (26), 718–721.

Clutton, R.E., Reed, F., Eddleston, M., Hulse, E.J. (Eds.), 2013. Prolonged Anaesthesia in Minipigs.

Cobo, A.A., Margallo, F.M.S., Diaz, C.B., Blazquez, V.B., Bueno, I.G., Crisostomo, V., 2020. Anesthesia protocols used to create ischemia reperfusion myocardial infarcts in swine. JAALAS 59 (5), 478–487.

Constable, P., Trefz, F.M., Stämpfli, H., 2019. Effects of pH and the plasma or serum concentrations of total calcium, chloride, magnesium, l-lactate, and albumin on the plasma ionized calcium concentration in calves. J. Vet. Intern. Med. 33 (4), 1822–1832.

CoRaAoP, 2009. Committee on recognition and alleviation of pain in laboratory Animals/NRC. Recognition and Alleviation of Pain in Laboratory Animals. National Academies Press (US), Washington (DC). https://doi.org/10.17226/125262009. https://www.ncbi.nlm.nih.gov/books/NBK32658/.

Cort, J.H., McCance, R.A., 1953. The neural control of shivering in the pig. J. Physiol. 120 (1–2), 115–121.

Daş, G., Vernunft, A., Görs, S., Kanitz, E., Weitzel, J.M., Brüssow, K.P., et al., 2016. Effects of general anesthesia with ketamine in combination with the neuroleptic sedatives xylazine or azaperone on plasma metabolites and hormones in pigs. J. Anim. Sci. 94 (8), 3229–3239.

De Witte, J., Sessler, D.I., 2002. Perioperative shivering: physiology and pharmacology. Anesthesiology 96 (2), 467–484. https://doi.org/10.1097/00000542-200202000-00036.

Dent, B.T., Stevens, K.A., Clymer, J.W., 2016. Forced-air warming provides better control of body temperature in porcine surgical patients. Vet. Sci. 3 (3).

Devitt, J.H., Rapanos, T., Kurrek, M., Cohen, M.M., Shaw, M., 1999. The anesthetic record: accuracy and completeness. Can. J. Anaesth. 46 (2), 122–128.

Dhondt, L., Croubels, S., De Paepe, P., Wallis, S.C., Pandey, S., Roberts, J.A., et al., 2020. Conventional pig as animal model for human renal drug excretion processes: unravelling the porcine renal function by use of a cocktail of exogenous markers. Front. Pharmacol. 11 (883).

Dukes, T.W., Szabuniewicz, M., 1969. The electrocardiogram of conventional and miniature swine (*Sus scrofa*). Can. J. Comp. Med. 33 (2), 118–127.

Dunbar, M.L., Walkowiak, K.J., Faustich, J.S., Rendahl, A.K., Graham, M.L., 2019. Preliminary evaluation of sustained-release compared with conventional formulations of meloxicam in sheep (*Ovis aries*). J. Am. Assoc. Lab. Anim. Sci. 58 (3), 339–345.

Duval, J.D., Pang, J.M., Boysen, S.R., Caulkett, N.A., 2018. Cardiopulmonary effects of a partial intravenous anesthesia technique for laboratory swine. J. Am. Assoc. Lab. Anim. Sci. 57 (4), 376–381.

Dyce, K.M., Sack, W.O., Wensing, C.J.G., 2009. Textbook of Veterinary Anatomy-E-Book. Elsevier Health Sciences.

Edelstein, C.L., 2008. Biomarkers of acute kidney injury. Adv. Chronic Kidney Dis. 15 (3), 222–234.

Ellegaard, L., Cunningham, A., Edwards, S., Grand, N., Nevalainen, T., Prescott, M., et al., 2010. Welfare of the minipig with special reference to use in regulatory toxicology studies. J. Pharmacol. Toxicol. Methods 62 (3), 167–183.

Ellenbroek, G.H., van Hout, G.P., Timmers, L., Doevendans, P.A., Pasterkamp, G., Hoefer, I.E., 2016. Primary outcome assessment in a pig model of acute myocardial infarction. J. Vis. Exp. 116.

Erdmann, E., Reuschel-Janetschek, E., 1991. Calcium for resuscitation? Br. J. Anaesth. 67 (2), 178–184.

Ettrup, K.S., Glud, A.N., Orlowski, D., Fitting, L.M., Meier, K., Soerensen, J.C., et al., 2011. Basic surgical techniques in the Göttingen minipig: intubation, bladder catheterization, femoral vessel catheterization, and transcardial perfusion. J. Vis. Exp. 52.

Fish, R.E., Brown, M.J., Danneman, P.J., Karaz, A.Z., 2008. Anesthesia and Analgesia in Laboratory Animals, 2nd. Elsevier, London.

Foley, P.L., 2014. Current options for providing sustained analgesia to laboratory animals. Lab. Anim. (NY) 43 (10), 364–371.

Forsling, M.L., Ingram, D.L., Stanier, M.W., 1980. Plasma antidiurectic hormone during hypoxia and anaesthesia in pigs. J. Endocrinol. 85 (2), 253–259.

Gay, C.C., Hinchcliff, D.C., Kenneth, W., Radostits, O.M., 2000. Veterinary Medicine; a Textbook of the Diseases of Cattle, Sheep, Pigs, Goats and Horses.

Glomset, D.J., Glomset, A.T., 1940. A morphologic study of the cardiac conduction system in ungulates, dog, and man: part II: the Purkinje system. Am. Heart J. 20 (6), 677–701.

Goebel, U., Siepe, M., Schwer, C.I., Schibilsky, D., Foerster, K., Neumann, J., et al., 2010. Inhaled carbon monoxide prevents acute kidney injury in pigs after cardiopulmonary bypass by inducing a heat shock response. Anesth. Analg. 111 (1), 29–37.

Goldmann, K., Kalinowski, M., Kraft, S., 2005. Airway management under general anaesthesia in pigs using the LMA-ProSealTM: a pilot study. Vet. Anaesth. Analg. 32 (5), 308–313.

Gomez de Segura, I.A., Tendillo, F.J., Mascias, A., Santos, M., Castillo-Olivares, J.L., Steffey, E.P., 1997. Actions of xylazine in young swine. Am. J. Vet. Res. 58 (1), 99–102.

Goutchtat, R., Chetboun, M., Wiart, J.F., Gaulier, J.M., Pattou, F., Allorge, D., et al., 2021. Long-term analgesia following a single application of fentanyl transdermal solution in pigs. Eur. Surg. Res. 62 (2), 115–120.

Gregson, R., Greenhalgh, S., Cox, B., Cochrane, S., Clutton, R.E., 2021. Feeding management before gastrointestinal studies in pigs. Lab. Anim. 55 (2), 177–180.

Guerra, R., De Monte, A., Girardis, M., 2012. A new technique for percutaneous dilatational tracheostomy (G-Trach): preliminary experience in pigs. Anaesthesia 67 (9), 968–972.

Gutierrez, K., Dicks, N., Glanzner, W.G., Agellon, L.B., Bordignon, V., 2015. Efficacy of the porcine species in biomedical research. Front. Genet. 6, 293.

Gyrd-Hansen, N., 1969. The effects of diuretics on renal clearances in pigs. Acta Vet. Scand. 10 (4), 345–358.

Hafer, A.L., Langley, R.L., Morrow, W.E.M., Tulis, J.J., 1996. Occupational hazards reported by swine veterinarians in the United States. Swine Health Prod. 4 (3).

Haga, H.A., Lervik, A., Nordgreen, J., 2018. Fentanyl causes shivering in isoflurane anaesthetised piglets, dexmedetomidine reduces muscular activity. In: 13th World Congress of Veterinary Anaesthesia. Venice.

Haga, H.A., Tevik, A., Moerch, H., 1999. Bispectral index as an indicator of anaesthetic depth during isoflurane anaesthesia in the pig. J. Vet. Anaesth. 26 (1), 3–7.

Hannon, J.P., Bossone, C.A., Wade, C.E., 1990. Normal physiological values for conscious pigs used in biomedical research. Lab. Anim. Sci. 40 (3), 293–298.

Harvey-Clark, C.J., Gilespie, K., Riggs, K.W., 2000. Transdermal fentanyl compared with parenteral buprenorphine in post-surgical pain in swine: a case study. Lab. Anim. 34 (4), 386–398.

Hawkins, P., Morton, D.B., Burman, O., Dennison, N., Honess, P., Jennings, M., et al., 2011. A guide to defining and implementing protocols for the welfare assessment of laboratory animals: eleventh report of the BVAAWF/FRAME/RSPCA/UFAW Joint Working Group on Refinement. Lab. Anim. 45 (1), 1–13.

Health USDoHHSNIo, 2010. How Loud Is Too Loud? How Long Is Too Long? Available from: https://www.nidcd.nih.gov/sites/default/files/Documents/health/hearing/Factsheet_HowLoudHowLong.pdf.

Herskin, M.S., Bundgaard, C., Ottesen, J.L., Sørensen, D.B., Marchant-Forde, J.N., 2021. The laboratory pig. In: Sørensen, D.B., Cloutier, C.J., Gaskill, B.N. (Eds.), Animal-Centric Care and Management Enhancing Refinement in Biomedical Research, first ed. CRC Press, pp. 173–186.

Hohlbaum, K., Bert, B., Dietze, S., Palme, R., Fink, H., Thone-Reineke, C., 2017. Severity classification of repeated isoflurane anesthesia in C57BL/6JRj mice-assessing the degree of distress. PLoS ONE 12 (6), e0179588.

Holliman, C.J., Kenfield, K., Nutter, E., Saffle, J.R., Warden, G.D., 1982. Technique for acute suprapubic catheterization of urinary bladder in the pig. Am. J. Vet. Res. 43 (6), 1056–1057.

Houpert, P., Combrisson, H., Le Nain, S., Autefage, A., Toutain, P.L., 1993. Intra- vs intermuscular injections in swine. Vet. Res. 24 (3), 278–285.

Isbell, C.L., Batchinsky, A.I., Hetz, K.M., Baker, W.L., Cancio, L.C., 2012. Correlation between capnography and arterial carbon dioxide before, during, and after severe chest injury in swine. Shock 37 (1), 103–109.

Ison, S.H., Clutton, R.E., Di Giminiani, P., Rutherford, K.M., 2016. A review of pain assessment in pigs. Front. Vet. Sci. 3, 108.

Izer, J., Wilson, R., Hernon, K., Ündar, A., 2017. Ultrasound-guided vessel catheterization in adult Yorkshire cross-bred pigs. Vet. Anaesth. Analg. 44 (1), 133–137.

Jaber, S.M., Sullivan, S., Hankenson, F.C., Kilbaugh, T.J., Margulies, S.S., 2015. Comparison of heart rate and blood pressure with toe pinch and bispectral index for monitoring the depth of anesthesia in piglets. JAALAS 54 (5), 536–544.

Jivegård, L., Frid, I., Haljamäe, H., Holm, J., Holm, S., Wickström, I., 1990. Cardiac output determinations in the pig-thoracic electrical bioimpedance versus thermodilution. Crit. Care Med. 18 (9), 995–998.

Jonholt, L., Bundgaard, C.J., Carlsen, M., Sorensen, D.B., 2021. A case study on the behavioural effect of positive reinforcement training in a novel task participation test in Gottingen mini pigs. Animals (Basel) 11 (6).

Jonna, S.P., Hauser, G.J., Heretzog, J.H., Dalton, H.J., 1998. Heparin lowers ionized calcium (iCa) measurements by blood gas analyzer† 206. Pediatr. Res. 43 (4), 38.

Joo, H.S., Kataoka, M.T., Chen, R.J., Doyle, J., Mazer, C.D., 2002. PVC tracheal tubes exert forces and pressures seven to ten times higher than silicone or armoured tracheal tubes—an in vitro study. Can. J. Anaesth. 49 (9), 986–989.

Jorquera-Chavez, M., Fuentes, S., Dunshea, F.R., Warner, R.D., Poblete, T., Unnithan, R.R., et al., 2021. Using imagery and computer vision as remote monitoring methods for early detection of respiratory disease in pigs. Comput. Electron. Agric. 187.

Junot, S., Troncy, E., Keroack, S., Gauvin, D., del Castillo, J.R., Boivin, R., et al., 2008. Renal effect of meloxicam versus ketoprofen in anaesthetized pseudo-normovolaemic piglets. Can. J. Physiol. Pharmacol. 86 (1–2), 55–63.

Kaiser, G.M., Heuer, M.M., Fruhauf, N.R., Kuhne, C.A., Broelsch, C.E., 2006. General handling and anesthesia for experimental surgery in pigs. J. Surg. Res. 130 (1), 73–79.

Kamiya, S., Nakamura, R., Saeki, N., Kondo, T., Miyoshi, H., Narasaki, S., et al., 2021. Prediction of blood pressure change during surgical incision under opioid analgesia using sympathetic response evoking threshold. Sci. Rep. 11 (1), 9558.

Keita, A., Pagot, E., Prunier, A., Guidarini, C., 2010. Pre-emptive meloxicam for postoperative analgesia in piglets undergoing surgical castration. Vet. Anaesth. Analg. 37 (4), 367–374.

Kilkenny, C., Browne, W.J., Cuthill, I.C., Emerson, M., Altman, D.G., 2010. Improving bioscience research reporting: the arrive guidelines for reporting animal research. PLoS Biol. 8 (6).

Kissin, I., 2000. Preemptive analgesia. Anesthesiology 93 (4), 1138–1143.

Kittleson, M.D., Olivier, N.B., 1983. Measurement of systemic arterial blood pressure. Vet. Clin. N. Am. Small Anim. Pract. 13 (2), 321–336.

Klein, C., Reinhold, P., 2001. Analysis of respiratory mechanics by impulse oscillometry in non-sedated and diazepam-sedated swine. Res. Vet. Sci. 70 (3), 181–189.

Klein, P., Nalos, L., Dejmek, J., Soukup, M., 2019. The method of long-term catheterization of the vena jugularis in pigs. J. Pharmacol. Toxicol. Methods 98.

Laber-Laird, K., Smith, A., Swindle, M., Colwell, J., 1992. Effects of isoflurane anesthesia on glucose tolerance and insulin secretion in Yucatan minipigs. Lab. Anim. Sci. 42 (6), 579–581.

Lervik, A., Toverud, S.F., Bohlin, J., Haga, H.A., 2021. Macrocirculatory parameters and oxygen debt indices in pigs during propofol or alfaxalone anesthesia when subjected to experimental stepwise hemorrhage. Front. Vet. Sci. 8.

Lesser, T., Braun, C., Wolfram, F., Gottschall, R., 2020. A special double lumen tube for use in pigs is suitable for different lung ventilation conditions. Res. Vet. Sci. 133, 111–116.

Li, D.-P., Zhang, W.-H., Yang, M.-L., Liu, C.-B., Zhang, X., Cai, C., et al., 2017. An improved urethral catheterization in female pigs: a pilot study. Chin. Med. J. (Engl.). 130 (15), 1880–1881.

Lindqwister, A.L., Lampe, J.W., Gould, J.R., Kaufman, C.L., Moodie, K.L., Paradis, N.A., 2020. Intravenous calcium as a pressor in a swine model of hypoxic pseudo-pulseless electrical mechanical activity—a preliminary report. Intensive Care Med. Exp. 8 (1), 50.

Linkenhoker, J.R., Burkholder, T.H., Linton, C.G.G., Walden, A., Abusakran-Monday, K.A., Rosero, A.P., et al., 2010. Effective and safe anesthesia for Yorkshire and Yucatan swine with and without cardiovascular injury and intervention. JAALAS 49 (3), 344–351.

Litton, E., Morgan, M., 2012. The PiCCO monitor: a review. Anaesth. Intensive Care 40 (3), 393–409.

Lumb, W.V., Tranquilli, W.J., Jones, E.W., Thurmon, J.C., Grimm, K.A., 2007. Lumb & Jones' Veterinary Anesthesia and Analgesia. Blackwell.

Luna, S.P.L., de Araujo, A.L., da Nobrega Neto, P.I., Brondani, J.T., de Oliveira, F.A., Azeredo, L., et al., 2020. Validation of the UNESP-Botucatu pig composite acute pain scale (UPAPS). PLoS ONE 15 (6), e0233552.

Mainau, E., Ruiz-de-la-Torre, J.L., Dalmau, A., Salleras, J.M., Manteca, X., 2012. Effects of meloxicam (Metacam®) on post-farrowing sow behaviour and piglet performance. Animal 6 (3), 494–501.

Malavasi, L.M., Nyman, G., Augustsson, H., Jacobson, M., Jensen-Waern, M., 2006. Effects of epidural morphine and transdermal fentanyl analgesia on physiology and behaviour after abdominal surgery in pigs. Lab. Anim. 40 (1), 16–27.

Manell, E., Jensen-Waern, M., Hedenqvist, P., 2017. Anaesthesia and changes in parameters that reflect glucose metabolism in pigs—a pilot study. Lab. Anim. 51 (5), 509–517.

Martín-Cancho, M.F., Lima, J.R., Luis, L., Crisóstomo, V., Ezquerra, L.J., Carrasco, M.S., et al., 2003. Bispectral index, spectral edge frequency 95%, and median frequency recorded for various concentrations of isoflurane and sevoflurane in pigs. Am. J. Vet. Res. 64 (7), 866–873.

Martinez-Taboada, F., Leece, E.A., 2014. Comparison of propofol with ketofol, a propofol-ketamine admixture, for induction of anaesthesia in healthy dogs. Vet. Anaesth. Analg. 41 (6), 575–582.

Mawhinney, L.J., Mabourakh, D., Lewis, M.C., 2013. Gender-specific differences in the central nervous system's response to anesthesia. Transl. Stroke Res. 4 (4), 462–475.

McInnes, E.F., McKeag, S., 2016. A brief review of infrequent spontaneous findings, peculiar anatomical microscopic features, and potential artifacts in Gottingen minipigs. Toxicol. Pathol. 44 (3), 338–345.

Moon, P.F., Smith, L.J., 1996. General anesthetic techniques in swine. Vet. Clin. N. Am. Food Anim. Pract. 12 (3), 663–691.

Murison, P.J., Jones, A., Mitchard, L., Burt, R., Birchall, M.A., 2009. Development of perioperative care for pigs undergoing laryngeal transplantation: a case series. Lab. Anim. 43 (4), 338–343.

Murphy, C., Rooney, S.J., Maharaj, C.H., Laffey, J.G., Harte, B.H., 2011. Comparison of three cuffed emergency percutaneous cricothyroidotomy devices to conventional surgical cricothyroidotomy in a porcine model. Br. J. Anaesth. 106 (1), 57–64.

Musk, G.C., Zwierzchoniewska, M., He, B., 2015. Catheterization of the urethra in female pigs. Lab. Anim. 49 (4), 345–348.

Musk, G.C., Costa, R.S., Tuke, J., 2016. Body temperature measurements in pigs during general anaesthesia. Lab. Anim. 50 (2), 119–124.

NCSV, 1995. Occupational Hazards on Swine Farms. NCSV. Available from: https://projects.ncsu.edu/project/swine_extension/healthyhogs/book1995/langley.htm.

Nicholls, S.M., Mitchard, L.K., Murrell, J.C., Dick, A.D., Bailey, M., 2012. Perioperative socialization, care and monitoring of National Institutes of Health miniature swine undergoing ocular surgery and sampling of peripheral blood. Lab. Anim. 46 (1), 59–64.

Nishimura, R., Kim, H., Matsunaga, S., Sakaguchi, M., Sasaki, N., Tamura, H., et al., 1992. Antagonism of medetomidine sedation by atipamezole in pigs. J. Vet. Med. Sci. 54 (6), 1237–1240.

Nishimura, R., Kim, H., Matsunaga, S., Hayashi, K., Tamura, H., Sasaki, N., et al., 1993a. Comparison of sedative and analgesic/anesthetic effects induced by medetomidine, acepromazine, azaperone, droperidol and midazolam in laboratory pigs. J. Vet. Med. Sci. 55 (4), 687–690.

Nishimura, R., Kim, H., Matsunaga, S., Hayashi, K., Tamura, H., Sasaki, N., et al., 1993b. Sedative effect induced by a combination of medetomidine and midazolam in pigs. J. Vet. Med. Sci. 55 (5), 717–722.

Nishimura, R., Kim, H.Y., Matsunaga, S., Hayashi, K., Tamura, H., Sasaki, N., et al., 1994. Effects of medetomidine-midazolam on plasma glucose and insulin concentrations in laboratory pigs. J. Vet. Med. Sci. 56 (3), 559–561.

Nonneman, D.J., Brown-Brandl, T., Jones, S.A., Wiedmann, R.T., Rohrer, G.A., 2012. A defect in dystrophin causes a novel porcine stress syndrome. BMC Genom. 13, 233.

Nyman, G., Funkquist, B., Kvart, C., Frostell, C., Tokics, L., Strandberg, A., et al., 1990. Atelectasis causes gas exchange impairment in the anaesthetised horse. Equine Vet. J. 22 (5), 317–324.

Obernier, J.A., Baldwin, R.L., 2006. Establishing an appropriate period of acclimatization following transportation of laboratory animals. ILAR J. 47 (4), 364–369.

Ortiz-Prado, E., Dunn, J.F., Vasconez, J., Castillo, D., Viscor, G., 2019. Partial pressure of oxygen in the human body: a general review. Am. J. Blood Res. 9 (1), 1–14.

Osorio Lujan, S., Habre, W., Daali, Y., Pan, Z., Kronen, P.W., 2017. Plasma concentrations of transdermal fentanyl and buprenorphine in pigs (*Sus scrofa domesticus*). Vet. Anaesth. Analg. 44 (3), 665–675.

Otten, W., Kanitz, E., Puppe, B., Tuchscherer, M., Brüssow, K., Nürnberg, G., Stabenow, B., 2004. Acute and long term effects of chronic intermittent noise stress on hypothalamic-pituitary-adrenocortical and sympatho-adrenomedullary axis in pigs. Anim. Sci. 78 (2), 271–283.

Pandey, S., Kalwa, U., Kong, T., Guo, B.Q., Gauger, P.C., Peters, D.J., et al., 2021. Behavioral monitoring tool for pig farmers: ear tag sensors, machine intelligence, and technology adoption roadmap. Animals 11 (9).

Panepinto, L.M., Phillips, R.W., Norden, S., Pryor, P.C., Cox, R., 1983. A comfortable, minimum stress method of restraint for Yucatan miniature swine. Lab. Anim. Sci. 33 (1), 95–97.

Patil, V.U., Fairbrother, C.R., Dunham, B.M., 1997. Use of the laryngeal mask airway for emergency or elective airway management situations in pigs. JAALAS 36 (6), 47–49.

Patschke, D., Brückner, J.B., Gethmann, J.W., Tarnow, J., Weymar, A., 1975. Einfluss der Ketaminnarkose auf die Hämodynamik und den myokardialen Sauerstoffverbrauch narkotisierter Hunde [The effect of ketamine on haemodynamics and myocardial oxygen consumption in anaesthetized dogs]. Praktische Anästhesie 10, 325–334.

Pavlovsky, V.H., Corona, D., Hug, P.J., Kummerlen, D., Graage, R., Bettschart-Wolfensberger, R., 2021. Butorphanol induces anxiety-like-behaviour and distress in piglets. Schweiz. Arch. Tierheilkd. 163 (7), 485–491.

Phillips, C.E., Li, Y.Z., Johnston, L.J., Goplen, A.E., Shurson, G.C., 2012. Technical note: a technique for ear vein catheterization in group-housed sows. J. Anim. Sci. 90 (2), 501–504.

Pinkernelle, J., Raschzok, N., Teichgräber, U.K.M., 2009. Sonographically guided placement of intravenous catheters in minipigs. Lab. Anim. 38 (7), 241–245.

Ranheim, B.T., Toverud, S.F., Haga, H.A., 2013. Sedative effect of medetomidine related to bodyweight in growing Duroc boars. In: Association of Veterinary Anaesthetists Spring Meeting. Association of Veterinary Anaesthetists and the American College of Veterinary Anesthesia and Analgesia, London, pp. 15–16.

Reed, F.C., Shaw, D.J., McLean, K.A., Clutton, R.E., 2015. Influence of age and body mass on the response of adolescent male pigs to anaesthesia. Vet. Rec. 177 (4), 98.

Reed, R., Barletta, M., Grimes, J., Mumaw, J., Park, H.J., Giguère, S., et al., 2018. Accuracy of an oscillometric blood pressure monitor in anesthetized pigs. Lab. Anim. 52 (5), 490–496.

Ringer, S.K., Spielmann, N., Weiss, M., Mauch, J.Y., 2016. Fentanyl bolus induces muscle tremors in sevoflurane-anaesthetized piglets. Lab. Anim. 50 (4), 312–314.

Rivat, C., Bollag, L., Richebe, P., 2013. Mechanisms of regional anaesthesia protection against hyperalgesia and pain chronicization. Curr. Opin. Anaesthesiol. 26 (5), 621–625.

Rodriguez, J.M., Munoz-Rascon, P., Navarrete-Calvo, R., Gomez-Villamandos, R.J., Dominguez Perez, J.M., Fernandez Sarmiento, J.A., et al., 2012. Comparison of the cardiopulmonary parameters after induction of anaesthesia with alphaxalone or etomidate in dogs. Vet. Anaesth. Analg. 39 (4), 357–365.

Rosero, E.B., Joshi, G.P., 2014. Preemptive, preventive, multimodal analgesia: what do they really mean? Plast. Reconstr. Surg. 134 (4), 85s–93s.

Roughan, J.V., Flecknell, P.A., 2002. Buprenorphine: a reappraisal of its antinociceptive effects and therapeutic use in alleviating post-operative pain in animals. Lab. Anim. 36 (3), 322–343.

Royal, J.M., Settle, T.L., Bodo, M., Lombardini, E., Kent, M.L., Upp, J., et al., 2013. Assessment of postoperative analgesia after application of ultrasound-guided regional anesthesia for surgery in a swine femoral fracture model. J. Am. Assoc. Lab. Anim. Sci. 52 (3), 265–276.

Ruemmler, R., Ziebart, A., Ott, T., Dirvonskis, D., Hartmann, E.K., 2020. Flexible fibreoptic intubation in swine—improvement for resident training and animal safety alike. BMC Anesthesiol. 20 (1), 206.

Rydén, A., Jensen-Waern, M., Nyman, G., Olsén, L., 2021. Physiological and clinical responses in pigs in relation to plasma concentrations during anesthesia with dexmedetomidine, tiletamine, zolazepam, and butorphanol. Animals 11 (6), 1482.

Sahinovic, M.M., Struys, M., Absalom, A.R., 2018. Clinical pharmacokinetics and pharmacodynamics of propofol. Clin. Pharmacokinet. 57 (12), 1539–1558.

Sakaguchi, M., Nishimura, R., Sasaki, N., Ishiguro, T., Tamura, H., Takeuchi, A., 1992. Enhancing effect of butorphanol on medetomidine-induced sedation in pigs. J. Vet. Med. Sci. 54 (6), 1183–1185.

Sakaguchi, M., Nishimura, R., Sasaki, N., Ishiguro, T., Tamura, H., Takeuchi, A., 1996. Anesthesia induced in pigs by use of a combination of medetomidine, butorphanol, and ketamine and its reversal by administration of atipamezole. Am. J. Vet. Res. 57 (4), 529–534.

Santos, M., de Lis, B.T.B., Tendillo, F.J., 2016. Effects of intramuscular dexmedetomidine in combination with ketamine or alfaxalone in swine. Vet. Anaesth. Analg. 43 (1), 81–85.

Sare, H., Ambrisko, T.D., Moens, Y., 2011. Occupational exposure to isoflurane during anaesthesia induction with standard and scavenging double masks in dogs, pigs and ponies. Lab. Anim. 45 (3), 191–195.

Seidler, T., Alter, T., Kruger, M., Fehlhaber, K., 2001. Transport stress-consequences for bacterial translocation, endogenous contamination and bactericidal activity of serum of slaughter pigs. Berl. Munch. Tierarztl. Wochenschr. 114 (9–10), 375–377.

Silva, A., Antunes, L., 2012. Electroencephalogram-based anaesthetic depth monitoring in laboratory animals. Lab. Anim. 46 (2), 85–94.

Smith, A.C., Swindle, M.M., 2006. Preparation of swine for the laboratory. ILAR J. 47 (4), 358–363.

Smith, A.C., Spinale, F.G., Swindle, M.M., 1990. Cardiac function and morphology of Hanford miniature swine and Yucatan miniature and micro swine. Lab. Anim. Sci. 40 (1), 47–50.

Smith, A.C., Zellner, J.L., Spinale, F.G., Swindle, M.M., 1991. Sedative and cardiovascular effects of midazolam in swine. Lab. Anim. Sci. 41 (2), 157–161.

Smith, A.C., Ehler, W.J., Swindle, M.M., 1997. Anesthesia and Analgesia in Swine. Anesthesia and Analgesia in Laboratory Animals. Elsevier, pp. 313–336.

Smith, D.M., Newhouse, M., Naziruddin, B., Kresie, L., 2006. Blood groups and transfusions in pigs. Xenotransplantation 13 (3), 186–194.

Solem, J.O., Tengborn, L., Olin, C., Steen, S., 1986. Autotransfusion of whole-blood in massive bleeding—an experimental-study in the pig. Acta Chir. Scand. 152, 427–432.

Souba, W.W., Wilmore, D.W., 2001. Surgical Research. Elsevier.

Steinbacher, R., von Ritgen, S., Moens, Y.P., 2012. Laryngeal perforation during a standard intubation procedure in a pig. Lab. Anim. 46 (3), 261–263.

Svendsen, M.N., Koch, L., 2013. Potentializing the research piglet in experimental neonatal research. Curr. Anthropol. 54, 118–128.

Swindle, M.M., 2007. Swine in the Laboratory: Surgery, Anesthesia, Imaging, and Experimental Techniques. CRC Press.

Swindle, M.M., 2009. Anesthesia & Analgesia in Swine.

Swindle, M.M., Smith, A.C., 2013. Best practices for performing experimental surgery in swine. J. Invest. Surg. 26 (2), 63–71.

Swindle, M.M., Smith, A.C., 2015. Swine in the Laboratory: Surgery, Anesthesia, Imaging, and Experimental Techniques, 2nd ed. CRC Press, Boca Raton.

Tendillo, F.J., Mascías, A., Santos, M., Segura, I.A., San Roman, F., Castillo-Olivares, J.L., 1996. Cardiopulmonary and analgesic effects of xylazine, detomidine, medetomidine, and the antagonist atipamezole in isoflurane-anesthetized swine. Lab. Anim. Sci. 46 (2), 215–219.

Theisen, M.M., Maas, M., Hartlage, M.A., Ploner, F., Niehues, S.M., Van Aken, H.K., et al., 2009. Ventral recumbency is crucial for fast and safe orotracheal intubation in laboratory swine. Lab. Anim. 43 (1), 96–101.

Thiede, A.J., Garcia, K.D., Stolarik, D.F., Ma, J., Jenkins, G.J., Nunamaker, E.A., 2014. Pharmacokinetics of sustained-release and transdermal buprenorphine in Gottingen minipigs (*Sus scrofa domestica*). J. Am. Assoc. Lab. Anim. Sci. 53 (6), 692–699.

Thomsen, A.F., Kousholt, B.S., 2021. Transition of farm pigs to research pigs using a designated checklist followed by initiation of clicker training—a refinement initiative. J. Vis. Exp. 174.

Thomas, J., Lerche, P., 2016. Anesthesia and Analgesia for Veterinary Technicians-E-Book. Elsevier Health Sciences.

Varkey, J., Welliver, M., 2013. Debunking volatile anesthetic cost myths between sevoflurane and desflurane. Anesth. eJ. 1 (2).

Viscardi, A.V., Hunniford, M., Lawlis, P., Leach, M., Turner, P.V., 2017. Development of a piglet grimace scale to evaluate piglet pain using facial expressions following castration and tail docking: a pilot study. Front. Vet. Sci. 4, 51.

Vullo, C., Barbieri, S., Catone, G., Graic, J.M., Magaletti, M., Di Rosa, A., et al., 2020. Is the piglet grimace scale (PGS) a useful welfare indicator to assess pain after cryptorchidectomy in growing pigs? Animals 10 (3).

Weeks, C.A., Brown, S.N., Lane, S., Heasman, L., Benson, T., Warriss, P.D., 2009. Noise levels in lairages for cattle, sheep and pigs in abattoirs in England and Wales. Vet. Rec. 165 (11), 308–314.

Weidemann, F., Jamal, F., Sutherland, G.R., Claus, P., Kowalski, M., Hatle, L., et al., 2002. Myocardial function defined by strain rate and strain during alterations in inotropic states and heart rate. Am. J. Physiol. Heart Circ. Physiol. 283 (2), H792–H799.

Wemyss-Holden, S.A., Porter, K.J., Baxter, P., Rudkin, G.E., Maddern, G.J., 1999. The laryngeal mask airway in experimental pig anaesthesia. Lab. Anim. 33 (1), 30–34.

Wilkinson, A.C., Thomas, M.L., Morse, B.C., 2001. Evaluation of a transdermal fentanyl system in Yucatan miniature pigs. Contemp. Top. Lab. Anim. 40 (3), 12–16.

Wolf, E., Braun-Reichhart, C., Streckel, E., Renner, S., 2014. Genetically engineered pig models for diabetes research. Transgenic Res. 23 (1), 27–38.

Woolf, C.J., 1983. Evidence for a central component of post-injury pain hypersensitivity. Nature 306 (5944), 686–688.

Zambricki, E.A., Dalecy, L.G., 2004. Rat sex differences in anesthesia. Comp. Med. 54 (1), 49–53.

Zhang, H., Zhou, Z.-F., Zhang, J.-T., Zhang, S.-X., Wang, H.-B., 2014. Laparoscopic cystostomy in pigs: technique and comparison with traditional open cystostomy for surgical stress. Acta Vet. Brno 83 (4), 385–391.

Zucker, B.A., Kruger, M., 1998. Effect of transport stress on the content of endotoxin in blood of slaughter pigs. Berl. Munch. Tierarztl. Wochenschr. 111 (6), 208–210.

Chapter 18

Anesthesia and analgesia in nonhuman primates

Elizabeth A. Nunamaker[1], Carolyn M. Malinowski[2], Anna E. Goodroe[3], Kathryn A. Guerriero[4] and Monika A. Burns[5]

[1]Charles River Laboratories, Global Animal Welfare and Training, Wilmington, MA, United States; [2]The University of Texas MD Anderson Cancer Center, Bastrop, TX, United States; [3]Southwest National Primate Research Center at Texas Biomedical Research Institute, San Antonio, TX, United States; [4]National Institutes of Health, Bethesda, MD, United States; [5]Animal Welfare Compliance, Novartis Institutes for BioMedical Research, Cambridge, MA, United States

Chapter outline

Anesthesia and Analgesia in Laboratory Animals. https://doi.org/10.1016/B978-0-12-822215-7.00003-2

I. Introduction

Nonhuman primates are important models for a wide variety of biomedical and behavioral research investigations because of their close phylogenetic relationship to humans and the translatability of research outcomes. They serve as models for the advancement of surgical techniques, neuroscience applications, understanding of communicable diseases and aging, as well as vaccine and therapeutics development. Advances in methods of anesthesia, analgesia, and chemical restraint have played an important role in advancing the welfare of nonhuman primates. Of the approximate 190 species of nonhuman primates, the majority utilized as models in biomedical research are macaques (*Macaca* spp.), baboons (*Papio* spp.), African green monkeys (*Chlorocebus* sp.), squirrel monkeys (*Saimiri* spp.), and marmosets (*Callitrichidae*). Chimpanzees (*Pan troglodytes*) have been primarily excluded from the current written text, although drug dosages have been included in tables and charts. For in-depth information about chimpanzees, previous editions of this text and current literature may be referenced.

When considering options for anesthesia, analgesia, and chemical restraint, the diversity of the order primate must be considered. The wide range in body size and weight of nonhuman primates plays an important role in selecting appropriate agents, the route of administration, and dosage (Sainsbury et al., 1989). Extrapolation of analgesic or anesthetic doses from one primate species to another should be done with caution, because of differences in the responses of some species. Other criteria within the same species, such as age, gender, and breeding status of the animal, must be considered when determining appropriate analgesic or anesthetic regimens.

This chapter provides a review of the literature on techniques, methodologies, and agents that have been reported in commonly utilized nonhuman primate species. In some instances, in which there is little information available in the literature and for which the authors have had insufficient experience, information has been obtained from knowledgeable clinicians by personal communication. The goal is to provide veterinarians and investigators with information that will ensure the provision of optimal analgesia and anesthesia for nonhuman primates.

II. Preprocedural considerations

A. Health and safety

Since nonhuman primates may carry potentially hazardous zoonotic diseases, any discussion relative to the handling of these species must address personnel health, safety, and biosecurity. A plan that addresses safety concerns relative to infectious, noninfectious, and physical hazards associated with working with research nonhuman primates must be in place. This plan may require special training of personnel and demand unique management, engineering, or equipment needs to mitigate the risk of contamination or injury to both personnel and the research subject.

Numerous pathogenic organisms can be transmitted from nonhuman primates to humans, and several human pathogens are communicable to nonhuman primates. Since nonhuman primates and humans have a relatively close phylogenetic relationship, the risk of transmission is greater than with other laboratory animals (National Research Council, 2003). Naturally occurring zoonotic diseases, as well as experimentally induced infectious diseases in the nonhuman primate models, must be considered. All personnel involved in providing anesthesia, analgesia, chemical restraint, and perioperative care to nonhuman primates should be fully aware of means to prevent possible exposure to zoonotic diseases, and any other induced infectious or communicable hazards (Wallis and Lee, 1999).

Personnel should receive training in the use of personal protective clothing compliance with universal sharps precautions, and should be enrolled in an appropriate occupational health program (Blanchard and Russell-Lodrigue, 2012). Personnel should also be aware of hazards associated with nonhuman primate behavior that could lead to bites, scratches, and splashes of potentially harmful body fluids. Occupational health and safety must also identify other noninfectious hazards to personnel, such as volatile anesthetics and potentially harmful chemical exposures (oral/ocular exposure to disinfectants, ketamine, etc.).

Each anesthetized nonhuman primate should be protected from cross-transmission of infectious organisms from other nonhuman primates. This may require species or cohort separation, dedicated equipment or space, and other management factors to prevent transmission of pathogens that may not even be readily apparent, such as Herpes B virus, *Mycobacterium tuberculosis*, simian immunodeficiency virus, or simian hemorrhagic fever.

B. History, records, and patient evaluation

Preprocedure assessment includes a review of previous research use, clinical records, and the influence of the current experimental protocol on anesthetic management. Because of the limitations associated with performing a thorough physical examination on an awake nonhuman primate, a cage-side evaluation should be performed to identify important signs of illness such as unusual posture or behavior, anorexia, and abnormal urine or feces. Obtaining body weight and temperature, determining the body condition score, auscultation of heart rhythm and bilateral lung sounds, peripheral pulse palpation, and observation of the mucous membranes for color and perfusion during the preprocedure period will provide additional information on the physical status of the animal. Additionally, pregnancy diagnosis should be performed for females housed in breeding enclosures.

Routine laboratory tests (e.g., CBC, blood chemistries, and select serology) may be performed while nonhuman primates are in quarantine, prior to study enrollment, or at predefined regular intervals (Kramer et al., 2012). Variations in testing within an institution may reflect specific needs associated with the use of nonhuman primates.

Concomitant natural and experimental diseases may influence the selection of an appropriate anesthetic protocol. Particular anesthetics or analgesics may be contraindicated or require modified use in nonhuman primates that are pregnant, young, aged, or have abnormal cardiovascular dynamics, liver, or renal function, as such conditions may affect anesthetic distribution, metabolism, or excretion (Brambrink et al., 2012; Havton et al., 2020; Hom et al., 1999).

C. Risk assessment—transportation anesthesia and monitoring

Forethought should be given to transport plans for the animal while chemically restrained or under general anesthesia. Consider how animals will be transported, plans for moving animals through common spaces to mitigate exposure to passing personnel, and the need for animal monitoring during transport. There are many options available for monitoring an animal ranging from simple cage-side evaluations, pulse oximetry, or more in-depth procedures including capnography and oscillometric blood pressure monitoring. Monitoring practices depend on the length of transport and clinical condition of the animal.

D. Chemical restraint, anesthetic, and analgesic considerations

During the planning stage, it is essential to consider if the procedure can be accomplished under chemical restraint or whether anesthesia is required. While general anesthesia is required for more invasive procedures, many short or less invasive procedures, such as physical examination, phlebotomy, or wound repair, can be performed with chemical restraint and multimodal analgesia as needed. Professional judgment, personnel competence, and available resources should be accounted for during the decision-making process.

An important consideration is the method of delivery for the agent(s) being administered. Depending on the housing type, size, and age of the animal, there are a range of options. Almost all agents for initial sedation are delivered via the intramuscular route. Nonhuman primates possess unique behavioral characteristics and are relatively quick and strong for their size, so it is critical to consider how an anesthetic agent will be safely delivered. Delivery of agents in nonhuman primates generally begins with some effective means of restraint or cooperative training (Wolf and White, 2012). This may include one or a combination of methods, such as operant training (presenting a limb for intravenous or intramuscular injection), physical restraint (squeeze back cage, manual restraint, and chair/tube restraint), a remote injection system (dart delivery by blowpipe, hand-pump pistol, or CO_2 pistol/rifle) (Isaza, 2012), or oral baiting (Pulley et al., 2004). For very large animals, and those in large enclosures, dart systems are typically required. Blowpipes and pump air guns are generally preferred over CO_2 pistols, as they are quieter and produce less tissue damage with impact (Isaza, 2012; Fowler, 1986). These methods can cause injury to both personnel and animals and should be restricted to use by trained and experienced personnel. The more control the anesthetist has over the animal the less stress and risk of accident or injury during the procedure.

E. Fasting and antiemetics

Although the optimal fasting time in nonhuman primates has not been established, it is conventional practice to fast larger species for at least 12 hours in order to decrease the risk of pulmonary aspiration. Exceptions to this are primates belonging to the family Callitrichidae (marmosets and tamarins) and neonatal animals, which are generally fasted for a shorter period of time (4–6 hours) to avoid perioperative hypoglycemia. Fasting for chemical restraint is also common practice, although generally for a shorter period of time (2–4 hours). Animals should be given ad libitum access to water during the fasting period unless a research or clinical exception is identified.

An additional option to assist with the prevention of aspiration pneumonia in anesthetized patients is to include an antiemetic, such as ondansetron or maropitant, as part of the peri-anesthetic plan. These drugs are also useful in emergency situations where optimal fasting times may not be achieved. If an animal must be anesthetized or chemically restrained unexpectedly, always check the oral cavity and cheek pouches for food or objects to prevent aspiration.

F. Training and acclimation

The use of operant and classical conditioning, positive reinforcement training (PRT), and habituation to acclimate nonhuman primates to routine husbandry, clinical, and research procedures enables voluntary participation. The literature is rife with peer-reviewed articles documenting success in training many species of nonhuman primates to accomplish routine tasks, including squirrel monkeys, marmosets, owl monkeys, and macaques (Graham et al.,

2012; Harrison and Simmonds, 1984; McKinley et al., 2003; McMillan et al., 2014; Rogge et al., 2013). The use of PRT enhances the psychological well-being of animals by giving them choice and control over their environments as well as by desensitizing them to potentially stressful stimuli. This results in stress reduction for the animal and an overall increase in animal welfare. Consultation with behaviorists and animal trainers is essential when implementing these techniques.

III. Chemical restraint

A. Agents

The objectives of chemical restraint are to inhibit purposeful movements by the animal that could cause injury to the personnel or escape of the primate. Personnel should be specifically cautioned of the rapidity of return of consciousness in nonhuman primates restrained with ketamine alone. Furthermore, animals that have been given sedatives, analgesics, or tranquilizers without the use of ketamine can be aroused from apparent depression and are very dangerous to handle.

1. Dissociative anesthetics

The dissociative drugs, ketamine and tiletamine, have a wide margin of safety and are the most common choices for chemical restraint of nonhuman primates. Ketamine as a sole agent for chemical restraint is commonly employed in both old-world and new-world monkeys. In nonhuman primates, dissociative agents produce rapid induction, redistribution, and return to consciousness. Dissociative agents produce good somatic analgesia, minimal respiratory depression, and hemodynamic stability; however, used alone, they produce poor muscle relaxation and can produce hypersalivation in some species. Ketamine is a controlled substance and, as such, requires specific storage and recordkeeping as required by the Drug Enforcement Agency. Given that the use of ketamine for chemical restraint of nonhuman primates is so frequent and widespread, it may be useful to reiterate some advantages and possible unwanted effects of the use of this drug.

a. Ketamine

Ketamine is an analog of phencyclidine and has been widely used for chemical restraint and as an anesthetic agent in nonhuman primates since the 1970s. Ketamine produces dissociative anesthesia (lower doses produce sedation), where the thalamocortical and limbic systems are dissociated. The manifestation of this anesthetic state is quite different from that seen with other anesthetic drugs and reflects an effect mediated through the N-methyl-D-aspartate (NMDA) receptor, whereas most injectable anesthetics act through the $GABA_A$ receptor. Through its action on the NMDA receptor, it also provides some somatic analgesia. Animals have altered consciousness, where they do not respond to external stimuli (Grimm et al., 2015). It is used in doses varying from 5 mg/kg to 20 mg/kg IM in many species as an agent for restraint and induction for subsequent administration of other injectable or gaseous anesthetics. A single ketamine injection will provide chemical restraint for 15–30 minutes. Complete recovery occurs within 40–60 minutes, depending upon the dosage used. Nonhuman primates retain pharyngeal and palpebral reflexes after ketamine administration. Accordingly, laryngospasm is not uncommon during intubation after ketamine administration due to the pharyngeal reflex and irritation of the vocal cords. Animals have poor muscular relaxation, and in some instances, ketamine may induce tonic-clonic movements and emergence delirium, particularly in juveniles (Green et al., 1981). For this reason, if a procedure requires general anesthesia, another agent is typically administered in combination with ketamine.

Ketamine administration may also negatively impact food intake in some old-world species. In a clinical trial, administration of ketamine 10 mg/kg IM to rhesus and African green monkeys was observed to significantly reduce daily feed intake, especially at 24 hour post-administration (mean % intake reduction: African green monkeys 57%; rhesus males 48%; and rhesus females 40%) and at 48 hours postdose (African green monkeys 24%, rhesus males 14%, and rhesus females 13%) (Springer and Baker, 2007). The use of ketamine in individuals of these species may warrant consideration for alternatives, especially if the animal is debilitated or the study protocol requires frequent chemical restraint. Prolonged reduction of feed intake may negatively impact the animal's health and well-being. Alternatives may include reducing the dose of ketamine, using other agents alone or in combination, or transitioning to the use of PRT to gain animal cooperation for some procedures and removing the need for repeated sedations.

The effects of ketamine on hematologic and serum biochemical values in nonhuman primates have been examined. Differences in some indices are based on whether a nonhuman primate has been given ketamine, or physically restrained with or without conditioning. Loomis et al. (1980), Bennett et al. (1992), Kim et al. (2005), and Venkatesan et al. (2006) compared hemograms and biochemistries of macaques that were either ketamine-treated or physically restrained for venipuncture. They found that leukocyte and lymphocyte counts and total plasma protein levels were reduced in the ketamine-treated animals. Additionally, they also found alterations in glucose, sodium, potassium, and cholesterol concentrations. Such variations have been attributed to the stress of conscious restraint.

The effect that ketamine has on the cardiovascular system and on selected plasma hormone levels in macaques has been studied. Castro et al. (1981) and Hom et al. (1999) both found that ketamine administered at 0–20 mg/kg had no significant effect on mean arterial blood pressure when compared to awake animals. Castro et al. (1981) further found that ketamine did not affect plasma insulin, glucose, or cortisol concentrations. After the insulin challenge, plasma glucose concentrations, growth hormone, and cortisol responses were similar in both ketamine-treated and control monkeys, which suggests that ketamine does not alter the magnitude of many endocrine responses. In general, ketamine does not produce significant respiratory depression and induces minimal cumulative effects when given over several hours in healthy animals.

Ketamine is also widely used in new-world monkeys as a sole agent for chemical restraint and minor procedures. Advantages of the use of ketamine as a sole agent include the provision of reliable chemical restraint and a wide margin of safety when dosed at 5–50 mg/kg IM (Marini and Haupt, 2019). It is used in the context of restraint for brief procedures such as physical exams, phlebotomy, and diagnostic imaging. Ketamine is also routinely used as a premedication agent prior to intubation and inhalant anesthesia maintenance for surgeries or prolonged imaging sessions. A thorough review of the literature and discussion of clinical applications related to anesthesia and analgesia of common marmosets is presented elsewhere (Goodroe et al., 2021).

While many veterinary practitioners have extensive experience using ketamine as a sole agent in new-world monkeys, there are a number of disadvantages to its use alone, or in combination with other drugs, to consider when selecting an anesthetic plan. Due to the relatively small size of new-world monkey species compared to old-world species, care must be taken to avoid intramuscular injection- or injection volume-related trauma that could potentially cause myotoxicity and tissue damage (Davy et al., 1987). The authors (MB and KG) have observed a high incidence of hypersalivation and vomiting in marmosets postadministration and during recovery from ketamine anesthesia. The analgesia provided by ketamine is not sufficient for procedures involving stimulus greater than blood collection, and additional analgesic agents must be provided prior to surgical procedures. Recent work has demonstrated that the use of ketamine in combination with other anesthetic agents, including alfaxalone, rather than as a sole agent, results in a more rapid recovery postanesthesia (Miyabe-Nishiwaki et al., 2020). The general application of combination anesthetic regimens involving ketamine and other agents are discussed elsewhere in this chapter.

While common marmosets and squirrel monkeys are the most used new-world monkey species in biomedical research settings, there is a small body of literature related to the use of ketamine anesthesia in other species. When compared to anesthesia with tiletamine-zolazepam (5 mg/kg; all doses estimated weight) or ketamine-xylazine (15 mg/kg ketamine; 0.5 mg/kg xylazine) anesthesia, capuchins dosed with ketamine-midazolam (15 mg/kg ketamine; 0.5 mg/kg midazolam) and ketamine-dexmedetomidine (15 mg/kg ketamine; 0.005 mg/kg dexmedetomidine) combinations provided greater muscle relaxation and remained sedated for a longer period of time (Raposo et al., 2015). The use of all four combinations resulted in efficient immobilization. A separate small study found that medetomidine/ketamine administered IM at 150 μg/kg and 4 mg/kg, respectively, provided adequate anesthesia for handling and restraint in capuchins (Theriault et al., 2008). See Tables 18.1–18.3 for suggested anesthetic and analgesic dose ranges for new-world monkey species.

Since the impact of different sedation and anesthetic combinations on a multitude of physiologic parameters has not been well-defined for most species of new-world primates, investigators should consider the potential for variability in physiologic data induced by the method of sample collection. In addition to effects on physiologic parameters, the impact of each anesthetic regimen on study outcome variables should be considered. In squirrel monkeys, ketamine restraint to obtain blood samples was shown to elevate estradiol and luteinizing hormone when compared to samples obtained from animals conditioned for 3 weeks to manual restraint for blood retrieval. These results suggest a possible side effect due to the use of ketamine that could interfere with studies involving reproductive physiology in squirrel monkeys (Yeoman et al., 1988). Ketamine and other drugs are able to cross the human placenta, resulting in fetal exposure with maternal administration (Griffiths and Campbell, 2015). While progress has been made in recent years to refine anesthetic and analgesic protocols, the authors strongly encourage further development of evidence-based guidelines for anesthesia, analgesia, and perioperative support of new-world monkeys.

b. Ketamine combinations

N-methyl-D-aspartate antagonists combinations NMDA antagonists, such as ketamine, may be combined with other injectable anesthetic or sedative agents to produce a longer sedation or anesthesia. Anesthesia is difficult to achieve without the addition of another drug (Green et al., 1981). Depending on the drug combination selected, muscle relaxation, smoother recovery, a reduced volume of drug injected, and additional analgesia may result. Tiletamine is commercially available when combined with zolazepam (Telazol, Zoetis; Parsippany, NJ). Dissociative anesthetics are not

TABLE 18.1 Chemical restraint agents.

Drug(s)	Species	Dose	Duration	Antagonist	Comments
Dissociate agents and their combinations					
Ketamine	Multiple	5–25 mg/kg IM	30 minutes	None	Moderate sedation, immobilization, some analgesia
Ketamine: midazolam	Macaque	8–10 mg/kg IM: 0.2–1 mg/kg IM		Flumazenil	Light to moderate sedation (Authier et al., 2006; Furtado et al., 2010)
Ketamine: midazolam	Marmoset	10 mg/kg IM: 0.3 mg/kg IM			Butorphanol 0.015 mg/kg IM administered concurrently (Ishibashi, 2016)
Ketamine: diazepam	Macaques, baboons	5–25 mg/kg IM: 0.2–1 mg/kg IM	<45 minutes	Flumazenil	Mild to moderate sedation. Diazepam is acidic and IM injection should be avoided (Green et al., 1981; Vaughan et al., 2014; Woolfson et al., 1980)
Ketamine: xylazine	Macaques, Baboons	7–10 mg/kg IM: 0.25–0.6 mg/kg IM	30–45 minutes	Atipamezole or yohimbine	Moderate sedation to general anesthesia, appropriate for minor surgical procedures such as trauma repair (Bankneider et al., 1978; Reutlinger et al., 1980)
Ketamine: xylazine	Marmosets	10–15 mg/kg IM: 1.5 mg/kg IM		Atipamezole or yohimbine	Buchanan-Smith, (2010)
Ketamine: dexmedetomidine	Macaques	3–10 mg/kg IM: 0.015–0.05 mg/kg IM	30–45 minutes	Atipamezole	Moderate sedation to general anesthesia, appropriate for minor surgical procedures such as trauma repair (Jasien et al., 2019; Romagnoli et al., 2016; Young et al., 2021)
Tiletamine: zolazepam	Macaques	3–5 mg/kg IM	15–45 minutes		Moderate sedation to general anesthesia, appropriate for minor surgical procedures such as trauma repair (Vaughan et al., 2014; Young et al., 2021)
Ketamine: alphaxalone	Marmosets	2.5 mg IM: 1 mg IM	30 minutes		Miyabe-Nishiwaki et al. (2020)
Benzodiazepines and their combinations					
Diazepam	Multiple	1 mg/kg IM		Flumazenil	Light sedation, ineffective as sole agent
Midazolam: medetomidine	Macaque	3: 0.03 mg/kg IM	75 ± 40 minutes	Flumazenil, atipamezole	Deep sedation to light anesthesia
Neuroactive steroid					
Alfaxalone	Marmoset	10 mg/kg IM		None	Immobilization
Propofol	Macaque	CRI 0.16–1.0 mg/kg/min			Benveniste et al. (2003); Fowler et al. (2001); Liu et al. (2013)
Neuroleptanalgesia					
Fentanyl: droperidol	Multiple	0.05-0.01 mL/kg IM, IV		Naloxone: none	Heavy sedation, good analgesia
Barbituates					
Pentobarbital	Multiple	15–30 mg/kg IV (survival); 30–100 mg/kg IV (nonsurvival)	30–60 minutes		Respiratory depression, hypotension, prolonged recovery (Davenport et al., 2014; Hom et al., 1999)
Thiopental	Multiple	3–7 mg/kg IV (if other agents are used); 10–20 mg/kg IV (induction)	<20 minutes		Short-acting, induction (Choi et al., 2016)

TABLE 18.2 Anesthesia chart.

Drug(s)	Species	Dose	Duration	Antagonist	Comments
Premedication and induction agents					
Ketamine	Multiple Marmoset	5–20 mg/kg IM 5–50 mg/kg IM	30 minutes 30 minutes	None None	Moderate sedation, immobilization, some analgesia Wide margin of safety
Tiletamine-zolazepam	Macaque Marmoset Baboon	3.5–5.0 mg/kg IM 5 mg/kg IM 4 mg/kg IM	15–45 minutes 15 minutes	Flumazenil* Flumazenil* Flumazenil*	Sufficient for induction and IV catheter placement (Bentson et al., 2003; Marini and Haupt, 2019; Vaughan et al., 2014; Young et al., 2021) Sufficient for blood collection (Ludlage and Mansfield, 2003).
Alfaxalone	Marmoset	7.5–10 mg/kg IM		None	Sufficient to achieve endotracheal intubation (Wada et al., 2020)
Propofol	Multiple	2–5 mg/kg IV slow bolus + additional amounts		None	Provides smooth and reliable induction in many nonhuman primate species (Fowler et al., 2001; Sainsbury et al., 1991)
Ketamine + midzaolam	Multiple	5 mg/kg + 0.1 mg/kg IV		Flumazenil*	Used to achieve anesthetic induction in many species (Jacobs et al., 1993)
Inhalant anesthetic agents					
Isoflurane	Macaque	1.6%–1.75%		n/a	Provides satisfactory anesthesia for most surgical applications (Tinker et al., 1977)
Isoflurane + fentanyl	Macaque	1.2% + 8 μg/kg		Naloxone**	A transient but clinically important decrease in heart rate and MAP was observed with this protocol (Valverde et al., 2000)
Sevoflurane	Macaque	2%		n/a	Provides satisfactory anesthesia for most surgical applications (Soma, 1988)
Intravenous anesthesia					
Ketamine + midazolam	Macaque	(5–20 mg/kg/h) + (0.1–0.4 mg/kg/h)		Flumazenil*	Provides sufficient anesthesia for imaging or dental procedures.
Propofol	Macaque	6–18 mg/kg/h		none	Provides sufficient anesthesia for imaging or dental procedures (Benveniste et al., 2003; Enlund et al., 1997)
Propofol + fentanyl	Macaque	(0.3 mg/kg/min) + (10–20 μg/kg/h)		Naloxone**	Provides sufficient anesthesia for imaging (Liu et al., 2013)
Alfaxalone	Marmoset	2–5 mg/kg IV bolus + 0.17 mg/kg/min CRI		none	Facilitates imaging or surgery (Marini and Haupt, 2019)
Sufentanil	Marmoset	8 μg/kg/h			With nitrous oxide, provides immobilization sufficient for neuroscience studies after initial induction with alfaxalone and diazepam (Rajan et al., 2013)

*Reversal agent for benzodiazepine portion only of the protocol.
***Reversal agent for opioid portion only of the protocol.

TABLE 18.3 Analgesia chart.

Drug(s)[a]	Species	Dose	Duration	Antagonist	Comments
Opioids					
Butorphanol	Macaque Marmoset	0.003–0.1 mg/kg 0.2 mg/kg			
Buprenorphine	Old-world monkey Marmoset	0.01–0.03 mg/kg QID-BID 0.005–0.02 mg/kg	6–12 hours 6–12 hours		Macaque (Nunamaker et al., 2013) Marmoset (Fitz et al., 2021) Baboon (Allison et al., 2007)
Buprenorphine SR	Macaque Marmoset	0.2 mg/kg 0.2 mg/kg	3 days 3 days		ZooPharm (Nunamaker et al., 2013) Marmoset (Fitz et al., 2021)
Simbadol	Macaque	0.24–0.72 mg/kg	3 days		Highly concentrated buprenorphine solution. May cause somnolence and pruritus (Mackiewicz et al., 2019)
Buprenorphine patch	Macaque	10–20 ug/h	Up to 144h		Animal needs to be maintained in jacket to prevent removal of patch
Fentanyl	Macaque Marmoset	3–32 ug/kg 10 ug/kg/hr	1 hour	Naloxone (0.01 mg/kg IV)	IV administration Infusion
Fentanyl patch	Macaque	25 ug/h	Up to 96 hours	Naloxone (0.01 mg/kg IV)	Animal needs to be maintained in jacket to prevent removal of patch (Smith et al., 2019)
Nonsteroidal antiinflammatory drugs					
Carprofen	Old-world monkey	2.2 mg/kg BID or 4.4 mg/kg SID			Baboon (Allison et al., 2007)
Meloxicam	Macaque	0.1–0.2 mg/kg SC or PO q24h			cynomolgus (Bauer et al., 2014)
Meloxicam SR	Macaque	0.6 mg/kg SC q72h			ZooPharm (Bauer et al., 2014)
Local anesthetics					
Lidocaine	Multiple	1–1.5 mg/kg			Dose adapted from dogs, max dose of 5 mg/kg (Engel et al., 2019) In humans, max cumulative dose of is 4.4 mg/kg.
Bupivacaine	Multiple	1.5 mg/kg			Dose adapted from dogs, max dose of 2 mg/kg (Engel et al., 2019) In humans, max cumulative dose of bupivacaine with 1:200,000 epinephrine is 1.3 mg/kg.
Muscle relaxants					
Pancuronium	Old-world monkeys	0.04–0.1 mg/kg IV		Neostigmine (0.075 mg/kg IM every 2–4 hours) with atropine	Always reverse (De Boer et al., 2006)
Vecuronium	Old-world monkeys	0.025–0.06 mg/kg IV; 0.1–0.2 mg/kg/h CRI		Neostigmine (see above); Sugammadex (0.5–1.0 mg/kg IV)	Always reverse (Staals et al., 2011)

[a]*For additional agents, please see the Association of Primate Veterinarians Formulary.*

reversible via a drug antagonist, but the clinical effects of alpha- 2 agonists and benzodiazepines are reversible and may facilitate quicker recoveries. The following sections will discuss some of these dissociative anesthetic combinations. When selecting a drug protocol, consider species, length of procedure, pain associated with procedure, and potential impact on study outcome. An assessment of ketamine combinations on physiological and blood biochemistry values in male rhesus macaques is available (Hernandez-Godinez et al., 2019).

Ketamine–xylazine The addition of the alpha-2 adrenergic receptor agonist xylazine to ketamine provides sedation or anesthesia (dose-dependent), muscle relaxation, and additional analgesia sufficient for imaging, tissue collection, or minor surgical procedures. This combination has been used for over 40 years (Green et al., 1981). Bradycardia, reflex hypertension followed by compensatory hypotension, hypothermia, and increased urine production are common effects of xylazine in most primates. Yohimbine and atipamezole are antagonists that reverse the effects of xylazine via the α2-adrenergic receptor and reduce recovery time. IV atipamezole administration is associated with hypotension and may result in very rapid recovery, which may pose a personnel safety concern when handling larger nonhuman primates. IM administration of atipamezole is recommended (Grimm et al., 2015).

Ketamine 7 mg/kg and xylazine 0.6 mg/kg IM given to rhesus macaques, varying in weight from 1 to 11 kg, provided adequate anesthesia for minor clinical procedures, including digit amputations (Banknieder et al., 1978). The effects of various ratios of ketamine and xylazine in rhesus macaques have been tested (Naccarato and Hunter, 1979). For this study, anesthesia was defined only as a loss of response to a pinprick stimulus. Therefore, the dosages used cannot be correlated with their efficacy for more invasive procedures, but merely as a method for chemical restraint. Among the dosage combinations used, ketamine 10 mg/kg and xylazine 0.25 mg/kg produced a mean anesthesia time of 45 minutes; increasing the xylazine dosage up to 2 mg/kg increased the anesthesia duration to a mean of 138 minutes. Reutlinger et al. (1980) studied the effects that ketamine and xylazine have on cardiovascular and pulmonary values in rhesus macaques. Four groups of six adult males were given ketamine 7 mg/kg, xylazine 0.6 mg/kg, ketamine and xylazine, or saline. There were no significant differences among the three-drug regimens and saline control animals with regard to mean respiratory rate, acid–base status, or arterial blood gases. However, xylazine or xylazine combined with ketamine produced statistically significant decreases in mean arterial blood pressure and heart rate compared to animals given ketamine.

Ketamine 10 mg/kg and xylazine 0.5 mg/kg IM administered to olive baboons reduced heart rate and blood pressure for over 6 hours postadministration. Atipamezole 0.1 mg/kg IM administered 25 minutes postketamine and xylazine administration resulted in a reversal of sedative and cardiopulmonary depression effects compared to baboons that did not receive atipamezole (Langoi et al., 2009). Ketamine 10–15 mg/kg and xylazine 1.5 mg/kg IM hae been used in common marmosets (Buchanan-Smith, 2010).

Ketamine–dexmedetomidine Dexmedetomidine, an alpha-2 adrenergic agonist, is the dextrorotatory isomer of medetomidine and has largely replaced its use in veterinary medicine in North America (Grimm et al., 2015). The previous edition of this text contains more details on medetomidine use in nonhuman primates. Dexmedetomidine combined with ketamine produces muscle relaxation and additional analgesia. Similar to other species, when given alone, alpha-2 adrenergic agonists typically cause biphasic cardiovascular effects in nonhuman primates. The duration of cardiovascular changes is drug- and dose-dependent. Heart rates as low as 70 beats per minute have been reported (Killoran et al., 2021). IV atipamezole administration is associated with hypotension, and IM administration of reversal agents is recommended (Grimm et al., 2015).

Ketamine 5 mg/kg and dexmedetomidine 0.02 mg/kg IM with atipamezole 0.02 mg/kg IM/IV were used for a glucose tolerance test in rhesus macaques aged 13–21 years of age; blood glucose decreased and insulin level increased compared to animals receiving ketamine with diazepam or Telazol (Vaughan et al., 2014). Ketamine 3 mg/kg and dexmedetomidine 0.05 mg/kg IM provided sedation in rhesus macaques to allow induction and maintenance with isoflurane (Jasien et al., 2019). Ketamine 1.5 mg/kg and dexmedetomidine 0.03 mg/kg IM provided 30 minutes of anesthesia sufficient for procedures with mild to moderate pain in rhesus macaques (Killoran et al., 2021). Atipamezole 0.3 mg/kg IM was given when the macaque was returned to its enclosure. Compared to macaques receiving ketamine 10 mg/kg IM only, recovery was significantly faster in macaques that received ketamine combined with dexmedetomidine (45.5 minutes compared to 12 minutes). Ketamine 10 mg/kg and dexmedetomidine 0.015 mg/kg IM were sufficient for imaging in 12-month-old rhesus macaques. Reversal was achieved with atipamezole 0.15 mg/kg IV (Young et al., 2021). Ketamine 8 mg/kg and dexmedetomidine 0.02 mg/kg IM were used to induce cynomolgus macaques prior to maintenance with constant rate infusion of thiopental 3 mg/kg/h and dexmedetomidine 0.012 mg/kg/h for intracranial surgery. Atipamezole 0.1 mg/kg IM was given at the conclusion of the 204 ± 121.2-min intracranial surgeries (Romagnoli et al., 2016).

Ketamine–diazepam The addition of diazepam, a benzodiazepine, with ketamine can provide muscle relaxation without significant cardiorespiratory effects. Benzodiazepines may be metabolized at different rates than ketamine, which may result in dysphoric or anxious recoveries in some species. Flumazenil, a benzodiazepine antagonist, serves as a reversal agent (0.01−0.2 mg/kg IV) (Grimm et al., 2015). Diazepam is acidic and formulated with propylene glycol; therefore IM injection should be avoided. Active metabolites are cleared slowly, though they are not a clinical concern in healthy animals unless repeated doses (or IV infusions) are given (Grimm et al., 2015).

Ketamine 5−25 mg/kg and diazepam 1 mg/kg IM were used in multiple species of monkeys to produce dissociative sedation (Green et al., 1981). Ketamine 10 mg/kg and diazepam 1 mg/kg IM were evaluated for glucose tolerance tests lasting 60 minutes in rhesus macaques but were insufficient due to the need for additional ketamine to maintain appropriate sedation. Telazol 5 mg/kg IM was the favored sedation regimen (Vaughan et al., 2014). The combination of ketamine 10 mg/kg and diazepam 0.2−0.35 mg/kg given IM has been reported to produce an effective restraint in adult male baboons during a dental study (Woolfson et al., 1980). Diazepam 5 mg was given IV after initial sedation with ketamine 10 mg/kg IM to facilitate intubation in adult baboons (Undar et al., 2004). While these published studies administered diazepam IM, the authors strongly recommend that the reader pursue other drug combinations (e.g., ketamine-midazolam, described below), or give combination drugs separately so that diazepam is administered via the IV route.

Ketamine−midazolam Midazolam offers certain advantages over diazepam. Compared to diazepam, it is better absorbed after IM injection, is a more effective anxiolytic tranquilizer, and has a shorter elimination half-life (Jacobs et al., 1993). Flumazenil also serves as the reversal agent.

Ketamine 8 mg/kg and midazolam 0.2 mg/kg IM provided sedation in rhesus macaques undergoing endoscopic intraduodenal drug administration (Authier et al., 2006). At this dose, palpebral, corneal, and pharyngeal reflexes were preserved at all times. Following an intraduodenal dose of dextrose, the ketamine−midazolam group showed an inconsistent increase in glycemia when compared to the other two anesthetic regimes. Recovery from isoflurane and propofol was significantly faster than from ketamine−midazolam. Midazolam 3 mg/kg PO produced a mild sedation in rhesus macaques while midazolam 1 mg/kg and ketamine 20 mg/kg PO combined resulted in severe ataxia and is not recommended (Pulley et al., 2004). Ketamine 10 mg/kg and midazolam 1 mg/kg IM produces 38.6 ± 31.5 minutes of immobilization (Furtado et al., 2010). Midazolam 0.3 mg/kg, ketamine 10 mg/kg, and butorphanol 0.015 mg/kg IM followed by sevoflurane produced balanced anesthesia in 271 of 273 marmosets (Ishibashi, 2016).

Ketamine-alfaxalone Alfaxalone, a GABA-agonist steroid anesthetic, has gained popularity as a single agent for sedating marmosets. Alfaxalone combination with ketamine (2.5 mg ketamine and 1 mg alfaxalone IM per marmoset) produced an average sedation time of 26.4 minutes and full recovery in 43.4 minutes (Miyabe-Nishiwaki et al., 2020).

c. Tiletamine-zolazepam (Telozol)

Tiletamine (NMDA antagonist) and zolazepam (benzodiazepine) are available as a combination product (Telazol, Zoetis; Parsippany, NJ).

Approximately 5 mg/kg of Telazol was sufficient for tracheal intubation and IV catheter placement in 18-month-old rhesus macaques (Young et al., 2021). Telazol 5 mg/kg was also reported to have no effect on blood glucose levels, therefore making it more useful for glucose tolerance tests in rhesus macaques ages 13−21 years (Vaughan et al., 2014). Telazol 5 mg/kg IM produces approximately 15 minutes of sedation in marmosets (Ludlage and Mansfield, 2003). Telazol 4 mg/kg IM was used to sedate baboons for blood collection, and 5 mg/kg IM was used to sedate macaques (Bentson et al., 2003).

2. *Alfaxalone*

Alfaxalone is a neuroactive steroid agent with activity at $GABA_A$ receptors (Albertson et al., 1992; Harrison and Simmonds, 1984). It is used in a wide range of species for induction and maintenance of anesthesia and is used frequently in small animal practice. A limitation to the use of alfaxalone as a sole anesthetic agent for immobilization or brief sedation in larger nonhuman primates is that the volume of injection greatly exceeds the recommended maximum injection volume for the intramuscular route, and a multi-site injection approach may need to be performed to prevent muscle tissue damage. In cynomolgus macaques, lateral recumbency was achieved in all study subjects administered dosages of at least 5 mg/kg (10 mg/mL) of alfaxalone IM. In the same study, endotracheal intubation was achieved in all animals that received a 7.5−10 mg/kg dose of the agent (Wada et al., 2020). Rhesus macaques were chemically immobilized with alfaxalone 2 mg/kg, medetomidine 20 μg/kg, and midazolam 0.3 mg/kg given subcutaneously (Bertrand et al., 2017). Of note, alfaxalone has been shown to decrease cerebral blood flow and intrinsic neuronal activity similar to ketamine in rhesus monkeys (Li et al., 2021). Following ketamine sedation, a continuous rate infusion of alphaxalone-alphadolone at approximately 0.2 mg/kg/min resulted in an adequate surgical plane of anesthesia in baboons (Cookson and Mills, 1983). When using alfaxalone for sole agent anesthesia, animals may recover to mobility and alertness relatively suddenly from lateral recumbency. This should be considered when incorporating alfaxalone into sedation protocols for old-world species.

Alfaxalone can be used as a sole agent for premedication or brief sedation in new-world monkeys, such as common marmosets. Mean SpO_2 values of 13 marmosets given an intramuscular dose of 12 mg/kg alfaxalone remained under 90% for 15 minutes postinjection until supplemental oxygen was provided. This indicates that the use of alfaxalone for single-agent sedation can be expected to cause hypoxemia in some circumstances and supplemental oxygen should be available (Konoike et al., 2017). Alfaxalone is routinely used to provide anesthesia for 30–60 minutes in combination with other agents such as ketamine, medetomidine, buprenorphine, or butorphanol in common marmosets (Bakker et al., 2018; Goodroe et al., 2021; Miyabe-Nishiwaki et al., 2020). The use of alfaxalone alone to initiate anesthesia in common marmosets may be preferable to the use of ketamine or ketamine combinations. Recovery time from alfaxalone anesthesia is significantly faster and less likely to involve side effects than ketamine or combination anesthesia (Bakker et al., 2013). Alfaxalone has also been successfully used as the sole anesthetic agent in newborn to adult squirrel monkeys at a dose range of 11.5–30 mg/kg (Lögdberg, 1988). While alfaxalone is a useful agent for sedation or anesthesia, particularly as a sole agent for new-world primates, when administered at doses greater than 10–12 mg/kg, hypotension, hypoxemia, and hypothermia may occur. Clinicians should plan to have supportive measures such as heat support devices and supplemental oxygen readily available when high doses of alfaxalone are in use.

3. Propofol

Propofol provides a smooth induction with adequate muscle relaxation sufficient for procedures of short duration. Because rapid clearance of propofol contributes to a relatively fast awakening, repeated boluses of 2–5 mg/kg IV or a continuous infusion of 0.2–0.4 mg/kg/min can be administered to extend the duration of chemical restraint without delaying recovery. In cynomolgus macaques, the duration of anesthesia varied from about 5 to 40 minutes with propofol doses of 2.5–10 mg/kg IV. A noticeable side effect of propofol is the occurrence of apnea, at higher doses. Slow delivery (approx. one-quarter of the total calculated dose every 15 s) will minimize hypoventilation and reduce the risk of apnea. Apnea for 1–2 minutes occurred immediately after administration at dosages exceeding 5 mg/kg (Sainsbury et al., 1991).

Propofol is known to have cardiovascular effects that require monitoring during use. Fanton et al. (2000) studied cardiovascular responses to propofol in rhesus monkeys. Intravenously administered induction doses of propofol (2 mg/kg of body weight, followed by continuous infusion of propofol 0.2 mg/kg/min) resulted in significant decreases in blood pressure, heart rate, and myocardial contractility. These changes were accompanied by an increase in systemic arterial compliance. Only minimal changes in left ventricular diastolic pressure, cardiac output, and stroke volume were observed in this study. Hom et al. (1999) found that mean arterial blood pressure was lower in animals anesthetized with propofol. Hematology, serum chemistry, and blood gases were unaffected. However, because of its formulation, propofol was inappropriate for use in animals in which studies of triglyceride levels were conducted.

In the authors' experience, propofol given at a dosage of 2–4 mg/kg provides smooth induction with adequate muscle relaxation in macaques and baboons, and it is sufficient for procedures of short duration (e.g., catheter placement, wound suturing, dental prophylaxis, and radiography) or as an induction agent for inhalational anesthesia. Because rapid clearance of propofol contributes to a relatively fast recovery, repeated boluses of 2–4 mg/kg IV can be administered to extend the duration of anesthesia. Alternatively, maintaining animals on a continuous infusion of propofol (0.2–0.4 mg/kg/min) provides reliable chemical restraint for imaging procedures, such as MRI or PET, which require no movement for prolonged periods of time. Benveniste et al. (2003) reported that pregnant bonnet macaques were successfully maintained on propofol infusions of 0.16–0.3 mg/kg/min for PET and MRI to identify fetal organs and to measure maternal and fetal isotope distribution and perform whole-body imaging for up to 7 hours. However, Fowler et al. (2001) found that rhesus macaques required a higher dose of propofol infusion to maintain animals sedated during MRI. Propofol infusion ranged between 0.31 and 0.64 mg/kg/min, with a mean value of 0.51 mg/kg/min during the 60-minute scan. The authors also noted large individual variations in the dose-response to propofol that revealed no relationship between physiological parameters or body weight. None of the animals developed hypoxemia or cardiovascular instability.

Ouchi et al. (2006) evaluated the effects of a low dose (12 mg/kg/h) and a high dose (25 mg/kg/h) of propofol with 65% nitrous oxide, under normothermic temperatures and mildly hypothermic conditions; cerebral metabolism, cerebral blood flow (CBF), and their regional coupling were determined through direct measurement by PET. The authors concluded that propofol and mild hypothermia (35°C) has an additive effect on metabolism, and can be considered safe because none of the combinations impaired the coupling of cerebral metabolism and blood flow.

Unlike other IV agents, propofol is formulated in an emulsion of soybean oil, glycerol, and egg lecithin, which readily supports bacterial growth. Accordingly, it is important that the sterile technique be practiced when this agent is used in nonhuman primates as postoperative infections have been traced to contamination of IV propofol in a number of nonhuman primate species (Bennett et al., 1992). Discarding the unused portion of the bottle is recommended at the end of the day unless using PropoFlo 28 (Abbott Animal Health), which has an added preservative, benzyl alcohol, that extends the shelf life to 28 days.

4. BAM

The butorphanol–azaperone–medetomidine (BAM) combination was developed in 2003 for use in wildlife as an alternative to ultrapotent opioids. BAM is a combination of butorphanol tartrate (27.3 mg/mL), azaperone tartrate (9.1 mg/mL), and medetomidine hydrochloride (10.9 mg/mL). Butorphanol, an opioid agonist-antagonist, has variable analgesia, antitussive, and antiemetic properties. Azaperone, a butyrophenone tranquilizer, has antipsychotic, sedative, and antiemetic properties. Medetomidine, a potent α2-adrenergic agonist sedative, has analgesic, anxiolytic, and muscle-relaxant properties. Used in combination, these drugs have the benefits of small injection volumes, antiemetic, smooth induction and recovery, reversibility, mild soft tissue analgesia, muscle relaxation, and lack of ptyalism. A dose of 16–24 μL/kg IM provided reliable chemical restraint in juvenile macaques, but oxygen supplementation and monitoring of cardiovascular parameters are strongly recommended (Malinowski et al., 2019).

5. Barbiturates

a. Pentobarbital

Prior to the general use of inhalant anesthetics in veterinary medicine, pentobarbital was routinely used to anesthetize nonhuman primates. The major difficulties with pentobarbital are severe respiratory depression and hypotension at high doses necessary for adequate anesthesia, the inability to modulate the depth of anesthesia well, and a very long period of recovery. For these reasons, pentobarbital is commonly used at a dose range of 30–100 mg/kg for short-term nonsurvival procedures that require deep anesthesia, such as cardiac perfusion (Davenport et al., 2014).

The most common dosage in nonhuman primates for survival procedures is 15–30 mg/kg IV; however, there may be considerable variation among animals. Pentobarbital anesthesia is typically induced by delivering approximately one-half of the calculated dosage as a bolus, and then delivering additional amounts to effect. The duration of surgical anesthesia will vary between 30 and 60 minutes. Usually, animals have been chemically restrained with ketamine prior to administration of pentobarbital, and this may reduce the needed dosage of pentobarbital by about one-third required to achieve surgical anesthesia. There are applications for which pentobarbital may be useful. These include some neurosurgical and ocular procedures because pentobarbital induces minimal changes in cerebrospinal fluid pressure, and decreases cerebral blood flow, metabolic rate (Branston et al., 1979), and inhibits ocular movements (Kim et al., 2012). The administration of pentobarbital (20–25 mg/kg over 10–15 minutes) in rhesus monkeys significantly reduced ($P < .05$) basal mean arterial blood pressure. This is due to venodilation, as well as a decrease in myocardial contractility (Hom et al., 1999).

The effect of pentobarbital anesthesia on respiratory and heart rates, and body temperature, was studied in adult cynomolgus macaques anesthetized for 3–9 hours during neurosurgical studies (Zola-Morgan and Micheletti, 1986). After ketamine induction, the animals were given an initial bolus of pentobarbital IV at a mean dosage of 11 mg/kg. This was followed by additional periodic boluses to effect throughout the procedures. The mean recovery period was more than 3 hours. Pentobarbital may also be appropriate for long-term, nonsurvival procedures that do not require deep anesthesia with concomitant analgesia.

b. Thiopental

This ultrashort-acting barbiturate is used to facilitate intubation prior to induction of anesthesia with inhalation agents at 10–20 mg/kg IV; the dosage is less (3–7 mg/kg) if the animal has received ketamine or other chemical restraint agents. Thiopental bolus for induction has been documented to cause a moderate, but transient decrease in systolic blood pressure in rhesus macaques (Choi et al., 2016).

Slow infusion of thiopental at 15–17 mg/kg/h has been reported to provide satisfactory chemical restraint and stable physiological baseline values for 90 minutes in baboons with animals recovered within 20 minutes after discontinuation of the infusion (Goosen et al., 1984). This rate of infusion resulted in a lower heart rate, slower respiration, and a moderate decrease in body temperature. Of interest is that mean arterial blood pressure did not differ from the values obtained from awake animals. Concurrent thiopental (3 mg/kg/h) and dexmedetomidine (0.012 mg/kg/h) have been used for intracranial surgery in cynomolgus macaques with a 6-min recovery time following atipamezole (0.1 mg/kg IM) administration once both CRIs were discontinued (Romagnoli et al., 2016). Administration of thiopental typically produces a modest reduction in blood pressure due to peripheral vasodilation, reflecting barbiturate-induced depression of the vasomotor center and decreased sympathetic nervous system outflow (Bakoch and Eilers, 2017). The unaffected blood pressures observed in these baboons and cynomolgus macaques may be partially explained by the fact that they were given a slow infusion rather than being induced with a bolus of thiopental.

6. *Etomidate*

Etomidate is a $GABA_A$ receptor agonist. Administration has a minimal impact on the cardiovascular system, and use in patients with cardiovascular compromise is common in veterinary medicine. However, evaluation of etomidate in rhesus macaques found a decrease in heart rate, contractility, and mean arterial pressure (Fanton et al., 2000). Etomidate is administered intravenously, which limits its use as a sole induction agent in primates. Constant-rate infusions are not recommended due to adrenocortical suppression and erythrocyte damage (Grimm et al., 2015). Etomidate 1–2 mg/kg IV was used to facilitate intubation in rhesus macaques after sedation with ketamine 2 mg/kg and midazolam 1.3 mg/kg IM (Portier et al., 2012). Etomidate 3 mg/kg IV was used as part of a multidrug induction regimen in baboons after sedation with ketamine and xylazine (Giffard et al., 2005).

B. Monitoring

The degree and frequency of physiological monitoring for primates under chemical restraint or sedation are less than primates maintained under general anesthesia. Consider the animal's age, preexisting clinical condition, length of chemical restraint or sedation, drug protocol selected, predicted adverse effects, and clinical procedures when determining the frequency and which physiological variables are monitored. A baseline suggestion is checking heart rate (via peripheral palpation, cardiac auscultation, or with a monitor), respiratory rate, temperature, mucous membrane color and capillary refill time every 15 minutes. Heart rate and hemoglobin saturation may be continuously monitored with pulse oximetry. It is prudent to have oxygen available for flow-by-support, intubation, and catheter supplies, as well as emergency drugs available nearby in case of an unanticipated event.

IV. Anesthesia

A. Inhalation anesthetics

1. *Induction*

Induction of anesthesia in most nonhuman primate species is typically initiated with ketamine (5–10 mg/kg IM) or tiletamine–zolazepam (3.5–5.0 mg/kg) to provide chemical restraint and facilitate IV access. Propofol, given at 2–5 mg/kg IV as a slow bolus followed by additional amounts to effect provides for a reliable and smooth induction in many nonhuman primate species. Alternatively, a combination of ketamine (5 mg/kg) and midazolam (0.1 mg/kg) administered IV can be used to achieve anesthetic induction. The required dose of induction agent(s) will be greatly dependent on the depth of sedation following premedication. Once induced, the animal can be easily intubated, and the inhalational anesthetic agent administered. It should be noted that most inhalation agents do not provide analgesia, and analgesic agents should be utilized as necessary.

2. *Intubation*

Endotracheal intubation ensures a patent airway, delivers gas anesthetics while preventing environmental contamination, reduces the risk of aspirating regurgitated material or secretions, and provides an anesthetist with the ability to assist or control ventilation. Preoxygenation with 100% oxygen for several minutes prior to intubation helps prevent systemic desaturation in animals during the intubation process.

Nonhuman primates should be adequately anesthetized to reduce the risk of laryngospasm or vagally mediated bradycardia. Endotracheal intubation can be accomplished with the animal in either the ventral or dorsal recumbency. Placing the animal in a sitting position with its head extended toward the anesthetist has been found to be useful during intubation of pediatric baboons or macaques, and smaller species of NHPs such as African green monkeys. Hyperextension of the atlanto-occipital joint facilitates the placement of endotracheal tubes in the supine position. Intubation of animals in the prone position requires elevation of the head with the neck overextended. The goal of both techniques is to achieve good visualization of the glottis. Application of local anesthetic to the vocal folds may be necessary to prevent laryngospasm. Endotracheal tubes of various sizes are used for old-world nonhuman primates, ranging from 3.0 to 8.0 mm. In general, cuffed Murphy endotracheal tubes are utilized. Prior to intubation, the endotracheal tube length should be compared with the animal size, specifically from the incisors to the thoracic inlet. If the tube appears to be long enough to pass beyond the approximate area of the thoracic inlet, the endotracheal tube should be trimmed to a more appropriate size. Endotracheal tubes should be passed with the help of an appropriate laryngoscope through the vocal folds to the level of the mid-trachea. The cuff on the endotracheal tube is carefully inflated to prevent leaks when the animal is ventilated with an Ambu bag. Alternatively, the endotracheal tube is connected to an anesthetic breathing bag that is gently squeezed to a pressure of 15–20 cm H_2O. This allows for bilateral auscultation of the animal's chest for lung sounds. It is important to confirm correct tube placement by capnography or auscultating for bilateral lung sounds. Once proper placement is confirmed, the tube is secured via the application of a gauze tie, stay sutures or other secure methods.

As an alternative to face masks and endotracheal tube intubation, a laryngeal mask airway (LMA) is commonly used in human medicine and has been used successfully in macaques. The LMA is a reusable device that is inserted into the oropharynx and rests in the inferior recess of the hypopharynx above the esophageal sphincter, and against the base of the tongue. It requires closer position monitoring than an endotracheal tube since it can shift placement during the procedure, but it is less likely to stimulate an animal's gag reflex and cause laryngospasm. Since most nonhuman primates are sedated with ketamine or telazol, the gag reflex remains and endotracheal intubation can cause laryngospasm. Therefore, the LMA is minimally stimulating since it does not pass into the trachea. The LMA can even be used to maintain an open airway in a sedated animal that has a difficult airway, such as obese animals.

Endotracheal intubation of smaller primate species, such as common marmosets and squirrel monkeys, has been described in detail (Goodroe et al., 2021; Morris et al., 1997; Thomas et al., 2012). Small oral cavities make intubation challenging, and the key to successful intubation is correct animal positioning. A 0 or 00 Miller laryngoscope blade is required. String or gauze may be placed in the oral cavity and used by the holder to open the jaw while distancing their hands from the small oral cavity to allow visualization by the person intubating. Long- handle atraumatic forceps or cotton swabs can be used to secure the tongue. The marmoset larynx enters the trachea at approximately 137°; a stylet may help achieve the appropriate angle of the endotracheal tube. The proper placement of the tube is confirmed by bilateral movement of the chest with manual compression of the reservoir bag of a nonrebreathing circuit such as the Bain system, movement of the reservoir bag by the patient, or visualization of waveforms on a capnograph. 1.5−2.0 mm internal diameter endotracheal tubes are used in marmosets. Beware that the outer diameter of endotracheal tubes varies by manufacturer and may impact fit. 1.0−1.5 mm internal diameter endotracheal tubes vary in materials and may be too flexible and prone to kink occluding the airway. The weight of the breathing circuit should be supported so that inappropriate pressure is not placed on the endotracheal tube. Further guidance regarding intubation of common marmosets can be found in species-specific reference texts (Goodroe et al., 2021; Marini and Haupt, 2019).

3. Nitrous oxide

Nitrous oxide is occasionally used to anesthetize macaques, but its use is not recommended as this compound is a greenhouse gas and can contribute to global warming (Sherman et al., 2012). Unlike the potent volatile anesthetics, nitrous oxide has a relatively high MAC, 200% in macaques versus 105% in humans, which prevents its use as a complete surgical anesthetic. Nitrous oxide is sometimes used in combination with other volatile anesthetics, such as isoflurane, because it allows for a lower inhaled concentration. The advantage of the inclusion of nitrous oxide with other potent volatile anesthetics is a less pronounced circulatory depression, which may be seen with the sole administration of isoflurane. The minimal cardiovascular effects produced by nitrous oxide can be attributed to its stimulatory effects on the sympathetic nervous system, characterized by slight elevations in heart rate and systemic and pulmonary arterial pressures (McKay, 2017). Because of the rapid elimination of large volumes of nitrous oxide from the blood into the alveoli with a consequent diminution in alveolar oxygen concentrations, diffusion hypoxia may occur if an animal is only allowed to breathe room air at the end of anesthesia. As a result, the administration of 100% oxygen for at least 5 minutes at the end of anesthetic administration is recommended to prevent this occurrence.

4. Isoflurane

Isoflurane is a widely used inhalational agent in nonhuman primates and the anesthetic of choice of the authors for most applications. An advantage of isoflurane is that it is minimally metabolized due to its chemical stability and low solubility and is accordingly exhaled essentially unchanged (see Chapter 6 for full description). This characteristic makes it a particularly safe agent if the nonhuman primate has hepatic or renal deficits, or if the research objective is compromised by an agent that has potentially toxic metabolites. Maintaining nonhuman primates at about 1.3 MAC (1.6%−1.75%) provides satisfactory anesthesia for most surgical applications in macaques (Tinker et al., 1977).

Alternatively, balanced anesthesia consisting of 0.5% −0.7% isoflurane and fentanyl titrated to achieve an appropriate depth of anesthesia may be used in nonhuman primates. This inhalational agent and opioid combination is useful when cardiovascular stability is needed for a procedure. It is important to note that cardiovascular-sparing effects are attributable to a reduction in the dose of inhalant anesthetics because opioids cause minimal cardiovascular depression. A transient but clinically important decrease in heart rate and MAP was observed with fentanyl administration (8 μg/kg) when end-tidal isoflurane concentration was maintained at 1.2% in rhesus monkeys (Valeverde et al., 2000).

The effects of isoflurane on brain metabolism and cerebral blood flow have been investigated in rhesus monkeys (Endlund et al., 1997). Because isoflurane induces dose-dependent hypotension with concomitant hypocapnia, cerebral oxygenation and blood flow may be affected. As expected, Endlund et al. (1997) noted that cerebral blood flow was reduced during isoflurane-induced hypotension. The cerebral metabolic rate of oxygen decreased globally in a dose-dependent manner, leading to higher oxygen extraction ratios in rhesus macaques. The authors concluded that, although isoflurane-induced hypotension reduced cerebral blood flow, it did not result in hypoxia.

5. *Sevoflurane*

Sevoflurane has minimal odor and is a potent bronchodilator (Ebert and Naze, 2017). These attributes make sevoflurane an excellent candidate for administration via a face mask to induce general anesthesia. It offers an advantage over mask induction with isoflurane in nonhuman primates. Lower pungency and airway irritation may provide a smoother anesthetic event and decrease the potential for injury to the animal or anesthetist.

MAC for cynomolgus monkeys has been determined at 2% (Soma, 1988). It has been shown to be unstable when exposed to soda lime. This instability was a concern because of potential nephrotoxicity for nonhuman primates (Iyer and Anders, 1996). However, multiple administrations of sevoflurane to cynomolgus monkeys did not detect any adverse effects on the animal's renal function (Soma et al., 1995). In this study, cynomolgus monkeys were anesthetized with sevoflurane at 1, 1.6, and 2 times the MAC for 3 hours/day and 3 days/week for 8 weeks. Reduction in total erythrocyte and leukocyte counts and increase in serum enzymes [aspartate aminotransferase, alanine aminotransferase, lactate dehydrogenase, and creatine kinase)] were the only changes noted. Changes were dose-dependent and returned to baseline values by week 2 in the lowest MAC group. The multiple administration of 1.0 and 1.6 MAC sevoflurane anesthesia was well tolerated by monkeys; however, at 2.0 MAC, some deaths occurred. Apart from the reduction of the thymus in the anesthetized monkeys, there were no gross, histopathologic, or ultrastructural changes found in any of the groups of monkeys.

As with other inhalant anesthetics, sevoflurane causes a dose-dependent increase in CBF, and in *M. mulatta*, the autoregulation of CBF is compromised at 2.0% sevoflurane anesthesia (Kaneko et al., 1997). However, the degree of change is less than that with other compounds.

6. *Halothane*

Although halothane was previously widely used in nonhuman primates for several decades and has proven to be, in most applications, a safe and effective inhalational agent, its production in the United States has been discontinued, and it has not been used in the past 20 years. Please see previous editions of this text for a full description of its use.

B. Intravenous anesthesia

Intravenous anesthesia is a viable option in nonhuman primates. Partial IV anesthesia (PIVA) is the IV administration of one or more drugs in addition to inhalants. Total IV anesthesia (TIVA) achieves anesthesia without the use of inhalants. PIVA and TIVA may provide a balanced plane of anesthesia as lower doses of drugs may be used when in combination, and this may reduce individual drug adverse effects. Drug doses can be reduced to achieve various levels of sedation or anesthesia based on procedure requirements. These protocols may also be advantageous for research procedures that restrict which drugs may be used. Drugs can be administered IV as repeated boluses or as a CRI. Providing drugs as a CRI prevents variable levels of anesthesia associated with repeated dosing (Goodroe et al., 2021).

PIVA and TIVA have a long history of use in macaques. Ketamine (5–20 mg/kg/h) can be used in combination with midazolam (0.1–0.4 mg/kg/h) to facilitate imaging or dental cleaning. Similarly, propofol (6–18 mg/kg/h) can also be used for these applications (Benveniste et al., 2003; Enlund et al., 1997). In the author's experience (EN), either the ketamine and midazolam combination or propofol infusions can be used in conjunction with fentanyl (10–20 μg/kg/h) to achieve a surgical plane of anesthesia for invasive dental procedures with ventilation support.

Total volumes infused, especially during longer procedures, must be considered when using PIVA or TIVA in marmosets. These nonhuman primates only have a total blood volume of 20–35 mL of blood (70 mL/kg) (Buchanan-Smith, 2010). Total fluid rates of <5 mL/kg/h are advisable, but further reduction should be considered for longer procedures. Attention should be paid to urine production, hematocrit, and electrolyte levels to guide fluid volumes administered in long procedures. A fluid pump capable of administering small volumes over extended lengths of time is highly recommended to ensure appropriate dosing. An anesthetic protocol of propofol administered at 0.6–1.0 mg/kg/min has been used to facilitate imaging. A lower propofol dose (0.3 mg/kg/min) can be used in conjunction with fentanyl at 10–20 μg/kg/h (Liu et al., 2013). An IV bolus of 2–5 mg/kg alfaxalone followed by a 0.17 mg/kg/min CRI facilitates imaging or surgery (Marini and Haupt, 2019). Sufentanil, 8 μg/kg/h, with nitrous oxide inhalant provides immobilization for neuroscience studies after initial induction with alfaxalone and diazepam (Rajan et al., 2013).

C. Anesthetic monitoring and management

Anesthetic monitoring provides the means to assess physiological function during anesthesia and ascertain the proper functioning of anesthetic equipment. It allows prompt recognition of adverse drug effects and guides the use of therapeutic interventions. However, the use of monitoring equipment is intended to enhance but not substitute for the awareness on the part of the anesthetist.

1. Cardiovascular monitoring

Heart rate can be monitored in nonhuman primates with a pulse oximeter and electrocardiogram (EKG), and EKG can also be utilized for heart rhythm monitoring. Electrocardiographic data in healthy baboons, capuchins, macaques, and squirrel monkeys has been documented (de Souza et al., 2018; Osborne and Roberts, 1972; Singh et al., 1970; Wolf et al., 1969; Yamaoka et al., 2013). In larger nonhuman primates, the insertion of an esophageal stethoscope during anesthesia can also be utilized to facilitate early detection of changes in heart rate and provides information on the adequacy of ventilation. Lead II is commonly used for the detection of cardiac dysrhythmias because it produces an easily recognizable P wave and establishes the relationship between atrial and ventricular depolarization. Indirect arterial blood pressure can be measured by placing the cuff on the nonhuman primate's distal arm or leg, as well as the tail in smaller primates. Noninvasive blood pressure reference values and techniques have been previously established for macaques, marmosets, baboons, and chimpanzees (Brownlee et al., 2020; Ely et al., 2011; France et al., 2018; Mietsch and Einspanier, 2015; Schmelting et al., 2009; Yeung et al., 2014).

Direct arterial pressure monitoring is achieved by percutaneous cannulation of the saphenous or radial artery using a 20- or 22-gauge catheter in macaques (France et al., 2018). Surgical cutdown of the femoral artery in nonhuman primates can also be performed for direct arterial pressure measurement. To cannulate the femoral artery, an 18-gauge catheter can be inserted in animals over 10 kg, and a 20-gauge Teflon catheter for smaller macaques. To avoid accidental displacement of the arterial catheter during the procedure, a Seldinger technique can be used. The catheter-over-the-needle (Angiocath) is used for percutaneous cannulation of the femoral artery. The skin at the cannulation site is pierced with the catheter's stylet to facilitate the advancement of the catheter and prevent a skin plug from occluding the stylet. After obtaining pulsatile blood flow from the cannulation site, a stylet is removed, and a guide wire is placed through the catheter and into the vessel. The catheter used for monitoring is then threaded over the wire into the artery. The placement of a three-way stopcock between the catheter and the arterial tubing allows for frequent blood sampling to determine arterial blood gas concentrations. Direct arterial pressure monitoring is usually reserved for animals with cardiac and respiratory dysfunction and cardiovascular research models.

For the management of fluid replacement, the femoral, axillary, or external jugular veins are accessible for cannulation. Caution should be used when attempting to cannulate the jugular vein due to the prominence and proximity of the air sacs in some nonhuman primate species, such as pigtail macaques, owl monkeys, and baboons. A 20-gauge polyurethane indwelling catheter is well suited for medium- and large-size macaques and baboons. Following initial cannulation, a J-wire is inserted through the catheter and advanced into the central vein. It is used as a guide for the placement of a longer venous catheter. Cannulation of the internal jugular vein usually requires a cutdown. Measurements of cardiac output and calculations of systemic and pulmonary vascular resistance can be obtained with a pulmonary artery catheter (Swan-Ganz). Placement of the pulmonary artery catheter into the right internal jugular vein represents the most direct approach to the right heart. Catheterization via the femoral vein is also commonly performed but usually requires fluoroscopic guidance. A 5-French pediatric Swan-Ganz catheter can be successfully inserted in adult macaques (4–8 kg), whereas in larger primates (e.g., 15–20 kg baboons), a 7.5-French pulmonary catheter is used.

2. Respiratory monitoring

Assessment of oxygenation and ventilation during the administration of anesthetics is essential. While insensitive, the color of the mucous membranes is the simplest method to ascertain the adequacy of oxygenation. Quantitative noninvasive pulmonary evaluation can be achieved with pulse oximetry, capnography, and arterial blood gas analysis. Reference values for arterial blood gas concentrations have been published in several nonhuman primate species (Binns et al., 1972; Cissik et al., 1986; Lee et al., 2012; Manning et al., 1969; Nakayama et al., 2017). Pulse oximetry provides continuous measurement of arterial oxygen saturation with the probe placed on a digit, ear, or tongue, as well as the scrotum in males. Dark or pigmented skin may interfere with the pulse oximeter signal and result in inaccurate or poor readings. Administration of specific drugs, such as alpha-2- adrenergic, that can cause vasoconstriction, will affect readings from oscillometric blood pressure monitors. In smaller new-world primates, such as common marmosets, a pediatric finger probe attached to a shaved footpad provides reliable and continuous monitoring of oxygen saturation and heart rate data.

3. Depth of anesthesia

Anesthetic depth is usually assessed by monitoring a variety of parameters. Loss of palpebral and corneal reflexes, degree of muscle relaxation, rate and depth of breathing, and lack of somatic response to surgical stimuli are most commonly used to ascertain the adequacy of anesthesia. If muscle relaxants are used during the maintenance of anesthesia, monitoring autonomic responses to surgical events must be done to assess the depth of anesthesia. Increases in heart rate and systolic blood pressure of 20% or more over baseline values can be interpreted as indications of an inadequate depth of anesthesia or a response to noxious stimulation, or both. Lacrimation and attempts to breathe out of synchrony with a ventilator might also be indicative of a light plane of anesthesia.

The degree of anesthetic depth is crucial to avoiding complications and maximizing experimental success. Traditional signs of anesthetic depth, such as heart rate and blood pressure, may be inadequate, depending on the anesthetic and species. As an adjunct to these monitoring methods, electroencephalography, which evaluates electrical brain activity, should be considered, particularly when muscle relaxants are utilized. Diverse opinions regarding what constitutes acceptable anesthetic depth exist among human and veterinary anesthesiologists, and an in-depth discussion of this evolving issue is beyond the scope of this chapter. However, researchers should be aware that animal movement during surgical and experimental procedures may not necessarily indicate that the animal is "under anesthetized" from the standpoint of awareness or discomfort (Antognini et al., 2005). This is because the dose of anesthetic required to cause loss of consciousness is lower than that required to prevent movement (at least for volatile anesthetics). Anesthesiologists use "MAC," the minimum alveolar anesthetic concentration required to prevent "gross and purposeful" movement. Patients generally lose consciousness and memory at around 0.25–0.4 MAC. Because MAC awake is a fraction of MAC for movement, animals can be anesthetized at depths that produce unconsciousness and amnesia, yet do not abolish movement. As a general guideline, evaluation of the depth of anesthesia should not be reliant upon any single value or observation but should be based on the integrated assessment of several physiological parameters by the anesthetist. Nevertheless, should an animal move under anesthesia, appropriate initial responses include assuming that the depth is inadequate and checking the function of equipment.

4. *Body temperature*

It is not uncommon for a nonhuman primate to become hypothermic during anesthesia and surgery. Very young and small-size animals (marmosets and squirrel monkeys) are particularly at risk of becoming hypothermic. Intraoperative monitoring of body temperature is routinely performed by inserting a temperature probe into either the esophagus or the rectum and connecting it to the monitor. The drawback of rectal temperature is that it does not accurately reflect blood or "core" temperature when changes in temperature are very rapid. Deep hypothermia induced for central nervous system surgery is an example that calls for monitoring core temperature by an esophageal probe inserted into the lower third of the esophagus. A tympanic probe placed in the external auditory canal will reflect brain temperature by measuring the temperature of blood perfusing the brain and is useful during cerebral cooling procedures. Thermal sensor microchips can also be placed in the subcutaneous space or intra-abdominally in the primate for comparison between the pre, peri, and postoperative states.

5. *Urinary output*

Urinary output is a direct indicator of renal function and serves as a useful guide for fluid therapy, keeping in mind that administered agents may affect urine output (Burchardi and Kackmarczyk, 1994). In female macaques and baboons, bladder catheterization is usually performed by inserting a soft rubber Foley catheter through the urethral meatus, located between two papillary folds posterior to the clitoris, into the bladder, and then connecting it to a urinary drainage bag. Transurethral catheterization in male macaques can be challenging due to the anatomical conformation of the ischial arch, resistance at the sigmoid flexure, and narrow urethra, but a successful transurethral approach has been described (Wickham et al., 2011).

D. Anesthetic support

1. *Fluid therapy*

IV infusion of crystalloid solutions during surgery helps to maintain normovolemia necessary for adequate tissue perfusion. Intraoperative fluid and blood loss replacement is usually determined by the site and duration of surgery. For minor procedures in nonhuman primates, administration of isotonic electrolyte solutions such as lactated Ringer's solution at the rate of 5–10 mL/kg/h is sufficient to maintain normal fluid composition. Because of their small intravascular volumes, marmosets and squirrel monkeys are especially at an increased risk of hypovolemia and electrolyte disturbances.

Significant intraoperative blood loss warrants serial determination of a nonhuman primate's hematocrit. If the hematocrit falls below 20%, rapidly decreases by >20%, or estimated circulating blood losses are >20%, then a blood transfusion should be considered. Initial blood transfusions in macaques and baboons do not normally cause any of the symptoms associated with an acute transfusion reaction because preformed isoantibodies to erythrocyte antigens are absent (Socha et al., 1982). For procedures with a high risk of significant blood loss, prior cross-matching of the blood between the same species of nonhuman primates is recommended to prevent transfusion reactions. Autologous blood transfusions can also be performed on study animals where significant blood loss is anticipated. Up to 10% of the nonhuman primate's blood is collected 10–14 days prior to the procedure and stored in a blood collection bag (with citrate-phosphate-dextrose as an anticoagulant) at

1–6°C until the day of surgery. Detailed methods and procedures for blood transfusions in nonhuman primates have been previously published (Cital et al., 2016).

A urinary catheter should be used to evaluate the adequacy of fluid therapy whenever surgery is prolonged (>4 hours) or if significant changes in intravascular volume are anticipated. Minor-to-moderate blood loss can be replaced with crystalloid solutions given in amounts equal to about three times the amount of blood loss. Monitoring blood pressure and urinary output allows one to determine whether intravascular fluid volume is being adequately replaced.

2. *Anticholinergics*

Anticholinergics, such as atropine and glycopyrrolate, are used to diminish salivary and bronchial secretions in nonhuman primates during anesthesia and to prevent the reflex bradycardia that may be experienced during ocular or deep neck surgery (oculocardiac and vasovagal reflexes). Bradycardia is of great significance in young nonhuman primates because their cardiac output is heart rate-dependent. The addition of atropine (0.02–0.05 mg/kg IM) will effectively reduce bradycardia induced by alpha-agonists and opiates. When an antisialogogue effect is desired, glycopyrrolate (0.005–0.01 mg/kg IM) is selected rather than atropine because it is twice as potent and has a longer duration of action. Additionally, glycopyrrolate does not cross the blood-brain barrier, which may be advantageous for neurophysiology studies. Nevertheless, the inclusion of an anti-cholinergic as part of premedication is not always necessary or indicated. It is noteworthy that atropine possesses arrhythmogenic properties and may predispose nonhuman primates to ventricular tachycardia and bigeminal patterns at the above-mentioned reference dose (Sedgwick, 1986). Because of this, atropine premedication should be avoided as part of the protocols for cardiac surgery.

3. *Antiemetics*

Many anesthetic agents can cause nausea within minutes to hours after administration. Antiemetics are recommended for all nonhuman primates undergoing anesthesia to reduce the risk of aspiration and facilitate a smoother recovery. Commonly used antiemetics in nonhuman primates include ondansetron, maropitant citrate, and metoclopramide, with doses and routes based on reports in humans and companion animals. Preoperative maropitant citrate at 1 mg/kg administered subcutaneously prior to anesthesia for neurosurgeries has been shown to decrease postoperative vomiting in rhesus and cynomolgus macaques (Steinbach et al., 2018). From the authors' experience, ondansetron administered intravenous or intramuscular route at 0.25–1 mg/kg is adequate to prevent peri and postoperative nausea/vomiting in macaques. Metoclopramide has both antiemetic and prokinetic properties and may be useful in nonhuman primates to facilitate gastric emptying prior to anesthesia. In cynomolgus monkeys, 2 mg/kg of intravenous metoclopramide significantly increased gastric emptying (Amrani et al., 2012). Additional studies are needed to validate the efficacy of antiemetics in nonhuman primates.

4. *Heat support*

The use of forced-air warming systems (e.g., Bair Hugger) is a simple and effective means of providing temperature support. Bair Hugger blankets are available in a variety of shapes and sizes to optimize convective warming for the large size range of nonhuman primates encountered in research. Recirculating water pads, heated discs, and other heated devices have also been used. Skin contact and temperature should be carefully monitored when heating devices are used to prevent thermal burns and hyperthermia. Warming of IV fluids generally does not contribute to the maintenance of normothermia. However, if large volumes of fluid are to be administered, this measure is recommended, as it would help to prevent fluid-induced hypothermia. Continuous monitoring of body temperature will allow for the prevention of intraoperative hyperthermia as well, which can occur especially in smaller species such as marmosets.

V. Analgesia

Pain assessments provide the foundation for the provision of analgesia through the evaluation of behavior and the clinical presentation of the animal (Association of Primate Veterinarians, 2019). Common clinical indications for the administration of analgesia to nonhuman primates include events such as trauma related to conspecific interactions in social housing, self-injurious behavior (SIB), or injury from activity in the animal's primary enclosure. Analgesia may also be indicated in conjunction with a study design that anticipates or produces a potentially painful situation.

Analgesia may be in the form of both pharmacologic and nonpharmacologic modalities. Regardless of the species, multimodal analgesia is recommended to facilitate the management of pain at multiple locations in the pain pathway. Opioids are most effective at decreasing pain transmitted by C-fiber nociceptors and are best combined with nonsteroidal antiinflammatory drugs (NSAIDs) for surgical procedures that may also elicit pain from A-β fibers (Grimm et al., 2015). Additionally, nonpharmacological methodologies may be utilized as an adjuvant to pharmacological agents. While often used together, each analgesic agent and modality will be discussed individually.

The most common analgesic agents employed in nonhuman primates include NSAIDs and opioids. Management of pain in animals requires that pain either be anticipated and prevented (preemptive) or be recognized and alleviated (postinductive). Preventive analgesia presumes that the pain will result from the procedure and that nonpharmacological and pharmacological protocols would be instituted prior to the induction of pain. Preemptive techniques include parenteral administration of systemic analgesics, including sustained release compounds, infiltration of a suture line with local anesthetics, and epidural administration of analgesics. Parenteral analgesia with an opioid or NSAID should be administered prior to making a surgical incision. Postinductive management is used to decrease an animal's experience of a noxious stimulus, and to maintain normal physiological and cardiovascular stability.

A. Pain assessments

Pain recognition is the cornerstone to effective pain assessment and management in nonhuman primates (Association of Primate Veterinarians, 2019), but can be challenging, especially if the observer is not confident in their skills (Miyabe-Nishiwaki et al., 2021). Due to the nature of many species of nonhuman primates, assessment is commonly limited to cage-side observation only. These observations can be performed directly or indirectly using video monitoring equipment. Direct cage-side observations are easy to perform and inexpensive because the animal is in clear view and can respond directly to the observer. However, the evaluation outcome may be skewed by the animal masking signs of pain to a human observer or through incorrect assessment of submissive postures as pain. An extended observation period is often required to allow the animal to habituate to the observer and allow accurate assessment. Limited interactions between observer and animal, such as offering a food treat or grooming through the bars, may be useful for assessment but the animal's familiarity with the observer will likely affect the assessment. The best observation outcomes are achieved if the observer is knowledgeable about the signs of pain in NHPs and very familiar with the individual animal being assessed. Because of the negative associations that animals may have developed in relation to veterinary personnel, the inclusion of the behavioral management team in performing pain assessments and observations is recommended.

Indirect video monitoring has the advantage of not disturbing the animal's natural behavior, but it can be technically challenging and labor-intensive to perform. Because the animal remains undisturbed, masking of pain is less likely to occur, making pain easier to recognize (Allison et al., 2007; Bourgeois et al., 2007; Gaither et al., 2014). Optimally, the camera is set up such that the animal can be visualized regardless of its location in the cage or its activity. The observer may need to watch extended periods of live feed or video recordings to identify pain in the animal(s) of interest, especially if the animal is not presenting to the camera in a way that facilitates assessment. If video recording is used, the observer needs to watch the video in a timely manner to allow for changes to the analgesic regimen in a relevant and beneficial period. Whether a live or recorded feed is used, the security of these materials is imperative.

Regardless of the method of observation, pain assessment should include observing for general signs of well-being, as well as a procedure- or injury-related clinical signs. General signs of pain observed across species include changes in food and water consumption, urination and defecation, and posture and appearance, such as an unkempt hair coat, piloerection, hunching, or arching of the back (Carstens and Moberg, 2000; National Research Council, 2009). Painful animals may be reluctant to move, may appear restless with difficulty achieving a comfortable position, or may assume an abnormal location within their enclosure. There may be guarding, increased attention (e.g., licking, rubbing, scratching, and biting), changes in mobility (Magden et al., 2013), or withdrawal of the painful part of the body or body area (Alreja et al., 1984; Sukhtankar et al., 2014). Socially housed animals may fail to interact with or may maintain an abnormal distance from cage mates (Arnold et al., 2011). Alternatively, painful primates may behave more aggressively toward conspecifics or handlers. Vocalization and teeth grinding may be observed in some animals.

A baseline understanding of an individual animal's normal behavior and its interaction with conspecifics and human care staff when not experiencing pain or distress is critical when conducting subsequent pain assessments. An important caveat is that many clinical signs are not specific to pain and instead could indicate a health issue that may or may not include pain as a component. It is also important to not misinterpret the degree of pain and provide inadequate or inappropriate analgesia.

The frequency of pain assessment to ensure adequate pain management is highly variable and relies on multiple factors, such as species-specific behaviors, the severity or invasiveness of the surgery or injury, the type of assessment (e.g., cage side vs. indirect), and variables related to the analgesic(s) administered. Regarding the analgesic(s), considerations for the frequency of assessments should include the specific type and method of analgesia (i.e., single drug vs. multimodal), the pharmacokinetics of analgesic agents used with attention to the expected duration of effectiveness, recent changes to the analgesic plan, and previous clinician experience with the analgesic plan. Veterinarians should use their professional judgment to determine the frequency of monitoring and be prepared to change the plan based on clinical signs. Particular attention should be placed on performing assessments prior to changing the pain management plan. A reassessment after a change should be performed within an appropriate timeline to ensure the new pain management plan is providing adequate analgesia to alleviate pain. When evaluating research protocols for adequacy of analgesia, the IACUC should consider whether the frequency of observations is adequate. Researchers and IACUCs should consult with the veterinarian to reconcile any doubt regarding whether the proposed plan ensures adequate monitoring.

B. Opioids

Opioids have been used in nonhuman primates for analgesia as well as to reduce the minimal alveolar concentration of inhalational anesthetics and to enhance intraoperative analgesia during balanced anesthesia. The main advantage of opioid use in anesthesia is that it has minimal impact on cardiovascular function, and effectively suppresses the sympathetic nervous system responses to surgical stress (Sofianos et al., 1985). Postoperative IM administration of opioids results in variable absorption, especially in severely hypotensive and hypothermic animals, and this may reflect a considerable delay between the administration of the drug and effective analgesia. Among the opioids available, buprenorphine is the most used in nonhuman primates for postoperative analgesia, and fentanyl is most often used as the analgesic component for balanced anesthesia.

Buprenorphine is a favored analgesia treatment due to its long duration of action compared with other opioids. Buprenorphine has been administered to many old-world primate species at a dose range of 0.005–0.03 mg/kg IM. A pharmacokinetic study performed in macaques demonstrated that buprenorphine dosed at 0.01 mg/kg IM required a dosing frequency of every 6–8 hours or 0.03 mg/kg IM be administered every 12 hours to maintain therapeutic plasma concentrations (Nunamaker et al., 2013). Additional pharmacokinetic studies have found no adverse effects of the buprenorphine when dosed with up to 0.03 mg/kg in macaques (Kelly et al., 2014; Nunamaker et al., 2013). While these clinically used doses are supported by pharmacokinetic studies, there are currently no supporting studies of efficacy in nonhuman primates. As such, it is important to closely monitor animals for the pain to ensure appropriate analgesia is provided.

Similar to old-world primate species, buprenorphine has been administered at 0.005–0.02 mg/kg IM or SC to marmosets every 6–12 hours. To facilitate administration to marmosets, it is best practice to dilute buprenorphine to 0.03 mg/mL (Mundinano et al., 2016). A pharmacokinetic study performed in marmosets demonstrated that buprenorphine dosed at 0.02 mg/kg IM required a dosing frequency of every 6–8 hours to maintain therapeutic plasma concentrations (Fitz et al., 2021). Another pharmacokinetic study in marmosets showed that both IM and subcutaneous routes of dosing provided a rapid increase in plasma concentration of buprenorphine (Fabian et al., 2021). Regardless of the species, these pharmacokinetic studies demonstrated the significant variation in buprenorphine plasma levels among individuals and emphasize the need for individual animal assessments to ensure adequate analgesia. Therapeutic plasma concentrations have not been established for nonhuman primate species.

Epidural anesthesia consisting of buprenorphine 0.005 mg/kg and lidocaine 2 mg/kg with the administered volume of 0.1–0.2 mL/kg in conjunction with isoflurane has been reported in the literature in marmosets (Goodroe et al., 2021) and used by an author (EN) in macaques. In both species, the combination produced balanced anesthesia with good pain control.

Although side effects such as respiratory depression, nausea, and constipation have been described for morphine and its derivatives, none of these adverse effects were observed in a large cohort of unsedated macaques that received buprenorphine doses increasing from 20 to 100 μg/kg IM (Vierboom et al., 2017). However, respiratory depression and apnea are common adverse effects associated with buprenorphine administered concomitantly with anesthetics in marmosets. Buprenorphine dosed at 0.02–0.03 mg/kg IM given in combination with ketamine IM (Allen et al., 2013) or alfaxalone IM (Bakker et al., 2018) resulted in apnea requiring artificial ventilation and led to several deaths in marmosets.

Butorphanol is also indicated for the treatment of mild-to-moderate pain in nonhuman primates. In macaques, butorphanol (0.003–0.1 mg/kg) produces mild to moderate analgesia and variable respiratory depression, but it does not produce significant sedation or muscle relaxation (Butelman et al., 1995). In marmosets, butorphanol (0.2 mg/kg IM) has also been used for postoperative analgesia, but it has been associated with apnea (Bakker et al., 2018).

Fentanyl is a valuable supplement to inhalational anesthesia for cardiovascular and neurosurgical procedures in old-world primates. Fentanyl produces minimal changes in MAP, cardiac output, pulmonary and central venous pressures, and systemic vascular resistance in doses not exceeding 16 μg/kg IV (Nussmeier et al., 1991). For cardiac surgeries, it can be administered either as a bolus (5–10 μg/kg) or as a continuous infusion (10–25 μg/kg/h) in combination with isoflurane.

Fentanyl and other potential pure mu-agonists have been evaluated for their analgesic and respiratory effects in macaques. An IV bolus of alfentanil (3–32 μg/kg) and ultrashort-acting remifentanil (3.2–5.6 μg/kg) had a shorter duration of analgesia than IV fentanyl (3–32 μg/kg) (Ko et al., 2002). In particular, 16 μg/kg IV fentanyl produced analgesia that lasted 60 minutes, but only 15 minutes at the same dose of alfentanil, and less than 15 minutes for remifentanil (Ko et al., 2002). The onset of action did not differ among the three mu agonists, and all produced a dose-dependent depression of respiration that returned to normal within 1 hour (Ko et al., 2002). A significant decrease in respiratory rates has been observed in rhesus macaques after a 2 μg/kg fentanyl dosage, whereas $PaCO_2$ increased significantly after 4 μg/kg and apnea occurred after a 64 μg/kg fentanyl bolus (Nussmeier et al., 1991).

There have also been reports on the use of fentanyl in marmosets (Goodroe et al., 2021). A bolus of 1 μg/kg fentanyl followed by an IV infusion (1–20 μg/kg/h) was used during general anesthesia with isoflurane. An infusion rate of 10 μg/kg/h was found to reduce the concentration of isoflurane required to maintain surgical anesthesia, but 15–20 μg/kg/h was associated with respiratory depression.

In case of potential overdose with opiate analgesics, naloxone can be of invaluable assistance. When administered intravenously it effectively reverses respiratory depression induced by opioids. The usual dose of naloxone is 0.01 mg/kg IV, repeated as needed. Naloxone is a short-acting antagonist, and a second dose may be necessary to avoid the return of respiratory depression. This may be of importance in trying to antagonize respiratory depression caused by the administration of long-lasting buprenorphine. Additionally, naloxone should be administered in nonhuman primates before extubation to counteract any elevation of $PaCO_2$ induced by opioids. Additional treatments for apnea include stimulation of the GV26 acupuncture point on the nasal plenum.

C. Nonsteroidal antiinflammatory drugs

Many NSAIDs used both historically and currently in nonhuman primates are nonselective COX inhibitors, blocking both isoforms of cyclooxygenase. This category includes aspirin, ibuprofen, ketoprofen, and ketorolac. Alternatively, there is a subset of NSAIDs available for veterinary use that selectively inhibit COX-2, providing antiinflammatory action with reduced potential for negative side effects related to prostaglandin inhibition. Carprofen is primarily a COX-2 inhibitor with some COX-1 activity. Meloxicam has been demonstrated to inhibit COX-2 to a greater extent than COX-1 in vitro and in vivo (Boehringer Ingelheim, 2021). A study evaluating analgesic and anesthetic administration in nonhuman primates undergoing surgery that evaluated a data set including predominantly macaque studies found that carprofen was the most commonly used perioperative NSAID, with meloxicam following as the second most commonly used agent (Bertrand et al., 2018). A treatment regimen of one or 4 days of 0.3 mg/kg meloxicam administered PO or SC once daily given along with 20 mg/kg aspirin PO twice a day to rhesus macaques found no effect on platelet aggregation when compared to baseline and is unlikely to result in clinically significant postoperative hemorrhage (Anderson et el., 2013). In cynomolgus macaques, a sustained-release formulation of meloxicam injected subcutaneously once at 0.6 mg/kg can reach a steady-state plasma concentration adequate to reach therapeutic levels for 2–3 days while standard intramuscular formulation given at 0.2 mg/kg given once daily IM provides adequate plasma concentrations for 12–24 hours (Bauer et al., 2014). Dosing with the oral formulation of meloxicam at 0.1 mg/kg PO once daily yielded lower plasma levels of the drug with a shorter duration in plasma than injectable formulations. In this study, three animals experienced injection site reactions initially, but no reactions were noted during a second round of dosing when the solution matrix was reformulated. A dose of 0.1 mg/kg of meloxicam given orally once daily has been used as part of a multimodal perioperative analgesia regimen for marmosets undergoing stereotaxic brain surgery (Mundiano et al., 2016). Oral administration of meloxicam at 0.5 mg/kg daily for 5 days has been found to block ovulation in adult female cynomolgus macaques (Hester et al., 2010). A number of new Cox-2 selective NSAIDs have been introduced to the veterinary market in recent years, including deracoxib, firocoxib, robenacoxib, and others. There is little literature on the use of the newer generation of NSAIDs in nonhuman primates (Bergh and Budsberg, 2005).

Flunixin meglumine, a nonspecific COX inhibitor, has been used in primate analgesia protocols since the 1970s. In a tail-shock test of rhesus macaques, analgesia provided by flunixin meglumine at 10 mg/kg IM was comparable to that provided by a 0.3 mg/kg IM dose of morphine (Ciofalo et al., 1977). Given the nonspecific COX inhibition of the drug, practitioners should note that significant side effects are more likely to be noted with the use of this agent.

Ibuprofen (7 mg/kg PO) has been used in both old-world and new-world nonhuman primates. It should be noted that ibuprofen is a mild analgesic, and as such may only be sufficient for alleviation of mild pain. While primates have a higher tolerance than dogs for naproxen, microscopic renal changes were observed in naproxen sodium-dosed cynomolgus macaques when dosed at 44, 88, or 176 mg/kg for 2 weeks via oral gavage (Leach et al., 1999).

D. Sustained release formulations

The use of sustained-release analgesic compounds is advantageous in nonhuman primate medicine because it allows for the ongoing provision of pain relief and rapid return to group housing. Decreased animal handling for analgesia administration may also result in a faster recovery and reduced animal stress. There are currently sustained-release formulations of both opioid and NSAIDs that are successfully used clinically.

Sustained release formulations of buprenorphine, Buprenorphine SR (0.2 mg/kg SC, ZooPharm, Nunamaker et al., 2013) and Simbadol (0.24–0.72 mg/kg SC, Zoetis, Mackiewicz et al., 2019) have demonstrated utility to provide 2–3 days of analgesia in macaques, based on pharmacokinetic studies. Buprenorphine SR has also demonstrated utility in marmosets, with 0.2 mg/kg SC providing up to 3 days of plasma concentrations associated with analgesia in other species (Fitz et al., 2021). The authors (AG and KG) have also had clinical success when using 0.1 mg/kg SC in marmosets. It remains important to perform pain assessments in animals who receive sustained-release formulations of buprenorphine as no efficacy studies have been performed. While Buprenorphine SR clinically seems to work well, its use can be associated with self-limiting injection site reactions, most commonly sterile abscesses, in macaques (Haertel et al., 2021; Nunamaker et al., 2013). It is also recommended to perform the injection under sedation or anesthesia as it can be painful.

Transdermal opioid patches have been used with mixed success in macaques. The transdermal buprenorphine patch (10–20 μg/h) has been shown to reach therapeutic plasma concentrations at 24 hours postapplication that lasts up to 6 days in macaques (Smith et al., 2019). Similarly, transdermal fentanyl patches (25 μg/h) reached a therapeutic plasma concentration at 8 hours postapplication that lasted up to 4 days in macaques (Carlson et al., 2016; Smith et al., 2019). However, there is concern about the inconsistent and unreliable pharmacokinetic properties leading the authors to not recommend fentanyl patch use (Carlson et al., 2016). When using opioid patches, it is best practice to clip the area first and maintain the animal in a jacket to prevent the removal of the patch. Due to the potential for abuse by humans, some facilities will require that access to these animals be limited through the use of special cage locks or controlled room access.

A transdermal fentanyl solution (Recuvyra, Elanco) has also been evaluated in macaques, and a pharmacokinetic study of 1.3–2.6 mg/kg found that therapeutic plasma concentrations could be maintained for 7–10 days (Salyards et al., 2017). However, Carlson et al. (2016) found that macaques experienced severe respiratory depression, unresponsiveness, hypothermia, and bradycardia when dosed at 2.6 mg/kg, but that these adverse effects were not seen in animals dosed at 1.95 mg/kg. Due to the unreliable pharmacokinetic properties, the authors did not recommend the use of transdermal fentanyl solutions in macaques (Carlson et al., 2016).

There is additionally a sustained-release formulation of a NSAID that has been evaluated in nonhuman primates. Meloxicam SR (0.6 mg/kg SC, ZooPharm) can be effectively used in both macaques (Bauer et al., 2014) and marmosets (Goodroe et al., 2021), providing 2–3 days of analgesia for mild pain.

E. Local anesthetics

To date, although little is published on the use of regional anesthesia in nonhuman primates, it is common practice to utilize this modality when clinically indicated. Guidance for local anesthesia is generally based on the canine or human literature. Lidocaine, bupivacaine, and mepivacaine are the most commonly used agents. Because so little is known about these drugs specifically in nonhuman primates, the general safety margins for dogs and humans are observed. Specifically, lidocaine is limited to 5 mg/kg and bupivacaine to 2 mg/kg, which are both well below the seizure threshold for adult rhesus macaques of 22.5 mg/kg and 4.4 mg/kg, respectively (Munson et al., 1975).

The use of regional anesthesia for dental blocks is the one area of use that has been documented in the literature (Engel et al., 2019). Engel and colleagues provided visual guides for regional anesthesia of the maxillary, greater palatine, nasopalatine (Fig. 18.1), infraorbital, inferior alveolar (Fig. 18.2), mental, lingual, and long buccal nerves (Fig. 18.3) in the rhesus macaque. In the authors' experience, an injection volume of 0.1–0.2 mL bupivacaine or lidocaine with a 1.5-inch, 25-gauge needle is generally adequate to achieve a nerve block in these locations. This agrees with the findings of Engel and colleagues that 0.1 mL of thiazine dye was sufficient for diffusion in all sites apart from infraorbital and superior alveolar nerves (0.4 mL), inferior alveolar nerves (0.2 mL in females, 0.4 mL in males), and the lingual nerve (0.2 mL). Please see Table 18.3 for dose recommendations.

F. Other agents

1. Gabapentin

Gabapentin is classified as a calcium channel blocker but its mechanism of action is not completely understood. Previous studies in various species have suggested that gabapentin has an analgesic effect on neuropathic pain; however, there are few studies investigating its analgesic use in nonhuman primates. Gabapentin (50–150 mg/kg, SC) had no effect on heat nociception in rhesus macaques subjected to the tail withdrawal assay; however, it did decrease capsaicin-induced allodynia (Henze and Urban, 2010). More studies are needed to understand its effects against neuropathic pain in nonhuman primates.

2. Anxiolytics

Several classes of anxiolytics, including benzodiazepines, selective serotonin reuptake inhibitors, and azapirones, have

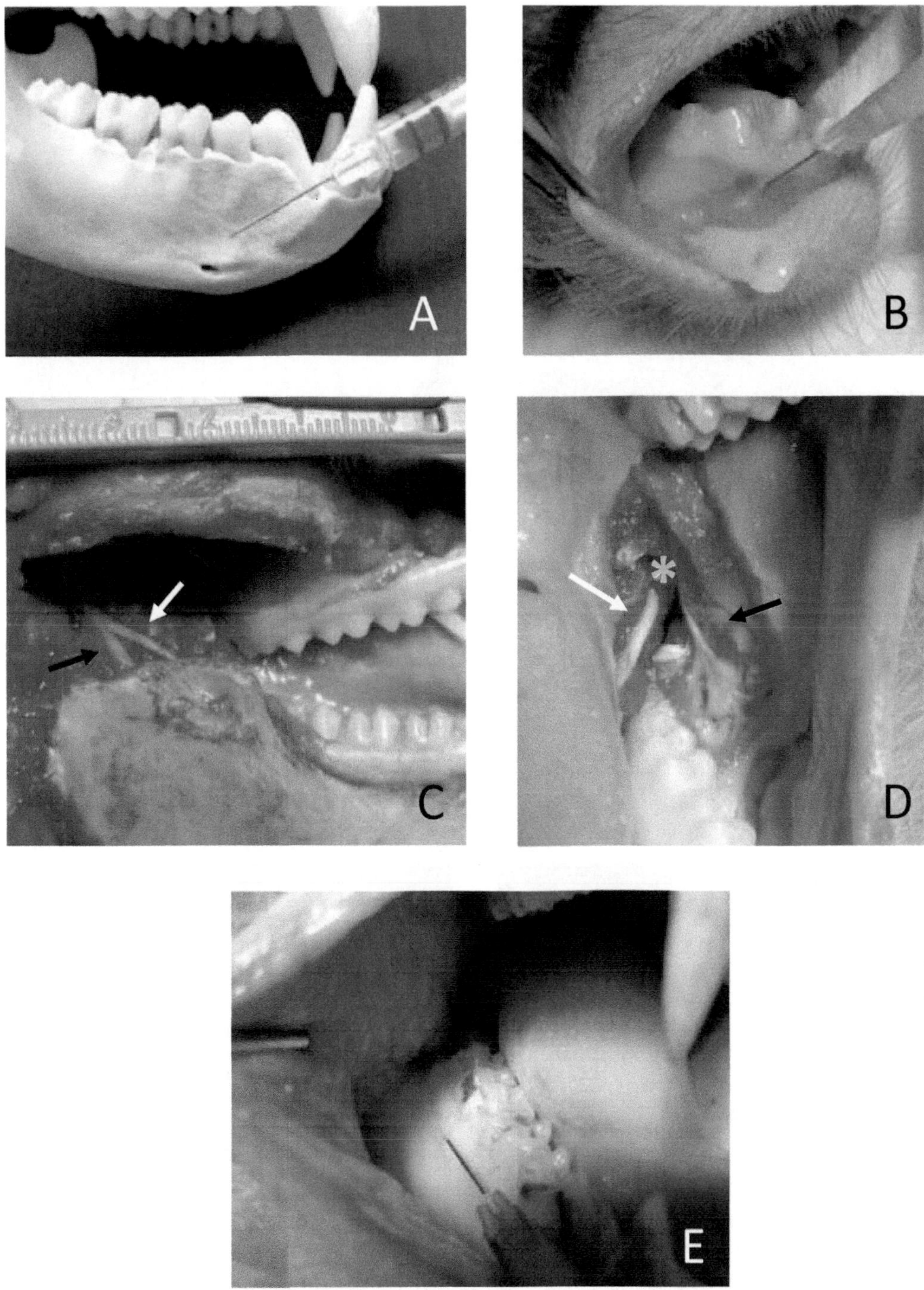

FIGURE 18.1 Blocks of the maxillary, greater palatine, and nasopalatine nerves in rhesus macaques. (A) The arrow points to the pterygomaxillary fissure and shows the approximate path of the needle from the mucobuccal fold dorsal to M2. (B) Injection angle to access the maxillary nerve via the pterygomaxillary fissure shown on a cadaver. (C) Arrow points to the greater palatine foramen medial to M3. (D) Injection angle to saturate the greater palatine nerve as it exits the greater palatine foramen shown on a cadaver. (E) Incisive foramina. The dotted line shows ideal placement of local anesthetic between the cranial edge of the canines. (F) Injection lateral to the incisive papilla shown on a cadaver. *Reprinted with permission (Engel et al., 2019).*

been therapeutically evaluated for efficacy against SIB in nonhuman primates (Novak et al., 2014). The etiology of SIB is complex and multifactorial, and the efficacy of anxiolytics for SIB is variable, suggesting that a "one size fits all" approach to therapy is impractical. Refer to the Handbook of Primate Behavioral Management (Schapiro, 2017) for a more detailed review and information on assessing and addressing behavioral abnormalities.

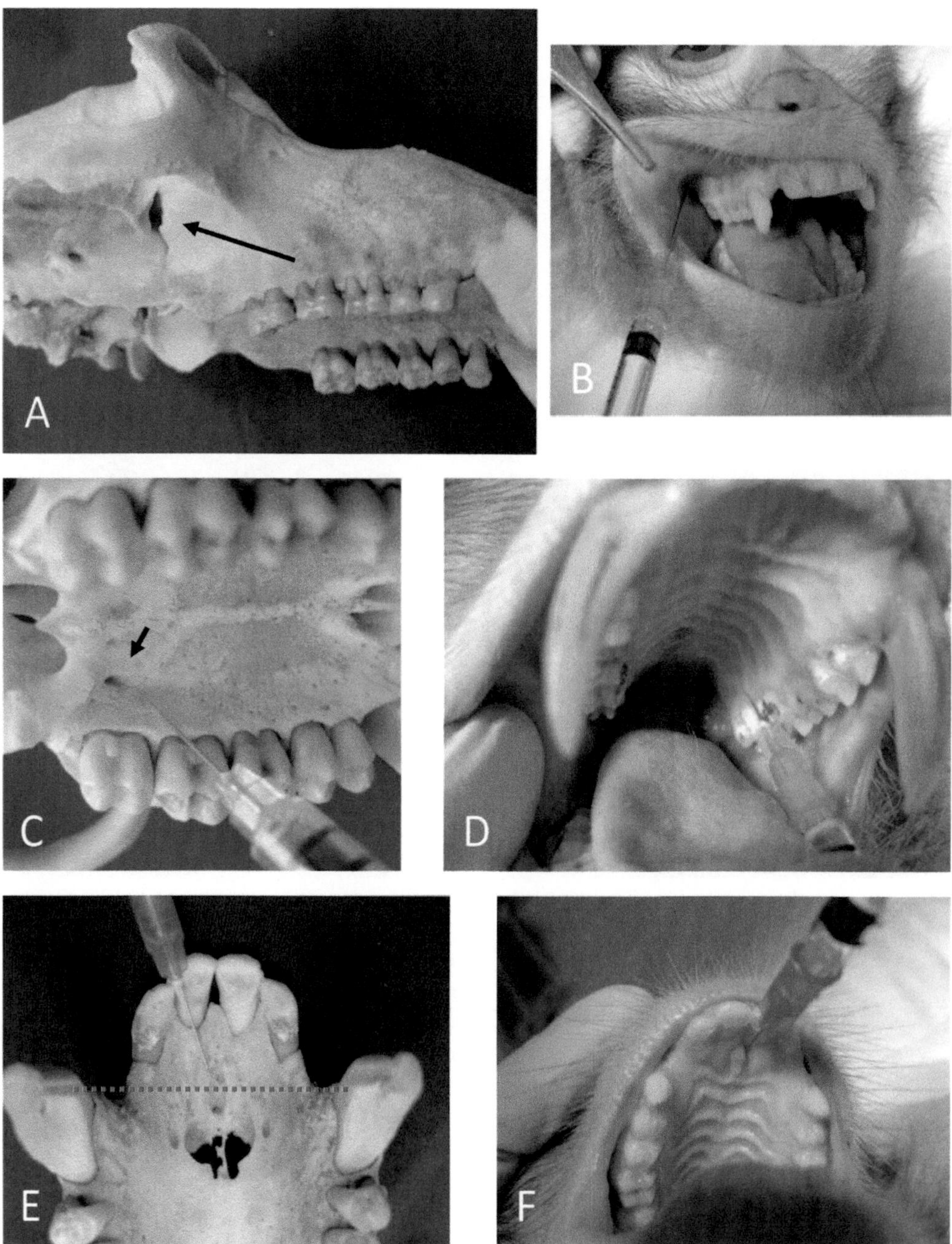

FIGURE 18.2 Blocks of the infraorbital and inferior alveolar nerves. (A) Injection angle aimed at the largest infraorbital foramen. (B) Multiple infraorbital foramina. (C) Infraorbital block injection shown on cadaver. The yellow-hubbed needle is inserted into the largest infraorbital foramen for reference. (D) Inferior alveolar injection shown on intact head; yellow-hubbed needles mark the caudal and cranial margins of the vertical mandibular ramus. The red line marks the occlusal plane of the mandibular molars. The X marks the midpoint of the line and approximate location of the mandibular foramen. (E) Medial surface of the mandible showing the mandibular foramen. The red dotted arrow shows the path of the needle during injection. *Reprinted with permission (Engel et al., 2019).*

3. Muscle relaxants

Spasmolytics, such as methocarbamol, have been used to treat muscle spasticity and associated musculoskeletal pain. Their mechanism of action is not fully understood but is thought to inhibit acetylcholinesterase at synapses in the central nervous system and neuromuscular junctions. While there are several studies evaluating its efficacy in musculoskeletal pain in humans and companion animals, there are no similar studies published in nonhuman primates to date.

Nondepolarizing muscle relaxants are not anesthetics or analgesics and should only be used in fully anesthetized animals. These agents reduce skeletal tone during surgery and are

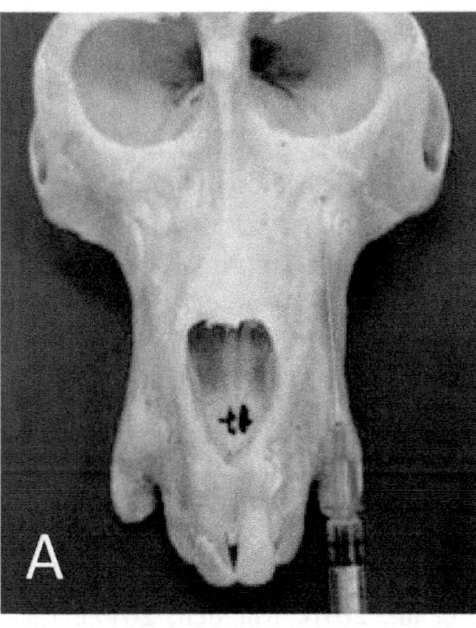

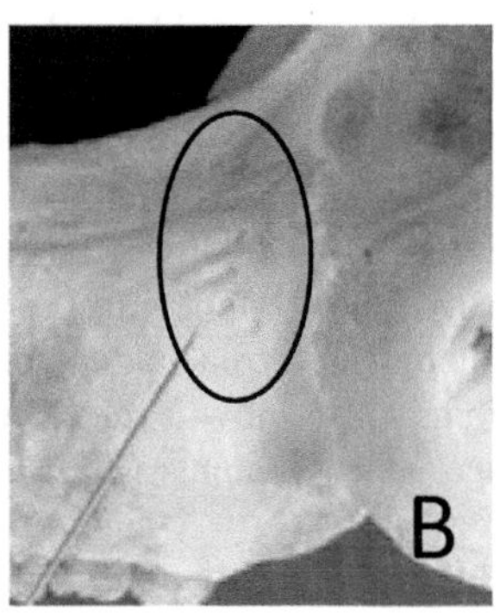

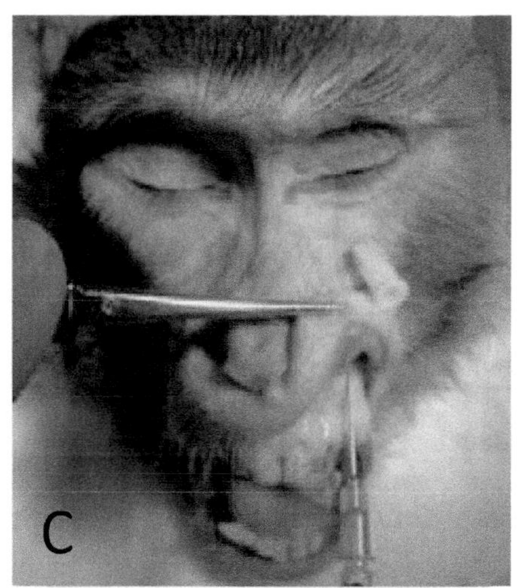

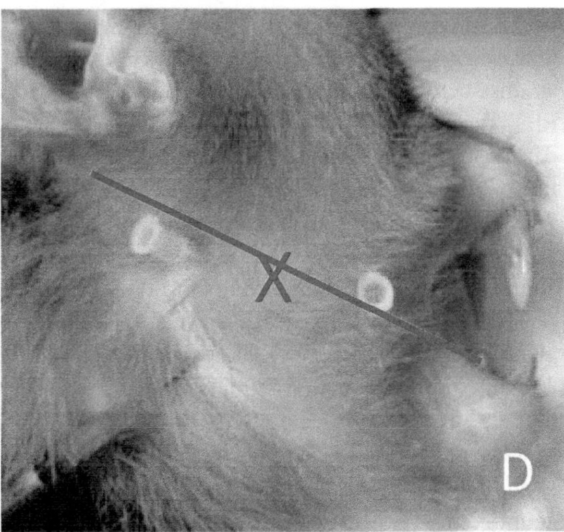

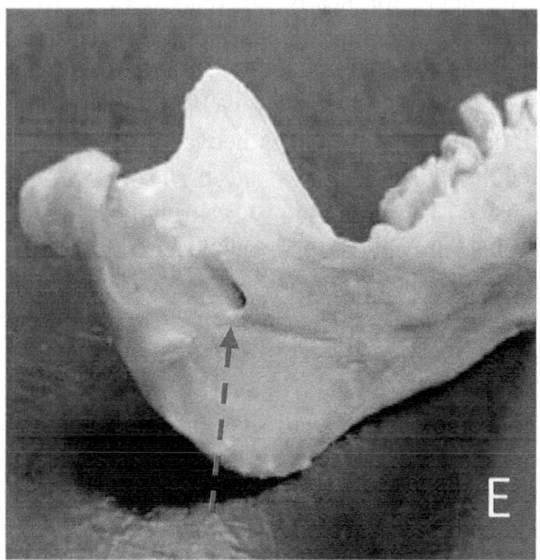

FIGURE 18.3 Blocks of the mental, lingual, and long buccal nerves. (A) Mental foramen and injection angle. (B) Mental injection on cadaver. Yellow-hubbed needle is inserted into mental foramen for reference. (C) Cadaver with vertical mandibular ramus removed. The black arrow indicates the inferior alveolar nerve; the white arrow indicates lingual nerve. (D) Lingual nerve shown passing over the mandible at the mandibular notch (green asterisk). The white arrow indicates the lingual nerve; the black arrow indicates the long buccal nerve. (E) Long buccal block injection into the buccal gingiva adjacent to the mandibular molars. *Reprinted with permission (Engel et al., 2019).*

often utilized for neuroimaging studies that require complete and prolonged immobilization; however, their use requires mechanical ventilation. Pancuronium (0.04–0.1 mg/kg IV) and vecuronium (0.025–0.06 mg/kg IV or 0.1–0.2 mg/kg/h CRI) can be used to produce muscle relaxation during maintenance of inhalational anesthesia in old-world species. Pancuronium is a long-acting muscle relaxant. It produces a moderate elevation in heart rate and blood pressure, while vecuronium has no hemodynamic effects and is a viable alternative to pancuronium for cardiovascular procedures. These muscle relaxants should always be reversed prior to anesthetic recovery to prevent distress and anesthetic complications. Neostigmine (0.075 mg/kg IM every 2–4 hours) is a reversal agent for nondepolarizing muscle relaxants and is typically given in combination with atropine (0.02–0.04 mg/kg IV or IM; de Boer et al., 2006). Sugammadex (0.5–1.0 mg/kg IV) has also been shown to reverse vecuronium in a dose-dependent manner in rhesus macaques (Staals et al., 2011).

G. Nonpharmacological agents

Mitigating pain through nonpharmacological methodologies serves as an adjuvant to traditional pharmacological modalities and should be utilized to maximize the analgesic effect. In addition to the techniques described below (laser therapy, acupuncture), other supportive therapies may be implemented to assist the animal in maintaining a positive affective state. One of the best methods for maintaining a positive affective state in nonhuman primates is the use of social housing whenever possible, as dictated by clinical and project needs. If social housing is not an option, conspecific protected contact (e.g., mesh or grooming bars) is recommended as a minimum standard. A quiet room with few human disturbances is the ideal setting for animals recovering from procedures. The use of additional enrichment devices to redirect attention and encourage occupational manipulations is recommended. Additionally, the provision of highly palatable, high-value food items is recommended to encourage weight maintenance along with the use of electrolytes or flavor mixes to encourage water consumption.

1. Laser therapy

Low-level laser light therapy (LLLT), also termed cold laser therapy or photobiomodulation, has been used as an alternative medicine for nearly 50 years. LLLT triggers biochemical changes at the cellular level by stimulating mitochondrial metabolism, which releases multiple signaling molecules and ultimately facilitates vasodilation, decreases inflammation, promotes neovascularization, and increases collagen synthesis to aid in healing wounds. Higher-intensity LLLT, in contrast, can inhibit mitochondrial metabolism in c-fibers and a-delta fibers, leading to nerve blockage (Colter et al., 2015). For more information on laser therapy principles and safety, refer to Chung et al. (2012) and the Occupational Health and Safety in the Care and Use of Research Animals Manual (1997).

While LLLT has been more extensively documented in humans and companion animals as an alternative therapy for diseases causing pain and inflammation, as well as for tissue healing, there are very few documented reports or studies evaluating LLLT in nonhuman primates. Simultaneous use of LLLT and acupuncture in a chimpanzee (*Pan troglodytes*) with frequent ventricular premature complexes (VPCs) suspected to be due to myocardial fibrosis was found to decrease the frequency of these VPCs (Magden et al., 2016). Of note, PRT was used to acclimate the chimpanzee to these treatments without the need for anesthesia or other type of restraint. More reports and hypothesis-driven studies evaluating the use and methods of LLLT for nonhuman primates as an alternative therapy are needed, especially as the scientific objectives of research studies often preclude the use of traditional methods (i.e., NSAIDs) for relief of pain and inflammation.

2. Acupuncture

The practice of acupuncture dates back to over a 1000 years ago, yet only in the last century has there been a focus on studies evaluating the efficacy and mechanisms of action of acupuncture in veterinary patients. Acupuncture is performed by inserting thin needles into defined points on the body that stimulate neural signaling. Acupuncture points typically correspond to nerve endings or blood vessel plexuses, and result in the release of endogenous opioids to provide analgesia, as well as vasodilation and the release of immune and antiinflammatory cytokines to facilitate circulation and tissue healing. These points are based on human anatomy, and therefore, the location of these points is relatively comparable in nonhuman primates because of the similar anatomy. To elicit a more intense response, electroacupuncture may be alternatively performed, in which a low-level electrical current is applied to the acupuncture points (Zhao et al., 2010).

A handful of reports in the literature have detailed the benefits of acupuncture and electroacupuncture in nonhuman primates. In chimpanzees and owl monkeys, acupuncture has been documented as a treatment for osteoarthritis (Magden et al., 2016; Magden, 2017). Electroacupuncture in rhesus monkeys can improve movement speed in animals with experimentally-induced Parkinson's disease (Zhao et al., 2010) and has neuroprotective effects against cerebral ischemia (Gao et al., 2002). Moreover, a PET scan of brain regions activated by neural pain demonstrated that electroacupuncture decreases activity in those brain regions in rhesus monkeys (Maenaka et al., 2006). In this study, the withdrawal response to heating the tail was also prolonged in animals undergoing electroacupuncture, further supporting its analgesic effect.

The overall risk for adverse effects of acupuncture and electroacupuncture is low, but on rare occasions, minor bleeding, infection, and foreign body (i.e., needle breaks off into the tissue) can occur. Because of the central nervous system's responses to acupuncture, sedation and anesthesia should be avoided in order to optimize the benefits of acupuncture. However, potential safety risks to the handler performing the acupuncture must be determined prior to working with any awake nonhuman primate, and a plan for acclimation to the needles and PRT is strongly recommended. Finally, while there is an increasing number of studies supporting the use of acupuncture and electroacupuncture in veterinary patients, because of the physiological mechanisms of action induced by acupuncture, careful consideration as to whether acupuncture may act as a confounding variable for the planned research must be evaluated.

VI. Special considerations

A. Obstetrics

Physiological changes during pregnancy influence the anesthesia management for obstetric surgery. A plasma volume increase of about 40% leading to dilutional anemia, increased heart rate, and stroke volume, increased alveolar ventilation, induction of a physiological hypercoagulable state, increase in oxygen demand, physical displacement of the stomach by the gravid uterus, prolonged gastric emptying with a corresponding increased rate of both passive and active regurgitation, and decreased requirements for inhaled anesthetics are among the most common physiological alterations (Pariente et al., 2016; Raffe, 2015; Soma-Pillay et al., 2016). Pregnancy also affects all aspects of the metabolism of anesthetic agents. MAC is reduced for all agents, and induction of anesthesia with inhalation agents is more rapid in pregnant than nonpregnant patients (Raffe, 2015).

Most anesthetic agents are fat-soluble and easily cross the placental barrier. In general, the fetus experiences anesthesia passively, and the anesthetic effects in the fetus are proportional to those observed in the mother (Raffe, 2015). However, as a result of exposure to anesthetic agents, the fetus may be negatively impacted by intraoperative hypoxemia caused by reduced uterine blood flow, exposure to teratogenic drugs, and an elevated risk for preterm delivery. The risk of fetal death and spontaneous abortion is higher during maternal anesthetic events in the first trimester of pregnancy, and exposure to anesthesia during the final weeks of pregnancy may risk premature labor and fetal death (Raffe, 2015). Maternal hypotension is the most common complication encountered during anesthesia, thus it is important to routinely monitor blood pressure and provide support as needed. Indirect blood pressure is monitored with the proper-size cuff placed around the area of the tibial or radial artery. Measuring indirect blood pressure in the arm may not provide correct information due to arterial hypotension occurring only in the lower extremities in the pregnant animal.

After ketamine sedation, propofol (2–5 mg/kg) IV can be used for induction of general anesthesia, with an inhalational agent for maintenance of anesthesia for cesarean section. Opioid use should be limited preoperatively to avoid any potential depressive impact on the fetal heart rate. For surgical procedures involving laparotomies or other major manipulations, maintenance of airway access for inhalant anesthesia via endotracheal intubation is necessary. To avoid maternal hypotension caused by inhalant anesthetic agents such as isoflurane or sevoflurane, anesthesia with propofol and/or the use of epidural anesthesia should be employed. In humans, pregnancy is associated with decreased anesthetic requirements, including decreased MAC (Rosen, 1999). Epidural administration of drugs allows for an extended duration of surgical anesthesia and pain management in the early recovery period. A 1:1 mixture (volume) of lidocaine and bupivacaine has been used successfully to provide regional anesthesia in small animal obstetric patients (Raffe, 2015).

Placing the pregnant nonhuman primate in a supine position may contribute to hypotension due to compression of the caudal vena cava and abdominal aorta by the gravid uterus. Tilting the pregnant animal to the left by elevating the right sacral area helps to prevent maternal hypotension. Maternal hypotension from any cause requires immediate volume restoration and, if needed, careful vasopressor therapy. Adequate uteroplacental circulation is crucial to both fetal and maternal homeostasis (Raffe, 2015). Hydration is maintained by intravenous infusion of lactated Ringer's solution at the rate of 5–10 mL/kg/h, and fluid boluses may be given to account for loss or low blood pressure. If hypotension persists, vasopressor therapy should be considered. Recently, among human anesthetists, consensus indicates that α-agonist drugs such as phenylephrine are the most appropriate first-line agents to treat or prevent maternal hypotension following spinal anesthesia (Kinsella et al., 2018). Maternal normocapnia should be maintained during the intraoperative period. Isoflurane and sevoflurane anesthesia are commonly used inhalant anesthetics for surgical procedures in macaques and other species of nonhuman primates.

Laparotomy performed on pregnant rhesus monkeys and baboons during the last third of gestation is often followed by pronounced uterine contractions, especially in the first few postoperative days, which may predispose to premature delivery (Taylor et al., 1983). Close attention to the level of postoperative analgesia may help to reduce postoperative myometrial contraction activity and enhance success after spontaneous parturition in pregnant nonhuman primates (Tame et al., 1999). Tame et al. administered a continuous infusion of buprenorphine at either 15 or 30 μg/kg/day for 48 hours through an intraarterial catheter protected by the tether system. Higher doses of buprenorphine resulted in the inhibition of postoperative myometrial contractions, as well as lower maternal estradiol and cortisol concentrations. Similarly, there were decreases in myometrial contractions and maternal plasma catecholamine concentrations with the use of a single injection of epidural morphine at 0.15 mg/kg) or a continuous infusion of morphine at 0.5 mg/h/day for 48 hours (Popilskis et al., 1994). Prevention of hypothermia is also an important factor in anesthesia management for obstetric surgery, especially during laparotomy procedures when the abdominal cavity is exposed to cool room air. As discussed previously, the use of forced-air warming systems (e.g., Bair Hugger) is strongly recommended. Warmed intravenous fluids can also be provided to prevent hypothermia.

During cesarean section procedures, surgery should be initiated as soon as possible after induction of anesthesia to avoid depressive impact of anesthesia on the fetus. Multimodal analgesia, most commonly involving a combination of meloxicam and buprenorphine (administered postoperatively) should always be provided during cesarean births.

After the cesarean section is completed, a specific plan to introduce the infant to the dam should be followed by well-trained staff to allow for optimal postoperative introduction of the infant to the dam. While dam-infant introductions can be successful under a variety of conditions, an optimal duration of initial introductory period for infants and dams postcesarean-section has been reported to be 2–3.5 hours in pigtail macaques (Bellanca et al., 2006).

B. Pediatrics

Successful pediatric anesthesia management requires an understanding of the physiologic and pharmacologic differences between adult, neonatal, and pediatric animals. There are a number of physiologic characteristics unique to neonates and pediatrics that must be considered when designing anesthetic protocols for this group, including relative hypoalbuminemia, increased permeability of the blood-brain barrier, increased percentage of body water content, a fixed circulating fluid volume, low body fat percentage, and a high metabolic rate with a high rate of oxygen consumption (Grubb et al., 2015). Cardiac output is heart rate dependent in pediatric animals since stroke volume is relatively fixed due to the noncompliant left ventricle in young nonhuman primates. The autonomic nervous system is also immature, leading to blunted responses to hypovolemia and drug-induced vasodilation. ECG, indirect blood pressure, oxygen saturation, and body temperature should routinely be monitored in pediatric cases. Indirect blood pressure is obtained by placing a proper-size cuff around the radial artery. The pulse oximetry transducer is best attached to the tongue or to the palm of the hand in the neonate. The high heart rate makes ECG monitoring difficult with routine electrocardiograph units. Monitoring equipment with probes sized for pediatric patients is widely available and should be used whenever possible to enhance the reliability of readings; arterial blood pressure is lower than that in adults. Accurate measurement of blood pressure can be a problem if adult human blood pressure cuffs are used. The authors have successfully used pediatric (size one) blood pressure cuffs for small (<1 kg) nonhuman primates.

Premedication for pediatric patients can be achieved with IM administration of ketamine (5 mg/kg) in macaques. In the author's experience, a low dose (3–5 mg/kg) of alfaxalone given IM can be used to sedate neonatal and pediatric common marmosets. The effects of ketamine may be prolonged in patients that have immature hepatic and renal systems (Wright, 1982). Exposure to alfaxalone can result in cardiovascular and respiratory depression (Amengual et al., 2013; Maney et al., 2013). This may also be exacerbated in neonates due to the relative large tongue size and the risk of airway obstruction. Another disadvantage of these two protocols is that they are not reversible and nontitratable. Benzodiazepines may be used as a reversible form of light sedation for pediatric patients. In some species, such as macaques and baboons, it is often necessary to sedate the dam in order to retrieve the neonate. Inhalational mask induction has historically been used for pediatric patients; however, the use of inhalant induction is no longer recommended as a routine induction technique for pediatric animals due to an associated increased risk of anesthesia-related mortality. Neonatal primates are usually allowed to nurse until anesthesia time, thus assisted ventilation during mask induction should be avoided. Assisted ventilation may lead to the insufflation of the stomach with gas and place the neonate at risk of aspiration. For the same reason, the authors often induce neonatal primates with propofol (2–4 mg/kg) IV. The suckling reflex is used as one of the indicators for the depth of anesthesia in neonatal nonhuman primates. This is done by placing a finger into the neonate's mouth, which elicits sucking. The loss of this reflex serves as a reliable indicator of adequate depth of anesthesia.

Intubation of pediatric nonhuman primates can be done with the use of either uncuffed or cuffed endotracheal tubes. Endotracheal tubes with 2.5–3.5 mm internal diameter have been used successfully for neonatal and juvenile baboons and macaques.

Small tidal volumes in pediatric animals require the use of nonrebreathing circuits such as modified Jackson Rees and Bain systems. A fresh gas flow of 1.5–2.0 L/min is adequate to prevent rebreathing during spontaneous ventilation. Pediatric animals have a larger surface area per kg of body weight than adults, resulting in increased heat loss to the environment. This, together with an increased metabolic rate and lack of body fat, increases the potential for significant hypothermia in pediatric nonhuman primates. The use of warming lights, forced-air warming systems (e.g., Bair Hugger), and warm IV fluids minimizes the severity of hypothermia. Caution should be taken to avoid overheating and hyperthermia as well.

Three different anesthetic regimens have been directly compared in neonatal macaques. When macaques of 5–7 days of age were exposed to isoflurane, ketamine, propofol, or no anesthesia for 5 hours, compared with ketamine anesthesia, neonatal macaques exposed to isoflurane anesthesia experienced more hypotensive events and required greater support in the form of intravenous fluids to maintain adequate blood pressure during the duration of anesthesia (Martin et al., 2014). No differences were noted between the isoflurane and propofol groups. Isoflurane and other halogenated ethers such as sevoflurane are still an appropriate choice for pediatric animals; however, care must be taken to prevent significant hypotension. Hypotension accompanying isoflurane anesthesia is not uncommon in pediatric baboons. It is important to monitor blood pressure and focus on reducing anesthetic depth where appropriate. Intravenous fluids should be provided intraoperatively for pediatric patients to treat hypotension, and additional pharmacologic interventions can be reserved for patients unresponsive to fluid therapy. Fluid requirements in neonatal patients are a greater due to a greater body surface area, immature renal function, greater percentage of body water, and higher respiratory rates (Boothe and Tannert, 1992). Blood glucose levels should be checked at a regular interval, and dilute dextrose solution added to intravenous fluids should be used to treat hypoglycemia.

The neurophysiological impact of repeat exposure to anesthetic agents in pediatric nonhuman primate patients should be considered when anesthetic events are planned. There is a growing body of literature available that examines the impact of exposure to different anesthetic agents, particularly inhalant anesthetics, on the fetal and infant nonhuman primate. Rhesus macaques exposed to sevoflurane anesthesia on three occasions for 4 h each time within the first 6 weeks of life showed exaggerated self-directed behaviors on the human intruder task at 1 and 2 years of age (Raper et al., 2018). Exposure of both fetal macaques to ketamine anesthesia for 24 hours and neonatal macaques to ketamine anesthesia for 9 hours induced neuroapoptosis in the brain (Brambrink et al., 2012).

Neonatal and pediatric animals experience pain in a manner similar to human pediatric patients. Due to differences in drug metabolism from adult patients, analgesics should be dosed to effect in pediatric and neonatal patients. Since opioid analgesics are reversible, they are often a good choice for analgesia in neonatal and pediatric patients (Grimm et al., 2015). NSAIDs can be reserved for older pediatric patients.

C. Geriatrics

Geriatric animals are generally considered to have reached 75% of their expected life span (Grimm et al., 2015). Rhesus macaques are considered geriatric at 20–25 years of age and aged when greater than 25 years of age (Simmons, 2016). Nonhuman primates maintained for aging studies or breeding colonies commonly achieve geriatric status. Age brings on physiologic and pathologic changes that impact anesthesia and analgesia management. Overall, organs have a decreased capacity for adaptation and response to external stress with age (Grimm et al., 2015). Cardiovascular changes, such as myocardial fibrosis, valvular fibrocalcification, and cardiac hypertrophy, may result in decreased pump capacity and cardiac output (Simmons, 2016). Echocardiographic parameters are available for rhesus macaques greater than 18 years of age (Ueda et al., 2017). Lung elasticity reduction and less compliant thoracic muscles may reduce oxygen exchange. Decreased skeletal muscle and body fat impair thermoregulation (Simmons, 2016). Decreased glomerular filtration rates can affect drug excretion, and decreased hepatic mass may reduce drug metabolism (Grimm et al., 2015). Patient positioning must accommodate osteoarthritic changes that impair joint mobility. Age-related changes affect all organs and are not limited to those listed here.

Suggestions to account for decreased organ capacity include the following: reduction of anesthetic or analgesic drug doses to account for changes in drug metabolism and excretion, available oxygen and ventilation support, monitoring intravascular fluid volumes administered, monitoring cardiovascular output (heart rate, blood pressure, hemoglobin oxygenation) and provide chronotropic or inotropic support as needed), and thermal support. Clinical records should always be reviewed prior to anesthetic events and any known clinical concerns addressed.

D. Laparoscopic and thoracoscopic procedures

Endoscopic surgeries have increased in popularity due to reductions in incision size, hemorrhage, pain, and procedure time, ultimately decreasing surgical morbidity and improving postoperative recovery. In addition, it reduces the number of animals required for certain studies because of the ability to retrieve serial samples (Liao et al., 2004). This, in turn, allows performing minimally invasive procedures on a single animal without the need for an additional animal for each collection point. Scopic procedures for various species of nonhuman primates have been described (de Queiroz et al., 2017; Gaglio et al., 2000; Liao et al., 2004; Perret-Gentil et al., 2000; Rawlings et al., 2000). For research purposes, it has been performed in baboons to obtain liver and splenic biopsy specimens (Rawlings et al., 2000), in rhesus for the study of hepatectomy and liver regeneration (Gaglio et al., 2000), for intra-abdominal biopsy in obese rhesus monkeys (Liao et al., 2004), and serial abdominal tissue samples for HIV studies in macaques (Perret-Gentil et al., 2000; Zevin et al., 2017).

A majority of laparoscopic procedures are performed under inhalational anesthetics, such as isoflurane or sevoflurane. In addition to routine monitors such as ECG and pulse oximeter, it is essential to incorporate capnography for continuous assessment of end-tidal CO_2. Because the pneumoperitoneum is created using CO_2 insufflation to a pressure of 8–12 mmHg, high abdominal pressure may induce adverse physiologic changes, including the retention of CO_2, hypotension (reduced venous return), and reduced visceral perfusion. This especially may be important to older and obese monkeys, with potentially greater medical risks associated with these conditions (Liao et al., 2004). Nevertheless, laparoscopy greatly reduces the likelihood of adhesions that are more common for open surgical procedures.

Bohm et al. (2000) describe the thoracoscopic collection of thymic tissues in rhesus monkeys. After premedication with acepromazine 0.02 mg/kg and butorphanol 0.013 mg/

kg IM, anesthesia was induced and maintained with isoflurane, and positive pressure ventilation was instituted throughout the procedure. Insufflation was performed with carbon dioxide at the rate of 2–5 L/min. Only minor complications, such as self-limiting bleeding and avascular adhesions that were easily broken, were observed. It should be noted that insufflation pressures should be maintained as low as possible and the CO_2 inflow rate kept preferably less than 2 L/min (Ebert, 2005). Higher pressures can cause a mediastinal shift, hemodynamic compromise, and an increase in end-tidal CO_2. Hypotension and tachycardia could be present, especially at pressures above 5 mmHg (Sato et al., 2005).

E. Magnetic resonance imaging

Magnetic resonance imaging (MRI) machines produce a strong magnetic field. Equipment must be MRI-compatible for the strength of the magnet being used. Staff should be aware of the MRI safety zone and vigilant regarding equipment brought into this zone. Ferromagnetic objects, such as stethoscopes or laryngoscopes, can become projectiles if brought within the magnetic field, with numerous reports of patient injury in the literature. Microchips should be verified to be MRI compatible, and anatomical location impact on desired images should be considered. MRI-compatible anesthesia machines and monitors are available, but it is still important to check exactly how close this equipment can be brought to the magnetic field. In the absence of MRI-compatible monitors, long sampling tubes can be connected to anesthesia monitors maintained outside the imaging room (Grimm et al., 2015).

Reliable sedation and anesthesia are essential to avoid gross movement during imaging. The drug selected to produce sedation or anesthesia is dependent on the planned length of the scan. Scans under 30 minutes may be feasible under ketamine and dexmedetomidine or Telazol (see "Ketamine Combinations" in this chapter). Scans of greater length will require a constant rate infusion (CRI) of an injectable drug or inhalant anesthesia.

Inhalant anesthesia may be administered at doses that produce sedation instead of general anesthesia since scans are not painful. Baboons were maintained under isoflurane anesthesia delivered via endotracheal tube; optimal concentration was 0.95%–1.45% (Miller et al., 2013). Propofol is commonly used as a CRI for imaging studies.

Fowler et al. (2001) used propofol CRI to obtain high-resolution MRIs in 27 rhesus macaques. Animals were sedated with tiletamine–zolazepam 3–5 mg/kg IM and induced with propofol 1 mg/kg IV. Animals were intubated to provide assisted ventilation and supplemental oxygen. Propofol infusion ranged between 0.31 and 0.64 mg/kg/min, with a mean value of 0.51 mg/kg/min during the 60-min scan. Benveniste et al. (2003) used propofol CRIs for up to 7 hours in pregnant bonnet macaques. Animals were sedated with ketamine 10 mg/kg IM and maintained on propofol 0.16–0.30 mg/kg/min. Rapid and uncomplicated recovery was observed postimaging; all mothers delivered normal, full-term babies. Propofol 0.3 mg/kg/min combined with fentanyl 10–20 ug/kg/h or just propofol 0.6–1.0 mg/kg/min has been used as a CRI to maintain sedation for marmosets undergoing MRI (Liu et al., 2013).

Hypothermia may occur secondary to the MRI room temperature, length of immobilization, and drug effect. Warm water blankets may be MRI-compatible, but compatibility with individual machines must be verified (Grimm et al., 2015).

Alternatively, animals may be acclimated to restraint devices that are MRI-compatible. Marmosets were lightly sedated with ketamine 2 mg and medetomidine 0.02 mg IM prior to placement in an MRI-compatible head and body restraint device. Atipamezole at 0.1 mg IM was administered and imaging was conducted after animals were fully recovered less than 30 minutes postreversal administration. Marmosets were acclimated to the restraint device prior to use (Tenney et al., 2004). Marmosets have also been acclimated to restraint in individual custom-built helmets within a restraint device and required no sedation to be placed in the device (Liu et al., 2013). The use of restraint devices may be especially helpful for functional MRI studies.

F. Neurological procedures

The ideal anesthetic for neurological procedures should protect against cerebral ischemia, not cause neuronal damage or degeneration, not increase intracranial pressure or affect cerebral blood flow, not be epileptogenic, and can be readily reversible and/or metabolized for a quick recovery and neurological evaluation of the patient. There is currently no widely accepted drug or anesthetic technique that has been shown to meet all of these criteria, and the most appropriate anesthetic regimen for a particular neurological procedure will depend on the individual animal's clinical/health status, the type of procedure, and the anesthetic goals of the procedure.

There is widespread evidence indicating that gas anesthetics, such as isoflurane and sevoflurane, can cause short-term toxic effects and long-lasting neurodevelopmental changes, even when short bouts of these gases are administered. Neonatal rhesus macaques exposed to three or more hours of isoflurane to maintain a surgical plane of anesthesia exhibited apoptosis of neurons in the cerebral cortex (Brambrink et al., 2010; Noguchi et al., 2017), and repeated exposure to 3 hours of isoflurane in neonatal macaques resulted in increased anxiety at 1 year of age (Coleman et al., 2017). Sevoflurane exposure in neonatal rhesus macaques altered gene expression, cytokine levels, and lipid metabolism, resulting in neuronal degeneration in the frontal cortex (Liu et al., 2015).

In contrast, injectable anesthetics may be neurotoxic or neuroprotective, depending on the drug class and length of anesthetic exposure. Long exposure to ketamine and propofol in prenatal and neonatal rhesus and cynomolgus macaques correlates with increased neuroapoptosis in the frontal cortex (Creeley et al., 2013; Koo et al., 2014; Slikker et al., 2007). In contrast, shorter (3 hours) length of exposure to ketamine in neonatal macaques was not associated with neuronal cell death (Slikker et al., 2007). Moreover, 12-h dexmedetomidine infusion in prenatal cynomolgus macaques caused minimal to no neuronal apoptosis (Koo et al., 2014). Alfaxalone appears to significantly suppress cerebral blood flow and intrinsic neuronal activity compared to ketamine (Li et al., 2021). Alternatives to ketamine should be considered for neuroscience studies evaluating NMDA receptor activity.

G. Prolonged anesthesia

Prolonged anesthesia (>24 hours) in nonhuman primates has been utilized for various research purposes, including neurophysiological studies (Huang et al., 2000; Smith et al., 2002), sepsis models (Poliquin et al., 2017, 2019), and elucidating the mechanisms of neurotoxic effects of anesthetics, particularly in the developing brain (Paule et al., 2011). Careful preprocedural planning is critical to prevent and address complications associated with prolonged anesthesia through monitoring and supportive care.

Periodic monitoring of the body temperature and adequate heat support is critical. To prevent reperfusion injury, rotation of the body and limbs should occur every 30–60 minutes. If rotation is not possible, then the limbs should be gently massaged every 30–60 minutes to facilitate adequate blood flow. Blood glucose should be monitored every 2–4 hours and intravenous dextrose can be used to prevent hypoglycemia. Supplementation with parenteral nutrition may be necessary. Paralytic ileus may develop under extremely prolonged (greater than 24 hours and up to 7 days) anesthesia and may be influenced by the study model (Poliquin et al., 2017). Administration of atropine or glycopyrrolate every 4–6 hours is recommended to reduce salivary secretions, in conjunction with careful suctioning of the endotracheal tube. A tracheostomy may also be performed to facilitate the removal of bronchial sections that build up over time and cannot be removed through coughing in the anesthetized patient, but the tracheostomy site may be prone to bleeding, irritation, or infection (Poliquin et al., 2017). Blood gas monitoring may also be useful to monitor acid-base disturbances. Venous O_2 saturation and venous pO_2 were significantly increased in infant and pregnant rhesus macaques subjected to 24 hours of continuous ketamine anesthesia compared to control animals (Hotchkiss et al., 2007; Paule et al., 2011).

VII. Responding to emergencies

The context of the emergency will dictate the response to the situation. Human safety takes priority in emergency situations, and each situation should be assessed in terms of human safety before actions are taken. Situational responses will differ greatly based on where the emergency occurs. For example, a quick response can take place if an animal encounters an emergency while already sedated or anesthetized. If safe, it may be ideal to either reverse injectable anesthesia or reduce/turn off gas anesthesia. In contrast, if an emergency occurs in group-housed animals much more thought and coordination must go into accessing, sedating, removing, and transporting the animal in a safe manner before emergency triage happens. It should be remembered that even an animal that is recumbent in an enclosure can cause significant harm to a human; professional judgment should be applied to the safety of each individual situation. In group housing situations, the behavior management team should assess and make recommendations to ensure group stability when an animal is removed for clinical reasons.

Triage of the situation should occur immediately once the situation has been deemed safe, and standard veterinary emergency practices should be implemented adhering to the ABCs of emergency care: airway, breathing, and circulation; ensure a patent airway, assess the respiratory parameters of the animal, and assess the function of the circulatory system (Aiello et al., 2016). Once triage and stabilization have occurred, further treatment can proceed based on the presentation of clinical signs.

VIII. Postprocedural recovery and care

A. Recovery period

Postprocedural monitoring ensures prompt recognition of potential complications and helps provide for an overall safe recovery from sedation and anesthesia. Physiological disorders most commonly encountered during postoperative recovery include pulmonary and circulatory complications, hypothermia, nausea, and pain.

As with any species, it is recommended to monitor general physiological parameters including respiratory pattern and rate, heart rhythm and rate, perfusion and tissue oxygenation, reflexes, and mentation. However, postprocedural monitoring in nonhuman primates depends largely on the procedure itself, the context under which the sedation or anesthetic event occurs, and the safety of the situation when performing the monitoring. At a minimum, respiratory rates and mentation should be monitored, as these can easily be observed from a safe distance during the recovery period.

It is not uncommon for nonhuman primates to exhibit signs of nausea (e.g., ptyalism, rubbing face on enclosure) or vomit when they emerge from sedation or anesthetic events. Animals with known histories of nausea and vomiting should receive antiemetics. If the animal is intubated, extubation should be delayed until the animal regains the swallowing reflex or other signs of voluntary movement occur (e.g., head movement and chewing). If vomiting occurs after extubation, the animal should be placed in a prone position with its head lowered to avoid aspiration of the vomitus. If a catheter is in place, it should be maintained while it is safe to remove it to allow for venous access should an emergency occur.

Hypothermia is frequently encountered during recovery from sedation and anesthesia. Smaller and younger nonhuman primate species are particularly at risk of developing severe hypothermia because of their large body surface area, which increases heat loss to the environment. The consequences of hypothermia include prolonged duration of action of administered drugs, patient discomfort, coagulopathies, impairment of immune system responses to infection, and reduced tissue healing (Sessler, 2016). Hypothermia should be treated with active and passive heating from blankets or towels, warming lights, heating blankets, and warm saline bags to raise the body temperature. It is important to prevent burns and avoid placing heat sources too close to the animal. Space heaters may be used to pre-heat the recovery area. The use of forced-air warming blankets (e.g., Bair Hugger) or heated water pads is a safe and effective means of providing temperature support during the recovery period.

Hypoglycemia is not uncommon among smaller and younger nonhuman primates. Very palatable foods should be offered as soon as the animal is fully awake. Alternatively, dextrose can be dripped onto oral mucous membranes during recovery.

In general, the recovery of all nonhuman primates should be accomplished in quiet areas with low noise levels and reduced traffic. Extraneous noise may result in unnecessary stress, especially among marmosets and owl monkeys.

B. Return to group or pair housing

The return of animals to group or pair housing situations after a sedation or anesthetic event is dependent on the professional opinions of both the veterinarian and the behavioral management team. The invasiveness of the procedures performed will also factor into the decision. Each situation is unique. Considering the clinical condition of the animal, length of time away from the social pair or group, social rank of the animal, and the behavioral history of the animal will help predict the outcome of the reintroduction of the animal to its pair mate or group.

References

Aiello, S.E., Moses, M.A., Allen, D.G. (Eds.), 2016. The Merck Veterinary Manual. Merck et Co., Inc, p. 3325.

Albertson, T.E., Walby, W.F., Joy, R.M., 1992. Modification of GABA-mediated inhibition by various injectable anesthetics. Anesthesiology 77 (3), 488–499.

Allen, P., Liechty, E., Howland, M., Bergin, I., October 27–31, 2013. Severe respiratory depression following buprenorphine administration in *Callithrix jacchus* [Conference presentation]. In: 64th AALAS National Meeting, Baltimore, MD, United States.

Allison, S.O., Halliday, L.C., French, J.A., Novikov, D.D., Fortman, J.D., 2007. Assessment of buprenorphine, carprofen, and their combination for postoperative analgesia in olive baboons (*Papio anubis*). J. Am. Assoc. Lab. Anim. Sci. JAALAS 46 (3), 24–31.

Alreja, M., Mutalik, P., Nayar, U., Manchanda, S.K., 1984. The formalin test: a tonic pain model in the primate. Pain 20 (1), 97–105.

Amengual, M., Flaherty, D., Auckburally, A., Bell, A.M., Scott, E.M., Pawson, P., 2013. An evaluation of anaesthetic induction in healthy dogs using rapid intravenous injection of propofol or alfaxalone. Vet. Anaesth. Analg. 40 (2), 115–123.

Amrani, A., Michaud, R., Loriot, S., Bétat, A., Aubert, N., Forster, R., Legrand, J., 2012. Evaluation of gastric emptying in the cynomolgus monkey. J. Pharmacol. Toxicol. Methods 66, 204–205.

Anderson, K.E., Austin, J., Escobar, E.P., Carbone, L., 2013. Platelet aggregation in rhesus macaques (*Macaca mulatta*) in response to short-term meloxicam administration. J. Am. Assoc. Lab. Anim. Sci. JAALAS 52 (5), 590–594.

Antognini, J.F., Barter, L., Carstens, E., 2005. Overview movement as an index of anesthetic depth in humans and experimental animals. Comp. Med. 55 (5), 413–418.

Arnold, C., Lamp, J., Lamp, O., Einspanier, A., 2011. Behavioral tests as indicator for pain and distress in a primate endometriosis model. J. Med. Primatol. 40 (5), 317–326.

Association of Primate Veterinarians, 2019. Guidelines for assessment of acute pain in nonhuman primates. J. Am. Assoc. Lab. Anim. Sci. JAALAS 58 (6), 748–749.

Authier, S., Chaurand, F., Legaspi, M., Breault, C., Troncy, E., 2006. Comparison of three anesthetic protocols for intraduodenal drug administration using endoscopy in rhesus monkeys (*Macaca mulatta*). J. Am. Assoc. Lab. Anim. Sci. JAALAS 45 (6), 73–79.

Bakker, J., Uilenreef, J.J., Pelt, E.R., Brok, H.P., Remarque, E.J., Langermans, J.A., 2013. Comparison of three different sedative-anaesthetic protocols (ketamine, ketamine-medetomidine and alphaxalone) in common marmosets (*Callithrix jacchus*). BMC Vet. Res. 9, 113. https://doi.org/10.1186/1746-6148-9-113.

Bakker, J., Roubos, S., Remarque, E.J., Arndt, S.S., Kronen, P.W., Langermans, J.A., 2018. Effects of buprenorphine, butorphanol or tramadol premedication on anaesthetic induction with alfaxalone in common marmosets (*Callithrix jacchus*). Vet. Anaesth. Analg. 45 (3), 309–319. https://doi.org/10.1016/j.vaa.2017.06.009.

Bakoch, M.P., Eilers, H., 2017. Intravenous anesthetics. In: Pardo, M., Miller, R.D. (Eds.), Basics of Anesthesia E-Book, seventh ed. Elsevier Health Sciences, pp. 104–122.

Banknieder, A.R., Phillips, J.M., Jackson, K.T., Vinal Jr., S.I., 1978. Comparison of ketmine with the combination of ketamine and xylazine for effective anesthesia in the rhesus monkey (*Macaca mulatta*). Lab. Anim. Sci. 28 (6), 742–745.

Bauer, C., Frost, P., Kirschner, S., 2014. Pharmacokinetics of 3 formulations of meloxicam in cynomolgus macaques (*Macaca fascicularis*). J. Am. Assoc. Lab. Anim. Sci. JAALAS 53 (5), 502–511.

Bellanca, R.U., Koberstein, D.R., Delio, P.J., Kelley, S.T., Crockett, C.M., 2006. Successful introduction of *Macaca nemestrina* infants to their mothers after cesarean delivery. J. Am. Assoc. Lab. Anim. Sci. JAALAS 45 (3), 27–32.

Bennett, J.S., Gossett, K.A., McCarthy, M.P., Simpson, E.D., 1992. Effects of ketamine hydrochloride on serum biochemical and hematologic variables in rhesus monkeys (*Macaca mulatta*). Vet. Clin. Pathol. 21 (1), 15–18. https://doi.org/10.1111/j.1939-165x.1992.tb00576.x.

Bentson, K.L., Capitanio, J.P., Mendoza, S.P., 2003. Cortisol responses to immobilization with Telazol or ketamine in baboons (*Papio cynocephalus/anubis*) and rhesus macaques (*Macaca mulatta*). J. Med. Primatol. 32 (3), 148–160. https://doi.org/10.1034/j.1600-0684.2003.00018.x.

Benveniste, H., Fowler, J.S., Rooney, W.D., Moller, D.H., Backus, W.W., Warner, D.A., Carter, P., King, P., Scharf, B., Alexoff, D.A., Ma, Y., Vaska, P., Schlyer, D., Volkow, N.D., PET study, MRI study, 2003. Maternal-fetal in vivo imaging: a combined PET and MRI study. J. Nucl. Med. Off. Publ. Soc. Nucl. Med. 44 (9), 1522–1530.

Bergh, M.S., Budsberg, S.C., 2005. The coxib NSAIDs: potential clinical and pharmacologic importance in veterinary medicine. J. Vet. Intern. Med. 19 (5), 633–643. https://doi.org/10.1892/0891-6640(2005)19[633:tcnpca]2.0.co;2.

Bertrand, H., Sandersen, C., Murray, J., Flecknell, P.A., 2017. A combination of alfaxalone, medetomidine and midazolam for the chemical immobilization of Rhesus macaque (*Macaca mulatta*): preliminary results. J. Med. Primatol. 46 (6), 332–336. https://doi.org/10.1111/jmp.12315.

Bertrand, H., Sandersen, C., Flecknell, P.A., 2018. Reported analgesic and anaesthetic administration to non-human primates undergoing experimental surgical procedure: 2010-2015. J. Med. Primatol. https://doi.org/10.1111/jmp.12346. Advance online publication.

Binns, R., Clark, G.C., Simpson, C.R., 1972. Lung function and blood gas characteristics in the rhesus monkey. Lab. Anim. 6 (2), 189–198. https://doi.org/10.1258/002367772781006248.

Blanchard, J.L., Russell-Lodrigue, K.E., 2012. Biosafety in laboratories using nonhuman primates. In: Abee, C.R., Mansfield, K., Tardif, S.D., Morris, T. (Eds.), Nonhuman primates in biomedical research: Biology and Management, 1. Academic Press, pp. 437–492.

Bohm Jr., R.P., Rockar, R.A., Ratterree, M.S., Blanchard, J.L., Harouse, J., Gettie, A., Cheng-Mayer, C., 2000. A method of video-assisted thoracoscopic surgery for collection of thymic biopsies in rhesus monkeys (*Macaca mulatta*). Contemp. Top. Lab. Anim. Sci. 39 (6), 24–26.

Boothe M, D, Tannert, K, 1992. Special considerations for drug and fluid therapy in the pediatric patient. Compend. Continuing Educ. Pract. Vet. 14 (3), 313–329.

Bourgeois, S.R., Vazquez, M., Brasky, K., 2007. Combination therapy reduces self-injurious behavior in a chimpanzee (*Pan Troglodytes*): a case report. J. Appl. Anim. Welfare Sci. JAAWS 10 (2), 123–140. https://doi.org/10.1080/10888700701313454.

Brambrink, A.M., Evers, A.S., Avidan, M.S., Farber, N.B., Smith, D.J., Zhang, X., Dissen, G.A., Creeley, C.E., Olney, J.W., 2010. Isoflurane-induced neuroapoptosis in the neonatal rhesus macaque brain. Anesthesiology 112 (4), 834–841. https://doi.org/10.1097/ALN.0b013e3181d049cd.

Brambrink, A.M., Evers, A.S., Avidan, M.S., Farber, N.B., Smith, D.J., Martin, L.D., Dissen, G.A., Creeley, C.E., Olney, J.W., 2012. Ketamine-induced neuroapoptosis in the fetal and neonatal rhesus macaque brain. Anesthesiology 116 (2), 372–384. https://doi.org/10.1097/ALN.0b013e318242b2cd.

Branston, N.M., Hope, D.T., Symon, L., 1979. Barbiturates in focal ischemia of primate cortex: effects on blood flow distribution, evoked potential and extracellular potassium. Stroke 10 (6), 647–653. https://doi.org/10.1161/01.str.10.6.647.

Brownlee, R.D., Kass, P.H., Sammak, R.L., 2020. Blood pressure reference intervals for ketamine-sedated rhesus macaques (*Macaca mulatta*). J. Am. Assoc. Lab. Anim. Sci. JAALAS 59 (1), 24–29. https://doi.org/10.30802/AALAS-JAALAS-19-000072.

Buchanan-Smith, H.M., 2010. Marmosets and tamarins. In: Hubrecht, R., Kirkwood, J. (Eds.), The UFAW Handbook on the Care and Management of Laboratory and Other Research Animals, eighth ed. Wiley-Blackwell, pp. 543–563.

Burchardi, H., Karczmarczyk, G., 1994. The effects of anesthesia of renal function. Eur. J. Anesthesiol. 11 (3), 163–168.

Butelman, E.R., Winger, G., Zernig, G., Woods, J.H., 1995. Butorphanol: characterization of agonist and antagonist effects in rhesus monkeys. J. Pharmacol. Exp. Therapeut. 272 (2), 845–853.

Carlson, A.M., Kelly III, R., Fetterer, D.P., Rico, P.J., Bailey, E.J., 2016. Pharmacokinetics of 2 formulations of transdermal fentanyl in cynomolgus macaques (*Macaca fascicularis*). J. Am. Assoc. Lab. Anim. Sci. JAALAS 55 (4), 436–442.

Carstens, E., Moberg, G.P., 2000. Recognizing pain and distress in laboratory animals. ILAR J. 41 (2), 62–71. https://doi.org/10.1093/ilar.41.2.62.

Castro, M.I., Rose, J., Green, W., Lehner, N., Peterson, D., Taub, D., 1981. Ketamine-HCI as a suitable anesthetic for endocrine, metabolic, and cardiovascular studies in *Macaca fascicularis* monkeys. Proc. Soc. Exp. Biol. Med. (New York, N.Y.) 168 (3), 389–394. https://doi.org/10.3181/00379727-168-41292.

Choi, Y.J., Park, H.J., Kim, H.H., Lee, Y.J., Jung, K.C., Park, S.H., Lee, J.I., 2016. Cardiopulmonary effects of thiopental versus propofol as an induction agent prior to isoflurane anesthesia in chair trained rhesus macaques (*Macaca mulatta*). Lab.Anim. Res. 32 (1), 8–15. https://doi.org/10.5625/lar.2016.32.1.8.

Chung, H., Dai, T., Sharma, S.K., Huang, Y.Y., Carroll, J.D., Hamblin, M.R., 2012. The nuts and bolts of low-level laser (light) therapy. Ann. Biomed. Eng. 40 (2), 516–533. https://doi.org/10.1007/s10439-011-0454-7.

Ciofalo, V.B., Latranyi, M.B., Patel, J.B., Taber, R.I., 1977. Flunixin meglumine: a non-narcotic analgesic. J. Pharmacol. Exp. Therapeut. 200 (3), 501–507.

Cissik, J.H., Hankins, G.D., Hauth, J.C., Kuehl, T.J., 1986. Blood gas, cardiopulmonary, and urine electrolyte reference values in the pregnant yellow baboon (*Papio cynocephalus*). Am. J. Primatol. 11 (3), 277–284. https://doi.org/10.1002/ajp.1350110310.

Cital, S., Colagross-Schouten, A., Summers, L., 2016. Primate transfusion medicine. In: Yagi, K., Holowaychuk, M.K. (Eds.), Manual of Veterinary Transfusion Medicine and Blood Banking, first ed. John Wiley and Sons, pp. 366–375.

Coleman, K., Robertson, N.D., Dissen, G.A., Neuringer, M.D., Martin, L.D., Cuzon Carlson, V.C., Kroenke, C., Fair, D., Brambrink, A.M., 2017. Isoflurane anesthesia has long-term consequences on motor and behavioral development in infant rhesus macaques. Anesthesiology 126 (1), 74–84. https://doi.org/10.1097/ALN.0000000000001383.

Cookson, J.H., Mills, F.J., 1983. Continuous infusion anaesthesia in baboons with alphaxolone-alphadolone. Lab. Anim. 17 (3), 196–197. https://doi.org/10.1258/002367783781070623.

Cotler, H.B., Chow, R.T., Hamblin, M.R., Carroll, J., 2015. The use of low level laser therapy (LLLT) for musculoskeletal pain. MOJ Orthop. Rheumatol. 2 (5), 00068. https://doi.org/10.15406/mojor.2015.02.00068.

Creeley, C., Dikranian, K., Dissen, G., Martin, L., Olney, J., Brambrink, A., 2013. Propofol-induced apoptosis of neurones and oligodendrocytes in fetal and neonatal rhesus macaque brain. Br. J. Anaesthesia 110 (Suppl. 1), i29–i38. https://doi.org/10.1093/bja/aet173.

Davenport, A.T., Grant, K.A., Szeliga, K.T., Friedman, D.P., Daunais, J.B., 2014. Standardized method for the harvest of nonhuman primate tissue optimized for multiple modes of analyses. Cell Tissue Bank. 15 (1), 99–110. https://doi.org/10.1007/s10561-013-9380-2.

Davy, C.W., Trennery, P.N., Edmunds, J.G., Altman, J.F., Eichler, D.A., 1987. Local myotoxicity of ketamine hydrochloride in the marmoset. Lab. Anim. 21 (1), 60–67. https://doi.org/10.1258/002367787780740725.

de Boer, H.D., van Egmond, J., van de Pol, F., Bom, A., Booij, L.H., 2006. Chemical encapsulation of rocuronium by synthetic cyclodextrin derivatives: reversal of neuromuscular block in anaesthetized Rhesus monkeys. Br. J. Anaesth. 96 (2), 201–206.

de Queiroz, F.F., Kristosch, G.C., Soffiati, F.L., Luz, M.J., de Abreu Oliveira, A.L., Borges, T., Miranda, C., da Silveira, L.S., 2017. Sterilization of hybrid marmoset (*Callithrix* Sp.) females: an evaluation of tow surgical methods. J. Zoo Wildl. Med. Off. Publ. Am. Assoc. Zoo Vet. 48 (4), 1095–1101. https://doi.org/10.1638/2016-0093.1.

de Souza, A.B., Rodrigues, R., Pessoa, G.T., da Silva, A.B., Moura, L.S., Sousa, F.C., da Silva, E.G., Diniz, A.N., Barbosa, M.A., Araújo, J.R., Santos, I.C., Guerra, P.C., Alves, J.J., Macedo, K.V., Diniz, B.L., Marques, D.C., Alves, F.R., 2018. Standard electrocardiographic data from capuchin monkeys (*Cebus apella,* Linnaeus, 1758). J. Am. Assoc. Lab. Anim. Sci. JAALAS 57 (1), 13–17.

Ebert, T.J., 2005. Inhalation anesthesia. In: Barash, P.G., Cullen, B.F., Stoelting, R.K. (Eds.), Clinical Anesthesia, fifth ed. Lippincott Williams & Williams, p. 396.

Ebert, T.J., Naze, S.A., 2017. Inhaled anesthetics. In: Barash, P.G. (Ed.), Clinical Anesthesia, 8e: eBook without Multimedia. Lippincott Williams & Wilkins, pp. 459–485.

Ely, J.J., Zavaskis, T., Lammey, M.L., Rick Lee, D., 2011. Blood pressure reference intervals for healthy adult chimpanzees (*Pan troglodytes*). J. Med. Primatol. 40 (3), 171–180. https://doi.org/10.1111/j.1600-0684.2011.00467.x.

Engel, R.M., Thomas 3rd, M.L., Banks, R.E., 2019. Regional anesthesia for dentistry and orofacial surgery in rhesus macaques (*Macaca mulatta*). J. Am. Assoc. Lab. Anim. Sci. JAALAS 58 (2), 223–230. https://doi.org/10.30802/AALAS-JAALAS-18-000068.

Enlund, M., Andersson, J., Hartvig, P., Valtysson, J., Wiklund, L., 1997. Cerebral normoxia in the rhesus monkey during isoflurane- or propofol-induced hypotension and hypocapnia, despite disparate blood-flow patterns. A positron emission tomography study. Acta Anaesthesiol. Scand. 41 (8), 1002–1010. https://doi.org/10.1111/j.1399-6576.1997.tb04827.x.

Fabian, N.J., Moody, D.E., Averin, O., Fang, W.B., Jamiel, M., Fox, J.G., Burns, M.A., Haupt, J.L., 2021. Pharmacokinetics of single-dose intramuscular and subcutaneous injections of buprenorphine in common marmosets (*Callithrix jacchus*). J. Am. Assoc. Lab. Anim. Sci. JAALAS. https://doi.org/10.30802/AALAS-JAALAS-20-000151. Advance online publication.

Fanton, J.W., Zarr, S.R., Ewert, D.L., Woods, R.W., Koenig, S.C., 2000. Cardiovascular responses to propofol and etomidate in long-term instrumented rhesus monkeys (*Macaca mulatta*). Comp. Med. 50 (3), 303–308.

Fitz, C.B., Goodroe, A.E., Moody, D.E., Fang, W.B., Capuano III, S.V., 2021. Pharmacokinetics of buprenorphine and sustained-release buprenorphine in common marmosets (*Callithrix jacchus*). J. Am. Assoc. Lab. Anim. Sci. JAALAS 60 (2), 188–194. https://doi.org/10.30802/AALAS-JAALAS-20-000082.

Fowler, M.E., 1986. Restraint. In: Folwer, M.E. (Ed.), Zoo and Wild Animal Medicine, second ed. Saunders, pp. 44–47.

Fowler, K.A., Huerkamp, M.J., Pullium, J.K., Subramanian, T., 2001. Anesthetic protocol: propofol use in Rhesus macaques (*Macaca mulatta*) during magnetic resonance imaging with stereotactic head frame application. Brain Res. Protocols 7 (2), 87–93. https://doi.org/10.1016/s1385-299x(00)00051-9.

France, L.K., Vermillion, M.S., Garrett, C.M., 2018. Comparison of direct and indirect methods of measuring arterial blood pressure in healthy male rhesus macaques (*Macaca mulatta*). J. Am. Assoc. Lab. Anim. Sci. JAALAS 57 (1), 64–69.

Furtado, M.M., Nunes, A.L., Intelizano, T.R., Teixeira, R.H., Cortopassi, S.R., 2010. Comparison of racemic ketamine versus (S+) ketamine when combined with midazolam for anesthesia of *Callithrix jacchus* and *Callithrix penicillata*. J. Zoo Wildl. Med. Off. Publ. Am. Assoc. Zoo Vet. 41 (3), 389–394. https://doi.org/10.1638/2008-0016.1.

Gaglio, P.J., Baskin, G., Bohm Jr., R., Blanchard, J., Cheng, S., Dunne, B., Davidson, J., Liu, H., Dash, S., 2000. Partial hepatectomy and laparoscopic-guided liver biopsy in rhesus macaques (*Macaca mulatta*): novel approach for study of liver regeneration. Comp. Med. 50 (4), 363–368.

Gaither, A.M., Baker, K.C., Gilbert, M.H., Blanchard, J.L., Liu, D.X., Luchins, K.R., Bohm, R.P., 2014. Videotaped behavior as a predictor of clinical outcome in rhesus macaques (*Macaca mulatta*). Comp. Med. 64 (3), 193–199.

Gao, H., Guo, J., Zhao, P., Cheng, J., 2002. The neuroprotective effects of electroacupuncture on focal cerebral ischemia in monkey. Acupuncture Electro-therapeut. Res. 27 (1), 45–57. https://doi.org/10.3727/036012902816026112.

Giffard, C., Young, A.R., Mézenge, F., Derlon, J.M., Baron, J.C., 2005. Histopathological effects of delayed reperfusion after middle cerebral artery occlusion in the anesthetized baboon. Brain Res. Bull. 67 (4), 335–340. https://doi.org/10.1016/j.brainresbull.2005.08.001.

Goodroe, A., Fitz, C., Bakker, J., 2021. Current Topics in marmoset anesthesia and analgesia. ILAR J. ilab001. https://doi.org/10.1093/ilar/ilab001. Advance online publication.

Goosen, D.J., Davies, J.H., Maree, M., Dormehl, I.C., 1984. The influence of physical and chemical restraint on the physiology of the chacma baboon (*Papio ursinus*). J. Med. Primatol. 13 (6), 339–351.

Graham, M.L., Rieke, E.F., Mutch, L.A., Zolondek, E.K., Faig, A.W., Dufour, T.A., Munson, J.W., Kittredge, J.A., Schuurman, H.J., 2012. Successful implementation of cooperative handling eliminates the need for restraint in a complex non-human primate disease model. J. Med. Primatol. 41 (2), 89–106. https://onlinelibrary.wiley.com/doi/10.1111/j.1600-0684.2011.00525.x.

Green, C.J., Knight, J., Precious, S., Simpkin, S., 1981. Ketamine alone and combined with diazepam or xylazine in laboratory animals: a 10 year experience. Lab. Anim. 15 (2), 163–170. https://doi.org/10.1258/002367781780959107.

Grimm, K.A., Lamont, L.A., Tranquilli, W.J., Greene, S.A., Robertson, S.A., 2015. Veterinary Anesthesia and Analgesia. Wiley Blackwell.

Griffiths, S.K., Campbell, J.P., 2015. Placental structure, function and drug transfer. Cont. Educ. Anaesth. Crit. Care Pain 15 (2), 84–89.

Grubb, T.L., Perez Jimenez, T.E., Pettifer, G.R., 2015. Neonatal and pediatric patients. In: Grimm, K.A., Lamont, L.A., Tranquilli, W.J., Greene, S.A., Robertson, S.A. (Eds.), Veterinary Anesthesia and Analgesia, fifth ed. Wiley Blackwell, pp. 983–988.

Haertel, A.J., Schultz, M.A., Colgin, L.M., Johnson, A.L., 2021. Predictors of subcutaneous injection site reactions to sustained-release buprenorphine in rhesus macaques (*Macaca mulatta*). J. Am. Assoc. Lab. Anim. Sci. JAALAS 60 (3), 329–336. https://doi.org/10.30802/AALAS-JAALAS-20-000118.

Harrison, N.L., Simmonds, M.A., 1984. Modulation of the GABA receptor complex by a steroid anaesthetic. Brain Res. 323 (2), 287–292. https://doi.org/10.1016/0006-8993(84)90299-3.

Havton, L.A., Biscola, N.P., Christe, K.L., Colman, R.J., 2020. Ketamine-induced neuromuscular reactivity is associated with aging in female rhesus macaques. PLoS One 15 (9), e0236430. https://doi.org/10.1371/journal.pone.0236430.

Henze, D.A., Urban, M.O., 2010. Large animal models for pain therapeutic development. In: Kruger, L., et al. (Eds.), Translational Pain Research: From Mouse to Man. CRC Press/Taylor & Francis.

Hernández-Godínez, B., Bonilla Jaime, H., Poblano, A., Arteaga-Silva, M., Medina Hernández, A., Contreras-Uribe, A., Ibáñez-Contreras, A., 2019. Effect of different anesthetic mixtures-ketamine-xylazine, ketamine-acepromazine and tiletamine-zolazepam-on the physiological and blood biochemistry parameters of male rhesus monkeys (*Macaca mulatta*) at different ages. Anim. Models Exp. Med. 2 (2), 83–97. https://doi.org/10.1002/ame2.12062.

Hester, K.E., Harper, M.J., Duffy, D.M., 2010. Oral administration of the cyclooxygenase-2 (COX-2) inhibitor meloxicam blocks ovulation in non-human primates when administered to simulate emergency contraception. Human Reprod. (Oxford, England) 25 (2), 360–367. https://doi.org/10.1093/humrep/dep424.

Hom, G.J., Bach, T.J., Carroll, D., Forrest, M.J., Mariano, M.A., Trainor, C.E., Wang, P.R., MacIntyre, D.E., 1999. Comparison of cardiovascular parameters and/or serum chemistry and hematology profiles in conscious and anesthetized rhesus monkeys (*Macaca mulatta*). Contemp. Top. Lab. Anim. Sci. 38 (2), 60–64.

Hotchkiss, C.E., Wang, C., Slikker Jr., W., 2007. Effect of prolonged ketamine exposure on cardiovascular physiology in pregnant and infant rhesus monkeys (*Macaca mulatta*). J. Am. Assoc. Lab. Anim. Sci. JAALAS 46 (6), 21–28.

Huang, J., Mocco, J., Choudhri, T.F., Poisik, A., Popilskis, S.J., Emerson, R., DelaPaz, R.L., Khandji, A.G., Pinsky, D.J., Connolly Jr., E.S., 2000. A modified transorbital baboon model of reperfused stroke. Stroke 31 (12), 3054–3063. https://doi.org/10.1161/01.str.31.12.3054.

Ingelheim, B., 2021. Metacam (meloxicam) solution for injection. https://www.bi-vetmedica.com/species/pet/products/metacam/metacam_injectable.html.

Isaza, R., 2012. Chapter 11: Remote drug delivery. In: West, G., Heard, D., Caulkett, N. (Eds.), Zoo Animal and Wildlife Immobilization and Anesthesia, second ed. John Wiley & Sons, Inc, pp. 115–169.

Ishibashi, H., 2016. More effective induction of anesthesia using midazolam-butorphanol-ketamine-sevoflurane compared with ketamine-sevoflurane in the common marmoset monkey (*Callithrix jacchus*). J. Vet. Med. Sci. 78 (2), 317–319. https://doi.org/10.1292/jvms.15-0099.

Iyer, R.A., Anders, M.W., 1996. Cysteine conjugate beta-lyase-dependent biotransformation of the cysteine S-conjugates of the sevoflurane degradation product compound A in human, nonhuman primate, and rat kidney cytosol and mitochondria. Anesthesiology 85 (6), 1454–1461. https://doi.org/10.1097/00000542-199612000-00028.

Jacobs, B., Harris, G.C., Allada, V., Chugani, H.T., Pollack, D.B., Raleigh, M.J., 1993. Midazolam as an effective intravenous adjuvant to prolonged ketamine sedation in young rhesus (*Macaca mulatta*) and Vervet (*Cercopithecus aethiops sabaeus*) monkeys: a preliminary report. Am. J. Primatol. 29 (4), 291–298. https://doi.org/10.1002/ajp.1350290406.

Jasien, J.V., Girkin, C.A., Downs, J.C., 2019. Effect of anesthesia on intraocular pressure measured with continuous wireless telemetry in nonhuman primates. Invest. Ophthalmol. Vis. Sci. 60 (12), 3830–3834. https://doi.org/10.1167/iovs.19-27758.

Kaneko, T., Ochiai, R., Yoshikawa, T., Takeda, J., Fukushima, K., Tsukada, H., Okada, H., Seki, C., Kakiuchi, T., 1997. The effect of cerebral perfusion pressure on cerebral blood flow in the rhesus monkey during sevoflurane anesthesia. Masui Jpn. J. Anesthesiol. 46 (2), 166–172.

Kelly, K.R., Pypendop, B.H., Christe, K.L., 2014. Pharmacokinetics of buprenorphine following intravenous and intramuscular administration in male rhesus macaques (*Macaca mulatta*). J. Vet. Pharmacol. Therapeut. 37 (5), 480–485. https://doi.org/10.1111/jvp.12113.

Killoran, K.E., Walsh, C.A., Asher, J.L., Tarleton, M.B., Wilson, S.R., 2021. Rapid recovery and short duration anesthesia after low dose ketamine and high dose dexmedetomidine in rhesus macaques (*Macaca mulatta*). J. Am. Assoc. Lab. Anim. Sci. JAALAS 60 (3), 337–340. https://doi.org/10.30802/AALAS-JAALAS-20-000112.

Kim, C.Y., Lee, H.S., Han, S.C., Heo, J.D., Kwon, M.S., Ha, C.S., Han, S.S., 2005. Hematological and serum biochemical values in cynomolgus monkeys anesthetized with ketamine hydrochloride. J. Med. Primatol. 34 (2), 96–100. https://doi.org/10.1111/j.1600-0684.2005.00097.x.

Kim, C.B., Ver Hoeve, J.N., Nork, T.M., 2012. The effect of pentobarbital sodium and propofol anesthesia on multifocal electroretinograms in rhesus macaques. Documenta ophthalmologica. Adv. Ophthalmol. 124 (1), 59–72. https://doi.org/10.1007/s10633-011-9306-x.

Kinsella, S.M., Carvalho, B., Dyer, R.A., Fernando, R., McDonnell, N., Mercier, F.J., Palanisamy, A., Sia, A., Van de Velde, M., Vercueil, A., Consensus Statement Collaborators, 2018. International consensus statement on the management of hypotension with vasopressors during caesarean section under spinal anaesthesia. Anaesthesia 73 (1), 71–92. https://doi.org/10.1111/anae.14080.

Ko, M.C., Terner, J., Hursh, S., Woods, J.H., Winger, G., 2002. Relative reinforcing effects of three opioids with different durations of action. J. Pharmacol. Exp. Therapeut. 301 (2), 698–704. https://doi.org/10.1124/jpet.301.2.698.

Konoike, N., Miwa, M., Ishigami, A., Nakamura, K., 2017. Hypoxemia after single-shot anesthesia in common marmosets. J. Med. Primatol. 46 (3), 70–74. https://doi.org/10.1111/jmp.12262.

Koo, E., Oshodi, T., Meschter, C., Ebrahimnejad, A., Dong, G., 2014. Neurotoxic effects of dexmedetomidine in fetal cynomolgus monkey brains. J. Toxicol. Sci. 39 (2), 251–262. https://doi.org/10.2131/jts.39.251.

Kramer, J.A., Ford, E.W., Capuano, S., 2012. Preventative medicine in nonhuman primates. In: Abee, C.R., Mansfield, K., Tardif, S.D., Morris, T. (Eds.), Nonhuman Primates in Biomedical Research: Biology and Management, , second ed.1. Academic Press, pp. 437–492.

Langoi, D.L., Mwethera, P.G., Abelson, K.S., Farah, I.O., Carlsson, H.E., 2009. Reversal of ketamine/xylazine combination anesthesia by atipamezole in olive baboons (*Papio anubis*). J. Med. Primatol. 38 (6), 404–410. https://doi.org/10.1111/j.1600-0684.2009.00378.x.

Leach, M.W., Frank, D.W., Berardi, M.R., Evans, E.W., Johnson, R.C., Schuessler, D.G., Radwanski, E., Cartwright, M.E., 1999. Renal changes associated with naproxen sodium administration in cynomolgus monkeys. Toxicol. Pathol. 27 (3), 295–306. https://doi.org/10.1177/019262339902700305.

Lee, J.I., Shin, J.S., Lee, J.E., Jung, W.Y., Lee, G., Kim, M.S., Park, C.G., Kim, S.J., 2012. Reference values of hematology, chemistry, electrolytes, blood gas, coagulation time, and urinalysis in the Chinese rhesus macaques (*Macaca mulatta*). Xenotransplantation 19 (4), 244–248. https://doi.org/10.1111/j.1399-3089.2012.00713.x.

Li, C.X., Kempf, D., Howell, L., Zhang, X., 2021. Effects of alfaxalone on cerebral blood flow and intrinsic neural activity of rhesus monkeys: a comparison study with ketamine. Magnetic Resonance Imaging 75, 134–140. https://doi.org/10.1016/j.mri.2020.10.011.

Liao, P., Bodkin, N., Cho, E., Alexander, T., Ortmeyer, H., 2004. Minimally invasive surgery via laparoscopy for intra-abdominal biopsy in obese rhesus macaques (*Macaca mulatta*). Comp. Med. 54 (2), 159–164.

Liu, J.V., Hirano, Y., Nascimento, G.C., Stefanovic, B., Leopold, D.A., Silva, A.C., 2013. fMRI in the awake marmoset: somatosensory-evoked responses, functional connectivity, and comparison with propofol anesthesia. Neuroimage 78, 186–195. https://doi.org/10.1016/j.neuroimage.2013.03.038.

Liu, F., Rainosek, S.W., Frisch-Daiello, J.L., Patterson, T.A., Paule, M.G., Slikker Jr., W., Wang, C., Han, X., 2015. Potential adverse effects of prolonged sevoflurane exposure on developing monkey brain: from abnormal lipid metabolism to neuronal damage. Toxicol. Sci. Off. J. Soc. Toxicol. 147 (2), 562–572. https://doi.org/10.1093/toxsci/kfv150.

Lögdberg, B., 1988. Alphaxolone-alphadolone for anesthesia of squirrel monkeys of different ages. J. Med. Primatol. 17 (3), 163–167.

Loomis, M.R., Henrickson, R.V., Anderson, J.H., 1980. Effects of ketamine hydrochloride on the hemogram of rhesus monkeys (*Macaca mulatta*). Lab. Anim. Sci. 30 (5), 851–853.

Ludlage, E., Mansfield, K., 2003. Clinical care and diseases of the common marmoset (*Callithrix jacchus*). Comp. Med. 53 (4), 369–382.

Mackiewicz, A.L., Salyards, G.W., Knych, H.K., Hill, A.E., Christe, K.L., 2019. Pharmacokinetics of a long-lasting, highly concentrated buprenorphine solution after subcutaneous administration in rhesus macaques (*Macaca mulatta*). J. Am. Assoc. Lab. Anim. Sci. JAALAS 58 (4), 501–509. https://doi.org/10.30802/AALAS-JAALAS-18-000115.

Maenaka, T., Tano, K., Nakanishi, S., Tsukada, H., Ishida, T., 2006. Positron emission tomography analysis of the analgesic effects of acupuncture in rhesus monkeys. Am. J. Chinese Med. 34 (5), 787–801. https://doi.org/10.1142/S0192415X06004296.

Magden, E.R., 2017. Spotlight on acupuncture in laboratory animal medicine. Vet. Med. 8, 53–58. https://doi.org/10.2147/VMRR.S125609.

Magden, E.R., Haller, R.L., Thiele, E.J., Buchl, S.J., Lambeth, S.P., Schapiro, S.J., 2013. Acupuncture as an adjunct therapy for osteoarthritis in chimpanzees (*Pan troglodytes*). J. Am. Assoc. Lab. Anim. Sci. JAALAS 52 (4), 475–480.

Magden, E.R., Sleeper, M.M., Buchl, S.J., Jones, R.A., Thiele, E.J., Wilkerson, G.K., 2016. Use of an implantable loop recorder in a chimpanzee (*Pan troglodytes*) to monitor cardiac arrhythmias and assess the effects of acupuncture and laser therapy. Comp. Med. 66 (1), 52–58.

Malinowski, C.M., Cameron, A.I., Burnside, W.M., West, S.E., Nunamaker, E.A., 2019. Butorphanol-azaperone-medetomidine for the immobilization of rhesus macaques (*Macaca mulatta*). J. Am. Assoc. Lab. Anim. Sci. JAALAS 58 (3), 346–355. https://doi.org/10.30802/AALAS-JAALAS-18-000088.

Maney, J.K., Shepard, M.K., Braun, C., Cremer, J., Hofmeister, E.H., 2013. A comparison of cardiopulmonary and anesthetic effects of an induction dose of alfaxalone or propofol in dogs. Vet. Anaesth. Analg. 40 (3), 237–244. https://doi.org/10.1111/vaa.12006.

Manning, P.J., Lehner, N.D., Feldner, M.A., Bullock, B.C., 1969. Selected hematologic, serum chemical, and arterial blood gas characteristics of squirrel monkeys (*Saimiri sciureus*). Lab. Anim. Care 19 (6), 831–837.

Marini, R.P., Haupt, J., 2019. Anesthesia and select surgical procedures. In: Marini, R.P., Wachtman, L.M., Tardif, S.D., Mansfield, K., Fox, J.G. (Eds.), The Common Marmoset in Captivity and Biomedical Research, first ed. Academic Press, pp. 177–193.

Martin, L.D., Dissen, G.A., McPike, M.J., Brambrink, A.M., 2014. Effects of anesthesia with isoflurane, ketamine, or propofol on physiologic parameters in neonatal rhesus macaques (*Macaca mulatta*). J. Am. Assoc. Lab. Anim. Sci. JAALAS 53 (3), 290–300.

McKay, R.E., 2017. Inhaled anesthetics. In: Pardo, M., Miller, R.D. (Eds.), Basics of Anesthesia E-Book, seventh ed. Elsevier Health Sciences, pp. 83–103.

McKinley, J., Buchanan-Smith, H.M., Bassett, L., Morris, K., 2003. Training common marmosets (*Callithrix jacchus*) to cooperate during routine laboratory procedures: ease of training and time investment. J. Appl. Anim. Welfare Sci. JAAWS 6 (3), 209–220. https://doi.org/10.1207/S15327604JAWS0603_06.

McMillan, J.L., Perlman, J.E., Galvan, A., Wichmann, T., Bloomsmith, M.A., 2014. Refining the pole-and-collar method of restraint: emphasizing the use of positive training techniques with rhesus macaques (*Macaca mulatta*). J. Am. Assoc. Lab. Anim. Sci. JAALAS 53 (1), 61–68.

Mietsch, M., Einspanier, A., 2015. Non-invasive blood pressure measurement: values, problems and applicability in the common marmoset (*Callithrix jacchus*). Lab. Anim. 49 (3), 241–250. https://doi.org/10.1177/0023677214565843.

Miller, B., Marks, L.A., Koller, J.M., Newman, B.J., Bretthorst, G.L., Black, K.J., 2013. Prolactin and fMRI response to SKF38393 in the baboon. PeerJ 1, e195. https://doi.org/10.7717/peerj.195.

Miyabe-Nishiwaki, T., Miwa, M., Konoike, N., Kaneko, A., Ishigami, A., Natsume, T., MacIntosh, A., Nakamura, K., 2020. Evaluation of anaesthetic and cardiorespiratory effects after intramuscular administration of alfaxalone alone, alfaxalone-ketamine and alfaxalone-butorphanol-medetomidine in common marmosets (*Callithrix jacchus*). J. Med. Primatol. 49 (6), 291–299. https://doi.org/10.1111/jmp.12482.

Miyabe-Nishiwaki, T., Gris, V.N., Muta, K., Nishimura, R., Mills, D.S., 2021. Primate veterinarians' knowledge and attitudes regarding pain in macaques. J. Med. Primatol. 50 (5), 259–269. https://doi.org/10.1111/jmp.12537.

Morris, T.H., Jackson, R.K., Acker, W.R., Spencer, C.K., Drag, M.D., 1997. An illustrated guide to endotracheal intubation in small nonhuman primates. Lab. Anim. 31 (2), 157–162. https://doi.org/10.1258/002367797780600143.

Mundinano, I.C., Flecknell, P.A., Bourne, J.A., 2016. MRI-guided stereotaxic brain surgery in the infant and adult common marmoset. Nat. Protoc. 11 (7), 1299–1308. https://doi.org/10.1038/nprot.2016.076.

Munson, E.S., Tucker, W.K., Ausinsch, B., Malagodi, M.H., 1975. Etidocaine, bupivacaine, and lidocaine seizure thresholds in monkeys. Anesthesiology 42 (4), 471–478. https://doi.org/10.1097/00000542-197504000-00018.

Naccarato, E.F., Hunter, W.S., 1979. Anaesthetic effects of various ratios of ketamine and xylazine in rhesus monkeys (*Macacca mulatta*). Lab. Anim. 13 (4), 317–319. https://doi.org/10.1258/002367779780943314.

Nakayama, S., Koie, H., Kanayama, K., Katakai, Y., Ito-Fujishiro, Y., Sankai, T., Yasutomi, Y., Ageyama, N., 2017. Establishment of reference values for complete blood count and blood gases in cynomolgus monkeys (*Macaca fascicularis*). J. Vet. Med. Sci. 79 (5), 881–888. https://doi.org/10.1292/jvms.16-0638.

National Research Council (US) Committee on Occupational Health and Safety in the Care and Use of Nonhuman Primates, 2003. Occupational Health and Safety in the Care and Use of Nonhuman Primates. National Academies Press (US).

National Research Council (US) Committee on Recognition and Alleviation of Pain in Laboratory Animals, 2009. Recognition and Alleviation of Pain in Laboratory Animals. National Academies Press (US).

Noguchi, K.K., Johnson, S.A., Dissen, G.A., Martin, L.D., Manzella, F.M., Schenning, K.J., Olney, J.W., Brambrink, A.M., 2017. Isoflurane exposure for three hours triggers apoptotic cell death in neonatal macaque brain. Br. J. Anaesthesia 119 (3), 524–531. https://doi.org/10.1093/bja/aex123.

Novak, M.A., El-Mallah, S.N., Menard, M.T., 2014. Use of the cross-translational model to study self-injurious behavior in human and nonhuman primates. ILAR J. 55 (2), 274–283. https://doi.org/10.1093/ilar/ilu001.

Nunamaker, E.A., Halliday, L.C., Moody, D.E., Fang, W.B., Lindeblad, M., Fortman, J.D., 2013. Pharmacokinetics of 2 formulations of buprenorphine in macaques (*Macaca mulatta* and *Macaca fascicularis*). J. Am. Assoc. Lab. Anim. Sci. JAALAS 52 (1), 48–56.

Nussmeier, N.A., Benthuysen, J.L., Steffey, E.P., Anderson, J.H., Carstens, E.E., Eisele Jr., J.H., Stanley, T.H., 1991. Cardiovascular, respiratory, and analgesic effects of fentanyl in unanesthetized rhesus monkeys. Anesth. Analg. 72 (2), 221–226. https://doi.org/10.1213/00000539-199102000-00015.

Osborne, B.E., Roberts, C.N., 1972. The electrocardiogram (ECG) of the baboon (*Papio* spp.). Lab. Anim. 6 (2), 127–133. https://doi.org/10.1258/002367772781006275.

Ouchi, T., Ochiai, R., Takeda, J., Tsukada, H., Kakiuchi, T., 2006. Combined effects of propofol and mild hypothermia on cerebral metabolism and blood flow in rhesus monkey: a positron emission tomography study. J. Anesth. 20 (3), 208–214. https://doi.org/10.1007/s00540-006-0411-z.

Pariente, G., Leibson, T., Carls, A., Adams-Webber, T., Ito, S., Koren, G., 2016. Pregnancy-associated changes in pharmacokinetics: a systematic review. PLoS Med. 13 (11), e1002160. https://doi.org/10.1371/journal.pmed.1002160.

Paule, M.G., Li, M., Allen, R.R., Liu, F., Zou, X., Hotchkiss, C., Hanig, J.P., Patterson, T.A., Slikker Jr., W., Wang, C., 2011. Ketamine anesthesia during the first week of life can cause long-lasting cognitive deficits in rhesus monkeys. Neurotoxicol. Teratol. 33 (2), 220–230. https://doi.org/10.1016/j.ntt.2011.01.001.

Perret-Gentil, M.I., Sinanan, M.N., Dennis, M.B., Anderson, D.M., Pasieka, H.B., Weyhrich, J.T., Birkebak, T.A., 2000. Video-endoscopic techniques for collection of multiple, serial intra-abdominal biopsy specimens in HIV-negative and HIV-positive pigtail macaques (*Macaca nemestrina*). J. Invest. Surg. Off. J. Acad. Surg. Res. 13 (4), 181–195. https://doi.org/10.1080/089419300416474.

Poliquin, P.G., Biondi, M., Ranadheera, C., Hagan, M., Bello, A., Racine, T., Allan, M., Funk, D., Hansen, G., Hancock, B.J., Kesselman, M., Mortimer, T., Kumar, A., Jones, S., Leung, A., Grolla, A., Tran, K.N., Tierney, K., Qiu, X., Kobasa, D., Strong, J.E., 2017. Delivering prolonged intensive care to a non-human primate: a high fidelity animal model of critical illness. Sci. Rep. 7 (1), 1204. https://doi.org/10.1038/s41598-017-01107-6.

Poliquin, G., Funk, D., Jones, S., Tran, K., Ranadheera, C., Hagan, M., Tierney, K., Grolla, A., Dhaliwal, A., Bello, A., Leung, A., Nakamura, C., Kobasa, D., Falzarano, D., Garnett, L., Bovendo, H.F., Feldmann, H., Kesselman, M., Hansen, G., Gren, J., Strong, J.E., 2019. Impact of intensive care unit supportive care on the physiology of Ebola virus disease in a universally lethal non-human primate model. Intensive Care Med. Exp. 7 (1), 54. https://doi.org/10.1186/s40635-019-0268-8.

Popilskis, S., Daniel, S., Smiley, R., August 21-25, 1994. Effects of epidural versus intravenous morphine analgesia on postoperative catecholamine response in baboons [Conference presentation]. In: 5th Proceedings of International Congress on Veterinary Anesthesia, Guelph, Canada.

Portier, K.G., Broillet, A., Rioufol, G., Lepage, O.M., Depecker, M., Taborik, F., Tranquart, F., Contamin, H., 2012. A novel minimal invasive closed chest myocardial ischaemia reperfusion model in rhesus monkeys (*Macaca mulatta*): improved stability of cardiorespiratory parameters. Lab. Anim. 46 (2), 129–135. https://doi.org/10.1258/la.2011.011037.

Pulley, A.C., Roberts, J.A., Lerche, N.W., 2004. Four preanesthetic oral sedation protocols for rhesus macaques (*Macaca mulatta*). J. Zoo Wildl. Med. Off. Publ. Am. Assoc. Zoo Veterinarians 35 (4), 497–502. https://doi.org/10.1638/03-092.

Raffe, M.R., 2015. Anesthetic considerations during pregnancy and for the newborn. In: Grimm, K.A., Lamont, L.A., Tranquilli, W.J., Greene, S.A., Robertson, S.A. (Eds.), Veterinary Anesthesia and Analgesia, fifth ed. Wiley Blackwell, pp. 708–722.

Rajan, R., Dubaj, V., Reser, D.H., Rosa, M.G., 2013. Auditory cortex of the marmoset monkey - complex responses to tones and vocalizations under opiate anaesthesia in core and belt areas. Eur. J. Neurosci. 37 (6), 924–941. https://doi.org/10.1111/ejn.12092.

Raper, J., De Biasio, J.C., Murphy, K.L., Alvarado, M.C., Baxter, M.G., 2018. Persistent alteration in behavioural reactivity to a mild social stressor in rhesus monkeys repeatedly exposed to sevoflurane in infancy. Br. J. Anaesthesia 120 (4), 761–767. https://doi.org/10.1016/j.bja.2018.01.014.

Raposo, A.C., Ofri, R., Schaffer, D.P., Gomes Júnior, D.C., Libório, F.A., Martins Filho, E.F., Oriá, A.P., 2015. Evaluation of ophthalmic and hemodynamic parameters in capuchin monkeys (*Cebus* sp.) submitted to dissociative anesthetic protocols. J. Med. Primatol. 44 (6), 381–389. https://doi.org/10.1111/jmp.12200.

Rawlings, C.A., Van Lue, S., King, C., Freeman, L., Damian, R.T., Greenacre, C., Chernosky, A., Mohamed, F.M., Chou, T.M., 2000. Serial laparoscopic biopsies of liver and spleen from Schistosoma-infected baboons (*Papio* spp.). Comp. Med. 50 (5), 551–555.

Reutlinger, R.A., Karl, A.A., Vinal, S.I., Nieser, M.J., 1980. Effects of ketamine HCl-xylazine HCl combination on cardiovascular and pulmonary values of the rhesus macaque (*Macaca mulatta*). Am. J. Vet. Res. 41 (9), 1453–1457.

Rogge, J., Sherenco, K., Malling, R., Thiele, E., Lambeth, S., Schapiro, S., Williams, L., 2013. A comparison of positive reinforcement training techniques in owl and squirrel monkeys: time required to train to reliability. J. Appl. Anim. Welfare Sci. JAAWS 16 (3), 211–220. https://doi.org/10.1080/10888705.2013.798223.

Romagnoli, N., Buonacucina, A., Lambertini, C., Ventrella, D., Peli, A., 2016. Constant-rate infusion of dexmedetomidine to manage thiopental anesthesia during intracranial surgery in cynomolgus macaques (*Macaca fascicularis*). J. Am. Assoc. Lab. Anim. Sci. JAALAS 55 (6), 801–804.

Rosen, M.A., 1999. Management of anesthesia for the pregnant surgical patient. Anesthesiology 91 (4), 1159–1163. https://doi.org/10.1097/00000542-199910000-00033.

Sainsbury, A.W., Eaton, B.D., Cooper, J.E., 1989. Restraint and anaesthesia of primates. Vet. Rec. 125 (26–27), 640–644.

Sainsbury, A.W., Eaton, B.D., Cooper, J.E., 1991. An investigation into the use of propofol (Rapinovet) in long-tailed macaques (*Macaca fascicularis*). J. Vet. Anaesthesia 18 (1), 38–41.

Salyards, G.W., Lemoy, M.J., Knych, H.K., Hill, A.E., Christe, K.L., 2017. Pharmacokinetics of a novel, transdermal fentanyl solution in rhesus macaques (*Macaca mulatta*). J. Am. Assoc. Lab. Anim. Sci. JAALAS 56 (4), 443–451.

Sato, M., Hamada, Y., Takada, K., Tanano, A., Tokuhara, K., Hatano, T., 2005. Thoracoscopic diaphragmatic procedures under artificial pneumothorax. Pediatr. Surg. Int. 21 (1), 34–38. https://doi.org/10.1007/s00383-004-1259-7.

Schapiro, S.J., 2017. Handbook of Primate Behavioral Management. CRC Press.

Schmelting, B., Niehoff, M., Egner, B., Korte, S.H., Weinbauer, G.F., 2009. High definition oscillometry: a novel technique for non-invasive blood pressure monitoring in the cynomolgus monkey (*Macaca fascicularis*). J. Med. Primatol. 38 (5), 293–301. https://doi.org/10.1111/j.1600-0684.2009.00344.x.

Sedgwick, C.J., 1986. Scaling and anesthesia for primates. In: Benirschke, K. (Ed.), Primates: The Road to Self-Sustaining Populations. Springer-Verlag, pp. 815–823.

Sessler, D.I., 2016. Perioperative thermoregulation and heat balance. Lancet (London, England) 387 (10038), 2655–2664. https://doi.org/10.1016/S0140-6736(15)00981-2.

Sherman, J., Le, C., Lamers, V., Eckelman, M., 2012. Life cycle greenhouse gas emissions of anesthetic drugs. Anesth. Analg. 114 (5), 1086–1090.

Simmons, H.A., 2016. Age-associated pathology in rhesus macaques (*Macaca mulatta*). Vet. Pathol. 53 (2), 399–416. https://doi.org/10.1177/0300985815620628.

Singh, R., Chakravarti, R.N., Chhuttani, P.N., Wahi, P.L., 1970. Electrocardiographic studies in rhesus monkeys. J. Appl. Physiol. 28 (3), 346–349. https://doi.org/10.1152/jappl.1970.28.3.346.

Slikker Jr., W., Zou, X., Hotchkiss, C.E., Divine, R.L., Sadovova, N., Twaddle, N.C., Doerge, D.R., Scallet, A.C., Patterson, T.A., Hanig, J.P., Paule, M.G., Wang, C., 2007. Ketamine-induced neuronal cell death in the perinatal rhesus monkey. Toxicol. Sci. Off. J. Soc. Toxicol. 98 (1), 145–158. https://doi.org/10.1093/toxsci/kfm084.

Smith, M.A., Bair, W., Movshon, J.A., 2002. Signals in macaque striate cortical neurons that support the perception of glass patterns. J. Neurosci. Off. J. Soc. Neurosci. 22 (18), 8334–8345. https://doi.org/10.1523/JNEUROSCI.22-18-08334.2002.

Smith, A.A., Halliday, L.C., Lindeblad, M.O., Fortman, J.D., 2019. Evaluation of analgesic patches in cynomolgus macaques (*Macaca fascicularis*). J. Am. Assoc. Lab. Anim. Sci. JAALAS 58 (3), 356–361. https://doi.org/10.30802/AALAS-JAALAS-18-000101.

Socha, W.W., Rowe, A.W., Lenny, L.L., Lasano, S.G., Moor-Jankowski, J., 1982. Transfusion of incompatible blood in rhesus monkeys and baboons. Lab. Anim. Sci. 32 (1), 48–56.

Sofianos, E., Alevizou, F., Zissis, N., Kostaki, P., Balamoutsos, N., 1985. Hormonal response in thoracic surgery. Effects of high-dose fentanyl anesthesia, compared to halothane anesthesia. Acta Anaesthesiol. Belg. 36 (2), 89–96.

Soma, L.R., 1988. Sevoflurane anesthesia in the monkey: the effects of multiples of MAC. Hiroshima J. Anesth. 24, 3–14.

Soma-Pillay, P., Nelson-Piercy, C., Tolppanen, H., Mebazaa, A., 2016. Physiological changes in pregnancy. Cardiovasc. J. Afr. 27 (2), 89–94. https://doi.org/10.5830/CVJA-2016-021.

Soma, L.R., Tierney, W.J., Hogan, G.K., Satoh, N., 1995. The effects of multiple administrations of sevoflurane to cynomolgus monkeys: clinical pathologic, hematologic, and pathologic study. Anesth. Analg. 81 (2), 347–352. https://doi.org/10.1097/00000539-199508000-00024.

Staals, L.M., van Egmond, J., Driessen, J.J., de Boer, H.D., van de Pol, F., Bom, A.H., Booij, L.H., 2011. Sugammadex reverses neuromuscular block induced by 3-desacetyl-vecuronium, an active metabolite of vecuronium, in the anaesthetised rhesus monkey. Eur. J. Anaesthesiol. 28 (4), 265–272. https://doi.org/10.1097/EJA.0b013e328340894f.

Steinbach, J.R., MacGuire, J., Chang, S., Dierks, E., Roble, G.S., 2018. Assessment of pre-operative maropitant citrate use in macaque (*Macaca fasicularis* & *Macaca mulatta*) neurosurgical procedures. J. Med. Primatol. 47 (3), 178–184. https://doi.org/10.1111/jmp.12343.

Sukhtankar, D.D., Lee, H., Rice, K.C., Ko, M.C., 2014. Differential effects of opioid-related ligands and NSAIDs in nonhuman primate models of acute and inflammatory pain. Psychopharmacology 231 (7), 1377–1387. https://doi.org/10.1007/s00213-013-3341-0.

Tame, J.D., Abrams, L.M., Ding, X.Y., Yen, A., Giussani, D.A., Nathanielsz, P.W., 1999. Level of postoperative analgesia is a critical factor in regulation of myometrial contractility after laparotomy in the pregnant baboon: implications for human fetal surgery. Am. J. Obstet. Gynecol. 180 (5), 1196–1201. https://doi.org/10.1016/s0002-9378(99)70616-2.

Taylor, N.F., Martin, M.C., Nathanielsz, P.W., Seron-Ferre, M., 1983. The fetus determines circadian oscillation of myometrial electromyographic activity in the pregnant rhesus monkey. Am. J. Obstet. Gynecol. 146 (5), 557–567. https://doi.org/10.1016/0002-9378(83)90803-7.

Tenney, J.R., Marshall, P.C., King, J.A., Ferris, C.F., 2004. fMRI of generalized absence status epilepticus in conscious marmoset monkeys reveals corticothalamic activation. Epilepsia 45 (10), 1240–1247. https://doi.org/10.1111/j.0013-9580.2004.21504.x.

Theriault, B.R., Reed, D.A., Niekrasz, M.A., 2008. Reversible medetomidine/ketamine anesthesia in captive capuchin monkeys (*Cebus apella*). J. Med. Primatol. 37 (Suppl. 1), 74–81. https://doi.org/10.1111/j.1600-0684.2007.00267.x.

Thomas, A.A., Leach, M.C., Flecknell, P.A., 2012. An alternative method of endotracheal intubation of common marmosets (*Callithrix jacchus*). Lab. Anim. 46 (1), 71–76. https://doi.org/10.1258/la.2011.011092.

Tinker, J.H., Sharbrough, F.W., Michenfelder, J.D., 1977. Anterior shift of the dominant EEG rhythm during anesthesia in the Java monkey: correlation with anesthetic potency. Anesthesiology 46 (4), 252–259. https://doi.org/10.1097/00000542-197704000-00005.

Ueda, Y., Gunther-Harrington, C.T., Cruzen, C.L., Roberts, J.A., Stern, J.A., 2017. Echocardiographic parameters of clinically normal geriatric rhesus macaques (*Macaca mulatta*). J. Am. Assoc. Lab. Anim. Sci. JAALAS 56 (4), 361–368.

Undar, A., Eichstaedt, H.C., Clubb Jr., F.J., Lu, M., Bigley, J.E., Deady, B.A., Porter, A., Vaughn, W.K., Fung, M., 2004. Anesthetic induction with ketamine inhibits platelet activation before, during, and after cardiopulmonary bypass in baboons. Artif. Organs 28 (10), 959–962. https://doi.org/10.1111/j.1525-1594.2004.07377.x.

Valverde, C.R., Mama, K.R., Kollias-Baker, C., Steffey, E.P., Baggot, J.D., 2000. Pharmacokinetics and cardiopulmonary effects of fentanyl in isoflurane-anesthetized rhesus monkeys (*Macaca mulatta*). Am. J. Vet. Res. 61 (8), 931–934. https://doi.org/10.2460/ajvr.2000.61.931.

Vaughan, K.L., Szarowicz, M.D., Herbert, R.L., Mattison, J.A., 2014. Comparison of anesthesia protocols for intravenous glucose tolerance testing in rhesus monkeys. J. Med. Primatol. 43 (3), 162–168. https://doi.org/10.1111/jmp.12104.

Venkatesan, R., Nagarajan, P., Rajaretnam, R.S., Majumdar, S.S., 2006. Hematologic and serum biochemical values in aged female bonnet macaques (*Macaca radiata*) anesthetized with ketamine hydrochloride. J. Am. Assoc. Lab. Anim. Sci. JAALAS 45 (2), 45–48.

Vierboom, M., Breedveld, E., Keehnen, M., Klomp, R., Bakker, J., 2017. Pain relief in nonhuman primate models of arthritis. Methods Mol. Biol. 1559, 411–417. https://doi.org/10.1007/978-1-4939-6786-5_28.

Wada, S., Koyama, H., Yamashita, K., 2020. Sedative and physiological effects of alfaxalone intramuscular administration in cynomolgus monkeys (*Macaca fascicularis*). J. Vet. Med. Sci. 82 (7), 1021–1029. https://doi.org/10.1292/jvms.20-0043.

Wallis, J., Lee, D.R., 1999. Primate conservation: the prevention of disease transmission. Int. J. Primatol. 20 (6), 803–826.

Wickham, L.A., Kulick, A.A., Gichuru, L., Donnelly, M.J., Gai, C.L., Johnson, C.V., Hickey, E.J., Nagabukuro, H., 2011. Transurethral bladder catheterization of male rhesus macaques: a refinement of approach. J. Med. Primatol. 40 (5), 342–350. https://doi.org/10.1111/j.1600-0684.2011.00494.x.

Wolf, R.F., White, G.L., 2012. Clinical techniques used for nonhuman primates. In: Abee, C.R., Mansfield, K., Tardif, S.D., Morris, T. (Eds.), Nonhuman Primates in Biomedical Research: Biology and Management, 1. Academic Press, pp. 323–338.

Wolf, R.H., Lehner, N.D., Miller, E.C., Clarkson, T.B., 1969. Electrocardiogram of the squirrel monkey, *Saimiri sciureus*. J. Appl. Physiol. 26 (3), 346–351. https://doi.org/10.1152/jappl.1969.26.3.346.

Woolfson, M.W., Foran, J.A., Freedman, H.M., Moore, P.A., Shulman, L.B., Schnitman, P.A., 1980. Immobilization of baboons (*Papio anubis*) using ketamine and diazepam. Lab. Anim. Sci. 30 (5), 902–904.

Wright, M., 1982. Pharmacologic effects of ketamine and its use in veterinary medicine. J. Am. Vet. Med. Assoc. 180 (12), 1462–1471.

Yamaoka, A., Koie, H., Sato, T., Kanayama, K., Taira, M., 2013. Standard electrocardiographic data of young Japanese monkeys (*Macaca fusucata*). J. Am. Assoc. Lab. Anim. Sci. JAALAS 52 (4), 491–494.

Yeoman, R.R., Williams, L.E., Hazelton, J.M., Ricker, R.B., Abee, R.C., 1988. The effects of brief manual restraint, prior conditioning and ketamine sedation on lutenizing hormone and estradiol levels in the female Bolivian squirrel monkey. Am. J. Primatol. 14 (4), 454–455.

Yeung, K.R., Lind, J.M., Heffernan, S.J., Sunderland, N., Hennessy, A., Makris, A., 2014. Comparison of indirect and direct blood pressure measurements in baboons during ketamine anaesthesia. J. Med. Primatol. 43 (4), 217–224. https://doi.org/10.1111/jmp.12113.

Young, J.T., Vlasova, R.M., Howell, B.R., Knickmeyer, R.C., Morin, E., Kuitchoua, K.I., Lubach, G.R., Noel, J., Hu, X., Shi, Y., Caudill, G., Alexander, A.L., Niethammer, M., Paule, M.G., Coe, C.L., Sanchez, M., Styner, M., 2021. General anaesthesia during infancy reduces white matter micro-organisation in developing rhesus monkeys. Br. J. Anaesthesia 126 (4), 845–853. https://doi.org/10.1016/j.bja.2020.12.029.

Zevin, A.S., Moats, C., May, D., Wangari, S., Miller, C., Ahrens, J., Iwayama, N., Brown, M., Bratt, D., Klatt, N.R., Smedley, J., 2017. Laparoscopic technique for serial collection of liver and mesenteric lymph nodes in macaques. JoVE 123, 55617. https://doi.org/10.3791/55617.

Zhao, F., Fan, X., Grondin, R., Edwards, R., Forman, E., Moorehead, J., Gerhardt, G., Wang, X., Zhang, Z., 2010. Improved methods for electroacupuncture and electromyographic recordings in normal and parkinsonian rhesus monkeys. J. Neurosci. Methods 192 (2), 199–206. https://doi.org/10.1016/j.jneumeth.2010.07.016.

Zola-Morgan, S., Micheletti, C., 1986. Respiration rate, heart rate, and body temperature values in cynomolgus monkeys (*Macaca fascicularis*) during barbiturate anesthesia. J. Med. Primatol. 15 (6), 399–408.

Chapter 19

Anesthesia and analgesia in dogs and cats

Jennifer Davis[1,2] and Gabrielle C. Musk[1,3]
[1]*School of Veterinary Medicine, Murdoch University, Murdoch, WA, Australia;* [2]*Animalius Vet, Bayswater, WA, Australia;* [3]*Animal Care Services, University of Western Australia, Crawley, WA, Australia*

Chapter outline

Anesthesia and Analgesia in Laboratory Animals. https://doi.org/10.1016/B978-0-12-822215-7.00020-2

I. Introduction

Although dogs and cats represent a small proportion of the animals used for scientific purposes, both random sourced and bred for purpose dogs and cats are used for research and teaching around the world. In 2017, in Europe, a total of 9,388,162 animals were involved in research (European Commission, 2020). The number of dogs involved was 13,688 (0.15%), and the number of cats involved was 1879 (0.02%) (European Commission, 2020). Nevertheless, these species tend to attract special attention from the public when they are involved in research and teaching as they are popular pets and many people have strong emotional bonds with these species.

Dogs and cats involved in research and teaching are likely to be a relatively heterogeneous group of animals when compared to classic laboratory animals. This potential variation in genetics and demographics may require an approach to anesthesia and analgesia that is tailored to the individual animal as opposed to a strictly standardized protocol. The evidence base of anesthesia and analgesia is large, for both dogs and cats, as they are common species in veterinary practice and in veterinary clinical research. Furthermore, most veterinarians choosing a career in veterinary anesthesia and analgesia will, at least in their specialist training, work primarily with these two species. The vast knowledge and skills of such veterinarians provide an invaluable resource for ensuring a high standard of care for dogs and cats requiring anesthesia and/or analgesia in research and teaching.

II. Preprocedural considerations

A. Planning

1. Health and safety

Personnel working with dogs and cats should be appropriately trained in handling these species. Animals with a quiet and calm temperament should be selected above those that are easily distressed and nervous, as injury to both animals and personnel is more likely if animals do not cooperate when restrained. Personal protective equipment should always be worn and must be appropriate for the physical or biological containment level within which the animals are housed. Acclimatizing dogs and cats to a research and/or teaching environment is especially rewarding as these domestic species will adapt to a new environment if efforts are made to familiarize them with routines, procedures, and personnel.

2. Animal assessment

When formulating a sedation or general anesthesia plan, it is important to consider animal factors such as signalment and health status, as well as the procedure to be performed.

a. Species and breed considerations

There are several important differences between dogs and cats that are relevant to anesthesia and pain management. For example, the pharmacokinetics of some commonly used drugs, and the relative risk of certain complications. These species-related differences will be discussed in more detail in the relevant sections of this chapter.

Breed-specific concerns must also be considered. Some breeds of cats and dogs are more susceptible to certain diseases or malformations that may affect anesthesia, while others metabolize certain drugs differently. Large and giant dog breeds generally require lower doses of sedative and anesthetic drugs compared to the smaller breeds of dogs and cats, while toy dog breeds and cats are more at risk of hypothermia due to their relatively large body surface area. Specific breed related considerations are listed in Table 19.1.

b. History and records

Prior to anesthesia or sedation, an animal's history must be reviewed. Previous medical problems, and/or recent changes in appetite, thirst, urination, or defecation may alert the anesthetist to underlying medical conditions. Records from previous procedures should be reviewed with particular interest paid to the effects of administered drugs and any complications.

c. Physical examination

A thorough physical examination should be performed for every animal prior to sedation or anesthesia. Prior to touching the animal, an assessment for abnormal behaviors that might indicate fear, stress, anxiety, or pain should be performed at a distance. Cats and dogs that are extremely

TABLE 19.1 Breed-specific considerations for sedation and anesthesia of cats and dogs.

Breed	Consideration
Boxers	Anecdotal reports of sensitivity (bradycardia, hypotension, excessive sedation) to acepromazine. May affect certain lines of boxers. Consider avoiding acepromazine or using lower end of dose range
Brachycephalic breeds (e.g., bulldogs, pugs, Persian cats)	Increased risk of upper airway obstruction due to any combination of hypoplastic trachea, elongated soft palate, everted laryngeal saccules, and stenotic nares. Increased risk of gastroesophageal regurgitation due to frequent incidence of hiatal hernia.
Collies, Australian/Old English/Shetland sheepdogs, German shepherds	Increased incidence of multidrug resistance gene (MDR1) mutation leading to reduced elimination, and increased passage across the blood brain barrier, of certain drugs, including acepromazine and butorphanol. Consider testing for gene mutation prior to anesthesia, and/or avoid acepromazine and butorphanol.
Sighthounds and greyhounds	Slow recovery following barbiturate (and to a lesser extent, propofol) anesthesia due to low body fat and cytochrome P450 deficiency.
Dobermann	Increased incidence of von Willebrand's factor deficiency and therefore risk of bleeding during surgery.
Miniature schnauzer	Increased incidence of sick sinus syndrome.

fearful and difficult to handle may require sedation before a full physical examination can safely be performed.

d. Laboratory testing

Adult, nongeriatric, dogs, and cats that are assessed as healthy based on history and physical examination usually require no further diagnostic testing prior to anesthesia or sedation. However, the collection of blood for baseline packed cell volume (PCV) and total solids (TS) measurements to assess hydration status should be considered as the minimum data base for every animal undergoing anesthesia. If abnormalities are detected during the assessment of the history and physical examination, further laboratory investigations or diagnostic imaging may be required to further diagnose and determine anesthetic risk. Pediatric cats and dogs have an increased risk of hypoglycemia (especially following preanesthetic fasting), so a blood glucose measurement should be taken prior to anesthesia to guide the need for glucose supplementation. A serum biochemistry profile and complete blood count may be beneficial in geriatric animals to identify early renal or hepatic dysfunction and other chronic diseases that may affect anesthesia, such as anemia. Additional testing should be considered based on existing disease(s), breed predispositions (Table 19.1) and the nature of the planned procedure (e.g., preparation for a potential blood transfusion when there is a risk of hemorrhage).

B. Fasting

Traditionally, withdrawal of food 8–12 hours prior to sedation and general anesthesia has been recommended in dogs and cats to lessen the risk of vomiting, gastroesophageal regurgitation (GER), and aspiration. However, it is increasingly recognized that prolonged fasting may increase the risk of reflux, and reduce the pH of gastric contents and promote ileus. Additionally, as a large percentage of water intake occurs at mealtimes in dogs and cats, prolonged fasting increases the risk of dehydration. Prolonged fasting of very young and/or thin animals may lead to hypoglycemia. Based on current evidence, fasting from food for 4–6 hours prior to anesthesia appears appropriate, with provision of water until the time of sedation or premedication (Grubb et al., 2020). Ideally, the last meal given prior to fasting should be soft, easily digestible food (e.g., avoid dry kibble) that will not remain in the stomach at the time of induction of anesthesia.

C. Need for analgesia

It is well recognized that nociception occurs in cats and dogs and that they are capable of the cognitive and emotional experience of pain, thus analgesia forms an important part of peri-anesthetic care. Additionally, maladaptive (or chronic) pain that outlives or is out of proportion to the expected healing/duration of the initial nociceptive stimulus is recognized in these species and must be identified and managed.

D. Balanced anesthesia

Balanced anesthesia refers to the combination of antinociception (provision of analgesia), the unconscious state, and muscle relaxation. There is no single anesthetic drug that creates these conditions, so a combination of drugs must be administered to ensure a balanced anesthetic is achieved. Anesthetic drugs are almost always administered with analgesic drugs to meet this aim.

The concept of *preventive analgesia* should be considered when formulating an anesthetic plan for a cat or dog undergoing a procedure that is expected to produce nociception and pain. This concept involves the provision of analgesia throughout the perioperative period from prior to the initiation of nociception (i.e., at premedication), during the procedure itself, and during the recovery period (Clark, 2014). This approach leads to milder postoperative pain that is easier to manage, and potentially to an overall reduced consumption of analgesic drugs postoperatively.

The other important concept to consider is a *multimodal* approach to analgesia, where two or more analgesic drugs, with differing mechanisms of action, are used in combination. The benefits of this approach are better overall analgesia, with reduced doses of individual drugs, and therefore less chance of adverse effects.

Finally, acute perioperative pain management strategies should be developed to ensure that analgesic therapy is administered for an adequate duration of time after the procedure is performed. It may be that analgesia should be administered for multiple days after the procedure. This duration can be predicted to some extent, based on experience with the model, but should be informed by regular pain assessments.

III. Chemical restraint (sedation)

For minor or noninvasive procedures, heavy sedation may be sufficient to ensure the dog or cat is adequately restrained. Sedation is defined as a state of calm or sleep; however, a sedated animal should retain a gag reflex and therefore the ability to protect their airway from aspiration of gastric contents. The benefits of heavy sedation versus general anesthesia include reduced preparation time, a more rapid recovery (particularly if reversible agents are used), and a lack of intubation related complication (e.g., laryngospasm, cough). However, most sedative agents produce dose-dependent cardiorespiratory depression, which may be more difficult to identify and manage as sedated patients usually have a lower level of monitoring and vascular access compared to an anesthetized animal. Furthermore, heavy sedation without airway protection is contraindicated for certain animals including brachycephalic dog breeds and animals at increased risk of GER. Heavy sedation should be reserved for healthy, non-brachycephalic animals. Procedures that may be performed under sedation include a thorough physical examination and minor diagnostic procedures (e.g., venepuncture, ultrasonography) in animals that are difficult to handle. Minor surgical procedures in combination with loco-regional anesthesia techniques (e.g., cutaneous surgery), may also be performed under sedation. In projects where serial sampling or imaging is required, training animals to cooperate for the procedure may be worthwhile, to avoid the need for chemical restraint and the associated physiological side effects.

A. Agents: pharmacological options for sedation

Administration of sedative agents is ideally provided via the intramuscular (IM) or intravenous (IV) route as these drugs will most reliably and predictably produce a therapeutic plasma concentration of drug. In general, the higher end of a dose range is selected for IM administration, and the lower end for IV administration. Administration of a combination of more than one drug is usually recommended as this approach provides sedation with a lower dose of each drug. Most commonly, an opioid agonist is used in combination with another sedative drug from a different class (Table 19.2).

1. Opioids

Opioids provide analgesia, produce dose-dependent sedation, and are synergistic with most other sedative agents, allowing lower doses of those agents and more reliable and predictable sedation. These drugs have agonist or antagonist effects on opioid receptors including mu and kappa receptors. While pure mu-receptor agonists (e.g., morphine, methadone, and fentanyl) cause a dose-dependent reduction in heart rate and minute ventilation, their cardiovascular effects are milder than many other sedative agents. Pure mu receptor agonists, particularly when administered over days to weeks, have the potential to produce adverse effects in many body systems, for example, gastrointestinal ileus, and urinary retention. Opioids produce dose-dependent respiratory depression and assisted ventilation may be necessary when used in high doses during anesthesia. Opioid administration also disrupts thermoregulation; in dogs, this usually manifests as hypothermia, while hyperthermia may be observed in cats. Butorphanol (a kappa-receptor agonist) produces good sedation, both alone and in combination with other sedative agents, but only mild and short-lived analgesia (up to 2 hours), so it is best reserved for use during procedures not expected to cause nociception or

TABLE 19.2 Suitable sedative (or premedication[a]) drug combinations for use in cats and dogs.

Drug(s)	Species	Dose	Route	Duration	Antagonist	Comments
Phenothiazines and their combinations						
Acepromazine alone	Cat, dog	0.01–0.1 mg/kg	IM, IV (lower end dose range)	6–8 hours	None	Mild—moderate sedation (often poor effect as sole agent), slow onset (up to 45 minutes to peak effect) no analgesia. Use lower end of dose range in large and giant dogs; to a maximum total dose of 1 mg.
Acepromazine + opioid	Cat, dog	Acepromazine 0.1–0.05 mg/kg + Opioid agonist (see Table 19.10)	IM, IV (lower end dose range)	4–6 hours (analgesic duration depends on opioid choice)	Naloxone for full mu opioids only	Moderate sedation, mild-moderate analgesia (depends on opioid choice)
Acepromazine + opioid + ketamine	Cat, dog	Acepromazine 0.1–0.05 mg/kg + Opioid agonist (see Table 19.10) + Ketamine 1–5 mg/kg	IM	6–8 hours (analgesic duration depends on opioid choice)	Naloxone for full mu opioids only	Moderate—heavy sedation, moderate analgesia, higher doses of ketamine may result in anesthesia. Useful for dogs and cats that are difficult to handle and potentially dangerous.
Acepromazine +opioid + alpha 2 agonist	Cat, dog	Acepromazine 0.1–0.03 mg/kg + Opioid agonist (see Table 19.10) + Medetomidine 5–10 ug/kg Dexmedetomidine 2.5–5 ug/kg	IM	6–8 hours (analgesic duration depends on opioid choice)	Naloxone for full mu opioids only, atipamezole	Moderate—heavy sedation, moderate analgesia. Useful for dogs and cats that are difficult to handle and potentially dangerous.
Acepromazine + midazolam + ketamine	Cats	Acepromazine 0.03–0.05 mg/kg + Midazolam 0.25 mg/kg + Ketamine 2.5–5 mg/kg	IM	6–8 hours	Flumazenil for midazolam only	Useful for cats that are difficult to handle and potentially dangerous

Continued

TABLE 19.2 Suitable sedative (or premedication[a]) drug combinations for use in cats and dogs.—cont'd

Drug(s)	Species	Dose	Route	Duration	Antagonist	Comments
Alpha$_2$-adrenoreceptor agonists and their combinations						
Medetomidine alone Dexmedetomidine alone		5–20 μ/kg 3–10 μ/kg	IM, IV (lower end dose range) IM, IV (lower end dose range)		Atipamezole	
Medetomidine/ dexmedetomidine + opioid	Cats, dogs	Medetomidine 5–10 μ/kg or dexmedetomidine 3–6 μ/kg Opioid agonist (see Table 19.10)	IM, IV (lower end dose range)		Atipamezole, plus naloxone if pure mu agonist used	Can add midazolam 0.25 mg/kg or ketamine 1–5 mg/kg to this combination in cats for profound sedation of longer duration
Benzodiazepine combinations						
Midazolam/diazepam + opioid	Cats, dogs	Midazolam (or diazepam) 0.1–0.4 mg/kg + Opioid agonist (see Table 19.10)	IM, IV	Up to 2 hours	Flumazenil, naloxone if pure mu agonist	Good option for sick or very old animals. Likely to cause excitement and poor sedation in healthy dogs and cats.
Midazolam/diazepam + ketamine	Cats	Midazolam (or diazepam) 0.1–0.4 mg/kg + Ketamine 2–5 mg/kg	IM, IV	Up to 2 hours	Flumazenil	Produces heavy sedation/ anesthesia
Alfaxalone + opioid	Cats, dogs	Alfaxalone 1–2 mg/kg + Opioid agonist (see Table 19.10)	IM	~30 minutes		IM doses impractical in dogs >10 kg due to injection volume, moderate-heavy sedation, anesthesia may occur (must be ready to intubate). Onset of sedation can be within a few minutes. Monitoring oxygenation (pulse oximetry) and ability to provide oxygen recommended.
Propofol + fentanyl	Cats, dogs	Propofol 0.5 mg/kg increments Fentanyl 2–5 ug/kg	IV	~15 minutes	Naloxone for fentanyl only	IV route only, heavy sedation, anesthesia may occur (must be ready to intubate)

[a]When used for premedication prior to general anesthesia, the lower end of the dose ranges specified should be used. For opioid agonist doses please refer to Table 19.10.

pain. Buprenorphine is a weak agonist with high affinity (i.e., it has a long-lasting but not maximal effect) at mu-receptors and an antagonist at kappa-receptors. Buprenorphine can enhance sedation when used in combination with other agents and provides long duration (up to 12 hours), albeit mild, analgesia, so it should be reserved for procedures associated with no or mild pain. The factors to consider when selecting an opioid include the expected severity of pain associated with a procedure, the desired duration of action (Table 19.10), the route of administration (e.g., pethidine should not be given IV), and whether antagonism (reversal) is required (naloxone can be used to reverse full mu agonists only).

2. Acepromazine

Acepromazine produces tranquillization via dopamine receptor antagonism. Sedation is dose-dependent, although in some animals a "ceiling" effect may be observed. Although the onset of action is relatively slow (approximately 30 minutes), sedation is long-lasting (approximately 6 hours). When acepromazine is used alone, the sedative effects are unreliable, although they may be enhanced by the addition of an opioid. Other features of acepromazine include a mild antiemetic effect and antiarrhythmic effects. The main adverse effect of acepromazine is vasodilation, which may result in hypotension, reduced hematocrit, and hypothermia. Historically, there have been anecdotal reports of increased sensitivity to acepromazine in Boxers (associated with cardiovascular collapse), though this appeared limited to specific breeding lines and does not appear widespread (Table 19.1). Consequently, acepromazine is not contraindicated in this breed when its use is warranted. Acepromazine provides no analgesia, and the sedative effects cannot be antagonized.

3. Alpha$_2$-adrenoreceptor agonists

Alpha$_2$-adrenoreceptor agonists provide dose-dependent sedation in small animals via interactions with a_2 receptors in the brainstem. While the sedative effects of this class of drugs are generally reliable, a ceiling effect might be reached in some individuals, and occasionally an animal that appears heavily sedated can rouse unexpectedly. The combination of an alpha$_2$-adrenoreceptor agonist with an opioid agonist enhances sedation and reduces the likelihood of sudden arousal. The most commonly used alpha$_2$-adrenoreceptor agonist drugs in cats and dogs are medetomidine and dexmedetomidine. Xylazine is no longer recommended for routine use in these species due to its poorer cardiovascular safety compared to medetomidine (likely due to less selectivity for a_2 vs. a_1 receptors), and evidence that its use increases anesthetic mortality in cats and dogs (Clarke and Hall, 1990). Medetomidine is an equal mixture of two optical enantiomers, dexmedetomidine, and levomedetomidine, of which dexmedetomidine is the active enantiomer. Pharmacologically, the use of dexmedetomidine alone, rather than medetomidine, is theorized to produce more reliable sedation and analgesia and a more rapid metabolism. However, no clear clinical benefit of an equipotent dose of dexmedetomidine over medetomidine has been demonstrated, and in the authors' experience, the level of sedation provided by medetomidine is more reliable. Both agents produce significant minimum alveolar concentration (MAC) sparing effects with volatile anesthetics in cats and dogs, and so it should be remembered that lower doses of volatile anesthetic agents (by up to 70%) are required when these drugs have been administered. Medetomidine and dexmedetomidine have been shown to have an antinociceptive effect in dogs (Siegenthaler et al., 2020), and it is likely a similar effect occurs in cats. Both medetomidine and dexmedetomidine produce significant cardiovascular effects: an initial phase of bradycardia and peripheral vasoconstriction, followed by a fall in blood pressure as vasoconstriction wanes and bradycardia remains. A significant reduction in cardiac output occurs, mainly due to bradycardia, making it sensible to reserve these drugs for healthy animals. Alpha$_2$-adrenoreceptor agonists also produce a diuretic effect, so urine output should be monitored. A benefit of including medetomidine or dexmedetomidine in a sedation protocol is the availability of a specific antagonist: atipamezole. Atipamezole should be administered at 5 times the dose (mg/kg) of medetomidine/dexmedetomidine in dogs and 2.5 times the dose (mg/kg) of medetomidine/dexmedetomidine in cats. While atipamezole may be administered IV (0.1 mg/kg) during cardiopulmonary arrest (CPA) when alpha$_2$-adrenoreceptor agonist drugs have been administered, the IM route is recommended for routine use as large IV doses may result in sudden awakening (due to reversal of sedation and analgesia), and vasodilation that may cause cardiovascular collapse in the face of ongoing bradycardia. For these reasons, IV use is not a licensed route of administration.

4. Benzodiazepines

Diazepam or midazolam may be used to enhance the sedation provided by other drugs. However, use of these agents alone is not recommended, particularly in young, healthy dogs and cats, as they can cause excitement, disinhibition, and dysphoria in these species. Combinations of benzodiazepines and opioids may provide adequate sedation in geriatric, pediatric, or sick animals, with the benefit of minimal cardiovascular depression. However, while these drugs produce only mild cardiorespiratory depression, they may enhance respiratory depression produced by other agents, such as opioids. A specific antagonist is available: flumazenil (0.01−0.03 mg/kg IV).

5. *Injectable anesthetic drugs for sedation*

Administration of injectable anesthetics such as alfaxalone and propofol by the IV route may be useful when heavy sedation is required to facilitate certain procedures. Alfaxalone may also be administered IM, though it is usually reserved for use in cats and small dogs by this route due to the injection volume required. Ketamine is commonly used in combination with other sedative drugs to enhance sedation and provide additional analgesia, and it is often a good choice in difficult-to-handle cats and dogs. Readers should consult the anesthetic induction section of this chapter for further information on these drugs. It is important to note that these drugs can result in unpredictably deep sedation that progresses to anesthesia, so equipment to perform intubation and provide oxygen supplementation should always be available. Additionally, these drugs lack specific antagonists.

B. Monitoring and supportive care

It is important that cats and dogs are monitored appropriately during sedation. Although the reported rate of mortality associated with sedation is lower than during or after general anesthesia; at 0.12% and 0.07% in cats and dogs, respectively, this risk is still significantly higher than mortality rates for anesthesia in healthy people (<0.00001%) (Brodbelt et al., 2008). The heart rate and respiratory rate should be monitored at least every 5 minutes, ideally continuously. Noninvasive blood pressure monitoring and pulse oximetry are recommended during heavy sedation. Most sedative combinations produce dose-dependent respiratory depression that could result in hypoxemia, so oxygen supplementation (e.g., flow by using a mask) should be considered, particularly during heavy sedation. Most sedative drugs reduce lower esophageal sphincter tone, making regurgitation of gastric contents more likely. If heavy sedation abolishes the gag reflex, tracheal intubation should be performed.

IV. General anesthesia

A. Premedication

The main aims of premedication are to relieve animal anxiety and stress, making handling easier for placement of an IV catheter and anesthetic induction, and allowing lower doses of subsequent anesthetic drugs for induction and maintenance of anesthesia. Additionally, premedication should provide some preemptive analgesia, particularly if the planned procedure is likely to cause pain. Drugs used for premedication are the same as those detailed for chemical restraint (sedation), though usually in lower doses (i.e., the lower end of the dose ranges listed) to minimize cardiorespiratory depression that is likely to be exacerbated by anesthetic induction and maintenance drugs (Table 19.2).

As all premedications have the potential to result in cardiorespiratory depression, it is important that animals are moved to an area where they can be constantly observed following drug administration. Water should be removed from the cage/kennel following premedication to avoid gastroesophageal reflux (GER) and aspiration. Premedicated animals may lose body heat due to inactivity, a reduced metabolic rate, and vasodilation; so, prewarming may be considered to minimize the risk of hypothermia during anesthesia. This approach is particularly relevant in dogs and cats that are young, small, have a poor/thin fur coat, or are cachexic. Prewarming may be provided by using a forced air warmer within the animal's cage.

B. Induction of anesthesia

The steps from initiation of anesthetic drug administration until loss of consciousness, intubation of the trachea, and connection to an anesthetic breathing system (or transitioning to the maintenance phase of anesthesia) are referred to as induction of anesthesia. This period is a time when significant depression of the central nervous, cardiovascular, and respiratory systems occurs, and the anesthetist has limited capacity to monitor these physiological changes as they occur. Simultaneously, the anesthetist is prioritizing acquiring and securing control of a patent airway. For this reason, it is vital to be prepared for all eventualities prior to induction of anesthesia (Box 19.1). Additionally, safety checklists are increasingly being utilized in veterinary anesthesia as a tool to reduce human errors that could lead to patient morbidity or mortality. While many versions of safety checklists exist, most are based on the World Health Organization Surgical Safety Checklist and involve three time points where the entire team pauses and addresses the checklist: preinduction, preprocedure, prerecovery. An example of a checklist is included (Fig. 19.1) and the Association of Veterinary Anaesthetists provides checklists that are free to download (https://ava.eu.com/resources/checklists/). For dogs at an increased risk of hypoxemia (e.g., brachycephalic breeds), and all cats, it is advisable to preoxygenate the lungs prior to induction of anesthesia. The aim of preoxygenation is to increase the arterial partial pressure of oxygen to delay the development of hypoxemia (i.e., due to a delay or difficulty

BOX 19.1 Items that should be prepared prior to initiating induction of anesthesia in dogs and cats

Intravenous cannula placed and secured

Induction drug dose calculated and prepared in labeled syringe(s)

Intubation equipment (ETT, laryngoscope, topical local anesthetic spray) is ready and suitable for use

Oxygen source available

Emergency drugs easily accessible, doses precalculated

Anesthetic delivery equipment was assembled and tested

Monitors switched on and ready to use (e.g., correct NIBP cuff size selected)

UCVM
Pre-induction checklist

When should this be used?
Before induction of general anesthesia.
Who should be present?
All members of anesthesia team.

☐ **CONFIRM VERBALLY** with all team members: patient ID, owner consent, procedure & site

☐ **IV ACCESS** patent
☐ **AIRWAY EQUIPMENT** prepared and tested:
ET tubes [3], cuffs tested, tube tie, laryngoscope, lube, gauze
☐ **ET TUBE** insertion depth **PRE-MEASURED**

☐ **ANAESTHETIC MACHINE** checked today
☐ Breathing system **LEAK TESTED** for this case
☐ **APL VALVE** open
☐ **OXYGEN** pipeline supply **CONNECTED**
☐ **ADEQUATE OXYGEN** in E cylinder

☐ **DISTRIBUTION OF TASKS** between team members

☐ Patient/procedureal **RISKS IDENTIFIED & COMMUNICATED**

☐ **EMERGENCY INTERVENTIONS** available

Used in conjunction with: 1) pre-anesthesia checkout procedure, 2) pre-anesthesia equipment checklist

Adapted from: The Association of Veterinary Anaesthetists Anaesthetic Safety Checklist

Designed by: DSJ Pang (2019), VSY Leung

FIGURE 19.1 An example of a preinduction checklist (University of Calgary, Canada). *APL*, adjustable pressure limiting valve.

in intubation of the trachea, or preexisting pulmonary disease). Ideally, 100% oxygen is provided for 3–5 minutes using a well-fitting mask (Ambros et al., 2018). Adequate premedication assists with ensuring the animal tolerates the facemask.

C. Pharmacological options

1. Injectable agents

In most situations, the IV route of administration is preferred for the induction of anesthesia, to provide a smooth, rapid, and controllable loss of consciousness. However, in some situations where venous access cannot be obtained in a conscious animal (e.g., aggressive dog or cat), IM administration may be considered (Table 19.3).

a. Propofol

The phenol derivative propofol is currently one of the most common IV induction agents used in dogs and cats. Propofol may be cleared more slowly in cats due to their reduced ability to perform glucuronidation, a phase 2 biotransformation reaction (conjugation) required during the hepatic metabolism of certain drugs. Repeated doses or prolonged infusions of propofol should be avoided in cats due to slow recoveries and a risk of anemia. Propofol causes dose-dependent vasodilation and negative inotropy. Propofol commonly produces transient hypoventilation and apnea may occur if it is injected too quickly, or a large total dose is given. For induction of anesthesia, propofol should be administered over 60 seconds by injecting one quarter of the calculated dose every 15–20 seconds and assessing the level of consciousness after each incremental dose. A 1:1 (v:v) mixture of propofol and ketamine ("ketofol") has been used to induce anesthesia in dogs, resulting in better maintenance of heart rate and blood pressure, but a reduced respiratory rate (Martinez-Taboada and Leece, 2014).

b. Alfaxalone

Like propofol, the steroid anesthetic alfaxalone is now a commonly used IV anesthetic induction agent for dogs and cats due to its rapid and smooth provision of anesthesia for

TABLE 19.3 Injectable anesthetic agents used for induction of general anesthesia in cats and dogs.

Drug(s)	Species	Dose	Onset	Duration	Comments
Propofol	Cats and dogs	1–10 mg/kg IV (depending on premedication drugs and their effect)	60–90 seconds	10 minutes	Some animals experience pain on IV injection of propofol, in **dogs** this may be counteracted with a small dose of lignocaine IV immediately prior to administration of propofol (0.5–1.0 mg/kg).
Alfaxalone	Cats	Up to 5 mg/kg IM or IV	60–90 seconds (up to 10 minutes IM)	10 minutes	Consider coinduction with midazolam to reduce alfaxalone dose requirement (Zapata et al., 2018)
	Dogs	Up to 3 mg/kg IV			
Ketamine-diazepam	Cats and dogs	5 mg/kg ketamine + 0.25 mg/kg diazepam IV or IM	3 minutes (up to 10 minutes IM)	Up to 60 minutes	Can mix ketamine (100 mg/mL) with diazepam (5 mg/mL) at 1:1 (v:v) and administer at 1 mL per 10 kg lean body weight (or in increments to effect.) Midazolam can be used in place of diazepam.
Tiletamine-zolazepam	Cats and dogs	1–4 mg/kg IV 3–10 mg/kg IM			Provide adequate premedication to avoid rough and dysphoric recoveries
Thiopentone	Cats and dogs	2–10 mg/kg IV (up to 30 mg/kg if no premedication)	60–90 seconds	20–30 minutes	
Etomidate	Cats and dogs	Up to 3 mg/kg IV	60–90 seconds	10 minutes	Use with midazolam to offset myoclonus

a short duration. While excitement has been reported during recovery from alfaxalone in dogs and cats, in the authors' experience this is uncommon if animals are premedicated and provided with appropriate analgesia. For induction of anesthesia, alfaxalone should be administered over 60 seconds by injecting one quarter of the calculated dose every 15–20 seconds and assessing level of consciousness after each incremental dose. A benefit of alfaxalone is that it can be administered IM in animals where venous access is not possible. This route of administration is useful in fractious cats, where doses of up to 5 mg/kg IM may induce anesthesia. However, IM induction of anesthesia using alfaxalone is impractical in larger dogs due to the excessive injection volume required.

c. Dissociative anesthetics

Ketamine and tiletamine are dissociative anesthetics that produce anesthesia via interactions with various receptors in the brain and spinal cord that result in functional "disorganization" of the CNS. Anesthesia following a single IV injection of ketamine lasts slightly longer than that of propofol or alfaxalone. Like alfaxalone, ketamine can be administered via the IM route if venous access is not possible, however; pain on injection may occur. Tiletamine is available as a proprietary mixture with the benzodiazepine zolazepam (1:1 ratio) in many countries. Tiletamine has similar properties to ketamine, but the adverse effects are usually more pronounced, and the duration of sedative/anesthetic action is prolonged (up to 5 hours), with unpredictable recoveries and potential unfavorable emergence reactions. Repeated dosing is not recommended, as this approach may prolong the recovery period and contribute to a poor quality of recovery. The benefits of tiletamine include a long shelf life and small injection volumes.

d. Barbiturates

Barbiturates are a large family of anesthetic drugs that are derived from barbituric acid and produce dose-dependent hypnotic effects via interactions with $GABA_A$ receptors in the CNS. Thiopentone is the only barbiturate commonly used during the anesthesia of dogs and cats. The onset of action following an IV dose of thiopentone is rapid, with the duration of anesthesia being slightly longer than that of propofol or alfaxalone: 20–30 minutes. Following initial rapid uptake in the brain and other well-perfused tissues, thiopentone is redistributed to poorly perfused tissues such as fat, which has a large storage ability for lipid-soluble drugs like barbiturates. This pharmacokinetic feature means that residual sedation may persist for several hours following the administration of a single dose, particularly in animals with low body fat and/or reduced ability for metabolism via the P450 cytochrome system (e.g., sighthounds). Repeated doses will have a cumulative effect, so thiopentone should be used as a single dose for induction of anesthesia only. Thiopentone produces dose-dependent cardiorespiratory depression, including myocardial depression, vasodilation, and hypoventilation. Barbiturates do not provide any direct analgesic effects but do produce good muscle relaxation. Thiopentone produces a solution of very alkaline pH, which is a tissue irritant and, if administered peri-vascularly, may produce skin necrosis and sloughing. For this reason, solutions of a concentration no higher than 2.5% should be used in dogs and cats, and administration must be via a preplaced and secure IV catheter that has recently been flushed and checked for patency. When used without premedication, some clinicians advocate the use of an initial rapid bolus of ~1/2 of the calculated dose to overcome excitement reactions, followed by a slower injection "to effect". However, in the authors' experience, this is rarely necessary if the animal has been adequately premedicated.

e. Etomidate

Etomidate is an imidazole derivative that produces anesthesia via effects on $GABA_A$ receptors in the CNS. Etomidate produces anesthesia of a similar onset and duration to propofol and alfaxalone. Etomidate has no analgesic effects and provides poor muscle relaxation, so should be used with drugs that have a muscle relaxant effect, such as the benzodiazepines and opioid agonists. Etomidate produces minimal cardiovascular depression making it a popular choice in situations where cardiovascular stability is important; however, it suppresses cortisol production by the adrenal gland, which may be of concern in critically ill animals or following prolonged administration.

f. Coinduction of anesthesia

Coinduction of anesthesia is a technique by which an adjunct agent is administered IV with an injectable anesthetic induction agent to reduce the dose of that agent (thus minimizing cardiorespiratory depression) and/or enhance muscle relaxation. Agents commonly used for coinduction include the benzodiazepines (e.g., midazolam 0.1–0.2 mg/kg) and the short-acting opioid agonist fentanyl (2 μ/kg). When benzodiazepines are used for coinduction with propofol or alfaxalone in cats and dogs, it is recommended to administer ~¼ of the calculated induction dose of the anesthetic agent prior to administering the benzodiazepine to avoid dysphoria-like reactions. Hence, a small proportion of the dose of propofol or alfaxalone is administered initially, and followed by the dose of benzodiazepine, before anesthesia is induced with propofol or alfaxalone.

2. *Inhalational induction*

While induction of anesthesia in dogs and cats is possible with inhalational anesthetic agents delivered by facemasks or in specially designed induction chambers, this approach is discouraged. Firstly, this practice carries the risk of exposure of personnel to high levels of volatile anesthetics, as it is often difficult to find a well-fitting facemask, and opening an induction chamber to retrieve the animal will result in anesthetic vapor escaping. In addition, even sedated dogs and cats will generally find the process of inhalational induction stressful, and ethical concerns aside, this technique may result in cardiovascular instability during anesthesia and catecholamine-induced arrhythmias. As mentioned above, the time when an animal is losing consciousness, but the anesthetist does not yet have control of their airway, is one of the riskiest periods of anesthesia. Inhalational induction of anesthesia tends to take longer and the anesthetist's access to the animal is limited, meaning the likelihood of respiratory complications such as airway obstruction or aspiration of regurgitated stomach contents is higher. If inhalational induction is the only available option, it is important that an agent of low solubility yet high potency, such as isoflurane or sevoflurane, is chosen to allow for rapid induction of anesthesia. Sevoflurane is generally preferred over isoflurane as it has a less pungent odor and is less irritant to the airway than isoflurane. Desflurane is not a good choice for inhalational induction given its low potency, airway irritability, and high environmental impact as a greenhouse gas if released to the atmosphere.

If this technique is employed, it is important to manage the aforementioned risks by ensuring the animals are adequately sedated prior to induction of anesthesia. It is generally recommended to familiarize the animal with the mask or chamber by delivering 100% oxygen initially, then gradually increasing the percentage of inhalational agent administered over a couple of minutes. It is important that masks and chambers have a facility for the removal of waste gases so that rebreathing of carbon dioxide does not occur. In some instances, training and acclimatization of the dog or cat to the equipment for inhaled anesthesia (a facemask or chamber) may enable a smooth induction of anesthesia, but this approach would only be warranted in projects where repeated anesthesia is required and where there are contraindications to the use of injectable anesthetic drugs.

D. Endotracheal intubation

Following induction of anesthesia, endotracheal intubation is recommended, regardless of whether anesthesia will be maintained with injectable or inhalational agents, to maintain a patent and "sealed" airway for delivery of oxygen and ventilatory support, and avoidance of pulmonary aspiration of regurgitated gastric contents. If anesthesia is to be maintained with inhalational agents, then an ETT also serves as a delivery route and avoids environmental contamination with anesthetic agents (Fig. 19.2).

1. Preparation and equipment

As all induction agents have the potential to cause hypoventilation or transient apnoea, and reduce esophageal sphincter tone while abolishing the gag reflex, it is important to perform tracheal intubation promptly following the induction of anesthesia; thus, all equipment necessary for intubation should be prepared prior to anesthetic induction (Box 19.2).

A laryngoscope provides both an external light source and serves to retract the tongue and pharyngeal tissues to help visualize the larynx during tube placement. While laryngoscopes are particularly useful where visualization and intubation are difficult (e.g., laryngeal pathology, brachycephalic breeds), it is recommended to use them for every anesthetic so that the anesthetist becomes familiar with their handling and use. Veterinary-specific laryngoscopes are available and are easier to use than those intended for humans. Blades may be straight (e.g., Miller) or curved (e.g., Macintosh) and are selected based on personal preference or determined by the morphology of the animal.

Clear PVC-cuffed endotracheal tubes (ETT) are generally preferred for dogs and cats. However, some advocate the use of uncuffed tubes for cats given the risk of tracheal damage from an inflated cuff. When selecting an ETT, attention should be paid to both the diameter and length of the tube. The diameter should be the widest that can pass through the larynx and trachea without causing trauma. The tracheal diameter can be estimated by tracheal palpation. A guide to ETT size selection is provided in Table 19.4; however, readers should bear in mind that there is much variation between breeds, for example, brachycephalic breeds often have a hypoplastic (narrowed) trachea. While the ETT must be long enough that, when inserted, the cuff is distal to the larynx and the breathing system connector is just beyond the level of the incisors, it is important that an excessively long tube is not used. An ETT that is too long will increase the work of breathing, the risk of endobronchial intubation, and apparatus dead space. The ETT should be premeasured against the awake animal's body; ensuring the tip is level with the point of the shoulder, and the connector is level with the incisor teeth.

Alternatives to ETTs are supraglottic airway devices such as laryngeal mask airways (LMAs). These devices carry the advantages of being quick and easy to insert (once the technique is learned), with less irritation to the larynx and trachea. They may be useful in situations where

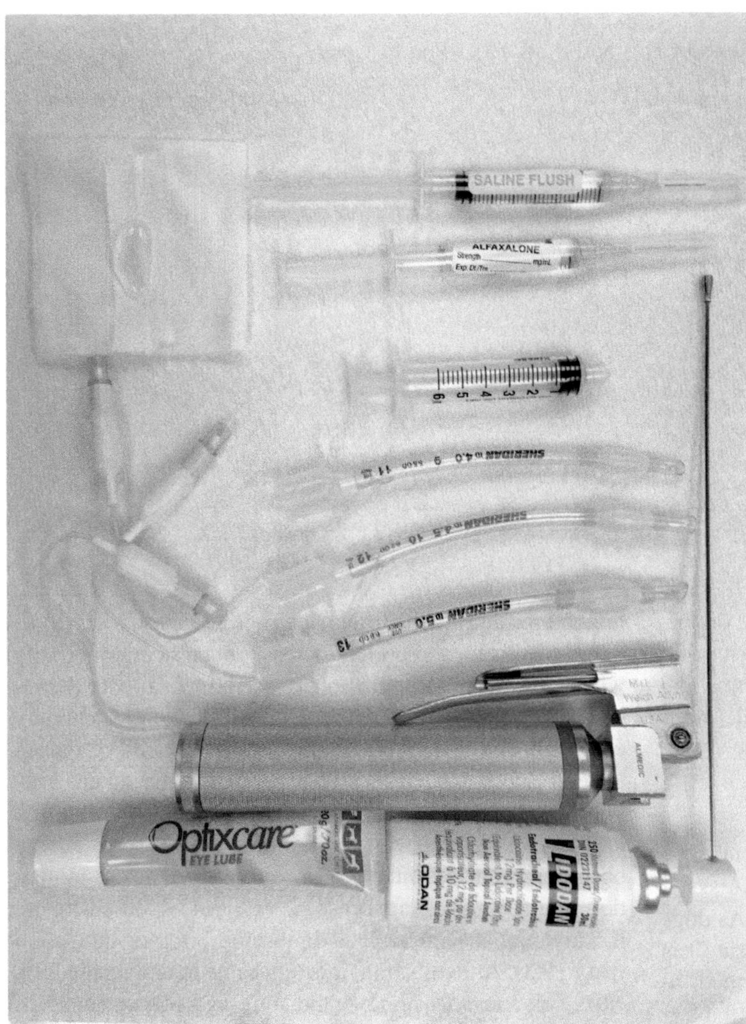

FIGURE 19.2 Materials prepared for endotracheal intubation in a cat. From *top to bottom*: gauze with lubricant and gauze to hold tongue (underneath), saline flush and intravenous induction agent, cuff syringe, 3 sizes of ETT, laryngoscope, lidocaine spray, eye lubricant. Note: the cuffs of the ETTs have been inflated for leak testing and will be deflated before induction of general anesthesia. In small cats, care should be taken that the combined dose of local anesthetic from the laryngeal spray (12 mg per dose, pictured) and any locoregional anesthesia techniques used does not exceed the toxic dose.

BOX 19.2 Items that should be prepared prior to endotracheal intubation in dogs and cats

Endotracheal tubes:

- minimum of three different sizes (internal diameters)
- trimmed to appropriate length to avoid excessive equipment dead space
- cuffs checked for patency

Laryngoscope:

- appropriate blade length and shape
- light checked

Tube tie (length of narrow gauze/bandage, or plastic tie)
Gauze swab (to hold the tongue)
Cuff inflation syringe
Sterile lubricant
Topical local anesthetic (cats): either lignocaine spray, or 0.1 mL lignocaine 2% injection in a 1 mL syringe (maximum total dose 6 mg/kg).

endotracheal intubation is difficult and persistence with attempts to intubate may result in hypoxemia and/or laryngeal trauma. However, they do not provide the same degree of airway protection as an ETT, so they carry a higher risk of aspiration environmental contamination with anesthetic gases. These devices may also increase airway resistance as a result of partial laryngeal compression, which may contribute to hypoxemia in prolonged procedures (Wenger et al., 2017). Additionally, the use of capnography to confirm correct positioning during anesthesia is vital due to the risk of them becoming displaced and potentially obstructing the airway. These devices are more

TABLE 19.4 Suggested endotracheal tube diameters for cats and dogs according to weight.

Species	Lean body weight (kg)	ETT size (internal diameter; mm)
Cat	<2	2.0–3.5
	2–4	3.0–4.5
	>4	3.5–5.0
Dog	<5	2.0–6.0
	5–10	5.0–8.0
	10–15	7.0–9.0
	15–20	8.0–10.0
	20–30	10.0–12.0
	>30	11.0–13.0

Note: predicting ET tube size in brachycephalic dog breeds is difficult and it is recommended to prepare a large selection of tubes.

likely to be used in cats given their higher risk of laryngospasm in this species. Indeed, veterinary-specific LMAs for cats (Cat v-gelÒ) are available and may be useful for short procedures in healthy, fasted, non-brachycephalic cats where capnography is available.

2. Dogs

Dogs are a relatively easy species to intubate as, in most breeds, the trachea is easy to visualize, and the risk of laryngospasm is low, compared to cats (Box 19.3). As dogs have a relatively high risk of GER during anesthesia, it is important that cuff inflation is carefully performed to ensure a good seal, and cuff deflation is delayed until a gag reflex is present.

3. Cats

Cats are a more challenging species to intubate given a relatively high risk of laryngospasm, endobronchial intubation, and tracheal damage/rupture. This is the most likely reason for a reported increase in anesthetic mortality when endotracheal intubation is performed in cats (Brodbelt et al., 2008). As the benefits of intubation generally outweigh the risks, intubation is recommended during general anesthesia in cats, but care must be taken. Laryngospasm in this species is easily triggered by manipulation of the larynx with the ETT and may lead to airway obstruction during intubation or recovery. During intubation, the risk of laryngospasm is reduced by desensitizing the arytenoids with topical lignocaine prior to intubation (Box 19.3). At extubation, it is advisable to deflate the ETT cuff early, and to remove the tube as soon as signs of increasing consciousness (e.g., ear flick, palpebral reflex) return to mitigate the risk of laryngeal trauma when the tube is removed. Endobronchial intubation will result in ventilation of only one lung, potentially causing hypoxemia, hypercapnia, and unstable anesthetic depth if using inhalational agents. Trimming the ETT to an appropriate length

BOX 19.3 Endotracheal intubation technique for cats and dogs

1. Position the animal in sternal recumbency. Assistant holds upper jaw open with one hand, other placed behind head to extend head and neck.
2. Operator opens the mouth and pulls out the tongue, using a gauze swab for grip.
3. The laryngoscope and tongue are both held in the nondominant hand—the laryngoscope is used to depress the tongue and allow visualization of the larynx. The laryngoscope should not touch the larynx.
4. CATS: apply topical lignocaine to the arytenoid cartilages (without touching them) and wait for at least 30 seconds before intubating (provide oxygen via mask or flow-by).
5. Pass the ETT over the epiglottis and through the larynx between the arytenoid cartilages, into the trachea. Do not attempt to force the tube through a closed larynx (especially cats); wait with the tip of the ETT close to the epiglottis and advance gently as soon as the larynx opens.
6. Tie the tube in place by securing the tube tie around the tube and then tying it around the mandible or maxilla, behind the canine teeth, or behind the ears.
7. Confirm placement in the trachea (i.e., direct visualization, capnography, palpation).
8. Connect the ETT to the breathing system with oxygen flowing.
9. Gradually inflate the cuff with air until no leaks are audible when a manual positive pressure breath at an inflation pressure of 15–20 cmH_2O is delivered.

prior to insertion will reduce the risk of endobronchial intubation. Cats' fragile tracheas put them at increased risk of tracheal mucosal damage and even tracheal rupture. Care must be taken to avoid excessive cuff inflation (Box 19.3), and some clinicians choose to use uncuffed tubes to intubate cats (however, this approach increases the risk of aspiration and environmental contamination by anesthetic agents). The ETT must always be disconnected from the breathing system prior to moving an anesthetized cat to avoid accidental tracheal damage (Fig. 19.3).

E. Maintenance of anesthesia

1. *Inhalational anesthesia*

a. Pharmacological options

The volatile anesthetic agents most often used for maintenance of anesthesia in dogs and cats are isoflurane and sevoflurane. Despite sevoflurane theoretically producing a faster recovery due to lower solubility compared to isoflurane, clinically, anesthesia and recovery characterises are similar between the two (Bennett et al., 2008). Halothane is less commonly used due to reduced availability and a higher incidence of adverse cardiovascular effects (e.g., cardiac arrhythmias). The theoretical benefits of desflurane (faster onset/offset) are usually outweighed by its cost and negative environmental impact. However, if a particularly rapid recovery from anesthesia is desirable, desflurane may be the best choice (Lopez et al., 2009). All fluorinated volatile agents produce dose dependent cardiovascular and respiratory depression in dogs and cats. If volatile agents are used alone, 1.25–1.5 times MAC is generally required to maintain general anesthesia (Table 19.5); however, the use of long-lasting agents for premedication, infusions of analgesic and anesthetic agents during anesthesia, and loco-regional anesthesia techniques can dramatically reduce inhalational anesthetic requirements (Reed and Doherty, 2018a, 2018b).

b. Delivery equipment

Volatile anesthetics should be delivered by precision vaporizers incorporated into an anesthetic machine. Anesthetic machines and workstations incorporating ventilators designed for use in people are suitable for use in dogs and cats; however, veterinary-specific workstations are now available with ventilators that offer lower minimum tidal

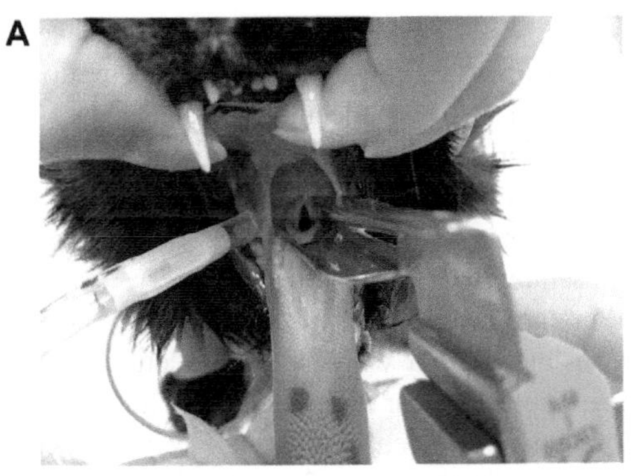

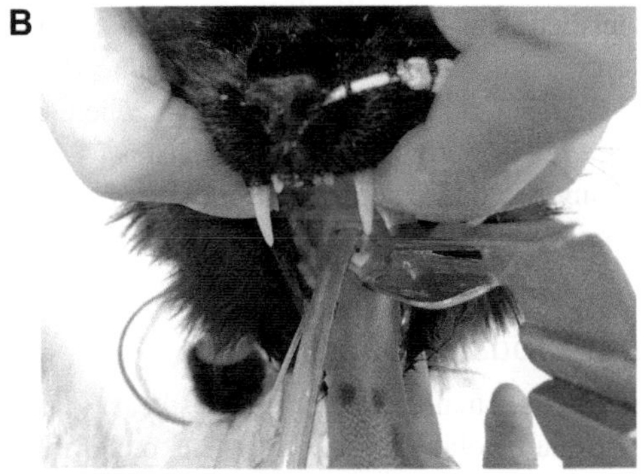

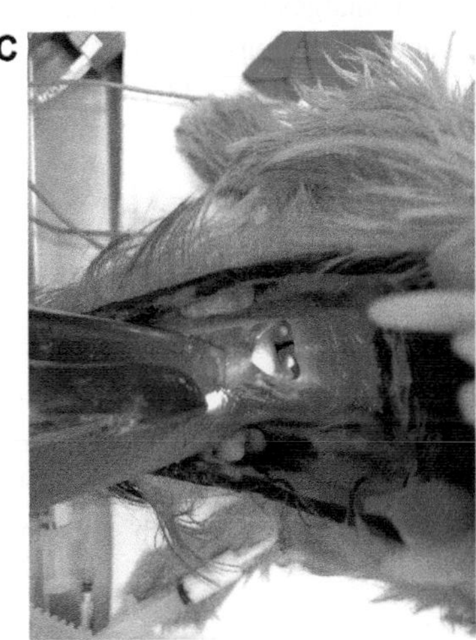

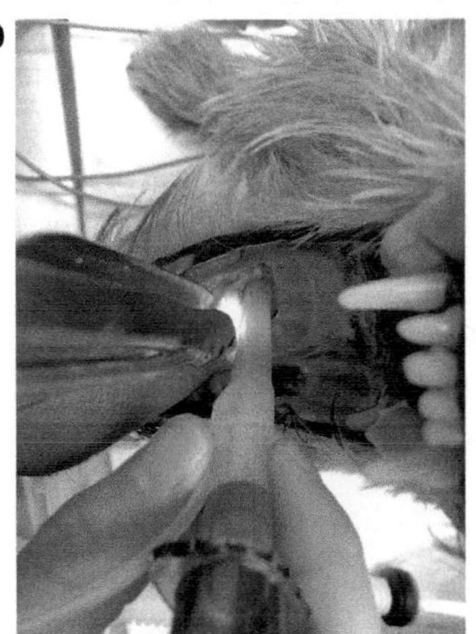

FIGURE 19.3 (A) View of the epiglottis and larynx of a cat in position for orotracheal intubation. (B) View of the ETT passing into the larynx of a cat. (C) View of the epiglottis and larynx of a dog in position for orotracheal intubation. (D) View of the ETT passing into the larynx of a dog.

TABLE 19.5 Minimum alveolar concentration (MAC) of volatile anesthetic agents in dogs and cats—data in table is range of values reported in various studies (Steffey et al., 2015).

	MAC dogs (%)	MAC cats (%)
Halothane	0.86–0.93	0.99–1.19
Isoflurane	1.28–1.50	1.28–2.21
Sevoflurane	2.10–2.36	2.58–3.41
Desflurane	7.2–10.3	9.8–10.3

volumes (e.g., Mindray VETA 5). Nonrebreathing or pediatric circle rebreathing systems should be used for cats and dogs <10 kg, while circle rebreathing systems are suitable for dogs >10 kg. When nonrebreathing systems (e.g., Bain, T-piece) are used, it is recommended that gas flow rates above minute volume are used to avoid rebreathing of carbon dioxide; 200 mL/kg/minute is a suitable starting point for dogs and cats. For circle systems, flow rates of 2–4 L/minute should be used for the first 5–10 minutes of anesthesia to allow concentrations of oxygen and anesthetic gas to equilibrate within the system (denitrogenation), then flow rates can be reduced to 0.5–1.0 L/minute. Flow rates lower than these may be used with rebreathing systems, provided the anesthetist is trained in low-flow techniques and end-tidal anesthetic agent and oxygen monitoring are available.

2. *Total intravenous anesthesia*

In certain situations, maintenance of anesthesia with injectable rather than volatile agents may be preferable. These situations include those where access to an anesthetic machine and oxygen is limited, or when the side effects of volatile anesthetic agents are undesirable (e.g., animals with elevated intracranial pressure (ICP)). Although an anesthetic machine is not necessary for total intravenous anesthesia (TIVA) delivery, it is important to remember that injectable anesthetic drugs all cause dose-dependent cardiorespiratory depression. Thus, tracheal intubation should always be performed, and oxygen supplementation should be provided wherever possible. Anesthetic monitoring requirements during TIVA are the same as during inhaled anesthesia.

a. Pharmacological options

<30 minutes For short procedures, repeated top-up doses of injectable anesthetic agents that do not have a significant cumulative effect are possible. Drugs with this favorable pharmacokinetic profile include propofol, alfaxalone, and ketamine. Doses of ~1/4 of the induction dose may be administered when required (to ensure an adequate depth of anesthesia). If ketamine dosing is repeated, it is important that repeat dosing of a muscle relaxant drug such as midazolam or diazepam is also considered. Intermittent IV dosing will lead to peaks and troughs in the plasma concentration of the drug and result in the same pattern of peaks and troughs in anesthetic depth, which may also lead to cardiorespiratory depression following each repeated dose.

>30 minutes For TIVA of longer duration, variable-rate infusions of injectable anesthetic agents are recommended—to produce smoother (avoiding peaks and troughs of plasma concentration of drug and anesthetic depth) anesthesia with a lower overall dose of drug and subsequently a more rapid recovery. Propofol and alfaxalone are most suited to TIVA as they are rapidly cleared from the plasma with minimal accumulation in the body. See Table 19.6 for infusion rates. The addition of analgesic infusions (e.g., fentanyl) to a TIVA protocol allows for a reduction in the dose of an anesthetic agent as well as the provision of analgesia. Target-controlled infusion of propofol is reported in dogs and is a good option for TIVA in this species (Beths et al., 2001; Musk et al., 2005).

TABLE 19.6 Total IV anesthesia drugs and doses for use in cats and dogs.

Drug	Species	Intravenous infusion rate for maintenance of general anesthesia	Comment
Alfaxalone	Cat	6–10 mg/kg/hour	
	Dog	4–9 mg/kg/hour	Respiratory depression commonly reported during alfaxalone TIVA in dogs; oxygen supplementation advised.
Propofol	Cat	12 mg/kg/hour	Limit propofol infusions to <60 minutes in this species.
	Dog	12–30 mg/kg/hour	

3. Partial intravenous anesthesia

Partial IV anesthesia involves the use of anesthetic or analgesic infusions in addition to a volatile agent for the maintenance of anesthesia. The theory behind this practice is that it allows for the administration of lower doses of all drugs, and therefore potentially a lower incidence of adverse effects. Ultimately, this approach provides balanced anesthesia. The concept of *balanced anesthesia* involves the use of more than one drug to provide all the important elements of general anesthesia: unconsciousness, muscle relaxation, and analgesia. Traditionally, this method has involved the addition of opioid infusions to volatile anesthesia to reduce the dose of the volatile agent and provide analgesia. However, it is becoming more common to use a *multimodal* approach to anesthesia whereby multiple IV agents are used in addition to a volatile agent: for example, an infusion of both an opioid and an alpha-2 adrenoreceptor agonist. Options for analgesic infusions that might be used in a multimodal anesthetic regime are in Table 19.10.

F. Neuromuscular blocking agents

Neuromuscular blocking agents are rarely required during anesthesia of dogs and cats as, unlike people, these species are generally easy to intubate and tolerate assisted ventilation readily. Specific indications include during thoracotomy to facilitate controlled mandatory ventilation, to aid surgical access during certain procedures (though the benefit is controversial), to maintain a central eye position during ocular surgery, and to ensure lack of patient movement during procedures where any movement could have devastating consequences (e.g., some neurological or cardiac surgeries). Depolarizing neuromuscular blocking agents that can be used in dogs and cats and their doses are listed in Table 19.7. For more detail on the pharmacology of each agent, refer to Chapter 8. As these agents produce paralysis of respiratory muscles, ventilatory support must be provided until adequate spontaneous respiration returns. The use of neuromuscular blocking agents makes monitoring anesthetic depth more difficult as these drugs abolish the peripheral reflexes commonly used to assess depth. Therefore, close attention should be paid to physiological parameters and the use of anesthetic agent concentration is recommended. Anesthetists must receive specific training and initial supervision in the use of these agents. Ideally, neuromuscular blockade should be monitored using a peripheral nerve stimulator (e.g., using a train-of-four stimulus pattern). In most cases, neuromuscular blockading agents should be reversed prior to recovery from anesthesia, even if there is evidence of the return of neuromuscular function, using reversal agents as listed in Table 19.7. Reversal ensures that there is no residual blockade of the respiratory muscles that may cause hypoventilation during recovery or of the laryngeal muscles, which could result in laryngeal paralysis.

V. Anesthetic management and monitoring

A. Monitoring during anesthesia

The overall aims of anesthetic monitoring are to ensure adequate oxygen delivery to vital tissues and ensure appropriate anesthetic depth. Anesthetic mortality rates reported in healthy cats and dogs are 0.11% and 0.05%, respectively, again, far higher than those reported in people despite similar anesthetic drugs and equipment being used (Brodbelt et al., 2008). The primary cause of death in >70% of these cases was a cardiovascular and/or respiratory cause; thus, continuous monitoring of these body systems is vital. Identifying trends in monitoring parameters is important so that abnormalities can be identified and managed early. For this reason, having a trained team member dedicated to monitoring anesthesia and noting each parameter at 5-minute intervals on an anesthetic record is an essential part of mitigating anesthetic risk.

1. Depth of anesthesia

Anesthetic depth can be estimated in dogs and cats by assessing the loss of reflexes, muscle relaxation, ocular position changes, autonomic nervous system activity, and electroencephalography (EEG). Assessment of changes in these various features helps the person responsible for anesthesia determine the extent of central nervous system depression and the adequacy of anesthesia and analgesia. In these species, the most common subjective methods to monitor anesthetic depth are assessment of the palpebral reflex, pedal withdrawal reflex, and jaw tone. However, bear in mind that frequent checking of the palpebral reflex may lead to overstimulation, and that jaw tone may be misleading in certain breeds with large facial musculature (e.g., bulldogs) or in kittens and puppies where jaw tone is naturally lax. If access to the head is not possible during a procedure, assessment of the perineal reflex (anal tone) may be useful. Eyeball position is a relatively reliable indicator of anesthetic depth in dogs and cats; the eye rotates ventromedially as anesthesia deepens but becomes central again at excessive anesthetic depth, and as the animal wakes up. Objective measurements that help interpret whether an animal is adequately anesthetized are related to the cardiovascular and respiratory systems. Generally, increased or unstable heart rate, blood pressure, and respiratory rate indicate lightning anesthetic depth. However, some animals will hold their breath when too lightly anesthetized, and occasionally, a light anesthetic depth

TABLE 19.7 Neuromuscular blocking drugs and reversal agents suitable for use in cats and dogs during anesthesia.

Agent	Dose	Duration of effect	Comment
Nondepolarizing neuromuscular blocking agents			
(Cis)Atracurium	Loading/intermittent IV: 0.25–0.5 mg/kg IV IV infusion: 0.4–0.5 mg/kg/hour IV infusion	20–40 minutes	Administer slowly due to risk of histamine release
Rocuronium-cats	0.3–0.6 mg/kg IV	15 minutes	Doses of 1–1.5 mg IV have been used during difficult tracheal intubation (Doodnaught and Pang, 2017)
Rocuronium-dogs	Loading/intermittent IV: 0.5–0.6 mg/kg IV IV infusion: 0.2 mg/kg/hour IV infusion	15–30 minutes	
Vecuronium	Loading/intermittent IV: 0.1 mg/kg IV infusion: 0.1 mg/kg/hour	20 minutes	
Antagonists to neuromuscular blocking agents			
Edrophonium	0.1–0.5 mg/kg IV		Preferred choice for atracurium reversal. Combine with atropine 0.04 mg/kg IV and administer slowly to effect.
Neostigmine	0.05–0.1 mg/kg IV		Preferred choice for vecuronium and rocuronium reversal. Precede with glycopyrrolate 0.01–0.02 mg/kg IV.
Sugammadex	2–8 mg/kg IV		Use to antagonize rocuronium or vecuronium (ineffective for benzylisoquinolones, such as atracurium)

produces a "vagal" response, leading to a fall in heart rate. Also, changes in heart rate and blood pressure may occur because of other factors such as altered fluid balance or in response to drug administration. Direct assessment of central nervous system depression is possible with EEG to monitor anesthetic depth, but this technique is not commonly utilized due to the cost of equipment, the requirement for considerable expertize, and a lack of species-specific evidence and devices.

2. Cardiovascular system

Most anesthetic agents, and many sedative and analgesic drugs, produce dose-dependent cardiovascular depression; hence, it is vital that the cardiovascular system is continuously monitored during general anesthesia. Cardiac output and arterial blood pressure are the main cardiovascular determinants of tissue oxygen delivery. While cardiac output may be measured in small animals using methods such as thermodilution, lithium dilution, and pulse contour analysis, continuous cardiac output monitoring is generally not practical in these species. However, heart rate and arterial blood pressure are major determinants of cardiac output that can easily be monitored. At a very minimum, heart rate should be monitored continuously during anesthesia. This is achieved by cardiac auscultation with a regular or esophageal stethoscope, pulse palpation, pulse oximetry, or ECG. Use of a pulse oximeter to measure the pulse rate has repeatedly been associated with reduced mortality in cats during anesthesia (Brodbelt et al., 2007; Matthews et al., 2017). For the continuous and most accurate measurement of arterial blood pressure, invasive measurements are acquired by attaching an arterial cannula (usually placed in the dorsal metatarsal artery in dogs and cats) to an electronic pressure transducer. However, placement of arterial cannula in these species, especially small dogs and cats, requires some experience to master, and it is not without risk (e.g., thrombosis, infection, hemorrhage). Noninvasive blood pressure monitoring can be performed using either an oscillometric device or Doppler-assisted sphygmomanometry. While oscillometry may be preferred as it measures systolic, diastolic, and mean pressures and is more "automatic", it is important to select a device that has passed validation criteria (e.g., ACVIM guidelines) for use in dogs or cats. While some devices have been shown to correlate well to invasive blood pressure measurements, others appear to be inaccurate in these species. Devices using high-definition oscillometry may be more accurate, particularly during bradycardia or other arrhythmias. The use of a Doppler flow probe with a sphygmomanometer can be used to measure arterial pressure, as well as to provide a continuous audible pulse sound. The probe is usually placed over the palmar aspect of the distal limb just proximal to the central pad, and the palmar metacarpal/metatarsal artery is auscultated. The probe may be secured in place to allow easy repeated measurements and continuous audible pulse rate monitoring. A cuff is placed proximal to the probe and inflated until the pulse sound is lost. The pressure at which the pulse sound returns approximates systolic arterial pressure in dogs. In cats, the Doppler technique underestimates systolic pressure and may represent a value closer to mean arterial pressure (Caulkett et al., 1998). For both oscillometric and Doppler techniques, best results are achieved if the cuff width is approximately 0.4 times the circumference of the limb (or tail) on which it is to be placed. In addition to blood pressure measurement, an estimate of perfusion and vascular tone may be made by assessment of capillary refill time and oral mucous membrane color, and palpation of peripheral pulses. Peripheral arterial pulses that may be palpated in dogs and cats include the dorsal metatarsal artery (dorsomedial aspect of metatarsus), palmar metacarpal artery (palmar aspect of fore-paws just proximal to central pad), and the lingual artery (ventral aspect of tongue, just off midline).

3. Respiratory system

Most anesthetic, sedative, and many analgesic drugs produce dose-dependent respiratory depression. The use of capnography allows rapid identification of hypoventilation (i.e., hypercapnia), as well as identifying equipment problems such as rebreathing or airway obstruction. As a minimum, the respiratory rate should be monitored continuously during general anesthesia. This measurement can be achieved by observing chest or breathing bag excursions, or ideally, with capnography. Monitoring oxygen saturation via pulse oximetry is a late indicator of respiratory depression in animals receiving oxygen supplementation, however, may assist in identification of sudden interruptions in oxygen supply and is useful during induction of anesthesia and recovery periods where oxygen supplementation is not being provided and hypoxemia is more likely. Additionally, as mentioned above, the use of pulse oximetry in cats is associated with a reduced risk of peri-anesthetic mortality (Brodbelt et al., 2007; Matthews et al., 2017). Pulse oximeter clips may be placed on the tongue, unpigmented toes, or other nonhairy, unpigmented areas such as the prepuce, vulva, ear flap, etc. In animals with pigmented skin where the tongue is inaccessible or too thin/small to obtain good contact (some cats), tail base or rectal reflectance probes may be of use.

4. Temperature

Hypothermia is one of the most frequently encountered anesthetic complications in dogs and cats, thus it is important to monitor temperature (Redondo et al., 2012a, 2012b). Ideally, core temperature is monitored continuously using an esophageal thermistor probe. Alternatively, digital thermometers can be used intermittently (every 10–15 minutes) to obtain a rectal temperature. In cats, auricular temperature measurements may be collected as an alternative to rectal measurements; while in dogs, auricular temperature measurement often underestimates core temperature (Greer et al., 2007; Sousa et al., 2013).

B. Peri-anesthetic support

Due to the dose-dependent cardiorespiratory depression induced by all anesthetic agents and the high risk of hypothermia during anesthesia; provision of oxygen, ventilation, fluid therapy, and warming are important support methods that should be considered for all anesthetized, or heavily sedated dogs and cats

1. Oxygen supplementation

Hypoventilation induced by anesthetic agents, and high doses of many sedative and analgesic drugs may lead to hypoxemia when breathing air at an oxygen concentration of 21%. It is recommended that during general anesthesia, a gas mixture containing at least 30% oxygen is provided via an ETT connected to an anesthetic machine. Facemasks or flow-by (tubing placed near to the face) oxygen delivered at 100–200 mL/kg/minute can increase the inspired oxygen concentration to up to 50% for animals that do not have an ETT in place (e.g., during recovery of sedation). It is important to ensure that the provision of oxygen to conscious animals does not lead to excessive stress and anxiety, as this can lead to increased oxygen demand and compromised ventilation (e.g., breath holding, airway obstruction). An oxygen cage may be a useful way to provide oxygen to stressed cats and small dogs during preanesthetic and recovery periods. However, such cages must have a mechanism for removal of CO_2 and control of temperature and humidity.

2. Ventilation

Indications for assisted ventilation during anesthesia include apnoea (common immediately postinduction in dogs and cats) and hypercapnia. Manual positive pressure may be administered by squeezing a rebreathing bag to generate inspiratory pressures of 5–15 cmH_2O until the animal resumes adequate spontaneous ventilation. Alternatively, automatic ventilators may be used. Initial settings in dogs and cats are tidal volume 8–15 mL/kg, peak inspiratory pressure 8–15 cmH_2O, frequency 8–20 breaths per minute, and inspiratory:expiratory ratio 1:2. Ventilators intended for use in adult humans may not allow setting of tidal volumes low enough to ventilate very small dogs and cats. Dogs and cats generally tolerate assisted ventilation well, and rarely require neuromuscular blocking agents to facilitate controlled mandatory ventilation.

3. Fluid therapy

The provision of intravenous fluid therapy during anesthesia is important for dogs and cats. Subclinical dehydration prior to anesthetic induction is common due to fasting (dogs and cats consume most of their daily water intake in and with food) and environmental stress (reluctance to drink, and loss via panting in dogs in a novel environment) (Costa et al., 2015). Additionally, fluid losses may occur due to drug administration (e.g., medetomidine/dexmedetomidine-induced diuresis) or surgical hemorrhage. Agreement upon intraoperative fluid rates that provide sufficient circulatory support without the risk of fluid overload in cats and dogs is controversial. Cats appear to be at a high risk of developing fluid overload, and the provision of fluids in this species has been associated with an increased risk of anesthetic mortality (Brodbelt et al., 2007). Regardless, in most animals, the circulatory-support benefits of fluid therapy outweigh the risk of fluid overload, and fluid therapy should be provided for all anesthetics over 30–60 minutes duration. Recommendations for dogs range from 5 to 10 mL/kg/hour and 3–5 mL/kg/hour for cats. A starting rate of 5 mL/kg/hour of a balanced isotonic crystalloid fluid such as lactated ringers' solution is a sensible approach for both dogs and cats. Animals assessed as dehydrated prior to anesthesia, or that suffer significant fluid losses during anesthesia may require higher fluid administration rates. High rate, bolus, and administration of fluids may be required to manage hypotension during anesthesia (see below).

4. Warming

Dogs and cats, particularly those of small body size and poor/thin fur coat are at particular risk of hypothermia during anesthesia due to drug-related depression of thermoregulation and peripheral vasodilation. As it can be difficult to warm an animal that is already hypothermic, one should aim to maintain body temperature >37.5°C from the beginning of anesthesia by means of active warming devices such as forced warm air blowers or thermostat-controlled patient warming blankets. Other types of heating pads (e.g., electric table pads or wheat bags/hot water bottles) are less effective, and when using these, it is important to ensure that thermal burns do not occur, by regularly checking the temperature of the blanket and placing a towel or blanket between the device and the animal. Exceeding a temperature setting of 42°C with warming devices is not recommended as the risk of thermal injury increases. When any active warming device is used, body temperature must be monitored to ensure that hyperthermia is avoided.

VI. Common anesthetic emergencies

A. Cardiovascular complications

Common cardiovascular complications encountered during anesthesia of dogs and cats are alterations in cardiac rate and/or rhythm, and hypotension.

Tachycardia most commonly occurs during anesthesia as a result of light anesthetic depth or in response to nociceptive stimulation. In these situations, the increase in heart rate is managed by treatment of the underlying cause: the provision of increases dose of anesthetic or analgesic agents, respectively. Tachycardia also occurs as compensation for low circulating blood volume or vasodilation. In these cases, the blood pressure will be low, and the correction of hypotension usually returns the heart rate to normal. Other causes of tachycardia include hypercapnia and hyperthermia. With the use of modern anesthetic agents, tachyarrhythmias are rare during anesthesia of healthy dogs and cats; however, these may be encountered in animals with underlying cardiomyopathy or electrolyte imbalances. Hypertrophic cardiomyopathy is relatively common in older cats and may be present without obvious clinical signs. Likewise, subclinical dilated cardiomyopathy may be present in certain dog breeds, including Doberman Pinscher, Great Dane, and Boxer breeds. Sustained or complex tachyarrhythmias, and those causing hemodynamic instability should be treated with an appropriate antiarrhythmic drug (Table 19.8).

Bradycardia is a common finding in small animal anesthesia and is often related to the administration of drugs that increase vagal activity, such as alpha-2 adrenoceptors agonists and mu receptor opioid agonists. Bradycardia in combination with a normal or high blood pressure is usually tolerated as it reflects a reflex mechanism to avoid excessive myocardial workload and oxygen consumption. If bradycardia leads to hypotension or if a significant bradyarrhythmia is present (e.g., high-degree AV block), then treatment with an antimuscarinic agent such as atropine or glycopyrrolate is advisable (Table 19.9). Administration of atropine to treat a_2-adrenoreceptor agonist induced bradycardia is usually contraindicated due to the risk of excessive myocardial workload due to high afterload and potential for serious cardiac arrhythmias. In this case, the bradycardia is usually tolerated if blood pressure is adequate. If blood pressure falls and it is >1 hour since a_2-adrenoreceptor agonist administration or if the patient has been receiving volatile anesthetic for >20 minutes, a small dose of an antimuscarinic may be trialled. Alternatively, atipamezole may be used to reverse the effects of the a_2 agonist (but beware potential hypotension due to vasodilation) or, in dogs, lignocaine may be used to offset the vagally medicated bradycardia (Tisotti et al., 2021). Bradycardia may also occur as a result of severe hypothermia, deep anesthesia, hypoxemia, hypervolemia, and hyperkalemia.

Hypotension (usually defined as MAP <60 mmHg, or SAP <80 mmHg) may arise during general anesthesia due to drug-induced cardiovascular depression, specifically myocardial depression, vasodilation, or bradycardia. The loss of circulating blood volume, for example due to intraoperative hemorrhage, may also lead to hypotension. Hypotension is a common complication even in healthy dogs and cats, with a reported frequency of up to 70% in young dogs undergoing sterilization (Costa et al., 2015). To treat hypotension, it is ideal to address the underlying cause; however, as this is often difficult to determine, a stepwise approach to managing hypotension is sensible (Fig. 19.4).

B. Regurgitation

In addition to cardiorespiratory depression and hypothermia, another common peri-anesthetic complication, in dogs particularly, is regurgitation of gastric contents into the esophagus. The frequency of GER in anesthetized dogs is reported to be up to 17%, and up to 33% in cats (Garcia et al., 2017; Torrente et al., 2017). Most anesthetic and

TABLE 19.8 Acceptable ranges for physiological parameters in anesthetized cats and dogs.

Parameter	Acceptable range of values for cats and dogs during anesthesia
Arterial blood pressure Systolic pressure Mean pressure Diastolic pressure	90–120 mmHg 60–100 mmHg 55–90 mmHg
End-tidal carbon dioxide	35–55 mmHg
Heart rate Cats Small-medium breed dogs Large/giant breed dogs	90–200 beats/minute 80–190 beats/minute 60–150 beats/minute
Peripheral hemoglobin oxygen saturation (Spo2)	>95%
Respiratory rate	6–40 breaths/minute
Temperature	37.5–39.0 °C

TABLE 19.9 Drugs used to manage cardiovascular complications during general anesthesia in cats and dogs.

Drug(s)	Action	Dose	Comments
Antimuscarinics			
Atropine	Increased heart rate via parasympatholytic effect	0.01–0.04 mg/kg IV	Duration of action 20–30 minutes. Higher doses likely to cause tachycardia. Lower doses may cause initial worsening of bradycardia.
Glycopyrrolate	Increased heart rate via parasympatholytic effect	0.005–0.02 mg/kg IV	Slightly slower onset compared to atropine, but duration of effect 2–3 hours. Less likely to cause severe tachycardia or paradoxical bradycardia than atropine.
Sympathomimetics			
Dopamine	Positive inotropy at lower doses via b_1 adrenergic agonism, peripheral vasoconstriction at higher doses via a_1 adrenergic agonism	5–20 μ/kg/minute IV	First-line sympathomimetic agent for management of hypotension in healthy dogs and cats. Rapid onset/offset—must be administered via constant rate infusion (usually diluted to 0.4 mg/mL).
Dobutamine	Positive inotropy via b_1 adrenergic agonism	2–10 μ/kg/minute IV (dogs) 1–5 μ/kg/minute IV (cats)	Rarely used to manage hypotension in healthy dogs and cats. May cause vasodilation due to b_2 adrenergic agonism at higher doses.
Ephedrine	Positive inotropy via direct b_1 adrenergic agonism, and peripheral vasoconstriction via indirect a_1 adrenergic agonism (upregulates presynaptic noradrenaline release)	0.05–0.1 mg/kg IV	Single dose lasts up to 20 minutes. Effect wanes over repeated doses due to depletion of noradrenaline stores (tachyphylaxis).
Norepinephrine (noradrenaline)	Predominantly vasoconstriction via a_1 adrenergic agonism, minimal b_1 effect	0.1–1 μ/kg/minute IV infusion	
Phenylephrine	Predominantly vasoconstriction via a_1 adrenergic agonism	2– 20 μ/kg IV 0.1–0.5 μ/kg/minute IV infusion	
Antiarrhythmics			
Esmolol	Type 2 antiarrhythmic: b_1 adrenergic antagonism	0.05–0.5 mg/kg slowly IV 25– 100 μ/kg/minute	Treatment for supraventricular tachyarrhythmias.
Lidocaine (lignocaine)	Type 1B antiarrhythmic: sodium channel blocker	1–2 mg/kg IV (dogs, and for emergencies only in cats). 25–100 μ/kg/minute IV infusion (dogs only)	First-line treatment for ventricular tachyarrhythmias. Useful for some supraventricular tachyarrhythmias. Use with great care in cats, and do not use by infusion in this species.
Magnesium	Effects on various ion channels/pumps	30 mg/kg IV over ~10–15 minutes	Used to treat refractory ventricular arrhythmias, and hypomagnesemia

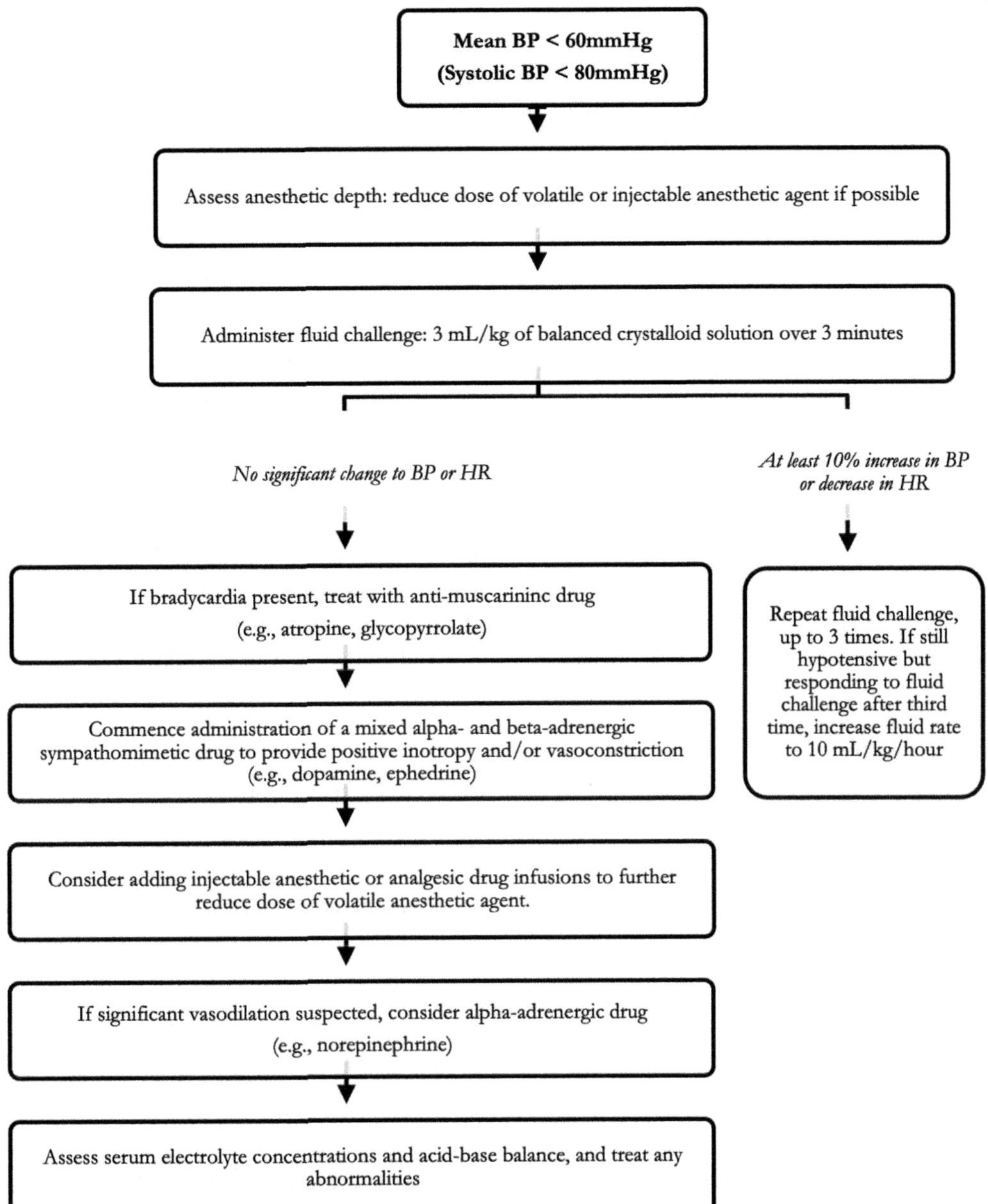

FIGURE 19.4 Stepwise approach to managing hypotension during general anesthesia in cats and dogs. *BP*, blood pressure; *HR*, heart rate.

sedative agents, and opioid agonists, reduce lower esophageal sphincter tone making GER more likely. The consequences of GER are damage to the esophageal mucosa by acidic gastric fluids and the potential for pulmonary aspiration, and the development of pneumonia. Tracheal intubation with a cuffed tube that is appropriately inflated is the best way to avoid aspiration pneumonia. To avoid aspiration during induction of anesthesia, dogs or cats at increased risk of GER should have their head extended above the level of their stomach until an ETTis placed and the cuff inflated. Suction should be available in case GER occurs during the induction of anesthesia. Small animals at increased risk of GER include brachycephalic dog breeds, those with a preexisting history of regurgitation and vomiting, pregnant animals, and those with gastrointestinal tract obstruction. During anesthesia, GER may be identified as the presence of colored fluid (frequently brown/green) in the animal's pharynx or nostrils, or on a table near the animal's head. In this case, the ETT cuff should be checked to ensure a seal is still present. The esophagus should then be suctioned to remove gastric fluid and can be lavaged with warm saline to increase the pH. However, many cases of GER in dogs are "silent"; regurgitant fluids do not reach the pharynx or nasal cavity and so go unnoticed. If regurgitation is noted to occur postextubation, during recovery, the animal's head should be lowered to allow drainage of fluid and avoid aspiration. Based on current evidence, it may be pertinent to pretreat animals at increased risk of GER with a proton pump inhibitor such as omeprazole (1 mg/kg orally) the evening before, and again, 3–4 hour prior to induction of anesthesia (Lotti et al., 2021; Panti et al., 2009; Garcia et al., 2017).

C. Cardiopulmonary arrest

Impending CPA in dogs and cats is usually identified by a rapid decrease in heart rate and end-tidal carbon dioxide. If CPA is suspected, time should not be wasted on attempts to palpate a pulse or commence additional monitoring; cardiopulmonary resuscitation (CPR) should be instigated immediately, and all anesthetic drug delivery ceased. For details on the provision of CPR, readers should refer to the most up-to-date version of the Reassessment Campaign on Veterinary Resuscitation (RECOVER) Initiative guidelines for dogs and cats (https://recoverinitiative.org/cpr-guidelines/current-recover-guideline/). The guidelines are summarized in Box 19.4. Asystole/pulseless electrical activity (PEA) is more commonly encountered than ventricular fibrillation during CPA in dogs and cats.

VII. Anesthesia for specific situations

A. Thoracotomy/thoracoscopy

Anesthesia of cats and dogs undergoing thoracotomy or thoracoscopy requires special consideration. The likelihood of hypoventilation and hypoxemia is increased due to altered intrathoracic pressure (i.e., the introduction of air into the thorax) and surgical manipulation of lung tissue. These procedures necessitate the application of positive pressure ventilation. Often, relatively complex ventilation strategies are required, for example, the provision of pressure-controlled ventilation and positive end-expiratory pressure (PEEP). It is recommended that mechanical ventilators are used and that personnel responsible for anesthesia have received special training. Additionally, neuromuscular blockade may be necessary to facilitate surgical access and effective positive pressure ventilation during these procedures. For certain procedures, it may be necessary to ventilate only one lung. This technique is a specialized procedure for which consultation with a specialist veterinary anesthesiologist is recommended. Surgical or interventional procedures within the thorax may also result in cardiovascular complications, for example, cardiac arrhythmias and/or rapid blood pressure changes due to manipulation of the heart or major blood vessels. Personnel responsible for anesthesia must be familiar with ECG identification of arrhythmias and their acute management and must be familiar with a range of treatments for intractable hypotension (e.g., positive inotropes, chronotropes, vasopressors).

B. Cardiac procedures

Anesthesia for interventional cardiovascular procedures or open-heart surgery in dogs and cats requires specialist consultation (both surgery and anesthesia) and planning. Significant cardiac arrhythmias and acute and severe hypotension are anticipated due to manipulation of the heart and major blood vessels. Personnel responsible for anesthesia must be familiar with the interpretation of the ECG and should be able to perform and interpret invasive blood

BOX 19.4 Approach to cardiopulmonary resuscitation in cats and dogs. Based on the 2012 RECOVER guidelines (Fletcher et al., 2012)

Basic life support (BLS)

1. Compressions: 100–120/minute; laterally @ 30%–50% chest width.
2. Ventilation: 10/minute; tidal volume 10 mL/kg, inspiratory time 1 second

Advanced life support (ALS)

3. Initiate monitoring ECG and end-tidal CO_2
4. Obtain vascular access
5. Administer reversal agents (e.g., naloxone, atipamezole, flumazenil)
6. Evaluate the animal and assess ECG. If no return of spontaneous circulation, continue BLS (1 cycle = 2 minutes), and specific therapy:

A. Asystole/pulseless electrical activity
Adrenaline (1:1000) 0.01 mg/kg IV (low dose), every other BLS cycles

Consider atropine 0.05 mg/kg IV, every other BLS cycle

For CPA >10 minutes, consider adrenaline (1:1000) 0.1 mg/kg (high dose) and bicarbonate therapy

B. Ventricular fibrillation (VF)/pulseless ventricular tachycardia (VT)
Defibrillation (or precordial thump).

If prolonged VF/VT consider amiodarone/lidocaine, adrenaline, increase defibrillator dose 50%.

pressure measurements. The ability to promptly provide appropriate treatment for cardiac arrhythmias and severe intractable hypotension is required. Cardio-pulmonary bypass is possible in dogs and cats but requires a collaborative approach from a highly specialized team, including specialist veterinary anesthesiologists.

C. Intracranial procedures

Anesthesia for dogs and cats that are undergoing intracranial procedures, or those with preexisting intracranial lesions poses a particular challenge. According to the Monroe-Kelly doctrine, the cranium is a fixed space consisting of brain tissue, cerebrospinal fluid, and blood vessels and their contents. An increase of any component leads to an increase in ICP and the potentially fatal consequence of brain herniation. As certain anesthetic drugs (e.g., inhalational anesthetic agents at doses above MAC, ketamine) and common anesthetic side effects (e.g., hypercapnia) elevate ICP, it is vital that these cases are carefully planned and managed. Additionally, intracranial surgery is associated with an increased risk of difficult-to-control hemorrhage, so the ability to provide an emergency blood transfusion must be available. The risk of serious complications, such as seizures and elevated ICP during the recovery is increased in these animals, so a recovery in a specialized intensive care unit is recommended. These procedures (surgery, anesthesia, and recovery) should only be performed by highly trained individuals.

D. Pregnancy

Anesthesia of pregnant dogs and cats brings two major challenges; overcoming the physiological changes of pregnancy that increase the risk of anesthetic complications for the mother, and consideration of fetal morbidity and mortality. Key physiological changes of pregnancy that affect anesthesia include reduced cardiac reserve (increased likelihood of hypotension), reduced functional residual capacity of the lungs (increased likelihood of hypoventilation and hypoxemia), reduced gastric motility and emptying, and reduced lower esophageal sphincter tone (risk of GER). Additionally, an altered response to anesthetic drugs must be anticipated as pregnancy leads to a decrease in MAC of inhalational anesthetics. To ensure the viability of fetuses, it is vital to maintain adequate uterine oxygenation and perfusion and to avoid using drugs that easily cross the placenta and may result in excessive sedation or anesthesia of the fetus. Pharmacological characteristics that favor placental transfer of drugs include low molecular weight, high lipid solubility, low plasma protein binding, and poor ionization. Unfortunately, most anesthetic, sedative, and analgesic drugs fulfill those criteria. A suggested anesthetic protocol for a pregnant dog or cat for a procedure other than whelping or caesarean section is premedication with an opioid alone (choice of full mu vs. butorphanol/buprenorphine depends on anticipated nociception and pain of procedure), induction of anesthesia with propofol or alfaxalone, and maintenance with isoflurane in oxygen. Where possible, additional analgesia should be provided using loco-regional anesthetic techniques to reduce systemic drug administration and so placental drug transfer.

For caesarean section, a similar protocol may be used; however, an additional challenge in this situation is the need for neonates to breathe spontaneously once delivered. Consequently, maternal administration of long-lasting agents that produce hypoventilation (e.g., barbiturates, some opioids) to the dam must be avoided. The use of opioids during caesarean section is an area of controversy with some veterinarians avoiding them until the puppies/kittens are birthed, and others using them with care. As opioids are arguably the main class of effective analgesic drugs to manage acute surgical pain in small animals, the authors recommend consideration of a low dose of a very short acting opioid as premedication prior to caesarean section, particularly for very anxious animals and/or in situations where the bitch/queen may have suffered pain associated with dystocia and attempted assisted birth prior to caesarean section. Epidural injection provides very effective analgesia for caesarean section, with minimal systemic absorption of drugs. However, it is important that the time between anesthetic induction and removal of puppies/kittens is kept to a minimum to avoid excessive sedation of neonates or harmful effects of reduced uterine perfusion/oxygenation. Thus, to minimize time, anesthetists must be skilled in the administration of epidural injection prior to their use in this setting. A suggested protocol for general anesthesia of a bitch or queen for caesarean section is as follows: no premedication, or low dose opioid (fentanyl 2–5 ug/kg IV) for anxious/painful animals (or where the epidural injection is not performed), induction with either propofol or alfaxalone (IV to effect), maintenance of anesthesia with isoflurane or sevoflurane in oxygen and lumbosacral (or sacrococcygeal) epidural injection of lignocaine (1 or 2%; 1 mL/7 kg to a maximum volume of 6 mL, note that lower volumes are used during pregnancy due to reduced volume of the epidural space) and morphine (0.1 mg/kg) prior to start of surgery. Inhalant anesthetic dose can often be significantly reduced following epidural injection. Rapid recovery of the mother and provision of adequate postoperative analgesia is vital to allow her to promptly feed and care for her puppies/kittens. Provision of adequate patient warming and oxygen supplementation assists with smooth anesthetic recovery. Postoperative analgesia may be provided with buprenorphine IV or IM.

Regardless of drug protocol used, for heavy sedation and anesthesia of pregnant animals, it is recommended to take additional steps to avoid hypoxemia, hypotension, and regurgitation. Preoxygenation should always be provided, with care taken to keep the head elevated until endotracheal intubation and cuff inflation is performed. Positive pressure ventilation should be commenced early to manage hypoventilation or apnoea, and fluid therapy must be administered to support the cardiovascular system.

Following delivery, a separate team of staff should be available to provide care, and resuscitation if needed, to the newborn animals. The neonate's head and mouth should be gently cleaned of membranes and fluid. Swinging the animal to remove fluid is not recommended due to the risk of traumatic injury. Suctioning of the mouth and nose may be necessary. Breathing can be stimulated by gentle rubbing of the newborn with a warm towel. Flow-by oxygen should be provided, and in some cases, intubation using an IV catheter may be attempted in order to provide positive pressure ventilation. If spontaneous ventilation is delayed and opioids were administered to the mother, 1−2 drops of naloxone may be administered sublingually, IM, or intranasally. The use of doxapram as a respiratory stimulant in newborns is controversial and is unlikely to be effective when used sublingually in depressed and hypoxemic newborns. In case of cardiac arrest, lateral chest compressions can be performed using a thumb and finger at a rate of 2 per second.

E. Neonate/pediatric

Dogs and cats are considered to be neonates for the first 6 weeks of life, and pediatric for the first 12 weeks. These young animals display certain physiological characteristics that may affect their anesthetic risk. Hypoalbuminemia, increased blood-brain barrier permeability, low body fat percentage, and immature renal and hepatic systems result in an exaggerated and potentially prolonged effect from the most sedative, analgesic, and anesthetic drugs. Thus, doses should be reduced, and long-acting agents (e.g., acepromazine) are best avoided. Very young animals have a reduced cardiac reserve (i.e., a reduced ability to compensate for the cardiovascular depressant effect of anesthetic drugs) due to a limited ability to increase myocardial contractility or vascular tone; these animals rely on heart rate and adequate preload to maintain cardiac output. Thus, maintenance of preanesthetic heart rate and the provision of fluid therapy is important. However, the risk of fluid overload is increased due to centralization of circulating volume. Respiratory reserve is reduced due to low pulmonary reserve, and a highly compliant chest wall coupled with a high oxygen requirement due to increased metabolic rate. Thus, the provision of oxygen supplementation and the ability to provide ventilatory support when needed is important. Young animals, particularly neonates, are at increased risk of hypoglycemia associated with fasting prior to anesthesia, so it is recommended to provide soft easily digestible food up to a few hours prior to anesthesia and to provide a meal as soon as possible following anesthetic recovery. An immature thermoregulatory system results in an increased likelihood of hypothermia, so particular care should be paid to patient warming, with strategies such as prewarming considered.

A suggested anesthetic drug protocol for a neonatal puppy or kitten is as follows: premedication with midazolam (0.1−0.2 mg/kg IV or IM) and an opioid (choice depends on the procedure to be performed, use lower end of dose range, may require glycopyrrolate/atropine to offset bradycardia), induction with propofol or alfaxalone (IV, to effect), intubation and maintenance with isoflurane or sevoflurane in oxygen.

F. Prolonged anesthesia

Prolonged anesthesia over many hours may be required in some experimental or educational settings. Regardless of whether recovery from the procedure is intended, it is important to take the approach that the animal will recover. Preservation of as close to normal physiology as possible is important to reduce the impact of anesthesia and procedures performed on the quality of the data that is collected. Hence, comprehensive monitoring of the cardiovascular and respiratory systems is essential and should include ECG, capnography, pulse oximetry, and invasive blood pressure measurement. In addition, the measurement and management of body temperature is vital. While hypothermia is likely to occur, prolonged use of active warming devices or the use of low flows with rebreathing anesthetic systems may cause hyperthermia. Fluid therapy must also be carefully tailored for prolonged procedures with special attention paid to care of the bladder, which will fill during the procedure. The placement of a urinary catheter may be appropriate at the start of the procedure, as passive emptying of the bladder is not a reliable method to avoid overdistension. Care should also be taken to prevent drying of the cornea. The regular application of ocular lubricant is important to avoid postoperative corneal ulceration and associated pain. With regards to nutrition, it may be necessary to monitor and manage blood glucose concentrations and consider the provision of calories during the procedure, especially if the animal will recover from the procedure. A team of people responsible for anesthesia is required to allow for continuous monitoring of animals anesthetized for prolonged periods so personnel can have a break to look after their own physiology. Careful planning for prolonged procedures is especially important to ensure that adequate supplies of drugs and consumables are on hand. Calculations of drug quantities should be performed and appropriately budgeted. Engagement with veterinary anesthesiologists for the planning and performance of these procedures is recommended.

VIII. Postprocedural recovery and care

A. Recovery period

The early recovery period following anesthesia is a high-risk period for cats and dogs. A multicentre study into peri-anesthetic mortality in small animals reported that two-thirds of feline deaths and one-third of canine deaths occurred in the first 3 hours postoperatively (Brodbelt et al., 2008). These statistics may be explained by the cessation of monitoring and support too early following the end of anesthesia. Removal of the ETT and oxygen supplementation at the end of anesthetic delivery carries the risk of hypoxemia if ventilation has not yet returned to normal. Endotracheal extubation is a high-risk period for laryngospasm in cats and airway obstruction in brachycephalic dog breeds.

1. Tracheal extubation—cats

As laryngospasm is a concern in cats, it is generally recommended that extubation is performed early during recovery, before the animal starts to move, so that there is minimal contact with the laryngeal tissue as the tube is removed. The presence of an ear flick when the inside of the pinna is gently touched generally indicates sufficient awakening for extubation in this species. Following extubation, the cat should be closely monitored for signs of laryngospasm (e.g., lack of airflow through mouth/nose, exaggerated chest movements). Should laryngospasm occur, the cat must be reanesthetized and reintubated immediately, for this reason, it is recommended to keep an induction dose of an injectable anesthetic and equipment for tracheal intubation close when recovering a cat from anesthesia.

2. Tracheal extubation—dogs

In contrast to cats, later extubation is generally recommended in dogs due to the risk of aspiration of regurgitated gastric fluids in this species. The presence of an ETT with an appropriately inflated cuff prevents pulmonary aspiration of fluid that might be present in the esophagus or pharynx until the animal has regained a sufficient gag reflex. Dogs should be extubated when swallowing has been observed. Brachycephalic breeds may be extubated even later to allow more time for muscle relaxation and sedation that may potentiate airway obstruction to resolve. These breeds often happily sit up and move around in their cage with an ETT in situ. However, extubation should be performed as soon as any chewing or distress is noted.

3. Emergence delirium/dysphoria

Sudden arousal following anesthesia in dogs and cats may result in distressed, dysphoric behavior including vocalization, paddling (in dogs), and excessive, uncoordinated motor activity. The likelihood of emergence delirium is lower when premedication was well managed and adequate analgesia provided. Ensuring an empty urinary bladder by palpation, and manual expression, prior to the end of anesthesia removes a full bladder as a potential cause of discomfort and stress. Dogs and cats should be recovered in quiet surroundings and should not be stimulated to wake up. Should delirium or dysphoria occur, it is important to distinguish it from pain. Gentle pressure around any surgical site or wound and the use of a species-specific acute pain scale (see below) will aid in identifying pain. Airway obstruction (e.g., laryngospasm in cats) may also appear like delirium. Once pain and airway obstruction have been ruled out, a small dose of a sedative agent, such as acepromazine (0.01−0.02 mg/kg IV) or medetomidine (1−2 μ/kg IV), may be administered. If sedated, appropriate monitoring and observation should be performed.

IX. Pain assessment and analgesia

A. Acute perioperative pain management

1. Pharmacological options

While there are many classes of drugs available for the management of acute pain in cats and dogs, well-established evidence for a clear beneficial effect exists only for three classes: NSAIDs, opioid agonists, and local anesthetics (when administered by a loco-regional route). These three classes of the drugs should form the mainstay of a perioperative analgesic plan, and other drug classes added as adjuncts where breakthrough pain is present and/or contraindications to any of these drugs exist (Table 19.10). A common, and sensible approach to perioperative analgesia, that incorporates both preventative and multi-modal concepts, is the use of a full mu opioid agonist (e.g., methadone) at premedication, a loco-regional block presurgery, and administration of an NSAID and repeated doses of opioid agonists postoperatively. For species-specific information on opioid agonists see "Chemical restraint" section above.

The use of NSAIDs in healthy dogs and cats is very common but the potential for adverse side effects from drugs in this class must be carefully considered. The administration of NSAIDs may result in adverse renal, gastrointestinal, and coagulopathic effects. For this reason, NSAIDs are contraindicated for use in animals with gastrointestinal symptoms such as vomiting (due to increased risk of gastrointestinal ulceration), those in which renal perfusion may be reduced, such as hypovolemia, and those at an increased risk of bleeding. Hepatotoxicity has been reported in Labrador retrievers after carprofen use, so this drug should be used carefully in this breed and in dogs

TABLE 19.10 Pharmacological agents used to provide an analgesic effect in cats and dogs.

Drug(s)	Species	Dose	Dosing interval	Comments
NSAIDs[a]				
Carprofen	Cats	4 mg/kg SQ	Once off (perioperative dose)	
	Dogs	4 mg/kg IV, SQ, or PO 2 mg/kg PO (maintenance dose)	Once off (loading dose) 12–24 hours	
Meloxicam	Cats	0.2 mg/kg SQ or PO **OR** 0.1 mg/kg PO	Once off (perioperative dose) 24 hours, for up to 3 days only	If required for >3 days, it is recommended that dose be tapered to the lowest possible (e.g., 0.05 mg/kg every other day).
	Dogs	0.2 mg/kg SQ or PO 0.1 mg/kg PO (maintenance dose)	Once off (loading dose) 24 hours	
Robenacoxib	Cats and dogs	2 mg/kg SQ 1 mg/kg (maintenance dose)	Once off (loading dose) 24 hours	
Grapiprant	Dogs	2 mg/kg PO	24 hours	NonCOX-inhibiting NSAID (specific prostaglandin receptor antagonist). For treatment of osteoarthritis in adult dogs. Do not use with NSAIDs or corticosteroids
Opioid agonists—full mu				
Methadone, morphine	Cats and dogs	0.1–0.5 mg/kg IV, IM, SQ	2–6 hours	Risk of histamine released with IV morphine—inject slowly (over 3–5 minutes). Morphine may cause vomiting. Sterile, preservative free morphine may also be administered epidurally or intraarticularly at 0.1 mg/kg)
		0.1 mg/kg hour IV infusion	n/a	
Hydromorphone	Cats and dogs	0.05–0.1 mg/kg IV, IM, SQ	4 hours	May cause vomiting.
		0.05–0.1 mg/kg/hour infusion	n/a	
Meperidine (pethidine)	Cats and dogs	3–5 mg/kg IM, SQ	1–1.5 hours	Do not use IV due to risk of histamine release. Heart rate is maintained or increased following pethidine administration due to an antimuscarinic effect
Fentanyl	Cats and dogs	1–2 μ/kg IV—loading dose 3–10 μ/kg/hour IV infusion	20–30 minutes n/a	Large interindividual variability is reported for transdermal update.
		Transdermal 3–5 μ/kg/hour	72 hours	
Opioid agonists—other				
Buprenorphine	Cats and dogs	0.01–0.03 mg/kg IV, IM, SQ, oral transmucosal (OTM)	4–12 hours	Duration is dose dependent (higher doses = longer duration of action). DOGS: OTM route is less reliable.
Butorphanol	Cats and dogs	0.1–0.4 mg/kg IV, IM, SQ	1.5–2 hours	Suitable for management of mild pain only. Infusion may be used for antitussive effect (e.g., following upper airway surgery)
		0.1–0.2 mg/kg/hour IV infusion	n/a	
Tramadol	Cats	1–4 mg/kg IV, IM, SQ, PO	12 hours	Also has nonopioid mechanisms of action (e.g., inhibition of serotonin and noradrenaline reuptake)

Local anesthetics				
Bupivacaine	Cats and dogs	*Dose depends on locoregional technique* Maximum safe dose: 2 mg/kg	Up to 12 hours, *depending on locoregional technique*	
Lidocaine (lignocaine)	Cats and dogs	*Dose depends on locoregional technique* Maximum safe dose: 6 mg/kg (cats), 10 mg/kg (dogs)	1–2 hours, *depending on locoregional technique*	Systemic lidocaine should not be used in cats due to increased risk of toxicity
	Dogs only	1–2 mg/kg IV—loading dose 25–50 μ/kg/minute infusion		
Ropivacaine	Cats and dogs	*Dose depends on locoregional technique* Maximum safe dose: 2 mg/kg (cats), 3 mg/kg (dogs)	Up to 8 hours, *depending on locoregional technique*	
Other (adjuncts)				
Amantadine	Cats and dogs	3–5 mg/kg PO	12–24 hours	NMDA antagonist, may be useful for chronic (maladaptive) pain; use for at least 21 days.
Ketamine	Cats and dogs	0.25–0.5 mg/kg IV, IM, SQ	Once off	Higher doses may cause dysphoria—use low end of dose range in awake animals
		0.1–0.6 mg/kg/hour IV infusion	n/a	
Gabapentin	Cats and dogs	5–20 mg/kg PO	8 hours	May cause sedation at higher doses
Paracetamol	Dogs only	10–15 mg/kg IV, PO	6–12 hours	Contraindicated in cats.
Bendinvetmab	Dogs	0.5–1.0 mg/kg SQ	Once monthly	Antinerve growth factor monoclonal antibodies, for alleviation of osteoarthritis pain in dogs
Frunevetmab	Cats	1 mg/kg SQ	Once monthly	Antinerve growth factor monoclonal antibodies, for alleviation of osteoarthritis pain in cats

Note: licensed doses vary by country and local licensing should be adhered to.
[a]*See text for contraindications/adverse effects.*

with significant liver disease. Cats are more prone to nephrotoxicity after NSAID use, but although additional care must be taken with their use this is not a reason to withhold NSAIDs in a healthy cat (Sparkes et al., 2010). Due to their inability to perform adequate hepatic glucuronidation, the use of paracetamol and systemic use of local anesthetics is contraindicated in cats due to increased risk of severe toxicity.

2. Loco-regional techniques

Loco-regional anesthesia is a particularly effective means of providing intraoperative, and potential postoperative analgesia, as the use of a local anesthetic applied appropriately has the potential to completely block nociceptive input to the central nervous system. Attention must be paid to toxicity limits of the local anesthetic agents, particularly in cats, as they are particularly sensitive to local anesthetic toxicity due to an inability to effectively metabolize these drugs (Table 19.10). Loco-regional anesthetic techniques have the additional benefit of reducing the amount of anesthetic agent required (i.e., MAC-sparing), which may enhance anesthetic stability and reduce the likelihood of adverse anesthetic events. In recent years, loco-regional techniques in dogs and cats have been a topic of vast and expanding research. Many techniques are performed using the guidance of peripheral nerve stimulators and/or ultrasound to increase the accuracy of their administration and their efficacy. Examples of loco-regional blocks appropriate for common surgical procedures are outlined in Table 19.11; however, readers are encouraged to reference specific texts for further information on specific blocks (Campoy and Read, 2013; Otero and Portela, 2018).

3. Acute pain assessment (see also Chapters 12 and 13)

As with all nonverbal species, identification and grading of pain can be challenging in dogs and cats. As the use of unidimensional scales is known to be highly subjective, it is recommended that validated, species-specific, multidimensional pain scales be used to assess postoperative pain where they are available. The most completely validated acute pain scale available for dogs is the Glasgow University Composite Measures Pain Scale-Short Form (CMPS-SF) (Reid et al., 2007). For cats, there are three validated acute pain scales available: the UNESP-Botucatu multidimensional composite pain scale (Brondani et al., 2013), the Glasgow University Composite Measure Pain Scale - Feline (www.newmetrica.com/) (Reid et al., 2017), and the Feline Grimace Scale (www.felinegrimacescale.com/) (Evangelista et al., 2019). Regardless of the scale chosen, it is important that it is used frequently in the postoperative period and that all staff involved in animal care are trained in its use. Most of these pain scales have intervention levels; scores at which analgesic (or additional analgesic) administration is recommended.

4. Chronic pain management (see also Chapters 13 and 27)

Types of chronic, or maladaptive pain, that may be encountered in dogs and cats include inflammatory pain conditions (e.g., osteoarthritis), cancer pain, and neurogenic pain (e.g., chronic postsurgical pain (CPSP)). In people, CPSP is well-recognized and arises due to maladaptive changes in the peripheral and central nervous systems. It has recently been acknowledged that CPSP may occur in animals that undergo painful procedures and is an important welfare issue that should be addressed in research settings (Clark, 2021). Although there are various, multifactorial risk factors for the development of CPSP, the severity of acute postoperative pain is a major determinant. Thus, careful attention to perioperative pain management (see above) is vital.

As for acute pain management, although there are many classes of analgesic drugs available to manage chronic pain in cats and dogs, only the use of NSAIDs and opioid agonists is supported by well-established evidence. Other agents may be used as adjuncts where these pain assessment reveals inadequate analgesia or when NSAIDs and/or opioids are contraindicated.

Regular pain assessment is important during the management of chronic pain and should be used to guide the choice of drugs, doses, and dosing intervals. Once a sufficient analgesic effect is obtained, doses and dosing intervals are often gradually reduced to the lowest level that provides sufficient therapeutic benefit. As mentioned above, the use of validated, species-specific pain scales is recommended where possible. Such scales include the Helsinki Chronic Pain Index (Hielm-Björkman et al., 2009) and Canine Brief Pain Inventory for dogs (Brown et al., 2007); and the Feline Musculoskeletal Pain Index (Benito et al., 2013) and the Cat Health and Wellbeing tool for cats (Freeman et al., 2016).

Nonpharmacologic methods that may be utilized as a part of a multimodal management plan for chronic pain in dogs and cats include nutraceuticals (e.g., glucosamine, chondroitin, omega-3 oils), rehabilitation therapies (e.g., cryotherapy, heat therapy, massage, passive range-of-motion exercise, hydrotherapy), and acupuncture (Chinese and/or Western). However, it must be noted that evidence for a beneficial analgesic effect is lacking for most of these therapies, so they should be considered adjuncts to the pharmacologic options mentioned above, and pain assessment should be regularly performed to assess for benefit.

TABLE 19.11 Examples of locoregional techniques that can be used to provide anesthesia for certain types of surgeries and pain in cats and dogs.

Procedure	Loco-regional techniques	Area desensitized	Level of difficulty
Oral surgery	Infraorbital nerve block	Maxillary teeth from first incisor to third premolar and associated soft tissues. *If needle tip is advanced into the canal, a caudal block to include the fourth premolar can be achieved.*	Easy
	Maxillary nerve block	All maxillary teeth and associated soft tissues. Skin of nose, cheek, and upper lip. Palatal and lateral nasal mucosa.	Easy
	Caudal alveolar nerve block	All mandibular teeth and associated soft tissues. Skin of rostral lower lip and rostral intermandibular region.	Easy
Nasal surgery/biopsies	Maxillary nerve block	As above	Easy
Aural surgery/pain	Great auricular nerve block	Pinna, vertical ear canal	Moderately easy
	Auriculo-temporal nerve block	Medial horizontal ear canal	Moderately easy
Thoracotomy	Epidural (lumbo-sacral, or more cranial)	Up to midthoracic level, depending on location performed and volume instilled	Moderately easy (lumbosacral) to difficult (cranial epidural injection)
	Intercostal nerve blocks	Lateral thoracic wall	Easy
	Intrapleural infiltration	Variable; thoracic wall and pleura	Easy (if chest drain in situ)
Abdominal surgery/pain	Lumbosacral epidural	Up to midthoracic level, depending on volume instilled	Moderately easy
	Transverse abdominis plane (TAP) block	Ventral and lateral abdominal wall (including skin, musculature, and mammary tissue)	Moderate (ultrasound guidance required)
Forelimb surgery	Cervical paravertebral block	Entire thoracic limb	Difficult
	Brachial plexus block	Distal to elbow (or from midhumerus if ultrasound guided approach)	Moderate
	Radial, ulnar, median, musculocutaneous (RUMM) block	Distal limb (carpus and below)	Moderate
	Digit (toe) block	Individual toes	Easy
	Intraarticular infiltration	Individual joints (e.g., for arthroscopy)	Depends on joint
Hindlimb surgery	Lumbosacral epidural	Entire pelvic limb, bilaterally	Moderately easy
	Psoas compartment block	Entire pelvic limb (unilateral)	Difficult
	Sciatic nerve block	Entire limb distal to femur when combined with femoral nerve block	Moderate
	Femoral nerve block	Entire limb distal to femur when combined with sciatic nerve block	Moderate
	Digit (toe) block	Individual toes	Easy
	Intraarticular infiltration	Individual joints (e.g., for arthroscopy)	Depends on joint
Perineal/tail surgery	Sacrococcygeal epidural	Perineum and tail (but may spread to pelvic limbs if large volume used)	Moderately easy

References

Ambros, B., Carrozzo, M.V., Jones, T., 2018. Desaturation times between dogs preoxygenated via face mask or flow-by technique before induction of anesthesia. Vet. Anaesth. Analg. 45, 452–458.

Benito, J., Depuy, V., Hardie, E., et al., 2013. Reliability and discriminatory testing of a client-based metrology instrument, feline musculoskeletal pain index (FMPI) for the evaluation of degenerative joint disease-associated pain in cats. Vet. J. (Lond., Engl.: 1997) 196, 368–373.

Bennett, R.C., Fancy, S.P.J., Walsh, C.M., et al., 2008. Comparison of sevoflurane and isoflurane in dogs anesthetised for clinical surgical or diagnostic procedures. J. Small Anim. Pract. 49, 392–397.

Beths, T., Glen, J.B., Reid, J., et al., 2001. Evaluation and optimisation of a target-controlled infusion system for administering propofol to dogs as part of a total intravenous anesthetic technique during dental surgery. Vet. Rec. 148, 198–203.

Brodbelt, D.C., Blissitt, K.J., Hammond, R.A., et al., 2008. The risk of death: the confidential enquiry into perioperative small animal fatalities. Vet. Anaesth. Analg. 35, 365–373.

Brodbelt, D.C., Pfeiffer, D.U., Young, L.E., et al., 2007. Risk factors for anesthetic-related death in cats: results from the confidential enquiry into perioperative small animal fatalities (CEPSAF). Br. J. Anaesth. 99, 617–623.

Brondani, J.T., Mama, K.R., Luna, S.P., et al., 2013. Validation of the English version of the UNESP-Botucatu multidimensional composite pain scale for assessing postoperative pain in cats. BMC Vet. Res. 9, 143.

Brown, D.C., Boston, R.C., Coyne, J.C., et al., 2007. Development and psychometric testing of an instrument designed to measure chronic pain in dogs with osteoarthritis. Am. J. Vet. Res. 68, 631–637.

Campoy, L.L.V., Read, M.R., 2013. Small Animal Regional Anesthesia and Analgesia, first ed. John Wiley & Sons, Inc.

Caulkett, N.A., Cantwell, S.L., Houston, D.M., 1998. A comparison of indirect blood pressure monitoring techniques in the anesthetized cat. Vet. Surg. 27, 370–377.

Clark, L., 2014. Pre-emptive or preventive analgesia—lessons from the human literature? Vet. Anaesth. Analg. 41, 109–112.

Clark, L., 2021. Chronic (or persistent) postsurgical pain: a veterinary problem? Vet. Anaesth. Analg. 48, 4–6.

Clarke, K.W., Hall, L.W., 1990. A survey of anesthesia in small animal practice: AVA/BSAVA report. Vet. Anesth. Analg. 17, 4–10.

Costa, R.S., Raisis, A.L., Hosgood, G., et al., 2015. Preoperative factors associated with hypotension in young anesthetised dogs undergoing elective desexing. Aust. Vet. J. 93, 99–104.

Doodnaught, G.M., Pang, D.S., 2017. Intubation following high-dose rocuronium in a cat with protracted laryngospasm. J. Feline Med. Surg. Open Rep. 3, 2055116917733642.

European Commission, 2020. 2019 Report on the Statistics on the Use of Animals for Scientific Purposes in the Member States of the European Union in 2015–2017 Brussels.

Evangelista, M.C., Watanabe, R., Leung, V.S.Y., et al., 2019. Facial expressions of pain in cats: the development and validation of a Feline Grimace Scale. Sci. Rep. 9, 19128.

Fletcher, D.J., Boller, M., Brainard, B.M., et al., 2012. RECOVER evidence and knowledge gap analysis on veterinary CPR. Part 7: clinical guidelines. J. Vet. Emerg. Crit. Care 22, S102–S131.

Freeman, L.M., Rodenberg, C., Narayanan, A., et al., 2016. Development and initial validation of the Cat HEalth and Wellbeing (CHEW) Questionnaire: a generic health-related quality of life instrument for cats. J. Feline Med. Surg. 18, 689–701.

Garcia, R.S., Belafsky, P.C., Della Maggiore, A., et al., 2017. Prevalence of gastroesophageal reflux in cats during anesthesia and effect of omeprazole on gastric pH. J. Vet. Intern. Med. 31, 734–742.

Greer, R.J., Cohn, L.A., Dodam, J.R., et al., 2007. Comparison of three methods of temperature measurement in hypothermic, euthermic, and hyperthermic dogs. J. Am. Vet. Med. Assoc. 230, 1841–1848.

Grubb, T., Sager, J., Gaynor, J.S., et al., 2020. 2020 AAHA anesthesia and monitoring guidelines for dogs and cats. J. Am. Anim. Hosp. Assoc. 56, 59–82.

Hielm-Björkman, A.K., Rita, H., Tulamo, R.M., 2009. Psychometric testing of the Helsinki chronic pain index by completion of a questionnaire in Finnish by owners of dogs with chronic signs of pain caused by osteoarthritis. Am. J. Vet. Res. 70, 727–734.

Lopez, L.A., Hofmeister, E.H., Pavez, J.C., et al., 2009. Comparison of recovery from anesthesia with isoflurane, sevoflurane, or desflurane in healthy dogs. Am. J. Vet. Res. 70, 1339–1344.

Lotti, F., Twedt, D., Warrit, K., et al., 2021. Effect of two different pre-anesthetic omeprazole protocols on gastroesophageal reflux incidence and pH in dogs. J. Small Anim. Pract. 62 (8), 677–682.

Martinez-Taboada, F., Leece, E.A., 2014. Comparison of propofol with ketofol, a propofol-ketamine admixture, for induction of anesthesia in healthy dogs. Vet. Anesth. Analg. 41, 575–582.

Matthews, N.S., Mohn, T.J., Yang, M., et al., 2017. Factors associated with anesthetic-related death in dogs and cats in primary care veterinary hospitals. J. Am. Vet. Med. Assoc. 250, 655–665.

Musk, G.C., Pang, D.S., Beths, T., et al., 2005. Target-controlled infusion of propofol in dogs—evaluation of four targets for induction of anesthesia. Vet. Rec. 157, 766–770.

Otero, P.E., Portela, D.A., 2018. Manual of Small Animal Regional Anesthesia, second ed. Editorial InterMedica SA.

Panti, A., Bennett, R.C., Corletto, F., et al., 2009. The effect of omeprazole on oesophageal pH in dogs during anesthesia. J. Small Anim. Pract. 50, 540–544.

Redondo, J.I., Suesta, P., Gil, L., et al., 2012a. Retrospective study of the prevalence of postanesthetic hypothermia in cats. Vet. Rec. 170, 206.

Redondo, J.I., Suesta, P., Serra, I., et al., 2012b. Retrospective study of the prevalence of postanesthetic hypothermia in dogs. Vet. Rec. 171, 374.

Reed, R., Doherty, T., 2018a. Minimum alveolar concentration: key concepts and a review of its pharmacological reduction in dogs. Part 1. Res. Vet. Sci. 117, 266–270.

Reed, R., Doherty, T., 2018b. Minimum alveolar concentration: key concepts and a review of its pharmacological reduction in dogs. Part 2. Res. Vet. Sci. 118, 27–33.

Reid, J., Nolan, A., Hughes, J., et al., 2007. Development of the Short-form Glasgow Composite Measure Pain Scale (CMPS-SF) and Derivation of an Analgesic Intervention Score. Animal Welfare.

Reid, J., Scott, E.M., Calvo, G., et al., 2017. Definitive Glasgow acute pain scale for cats: validation and intervention level. Vet. Rec. 180, 449.

Siegenthaler, J., Pleyers, T., Raillard, M., et al., 2020. Effect of medetomidine, dexmedetomidine, and their reversal with atipamezole on the nociceptive withdrawal reflex in beagles. Animals (Basel) 10, 1240.

Sousa, M.G., Carareto, R., Pereira-Junior, V.A., et al., 2013. Agreement between auricular and rectal measurements of body temperature in healthy cats. J. Feline Med. Surg. 15, 275–279.

Sparkes, A.H., Heiene, R., Lascelles, B.D., et al., 2010. ISFM and AAFP consensus guidelines: long-term use of NSAIDs in cats. J. Feline Med. Surg. 12, 521–538.

Steffey, E.P., Mama, K.R., Brosnan, R.J., 2015. Inhalation anesthetics. In: Grimm, K.A., Lamont, L.A., Tranquilli, W.J., et al. (Eds.), Veterinary Anesthesia and Analgesia: The Fifth Edition of Lumb and Jones, fifth ed. John Wiley & Sons, Inc., Iowa, USA, pp. 297–331.

Tisotti, T., Valverde, A., Hopkins, A., et al., 2021. Use of intravenous lidocaine to treat dexmedetomidine-induced bradycardia in sedated and anesthetized dogs. Vet. Anaesth. Analg. 48, 174–186.

Torrente, C., Vigueras, I., Manzanilla, E.G., et al., 2017. Prevalence of and risk factors for intraoperative gastroesophageal reflux and post-anesthetic vomiting and diarrhea in dogs undergoing general anesthesia. J. Vet. Emerg. Crit. Care 27, 397–408.

Wenger, S., Müllhaupt, D., Ohlerth, S., et al., 2017. Experimental evaluation of four airway devices in anaesthetized New Zealand White rabbits. Vet. Anaesth. Analg. 44, 529–537.

Zapata, A., Laredo, F.G., Escobar, M., et al., 2018. Effects of midazolam before or after alfaxalone for co-induction of anesthesia in healthy dogs. Vet. Anaesth. Analg. 45, 609–617.

Chapter 20

Anesthesia and analgesia in ruminants

Jenelle Izer[1], Cathy Dwyer[2] and Ronald P. Wilson[1]

[1]*Department of Comparative Medicine, College of Medicine, The Pennsylvania State University, Hershey, PA, United States;* [2]*Animal and Veterinary Sciences, Animal Welfare, Safe & Improved Food Challenge Centre, Scotland's Rural College, Edinburgh, United Kingdom*

Chapter outline

I. Introduction

Sheep, goats, and calves are the most common ruminants used in biomedical research, testing, or training and this review will be limited to those species. As large animal models, they are docile, adapt well to frequent handling, restraint, and chronic instrumentation that may be dictated by research needs. They are readily available either as purpose-bred or farm-raised, conditioned animals. Sheep of any age and size are the most common small ruminants encountered in the research setting. This species, and to a lesser extent, goats are utilized in cardiovascular research, medical device implantation and testing, pharmacokinetic studies, regenerative medicine, orthopedic research, fetal surgery, and pulmonary studies. With recent advances in gene editing technologies, especially CRISPR, genetically modified sheep and goats are becoming important translational animal models of human disease (Kalds et al., 2019, 2020; Menchaca et al., 2020; Rogers, 2016). Sheep and goats are often used for the production of biologics and reagents used in experimentation, including red blood cells, sera, and antibodies. Calves are most often used for testing medical devices, especially mechanical circulatory support devices.

Anesthesia and Analgesia in Laboratory Animals. https://doi.org/10.1016/B978-0-12-822215-7.00025-1

II. Preprocedural considerations

A. Anatomic and physiologic influences on anesthesia of ruminant species

Attention to the unique anatomical and physiologic characteristics of the ruminant and taking steps to minimize potential adverse effects these differences may have on anesthesia, surgery, and recovery is paramount to a successful anesthetic and surgical outcome in these species. The unique structure, function, and volume of the ruminant gastrointestinal system present challenges for anesthesia and surgery not encountered in monogastric species. Preventing bloating, minimizing regurgitation, reducing rumen volume by judicious fasting, and protecting the airway are key factors in successfully anesthetizing the ruminant animal. Common complications encountered in anesthetizing ruminants are directly associated with the effects of the digestive system on adequate ventilation and include regurgitation and aspiration, inadequate oxygenation, and bloating. Addressing these potential problems by proper preparation of the animal and preventive measures is the key to a successful surgical outcome irrespective of the anesthetic regimen used.

The stomach consisting of the rumen, reticulum, omasum, and abomasum is unique to ruminant species and is the site of the production of volatile fatty acids, the primary energy source, through microbial fermentation (Leek, 2004). The ruminant stomach occupies approximately 75% of the abdominal cavity, filling most of the left half of the cavity and extending into the right half of the abdomen (Habel, 1975). The relative sizes of the four compartments of the stomach develop and change with the age of the animal. In the newborn calf, the ruminoreticulum contains less than half the volume of the abomasum and remains functionless while the animal is on a milk diet (Habel, 1975; Nickel et al., 1973). The capacity of the ruminoreticulum is approximately equal to the abomasum by 8 weeks of age, double the capacity of the abomasum by 12 weeks, and in adults, the capacity is approximately 9:1 that of the abomasum (Habel, 1975). In lambs, the stomach represents 22% of total gastrointestinal wet tissue mass but increases to 49% in adult sheep (Valverde and Doherty, 2008). In cattle, the volume of the stomach is approximately 115–150 L while in sheep and goats stomach volume is 15–18 L (Habel, 1975; Valverde and Doherty, 2008). The size and volume of the ruminant stomach can impede respiration and ventilation in the anesthetized animal by interfering with diaphragmatic excursion resulting in a reduction in the functional residual capacity of the lung, thus interfering with effective pulmonary gas exchange (Greene, 2003; Lee and Swanson, 1996). Positioning of the anesthetized ruminant may further exacerbate hypoventilation as recumbency shifts the rumen mass, leading to the displacement of the diaphragm into the thoracic cavity. Cattle placed in lateral or dorsal recumbency developed significant hypoxemia and hypercapnia (Jorgensen and Cannedy, 1996; Wagner et al., 1990). Furthermore, the displaced rumen may interfere with venous return, predisposing to decreased cardiac output and low blood pressure (Jorgensen and Cannedy, 1996; Valverde and Doherty, 2008). For these reasons, a key to successful anesthetic management and surgery of the small ruminant is taking preventive measures to minimize the potential for regurgitation and aspiration of stomach contents, prevent bloating and ensure adequate ventilation during anesthesia and surgery.

1. *Fasting*

Withholding food and water prior to surgery decreases the rate of fermentation and the risk of regurgitation, and may decrease rumen volume (Swindle et al., 2002). Recommendations on the duration of fasting prior to surgery vary widely ranging from a few hours to 48 hours. Excessive fasting may lead to alterations in the rumen flora, reduced motility, and rumen stasis, resulting in a negative energy balance and complications during the postoperative period (Abrahamsen, 2009a, 2013). Furthermore, fasting may have adverse effects on acid-base status sufficient to cause cardiac arrhythmias (Abrahamsen, 2009a, 2013). In adult cattle, a 48-hour fast produced a 20%–30% reduction in heart rate, which persisted for 48 hours following recovery (Bednarski and McGuirk, 1986; McGuirk et al., 1990; Riebold, 2015). Fasting from food for 24–48 hours and withholding water for 12–24 hours in healthy sheep and goats resulted in better ventilation, less tympany, and reduced incidence of regurgitation (Carroll and Hartsfield, 1996). Other authors recommend shorter periods of no more than 12–18 hours fasting from food and either not withholding water or withholding for only 4–6 hours (Abrahamsen, 2009a, 2013; Swindle et al., 2002). In the authors' experience, withholding food and water from calves and adult sheep for 12–16 hours before surgery and supporting fluid balance with intravenous maintenance fluids supplemented with potassium decreases total rumen volume, and subsequently optimizing mechanical ventilation while avoiding the complications of prolonged fasting (Carney et al., 2009a, 2009b; Izer et al., 2018). Young animals that are transitioning from a functional monogastric to a ruminant should not fast for longer than 12 hours (Carroll and Hartsfield, 1996).

2. *Preventing regurgitation and bloat*

Regurgitation in the anesthetized ruminant may be either an active or passive process. Active regurgitation is most likely to occur due to inadequate or light anesthesia, whereas passive regurgitation results from increased transluminal pressure gradients and relaxed esophageal sphincters (Jorgensen and Cannedy, 1996; Steffey, 1986). In addition to fasting prior to anesthesia, induction techniques that quickly eliminate the gag reflex and position the animal in sternal recumbency with the head elevated reduce the risk of regurgitation during intubation (Abrahamsen, 2009a, 2013). Intubation with an appropriately sized endotracheal tube with the cuff inflated will protect the airway if regurgitation occurs during surgery.

In the ruminant animal, gases in the form of carbon dioxide (60%) and methane (30%–40%) are produced by the fermentation process in the rumen (Leek, 2004). The amount of gas production in adult cattle has been estimated to peak at a rate of 40 L/hour, 2–4 hours following a meal, and the accumulation of gas is normally eliminated by eructation, which occurs every 1–2 minutes (Leek, 2004). Heavy sedation or general anesthesia inhibits ruminoreticular motility and impairs eructation (Valverde and Doherty, 2008). The placement of an orogastric tube into the rumen at the time of anesthesia induction will minimize the accumulation of gas. A tube with an inflatable cuff, such as a foal urethral tube will assist in positioning the end of the tube at the gas-liquid interface in the rumen so that primarily gas and not rumen fluid will be suctioned off (Swindle et al., 2002). Removal of large amounts of liquid from the rumen will not eliminate gas production and is likely to result in a dry mass of ingesta that can impair the return to normal digestive function in the postoperative period. The orogastric tube may on occasion become clogged with ingesta or the wall of the rumen sucked onto the end of the tube causing it to no longer work. The authors' (JI and RW) have found that use of a low-pressure, intermittent vacuum is sufficient to minimize gas accumulation while avoiding the problems of clogging with solid food materials or suction of the rumen wall, thus occluding the tube. If the tube ceases to function and gas accumulates during surgery, the gas cap can be cannulated percutaneously with a large-bore (14–18 gauge) intravenous catheter connected to a sterile vacuum hose. The use of oral antibiotics such as neomycin prior to surgery to reduce fermentation will not significantly reduce the potential for regurgitation or bloating, can lead to problems with the return to normal gastrointestinal function following surgery, and is not recommended.

Detailed information on all aspects of anesthesia and analgesia for ruminants in the research setting is beyond the scope of this section; however, readers are referred to the excellent review of this topic by Valverde and Doherty (2008).

B. Animal welfare and the use of small ruminants in biomedical research

Animal welfare is generally considered to be the mental and physical well-being of an animal as it interacts with the environment. There have been many definitions and conceptions of animal welfare over the years, beginning with the Five Freedoms (Farm Animal Welfare Committee [FAWC], 1979), and considerations of the biological functioning, or feelings of the animal or the naturalness of the conditions under which it is kept (Fraser et al., 1997). However, more recently, this has been increasingly refined and centered on the capacity of the animal to feel or experience emotions, and therefore sentience. In this regard, the Five Domains concept (Mellor et al., 2020), which was initially developed specifically to assess welfare in biomedical research, is the most applicable to small ruminants used in research. The Five Domains framework, in this context, considers the impact of research practices on four physical or functional domains (nutrition, environment, health, and behavioral interactions; Mellor et al., 2020). Challenges in each domain influence the emotional state of the animal (positively and negatively), and these impacts provide information on the fifth domain, mental state. The cumulative balance of emotions elicited in the mental state domain leads to an overall welfare state assessment in the animal.

For small ruminants undergoing procedures potentially requiring anesthesia and analgesia, consideration of the welfare impact on the animal is critical to assess whether the costs to the animal of the procedure are acceptable when balanced against the benefits, and to address means to mitigate some of the impacts. For example, the costs to the animal of the withdrawal of food and water, up to 24 hours before anesthesia, will impact aspects of the nutrition domain (eliciting emotions of hunger, thirst, or frustration). Although small ruminants, particularly sheep, can cope with only small physiological impacts of food deprivation (Hogan et al., 2007), these species have evolved to spend large parts of their day searching for food and grazing. Thus, the behavioral motivation to feed is still present, and animals that are not fed show behavioral responses suggestive of negative affective states (Verbeek et al., 2011, 2014). Small ruminants are social species, and separation from conspecifics is associated with behavioral and physiological responses indicative of stress (Dwyer, 2004). Isolating an animal from conspecifics during recovery or to maintain a surgical site, thus affects the behavioral interaction domain, potentially eliciting emotions of fear, panic, anxiety, or boredom. Finally, surgical procedures are likely to cause at least transitory pain. Although some of these may be unavoidable or considered a necessary cost, consideration of whether they can be mitigated should always be part of experimental planning. For example, could an isolated animal be housed in sight and auditory communication with other animals, or a 'buddy' animal be housed with the experimental animal? For very young ruminants, being housed with their mothers can help reduce the impact of painful stimuli (Walker et al., 2003), and monitoring the potential presence of pain can ensure that these impacts are reduced.

C. The behavior of small ruminants

Ruminants are prey animals and have specific and highly motivated behavioral adaptations to deal with potential threats from predators. These are still maintained and expressed in the animal, regardless of whether a predator threat is present. For sheep, goats, and cattle, this involves highly organized social behavior, fear and anxiety when socially isolated, and flight from a threat (Dwyer, 2004). All species will also use aggression, particularly head threats and butting, particularly when cornered, although intact males will be more likely to attack than females. Sheep are generally the most fearful of the three species, although they are also the least likely to use aggression as a response, and, unless well-handled and trained from a young age, will regard humans as potential predators. Goats and young calves can be more curious and less fearful of human presence. All species are, however, very trainable, and if an animal is to be used in a study for a prolonged period, investing time in handling or 'gentling' the species, ideally with food rewards (Mellor, 2004), and habituating them to the experimental pens or apparatus can result in less stress and better cooperation from the animal and better experimental outcomes. All species respond well to stroking, hand feeding, and calm handling (Destrez et al., 2013), which can minimize the stress and difficulty of working with these species.

In agricultural practice, these species are almost always moved by driving away from the handler. All animals will tolerate the presence of humans (and indeed predators) at a distance but maintain a 'flight zone' around themselves, whereby encroachments into this space will elicit movement away (Grandin, 2014). The size of the flight zone will vary with species, experience, breed, and context, but for all species using low-stress handling techniques by working at the outer edge of the flight zone, such that the animal moves away slowly and calmly, is advised. Rapid movement into the flight zone will elicit panic and flight, which is counterproductive and can result in injury. As prey animals, these species have excellent peripheral vision, with the eyes located on the sides of the head, allowing 270° of vision, but with a blind spot directly behind (Piggins and Philips, 1996). The handler can speed up or slow down the movement of the animal by their position relative to the desired direction of travel (termed the 'point of balance' at the shoulder in cattle). Handlers positioned forward of the point of balance, in a 90° arc from the shoulder to the head, will slow down and stop movement, which can be started by moving caudally. When animals are in a chute or a confined space, moving backward along the line of animals will cause them to move forward. Calm and confident movement around animals is always advised, avoiding sudden or rapid movements which can elicit fear, panic, and flight. This is particularly relevant to larger males, which may carry horns, where a rapid movement toward the animal may result in charging and butting instead of flight, potentially causing serious injury to handlers. Although sheep and cattle will charge and butt with the head lowered, male goats rise on their hind legs and angle a head blow from above, so care must be taken when handling these animals.

In a laboratory setting, small ruminants can be trained to walk on a halter, and this can facilitate movement over short distances. Animals can also be easily trained to follow a bucket of feed, and this can be the simplest and least stressful method to move them. This method of encouraging movement makes use of the evolved following behavior, particularly of sheep, where the movement of another animal in front encourages other animals to follow. Designing movement routes to avoid dead-ends or sharp bends where the animal in front may suddenly disappear, and where there is only one easily observed route can facilitate animal movements (Starling et al., 2021). Unless specifically trained to tolerate handling and movements away from the social group, single animals are always difficult to move alone. Transporting these animals in a confined transporter may reduce the opportunity of a panicking animal injuring itself on obstructions.

1. *Restraint*

Any form of restraint and close confinement is stressful for small ruminants, eliciting fear, thus consideration of whether it is necessary and minimizing the time spent restrained is important. Sheep, goats and calves can often be caught and restrained manually by experienced animal handlers, as they are lightweight and, with training, relatively docile (Fonseca et al., 2019). Animals should be caught by gradually reducing the range of movement in the pen until the animal can be caught and restrained against the handler's legs or gently held against the side of the pen, usually by holding the chin with one hand, and pressing a knee against the lumbar vertebrae in front of the stifle. Animals should not be caught by the fleece, horns, ears, or tails, which can cause pain, bruising, and, in the case of horns, may break off and cause considerable bleeding.

Calves are usually restrained in a standing position, and for larger calves, this may require the use of a chute and head yoke to position the animal in a way that reduces the chance of injury. Sheep and goats can be cast (tipped onto their rump) if this is required for experimental procedures, but note that, although this usually causes the animal to remain still, this is still a stressful position for animals, and the time spent in this position should be minimized. Late pregnant ewes or does should not be cast.

Various forms of animal handling equipment, such as squeeze chutes, tilt tables, and rollover crates, are available which can make animal handling and restraint easier for the handler. These rely on physically restraining the animal within a crate or against a table, and then, for tilt tables and rollover crates, positioning the animal on its side or back as required. These have considerable benefits for the handler and may reduce the ability of the animal to struggle and injure themselves compared to manual restraint, but they are still associated with fear and stress in the animal. It is imperative that use of these devices is kept to a minimum in the conscious animal, which often cannot express its distress when restrained, and the ease for the handler should not be interpreted as a signal to keep animals restrained for longer than is necessary. Sheep or goats restrained on their backs are also susceptible to asphyxia, as fermentation in the rumen can put pressure on the lungs and impact the ability of the animal to breathe. Breathlessness has been identified as a significant cause of stress in ruminants (Beausoleil and Mellor, 2015), so avoiding the use of this position as much as possible will improve welfare.

III. Pain assessment and the need for analgesia

A. Pain assessment

In dealing with pain, the principles of the 3Ss (Suppress, Substitute, and Soothe) which have been developed for farm animals (Guatteo et al., 2012), should equally be employed when dealing with farm animals used in experiments. This approach is analogous to the 3Rs but focused on pain. It considers that those working with animals should suppress any source of pain that has no obvious advantage to the animal or those working with it. For example, consideration of whether common farming practices, such as castration or tail docking, are warranted in an experimental setting. Secondly, the substitution of a technique causing pain by another less painful method should be used wherever possible. This then requires a constant review of methods and consideration of less painful alternatives where these become available. Finally, in situations where a painful technique cannot be avoided then there is an expectation that all appropriate treatments to soothe that pain will be used. However, pain management in small ruminants is often inadequate, and this is frequently suggested to be because, as prey species, these animals may avoid showing overt signs of pain compared to other species (Anil et al., 2002). Studies of veterinarians in farm animal practice also suggest that some may believe that farm animals feel less pain than companion animals (Raekallio et al., 2003), perhaps due to an inability to adequately recognize signs that the animal is in pain. Experimentally, many studies have investigated methods to assess pain in ruminants, and a variety of different methods are used, often validated with the use of anesthesia or analgesia (Table 20.1). These suggest that there are well-validated and useful methods to assess pain, which can be applied when small ruminants are used in research.

The choice of which method of pain assessment, or combination, to use often depends on the type of pain expected or the type of procedure. Acutely painful stimuli, particularly those located in a somatic region, are often accompanied by well-defined behavioral and physiological responses, which can be readily scored or monitored. Changes in sensitivity to tactile stimulation of a specific site associated with injury or surgery can provide some information on the nociceptive responses of an animal, when associated with sensitive behavioral indicators of withdrawal, guarding, or other responses. However, chronic pain or more diffuse stimuli, which may be visceral in origin, are more challenging to assess, as they may be associated with alterations in daily time budgets, circadian rhythms of behavior, or physiological indicators, or more subtle changes in response. More recently the use of novel behavioral techniques, such as facial expressions, have been developed for use in ruminant species, following work on laboratory rodents (Table 20.1), and can give a more sensitive measure for assessing pain. An alternative approach, that of qualitative behavioral assessment (QBA), takes a holistic approach to assessing the whole animal, based on the dynamic expressivity of how that animal behaves, rather than what it does (Wemelsfelder et al., 2001). QBA has successfully provided a sophisticated understanding of the emotions associated with painful stimuli in sheep and cattle pain models, and further development of the use of this method in pain assessment is warranted. In general, however, while there is no one specific measure of pain, or pain assessment tool that works in all pain situations, there are a number of validated pain assessment scales that have greater value than single physiological measures, such as elevated heart rate. The use of a complementary combination of indicators, or a validated multidimensional or composite pain scoring system, can provide an accurate representation of the degree of pain experienced.

Pain, as an emotional state, can be experienced differently between different animals, and whereas some indicators in Table 20.1 attempt to understand the impact on

TABLE 20.1 A summary of the various types of behavioral and other indicators used to assess pain in small ruminants under different conditions.

Indicator or biomarker	Types of measures or responses	Examples of pain models where used	Example references
Specific pain-related behaviors	Kicking, stamping, rolling, looking at the site, head-shaking, vocalization	Castration, tail-docking, disbudding	Marini et al. (2017), Theurer et al. (2012) and Molony et al. (2002)
General behavioral changes	Daily activity budgets, feeding behavior, lying, social behavior	Chronic lameness, mastitis, metritis	Barragan et al. (2018)
Physiological indicators	Plasma or salivary cortisol, adrenaline/noradrenaline, substance P, haptoglobin, serum amyloid A, blood counts	Castration, tail-docking, disbudding	Sutherland et al. (2019), Kleinhenz et al. (2018) and Musk et al. (2017b)
Clinical indicators (often of SAM axis)	Blood pressure, respiratory rate, heart rate and heart rate variability, electromyography, EEG, assessment of lesions and healing	Castration, tail-docking, disbudding, surgical approaches	Harris et al. (2020), Sutherland et al. (2019), and Krohm et al. (2011)
Algometry	Von Frey hairs, thermal sensitivity, pressure plates	Castration, tail-docking, disbudding, lameness; reticuloperitonitis; keratoconjunctivitis	Troncoso et al. (2018), Kleinhenz et al. (2018), Musk et al. (2017c), and Dewell et al. (2014)
Facial expression	Orbital tightening, ear posture, shape of nares or muzzle, tension in cheeks	Lameness, mastitis, hot iron branding; osteotomy	Muller et al. (2019), McLennan et al. (2016) and Gleerup et al. (2015)
Qualitative behavioral assessment (QBA)	Terms associated with pain, irritation, uncomfortable, restlessness, anxiety and fear	Mastitis, castration	Maslowska et al. (2020), Grant et al. (2020), Vindevoghel et al. (2019) and des Roches et al. (2018)
Infrared thermography (IRT)	Surface eye temperature, inflammation	Castration in calves	Stewart et al. (2010), Kleinhenz et al. (2018) and Harris et al. (2021)
Numerical rating scales and visual analogue scales	Scores of perceived pain, such as gait scores for lameness, or more holistic assessments of pain	Lameness	Vieira et al. (2015), Kaler et al. (2009), Tuyttens et al. (2009) and Welsh et al. (1993)
Composite or multidimensional pain scoring systems	Multi-modal measures on various scales	Orchiectomy, stifle arthrotomy, thoracotomy	Izer et al. (2019), della Rocca et al. (2017), de Oliveira et al. (2014), Krohm et al. (2011) and Adami et al. (2011)

the animal at the emotional level (e.g., QBA), others, such as mechanical nociceptive threshold testing, for example, can be useful at understanding how stimuli are processed but do not provide an insight into the animal's perception of the painful stimuli. Pain can induce aversion to a place, people, or other stimuli because of the associations formed between the negative emotional state and another unconditioned stimulus. Pain-inducing stimuli may also affect the central processing of other stimuli, for example, resulting in more pessimistic-like behavior in cognitive or judgment bias testing in calves (Neave et al., 2014), or changes in responses to predator stimuli in fish (Ashley et al., 2009). Persistent or chronic pain can cause significant alterations in the central processing of stimuli, and more sophisticated assessments of behavioral responses may be required to understand the impact of chronic pain.

Relief of pain is a scientific imperative for any species used in biomedical research (National Research Council [NRC], 2011). Recognition and relief of pain are required by the Animal Welfare Regulations when these species are used in biomedical research (United States Department of Agriculture [USDA], 2008). In the research setting, anesthetic techniques and analgesic protocols often differ from those used in the field setting common to clinical practice, and certain experimental surgical procedures may require complex anesthetic and analgesic regimens. There is a growing body of literature on anesthesia, analgesia, and pain management specific to small ruminants (see, for example, Abrahamsen, 2009a, 2013; Carroll and Hartsfield, 1996; Carroll et al., 1998b; Coetzee, 2013; Gray and McDonell, 1986a, b; Greene, 2003; Lee and Swanson, 1996; Lin and Pugh, 2002; Lin and Walz, 2014; Riebold, 2015; Swindle et al., 2002; Valverde and Doherty, 2009). For some procedures, empirical use of anesthetics and analgesics reportedly used in humans, companion animals, or other species may be adopted and modified for the small ruminant. Cardiovascular studies in particular may require the use of cardiopulmonary bypass which is beyond the scope of clinical practice (see Carney et al., 2009b; Collan, 1970; Gerring and Scarth, 1974; Schauvliege et al., 2006). The attending veterinarian should be consulted for assistance in developing specific anesthetic protocols to meet study objectives.

B. Common husbandry procedures that cause pain

In normal agricultural practice, sheep, goats, and calves are subjected to painful procedures as part of routine management. These typically involve castration of all species, disbudding in calves and goat kids, and tail docking in sheep. In many cases, despite considerable research into methods to provide anesthesia and analgesia, these procedures can be done, legally, in many countries without the use of anesthesia or analgesia. When animals are used for biomedical research, as with all painful procedures, appropriate anesthesia and analgesia must be used, and justified on welfare, veterinary, or scientific grounds (Forbes et al., 2007).

Castration is usually carried out in agricultural practice within a few days of birth to reduce unplanned matings, to avoid taint or changes in other sensory characteristics of meat in postpubertal males, and/or to reduce the risk of injury to humans and other animals in managing intact male animals (Sutherland and Tucker, 2011). Several different techniques are routinely used, including the use of tight rubber rings (elastration), banding, instruments designed to crush the spermatic cords (known as bloodless castration), and surgical approaches. In many countries, the method or timing of the use of some of these methods without appropriate anesthesia or analgesia may be restricted. For example, in the UK, castration using tight rubber rings is only permitted for lambs or kids under 7 days of age, without anesthesia or analgesia, and is forbidden in some European countries. Castration by any method has been shown to be associated with behaviors indicative of pain (e.g., rolling, kicking, stamping, abnormal postures), and elevations of plasma cortisol and heart rate (Graham et al., 1997; Kells et al., 2020; Molony et al., 2002; Paull et al., 2009). These behaviors can persist for several hour after the procedure and can be significantly reduced using local anesthetics (lidocaine) injected into the testes and scrotal neck, but not completely abolished (Kells et al., 2020; Stewart et al., 2014). Subcutaneous, but not intramuscular, meloxicam reduced pain behaviors in the 12 hours after castration (Paull et al., 2012), although it did not affect acute pain responses (Kells et al., 2020). Topical application of local anesthetic has been shown to reduce the pain associated with surgical castration (Paull et al., 2009), but this method of castration is prohibited in many countries as it causes the greatest behavioral pain responses. More recently, formulations to deliver NSAIDs through a buccal route in small ruminants have been developed and can help to reduce pain expression to a greater degree than is achieved through local anesthetic alone (Small et al., 2018).

1. Disbudding

Disbudding is usually carried out in young calves or goat kids soon after birth but is rarely practiced with sheep. Dehorning refers to the removal of the developing or mature horn in older animals. In agriculture, this is done to avoid handler or between-animal injury, especially when animals are kept in confined spaces. This might be a relevant issue for research uses of animals. However, all species have several polled breeds; thus, unless there is a very specific and justifiable reason for using a horned breed, the use of polled varieties would be greatly encouraged to avoid the need for this procedure. When required, disbudding of the young animal (<2 months of age) is preferred over dehorning and should be in compliance with applicable regulations (ASAS, 2020).

Disbudding can be carried out using caustic paste, scoops, or thermal cautery (Brooks et al., 2021; Hempstead et al., 2018a). In general, pastes and scoops are not recommended methods due to the pain associated with these approaches, and with paste, the potential for causing burns to other parts of the animal. In many countries, disbudding can only be carried out by a veterinarian, and requires the use of at least local anesthesia, and often postoperative analgesia. In goat kids, the skull is thin around the site of the horn bud, and disbudding is often carried out under general anesthesia as the risk of inadvertently causing brain damage is considerable. Even with the use of local anesthesia and analgesia (such as lidocaine and flunixin meglumine) or general anesthetic and NSAIDs (isoflurane and meloxicam), there is evidence of pain in the animals, such as head shaking, a reduced growth rate, and pessimistic behavioral responses in cognitive bias testing for a number of days after the procedure (Ajuda et al., 2020; Hempstead et al., 2018b; Neave et al., 2014).

2. Tail-docking

This procedure is only commonly carried out on sheep in agricultural practice. For sheep, tail docking is routinely carried out to reduce the risk of fecal soiling of the breech area, which can be a risk factor for cutaneous myiasis (flystrike). This is a painful and unpleasant condition, which can cause distress and mortality in sheep if not treated (French et al., 1994). However, the evidence that tail-docking can reduce the incidence is unclear (Orihuela and Ungerfeld, 2019; Sutherland and Tucker, 2011), and the use of other practices, such as regular shearing of the perineal area, insecticides, and topical applications of deterrents, may be at least as effective.

Tail docking is generally carried out by the same methods as described for castration, but also using hot docking irons. Similar restrictions apply in many countries, and the procedure is associated with behavioral and physiological evidence of pain in the lamb, albeit at a lower level than seen for castration (Molony et al., 2002). The use of subcutaneous local anesthetic drugs, such as bupivacaine, administered immediately before docking is effective at reducing these responses (Graham et al., 1997).

IV. Sedation and premedication

Sedation of small ruminants prior to the induction of anesthesia is advantageous in that sedatives and tranquilizers may help minimize stress and anxiety and allow for better control of the animal. Often the dose of the induction agent(s) and the amount of maintenance anesthetic are reduced with the use of sedative premedications. Depending on the choice of sedative or tranquilizer selected, some drugs may provide analgesic effects as well. Common doses of sedatives and anesthetic induction agents used in calves and small ruminants are presented in Tables 20.2 and 20.3, respectively.

A. α_2 agonists and antagonists

In ruminants, α-2 adrenergic receptor agonists produce reliable, dose-dependent sedation that can range from mild sedation to complete recumbency (Valverde and Doherty, 2008). Xylazine can be used as a single agent or combined with an opioid for sedation prior to anesthesia, or alternatively, it may be administered with a dissociative agent such as ketamine or tiletamine-zolazepam to induce anesthesia (Flecknell et al., 2015). All α-2 agonists yield a quick onset of sedation with ruminants being particularly sensitive to the effects of xylazine. One-tenth or less of the xylazine dose used in other species is required to produce sedation in cattle and small ruminants (Valverde and Doherty, 2008). Goats appear to be more sensitive to the effects of xylazine than sheep (Taylor, 1991). The difference in sensitivity between species appears to be of pharmacodynamic origin and is likely due to G-protein binding affinity in ruminants species compared to nonruminant species (Törneke et al., 2003).

In sheep, hypoxemia and the formation of pulmonary edema are well-known adverse effects of α-2 agonists, with the exact pathophysiology largely unclear. These hypoxemic reactions appear to be highly variable, potentially individual- and breed-dependent, making it difficult to predict whether an individual animal will react adversely, and the degree of hypoxemia which may develop (Kästner, 2006; Kutter et al., 2006). In addition to the development of hypoxemia and pulmonary edema, bradycardia, hypercapnia, hypotension, hyperglycemia, hypoinsulinemia, and increased urine production have been reported following xylazine administration (Greene and Thurmon, 1988). Combining xylazine with methadone, morphine, or

TABLE 20.2 Common doses for sedative drugs in small ruminants.

Variable	Calf (mg/kg)	Sheep (mg/kg)	Goat (mg/kg)
Acepromazine	0.02; IV, IM	0.01–0.02; IV	0.01–0.02; IV
	0.04–0.09; IM	0.04–0.09; IM	
Medetomidine	0.03; IV, IM	0.001–0.007; IV	0.001–0.007; IV
	0.04; IM	0.04; IM	
Xylazine	0.05–0.3; IV, IM	0.01–0.02; IV	0.01–0.02; IV
	0.1–0.3; IM, SQ	0.1–0.3; IM, SQ	
Detomidine	0.03; IV, IM	0.001–0.007; IV	0.001–0.007; IV
	0.04; IM		
Dexmedetomidine		0.005; IV	
Diazepam	0.25–0.5; IV	0.25–0.5; IV	0.25–0.5; IV
Midazolam	0.1–0.3; IV, IM	0.1–0.5; IV, IM, SQ	0.1–0.5; IV, IM, SQ

Modified from Valverde and Doherty (2008).

TABLE 20.3 Common doses for induction drugs in small ruminants.

Variable	Calf (mg/kg)	Sheep (mg/kg)	Goat (mg/kg)
Propofol	4–6	4–6	4–6
Methohexital	3–5	3–5	3–5
Ketamine	5–10	5–10	10
Xylazine[a]/ketamine	0.05–0.1/3–5	0.03–0.05/3–5	0.05–0.1/3–5
Ketamine/midazolam	4/0.4	4/0.4	4/0.4
Ketamine/diazepam	4/0.4	4/0.4	4–5/0.4–0.5
Xylazine[a]/ketamine/diazepam	0.05/3/0.4	0.03/5/0.4	0.03/5/0.4
Tiletamine-zolazepam (1:1 mixture)	4	1–4	1–4
Xylazine[a]/tiletamine-zolazepam	0.05/2	0.05/2	0.05/2
Xylazine[a]/ketamine/guaifenesin	0.05/2/75	0.05/2/75	0.05/2/75

[a]*Can be substituted by equipotent dose of another alpha$_2$ agonist.*
Source. Valverde and Doherty, 2008.

tramadol resulted in cardiopulmonary changes similar to those induced by xylazine alone in sheep; however, these combinations produced enhanced sedation at 15 and 30 minutes following administration (de Carvalho et al., 2016). Xylazine also has an oxytocin-like effect in ruminants (Greene and Thurmon, 1988). Xylazine administered to ruminants in the final trimester of pregnancy may cause premature parturition and retention of fetal membranes (Rosenberger et al., 1968), which is important to note as sheep are often used as models in reproductive and fetal research studies. Increased myometrial tone and increased intrauterine pressure have been reported in cows following xylazine administration (Leblanc et al., 1984).

Detomidine may be used as a safer alternative to xylazine in pregnant sheep and goats as it is unlikely to induce abortion in pregnant ruminants (Jedruch and Gajewski, 1986; Pyörälä et al., 1986). While the pharmacologic effects of detomidine are comparable to those of xylazine, ruminants seem to be less sensitive to detomidine than to xylazine (Celly et al., 1997). Because detomidine is more α_2-specific than xylazine, a lower dose is required to achieve adequate sedation with less adverse effects (Singh et al., 1994). The severity of hypoxemia and pulmonary edema induced by detomidine is less in comparison to other α_2 agonists (Kästner, 2006). Detomidine administered at 20 µg/kg intravenously as a bolus dose followed by an infusion of 60 µg/kg/hour produced satisfactory sedation for minimally invasive procedures with no significant cardiorespiratory effects in sheep (de Moura et al., 2018).

Other α-2 agonists commonly used in small ruminants in a research setting include medetomidine and dexmedetomidine. Because α-2 agonists also have analgesic and muscle relaxant effects, they are often used as preanesthetics or as anesthetic adjuncts in ruminants (Lin, 2015). Medetomidine induces dose-dependent sedation, and when administered at a dose of 0.005 mg/kg, produces analgesia in sheep that is comparable to that of fentanyl dosed at 0.015 mg/kg (Muge et al., 1994). Intravenous xylazine produced significant decreases in pulmonary function in ventilated isoflurane-anesthetized sheep in comparison to an equipotent dose of medetomidine, suggesting that medetomidine may be the preferred α-2 agonist when optimal pulmonary function is essential (Raisis et al., 2021). The onset of sedation produced by medetomidine is more rapid and lasts longer than that produced by xylazine in calves and goats (Carroll et al., 2005; Rioja et al., 2008). Cardiopulmonary effects such as increases in heart rate, mean arterial blood pressure, and pulmonary arterial blood pressure have been reported following IV or IM administration of medetomidine in ruminants (Carroll et al., 2005; Kästner et al., 2003; Rioja et al., 2008). Medetomidine also results in increased cortisol and glucose levels in ruminants by having a profound effect on the stress response (Carroll et al., 1998, 2005; Ranheim et al., 2000).

While racemic medetomidine has a binding ratio of 1620:1 (α_1:α_2), its D-enantiomer, dexmedetomidine, is even more selective (Murrell and Hellebrekers, 2005; Virtanen et al., 1988). Dexmedetomidine is twice as potent as medetomidine, with a dose of 5 µg/kg IV being equipotent to 10 µg/kg IV of medetomidine for sedation in sheep (Kästner et al., 2001a). Cardiopulmonary depression and moderate-to-severe hypoxemia are adverse effects of dexmedetomidine administration, and similar cardiopulmonary and sedative effects have been reported in comparing dexmedetomidine and medetomidine in sheep (Kästner et al., 2001a, 2001b, 2005, 2007a, 2007b). Compared to the use of dexmedetomidine alone in sheep, combining dexmedetomidine with an opioid (butorphanol, methadone, morphine, or tramadol) resulted in the same degree of cardiopulmonary depression without a significant impact on the degree or duration of sedation achieved (Borges et al., 2016). In regards to sedation, these results suggest no real added benefit in combining an opioid with dexmedetomidine.

The sedative and adverse effects of α-2 agonists can be reversed with specific α-2 adrenergic antagonists. Atipamezole, yohimbine, tolazoline, and idazoxan have been used to reverse the effects of α-2 agonists and curtail recovery time. It is important to note that the use of α-2 adrenergic antagonists will also reverse the analgesic effects provided by the α-2 agonists, so supplemental analgesia should be provided as necessary upon reversal. Yohimbine dosed at 1 mg/kg IV will reverse the sedative effects of xylazine in sheep (Riebold, 2015). Yohimbine is less effective than other α-2 antagonists, as tolazoline dosed at 0.5–2 mg/kg IV has been shown to reverse the effects of xylazine in calves more rapidly than yohimbine (Thurmon et al., 1989; Valverde and Doherty, 2008; Young et al., 1989). Ketamine-medetomidine sedation can be successfully reversed using tolazoline (2.2 μg/kg IV) and atipamezole (20–60 μg/kg IV or IM) in calves (Lin et al., 1999; Raekallio et al., 1991). When administered rapidly, tolazoline has been reported to cause tachycardia, increased cardiac output, vasodilation, and coronary vasodilation (Yellin et al., 1975). The risk of central nervous system excitement and adverse cardiovascular effects are reduced when α-2 antagonists are administered intramuscularly (Abrahamsen, 2008).

B. Phenothiazines

Acepromazine maleate produces mild sedation and skeletal muscle relaxation in ruminants (Lemke, 2007). When administered at a dose of 0.02–0.1 mg/kg IV or SQ, acepromazine provides mild tranquilization with minimal respiratory depression (Swindle et al., 2002). Although acepromazine does not provide any analgesic effects, it does have a sparing effect on inhalant anesthetics and may protect against the arrhythmogenic effects of anesthetics (Flecknell et al., 2015). The drug has minimal effects on heart rate but may result in hypotension in volume-depleted animals due to its alpha-adrenergic blocking properties (Lin et al., 2012; Valverde and Doherty, 2008). When combined with an opioid as a preanesthetic, sedation and preemptive analgesia can be achieved prior to the induction of anesthesia. Acepromazine alone administered to sheep resulted in a level of sedation similar to that observed when administered in combination with the opioids methadone, morphine, and tramadol without causing clinical changes in cardiorespiratory function (Nishimura et al., 2017). The degree of sedation produced by the administration of acepromazine and buprenorphine compared to acepromazine combined with morphine is similar in sheep (Musk and Wilkes, 2018). These preanesthetic combinations did not produce observable adverse effects and were sufficient for restraint prior to anesthesia induction (Musk and Wilkes, 2018).

C. Benzodiazepines

Diazepam and midazolam are the most commonly used benzodiazepines in small ruminants due to their anxiolytic, anticonvulsant, and central muscle relaxant effects (Lin et al., 2012). These drugs have minimal cardiopulmonary depressant effects and may be used as alternatives to α_2-agonists for sedation and restraint in small ruminants and calves. Diazepam is frequently used for sedation and to decrease anxiety in high-risk animals and can be combined with ketamine to improve muscle relaxation during anesthesia (Gray and McDonell, 1986b). As a tissue irritant, diazepam should only be administered intravenously, while midazolam can be administered both IV and IM as it is water-soluble and nonirritating to tissues (Valverde and Doherty, 2008). In conscious sheep and goats, rapid IV administration of low doses of benzodiazepines may cause an initial excitement phase (Valverde and Doherty, 2008). Diazepam dosed at 0.2–0.5 mg/kg given slowly IV provides a short period of sedation and recumbency (Valverde and Doherty, 2008). The degree and duration of sedation produced may be enhanced when benzodiazepines are combined with an opioid, such as butorphanol or morphine. The effects of benzodiazepines can be reversed using flumazenil, but typically there is no need for a reversal of these agents (Valverde and Doherty, 2008).

D. Opioids

When administered alone as premedication, opioids do not produce reliable sedation and may cause unwanted behavioral changes in ruminants, such as agitation and chewing (Valverde and Doherty, 2008). However, when combined with other premedicant drugs, opioids may provide preemptive, multimodal analgesia, improved quality of sedation, as well as a reduction in the required anesthetic induction and maintenance doses. Adverse effects of ataxia and dysphoria have been reported following high doses of IV administration of butorphanol (0.1–0.2 mg/kg) in sheep (Waterman et al., 1991). To avoid these adverse effects, lower doses of butorphanol (0.02–0.05 mg/kg) should be used. Methadone (0.5 mg/kg), morphine (0.5 mg/kg), or tramadol (5 mg/kg) administered intravenously with acepromazine (0.05 mg/kg) were shown to produce sedation in sheep without clinically relevant cardiorespiratory changes (Nishimura et al., 2017). Acepromazine (0.03 mg/kg) administered with buprenorphine (0.02 mg/kg) or morphine (0.3 mg/kg) given IM as a premedication combination produced similar sedation in sheep without observed adverse effects (Musk and Wilkes, 2018). In comparison to conscious ruminants, opioids administered to anesthetized ruminants are less likely to cause excitement and are more beneficial due to their potent analgesic effects (Valverde and Doherty, 2008).

V. Anesthesia

A. Anesthetic induction

1. Barbiturates

Ultrashort-acting barbiturates, such as methohexital, are commonly used for rapid induction of anesthesia, followed by maintenance of anesthesia with inhalant anesthetics. Methohexital sodium (3–5 mg/kg IV) is a nonsulfur-containing, ultrashort-acting oxybarbiturate used to induce anesthesia and facilitate endotracheal intubation in sheep, calves, and goats (Carney et al., 2009b; Collan, 1970; Thurmon, 1986).

In comparison to the use of ketamine-combinations for anesthesia induction in sheep and calves, the authors (JI, RW) prefer methohexital as it produces significantly less salivary secretions, allowing for easier endotracheal intubation without the need to suction the oropharynx for improved visualization. In the authors' experience, rapid administration of methohexital often results in apnea, or a decreased respiratory rate, therefore necessitating prompt intubation and mechanical ventilation. Thiamylal (8–14 mg/kg IV) or thiopental (10–16 mg/kg IV) are thiobarbiturates previously used for induction of anesthesia; however, they are no longer available in the United States (Ewing, 1990). Because barbiturates are highly alkaline, they should be administered through a preplaced intravenous catheter to avoid tissue necrosis due to perivascular leakage of the agent (Swindle et al., 2002).

2. Propofol

Propofol (4–6 mg/kg IV) is commonly used for a smooth, rapid induction and/or maintenance of general anesthesia in sheep, goats, and calves (Alves et al., 2003; Carroll and Hartsfield, 1996; Prassinos et al., 2005; Reid et al., 1993; Riebold, 2015; Valverde and Doherty, 2008; Waterman, 1988). Because it is highly lipophilic, propofol distributes from blood to tissues and crosses the blood-brain barrier very rapidly, facilitating quick anesthesia induction with short-lasting effects (Cagnardi et al., 2009). Following induction, propofol may be administered as a constant rate infusion (0.5 mg/kg/minute IV) in sheep to produce light anesthesia (Lin et al., 1997). Calves induced with propofol (5 mg/kg IV) and maintained by continuous infusion of propofol (0.6–0.8 mg/kg/minute IV) developed no clinically significant hemodynamic changes (Deschk et al., 2016). In goats, the median minimum infusion rate of propofol required to prevent purposefu.l movement of the extremities in response to a noxious stimulus was determined to be 0.45 mg/kg/minute (Ferreira et al., 2016). In this study, no significant cardiopulmonary changes were observed, but clinically relevant hypoxemia was consistently present in the goats at 2 minutes following anesthesia induction (Ferreira et al., 2016). Apnea induced by propofol has been correlated more closely with dose rather than the rate of administration (Prassinos et al., 2005).

3. Ketamine

Ketamine, a dissociative anesthetic agent, is frequently used as an induction agent in ruminants. When used as a sole agent, ketamine increases muscle tone, peripheral reflexes are maintained, and even at the highest dose, ketamine is not a complete anesthetic (Valverde and Doherty, 2008). It is therefore not recommended to be used as the sole agent for induction or short-term anesthesia. Instead, ketamine is often administered following premedication with acepromazine or α2-agonist such as xylazine or dexmedetomidine. Ketamine may be coadministered with a benzodiazepine such as midazolam for greater analgesia, sedation, and muscle relaxation during anesthesia (Lin et al., 2012). Because ketamine is an N-methyl-D-aspartate (NMDA) receptor antagonist, its use often results in an apneustic breathing pattern, but may produce dose-dependent apnea during inspiration (Valverde and Doherty, 2008). Analgesia is also produced as a result of the effects of ketamine on the NMDA receptor (Himmelseher et al., 2005). However, the degree and duration of analgesia produced from ketamine utilized as a single agent are typically insufficient in effectively managing postoperative pain. As opposed to other anesthetics that cause cardiovascular depression, ketamine stimulates the sympathetic nervous system, leading to increased heart rate and arterial blood pressure (Lin et al., 2012). When ketamine is combined with an α_2-agonist, the cardiovascular stimulation induced by ketamine is offset by the cardiovascular depressive effects of the α_2-agonist. Small ruminants have been effectively induced or undergone a short duration of anesthesia with combinations of ketamine and xylazine, medetomidine, or dexmedetomidine (Caulkett et al., 1996; Coetzee et al., 2010; Gogoi et al., 2003; Kästner et al., 2001a; Lin et al., 1997; Raekallio et al., 1991; Singh et al., 2010; Swindle et al., 2002; Valverde and Doherty, 2008; Özkan et al., 2010). It is not recommended to use a combination of ketamine (2 mg/kg IV or 4 mg/kg IM) and xylazine (0.05–0.1 mg/kg IV or IM) for short-term anesthesia in clinically unhealthy ruminants with potential underlying cardiopulmonary disease due to the adverse effects on cardiopulmonary function associated with the large dose of xylazine (Abrahamsen, 2013). These IV and IM combinations should only be used in clinically healthy ruminants (Abrahamsen, 2013).

As an alternative to a ketamine-α_2-agonist combination, ketamine can be administered with diazepam or midazolam for induction of anesthesia with very minimal cardiopulmonary depression. Muscle relaxation provided by the benzodiazepines negates the muscle rigidity produced by ketamine. Equal volumes of ketamine (100 mg/mL) and diazepam (5 mg/mL) administered intravenously at 1 mL/18–22 kg will provide up to 20 minutes of surgical analgesia in small ruminants (Abrahamsen, 2013). Alternatively, ketamine (4 mg/kg) and midazolam (0.4 mg/kg) have been used to induce anesthesia in goats (Stegmann, 1998). In healthy small ruminants, anesthesia induction is commonly accomplished using a combination of ketamine (5 mg/kg IV), diazepam (0.3–0.5 mg/kg IV), and xylazine (0.03 mg/kg IM) (Valverde and Doherty, 2008). Xylazine is administered first to induce mild sedation and provide a more controlled induction, followed by IV administration of ketamine-diazepam, given to effect, to facilitate intubation (Valverde and Doherty, 2008).

4. *Tiletamine-zolazepam*

Telazol (tiletamine-zolazepam) is similar to ketamine-diazepam as a dissociative NMDA-antagonist (tiletamine) that is combined with a GABA-agonist benzodiazepine (zolazepam) (Valverde and Doherty, 2008). Telazol yields greater analgesic effects and muscle relaxation in comparison to ketamine (Valverde and Doherty, 2008). However, the degree and duration of analgesia provided by Telazol alone or ketamine alone, administered as single agents, are insufficient for adequately managing postoperative pain. Neither agent should be used for the sole purpose of providing analgesia. While it provides a rapid and smooth induction in ruminants, it often results in cardiovascular stimulation, hypoventilation, and hypothermia, necessitating oxygen and ventilatory support (Valverde and Doherty, 2008). A combination of Telazol (13.2 mg/kg IV) and xylazine (0.11 mg/kg IV) produced better muscle relaxation and a longer duration of anesthesia than Telazol alone (13.2 mg/kg IV) in sheep with a smooth and gradual recovery (Lin et al., 1993a).

VI. Maintenance of anesthesia

A. Endotracheal intubation of small ruminants and calves

Following the induction of anesthesia, it is crucial to intubate the airway of small ruminants as quickly as possible to prevent aspiration of salivary secretions and ruminal contents. Small ruminants and calves must be sufficiently

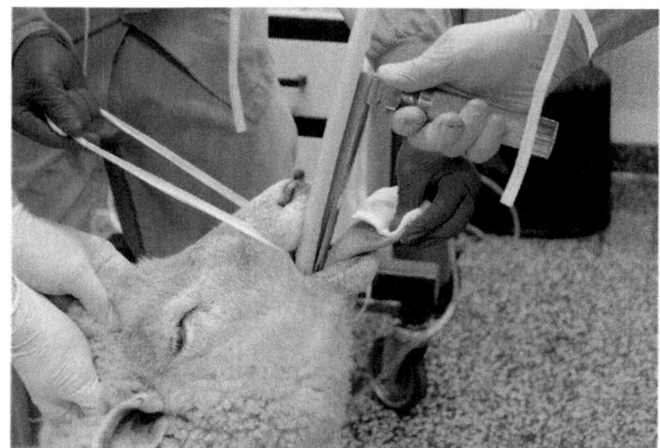

FIGURE 20.1 Endotracheal intubation of an adult sheet after induction of anesthesia with methohexital. Positioning of the anesthetized animal in sternal recumbency with the head and neck extended by an assistant permits visualization of the epiglottis and tracheal opening and aids rapid intubation. Larger animals may be positioned on the floor or a table.

anesthetized before trying to pass an endotracheal tube. The small ruminant should be positioned in sternal recumbency with the head and neck extended to allow for direct visualization of the larynx (Fig. 20.1). Depending on the size of the animal, the laryngoscope blade should be between 20 and 40 cm in length for small and larger animals, respectively, in order to reach the larynx (Valverde and Doherty, 2008). In comparison to goats, sheep have a slightly larger airway and typically require an endotracheal tube with an internal diameter of 8.5–14 mm (Valverde and Doherty, 2008). Calves typically require endotracheal tubes 11–14 mm in size (Valverde and Doherty, 2008). It is recommended to use the largest tube possible in order to prevent airway secretions and ruminal contents from entering the larynx (Valverde and Doherty, 2008). Use of a stylet is recommended in order to stiffen the tube to allow for easier passage through the larynx. Once placed, the cuff of the tube should be immediately inflated and the tube secured prior to moving or repositioning the animal (Valverde and Doherty, 2008). Alternatively, small ruminants can be intubated blindly in either sternal or lateral recumbency by an experienced individual (Valverde and Doherty, 2008).

B. Inhalant anesthetics

The most commonly used inhalant anesthetics to maintain general anesthesia in ruminants are isoflurane and sevoflurane. Halothane and methoxyflurane are older anesthetics that are no longer available in most countries (Flecknell et al., 2015). The minimum alveolar concentration (MAC) values of inhalants that are currently used in ruminants are presented in Table 20.4. The advantage of using inhalant anesthetics is the ability to quickly adjust anesthetic depth with a rapid and smooth anesthetic recovery (Flecknell et al., 2015). The disadvantage of using

TABLE 20.4 Minimum alveolar concentration (MAC) values (%) of commonly used inhalants in ruminants.

Inhalant	Cattle	Sheep	Goat
Isoflurane	1.27	1.19–1.53	1.14–1.43
Sevoflurane	N/A	3.3	2.33
Desflurane	N/A	9.81	N/A

Note: *N/A*, not available.
Sources: Vlaverde and Doherty, (2008), Columbano et al. (2018a, 2018b)

inhalant anesthetics is the significant cardiovascular depression associated with these agents. All inhalant anesthetics produce decreases in stroke volume, cardiac output, blood pressure, tidal volume, respiratory rate, minute volume, and increases in $PaCO_2$ that are dose-dependent (Lin et al., 2012; Valverde and Doherty, 2008). Isoflurane and sevoflurane produce vasodilation, which results in decreased arterial blood pressure (Hikasa et al., 1998).

Inhalant anesthetics do not possess analgesic properties. Preanesthetic medications, as well as preemptive and intraoperative analgesics, often lower the MAC and the amount of inhalant required to maintain a surgical plane of anesthesia (Flecknell et al., 2015; Valverde and Doherty, 2008). Administration of a propofol CRI has been shown to significantly reduce the isoflurane MAC in a dose-dependent manner in goats without significant cardiovascular effects (Dzikiti et al., 2011). Tiletamine-zolazepam used as a premedicant or induction agent, as well as acepromazine administered as a premedicant, have been shown to reduce the isoflurane MAC or concentration required to maintain anesthesia in goats (Doherty et al., 2002a, 2002b).

Because sevoflurane and desflurane are less soluble in blood than isoflurane, their ability to induce and alter the depth of anesthesia is more rapid in comparison to that of isoflurane. Similarly, ruminants recover more quickly following sevoflurane and desflurane anesthesia (Flecknell et al., 2015). The use of sevoflurane for anesthesia maintenance of ruminants in a research setting may be limited due to its high cost and higher MAC necessary to reach a surgical plane of anesthesia.

C. Total and partial intravenous anesthesia

A combination of injectable anesthetic, sedative, and tranquilizer drugs can be administered intravenously via intermittent boluses or, preferably, as a continuous rate infusion for the maintenance of general anesthesia. Use of total intravenous anesthesia (TIVA) may be advantageous in a research environment when inhalant agents cannot be used, such as during MRI imaging studies. The use of a "double drip" consisting of ketamine (1 mg/mL) and guaifenesin (50 mg/mL) is commonly used to induce and maintain a stable plane of anesthesia in small ruminants (Abrahamsen, 2013). Guaifenesin provides muscle relaxation as well as some sedation (Valverde and Doherty, 2008). The induction of anesthesia with double drip is achieved by infusing 1.7–2.2 mL/kg, followed by maintenance of anesthesia with a continued infusion rate of 2.6 mL/kg/hour (Abrahamsen, 2013). It is recommended not to exceed 60–90 minutes of continuous guaifenesin administration, as a residual accumulation of guaifenesin may result in adverse effects such as muscle weakness and prolonged anesthetic recovery. Use of an opioid, such as butorphanol (0.05–0.1 mg/kg IV or IM) or morphine (0.05–0.1 mg/kg IV or IM), can be considered to provide enhanced analgesia when a CRI of double drip is used for maintenance of anesthesia (Abrahamsen, 2013).

Alternatively, a continuous intravenous infusion of guaifenesin (50 mg/mL), ketamine (1–2 mg/mL), and xylazine (0.1 mg/mL), commonly known as "triple drip," can be used to induce and maintain anesthesia in healthy ruminants (Abrahamsen, 2013; Lin et al., 1993a, 1993b). While the addition of xylazine provides further analgesic effects, adverse effects include cardiopulmonary depression. An initial administration rate of 1–1.5 mL/kg of triple drip is required to induce anesthesia, followed by a maintenance rate of 2.6 mL/kg/hour without significant depression of the cardiopulmonary systems (Abrahamsen, 2013).

The effects of a propofol (12 mg/kg/hour) and fentanyl (0.02 mg/kg/hour) TIVA versus a propofol (12 mg/kg/hour) and midazolam (0.3 mg/kg/hour) TIVA were compared in spontaneously-breathing goats receiving supplemental oxygen (Dzikiti et al., 2010). Cardiopulmonary function was well maintained with both TIVA combinations, and the median propofol dose for maintenance was less with the propofol-fentanyl combination (12 mg/kg/hour) compared to propofol-midazolam (18 mg/kg/hour) (Dzikiti et al., 2010). Anesthetic recovery following propofol-fentanyl was not consistently smooth (Dzikiti et al., 2010).

Partial intravenous anesthesia (PIVA) uses a combination of inhalants and injectable anesthetics. Anesthetic, analgesic, and sedative drugs delivered by constant rate infusion can enhance analgesia and reduce the MAC of the inhalant, subsequently reducing cardiopulmonary depression (Valverde and Doherty, 2008). In goats, a low dose ketamine CRI (25–50 μg/kg/minute) with or without lidocaine (100 μg/kg/minute) produced a 30% reduction in the MAC of isoflurane (Doherty et al., 2007; Queiroz-Castro et al., 2006). Lidocaine infused at 50 μg/kg/minute reduced the isoflurane requirement by approximately 17% in calves undergoing umbilical surgery (Vesal et al., 2011).

VII. Anesthesia monitoring

Ruminants should be monitored continuously during anesthesia. Many research facilities have the capability to measure pulse rate, cardiac rhythm, invasive or noninvasive blood pressure, end-tidal CO_2, and O_2 saturation. The depth of anesthesia can be assessed via clinical evaluation and physiological indicators. The palpebral reflex gradually wanes as the depth of anesthesia increases and becomes absent or sluggish once a surgical plane of anesthesia has been reached (Valverde and Doherty, 2008). While eye position is often used to assess anesthetic depth in other species, it is not a reliable indicator of anesthetic depth in sheep and goats (Riebold, 2015). Upon induction, the eye is centrally located and then rotates ventrally as the anesthetic plane deepens (Abrahamsen, 2009a; Riebold, 2015). Upon reaching a surgical plane of anesthesia, the eye will move back to a central location and will return toward the ventral position at deep planes of anesthesia (Abrahamsen, 2009a; Riebold, 2015). Motor movement either spontaneously or resulting from surgical stimulation is a clear indicator of an inadequate plane of anesthesia (Valverde and Doherty, 2008). Physiologic indicators, such as changes in heart rate, blood pressure, and respiratory rate, may be used in conjunction with assessment of the palpebral reflex and jaw tone to evaluate the anesthetic plane.

Cardiovascular monitoring should include the use of an ECG for continuous assessment of heart rate and rhythm, as well as the measurement of arterial pressure. Direct blood pressure measurement via a catheter placed in a peripheral artery is the most accurate. The medial auricular branch of the rostral auricular artery, the saphenous artery, or the common digital artery can be catheterized in small ruminants (Flecknell et al., 2015; Riebold, 2015). The common digital artery courses between the dewclaws of the forelimbs and is easily accessible (Fig. 20.2).

Noninvasive blood pressure measurement is inaccurate in sheep, goats, and calves (Aarnes et al., 2014; Izer and Wilson, 2020; Trim et al., 2013). A jugular catheter can be used to measure central venous pressure (normal range is 5−10 cm H_2O, 3−7 mmHg), and cardiac output may be monitored during anesthesia if necessary for the research protocol (Riebold, 2015).

The use of capnography and pulse oximeters to monitor end-tidal CO_2 levels and O_2 saturation is essential to ensure adequate ventilation and gas exchange (Lin et al., 2012). Capnography is advantageous in that it provides a breath-by-breath analysis of changes in $EtCO_2$, while pulse oximetry provides a continuous approximation of oxygen saturation (Valverde and Doherty, 2008). The lingual artery of the tongue and the auricular artery of the ear are common sites for probe placement in sheep and goats (Lin et al., 2012). Most research facilities have point-of-care blood analyzers available, which are the most accurate means of determining the partial pressures of oxygen and carbon dioxide in the animal's blood (Valverde and Doherty, 2008).

VIII. Intraoperative support

A. Hypotension

A balanced electrolyte solution should be administered intravenously at 5−10 mL/kg/hour to support hydration during anesthesia (Lin et al., 2012). Perioperative intravenous fluid administration increases cardiac output and blood pressure with a subsequent increase in oxygen delivery to tissues (Valverde and Doherty, 2008).

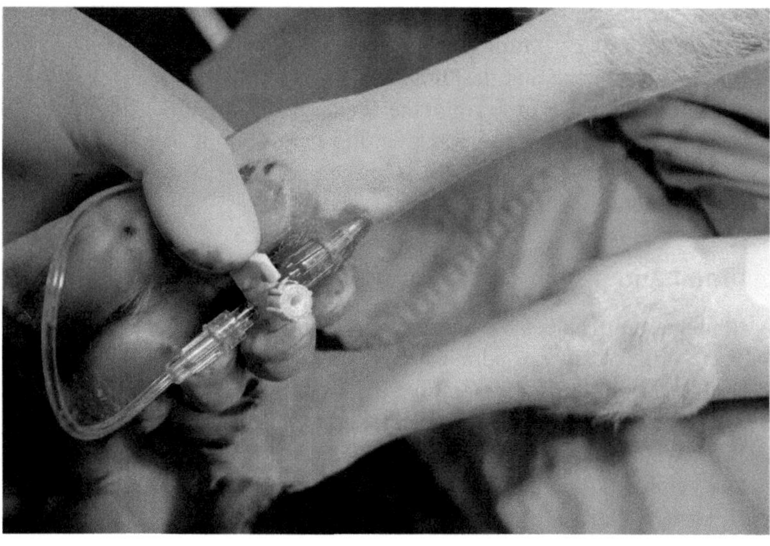

FIGURE 20.2 Catheterization of the palmar common digital artery of a calf for direct blood pressure measurement. Insertion point of a 20 gauge catheter in the common digital artery. The artery is most superficial just proximal to a point midway between the dewclaws of the forelimb. The artery courses in a slight lateral to medial direction.

Intraoperative hypotension is a common occurrence when anesthesia is maintained via inhalational anesthetics. Hypotension may also result from hypovolemia and decreased vascular resistance (Valverde and Doherty, 2008). Normotension can be achieved by correcting volume deficits and decreasing the anesthetic plane if the ruminant becomes too deep under anesthesia (Valverde and Doherty, 2008).

B. Mechanical ventilation

In addition to hypotension, inhalant anesthetics produce dose-dependent respiratory depression. When ruminants are placed in lateral or dorsal recumbency, pressure from the weight of the abdominal viscera pushes the diaphragm further into the thoracic cavity, reducing the functional residual capacity of the lung (Lin, 2015). The weight of the abdominal viscera will also compress the great vessels, such as the vena cava, which can result in decreased venous return, cardiac output, arterial blood pressure, and tissue perfusion (Klein and Fisher, 1988). Furthermore, gas produced as a byproduct of fermentation continues to accumulate in the rumen, increasing intragastric pressure. The subsequent decrease in tidal volume, lung compliance, and minute ventilation leads to increased ventilation/perfusion mismatch with significant hypoventilation, hypoxemia, and respiratory acidosis (Lin, 2015).

Mechanical ventilatory support is often needed with anesthetized ruminants as respiratory rate and tidal volume decrease with deeper anesthetic planes (Abrahamsen, 2009a). Many anesthesia systems used in the research setting offer the choice of either pressure- or volume-controlled ventilation when conventional positive pressure ventilation is utilized (Davis and Musk, 2014). Positive pressure ventilation using a tidal volume of 10–15 mL/kg, a respiratory rate of 8–12 breaths/minute, and a peak pressure not to exceed 30 cm H_2O is recommended for anesthetized small ruminants (Carney et al., 2009b Valverde and Doherty, 2008). In the authors' experience, the use of 5–12 cm H_2O positive end-expiratory pressure (PEEP) aids in preventing pulmonary atelectasis during thoracic surgery. Application of 10 cm H_2O of PEEP significantly improved lung aeration and gas exchange in adult laterally recumbent sheep anesthetized via a continuous rate infusion of propofol (Staffieri et al., 2010). Tidal volume should be adjusted to produce inspiratory pressures sufficient to maintain an end-tidal CO_2 of 35–45 mm Hg. In pregnant anesthetized ewes, both volume-controlled ventilation and pressure-controlled ventilation have been shown to produce adequate oxygenation, but pressure-controlled ventilation gave superior oxygenation at a lower peak inspiratory pressure (Davis and Musk, 2014). Regardless of the ventilation mode selected, the use of capnography with spirometry, along with arterial blood gas analyses, is recommended to best assess the adequacy of ventilation and oxygenation.

Because ruminants continue to produce a large amount of saliva while anesthetized, they should be positioned in such a way to facilitate saliva egress by placing a pad or a rolled-up towel under the neck so the opening of the mouth is below the level of the larynx (Abrahamsen, 2013). Doing so, along with the use of a cuffed endotracheal tube, will help protect the airway of the anesthetized ruminant from saliva and rumen contents. Preemptive treatment with atropine to reduce salivation is not recommended, as atropine merely reduces the water content of the saliva, causing it to become more viscous and therefore more likely to obstruct the endotracheal tube (Weaver, 1971). Passage of an orogastric tube into the rumen with intermittent suctioning of the mouth will help decrease the risk of aspiration. The use of an orogastric tube also minimizes the occurrence of free-gas bloat and ruminal tympany. Proper positioning and provision of adequate padding are important to prevent muscle and nerve damage during anesthesia. A 5 cm-thick foam pad is recommended to prevent nerve paralysis in calves and small ruminants (Lin, 2015).

C. Thermal support

Hypothermia frequently results in a major reduction of anesthetic requirement, prolonged anesthetic recovery, and adverse effects on wound healing and blood coagulation (Hall and Clarke, 1983; Valverde and Doherty, 2008). Thermal support can be provided by the use of a circulating warm water blanket or other commercial warming pads such as electronically conductive fabric (HotDog® Patient Warmer, Eden Prairie, MN). Forced air warming systems, IV fluid line warming devices, and maintenance of a warm environmental temperature can also be used to support normothermia during anesthesia and recovery. Like other species, ruminants should not be placed directly on radiant heat sources to avoid burns and overheating (Valverde and Doherty, 2008).

IX. Analgesia

To ensure animal welfare and a high standard of care, it is imperative for small ruminants to be routinely assessed for pain and distress, regardless of the analgesic regimen selected (Izer et al., 2019). Opioids, α-2 adrenergic receptor agonists, nonsteroidal antiinflammatory drugs (NSAIDs), and local anesthetics, either administered as sole agents, or preferably, in combination, are the analgesics most frequently used in small ruminants and calves. These agents can be administered via IV, IM, epidural, local infiltration, and intraarticular routes (Valverde and Doherty, 2008). As with other species, the use of preemptive and multimodal analgesia is recommended to produce effective, balanced analgesia. The use of several classes of analgesics together prevents pain transmission at multiple levels and decreases the adverse effects of each drug since a lower dose of each agent is required (Lin, 2014). Doses of systemic analgesics are presented in Table 20.5.

TABLE 20.5 Common routes and doses for analgesic drugs and NSAIDs in small ruminants.

Variable	Dose	Route
Morphine	0.1–0.5 mg/kg	IM
	0.5–1 mg/kg	IV
Butorphanol	0.05–0.5 mg/kg	IM, IV, SQ
Buprenorphine	0.005–0.01 mg/kg	SQ
	0.005–0.1 mg/kg	IM, IV
Fentanyl	2.5–5 mcg/kg	IV
	50 mcg/hour	Transdermal
Xylazine	0.05–0.2	IM, IV
Detomidine	0.003–0.01	IM, IV
Medetomidine	0.005–0.01	IM, IV
Lidocaine	2.5 mg/kg	IV
	0.05–0.1 mg/kg/minute	CRI
Ketamine	0.4–1.2 mg/kg/hour	CRI
	0.25–0.5 mg/kg	IM
Trifusion		CRI
Ketamine	0.6 mg/kg/hour	
Butorphanol (or alternatively morphine)	0.022 mg/kg/hour	
	0.025 mg/kg/hour	
Lidocaine	1.2 mg/kg/hour	
Pentafusion		CRI
Ketamine	0.6 mg/kg/hour	
Butorphanol	0.022 mg/kg/hour	
Lidocaine	1.2 mg/kg/hour	
Dexmedetomidine (or alternatively, detomidine)	0.0005 mg/kg/hour	
	0.004 mg/kg/hour	
Acepromazine	0.0022 mg/kg/hour	
Aspirin	50–100 mg/kg	PO
Flunixin meglumine	1–2.2 mg/kg	PO
	1–2.5 mg/kg	SQ
	1 mg/kg	IV
Ketoprofen	2–3 mg/kg	IV, IM
Phenylbutazone	5–10 mg/kg	PO
Carprofen	2–4 mg/kg	PO, SQ, IV

Source. Valverde and Doherty (2008).

A. Regulatory considerations

The use of many anesthetic and analgesic drugs in small ruminants may constitute "extra-label" use. Currently, there are no analgesic drugs approved for the alleviation of pain in livestock in the US (Coetzee, 2013; Smith, 2013; Stock and Coetzee, 2015). Only one anesthetic drug, 2% lidocaine is approved for use in cattle in the United States and one NSAID, flunixin meglumine, is approved for use in livestock for the relief of pyrexia and inflammation, but not pain (Smith, 2013; Smith and Modric, 2013). The Animal Medicinal Drug Use Act of 1994 permits the extra-label use of drugs for the alleviation of pain and suffering if all criteria for the extra-label use of such compounds in food-producing animals are met. Specifically, the animal must be identified and steps taken to assure the animal does not enter the food chain. This regulatory requirement must be considered if there is the potential for return of ruminants used in research into the food supply through practices such as adoption, resale, or rendering.

B. Opioids

Commonly used opioids for pain management in small ruminants are buprenorphine, butorphanol, meperidine, and fentanyl. Morphine, a full μ receptor agonist, should be used with caution due to the potential adverse effects on the GI system, such as decreased GI motility and reduced fecal output (Flecknell et al., 2015). Morphine has also produced behavioral side effects as a result of CNS stimulation and has poor analgesic properties in sheep and goats (Flecknell et al., 2015; Lin et al., 2012). Meperidine is a synthetic opioid that produces mild sedation with an analgesic potency of only 10%–50% that of morphine (Lin, 2014).

Fentanyl, a full μ receptor agonist, has a potency that is 75–100 times that of morphine and can be administered either parenterally or transdermally in small ruminants (Lin et al., 2012). Intravenous administration of fentanyl produces analgesia within 5 minutes and lasts for approximately 20 minutes (Lin et al., 2012). Intravenous administration of fentanyl in nonanesthetized farm animals has been associated with adverse effects including pica, hyperexcitability, ataxia, nystagmus, sedation, bradycardia, and respiratory depression (Carroll et al., 1999; George, 2003). With a half-life of 3 hours following IV administration in sheep, fentanyl is an effective peri-operative analgesia with minimal effects on GI function and rumen motility (Ahern et al., 2010; Flecknell et al., 2015). When placed 12 hours prior to general anesthesia, transdermal fentanyl patches (50 μg/hour) produced stable blood fentanyl concentrations for 40 hours in adult ewes (Ahern et al., 2010). For sheep undergoing orthopedic surgery, a preemptive fentanyl patch should be placed 24–36 hours prior to surgery, and 2 μg/kg/hour is an effective minimum therapeutic dose rate (Christou et al., 2015). Studies have shown high interindividual variability in absorption rates with the use of transdermal fentanyl patches in pregnant sheep models (Heikkinen et al., 2015; Musk et al., 2017a). Sheep displayed significant interanimal variation in plasma fentanyl concentrations after transdermal fentanyl solution dosing as well as adverse effects such as severe sedation, stereotypic pacing and head pressing, and drug-induced urinary retention necessitating naloxone reversal (Jen et al., 2017).

Buprenorphine hydrochloride, a partial μ agonist, has an analgesic potency that is 25 times that of morphine and is an effective analgesic in small ruminants and calves. In comparison to other species, it has a shorter duration of action in ruminants and requires more frequent dosing at 4–6 hours (Ahern et al., 2009; Swindle et al., 2002). Analgesia onset is approximately 45 minutes after IM administration (0.005–0.01 mg/kg) and lasts for 240 minutes (Lin et al., 2012). Reported adverse effects in sheep following buprenorphine administration include rapid and frequent head movements, propulsive walking, chewing, and heightened sensitivity to visual and auditory stimuli (Nolan et al., 1987). Buprenorphine (0.01 mg/kg IM) administered every 6 hours to goats after orthopedic surgery produced satisfactory analgesia (Lin, 2014). Others have reported agitation, rumen stasis, and increased plasma concentrations of cortisol and vasopressin following buprenorphine treatment (0.02 mg/kg IV or IM) in goats (Ingvast-Larsson et al., 2007). Therefore, buprenorphine should be used with caution in this species.

A sustained-release formulation of buprenorphine is now commercially available which has the advantage of minimizing restraint-induced stress associated with repeated injections and decreasing the probability of end-of-dose breakthrough pain (Walkowiak and Graham, 2015). A single dose of sustained-release (SR) buprenorphine (0.27 mg/kg IM or SQ) produced steady plasma concentrations and continuous analgesia assessed via thermal nociception for 72 hours without clinical adverse effects in a pilot study of adult sheep (Walkowiak and Graham, 2015). Another study found a long-lasting potential analgesic plasma level of buprenorphine following a single SQ dose of 0.1 mg/kg of SR buprenorphine in adult sheep starting 2 days after treatment, which lasted for 5 days (Zullian et al., 2016). These results were based on an effective analgesic plasma threshold determined in other species to be 0.1 ng/mL, but the authors acknowledge that a threshold specific to sheep has yet to be determined (Zullian et al., 2016).

Butorphanol is both a κ receptor agonist and a μ receptor antagonist. When dosed at 0.05–0.1 mg/kg IV, IM, or SQ every 4–6 hours, it can relieve mild to moderate pain in small ruminants (Abrahamsen, 2009b). When administered as a sole agent, it can produce light sedation in small ruminants (Lin et al., 2012). Adverse effects, including ataxia and excitement, have been reported with IV administration of butorphanol in sheep and goats (Doherty et al., 2002a; Waterman et al., 1991). Butorphanol combined with a sedative or a tranquilizer can effectively produce standing sedation and analgesia for minor surgery in small ruminants (Lin et al., 2012).

C. Nonsteroidal antiinflammatory drugs

NSAIDs including flunixin meglumine, carprofen, meloxicam, ketoprofen, phenylbutazone, and aspirin have been used in ruminants for the relief of pain (Anderson and Edmondson, 2013; Lin, 2014; Plummer and Schleining, 2013; Swindle et al., 2002; Valverde and Doherty, 2008). Although not labeled for use as an analgesic, flunixin meglumine (1.1−2.2 mg/kg) is often used for pain management in ruminants. Dosing should be limited to a maximum of four doses to minimize the adverse effects of renal toxicity and gastric hemorrhage (Swindle et al., 2002). Carprofen administered to sheep at 0.7 mg/kg and 4 mg/kg IV had therapeutic plasma concentrations of the drug for a duration of at least 72 hours (George, 2003). When compared to phenylbutazone and aspirin, carprofen is more potent and has less potential to induce GI ulceration (Delatour et al., 1996). In addition to reaching therapeutic plasma concentrations, studies have demonstrated the efficacy of NSAIDs in reducing pain-associated behaviors and physiological responses to painful husbandry procedures in sheep and calves (Colditz et al., 2009; Faulkner and Weary, 2000; Paull et al., 2007, 2009).

Meloxicam has provided effective analgesia to calves following castration and dehorning and has reportedly produced significant analgesic effects in pain models of sheep (Colditz et al., 2019; Heinrich et al., 2010; Marini et al., 2015; Theurer et al., 2012; Todd et al., 2010). An initial study of the use of sustained-release meloxicam in sheep following SQ administration demonstrated higher plasma levels of the drug than from the standard formulation throughout the initial 24 hours period (Dunbar et al., 2019). There was variability in plasma levels of sustained-release meloxicam thereafter, and presumed therapeutic levels of 400 ng/mL were not sustained for the full 72 hours across all animals in this preliminary investigation (Dunbar et al., 2019). Additional studies are needed to fully characterize the use of sustained-release meloxicam in sheep.

D. Ketamine

At subanesthetic and anesthetic doses, ketamine inhibits NMDA receptors and stimulates μ receptors to produce strong analgesic effects (Lin, 2014). There is increased acceptance of using low-dose ketamine either to manage acute or chronic pain in humans and animals (Chiz, 2007; Gorlin et al., 2016; Muir, 2010). In humans, subanesthetic doses (0.3 mg/kg or less IV) blunt central pain sensitization with negligible physiologic effects (Gorlin et al., 2016). Perioperative low-dose ketamine enhances analgesia and reduces opioid requirements in the postoperative period following a variety of surgical procedures in humans (Gorlin et al., 2016). Low-dose ketamine has been safely used for short- and long-term pain management in healthy conscious horses via continuous rate infusion at 1.5 mg/kg/hour, with excitability effects noted when plasma concentrations exceeded 0.280 mg/mL (Lankveld et al., 2006). Ketamine (0.6 mg/kg/hour) is useful as an adjunct to other perioperative analgesics to provide pain control and decrease the concentration of inhalant anesthetic required in dogs and cats (Bednarski, 2015). Similarly, ketamine (1.5 mg/kg IV loading dose followed by 50 μg/kg/minute) combined with lidocaine (2.5 mg/kg IV loading dose followed by 100 μg/kg/minute) resulted in a substantial reduction in the concentration of isoflurane required to maintain general anesthesia in goats (Doherty et al., 2007). Subanesthetic infusions of ketamine (20 μg/kg/minute) reduced postoperative pain following rumenotomy in goats; however, the low-dose ketamine infusion did not provide sufficient analgesia intraoperatively in the ketamine-diazepam anesthetized goats (Udegbunam et al., 2019). There is a potential for using low-dose ketamine for analgesia in sheep. Long-lasting analgesic effects have been reported in sheep undergoing orthopedic procedures (Guedes et al., 2006). Ketamine in combination with drugs active at other receptor sites, i.e., α2-adrenergic agonists is recommended for the control of severe pain in sheep (Lizarraga and Chambers, 2012). Ketamine combined with lidocaine and butorphanol ("trifusion") has been used by the authors to effectively manage postoperative pain following thoracotomy in sheep and calves, as discussed below.

E. Multimodal analgesic continuous rate infusions

Administration of analgesic combinations via continuous infusion allows low doses of analgesics to be used to maintain steady-state plasma concentrations and avoid breakthrough pain associated with peak and trough fluctuations of drug effects that occur with repeated injections (Lin, 2014). A continuous rate infusion of an opioid (butorphanol 0.022 mg/kg/hour or morphine 0.025 mg/kg/hour), lidocaine (1.2 mg/kg/hour), and ketamine (0.6 mg/kg/hour), commonly referred to as "trifusion," is effective in providing long-lasting analgesia in sheep and goats (Lin, 2014). The solution is prepared by adding 20 mg butorphanol, 1200 mg lidocaine, and 600 mg ketamine to a 1 L bag of 0.9% NaCl for final drug concentrations of 0.02 mg/mL butorphanol, 1.2 mg/mL lidocaine and 0.6 mg/mL ketamine. Before initiating the CRI, a loading dose of butorphanol (0.05−0.1 mg/kg IV or IM) should be administered to small ruminants to immediately increase the plasma concentration of the drug (Lin, 2014). A loading dose of lidocaine (1 mg/kg IV) may be administered slowly to prevent adverse cardiovascular and CNS effects (Lin, 2014); however, in the author's experience, is not necessary prior to initiating the CRI.

Detomidine (0.004 mg/kg/hour) and acepromazine (0.0022 mg/kg/hour) have been added to trifusion, creating a five-drug combination known as "pentafusion" (Abrahamsen, 2009b). The authors use a lower concentration of dexmedetomidine (0.0005 mg/kg/hour), which minimizes behavioral or GI side effects, to successfully alleviate postoperative pain in sheep and calves following thoracotomy and sternotomy. It is the authors' practice to administer dexmedetomidine and acepromazine as individual CRIs separate from the trifusion combination to allow for a gradual decrease and discontinuation of one analgesic at a time as the immediate postoperative period progresses and the need for severe pain management diminishes.

F. Local and regional anesthesia

Local anesthetics such as lidocaine, bupivacaine, and others can be used as sole agents for minor procedures or as supplements to anesthetic or analgesic regimens. Infusion of lidocaine alone or in combination with ketamine during surgery has an anesthetic-sparing effect, improving anesthetic stability (Raske et al., 2010; Vesal et al., 2011). When combined with other analgesics in a constant rate infusion, lidocaine acts in an additive or synergistic effect for the management of severe acute pain in the postoperative period (Abrahamsen, 2009b; Lin and Walz, 2014).

Local anesthetics injected or infiltrated subcutaneously (i.e., ring block) can be effectively used in the awake animal for minor procedures such as laceration repair. Intravenous regional anesthesia achieved by injection of local anesthetics in the vein of a distal limb after compression of the venous drainage, the eponymously named "Bier block", will effectively anesthetize the region of the limb below the point of venous occlusion (Edmondson, 2016; Campoy and Read, 2015). The technique is often used in the field for surgery on the foot, but one of the authors (RW) has used the technique for minor surgery of the distal limb in calves. The technique is well described and illustrated in the cited references.

Local anesthesia of specific nerves and administration of analgesics by the epidural route has long been used in the clinical management of various conditions in ruminants. These can be easily adopted to supplement the anesthesia and analgesia of ruminants in the biomedical research setting. Detailed description of the various techniques is beyond the scope of this chapter, and the reader is referred to any of the comprehensive veterinary anesthesia texts such as *Lumb and Jones Veterinary Anesthesia and Analgesia* (Grimm et al., 2015) and *Farm Animal Anesthesia* (Lin and Walz, 2014).

Delivery of local anesthetics directly to the wound is a common technique for providing additional analgesia postoperatively. Application of local anesthetics to the wound, so-called "splash blocks" are a simple method for providing additional analgesia in the immediate postoperative period. However, the duration of analgesia is short and unpredictable, being determined by the specific local anesthetic used, the rate of diffusion from the wound site, dilution by bodily fluids, etc. Continuous delivery of local anesthetic to the surgical wound through a diffusion ("soaker") catheter is a technique adopted from human medicine and widely used for supplemental analgesia following surgery in companion animals. The authors have routinely used wound catheters to deliver local anesthetics (lidocaine and bupivacaine) to thoracotomy incisions in calves and sheep. Following the closure of the thoracotomy incision, an 18 cm or 22.5 cm diffusion catheter (Mila International, Inc.) is placed along the suture line at the level of the ribs and intercostal muscles and the subcutaneous and skin are closed over the catheter (Fig. 20.3). Bupivacaine is administered every 4−6 hours using a dose extrapolated from the canine dosage (5 mL for lambs and 8 mL for adult sheep and calves). Assay of plasma bupivacaine levels have not detected concentrations associated with toxicity in sheep (unpublished data). Typically, the catheters are kept in place and local anesthetics are administered for 3−5 days postsurgery. Additional analgesia is administered if indicated. It is possible to administer local anesthetics through the diffusion catheter by CRI; however, experience with this administration route in dogs indicates periodic bolus administration provided superior drug concentrations at the wound site (Hansen et al., 2013). Delivery of local anesthetics to the surgical wound combined with systemic analgesics provides effective pain management for ruminants following surgeries involving thoracotomies (Izer et al., 2018, 2019).

A.

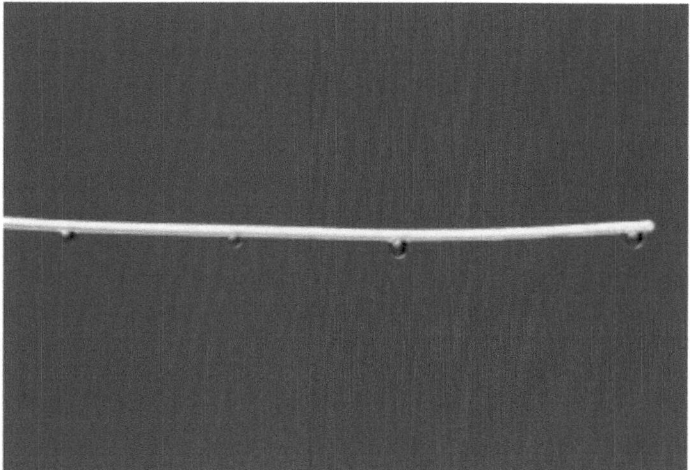

B.

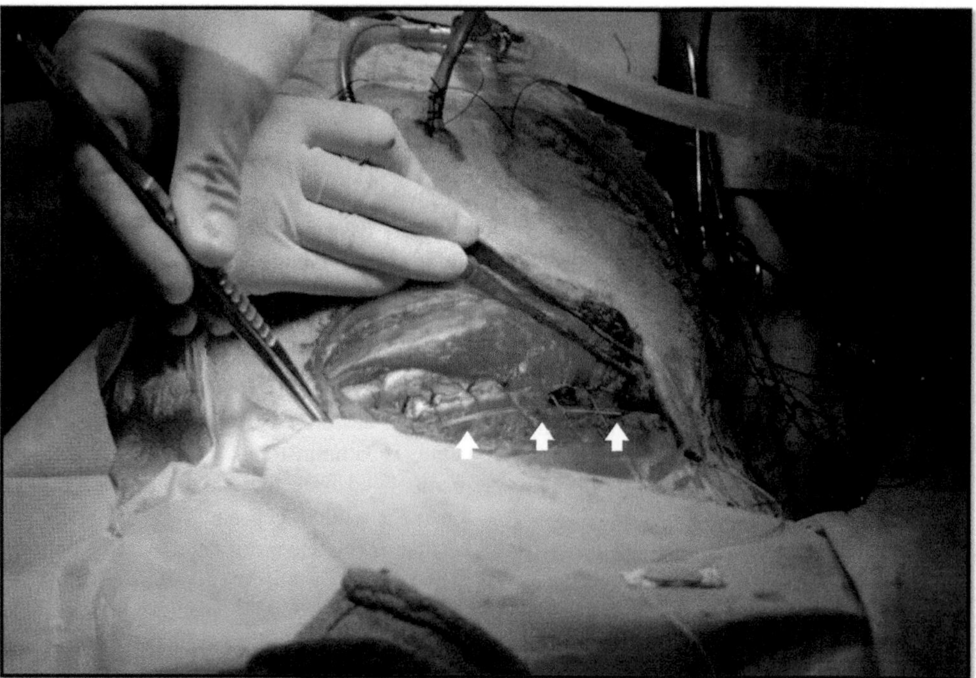

FIGURE 20.3 Placement of diffusion ("soaker") catheter at thoracotomy incision for delivery of local anesthetic. (A) 22.5 cm diffusion catheter. (B) The catheter (*arrows*) is placed after closure of the chest incision and before closure of the subcutaneous layers and skin. *(A) Photo courtesy of Mila International.*

References

Aarnes, T.K., Hubbell, J.A., Lerche, P., Bednarski, R.M., 2014. Comparison of invasive and oscillometric blood pressure measurement techniques in anesthetized sheep, goats, and cattle. Vet. Anaesth. Analg. 41 (2), 174–185.

Abrahamsen, E., 2009a. Inhalation anesthesia in ruminants. In: Anderson, D., Rings, D. (Eds.), Current Veterinary Therapy Food Animal Practice, fifth ed. Elsevier, pp. 559–569.

Abrahamsen, E., 2009b. Managing severe pain in ruminants. In: Anderson, D.E., Rings, D.M. (Eds.), Current Veterinary Therapy Food Animal Practice, fifth ed. Elsevier, pp. 570–575.

Abrahamsen, E.J., 2008. Ruminant field anesthesia. Vet. Clin. N. Am. Food Anim. Pract. 24 (3), 429–441.

Abrahamsen, E.J., 2013. Chemical restraint and injectable anesthesia of ruminants. Vet. Clin. N. Am. Food Anim. Pract. 29 (1), 209–227.

Adami, C., Bergadano, A., Bruckmaier, R.M., Stoffel, M.H., Doherr, M.G., Spadavecchia, C., 2011. Sciatic-femoral nerve block with bupivacaine in goats undergoing elective stifle arthrotomy. Vet. J. 188 (1), 53–57. https://doi.org/10.1016/j.tvjl.2010.02.008.

Ahern, B.J., Soma, L.R., Boston, R.C., Schaer, T.P., 2009. Comparison of the analgesic properties of transdermally administered fentanyl and intramuscularly administered buprenorphine during and following experimental orthopedic surgery in sheep. Am. J. Vet. Res. 70 (3), 418–422.

Ahern, B.J., Soma, L.R., Rudy, J.A., Uboh, C.E., Schaer, T.P., 2010. Pharmacokinetics of fentanyl administered transdermally and intravenously in sheep. Am. J. Vet. Res. 71 (10), 1127–1132.

Ajuda, I., Battini, M., Mattiello, S., Arcuri, C., Stilwell, G., 2020. Evaluation of pain mitigation strategies in goat kids after cautery disbudding. Animals 10, 277. https://doi.org/10.3390/ani10020277.

Alves, G., Hartsfield, S., Carroll, G., Santos, D., Zhang, S., Tsolis, R., et al., 2003. Use of propofol, isoflurane and morphine for prolonged general anesthesia in calves. Arq. Bras. Med. Vet. Zootec. 55 (4), 411–420.

American Society for Animal Science [ASAS], 2020. Guide for the Care and Use of Agricultural Animals in Research and Teaching, fourth ed. https://www.asas.org/docs/default-source/default-document-library/ag guide_4th.pdf?sfvrsn=56b44ed1_2.

Anderson, D.E., Edmondson, M.A., 2013. Prevention and management of surgical pain in cattle. Vet. Clin. N. Am. Food Anim. Pract. 29 (1), 157–184.

Anil, S.S., Anil, L., Deen, J., 2002. Challenges of pain assessment in domestic animals. J. Am. Vet. Med. Assoc. 220, 313–319.

Ashley, P.J., Ringrose, S., Edwards, K.L., Wallington, E., McCrohan, C.R., Sneddon, L.U., 2009. Effect of noxious stimulation upon antipredator responses and dominance status in rainbow trout. Anim. Behav. 77 (2), 403–410. https://doi.org/10.1016/j.anbehav.2008.10.015.

Barragan, A.A., Bauman, L.M., Schuenemann, G.M., Velez, J., Lakritz, J., Coetzee, J.F., et al., 2018. Administration of acetylsalicylic acid after parturition in lactating dairy cows under certified organic management: part II. Biomarkers of nociception, inflammation, and stress. J. Dairy Sci. 103 (12), 11713–11722. https://doi.org/10.3168/jds.2020-18389.

Beausoleil, N.J., Mellor, D.J., 2015. Introducing breathlessness as a significant animal welfare issue. N. Z. Vet. J. 63 (1), 44–51. https://doi.org/10.1080/00480169.2014.940410.

Bednarski, R.M., 2015. Dogs and cats. In: Grimm, K.A., Lamont, L.A., Tranquilli, W.J., Greene, S.A., Robertson, S.A. (Eds.), Veterinary Anesthesia and Analgesia: The Fifth Edition of Lumb and Jones, fifth ed. John Wiley & Sons, Inc, pp. 817–826.

Bednarski, R., McGuirk, S., 1986. Bradycardia associated with fasting in cattle. Vet. Surg. 15 (6), 458.

Borges, L.P., Nishimura, L.T., Carvalho, L.L., Cerejo, S.A., Auckburally, A., Mattos-Junior, E., 2016. Behavioral and cardiopulmonary effects of dexmedetomidine alone and in combination with butorphanol, methadone, morphine or tramadol in conscious sheep. Vet. Anaesth. Analg. 43 (5), 549–560. https://doi.org/10.1111/vaa.12339.

Brooks, K.S.M., Hempstead, M.N., Anderson, J.L., Parsons, R.L., Sutherland, M.A., Plummer, P.J., Millman, S.T., 2021. Characterization of efficacy and animal safety across four caprine disbudding methodologies. Animals 11, 430. https://doi.org/10.3390/ani11020430.

Cagnardi, P., Zonca, A., Gallo, M., Pravettoni, D., Morandi, N., Villa, R., Carli, S., 2009. Pharmacokinetics of propofol in calves undergoing abdominal surgery. Vet. Res. Commun. 33, 177–179. https://doi.org/10.1007/s11259-009-9281-9.

Campoy, L., Read, M., 2015. Local and regional anesthetic techniques. In: Gaynor, J.S., Muir, W.W. (Eds.), Handbook of Veterinary Pain Management, third ed. Mosby, pp. 224–265 https://doi.org/10.1016/B978-0-323-08935-7.00012-0.

Carney, E.L., Clark, J.B., Myers, J.L., Peterson, R., Wilson, R.P., Weiss, W.J., 2009a. Animal model development for the Penn State pediatric ventricular assist device. Artif. Organs 33 (11), 953–957. https://doi.org/10.1111/j.1525-1594.2009.00896.x.

Carney, E., Litwak, K., Weiss, W., 2009b. Animal Models Working Group. Animal models for pediatric circulatory support device preclinical testing: National Heart, Lung, and Blood Institute Pediatric Assist Device Contractor's Meeting Animal Models Working Group. Am. Soc. Artif. Intern. Organs J. 55 (1), 6–9. https://doi.org/10.1097/MAT.0b013e318198e11c.

Carroll, G.L., Hartsfield, S.M., 1996. General anesthetic techniques in ruminants. Vet. Clin. N. Am. Food Anim. Pract. 12 (3), 627–661. https://doi.org/10.1016/S0749-0720(15)30391-1.

Carroll, G.L., Hartsfield, S.M., Champney, T.H., Geller, S.C., Martinez, E.A., Haley, E.L., 2005. Effect of medetomidine and its antagonism with atipamezole on stress-related hormones, metabolites, physiologic responses, sedation, and mechanical threshold in goats. Vet. Anaesth. Analg. 32 (3), 147–157. https://doi.org/10.1111/j.1467-2995.2005.00187.x.

Carroll, G.L., Hartsfield, S.M., Champney, T.H., Slater, M.R., Newman, J.A., 1998. Stress-related hormonal and metabolic responses to restraint, with and without butorphanol administration, in preconditioned goats. Lab. Anim. Sci. 48 (4), 387–390.

Carroll, G.L., Hooper, R.N., Boothe, D.M., Hartsfield, S.M., Randoll, L.A., 1999. Pharmacokinetics of fentanyl after intravenous and transdermal administration in goats. Am. J. Vet. Res. 60 (8), 986–991.

Caulkett, N., Duke, T., Cribb, P., 1996. Cardiopulmonary effects of medetomidine-ketamine in domestic sheep (*Ovis ovis*) maintained in sternal recumbency. J. Zoo Wildl. Med. 27, 217–226.

Celly, C.S., McDonell, W.N., Young, S.S., Black, W.D., 1997. The comparative hypoxaemic effect of four alpha 2 adrenoceptor agonists (xylazine, romifidine, detomidine and medetomidine) in sheep. J. Vet. Pharmacol. Therapeut. 20 (6), 464–471.

Chiz, B.A., 2007. Low dose ketamine: a therapeutic and research tool to explore N-methyl-D-aspartate (NMDA) receptor-mediated plasticity in pain pathways. J. Psychopharmacol. 21 (3), 259–271. https://doi.org/10.1177/0269881105062484.

Christou, C., Oliver, R.A., Rawlinson, J., Walsh, W.R., 2015. Transdermal fentanyl and its use in ovine surgery. Res. Vet. Sci. 100, 252–256. https://doi.org/10.1016/j.rvsc.2015.04.006.

Coetzee, J.F., 2013. A review of analgesic compounds used in food animals in the united states. Vet. Clin. North Am. Food Anim. Pract. 29, 11–28.

Coetzee, J.F., Gehring, R., Tarus-Sang, J., Anderson, D.E., 2010. Effect of sub-anesthetic xylazine and ketamine ('ketamine stun') administered to calves immediately prior to castration. Vet. Anaesth. Analg. 37 (6), 566–578. https://doi.org/10.1111/j.1467-2995.2010.00573.x.

Colditz, I.G., Lloyd, J.B., Paull, D.R., Lee, C., Giraudo, A., Pizzato, C., Fisher, A., 2009. Effect of the non-steroidal antiinflammatory drug, carprofen, on weaned sheep following non-surgical mulesing by intradermal injection of cetrimide. Aust. Vet. J. 87 (1), 19–26. https://doi.org/10.1111/j.1751-0813.2008.00384.x.

Colditz, I.G., Paull, D.R., Lloyd, J.B., Johnston, L., Small, A.H., 2019. Efficacy of meloxicam in a pain model in sheep. Aust. Vet. J. 97 (1–2), 23–32. https://doi.org/10.1111/avj.12779.

Collan, R., 1970. Anesthetic and paraoperative management of sheep for total heart replacement. Anesth. Analg. 49 (2), 336–343.

Columbano, N., Duffee, L.R., Melosu, V., Scanu, A., Dore, S., Sotgiu, G., Driessen, B., Careddu, G.M., 2018a. Determination of minimum alveolar concentration and cardiovascular effects of desflurane in positive-pressure ventilated sheep. Am. J. Vet. Res. 79, 727–732. https://doi.org/10.2460/ajvr.79.7.727.

Columbano, N., Scanu, A., Duffee, L., Melosu, V., Sotgiu, G., Driessen, B., 2018b. Determination of the minimum alveolar concentration (MAC) and cardiopulmonary effects of sevoflurane in sheep. Vet. Anaesth. Analg. 45, 487–495. https://doi.org/10.1016/j.vaa.2018.01.007.

Davis, J., Musk, G.C., 2014. Pressure and volume controlled mechanical ventilation in anaesthetized pregnant sheep. Lab. Anim. 48 (4), 321–327. https://doi.org/10.1177/0023677214543842.

de Carvalho, L.L., Nishimura, L.T., Borges, L.P., Cerejo, S.A., Villela, I.O., Auckburally, A., de Mantos-Junior, E., 2016. Sedative and cardiopulmonary effects of xylazine alone or in combination with methadone, morphine or tramadol in sheep. Vet. Anaesth. Analg. 43 (2), 179–188. https://doi.org/10.1111/vaa.12296.

de Moura, R.S., Bittar, I.P., da Silva, L.H., Villela, A.C.V., Dos Santos Júnior, M.B., Borges, N.C., Franco, L.G., 2018. Sedative and cardiorespiratory effects of detomidine constant rate infusion in sheep. Lab. Anim. 52 (1), 51–58. https://doi.org/10.1177/0023677217714013.

de Oliveira, F.A., Luna, S.P.L., do Amaral, J.B., Rodrigues, K.A., Sant'Anna, A.C., Daolio, M., Brondani, J.T., 2014. Validation of the UNESP-Botucatu unidimensional composite pain scale for assessing postoperative pain in cattle. BMC Vet. Res. 10, 200. https://doi.org/10.1186/s12917-014-0200-0.

Delatour, P., Foot, R., Foster, A.P., Baggot, D., Lees, P., 1996. Pharmacodynamics and chiral pharmacokinetics of carprofen in calves. Br. Vet. J. 152 (2), 183–198.

della Rocca, G., Brondani, J.T., de Oliveira, F.A., Crociati, M., Sylla, L., Ngonput, A.E., et al., 2017. Validation of the Italian version of the UNESP-Botucatu unidimensional composite pain scale for the assessment of postoperative pain in cattle. Vet. Anaesth. Analg. 44 (5), 1253–1261. https://doi.org/10.1016/j.vaa.2016.11.008.

des Roches, A.B., Lussert, A., Faure, M., Herry, V., Rainard, P., Durand, D., et al., 2018. Dairy cows under experimentally-induced *Escherichia coli* mastitis show negative emotional states assessed through Qualitative Behavioural Assessment. Appl. Anim. Behav. Sci. 206, 1–11. https://doi.org/10.1016/j.applanim.2018.06.004.

Deschk, M., Wagatsuma, J.T., Araújo, M.A., Santos, G.G., Júnior, S.S., Abimussi, C.J., et al., 2016. Continuous infusion of propofol in calves: bispectral index and hemodynamic effects. Vet. Anaesth. Analg. 43 (3), 309–315. https://doi.org/10.1111/vaa.12302.

Destrez, A., Coulon, M., Deiss, V., Delval, E., Boissy, A., Boivin, X., 2013. The valence of the long-lasting emotional experiences with various handlers modulates discrimination and generalization of individual humans in sheep. J. Anim. Sci. 91 (11), 5418–5426. https://doi.org/10.2527/jas.2012-5654.

Dewell, R.D., Millman, S.T., Gould, S.A., Tofflemire, K.L., Whitley, R.D., Parsons, R.L., et al., 2014. Evaluating approaches to measuring ocular pain in bovine calves with corneal scarification and infectious bovine keratoconjunctivitis-associated corneal ulcerations. J. Anim. Sci. 92 (3), 1161–1172. https://doi.org/10.2527/jas.2013-7264.

Doherty, T.J., Rohrbach, B.W., Geiser, D.R., 2002a. Effect of acepromazine and butorphanol on isoflurane minimum alveolar concentration in goats. J. Vet. Pharmacol. Therapeut. 25 (1), 65–67. https://doi.org/10.1046/j.1365-2885.2002.00371.x.

Doherty, T.J., Rohrbach, B.W., Ross, L., Schultz, H., 2002b. The effect of tiletamine and zolazepam on isoflurane minimum alveolar concentration in goats. J. Vet. Pharmacol. Therapeut. 25 (3), 233–235. https://doi.org/10.1046/j.1365-2885.2002.00401.x.

Doherty, T., Redua, M.A., Queiroz-Castro, P., Egger, C., Cox, S.K., Rohrbach, B.W., 2007. Effect of intravenous lidocaine and ketamine on the minimum alveolar concentration of isoflurane in goats. Vet. Anaesth. Analg. 34 (2), 125–131. https://doi.org/10.1111/j.1467-2995.2006.00301.x.

Dunbar, M.L., Walkowiak, K.J., Faustich, J.S., Rendahl, A.K., Graham, M.L., 2019. Preliminary evaluation of sustained-release compared with conventional formulations of meloxicam in sheep (*Ovis aries*). JAALAS 58 (3), 339–345. https://doi.org/10.30802/AALAS-JAALAS-18-000076.

Dwyer, C.M., 2004. How has the risk of predation shaped the behavioural responses of sheep to fear and distress? Anim. Welf. 13 (3), 269–281.

Dzikiti, B.T., Stegmann, F.G., Dzikiti, L.N., Hellebrekers, L.J., 2010. Total intravenous anaesthesia (TIVA) with propofol-fentanyl and propofol-midazolam combinations in spontaneously-breathing goats. Vet. Anaesth. Analg. 37 (6), 519–525. https://doi.org/10.1111/j.1467-2995.2010.00568.x.

Dzikiti, B.T., Stegmann, F.G., Cromarty, D., Dzikiti, L.N., Hellebrekers, L.J., 2011. Effects of propofol on isoflurane minimum alveolar concentration and cardiovascular function in mechanically ventilated goats. Vet. Anaesth. Analg. 38 (1), 44–53. https://doi.org/10.1111/j.1467-2995.2010.00585.x.

Edmondson, M.A., 2016. Local, regional, and spinal anesthesia in Ruminants. Vet. Clin. North Am. Food Anim. Pract. 32 (3), 535–552. https://doi.org/10.1016/j.cvfa.2016.05.015.

Ewing, K.K., 1990. Anesthesia techniques in sheep and goats. Vet. Clin. N. Am. Food Anim. Pract. 6 (3), 759–778.

Farm Animal Welfare Committee, 2009. FAWC Report on Farm Animal Welfare in Great Britain: Past, Present and Future. Retrieved May 17, 2021, from. https://www.gov.uk/government/publications/fawc-report-on-farm-animal-welfare-in-great-britain-past-present-and-future.

Faulkner, P.M., Weary, D.M., 2000. Reducing pain after dehorning in dairy calves. J. Dairy Sci. 83 (9), 2037–2041. https://doi.org/10.3168/jds.s0022-0302(00)75084-3.

Ferreira, J.P., Ndawana, P.S., Dzikiti, L.N., Dzikiti, B.T., 2016. Determination of the minimum infusion rate of propofol required to prevent purposeful movement of the extremities in response to a standardized noxious stimulus in goats. Vet. Anaesth. Analg. 43 (5), 519–527. https://doi.org/10.1111/vaa.12327.

Flecknell, P., Lofgren, J., Dyson, M., Marini, R., Swindle, M., Wilson, R., 2015. Preanesthesia, anesthesia, analgesia and euthanasia. In: Fox, J.G., Anderson, L.C., Otto, G.M., Pritchett-Corning, K.R., Whary, M.T. (Eds.), Laboratory Animal Medicine, third ed. Academic Press, pp. 1135–1200. https://doi.org/10.1016/B978-0-12-409527-4.00024-9.

Fonseca, V.F.C., Saraiva, E.P., Maia, A.S.C., Costa, C.C.D., dos Santos, S.G.C.G., Morais, L.K.C., et al., 2019. Training sheep for indirect calorimetry trials. Small Rumin. Res. 177, 36–43. https://doi.org/10.1016/j.smallrumres.2019.06.010.

Forbes, D., Blom, H.J.M., Kostomitsopoulos, N., Moore, G., Perretta, G., 2007. Felasa Euroguide. On the Accomodation and Care of Animals Used for Experimental and Other Scientific Purposes.

Fraser, D., Weary, D.M., Pajor, E.A., Milligan, B.N., 1997. A scientific conception of animal welfare that reflects ethical concerns. Anim. Welf. 6, 187—205.

French, N.P., Wall, R., Morgan, K.L., 1994. Lamb tail docking—a controlled field study of the effects of tail amputation on health and productivity. Vet. Rec. 134 (18), 463—467.

Gray, P.R., McDonell, W.N., 1986a. Anesthesia in goats and sheep 1. Local analgesia Compendium on Continuing Education For the Practicing Veterinarian 8, S33—S39.

Gray, P.R., McDonell, W.N., 1986b. Anesthesia and analgesia in goats and sheep 2. General anesthesia Compendium on Continuing Education For the Practicing Veterinarian 8, S127—S135.

George, L., 2003. Pain control in farm animals. In: Steffey, E.P. (Ed.), Recent Advances in Anesthetic Management of Large Domestic Animals. International Veterinary Information Service (IVIS). https://www.ivis.org/node/85814.

Gerring, E.L., Scarth, S.C., 1974. Anesthesia for open-heart surgery in calf. Brit. J. Anaesthesia 46, 455—460.

Gleerup, K.B., Andersen, P.H., Munksgaard, L., Forkman, B., 2015. Pain evaluation in dairy cattle. Appl. Anim. Behav. Sci. 171, 25—32. https://doi.org/10.1016/j.applanim.2015.08.023.

Gogoi, S.R., Sarma, B., Lahon, D.K., 2003. Clinical evaluation of medetomidine and medetomidine ketamine in goats. Indian J. Anim. Sci. 73, 271.

Gorlin, A.W., Rosenfeld, D.M., Ramakrishna, H., 2016. Intravenous subanesthetic ketamine for perioperative analgesia. J. Anaesthesiol. Clin. Pharmacol. 32 (2), 160—167. https://doi.org/10.4103/0970-9185.182085.

Graham, M.J., Kent, J.E., Molony, V., 1997. Effects of four analgesic treatments on the behavioural and cortisol responses of 3-week-old lambs to tail docking. Vet. J. 153, 87—97.

Grandin, T., 2014. Behavioural principles of handling cattle and other grazing animals under extensive conditions. In: Grandin, T. (Ed.), Livestock Handling and Transport. CAB International, pp. 63—86. https://doi.org/10.1079/9781780643212.0039.

Grant, E.P., Wickham, S.L., Anderson, F., Barnes, A.L., Fleming, P.A., Miller, D.W., 2020. Preliminary findings on a novel behavioural approach for the assessment of pain and analgesia in lambs subject to routine husbandry procedures. Animals 10 (7), 1148. https://doi.org/10.3390/ani10071148.

Gray, P.R., McDonell, W.N., 1986. Anesthesia in goats and sheep, part II: general anesthesia. Compend. Continuing Educ. Pract. Vet. 8, S127—S135.

Greene, S., 2003. Protocols for anesthesia of cattle. Vet. Clin. North Am. Food Anim. Pract. 19, 679—693.

Greene, S.A., Thurmon, J.C., 1988. Xylazine—a review of its pharmacology and use in veterinary medicine. J. Vet. Pharmacol. Therapeut. 11 (4), 295—313.

Grimm, K.A., Lamont, L.A., Tranquilli, W.J., Greene, S.A., Robertson, S.A. (Eds.), 2015. Veterinary anesthesia and analgesia. John Wiley & Sons.

Guatteo, R., Levionnois, O., Fournier, D., Guemene, D., Latouche, K., Leterrier, C., et al., 2012. Minimising pain in farm animals: the 3S approach—'Suppress, Substitute, Soothe'. Animal 6 (8), 1261—1274. https://doi.org/10.1017/S1751731112000262.

Guedes, A.G.P., Pluhar, G.E., Daubs, B.M., Rude, E.P., 2006. Effects of preoperative epidural administration of racemic ketamine for analgesia in sheep undergoing surgery. Am. J. Vet. Res. 67 (2), 222—229. https://doi.org/10.2460/ajvr.67.2.222.

Habel, R.E., 1975. Ruminant digestive system. In: Getty, R. (Ed.), Sisson and Grossman's— The Anatomy of the Domestic Animals, fifth ed. W.B. Saunders Co, Philadelphia, PA, pp. 861—915.

Hall, L.W., Clarke, K.W., 1983. Accident and emergencies associated with anesthesia. In: Veterinary Anaesthesia, eighth ed. Bailliere Tindall, pp. 367—388.

Hansen, B., Lascelles, B.D.X., Thomson, A., DePuy, V., 2013. Variability of performance of wound infusion catheters. Vet. Anaesth. Analg. 40 (3), 308—315. https://doi.org/10.1111/vaa.12016.

Harris, C., White, P.J., Mohler, V.L., Lomax, S., 2020. Electroencephalography can distinguish between pain and anaesthetic intervention in conscious lambs undergoing castration. Animals 10 (3), 428. https://doi.org/10.3390/ani10030428.

Harris, C., White, P.J., Hall, E., van der Saag, D., Lomax, S., 2021. Evaluation of electroencephalography, behaviour and eye temperature in response to surgical castration in sheep. Animals 11 (3), 637. https://doi.org/10.3390/ani11030637.

Heikkinen, E.M., Voipio, H.M., Laaksonen, S., Haapala, L., Räsänen, J., Acharya, G., et al., 2015. Fentanyl pharmacokinetics in pregnant sheep after intravenous and transdermal administration to the ewe. Basic Clin. Pharmacol. Toxicol. 117 (3), 156—163. https://doi.org/10.1111/bcpt.12382.

Heinrich, A., Duffield, T.F., Lissemore, K.D., Millman, S.T., 2010. The effect of meloxicam on behavior and pain sensitivity of dairy calves following cautery dehorning with a local anesthetic. J. Dairy Sci. 93 (6), 2450—2457. https://doi.org/10.3168/jds.2009-2813.

Hempstead, M.N., Waas, J.R., Stewart, M., Cave, V.M., Sutherland, M.A., 2018a. Evaluation of alternatives to cautery disbudding of dairy goat kids using behavioural measures of post-treatment pain. Appl. Anim. Behav. Sci. 206, 32—38. https://doi.org/10.1016/j.applanim.2018.05.035.

Hempstead, M.N., Waas, J.R., Stewart, M., Zobel, G., Cave, V.M., Julian, A.F., Sutherland, M.A., 2018b. Pain sensitivity and injury associated with three methods of disbudding goat kids: cautery, cryosurgical and caustic paste. Vet. J. 239, 42—47. https://doi.org/10.1016/j.tvjl.2018.08.004.

Hikasa, Y., Okuyama, K., Kakuta, T., Takase, K., Ogasawara, S., 1998. Anesthetic potency and cardiopulmonary effects of sevoflurane in goats: comparison with isoflurane and halothane. Can. J. Vet. Res. 62 (4), 299—306.

Himmelseher, S., Durieux, M.E., Weiskopf, R.B., 2005. Ketamine for perioperative pain management. Anesthesiology 102 (1), 211—220. https://doi.org/10.1097/00000542-200501000-00030.

Hogan, J.P., Petherick, J.C., Phillips, C.J.C., 2007. The physiological and metabolic impacts on sheep and cattle of feed and water deprivation before and during transport. Nutr. Res. Rev. 20 (1), 17—28. https://doi.org/10.1017/S0954422407745006.

Ingvast-Larsson, C., Svartberg, K., Hydbring-Sandberg, E., Bondesson, U., Olsson, K., 2007. Clinical pharmacology of buprenorphine in healthy, lactating goats. J. Vet. Pharmacol. Therapeut. 30 (3), 249—256. https://doi.org/10.1111/j.1365-2885.2007.00858.x.

Izer, J., Wilson, R., 2020. Comparison of invasive and non-invasive blood pressure measurements in anesthetized female Dorset cross-bred lambs (*Ovis aries*). Res. Vet. Sci. 132, 257—261. https://doi.org/10.1016/j.rvsc.2020.07.004.

Izer, J.M., LaFleur, R.A., Weiss, W.J., Wilson, R.P., 2019. Development of a pain scoring system for use in sheep surgically implanted with ventricular assist devices. J. Invest. Surg. 32 (8), 706–715. https://doi.org/10.1080/08941939.2018.1457191.

Izer, J.M., Wilson, R.P., Clark, J.B., Myers, J.L., Weiss, W.W., Ündar, A., 2018. Animal models for pediatric mechanical circulatory support research at Penn State Health. Artif. Organs 42, 347–353. https://doi.org/10.1111/aor.13133.

Jedruch, J., Gajewski, Z., 1986. The effect of detomidine hydrochloride (Domosedan) on the electrical activity of the uterus in cows. Acta Vet. Scand. 82, S189–S192.

Jen, K.Y., Dyson, M.C., Lester, P.A., Nemzek, J.A., 2017. Pharmacokinetics of a transdermal fentanyl solution in Suffolk sheep (*Ovis aries*). JAALAS 56 (5), 550–557.

Jorgensen, J., Cannedy, A., 1996. Physiologic and pathophysiologic considerations for ruminant and swine anesthesia. Vet. Clin. North Am. Food Anim. Pract. 12, 481–500.

Kalds, P., Gao, Y., Zhou, S., Cai, B., Huang, X., Wang, X., Chen, Y., 2020. Redesigning small ruminant genomes with CRISPR toolkit: overview and perspectives. Theriogenology 147, 25–33. https://doi.org/10.1016/j.theriogenology.2020.02.015.

Kalds, P, Zhou, S, Cai, B, Liu, J, Wang, Y, Petersen, B, Sonstegard, T, Wang, X, Chen, Y, 2019. Sheep and Goat Genome Engineering: From Random Transgenesis to the CRISPR Era. Frontiers in Genetics 10, 750. https://doi.org/10.3389/fgene.2019.00750.

Kaler, J., Wassink, G.J., Green, L.E., 2009. The inter- and intra-observer reliability of a locomotion scoring scale for sheep. Vet. J. 180 (2), 189–194. https://doi.org/10.1016/j.tvjl.2007.12.028.

Kästner, S.B., 2006. A2-agonists in sheep: a review. Vet. Anaesth. Analg. 33 (2), 79–96. https://doi.org/10.1111/j.1467-2995.2005.00243.x.

Kästner, S.B., Boller, M., Kutter, A., Akens, M.K., Bettschart-Wolfensberger, R., 2001a. Clinical comparison of preanaesthetic intramuscular medetomidine and dexmedetomidine in domestic sheep. Dtsch. Tierärztliche Wochenschr. (DTW) 108 (10), 409–413.

Kästner, S.B., Von Rechenberg, B., Keller, K., Bettschart-Wolfensberger, R., 2001b. Comparison of medetomidine and dexmedetomidine as premedication in isoflurane anaesthesia for orthopaedic surgery in domestic sheep. J. Vet. Med. Ser. A 48 (4), 231–241. https://doi.org/10.1046/j.1439-0442.2001.00354.x.

Kästner, S.B., Wapf, P., Feige, K., Demuth, D., Bettschart-Wolfensberger, R., Akens, M.K., Huhtinen, M., 2003. Pharmacokinetics and sedative effects of intramuscular medetomidine in domestic sheep. J. Vet. Pharmacol. Therapeut. 26 (4), 271–276. https://doi.org/10.1046/j.1365-2885.2003.00492.x.

Kästner, S.B., Kull, S., Kutter, A.P., Boller, J., Bettschart-Wolfensberger, R., Huhtinen, M.K., 2005. Cardiopulmonary effects of dexmedetomidine in sevoflurane-anesthetized sheep with and without nitric oxide inhalation. Am. J. Vet. Res. 66 (9), 1496–1502. https://doi.org/10.2460/ajvr.2005.66.1496.

Kästner, S., Boller, J., Kutter, A., Pakarinen, S., Ramela, M., Huhtinen, M., 2007a. Comparison of cardiopulmonary effects of dexmedetomidine administered as a constant rate infusion without loading dose in sheep and goats anaesthetised with sevoflurane. Small Rumin. Res. 71 (1–3), 75–82. https://doi.org/10.1016/j.smallrumres.2006.05.001.

Kästner, S.B., Ohlerth, S., Pospischil, A., Boller, J., Huhtinen, M.K., 2007b. Dexmedetomidine-induced pulmonary alterations in sheep. Res. Vet. Sci. 83 (2), 217–226. https://doi.org/10.1016/j.rvsc.2006.11.015.

Kells, N.J., Beausoleil, N.J., Godfrey, A.J.R., Littlewood, K.E., Ward, R.N., Johnson, C.B., 2020. Effect of analgesic strategies on pain behaviour associated with combined ring castration and hot iron tail docking in Merino lambs. Appl. Anim. Behav. Sci. 222, 104914. https://doi.org/10.1016/j.applanim.2019.104914.

Klein, L., Fisher, N., 1988. Cardiopulmonary effects of restraint in dorsal recumbency on awake cattle. Am. J. Vet. Res. 49 (9), 1605–1608.

Kleinhenz, M.D., Van Engen, N.K., Smith, J.S., Gorden, P.J., Ji, J., Wang, C., et al., 2018. The impact of transdermal flunixin meglumine on biomarkers of pain in calves when administered at the time of surgical castration without local anesthesia. Livest. Sci. 212, 1–6. https://doi.org/10.1016/j.livsci.2018.03.016.

Krohm, P., Levionnois, O., Ganster, M., Zilberstein, L., Spadavecchia, C., 2011. Antinociceptive activity of pre- versus post-operative intra-articular bupivacaine in goats undergoing stifle arthrotomy. Vet. Anaesth. Analg. 38 (4), 363–373. https://doi.org/10.1111/j.1467-2995.2011.00623.x.

Kutter, A.P., Kästner, S.B., Bettschart-Wolfensberger, R., Huhtinen, M., 2006. Cardiopulmonary effects of dexmedetomidine in goats and sheep anaesthetised with sevoflurane. Vet. Rec. 159 (19), 624–629. https://doi.org/10.1136/vr.159.19.624.

Lankveld, D.P., Driessen, B., Soma, L.R., Moate, P.J., Rudy, J., Uboh, C.E., et al., 2006. Pharmacodynamic effects and pharmacokinetic profile of a long-term continuous rate infusion of racemic ketamine in healthy conscious horses. J. Vet. Pharmacol. Therapeut. 29 (6), 477–488. https://doi.org/10.1111/j.1365-2885.2006.00794.x.

Leblanc, M.M., Hubbell, J.A., Smith, H.C., 1984. The effects of xylazine hydrochloride on intrauterine pressure in the cow. Theriogenology 21 (5), 681–690.

Lee, D., Swanson, C., 1996. General principles of anesthesia and sedation in food animals. Vet. Clin. North Am. Food Anim. Pract. 12, 473–480.

Leek, B.F., 2004. Digestion in the ruminant stomach. In: Reece, W.O. (Ed.), Duke's Physiology of Domestic Animals, twelveth ed. Cornell University Press, Ithaca, NY.

Lemke, K., 2007. Anticholingerics and sedatives. In: Tranquilli, W., Thurmon, C., Grimm, K. (Eds.), Lumb and Jones' Veterinary Anesthesia and Analgesia, fourth ed. Blackwell Publishing, pp. 203–239.

Lin, H.C., 2014. Pain management in farm animals. In: Lin, H.C., Walz, P. (Eds.), Farm Animal Anesthesia: Cattle, Small Ruminants, Camelids, and Pigs. John Wiley & Sons, Inc, pp. 174–214. https://doi.org/10.1002/9781118886700.ch9.

Lin, H., 2015. Comparative anesthesia and analgesia of ruminants and swine. In: Grimm, K.A., Lamont, L.A., Tranquilli, W.J., Greene, S.A., Robertson, S.A. (Eds.), Veterinary Anesthesia and Analgesia: The Fifth Edition of Lumb and Jones, fifth ed. John Wiley & Sons, Inc, pp. 743–753.

Lin, H.C., Walz, P., 2014. Farm Animal Anesthesia: Cattle, Small Ruminants, Camelids, and Pigs. John Wiley & Sons, Inc.

Lin, H.C., Tyler, J.W., Wallace, S.S., Thurmon, J.C., Wolfe, D.F., 1993a. Telazol and xylazine anesthesia in sheep. Cornell Vet. 83 (2), 117–124.

Lin, H.C., Tyler, J.W., Welles, E.G., Spano, J.S., Thurmon, J.C., Wolfe, D.F., 1993b. Effects of anesthesia induced and maintained by continuous intravenous administration of guaifenesin, ketamine, and xylazine in spontaneously breathing sheep. Am. J. Vet. Res. 54 (11), 1913–1916.

Lin, H.C., Pugh, D.G., 2002. Anesthetic management. In: Pugh, D.G. (Ed.), Sheep and Goat Medicine. Saunders, Philadelphia, PA.

Lin, H.C., Purohit, R.C., Powe, T.A., 1997. Anesthesia in sheep with propofol or with xylazine-ketamine followed by halothane. Vet. Surg. 26 (3), 247–252. https://doi.org/10.1111/j.1532-950X.1997.tb01494.x.

Lin, H., Riddell, M., DeGraves, F., 1999. Comparison of three alpha-2 antagonists, yohimbine, tolazoline, or atipamezole for reversing the anesthetic effects of medetomidine and ketamine in dairy calves. Bov. Pract. (33), 21–28.

Lin, H.-C., Caldwell, F., Pugh, D.G., 2012. Anesthetic management. In: Pugh, D.G., Baird, A.N. (Eds.), Sheep and Goat Medicine, second ed. W. B. Saunders, pp. 517–538. https://doi.org/10.1016/B978-1-4377-2353-3.10018-6.

Lizarraga, I., Chambers, J.P., 2012. Use of analgesic drugs for pain management in sheep. N. Z. Vet. J. 60 (2), 87–94. https://doi.org/10.1080/00480169.2011.642772.

Marini, D., Colditz, I.G., Hinch, G., Petherick, J.C., Lee, C., 2017. Self-administration by consumption of flunixin in feed alleviates the pain and inflammation associated with castration and tail docking of lambs. Appl. Anim. Behav. Sci. 188, 26–33. https://doi.org/10.1016/j.applanim.2016.12.008.

Marini, D., Pippia, J., Colditz, I.G., Hinch, G., Petherick, J.C., Lee, C., 2015. Randomised trial of the bioavailability and efficacy of orally administered flunixin, carprofen and ketoprofen in a pain model in sheep. Aust. Vet. J. 93 (8), 265–270. https://doi.org/10.1111/avj.12351.

Maslowska, K., Mizzoni, F., Dwyer, C.M., Wemelsfelder, F., 2020. Qualitative behavioural assessment of pain in castrated lambs. Appl. Anim. Behav. Sci. 233, 105143. https://doi.org/10.1016/j.applanim.2020.105143.

McGuirk, S.M., Bednarski, R.M., Clayton, M.K., 1990. Bradycardia in cattle deprived of food. J. Am. Vet. Med. Assoc. 196 (6), 894–896.

McLennan, K.M., Rebelo, C.J.B., Corke, M.J., Holmes, M.A., Leach, M.C., Constantino-Casas, F., 2016. Development of a facial expression scale using footrot and mastitis as models of pain in sheep. Appl. Anim. Behav. Sci. 176, 19–26. https://doi.org/10.1016/j.applanim.2016.01.007.

Mellor, D.J., 2004. Taming and training of pregnancy sheep and goats and of newborn lambs, kids and calves before experimentation. Altern. Lab. Anim. 32 (Suppl. 1A), 143–146. https://doi.org/10.1177/026119290403201s22.

Mellor, D.J., Beausoleil, N.J., Littlewood, K.E., McLean, A.N., McGreevy, P.D., Jones, B., Wilkins, C., 2020. The 2020 five domains model—including human-animal interactions in assessments of animal welfare. Animals 10 (10), 1870. https://doi.org/10.3390/ani10101870.

Menchaca, A., dos Santos-Neto, P.C., Mulet, A.P., Crispo, M., 2020. CRISPR in livestock: from editing to printing. Theriogenology 150, 247–254. https://doi.org/10.1016/j.theriogenology.2020.01.063.

Molony, V., Kent, J.E., McKendrick, I.J., 2002. Validation of a method for assessment of an acute pain in lambs. Appl. Anim. Behav. Sci. 76 (3), 215–238. https://doi.org/10.1016/S0168-1591(02)00014-X.

Muge, D.K., Chambers, J.P., Livingston, A., Waterman, A.E., 1994. Analgesic effects of medetomidine in sheep. Vet. Rec. 135 (2), 43–44.

Muir, W.W., 2010. NMDA receptor antagonists and pain: ketamine. Vet. Clin. N. Am. Equine Pract. 26 (3), 565–578. https://doi.org/10.1016/j.cveq.2010.07.009.

Muller, B.R., Soriano, V.S., Bellio, J.C.B., Molento, C.F.M., 2019. Facial expression of pain in Nellore and crossbred beef cattle. J. Vet. Behav. (34), 60–65. https://doi.org/10.1016/j.jveb.2019.07.007.

Murrell, J.C., Hellebrekers, L.J., 2005. Medetomidine and dexmedetomidine: a review of cardiovascular effects and antinociceptive properties in the dog. Vet. Anaesth. Analg. 32 (3), 117–127. https://doi.org/10.1111/j.1467-2995.2005.00233.x.

Musk, G.C., Wilkes, G.J., 2018. Sedation of sheep following the administration of acepromazine with buprenorphine or morphine is similar. Res. Vet. Sci. 118, 41–42. https://doi.org/10.1016/j.rvsc.2018.01.013.

Musk, G.C., Catanchin, C.S.M., Usuda, H., Woodward, E., Kemp, M.W., 2017a. The uptake of transdermal fentanyl in a pregnant sheep model. Vet. Anaesth. Analg. 44 (6), 1382–1390. https://doi.org/10.1016/j.vaa.2017.05.001.

Musk, G.C., Jacobsen, S., Hyndman, T.H., Lehmann, H.S., Tuke, S.J., Collins, T., et al., 2017b. Objective measures for the assessment of post-operative pain in *Bos indicus* bull calves following castration. Animals 7 (10), 76. https://doi.org/10.3390/ani7100076.

Musk, G.C., Laurence, M., Collins, T., Tuke, J., Hyndman, T.H., 2017c. Mechanical nociceptive threshold testing in *Bos indicus* bull calves. Anim. Prod. Sci. 57 (3), 576–582. https://doi.org/10.1071/AN15441.

National Research Council [NRC], 2011. Guide for the Care and Use of Laboratory Animals. National Academies Press, Washington, DC.

Neave, H.W., Daros, R.R., Costa, J.H.C., von Keyserlingk, M.A.G., Weary, D.M., 2014. Pain and pessimism: dairy calves exhibit negative judgement bias following hot-iron disbudding. PLoS One 9 (4), e96135. https://doi.org/10.1371/journal.pone.0080556.

Nickel, R., Schummer, A., Seiferle, E., Sack, W.O., 1973. The Viscera of the Domestic Mammals. Springer-Verlag, New York, NY.

Nishimura, L.T., Villela, I.O.J., Carvalho, L.L., Borges, L.P.B., Silva, M.A.M., Mattos-Junior, E., 2017. The effect of acepromazine alone or in combination with methadone, morphine, or tramadol on sedation and selected cardiopulmonary variables in sheep. Vet. Med. Int. 2017, 7507616. https://doi.org/10.1155/2017/7507616.

Nolan, A., Livingston, A., Waterman, A.E., 1987. Investigation of the antinociceptive activity of buprenorphine in sheep. Br. J. Pharmacol. 92 (3), 527–533.

Orihuela, A., Ungerfeld, R., 2019. Tail docking in sheep (*Ovis aries*): a review on the arguments for and against the procedure, advantages/disadvantages, methods, and new evidence to revisit the topic. Livest. Sci. 230, 103837. https://doi.org/10.1016/j.livsci.2019.103837.

Özkan, F., Çakõr-Özkan, N., Eyibilen, A., Yener, T., Erkorkmaz, Ü., 2010. Comparison of ketamine-diazepam with ketamine-xylazine anesthetic combinations in sheep spontaneously breathing and undergoing maxillofacial surgery. Bosn. J. Basic Med. Sci. 10 (4), 297–302. https://doi.org/10.17305/bjbms.2010.2675.

Paull, D., Lee, C., Colditz, I., Atkinson, S., Fisher, A., 2007. The effect of a topical anaesthetic formulation, systemic flunixin and carprofen, singly or in combination, on cortisol and behavioural responses of Merino lambs to mulesing. Aust. Vet. J. 85 (3), 98–106. https://doi.org/10.1111/j.1751-0813.2007.00115.x.

Paull, D.R., Lee, C., Colditz, I.G., Fisher, A.D., 2009. Effects of a topical anaesthetic formulation and systemic carprofen, given singly or in combination, on the cortisol and behavioural responses of Merino lambs to castration. Aust. Vet. J. 87 (3), 230–237. https://doi.org/10.1111/j.1751-0813.2007.00115.x.

Paull, D.R., Small, A.H., Lee, C., Palladin, P., Colditz, I.G., 2012. Evaluating a novel analgesic strategy for ring castration of ram lambs. Vet. Anaesth. Analg. 39 (5), 539–549. https://doi.org/10.1111/j.1467-2995.2012.00716.x.

Piggins, D., Philips, C.J.C., 1996. The eye of the domesticated sheep with implications for vision. Anim. Sci. 62, 301–308.

Plummer, P.J., Schleining, J.A., 2013. Assessment and management of pain in small ruminants and camelids. Vet. Clin. N. Am. Food Anim. Pract. 29 (1), 185–208. https://doi.org/10.1016/j.cvfa.2020.12.005.

Prassinos, N.N., Galatos, A.D., Raptopoulos, D., 2005. A comparison of propofol, thiopental or ketamine as induction agents in goats. Vet. Anaesth. Analg. 32 (5), 289–296. https://doi.org/10.1111/j.1467-2995.2005.00204.x.

Pyörälä, E., Koppinen, J., Vainio, O., Alanko, M., 1986. Detomidine in pregnant cows. Nor. Veterinaertidsskr. 38 (4), 237–240.

Queiroz-Castro, P., Egger, C., Redua, M.A., Rohrbach, B.W., Cox, S., Doherty, T., 2006. Effects of ketamine and magnesium on the minimum alveolar concentration of isoflurane in goats. Am. J. Vet. Res. 67 (12), 1962–1966. https://doi.org/10.2460/ajvr.67.12.1962.

Raekallio, M., Heinonen, K.M., Kuussaari, J., Vainio, O., 2003. Pain alleviation in animals: attitudes and practices of Finnish veterinarians. Vet. J. 165 (2), 131–135. https://doi.org/10.1016/S1090-0233(02)00186-7.

Raekallio, M., Kivalo, M., Jalanka, H., Vainio, O., 1991. Medetomidine/ketamine sedation in calves and its reversal with atipamezole. Vet. Anaesth. Analg. (18), 45–47.

Raisis, A.L., Hosgood, G.L., Crawford, N., Kästner, S., Musk, G.C., Herrmann, P., Mosing, M., 2021. Comparison of pulmonary function in isoflurane anaesthetized ventilated sheep (*Ovis aries*) following administration of intravenous xylazine versus medetomidine. Lab. Anim. https://doi.org/10.1177/0023677220983366.

Ranheim, B., Horsberg, T.E., Søli, N.E., Ryeng, K.A., Arnemo, J.M., 2000. The effects of medetomidine and its reversal with atipamezole on plasma glucose, cortisol and noradrenaline in cattle and sheep. J. Vet. Pharmacol. Therapeut. 23 (6), 379–387. https://doi.org/10.1046/j.1365-2885.2000.00291.x.

Raske, T., Pelkey, S., Wagner, A., Turner, A.S., 2010. Effect of intravenous ketamine and lidocaine on isoflurane requirement in sheep undergoing orthopedic surgery. Lab. Anim. 39, 76–79. https://doi.org/10.1038/laban0310-76.

Reid, J., Nolan, A.M., Welsh, E., 1993. Propofol as an induction agent in the goat: a pharmacokinetic study. J. Vet. Pharmacol. Therapeut. 16 (4), 488–493.

Riebold, T.W., 2015. Ruminants. In: Grimm, K.A., Lamont, L.A., Tranquilli, W.J., Greene, S.A., Robertson, S.A. (Eds.), Veterinary Anesthesia and Analgesia. https://doi.org/10.1002/9781119421375.ch49.

Rioja, E., Kerr, C.L., Enouri, S.S., McDonell, W.N., 2008. Sedative and cardiopulmonary effects of medetomidine hydrochloride and xylazine hydrochloride and their reversal with atipamezole hydrochloride in calves. Am. J. Vet. Res. 69 (3), 319–329. https://doi.org/10.2460/ajvr.69.3.319.

Rogers, C.S., 2016. Genetically engineered livestock for biomedical models. Transgenic Res. 25 (3), 345–359. https://doi.org/10.1007/s11248-016-9928-6.

Rosenberger, G., Hempel, E., Baumeister, M., 1968. Contribution to the effects and use of Rompun in cattle. Dtsch. Tierärztliche Wochenschr. (DTW) 75 (22), 572–578.

Schauvliege, S., Narine, K., Bouchez, S., Desmet, D., Van Parys, V., Van Nooten, G., Gasthuys, F., 2006. Refined anaesthesia for implantation of engineered experimental aortic valves in the pulmonary artery using a right heart bypass in sheep. Lab. Anim. 40, 341–352.

Singh, A., Sharma, S., Adarsh, K., Amit, K., 2010. Atropine-medetomidine-ketamine as balanced anaesthesia for neonatal calves: sedative, clinical and haematobiochemical studies. Indian J. Vet. Surg. 31 (2), 113–115.

Singh, J., Singh, A., Peshin, P., Sharifi, D., Patil, D., 1994. Evaluation of detomidine as a sedative in sheep. Indian J. Anim. Sci. 64, 237–238.

Small, A.H., Marini, D., Dyall, T., Paull, D., Lee, C., 2018. A randomised field study evaluating the effectiveness of buccal meloxicam and topical local anaesthetic formulations administered singly or in combination at improving welfare of female Merino lambs undergoing surgical mulesing and hot knife tail docking. Res. Vet. Sci. 118, 305–311. https://doi.org/10.1016/j.rvsc.2018.03.006.

Smith, G., 2013. Extralabel use of anesthetic and analgesic compounds in cattle. Vet. Clin. North Am. Food Anim. Pract. 29, 29–46.

Smith, E., Modric, S., 2013. Regulatory considerations for the approval of analgesic drugs for cattle in the United States. Vet. Clin. North Am. Food Anim. Pract. 29, 1–10.

Staffieri, F., Driessen, B., Monte, V.D., Grasso, S., Crovace, A., 2010. Effects of positive end-expiratory pressure on anesthesia-induced atelectasis and gas exchange in anesthetized and mechanically ventilated sheep. Am. J. Vet. Res. 71 (8), 867–874. https://doi.org/10.2460/ajvr.71.8.867.

Starling, M.J., Payne, E., McgGreevy, P., 2021. Optimal flow: a pilot study balancing sheep movement and welfare in abattoirs. Animals 11, 344. https://doi.org/10.3390/ani11020344.

Steffey, E., 1986. Some characteristics of ruminants and swine that complicate management of general-anesthesia. Vet. Clin. North Am. Food Anim. Pract. 2, 507–516.

Stegmann, G.F., 1998. Observations on the use of midazolam for sedation, and induction of anaesthesia with midazolam in combination with ketamine in the goat. J. S. Afr. Vet. Assoc. 69 (3), 89–92.

Stewart, M., Beausoleil, N.J., Johnson, C.B., Webster, J.R., Schuetz, K.E., Cox, N., Stafford, K.J., 2014. Do rubber rings coated with lignocaine reduce the pain associated with ring castration of lambs? Appl. Anim. Behav. Sci. 160, 56–63. https://doi.org/10.1016/j.applanim.2014.08.007.

Stewart, M., Verkerk, G.A., Stafford, K.J., Schaefer, A.L., Webster, J.R., 2010. Non-invasive assessment of autonomic activity for evaluation of pain in calves, using surgical castration as a model. J. Dairy Sci. 93 (8), 3602–3609. https://doi.org/10.3168/jds.2010-3114.

Stock, M.L., Coetzee, J.F., 2015. Clinical pharmacology of analgesic drugs in cattle. Vet. Clin. North Am. Food Anim. Pract. 31, 113–138. https://doi.org/10.1016/j.cvfa.2014.11.002.

Sutherland, M.A., Bright, A.L., Schutz, K.E., 2019. Effect of a buccal meloxicam formulation on the behavioural response to ring castration of calves. Anim. Prod. Sci. 59 (3), 564–569. https://doi.org/10.1071/AN17641.

Sutherland, M.A., Tucker, C.B., 2011. The long and short of it: a review of tail docking in farm animals. Appl. Anim. Behav. Sci. 135 (3), 179–191. https://doi.org/10.1016/j.applanim.2011.10.015.

Swindle, M., Vogler, G., Fulton, L., Marini, R., Popilskis, S., 2002. Preanesthesia, anesthesia, analgesia, and euthanasia. In: Fox, J., Anderson, L., Loew, F., Quimby, F. (Eds.), Laboratory Animal Medicine, second ed. Elsevier, pp. 955–1003. https://doi.org/10.1016/B978-012263951-7/50025-9.

Taylor, P., 1991. Anaesthesia in sheep and goats. Practice 13 (1), 31–36. https://doi.org/10.1136/inpract.13.1.31.

Theurer, M.E., White, B.J., Coetzee, J.F., Edwards, L.N., Mosher, R.A., Cull, C.A., 2012. Assessment of behavioral changes associated with oral meloxicam administration at time of dehorning in calves using a remote triangulation device and accelerometers. BMC Vet. Res. 8, 48. https://doi.org/10.1186/1746-6148-8-48.

Thurmon, J.C., 1986. Injectable anesthetic agents and techniques in ruminants and swine. Vet. Clin. N. Am. Food Anim. Pract. 2 (3), 567–591.

Thurmon, J., Lin, H., Tranquilli, T., Benson, G., Olson, W., 1989. A comparison of yohimbine and tolazoline as antagonist of xylazine sedation in calves. Vet. Surg. 18, 170–171.

Todd, C.G., Millman, S.T., McKnight, D.R., Duffield, T.F., Leslie, K.E., 2010. Nonsteroidal anti-inflammatory drug therapy for neonatal calf diarrhea complex: effects on calf performance. J. Anim. Sci. 88 (6), 2019–2028. https://doi.org/10.2527/jas.2009-2340.

Törneke, K., Bergström, U., Neil, A., 2003. Interactions of xylazine and detomidine with alpha2-adrenoceptors in brain tissue from cattle, swine and rats. J. Vet. Pharmacol. Therapeut. 26 (3), 205–211. https://doi.org/10.1046/j.1365-2885.2003.00466.x.

Trim, C.M., Hofmeister, E.H., Peroni, J.F., Thoresen, M., 2013. Evaluation of an oscillometric blood pressure monitor for use in anesthetized sheep. Vet. Anaesth. Analg. 40 (6), e31–e39. https://doi.org/10.1111/vaa.12018.

Troncoso, R.J., Herzberg, D.E., Meneses, C.S., Muller, H.Y., Werner, M.P., Bustamante, H., 2018. Mechanical/thermal sensitivity and superficial temperature in the stump of long-term tail-docked dairy cows. PeerJ 6, e5213. https://doi.org/10.7717/peerj.5213.

Tuyttens, F.A.M., Sprenger, M., Van Nuffel, A., Maertens, W., Van Dongen, S., 2009. Reliability of categorical versus continuous scoring of welfare indicators: lameness in cows as a case study. Anim. Welf. 18 (4), 399–405.

Udegbunam, R.I., Ugwu, A.U., Onuba, A.C., Okereke, N.H., Udegbunam, S.O., 2019. Effects of sub-anaesthetic (low) dose ketamine infusion on intra-operative and postoperative pain in goats anaesthetized with diazepam-ketamine prior to rumenotomy. Sokoto J. Vet. Sci. 17 (1), 19–26. https://doi.org/10.4314/sokjvs.v17i1.3.

USDA, 2008. *Animal welfare act and animal welfare regulations.* USDA Animal and Plant Health Inspection Service.

Valverde, A., Doherty, T.J., 2008. Anesthesia and analgesia of ruminants. In: Fish, R.E., Brown, M.J., Danneman, P.J., Karas, A.Z. (Eds.), Anesthesia and Analgesia in Laboratory Animals, second ed. Academic Press, pp. 385–411.

Valverde, A., Doherty, T.J., 2009. Pain management in cattle and small ruminants. In: Anderson, D.E., Rings, D.M. (Eds.), Current Veterinary Therapy: Food Animal Practice, Fifth ed. Saunders Elsevier, St. Louis, Missouri.

Verbeek, E., Ferguson, D., Lee, C., 2014. Are hungry sheep more pessimistic? The effects of food restriction on cognitive bias and the involvement of ghrelin in its regulation. Physiol. Behav. 123 (17), 67–75. https://doi.org/10.1016/j.physbeh.2013.09.017.

Verbeek, E., Waas, J.R., McLeay, L., Matthews, L.R., 2011. Measurement of feeding motivation in sheep and the effects of food restriction. Appl. Anim. Behav. Sci. 132 (3–4), 121–130. https://doi.org/10.1016/j.applanim.2011.03.014.

Vesal, N., Spadavecchia, C., Steiner, A., Kirscher, F., Levionnois, O.L., 2011. Evaluation of the isoflurane-sparing effects of lidocaine infusion during umbilical surgery in calves. Vet. Anaesth. Analg. 38 (5), 451–460. https://doi.org/10.1111/j.1467-2995.2011.00636.x.

Vieira, A., Oliveira, M.D., Nunes, T., Stilwell, G., 2015. Making the case for developing alternative lameness scoring systems for dairy goats. Appl. Anim. Behav. Sci. 171, 94–100. https://doi.org/10.1016/j.applanim.2015.08.015.

Vindevoghel, T.V., Fleming, P.A., Hyndman, T.H., Musk, G.C., Laurence, M., Collins, T., 2019. Qualitative Behavioural Assessment of *Bos indicus* cattle after surgical castration. Appl. Anim. Behav. Sci. 211, 95–102. https://doi.org/10.1016/j.applanim.2018.11.004.

Virtanen, R., Savola, J., Saano, V., 1988. Characterization of the selectivity, specificity and potency of medetomidine as an alpha 2-adrenoceptor agonist. Eur. J. Pharmacol. 150 (1–2), 9–14. https://doi.org/10.1016/0014-2999(88)90744-3.

Wagner, A.E., Muir, W.W., Grospitch, B.J., 1990. Cardiopulmonary effects of position in conscious cattle. Am. J. Vet. Res. 51, 7–10.

Walker, C.D., Kudreikis, K., Sherrard, A., Johnston, C.C., 2003. Repeated neonatal pain influences maternal behavior, but not stress responsiveness in rat offspring. Dev. Brain Res. 140 (2), 253–261. https://doi.org/10.1016/S0165-3806(02)00611-9.

Walkowiak, K.J., Graham, M.L., 2015. Pharmacokinetics and antinociceptive activity of sustained-release buprenorphine in sheep. JAALAS 54 (6), 763–768.

Waterman, A.E., 1988. Use of propofol in sheep. Vet. Rec. 122 (11), 26.

Waterman, A.E., Livingston, A., Amin, A., 1991. Analgesic activity and respiratory effects of butorphanol in sheep. Res. Vet. Sci. 51 (1), 19–23. https://doi.org/10.1016/0034-5288(91)90024-I.

Weaver, A.D., 1971. Complications in halothane anaesthesia of cattle. Zentbl. Vetmed. Reihe A 18 (5), 409–416.

Wegner, K., 2008. Anesthesia and analgesia. In: Haskell, S.R.R. (Ed.), Blackwell's Five-Minute Veterinary Consult. Wiley-Blackwell, pp. 66–69.

Welsh, E.M., Gettinby, G., Nolan, A.M., 1993. Comparison of a visual analog scale and a numerical rating scale for assessment of lameness, using sheep as a model. Am. J. Vet. Res. 54 (6), 976–983.

Wemelsfelder, F., Hunter, T.E.A., Mendl, M.T., Lawrence, A.B., 2001. Assessing the 'whole animal': a free choice profiling approach. Anim. Behav. 62 (2), 209–220. https://doi.org/10.1006/anbe.2001.1741.

Yellin, T.O., Sperow, J.W., Buck, S.H., 1975. Antagonism of tolazoline by histamine H2-receptor blockers. Nature 253 (5492), 561–563.

Young, D., Shawley, R., Barron, S., 1989. Tolazoline reversal of xylazine-ketamine anesthesia in calves. Vet. Surg. 18 (2), 171.

Zullian, C., Lema, P., Lavoie, M., Dodelet-Devillers, A., Beaudry, F., Vachon, P., 2016. Plasma concentrations of buprenorphine following a single subcutaneous administration of a sustained release formulation of buprenorphine in sheep. Can. J. Vet. Res. 80 (3), 250–253.

Further reading

Edmonson, M.A., 2014. Local and regional anesthetic techniques. In: Lin, H.C., Walz, P. (Eds.), Farm Animal Anesthesia: Cattle, Small Ruminants, Camelids, and Pigs. John Wiley & Sons, Inc, pp. 136–154.

Hageri, C., Biernot, S., Buettner, M., Glage, S., Keubler, L.M., Held, N., et al., 2017. The Sheep Grimace Scale as an indicator of post-operative distress and pain in laboratory sheep. PLoS One 12 (4), e0175839. https://doi.org/10.1371/journal.pone.0175839.

Mohamadnia, A.R., Hughes, G., Clarke, K.W., 2008. Maintenance of anaesthesia in sheep with isoflurane, desflurane or sevoflurane. Vet. Rec. 163 (7), 210–215. https://doi.org/10.1136/vr.163.7.210.

Rezakhani, A., Edjtehadi, M., Szabuniewicz, M., 1977. Prevention of thiopental and thiopental/halothane cardiac sensitization to epinephrine in the sheep. Can. J. Comp. Med. 41 (4), 389–395.

Chapter 21

Analgesia and anesthesia in ferrets

Cathy Johnson-Delaney[1] and Angela Lennox[2]
[1]*Washington Ferret Rescue & Shelter, Everett, WA, United States;* [2]*Avian & Exotic Animal Clinic of Indianapolis, Indianapolis, IN, United States*

Chapter outline

I. Introduction

Ferrets are valuable small animal models in biomedical research and can be an economical carnivore to house and manage. They share many unique anatomical and physiological features with humans, which makes them ideal animal models for diseases such as influenza and SARS-CoV-19. They served as an animal model for Helicobacter sp.-induced gastritis and ulceration. Ferrets are also useful in pulmonary, dental, neurological, endocrinological, and reproductive studies. They have an oropharyngeal anatomy and size similar to a human neonate and are used to train medical personnel on neonatal intubation. They are used as an emetic model in assessments of new therapies. They have a relatively high metabolic rate, and there are significant differences in drug dosing, analgesic, and anesthetic management when compared to dogs and cats. This chapter will discuss sedation, anesthesia, and analgesics in ferrets, with emphasis on a multi-modal approach to providing effective analgesia and anesthesia. Supportive care, emergency resuscitation, monitoring, and adjunctive nonpharmacologic options will also be discussed.

II. Preprocedural considerations

A. Planning: careful planning helps reduce anesthetic risk

1. Health and safety

Both the health of ferrets as well as that of the personnel working with them must be considered. Personnel need to be trained in the handling of ferrets to prevent bites and injury to the ferret. Consider a didactic session to familiarize personnel with the anatomy, physiology, and behavior of the ferret along with training in proper handling followed by a hands-on session to learn safe handling and injection or oral drug administration techniques. Zoonotic precautions are primarily to keep the research colony

Anesthesia and Analgesia in Laboratory Animals. https://doi.org/10.1016/B978-0-12-822215-7.00026-3

disease-free: personnel working with ferrets must be free of influenza and COVID-19, as ferrets can become ill with either of these viral diseases. Personal protective equipment for working with ferrets should include fit-tested N95 or equivalent respirators, dedicated clothing, and procedure or surgery gloves. In rare instances where a ferret is aggressive, welder's gloves will provide hand protection.

2. History and record keeping

Records of colony animals should include date of arrival, vendor/breeder, sex, age, diet, body weight, and housing (social or individual). Reproductive status should be noted, especially if the ferret is pregnant or designated for breeding. Any previous health concerns should also be recorded. An anesthetic record for procedures should include notations of time, vitals such as heart rate, blood pressure, pulse oximetry, capnography, respiratory rate, temperature, peri-anesthetic agents, doses, and route of drug administration. Postoperative monitoring at a minimum should include temperature, heart and respiratory rates, and possibly pulse oximetry; supportive care and any additional medications or treatments should be recorded. Adverse events must also be part of the record.

3. Patient evaluation

1. Physical examination of the ferret is similar to that of other mammals. Palpation is relatively easy, and the major abdominal organs are easily identified. The oral examination can be done as an assistant scruffs and holds the ferret vertically—this positioning will usually elicit a yawn, allowing easy visualization of the mouth and teeth. An intact female (a jill) presenting with a swollen vulva needs to be assessed for anemia, particularly if estrus has been prolonged. Ferrets are copulatory ovulators, and jills can become critically anemic from prolonged hyperestrogenemia.
2. Laboratory evaluation usually consists of complete blood counts and serum chemistries. A minimal database would be a packed cell volume, total protein, blood urea nitrogen, and blood glucose (BG). Urinalysis or other diagnostics may be indicated, including imaging, depending on the project to be done, and baseline data needed. The BG reading needs to be interpreted based on the known last meal. If the ferret is normoglycemic (62–207 mg/dL, Morrisey and Johnston, 2018) 4 hours or more after eating, then it is unlikely the ferret has an insulinoma. A hypoglycemic reading less than 4 hours after feeding needs to be further investigated. Ferrets' BG levels are normally slightly lower than dogs or cats.

4. Preanesthetic fasting

As ferrets have a rapid gastrointestinal transit time of approximately 3–4 hours, it is unnecessary to fast or withhold water from a ferret for longer than a few hours, regardless of whether the ferret is on a solid or liquid diet (Johnson-Delaney, 2017a,b).

III. Chemical restraint (sedation) principles

When developing the research protocol, sedation or general anesthesia are options that should be carefully considered. Many procedures can be accomplished safely (for the personnel and the ferret) without general anesthesia. It should be kept in mind that a conscious, sedated patient can experience pain; therefore an appropriate analgesic plan must be developed as indicated.

IV. General anesthesia principles

The anesthetic event consists of premedication agents, induction agents, maintenance agents, and analgesics.

A. Goals of premedication

The goal of premedication is to reduce general anesthetic requirements and reduce anxiety and stress of induction. Appropriate drug combinations and analgesics may allow vascular access and other procedural preparation.

B. Premedication delivery

Premedications can be delivered via intramuscular, subcutaneous, intravenous, or intraosseous routes; however, IV/IO administration (and particularly catheter placement to facilitate IO administration) is stressful in the conscious patient and should be avoided (see Table 21.1, vascular access/blood draw sites). Subcutaneous injections can be given in the scapular area similar to other mammals. However, the skin of the ferret is the thickest in that location, and as restraint is usually by scruffing, injection near a person's hand can result in needlesticks, particularly if the ferret is fractious. SC injections and fluid administration are well tolerated in the flank area in the abundant loose skin. Intramuscular injections are usually given into the anterior thigh to avoid the sciatic nerve. The biceps or triceps are alternative IM sites. As muscles are relatively small, injection volume should be limited to a maximum of 0.5 mL.

C. Induction of general anesthesia

Induction agents can be injectable or inhalant. With proper premedication, induction facilitates safe, stress-free intubation. All induction agents must be used to effect, and the patient must be monitored carefully to detect hypoventilation, apnea, bradyarrhythmia, and other abnormalities.

TABLE 21.1 Selected ferret normative data (Johnson-Delaney, 2017a).

Parameter	Value
Body temperature	37.8–40°C
Blood pressure (awake)	140–164 mmHg systolic
	110–125 mmHg diastolic
Blood pressure (butorphanol/midazolam)	95–155 mmHg systolic
	52–89 mmHg diastolic
Heart rate	200–400 beats/minute
Respiration rate	33–36 breaths/minute
Cardiac output	139 mL/minute
Circulation time	4.5–6.8 seconds
Blood volume	75 mL/kg
Blood sampling maximum volume from a healthy adult ferret	7.5 mL/kg
Blood sampling sites	Cephalic, lateral saphenous, jugular, cranial vena cava
Vascular access (for catheter placement, drug delivery)	IV (cephalic, saphenous, jugular, cranial vena cava, tail), IO (tibia, femur)
Gastrointestinal transit time	3–4 hours

D. Intubation

Visual (direct observation of the glottis) intubation is easily performed in the ferret using a laryngoscope with a 0 or 1 Miller blade. Most smaller ferrets tolerate a 2.0–3.0 mm uncuffed endotracheal tube, while larger ferrets may require 3.0–4.0 cuffed tubes. Due to the short muzzle of the ferret, some operators find it more effective to secure the tube around the shoulder and thoracic limbs to prevent the ties from slipping.

E. Maintenance of anesthesia

Most ferret surgeries are maintained with inhalant agents. Careful titration of injectable agents can be considered, and total intravenous anesthesia using a pediatric syringe pump has been described (Hawkins and Pascoe, 2021).

V. Support and monitoring of the patient

A. Support

Support of the surgical patient is critically important, and anesthetics can produce or exacerbate, among other things hypovolemia and hypothermia.

1. Vascular access and fluid therapy

An IV catheter can easily be placed in the cephalic vein, or the lateral saphenous vein (Fig. 21.1). For smaller ferrets weighing less than 200 g, an intraosseous catheter placed in the proximal femur or proximal tibia is an alternative. IO catheter placement is painful, and a local block over the skin, within the subcutis, and the periosteum is recommended. Fluid therapy is routine for anesthetized and sedated patients. Most procedures in research are done on healthy ferrets, but fluid therapy can mitigate dangerous changes in blood pressure. Use crystalloid solutions such as Lactated Ringers or Normosol, or other fluid types as indicated. The standard surgical rate for healthy mammal patients is 8–10 mL/kg/hour, with additional fluid boluses as needed to correct hypovolemia from anesthesia or blood loss. The general guidelines for the treatment of hypovolemia are to reduce the level of

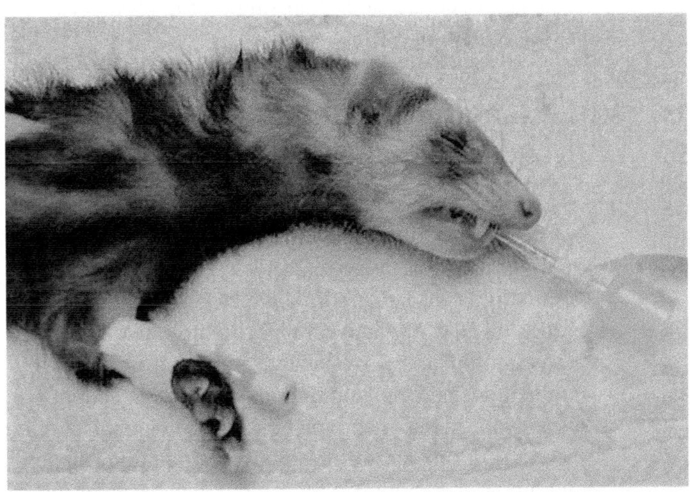

FIGURE 21.1 Ferret intubated with a 24 ga cephalic IV catheter, 2.0 endotracheal tube. *Copyright Johnson-Delaney (2017a, 2017b).*

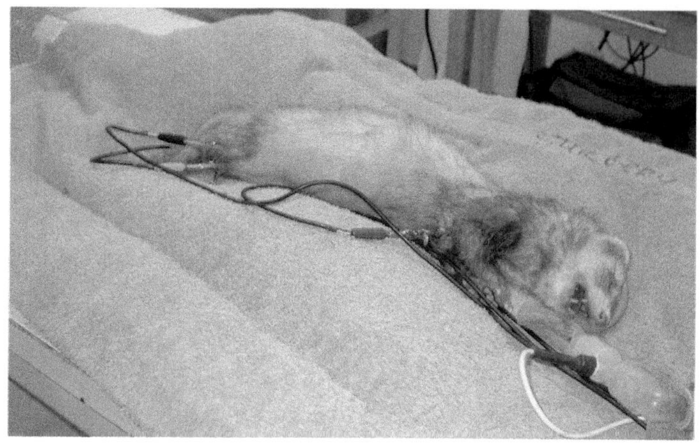

FIGURE 21.2 Ferret on a hot air blanket, intubated, ECG leads and capnography/respiration monitor attached to the endotracheal tube. *Copyright Johnson-Delaney (2017a, 2017b).*

general anesthesia and give crystalloids at 10 mL/kg in fluid boluses.

2. Maintenance of body heat

Active warming is provided using hot-air blanket systems or hot water circulating blankets; note the performance of hot water blankets should be assessed to minimize the risk of burns (Fig. 21.2).

B. Monitoring

i. Monitoring requirements for sedation versus anesthesia: the American Animal Hospital Association has developed guidelines for monitoring (Grubb et al., 2020). Monitoring of the anesthetized patient is continuous, while monitoring of the sedated patient uses the same parameters, but intermittently.

ii. Monitoring Equipment and Techniques: Monitor heart rate and rhythm via a small animal ECG monitor that is validated for rates over 250 beats per minute. Blood pressure (indirect and systolic) can be monitored using the ventral tail with a doppler ultrasound device and pediatric or small animal cuff (the choice depends on the tail circumference to cuff diameter) and a sphygmomanometer. Direct blood pressure monitoring could be considered using an available artery. Oscillometric devices validated for higher heart rates can also be used. Pulse oximetry and capnography equipment for small animals can be used for ferrets. A pulse oximetry clamp can be applied to the tongue or foot but may need to be moved multiple times due to eventual compression of the tissues. An SPO2 reading lower than 90% indicates hypoxia. An esophageal stethoscope is also an option for monitoring heart rate and respiratory sounds. A rectal thermometer probe should be inserted and taped in place. Even if heavily sedated or anesthetized, the insertion of this probe often causes defecation. Capnography can be used to assess ventilation and guide mechanical ventilation. A capnograph using a pediatric sampling chamber or one suitable for small mammals will generate acceptable waveforms. If the ferret is being maintained on a ventilator, it is usually set for 28–35 respirations per minute. Assessing the depth of anesthesia includes assessing muscle tone by testing the pedal withdrawal reflex as well as the loss of the righting reflex. The blink reflex and corneal reflex may not be as useful to assess depth if a face mask is used that covers the eyes, although the loss of both is usually associated with achieving a surgical anesthetic plane. Table 21.1 lists normal monitoring parameters for the ferret.

VI. Drugs used for sedation and anesthesia

Many drug protocols have been described for ferrets, and there is limited research on the determination of the best combinations resulting in optimal patient safety, comfort, and overall suitability. In general, drug combinations allow lower dosages and are safer than single-drug protocols. See Tables 21.2, 21.3 and 21.4.

VII. Common anesthetic emergencies and treatment

a. Anesthetic emergencies are often due to higher than optimal doses of anesthetic agents. Bradycardia, arrhythmias, apnea, hypoxia, and hypotension are often the first indicators that corrective steps should be taken. Ferrets have a very active vagal response, particularly if the epiglottis/larynx is irritated (repeated, unsuccessful intubations, neck manipulations) or if the abdominal viscera are being manipulated. To decrease histamine secretion during gastrointestinal manipulation, diphenhydramine at 0.5 mg/kg SC or PO can be given prior

TABLE 21.2 Emergency drugs, dosages, and routes for use in ferrets (Matchett et al., 2012; Johnson-Delaney, 2017a,b; Morrisey and Johnston, 2018).

Agent	Dosage	Route	Indications
Atropine	0.05 mg/kg	IV, SC, IM	May reverse bradycardia when given slowly during anesthetic event. Usually given preoperatively to counter excessive salivation caused by some agents.
Atipamezole	1 mg/kg	SC, IM	Reversal agent for xylazine, medetomidine, dexmedetomidine. Will lighten anesthesia plane if the ferret is too deep or at the end of the anesthesia event.
Dextrose 50%	0.25–2 mg/kg	IV to effect	Hypoglycemia with or without seizures
Diphenhydramine	0.5–2 mg/kg	IV, IM	Will counter histamine release if vagal reflex is triggered (severe bradycardia) associated with gastrointestinal manipulation. Also used in vaccine reactions.
Dobutamine (5 mg/mL)	0.01 mL/ferret	IV	As needed, counters hypotension and cardiovascular dysfunction
Doxapram	5–10 mg/kg	IV, IM	Respiratory stimulant
Epinephrine	1:10,000; use 0.2–0.5 mL	IV, intratracheal	Positive inotropic agent
Furosemide	1–4 mg/kg	IV, SC, IM	Diuretic.
Glycopyrrolate	0.01 mg/kg	SC, IM	Same effects as atropine, although less arrhythmogenic. Longer duration of action in the GI. Does not cross placental and blood-brain barriers.
Metoclopramide	0.2–1 mg/kg	PO, SC, IM	Antiemetic, motility enhancer
Naloxone	0.01–0.03 mg/kg	IV, SC, IM	Opioid reversal (avoid unless absolutely necessary). May lighten plane of anesthesia if depth due to opioid and decrease the level of analgesia.
Yohimbine	0.5 mg/kg	SC, IM	Reversal agent for xylazine.
Vitamin K	5 mg/kg	SC, IM	May increase coagulation, decrease hemorrhage

to surgery (Johnson-Delaney, 2005b). It may have a very slight sedative effect. Famotidine at 2.5 mg per ferret SC or PO prior to procedures or surgeries may decrease the likelihood of gastrointestinal ulceration (Johnson-Delaney, 2005b, 2017a). Drugs for use in CPR and anesthetic emergencies are listed in Table 21.5.

b. Emergency Preparedness: A ferret-specific emergency kit, which can be as simple as a clearly labeled fishing tackle box, allows rapid access to all important supplies in case of cardiopulmonary arrest or other anesthetic emergencies. The kit includes small vials of emergency drugs, plus a copy of all dosages in a prominent location. One author uses a specific form for each patient with emergency drugs precalculated (Johnson-Delaney, 2005a). The emergency kit also contains a laryngoscope, spare endotracheal tubes and stylet, a calculator and pen, a stethoscope, and appropriately sized syringes and needles. Other useful items include alcohol pads, bandage scissors, hemostats, #15 scalpel blades, suture material (for wounds or to suture a catheter in place), 24 ga intravenous catheters, caps, fluid infusion sets, and smaller bags of several types of fluids, e.g., LRS, 5% dextrose, masking or adhesive tape, roll gauze, and 2 × 2 and 3 × 3 gauze sponges. Each emergency kit should be clearly labeled, and sealed with a strip of tape that indicates the date the kit was checked and refilled and the initials of the person servicing the kit.

VIII. Postanesthetic considerations

Ferrets rarely interfere with incision sites and sutures. A cage mate, however, may chew a catheter plug or other protrusion, so if there is any apparatus remaining, wrapping it with a bandaging material is recommended. Most ferrets can be returned to their home cage and cage mates within a few hours of the procedure, provided all vitals have returned to normal. It is also advantageous to offer food and observe the ferret eating prior to placement back in its home environment.

TABLE 21.3 Sedation and premedication agents suggested for use in ferrets; note single agent protocols have been described for use but may be associated with increased risk of untoward effects at higher dosages.

Agent	Dose (mg/kg)	Route	Comments
Butorphanol + Midazolam ± Alfaxalone	0.2 0.25–0.5 1	SQ, IM	Butorphanol is particularly sedating in ferrets, and alfaxalone may not be required Preferred sedation protocol for aged or ill animals (AML, CAJD)
Butorphanol + Midazolam + Alfaxalone	0.1 1 6	IM	Dosages are higher than above, but may be more appropriate for healthy, often intact laboratory ferrets
Ketamine + Diazepam	10 + 0.5	IV	Deep sedation to general anesthesia. Endotracheal intubation may be possible.
Ketamine + Midazolam	5–10 + 0.25–0.5	IV	Deep sedation to general anesthesia. Endotracheal intubation may be possible.
The following are single-agent protocols described in the literature; drug combinations are preferred.			
Medetomidine	0.02–0.04 mg/kg	SC, IM	Available outside the United States. Has been largely replaced with dexmedetomidine due to availability. Often causes bradycardia, may cause apnea: provide oxygen, α_2 agonist, antagonize with atipamezole at 1 mg/kg SC or IM
Dexmedetomidine	0.04–0.1 mg/kg	IM	Sedation and analgesia for minor procedures. Higher dosages may cause bradycardia, apnea: provide oxygen, α_2 agonist, antagonize with atipamezole at 1 mg/kg SC or IM. May provide analgesia
Midazolam	0.25–0.3	SC, IM	Mild sedation, premedication
	0.25–0.5	SC, IM, IV	Deeper sedation, premedication
	0.5	IN	Intranasal delivery can provide slight sedation or calming, allowing for ease of examination or administration of other drugs.
Diazepam	0.5 mg/kg	PO, IM, IV	Relaxes smooth muscle in urethral obstruction
	2 mg/kg	SC, IM	Light sedation. Can be used in combination with ketamine for deeper sedation/general anesthesia.
	1–2 mg/kg	IN	Intranasal delivery can provide slight sedation or calming, allowing for ease of examination or administration of other drugs.
Ketamine	10–20 mg/kg	IM	Sedation or general anesthesia, depending on dose. Associated with paroxysmal sneezing when touched or picked up.
Xylazine	0.1–0.5	SC, IM	Sedation and some analgesia for minor procedures. May cause hypotension, bradycardia, and arrhythmias particularly in ill animals. Reverse with yohimbine at 0.5 mg/kg SC or IM
Xylazine	2 mg/kg	IV	Immobilization (decreased ability to ambulate/wiggle but can be roused with stimuli such as injections), rapid within 3–5 minutes: arrythmias, bradycardia, and hypotension. Reverse with yohimbine at 0.5 mg/kg SC or IM
Acepromazine	0.1–0.5	SC, IM	Rapid onset of good sedation when given IM usually within 3–5 minutes. Doses above 0.2 mg/kg associated with prolonged recovery time, hypothermia

Combinations allow lower dosages of individual drugs (Matchett et al., 2012; Morrisey and Johnston, 2018; Giral et al., 2014). Few controlled studies of drug combinations for onset of action and peak effects have been published in ferrets. Combinations with known time points are in Table 21.7.

TABLE 21.4 Induction agents (Matchett et al., 2012; Morrisey and Johnston, 2018; Johnson-Delaney, 2017b; Giral et al., 2014).

Agent	Route	Dosage	Comments
Isoflurane	Inhalation	Induce at 3%–4% (MAC: 1.52%), mask; oxygen flow: 2 L/minute (non-rebreathing circuit)	Decreases systolic blood pressure, heart rate, hematocrit, as a sole agent. Recommend for use with premedications.
Sevoflurane	Inhalation	Induce at 6.5% (MAC 1.52%), mask; oxygen flow: 2 L/minute (nonrebreathing circuit)	Lower blood solubility results in more rapid induction and recovery compared with isoflurane, although this may be difficult to assess clinically. Decreases systolic blood pressure, heart rate, hematocrit. Recommended for use with premedications.
Alfaxalone	IV	5 mg/kg	Anesthetic induction
Etomidate	IV	1 mg/kg	Inject slowly to effect, allows intubation
Ketamine, diazepam	IV	0.1 mL/kg of: equal volumes (0.05 mL of K 100 mg/mL and 0.05 mL of D 5 mg/mL)	Induction
Ketamine, midazolam	IV	0.1 mL/kg of: equal volumes (0.05 mL of K 100 mg/mL and 0.05 mL of M 5 mg/mL)	Induction
Propofol	IV	1–5 mg/kg (following premedication)	Induction. Provide supplemental oxygen by mask at 0.5–1 L/minute during propofol administration as propofol may cause bradypnea or apnea with hypoxia.
Alfaxalone + midazolam + butorphanol	IM	6 mg/kg (A) + 1 mg/kg (M) + 0.1 mg/kg (B)	Sometimes listed as a combination for anesthetic induction

A. The immediate postsurgical period

Most anesthetic losses in investigated species occur within 1–3 hours of the end of the anesthetic period (Brodbelt, 2009). Therefore, monitoring must be most vigilant during this period with a dedicated staff person assigned to monitor postoperative patients until full return to function. Any complications during the recovery period (slow recovery, evidence of pain, vocalizations, and seizures) should be addressed immediately.

B. Pain assessment in ferrets

Many texts repeat the idea that ferrets are stoic and do not show pain. This has been refuted in various studies (Reijgwart et al., 2017; McLennan et al., 2019; Mogil et al., 2020). Ferrets do show pain quite dramatically, via facial expressions, postures, and behaviors. Painful ferrets often remain curled up and hiding, may not eat or play, and may even be reluctant to use the litter box. Reactions to stimulation painful areas include muscle spasms, jerking, and even hissing or biting at the examiner. A grimace scale has been proposed for the ferret as well (Fig. 21.4). Administration of appropriate analgesics often results in a return to normal activities and behaviors.

IX. Analgesia

a. Ferrets are similar to dogs and cats in their physiological responses to noxious stimuli, including surgeries, trauma, and other types of discomfort. Consideration of the choice of analgesic agents must consider what type of pain is present, for how long duration the pain will be present, and how an agent can impact normal behaviors such as eating. Route of administration of the initial or peri/postoperative dosing may not be available for the entire recovery period. For example, preoperatively, an IM injection may be given. Intraoperatively and immediately postoperatively, an IV route is available, but following removal of the catheter, oral administration may be preferable. Analgesic selections should

TABLE 21.5 Specific injectable drug combinations described for use for anesthesia for ferrets when inhalant agents are not available or preferred.

Agent	Dose	Route	Comments
Ketamine	30–60 mg/kg	IV	Not recommended as a sole agent; may not provide adequate anesthesia/analgesia; high dosages may cause poor muscle relaxation, hyperreflexiveness, salivation, rough recoveries, and convulsions.
Ketamine-acepromazine	K: 30 mg/kg + A: 0.3 mg/kg	SC, IM	Mild anesthesia with superficial analgesia for minor procedures like blood draws, catheter placement. Effects: hypotension, hypothermia
Ketamine-diazepam	K: 10–20 mg/kg + D: 1–2 mg/kg	IM	Anesthesia but poor analgesia
Ketamine-dexmedetomidine	K: 5 mg/kg + Dexm: 0.03 mg/kg	IM	Dexmedetomidine may cause bradycardia, apnea
Ketamine-dexmedetomidine-butorphanol	K: 5 mg/kg + Dexm: 0.04 mg/kg + B: 0.2 mg/kg	IM	Allows for intubation, 60–80 minutes surgical plane of anesthesia
Ketamine-midazolam	K: 15 mg/kg + M: 0.4 mg/kg	SC, IM	Mild anesthesia, superficial analgesia. Midazolam better absorption than diazepam.
Ketamine-xylazine	K: 10–25 mg/kg + X: 1–2 mg/kg; K: 20–25 mg/kg + X: 2.0–2.5 mg/kg	SC, IM, IP	Anesthesia. Avoid in ill ferrets. Adequate analgesia, muscle relaxation, smooth recovery. At anesthesia (higher doses) ventricular premature contractions, sinus bradycardia, AV heart block, respiratory depression, hypotension, hypothermia (mainly related to xylazine). Use atropine preanesthetic. Reverse xylazine with atipamezole or yohimbine.
Ketamine-xylazine-butorphanol	K: 15 mg/kg + X: 2 mg/kg + B: 0.2 mg/kg	IM	Low blood oxygen, arrhythmias. Provide oxygen. Reverse xylazine with atipamezole or yohimbine.
Tiletamine/zolazepam	12–22 mg/kg	IM	Minor surgical procedures at 22 mg/kg; prolonged recovery time, poor muscle relaxation. Hypoxemia—provide oxygen. Note: rarely used alone.

Protocols are similar to those described for traditional mammal species. Oxygen must be provided for all anesthetized patients (Matchett et al., 2012; Morrisey and Johnston, 2018; Johnson-Delaney, 2009, 2017b; Kapaldo and Eshar, 2022; Ko and Marini, 2014; Lennox unpublished; Sladky et al., 2000).

be included in the animal care and use protocol and take into consideration routes available, level and type of pain anticipated, and for the duration, pain will need to be controlled.

i. Multimodal analgesia: Multimodal analgesia is a method that uses combinations of different agents, which pharmacologically have slightly different actions, but may synergistically provide more complete analgesia along with using lower doses of all agents than if just a single agent was used. Usually, this means using drugs from different drug classes, so pain is managed via different mechanisms. This is usually coupled with multi-modal anesthetic protocols, which also provide a better physiological plane of anesthesia while using lower doses of all the agents.

ii. Preemptive analgesia: Administering analgesics prior to a painful procedure has been demonstrated in many species to be superior to administration after pain is established. In order to prevent breakthrough pain, subsequent doses of analgesics should be timed to be effective just prior to when the previous dose would be wearing off. Knowing this can be difficult, as there are insufficient pharmacologic analgesic studies conducted in ferrets that establish dosing intervals. Much of the dosing schedules are extrapolated from dog/cat pharmacologic studies, clinical observations of ferrets, and clinical experience monitoring postoperatively. Even the number of days a ferret should receive analgesia postoperatively must be extrapolated from other species.

iii. Pharmacologic options: There are many pharmacologic options for analgesia in ferrets. While most have not undergone pharmacologic studies, anecdotal observations and experience with ferrets suggest efficacy. Tables 21.6 and 21.7 list pharmacologic

TABLE 21.6 Analgesic agents used in ferrets (Katzenbach et al., 2018; Matchett et al., 2012; Johnson-Delaney, 2017b; Ko and Marini, 2008, 2014; Morrisey and Johnston, 2018; Eshar and Wilson, 2010).

Agent	Dosage	Route	Frequency	Comments
Acetylsalicylic acid (aspirin)	0.5–22 mg/kg	PO	Q8–24 hours	NSAID. Antipyretic. Do not compound as molecule unstable in aqueous solution.
Amantadine	3–5 mg/kg	PO	Unknown	Thought to potentiate other analgesics via NMDA antagonist action
Bupivacaine	1–2 mg/kg	SC, dental block	Q8 hours although exact interval not documented	May be used with lidocaine to extend analgesia especially in dental nerve blocks
Buprenorphine	12 μg/kg	Epidural	Once	Analgesia, anesthesia
	0.04 mg/kg	IM	Q4–6 hours	PK study
	0.01–0.05 mg/kg	Oral transmucosal, SC, IM, IV	Q6–12 hours	Analgesia
Butorphanol	01–0.5 mg/kg	SC, IM	Q4–6 hours	Higher doses may cause sedation
Butorphanol	0.3 mg/kg	SC	Q2–4 hours	PK study
Butorphanol CRI	0.1–0.2 mg/kg/hour	IV	CRI	Loading dose: 0.02–0.06 mg/kg
Carprofen	4 mg/kg	SC	Q12 hours	NSAID. Use with caution—gastritis potential
Carprofen	1–5 mg/kg	PO	Q12 hours	
Fentanyl	1.25–5 μg/kg	IV	Constant rate infusion	Also for postoperative analgesia
Fentanyl CRI	10–30 μg/kg	IV	Constant rate infusion	Loading dose: 5–10 μg/kg IV
Fentanyl CRI	0.005–0.02 mg/kg/hour	IV	Constant rate infusion	Loading dose: 0.005 mg/kg, postop dose: 0.0025 mg/kg
Gabapentin	3–5 mg/kg	PO	Q12 hours	Neuropathic pain, may cause sedation at higher doses. Start with a lower dose and increase as needed.
Hydromorphone	0.1 mg/kg	SC	1–2 hours	PK study
Hydromorphone CRI	0.025–0.05 mg/kg/hour	IV		Loading dose 0.05 mg/kg IV
	0.1–0.2 mg/kg	SC, IM, IV	1–2 hours	
Ibuprofen	1 mg/kg	PO	Q12–24 hours	NSAID. Use children's over the counter oral solution (20 mg/mL), provide gastric protection during use.
Ketamine CRI	0.1–0.4 mg/kg/hour	IV	CRI	

Continued

TABLE 21.6 Analgesic agents used in ferrets (Katzenbach et al., 2018; Matchett et al., 2012; Johnson-Delaney, 2017b; Ko and Marini, 2008, 2014; Morrisey and Johnston, 2018; Eshar and Wilson, 2010).—cont'd

Agent	Dosage	Route	Frequency	Comments
Ketamine CRI	0.3–1.2 mg/kg/hour	IV	CRI	Loading dose: 2–5 mg/kg
Ketamine	0.4–1.0 mg/kg/hour	IV	CRI	Loading dose: 0.4–0.5 mg/kg, postop dose: 0.3–0.4 mg/kg
Ketamine + fentanyl + lidocaine CRI	K: 0.15 mg/kg/hour + F: 0.012 mg/kg/hour + L: 0.6 mg/kg/hour	IV	CRI	
Lidocaine	1–2 mg/kg total	SC, but usually infiltrated	Q12 hours	Use 1%–2% solution, duration of action 15–30 minutes
	Saturate cotton tipped applicator with 4%–5% dental gel	Topical, on gingiva/dental surgery site, intraoral	Q12 hours	Tastes bitter, may cause excessive salivation. If possible, give ferret a treat to remove bad taste.
Meloxicam	0.1–0.3 mg/kg	PO, SC, IM	Q24 hours	NSAID, monitor liver, kidney values if using long-term, provide gastric protection
Meperidine	5–10 mg/kg	SC, IM, IV	Q2–4 hours	Analgesia
Methadone	0.2 mg/kg	SC, IM	Once, duration of action not published	Good analgesia, poor sedation
Morphine	0.1 mg/kg	Epidural	Once	Analgesia for procedures hind quarters
	0.2–5 mg/kg	SC, IM	Q2–6 hours	SC may cause emesis, excitability, ptyalism
Nalbuphine	0.5–1.5 mg/kg	IM, IV	Q2–3 hours	Analgesia
Oxymorphone	0.06–0.2 mg/kg	SC, IM, IV	Q8–12 hours	Analgesia
Pentazocine	5–10 mg/kg	IM	Q4 hours	Analgesia
Tramadol	1–5 mg/kg	PO	Q12 hours	Anecdotal usage, however study showed no abolition of toe pinch at 5 or 10 mg/kg (Giral, Duval)
Epidural anesthesia/analgesia (Fig. 21.3)				
Bupivacaine	1 mg/kg	Epidural	Anesthesia/analgesia caudal body	Volume usually less than 0.25 mL/kg ferret
Morphine	0.1 mg/kg	Epidural	Primarily analgesia caudal body	
Local anesthetics				
Bupivacaine	1–1.5 mg/kg	SC infiltrate, dental block	Local anesthesia lasting several hours	
Lidocaine	1–2 mg/kg	SC using a 1% or 2% solution, dental block	Local anesthesia lasting 15–30 minutes	

Continued

TABLE 21.6 Analgesic agents used in ferrets (Katzenbach et al., 2018; Matchett et al., 2012; Johnson-Delaney, 2017b; Ko and Marini, 2008, 2014; Morrisey and Johnston, 2018; Eshar and Wilson, 2010).—cont'd

Agent	Dosage	Route	Frequency	Comments
Topical anesthetics				
Lidocaine 4%–5%	1–2 mg/kg total	On small skin area, or applied to gingiva on a cotton tip applicator	Topical anesthesia to allow IV catheter placement. On gingiva, allows for dental examination, or site for injectable anesthesia. Note: Lidocaine primarily for dental use is a gel; for skin: cream or lotion.	
Lidocaine 2.5%/prilocaine 2.5%	Dose for the lidocaine portion at 1–2 mg/kg total	Apply to skin	Allows for IV catheter placement, injections, etc.	Recommend cover application site with flexible bandage, may take up to 30 minutes for skin anesthesia (personal observation, CAJD)

TABLE 21.7 Analgesic durations of various anesthetic combinations in ferrets (Ko and Marini, 2008).

Drug combinations (IM route)	Toe pinch analgesia (minutes)	Skin pinch analgesia (minutes)	Tail clamp analgesia (minutes)
Acepromazine 0.1 mg/kg	0	0	0
Acepromazine 0.1 mg/kg + butorphanol 0.2 mg/kg	7 ± 14	2 ± 5	16 ± 19
Acepromazine 0.1 mg/kg + butorphanol 0.2 mg/kg + ketamine 15 mg/kg	8 ± 10	7 ± 10	30 ± 26
Diazepam 3 mg/kg	0	0	0
Diazepam 3 mg/kg + butorphanol 0.2 mg/kg	0	0	4 ± 9
Diazepam 3 mg/kg + butorphanol 0.2 mg/kg + ketamine 15 mg/kg	16 ± 23	10 ± 18	20 ± 25
Medetomidine 80 mg/kg or dexmedetomidine 40 mg/kg	10 ± 8	20 ± 19	16 ± 14
Medetomidine 80 mg/kg or dexmedetomidine 40 mg/kg + butorphanol 0.2 mg/kg	90 ± 4[a]	92 ± 4[a]	91 ± 8[a]
Medetomidine 80 mg/kg or dexmedetomidine 40 mg/kg + butorphanol 0.2 mg/kg + ketamine 5 mg/kg	93 ± 4[a]	91 ± 5[a]	95 ± 0[a]
Xylazine 2 mg/kg	40 ± 27	32 ± 18	35 ± 17
Xylazine 2 mg/kg + butorphanol 0.2 mg/kg	54 ± 11	43 ± 10	69 ± 5
Xylazine 2 mg/kg + butorphanol 0.2 mg/kg + ketamine 15 mg/kg	69 ± 12	63 ± 15	81 ± 19

Medetomidine may not be available commercially. Dexmedetomidine equivalent dosage has been added.
[a]*If not antagonized with atipamezole.*
All results modified from references Brown (1997), Canadian Pediatric Society (2000), Marini et al. (1994) and Ko et al. (1998).

analgesic agents. Many agents can be delivered orally, topically, or by injection. The major classes of analgesics that have been used in ferrets are:

1. Opioids: These include butorphanol, buprenorphine, hydromorphone, methadone, morphine, tramadol, and fentanyl. Butorphanol is more sedating than other opioids, which can be beneficial. Morphine-like drugs can be linked with emesis.
2. Alpha-2 adrenergic agonists: Dexmedetomidine and xylazine have some analgesic actions and are part of a multi-modal approach to anesthesia.
3. Topical anesthetic agents: Lidocaine, and bupivacaine can be used pre, intra, and postoperatively to anesthetize a local area and alleviate pain. There are anecdotal reports of the use of dental and local blocks using techniques described for canine and feline patients. An epidural injection is done at a site in between the wings of the ileum, pelvis, and on the midline between the last lumbar vertebral bodies (Fig. 21.3). Local lines analgesia/anesthetic is delivered once the ferret is anesthetized but before an incision is made (Johnson-Delaney, 2017a,b).
4. NSAIDs: These include meloxicam and carprofen, which are commonly used in ferrets, primarily postoperatively. However, like cats, ferrets are deficient in the glucuronidation pathway (Litchtenberger, 2006), so their metabolism may be slow. Renal failure can occur with prolonged use. It is recommended that a gastrointestinal protectant such as sucralfate, along with an acid reducer such as famotidine be used if NSAIDs are utilized. It is a common practice to administer one of the NSAIDs just as the ferret is regaining consciousness and the blood pressure and body temperature have returned to normal.
5. Gamma-aminobutyric acid analogs: Gabapentin is considered useful in treating primarily neurologic pain (Morrisey and Johnston, 2018), but it also has anticonvulsant properties, and in humans, some antianxiety effects. It is becoming widely used, particularly, postoperatively and in geriatric ferrets that may have chronic pain due to neurologic and corresponding musculoskeletal pain (CAJD personal experience).

b. Nonpharmacologic options: Several nonpharmacologic adjunctive or alternative therapies are being used in ferrets in clinical pet practice. Clinical studies proving effectiveness have not been done, but extrapolation of these techniques used in other animals and humans can lead to the conclusion that they will do no harm, and potentially may help. These include the use of therapeutic lasers, acupuncture, including the use of acupressure points, physical therapy, and massage. If necessary, housing should be adapted to allow easy access to food, water, and the latrine area. Social housing is often provided as ferrets seem more relaxed and more comfortable when housed with a conspecific. Nutraceuticals and supplements have been used anecdotally may be beneficial, but they should be compatible with research goals.

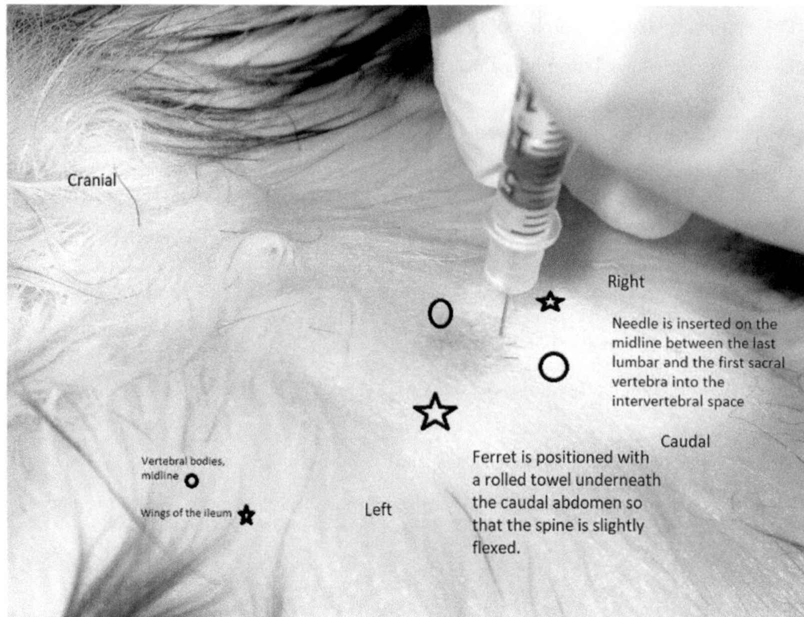

FIGURE 21.3 Landmarks for epidural injection. An insulin (25–29 ga) 0.5–1.0 syringe is used. *Copyright Johnson-Delaney (2017a, 2017b).*

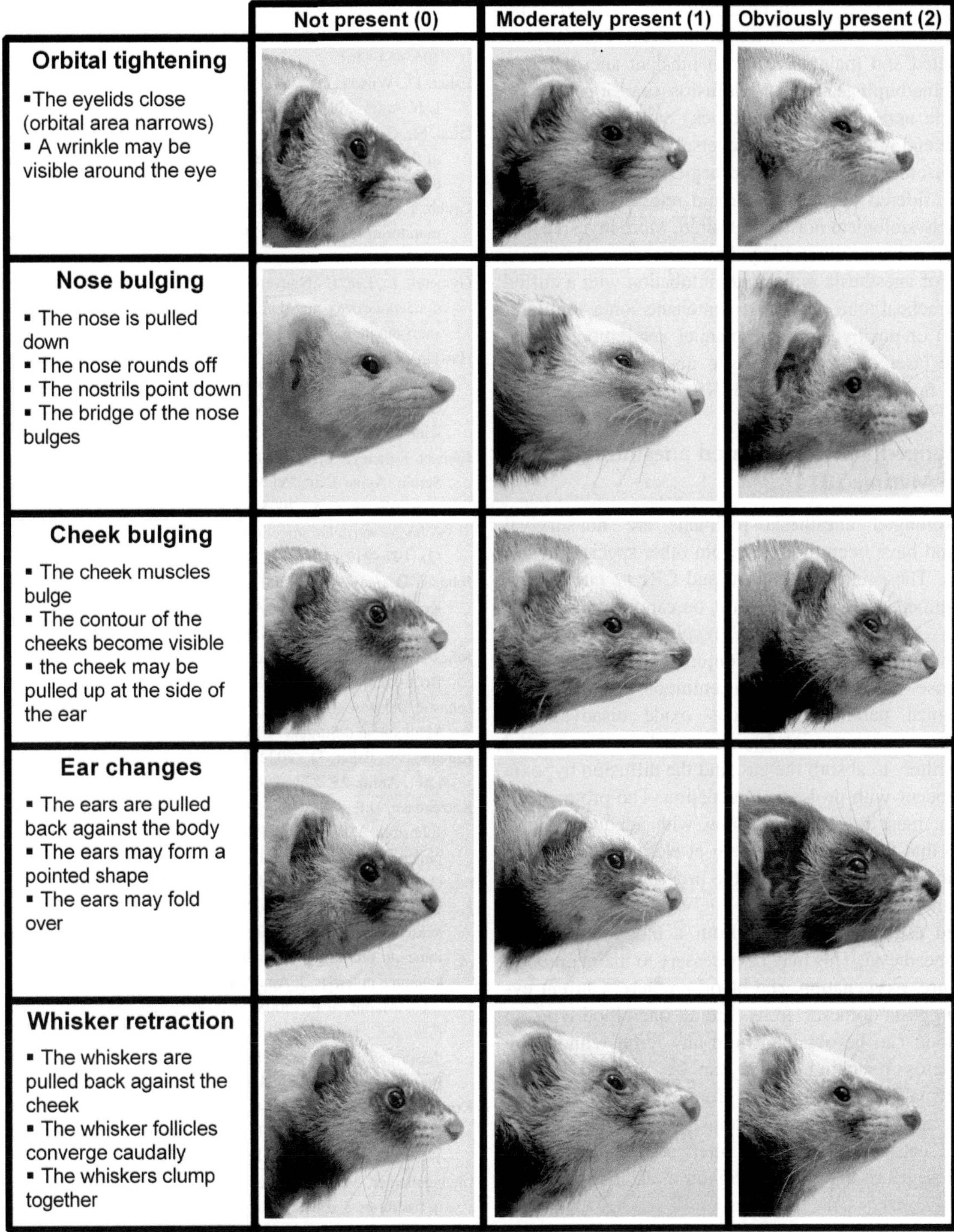

FIGURE 21.4 Ferret grimace scale. *From Reijgwart et al. (2017). Used by permission.*

X. Anesthesia and analgesia for specific situations

a. Common procedures done in ferrets include catheter placement for infusions, placement of vascular access ports and other implants for telemetry, laparotomy, and thoracotomy. In healthy ferrets, a preoperative regimen might include atropine, an opioid such as butorphanol or buprenorphine, and a benzodiazepine such as midazolam. This generally allows IV catheterization and patient preparation; stress-free induction; then proceeds with an inhalant. The ferret is intubated and maintained on an inhalant anesthetic. A lidocaine/bupivacaine local infusion (incisional block/ discrete nerve block/splash block) can be considered. At the end of the procedure, reversal of benzodiazepines (flumazenil) and alpha-2 adrenergic (atipamezole) may be considered to promote a rapid return to consciousness/physiological normal if desired. More invasive surgeries include thoracotomy; this procedure requires a plane of anesthesia to facilitate intubation with a cuffed endotracheal tube, and then maintenance on a ventilator (ideal) or positive pressure manual ventilation. Therapeutic laser of the incision site may help to promote blood flow (Avci et al., 2013; Ritzman et al., 2015).

A. Prolonged and complicated anesthesia (Ko and Marini, 2014)

Most prolonged anesthesia regimens are nonsurvival studies and have been modified from other species for use in ferrets. These include inhalant and CRI or intermittent bolus regimens; any protocol must be carefully titrated to minimize cardiovascular and respiratory depression. Nitrous oxide has been used in conjunction with isoflurane to decrease the isoflurane concentration and maintain physiological parameters. Nitrous oxide disadvantages include the cost, potential for abuse, failure of activated charcoal filters to absorb the gas, and the diffusion hypoxia that can occur with prolonged inhalation. The protocol for anesthesia must be designed along with adequate monitoring so that the ferret can remain at close to the physiological normal state throughout the procedure.

Anesthesia of anemic ferrets (PCV < 20) e.g., jills in prolonged estrus, may benefit from a blood transfusion prior to anesthesia. This may be necessary to maintain body temperature, oxygenation, and blood pressure. Current evidence suggests domestic ferrets are all one blood type, so donor blood can be obtained from any ferret without the need of cross-matching. Blood can be obtained from a donor (usually up to 20 mL from a ferret weighing >1.5 kg) and set up through a transfusion set as used for dogs and cats. Anemic ferrets often require lower than typical dosages of anesthetics (Pignon et al., 2014).

References

Avci, P., Gupta, A., Sadasivam, M., et al., 2013. Low-level laser (light) therapy (LLLT) in skin: sitmulating, healing, restoring. Semin. Cutan. Med. Surg. 32, 41–52.

Brodbelt, D., 2009. Perioperative mortality in small animal anaesthesia. Vet. J. 182, 152–161.

Brown, S.A., 1997. Clinical techniques in domestic ferrets. Semin. Avian Exot. Pet Med. 6, 75–78.

Canadian Pediatric Society, 2000. Fetus and newborn committee. Prevention and management of pain and stress in the neonate. Pediatrics 105, 454–461.

Eshar, D., Wilson, J., 2010. Epidural anesthesia and analgesia in ferrets. Lab. Anim. 39, 339–340.

Giral, M., Garcia-Olmo, D.C., Gomex-Juarex, M., 2014. Anesthetic effects in the ferret of alfaxalone alone and in combination with medetomidine or tramadol: a pilot study. Lab. Anim. 48 (4), 313–320.

Grubb, T., Sager, J., Gaynor, J.S., et al., 2020. 2020 AAHA anesthesia and monitoring guidelines for dogs and cats. J. Am. Anim. Hosp. Assoc. 56, 1–24.

Gymerek, L., Lee, C., Nguyen, N., 1999. Pharmacology of G-1-64, a new nondepolarizing neuromuscular blocking agent with rapid onset and short duration of action. Acta Anaesthesiol. Scand. 43, 651–657.

Hawkins, M.G., Pascoe, P.J., 2021. Anesthesia, analgesia, and sedation of small mammals. In: Quesenberry, K.E., Orcutt, C.J., Mans, C., Carpenter, J.W. (Eds.), Ferrets, Rabbits, and Rodents. Clinical Medicine and Surgery, fourth ed. Elsevier, St. Louis, MO, pp. 536–558.

Johnson-Delaney, C.A., 2005a. Ferret cardiopulmonary resuscitation. Semin. Avian Exot. Pet Med. 14 (2), 135–142.

Johnson-Delaney, C.A., 2005b. The ferret gastrointestinal tract and *Helicobacter mustelae* infection. Vet. Clin. N. Am. Exot. Anim. Pract. 8 (2), 197–212.

Johnson-Delaney, C.A., 2009. Ferrets: anaesthesia and analgesia. In: Keeble, E., Meredith, A. (Eds.), BSAVA Rodents and Ferrets. BSAVA, Quedgeley, UK, pp. 245–253.

Johnson-Delaney, C.A., 2017a. Ferret Medicine and Surgery. CRC Press, Boca Raton, FL.

Johnson-Delaney, C.A., 2017b. Analgesia and anaesthesia. In: Ferret Medicine and Surgery. CRC Press, Boca Raton, FL, pp. 377–387.

Kapaldo, N., Eshar, D., 2022. Ferret sedation and anesthesia. Vet. Clin. Exot. Anim. 25, 273–296.

Katzenbach, J.E., Wittenburg, L.A., Allweiler, S.I., Gustafson, D.L., Johnston, M.S., 2018. Pharmacokinetics of single-dose buprenorphine, butorphanol, and hydromorphone in the domestic ferret (*Mustela putorius furo*). J. Exot. Pet Med. 27, 95–102.

Ko, J.C.H., Smith, T.A., Kuo, W.C., Nicklin, C.F., 1998. Comparison of anesthetic and cardiorespiratory effects of diazepam-butorphanol-ketamine, acepromazine-butrophanol-ketamine, and xylazine-butorphanol-ketamine in ferrets. J. Am. Anim. Hosp. Assoc. 34, 407–416.

Ko, J.C., Marini, R.P., 2008. Anesthesia and analgesia in ferrets. In: Fish, R.E., Danneman, P.J., Brown, M.J., Karas, A.Z. (Eds.), Anesthesia and Analgesia in Laboratory Animals, second ed. Academic Press, Boston, pp. 443–456.

Ko, J.C., Marini, R.P., 2014. Anesthesia. Chapter 12. In: Fox, J.G., Marini, R.P. (Eds.), Biology and Diseases of the Ferret, third ed. Wiley Blackwell, Ames, IA, pp. 259–283.

Litchtenberger, M., 2006. Shock, fluid, therapy, anesthesia and analgesia in the ferret. Exot. DVM 7 (2), 24–30.

Marini, R.P., Esteves, M.I., Fox, J.G., 1994. A technique for catheterization of the urinary bladder in the ferret. Lab. Anim. 28, 155–157.

Matchett, C.A., Marr, R., Berard, F.M., Cawthon, A.G., Swing, S.P., 2012. The Laboratory Ferret. CRC Press, Boca Raton, FL.

McLennan, K.M., Miller, A.L., Dalla Costa, E., Stucke, D., Corke, M.J., Broom, D.M., Leach, M.C., 2019. Conceptual and methodological issues relating to pain assessment in animals: the development and utilisation of pain facial expression scales. Appl. Anim. Behav. Sci. 217, 1–15.

Mogil, J.S., Pang, D.S.J., Guanaes Silva Dutra, G., Chambers, C.T., 2020. The development and use of facial grimace scales for pain measurement in animals. Neurosci. Biobehav. Rev. 116, 480–493.

Morrisey, J.K., Johnston, M.S., 2018. Ferrets. In: Carpenter, J.W., Marion, C.J. (Eds.), Exotic Animal Formulary, fifth ed. Elsevier, St. Louis, pp. 32–557.

Pignon, C., Donnelly, T.M., Todeschini, C., Deschamps, J.Y., Roux, F.A., 2014. Assessment of a blood preservation protocol for use in ferrets before transfusion. Vet. Rec. 174 (11), 277.

Reijgwart, M.L., Schoemaker, N.J., Pascuzzo, R., et al., 2017. The composition and initial evaluation of a grimace scale in ferrets after surgical implantation of a telemetry probe. PLoS ONE 1211, e0187986.

Ritzman, T.K., Griffin, C., Kilgore, A., et al., 2015. Therapeutic laser treatment for exotic animal patients. J. Avian Med. Surg. 29, 69–73.

Sladky, K.K., Horne, W.A., Goodrowe, K.L., et al., 2000. Evaluation of epidural morphine for postoperative analgesia in ferrets (*Mustela putorius furo*). Contemp. Top. 30, 33–38.

Further reading

Allweiler, S.I., 2016. How to improve anesthesia and analgesia in small mammals. Vet. Clin. N. Am. Exot. Anim. Pract. 19, 361–377.

Boyce, S.W., Zingg, B.M., Lightfoot, T.L., 2001. Behavior of *Mustela putorius furo* (the domestic ferret). Vet. Clin. N. Am. Exot. Anim. Pract. 4 (3), 697–712.

Brietzke, S.E., Mair, E.A., 1990. Laryngeal mask versus endotracheal tube in a ferret model. Ann. Otol. Rhinol. Laryngol. 110, 827–833.

Duvall, A., 2017. Tramadol. J. Exot. Pet Med. 26, 74–77.

Evans, A.T., Springsteen, K.K., 1998. Anesthesia of ferrets. Semin. Avian Exot. Pet Med. 7, 48–52.

Flecknell, P., 2016. Analgesia and post-operative care. In: Flecknell, P. (Ed.), Laboratory Animal Anaesthesia, fourth ed. Academic Press, Waltham, MA, pp. 141–192.

Flecknell, P., 2018. Analgesics in small mammals. Vet. Clin. N. Am. Exot. Anim. Pract. 21, 83–103.

Grundy, D., 1990. The effect of surgical anaesthesia on antral motility in the ferret. Exp. Physiol. 75, 701–703.

Horn, C.C., Meyers, K., Pake, D., et al., 2012. Post-anesthesia vomiting: impact of isoflurane and morphine on ferrets and musk shrews. Physiol. Behav. 106, 562–658.

Johnston, M.S., 2005. Clinical approaches to analgesia in ferrets and rabbits. Semin. Avian Exot. Pet Med. 14 (4), 229–235.

Jones, E.J., Poole, K.C., Sollini, J., Town, S.M., Bizley, J.K., August 7, 2020. Seasonal weight changes in laboratory ferrets. PLoS ONE 15 (8), e0232733.

Kircher, S.S., Murray, L.E., Juliano, M.L., November 2009. Minimizing trauma to the upper airway: a ferret model of neonatal intubation. J. Am. Assoc. Lab. Anim. Sci. 48 (6), 780–784.

Kleine, S., Quandt, J.E., 2012. Anesthesia case of the month. Hypothermia and hypercarbia in a ferret during anesthesia. J. Am. Vet. Med. Assoc. 241, 1577–1580.

MacPhail, C.M., Monnet, E., Gaynor, J.S., Perini, A., 2004. Effect of sevoflurane on hemodynamic and cardiac energetic parameters of ferrets. Am. J. Vet. Res. 65, 653–658.

Marini, R.P., Callahan, R.J., Jackson, L.R., et al., 1997. Distribution of technetium 99 m labeled red blood cells during isoflurane anesthesia in ferrets. Am. J. Vet. Res. 58 (7), 781–785.

Olin, J.M., Smith, T.J., Talcott, M.R., 1997. Evaluation of noninvasive monitoring techniques in domestic ferrets (*Mustela putorius furo*). Am. J. Vet. Res. 58, 1065–1069.

Payton, A.J., Pick, J.R., 1989. Evaluation of a combination of tiletamine and zolazepam as an anesthetic for ferrets. Lab. Anim. Sci. 39, 243–246.

Phillips, B.E., Harms, C.A., Messenger, K.M., 2015. Oral transmucosal detomidine gel for the sedation of the domestic ferret (*Mustela putorius furo*). J. Exot. Pet Med. 24, 446–454.

Roe, A.W., Pallas, S.L., Kwon, Y.H., Sur, M., 1992. Visual projections routed to the auditory pathway in ferrets: receptive fields of visual neurons in primary auditory cortex. J. Neurosci. 12 (9), 3651–3664.

Schernthaner, A., Lendl, C.E., Hartmann, K., Pragst, I., Preissel, A.-K., Henke, J., 2011. Medetomidine/midazolam/ketamine anaesthesia in ferrets: effects on cardiorespiratory parameters and evaluation of plasma drug concentrations. Vet. Anaesth. Analg. 38, 439–450.

Simoneau, I.I., Hamza, M.S., Mata, H.P., et al., 2001. The cannabinoid agonist WIN55, 212-2 suppresses opioid-induced emesis in ferrets. J. Am. Soc. Anesthesiol. 94, 882–887.

Sylvina, T.J., Berman, N.G., Fox, J.G., 1990. Effects of yohimbine on bradycardia and duration of recumbency in ketamine/xylazine anesthetized ferrets. Lab. Anim. Sci. 40, 178–182.

van Oostrom, H., Schoemaker, N.J., Uilenreef, J.J., 2011. Pain management in ferrets. Vet. Clin. N. Am. Exot. Anim. Pract. 14 (1), 105–116.

Yu, H., Farley, B.J., Jin, D.Z., Sur, M., 2005. The coordinated mapping of visual space and response features in visual cortex. Neuron 47, 267–280.

Chapter 22

Anesthesia and analgesia in other mammals

Lucy Kennedy
Unit for Laboratory Animal Medicine, University of Michigan, Ann Arbor, MI, United States

Chapter outline

The discipline of comparative medicine contributes to a greater understanding of life through studies defining and comparing organisms and processes. Animals other than traditional laboratory species offer unique anatomical, physiological, behavioral, and developmental characteristics, making them valuable models for the study of human disease and disorders. Knowledge of anesthesia and analgesia for these nontraditional species is sometimes sparse, or more commonly found in the literature for zoo, wildlife, or pet medicine. This chapter attempts to gather that information and present what is known for the nontraditional species of laboratory mammals that have been found to be useful in biomedical research.

I. Marsupialia: marsupials

Marsupials, such as opossums and sugar gliders, have short gestations, undeveloped neonates, extended development and lactation in the pouch, metabolic rates 26%–35% lower than those of equivalently sized eutherian mammals, and lower core body temperatures, making them uniquely interesting for biomedical research applications (Holz,

Anesthesia and Analgesia in Laboratory Animals. https://doi.org/10.1016/B978-0-12-822215-7.00017-2

2003; Pye, 2001). The marsupials most commonly used in biomedical research are found in three families, including relatively small species compared to the more familiar macropods like kangaroos and wallabies found in zoos.

Order Marsupialia

Family Didelphidae (New World opossums)

Didelphis virginiana (Virginia opossum)

Monodelphis domestica (short-tailed opossum)

Family Phalangeridae (Australian opossums)

Trichosurus vulpecula (brushtail opossum)

Family Petauridae

Petaurus breviceps (sugar glider)

A. Manual restraint

Nest boxes can be helpful for transporting smaller marsupials to induction chambers (Ness and Johnson-Delaney, 2012). The small marsupials used in biomedical research may be firmly gripped behind the head and the tail base or hind legs for placement in an anesthetic induction chamber or administration of intramuscular injections (Holz, 2003; Pye, 2001). Sugar gliders may be restrained in a bag with their head exposed for mask induction with isoflurane or their legs exposed for IM injection (Pye, 2001). Virginia opossums are often wild-caught and may need thick gloves to handle, but can still be manually restrained with a towel over their heads for access to hind limbs for IM injections (personal communication with Allison Ostdiek, DVM, University of Chicago).

B. Chemical restraint

Although sugar gliders are a smaller species, IM injections can be performed safely in either the epaxial muscles of the neck and upper thorax or the biceps femoris in the anterior thigh (Ness and Johnson-Delaney, 2012). Preanesthetic fasting of 4–6 hours is recommended since regurgitation under anesthesia is possible (Holz, 2003). Isoflurane is the agent of choice for both inductions via a mask (3%–5%) or chamber as well as maintenance (1%–3%) for adults and neonates (Hernandez-Divers, 2004; Holz, 2003; Johnson-Delaney, 2021) (Fig. 22.1). Premedication of sugar gliders with butorphanol (0.2 mg/kg IM) contributes to a smooth induction when using a chamber or face mask for the delivery of isoflurane (Hernandez-Divers, 2004). Sevoflurane may be used to effect as an alternative to isoflurane (Johnson-Delaney, 2021). One group has had success sedating Virginia opossums with a combination of alfaxalone 7–10 mg/kg IM and midazolam 0.5 mg/kg IM, either for noninvasive procedures such as imaging or for further intubation for gas anesthesia. The midazolam can be reversed with flumazenil at 0.01–0.02 mg/kg. Prolonged sedation has been noted even with the reversal, so starting with the lower end of the alfaxalone range is preferable (personal communication with Allison Ostdiek, DVM, University of Chicago). Premedication with atropine 0.01–0.02 mg/kg IM, IV, SQ (Holz, 2003; Morrisey and Carpenter, 2020), or glycopyrrolate 0.01–0.02 mg/kg IM, IV, or SQ (Morrisey and Carpenter, 2020; Shima, 1999) can aid in the control of hypersalivation. Anesthetics, sedatives, and analgesics for marsupials can be found in Tables 22.1 and 22.2.

C. Vascular access

The jugular, femoral, lateral coccygeal, and cephalic veins are accessible for blood collection or catheterization in most marsupial species (Holz, 2003). The jugular vein and cranial vena cava are the most reliable sites for blood collection in sugar gliders, but small amounts can also be collected from peripheral vessels, including the cephalic, lateral saphenous, and ventral coccygeal veins (Ness and Johnson-Delaney, 2012). The ventral or lateral coccygeal veins of the Virginia opossum may be used for blood collection as well as catheterization (Johnson-Delaney, 2006). Fig. 22.2 shows

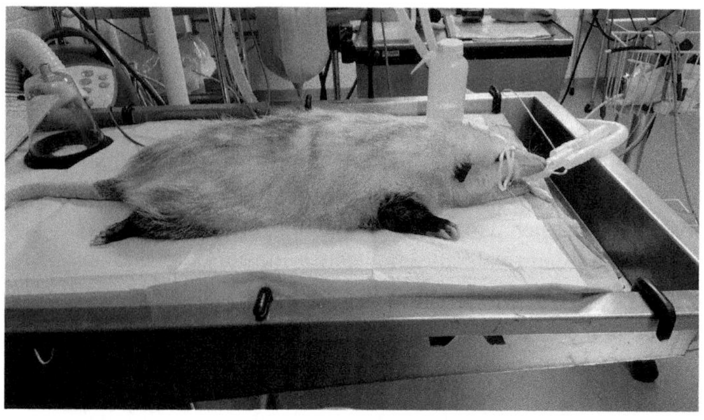

FIGURE 22.1 A Virginia opossum (*Didelphis virginiana*) intubated for general anesthesia with isoflurane. Intubation is a straight-forward procedure in this species. *Courtesy of University of Chicago.*

TABLE 22.1 Injectable anesthetics and sedatives for marsupials.

Species	Drug	Dosage and route	References
Short-tailed opossum	Ketamine plus dexmedetomidine	100 mg/kg IP; 0.1 mg/kg IP	Barnett et al. (2017)
Sugar gliders	Bupivacaine Diazepam Ketamine plus midazolam Ketamine plus xylazine Lidocaine Midazolam	1–2 mg/kg SQ—local 0.5–2.0 mg/kg IM, IV, PO—sedation 10–20 mg/kg SQ, IM; 0.35–0.5 mg/kg SQ, IM 10–25 mg/kg SQ, IM; 5 mg/kg SQ, IM 1–4 mg/kg SQ—local 0.25–0.5 mg/kg IM—sedation	Morrisey and Carpenter (2020) Morrisey and Carpenter (2020) Morrisey and Carpenter (2020) Brust and Mans (2018) Morrisey and Carpenter (2020) Morrisey and Carpenter (2020)
Virginia opossum	Ketamine plus medetomidine[a] Ketamine plus dexmedetomidine[a] Tiletamine/zolazepam (Telazol)	2–3 mg/kg IM; 0.05–0.1 mg/kg IM 4–6 mg/kg IM; 0.03–0.075 mg/kg IM 15 mg/kg IM	Vogelnest (2015) Ostdiek (2021) Vogelnest (2015)
Brushtail possum	Alfaxalone Diazepam Ketamine plus medetomidine[a] Ketamine plus xylazine	5–8 mg/kg IM 0.5–1.0 mg/kg IM—sedation 1–3 mg/kg IM; 0.02–0.1 mg/kg IM 50 mg/kg IM; 10 mg/kg IM	Vogelnest (2015) Vogelnest (2015) Vogelnest (2015) Bathgate et al. (1992)
	Tiletamine/zolazepam (Telazol)	10 mg/kg IM	Pye (2001)

[a]*Reversal with atipamezole 0.05–0.4 mg/kg IV.*

TABLE 22.2 Analgesics for small marsupial species.

Species	Drug	Dosage and route	References
Short-tailed opossum	Buprenorphine	0.01 mg/kg SQ, IM q 8 hours	Johnson-Delaney (2006)
	Butorphanol	0.1–0.5 mg/kg SQ, IM q 6–8 hours	Johnson-Delaney (2006)
	Carprofen	1.0 mg/kg PO, SQ q 12–24 hours	Johnson-Delaney (2006)
	Meloxicam	0.2 mg/kg PO SQ q 24 hours	Johnson-Delaney (2006)
Virginia opossum	Buprenorphine	0.1 mg/kg SQ, IM q 8–12 hours	Johnson-Delaney (2006)
	Butorphanol	0.1–0.5 mg/kg SQ, PO q 6–8 hours	Johnson-Delaney (2006)
	Carprofen	1.0 mg/kg PO, SQ q 12–24 hours	Johnson-Delaney (2006)
	Meloxicam	0.2 mg/kg PO, SQ q 24 hours	Johnson-Delaney (2006)
Sugar glider	Buprenorphine	0.01–0.03 mg/kg PO, SQ, IM q 8–12 hours	Brust and Mans (2018)
	Butorphanol	0.1–0.5 mg/kg SQ, IM q 6–8 hours	Morrisey and Carpenter, 2020
	Meloxicam	0.1–0.2 mg/kg PO, SQ q 12–24 hours	Brust and Mans (2018)

examples of catheterization in the Virginia opossum using either the lateral coccygeal or cephalic veins. Intraosseous catheterization into the femur or tibia is an appropriate choice for sugar gliders, as catheterization in other locations is difficult in this species (Johnson-Delaney, 2021).

D. Fluid therapy

For marsupials used in research, 50–100 mL/kg/day of crystalloid fluids may be administered subcutaneously using a butterfly catheter (Johnson-Delaney, 2006). Fluids given subcutaneously in the sugar glider can cause

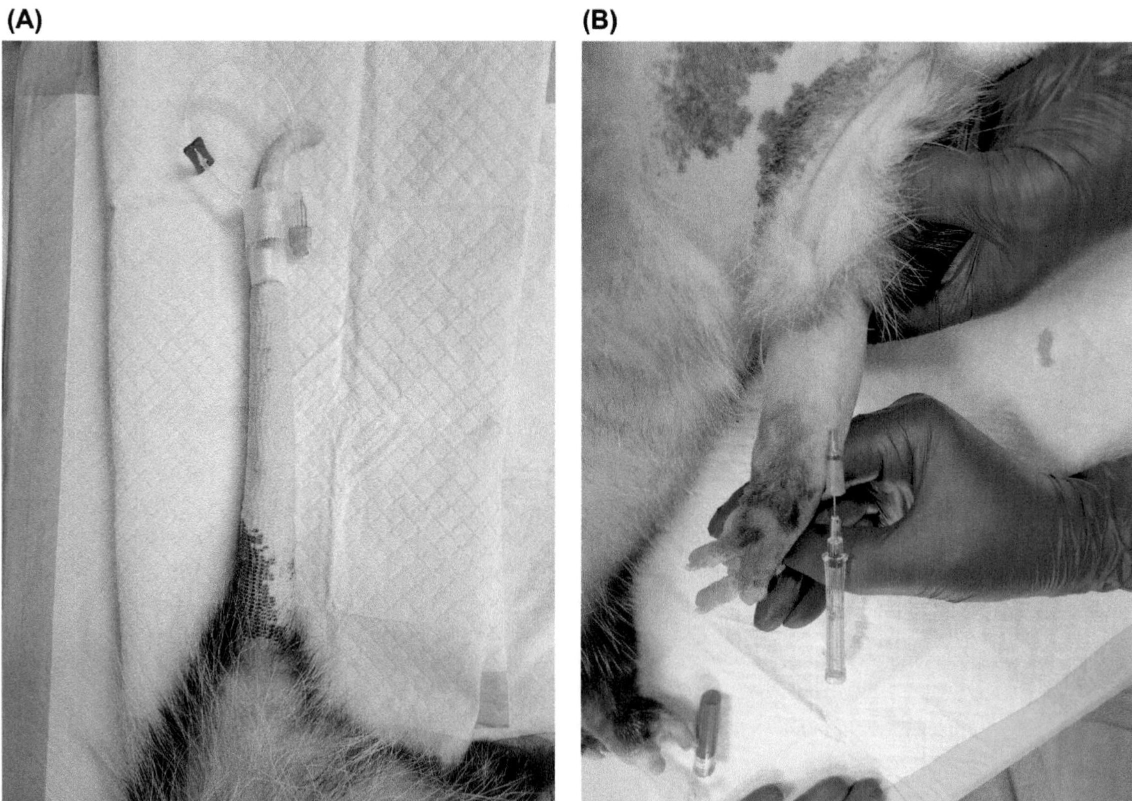

FIGURE 22.2 A Virginia opossum (*Didelphis virginiana*) with intravenous catheters placed for vascular access in the (A) lateral coccygeal vein and (B) cephalic vein. *Courtesy of University of Chicago.*

discomfort and distress if given in the patagium (the gliding membrane extending between the forelimb and the hindlimb), and care should be taken to avoid that area when possible (Johnson-Delaney, 2021). Fluids can be given intravenously through the ventral coccygeal vein in the Virginia opossum. A femoral intraosseous catheter may be used for fluid replacement in sugar gliders, short-tailed opossums, and Virginia opossums by first anesthetizing the animal and aseptically preparing the hip area as if for surgery. After an optional local skin block (2% lidocaine), a 1 inch, 18–22-gauge hypodermic or spinal needle is placed into the proximal aspect of the femur through a small skin incision. After taping the needle in place, administer warmed fluids at 5 mL/hour. Avoid fluids with glucose since marsupials develop cataracts and hepatic lipidosis with dextrose-containing fluids (Johnson-Delaney, 2006).

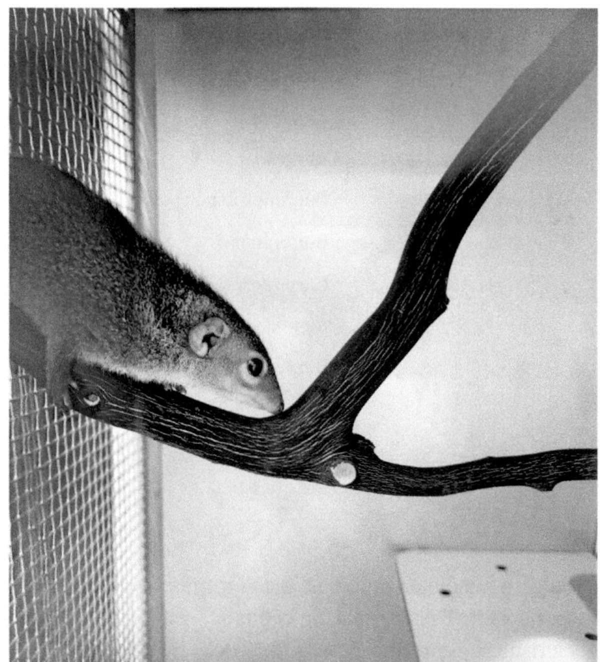

FIGURE 22.3 Example of a tree shrew (*Tupaia glis*) housed in a biomedical research setting. *Courtesy of Vanderbilt University Medical Center.*

II. Scandentia and Eulipotyphla: insectivores

Insectivores used in biomedical research include several families of shrews (*Sorex* sp., *Cryptotis* sp., *Suncus* sp., *Tupaia* sp.) (Fig. 22.3), all with rapid heart rates (up to 800 beats/minute), high metabolic rates, rod-prominent retinas, small brains with few fissures, low body temperatures 91–95°F (33–35°C) (outside of *Sorex* sp., which have a higher body temperature at 98–100°F (37–38°C)), and seasonal torpor or hibernation at temperatures less than 65°F (18°C) (Barbiers, 2003; D'Agostino, 2015).

Order Scandentia

Family Tupaiidae

Tupaia glis (common tree shrew)

Order Eulipotyphla

Family Soricidae

Suncus etruscus (Etruscan, pygmy shrew)

Suncus murinus (Asian house musk shrew)

Sorex araneus (long-tailed shrew)

Cryptotis parva (small-eared shrew)

A. Manual restraint

Clear acrylic tubes facilitate visual examination of shrews without the stress associated with manual restraint (D'Agostino, 2015; Isenbugel and Baumgartner, 1993). The Etruscan shrew is the smallest known mammalian species at 2–3 g and cannot be restrained by hand due to their size and their speed of movement. Instead, forceps with silicone tip covers can be used to pick the shrews up by the tail root for transfer into an induction box (Geyer et al., 2022).

B. Chemical restraint

Isoflurane is administered by face mask or induction chamber (3%–5%) with face mask maintenance (0.5%–3.0%) is the anesthetic of choice (Barbiers, 2003; Isenbugel and Baumgartner, 1993). Endotracheal intubation is difficult due to the small oral cavity (D'Agostino, 2015). Due to their rapid metabolism, a preanesthetic fasting period is not recommended, and they may be more susceptible to hypothermia and hypoglycemia (D'Agostino, 2015). Small shrews may be at risk of hyperthermia during stress (Barbiers, 2003). Preanesthetic treatment with atropine 0.01–0.04 mg/kg SQ or IM is recommended for hedgehogs (Morrisey and Carpenter, 2020) and should be considered for other insectivores. Analgesic doses are not published for shrew species; however, there is a large body of published information on hedgehogs, and some of these doses may be an appropriate starting place for other insectivores. Table 22.3 covers anesthetic and analgesic doses for insectivores.

TABLE 22.3 Injectable anesthetics, sedatives, and analgesics for Insectivores.

Drug	Dosage and route	Comments	References
Buprenorphine Butorphanol Carprofen Diazepam	0.01 mg/kg SQ, IM q 6–8 hours 0.05–0.4 mg/kg SQ q 6–8 hours 1 mg/kg PO, SQ q 12–24 hours 0.5–2.0 mg/kg IM	Hedgehog dose—analgesic Hedgehog dose—analgesic Hedgehog dose—analgesic Mild sedation	Morrisey and Carpenter, 2020 Morrisey and Carpenter, 2020 Morrisey and Carpenter, 2020 D'Agostino (2015)
Ketamine	5–20 mg/kg IM	Used in combinations with a benzodiazepine or α_2-agonist	D'Agostino (2015)
Ketamine plus medetomidine[a] Ketamine plus medetomidine plus midazolam[b]	5 mg/kg IM; 0.1 mg/kg IM 20 mg/kg SQ; 0.2 mg/kg SQ; 3 mg/kg SQ		D'Agostino (2015) D'Agostino (2015)
Ketamine plus xylazine	10 mg/kg IM; 2 mg/kg IM	For endotracheal intubation of tree shrew	Ohl et al. (1999)
Ketamine plus xylazine	10–20 mg/kg IM; 1 mg/kg IM	20–30 minutes anesthesia in shrews	Isenbugel and Baumgartner (1993)
Medetomidine[a] Meloxicam Tiletamine/zolazepam (Telazol)	0.05–0.1 mg/kg IM 0.2 mg/kg IM 0.5 mg/kg SQ q 12 hours 1–5 mg/kg IM	Light sedation Heavy sedation Hedgehog dose—analgesic Prolonged recovery	D'Agostino (2015) Morrisey and Carpenter, 2020 D'Agostino (2015)
Xylazine[c]	0.5–1.0 mg/kg IM	Given with ketamine	D'Agostino (2015)

[a]*Reverse with atipamezole 0.3–0.5 mg/kg IM.*
[b]*Reverse with atipamezole 1.0 mg/kg SQ and flumazenil 0.2 mg/kg SQ.*
[c]*Reverse with yohimbine 0.5–1.0 mg/kg IM.*

C. Vascular access

Intravenous access is challenging due to the small size of these species; however, intraosseous injections can be performed under anesthesia into the femur. Small samples may be collected from the lateral saphenous, cranial vena cava, cephalic, jugular, or femoral veins. Hematocrits may decrease significantly during hibernation (D'Agostino, 2015).

III. Rodentia: nontraditional species of laboratory rodents

Rodents other than *Rattus norvegicus*, *Mus musculus*, *Cavia porcellus*, *Mesocricetus auratus,* and *Meriones unguiculatus* described below offer unique anatomic, behavioral, and physiologic characteristics, making them valuable for scientific studies.

A. Suborders Castorimorpha and Myomorpha

This group of nontraditional rodents is the most similar to our commonly found laboratory mice and rats. For many of these species, specific doses of anesthetics and analgesics have not been published. Traditional doses used in *Mus musculus* and *Rattus norvegicus* can be useful starting doses when working with these species.

Suborder Castorimorpha

Family Geomyidae: pocket gophers (true gophers)

Family Heteromyidae: kangaroo rats and kangaroo mice

Suborder Myomorpha

Family Cricetidae: rice rat, pack rat, voles

Family Dipodidae: jerboas

Family Muridae: multimammate rat, sand rat, cotton rat, grass rat, jird

1. Manual restraint

Nontraditional species of laboratory rats, mice, voles, and gophers described above are commonly fractious and difficult to manually restrain (Fig. 22.4). In the species listed above, manual restraint techniques should be performed using gloves and with great caution to avoid tail injury (degloving or amputation) if the animal struggles (Cantwell, 2001; Donnelly et al., 2015; Sainsbury, 2003). For some species, clear plastic tubes or soft forceps can be used to help move the animal from one location to another (Yarto-Jaramillo, 2015).

2. Chemical restraint

Fasting is not routinely done for these species, as they are unable to vomit and can easily exhaust their glycogen stores when fasted (Yarto-Jaramillo, 2015). Isoflurane inhalation anesthesia via induction chamber (3%–5%) minimizes complications with manual restraint of wild or easily stressed rodents (Cantwell, 2001; Sainsbury, 2003) and is the anesthetic of choice for all nontraditional rodents (Mayer and Mans, 2018). For species that tolerate manual restraint, sedatives, and tranquilizers administered 30–60 minutes prior to a face mask (0.5%–3%) or chamber induction may ensure a smoother induction (Table 22.4). Midazolam at 0.1–2 mg/kg IM, IP, or SQ has minimal cardiopulmonary effects and is safe to use as a preanesthetic sedative even in sick or compromised rodents (Yarto-Jaramillo, 2015). Inhalation anesthetic administration in rodents that are difficult-to-handle may best be accomplished by placing the rodent

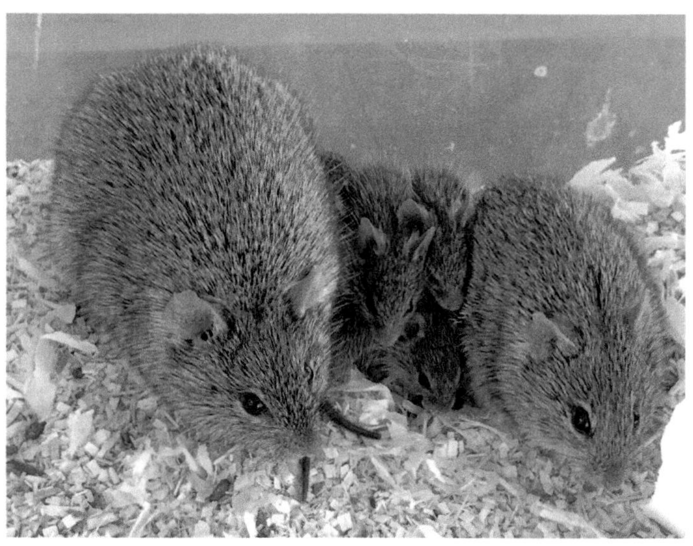

FIGURE 22.4 Most nontraditional species of rodents, such as these grass rats (*Arvicanthis niloticus*), are difficult to restrain and require thick gloves. *Courtesy of Katrina Linning-Duffy.*

TABLE 22.4 Sedatives and tranquilizers for all nontraditional mouse and rat species (especially useful 30–60 minutes prior to isoflurane mask or chamber induction).

Drug	Dosage
Acepromazine	0.5–5.0 mg/kg IM, SQ, PO—higher doses only PO
Diazepam	2.5–5.0 mg/kg IM
Midazolam	1.0–3.0 mg/kg IM

All dosages are from Mayer and Mans (2018).

TABLE 22.5 Injectable anesthetics for all nontraditional laboratory rat and mouse species.

Drug	Dose	Comments
Fentanyl/fluanisone (Hypnorm)	0.2–0.6 mL/kg IM, IP	
Ketamine plus acepromazine	50–150 mg/kg IP, IM; 2.5–5.0 mg/kg IP, IM	Lower end of doses preferred
Ketamine plus dexmedetomidine	2–4 mg/kg IM; 0.025 mg/kg IM	Sedation, atipamezole reversal
Ketamine plus xylazine	75 mg/kg IP; 0.5 mg/kg IP	Atipamezole reversal
Propofol	100 mg/kg IM, IP; 5 mg/kg IM, IP	Yohimbine reversal
	7.5–10 mg/kg IV	
Tiletamine/zolazepam (Telazol)	50–80 mg/kg IM	

All dosages are from Mayer and Mans (2018).

TABLE 22.6 Analgesics for nontraditional laboratory rodents.

Drug	Dosage
Buprenorphine	0.01–0.05 mg/kg SQ q 8–12 hours
Butorphanol	0.2–2 mg/kg SQ q 2–4 hours
Carprofen	2–5 mg/kg PO, SQ q 12–24 hours
Meloxicam	1–5 mg/kg PO, SQ q 24 hours
Morphine	2–5 mg/kg SQ, IM q 4 hours

All dosages are from Mayer and Mans (2018).

inside an opaque nest box or an extending tube from the home cage into an induction chamber. Frequent observations of the depth of anesthesia are required if the rodent cannot easily be seen inside the nest box. Dropbox techniques can be used but must be monitored carefully as dangerously high levels of anesthetic may be produced with cotton or gauze soaked in inhalant anesthetic (Sainsbury, 2003). Once the righting reflex is lost, anesthesia in nontraditional laboratory rodents may be maintained by inhalation anesthesia (face mask or intubation) or by injectable agents (Table 22.5). Maintenance with inhalational anesthesia should be done with a nonrebreathing anesthetic circuit for these small mammals (Yarto-Jaramillo, 2015). Some rodent species are prone to apnea under isoflurane anesthesia, which can be ameliorated with doxapram 5–10 mg/kg IV or IM (Hahn, 2019). Atropine administered at 0.04–0.4 mg/kg IM or SQ or glycopyrrolate at 0.01–0.02 mg/kg SQ (Mayer and Mans, 2018) reduces oral and respiratory mucus secretions. Systemic analgesic doses for all nontraditional laboratory animal rodents can be found in Table 22.6. In addition, local anesthetic options such as lidocaine at up to 4 mg/kg and bupivacaine at up to 2 mg/kg, given topically or through tissue infiltration, are effective at providing good (if brief) pain control that can contribute to a multi-modal analgesic plan in these species (Yarto-Jaramillo, 2015).

3. Vascular access

Intravenous catheterization in these small species is difficult. In general, the most frequent sites of blood collection include the jugular, cephalic, saphenous, femoral, cranial vena cava, and lateral tail veins in small rodents. Anesthesia may be needed to access some of these vessels (Yarto-Jaramillo, 2015).

4. Intraoperative management

For prevention of tissue trauma, hypovolemia, and hypothermia, nontraditional laboratory mouse, rat, and gopher species should be given the same attention as given to *M. musculus* and *R. norvegicus*. Eyes should be well lubricated to prevent corneal damage. Heat support should be used throughout all anesthetic procedures. Subcuticular, absorbable sutures or tissue adhesives can be used to reduce postoperative chewing of sutures and eliminate the need for handling for suture removal (Sainsbury, 2003).

4. Recovery

A recovery area for small rodents (<500 g) and larger rodents should be 35–37 and 25–35°C, respectively. The ambient temperature should be reduced to 20–25°C once the righting reflex returns. Dusty bedding should be avoided to prevent airway obstruction. Isotonic fluids (50–100 mL/kg) warmed to 37°C and administered subcutaneously may prevent postoperative dehydration (Sainsbury, 2003).

B. Suborder Sciuromorpha

Suborder Sciuromorpha

Family Gliridae: dormouse

Family Sciuridae: squirrels, woodchucks, prairie dogs

1. Family Gliridae—dormice (*Graphiurus kelleni*)

Kellen's African dormouse is a small rodent, weighing in at 18–23 g, originating from the sub-Saharan African region. This species came of interest to biomedical research in 2003, when an outbreak of human monkeypox occurred after transmission from imported African rodents. Graphiurus kelleni was developed into a model for this disease as it is highly susceptible to the virus (Schultz et al., 2009; Long and West, 2012).

a Manual restraint

Captive-bred dormice can be restrained by grasping the loose skin over the back of the neck, similar to in Mus sp. This species is susceptible to degloving injuries and stress from handling, and gentle methods of handling (such as gently encouraging them into a hut placed in the cage and moving the entire structure together with the animals) are encouraged (Long and West, 2012).

b Chemical restraint

Induction using isoflurane in a chamber (3%–5%) is ideal to minimize handling and stress of the animals. Anesthesia is maintained by administering isoflurane (1.5%–2.5%) via a mask. It's been noted by one group that dormice seem to have a prolonged recovery with isoflurane in comparison to the traditional laboratory mouse, but recovery was improved with heat support and manual stimulation (Kastenmayer et al., 2010). Tremors of the large muscle groups were also seen during recovery. Analgesic doses found in Table 22.6 can be used in this species as well.

c Vascular access

Blood collection can be performed with a 23-gauge needle in the mandibular region, approximately 0.5–1 cm ventral from the ear base (Kastenmeyer et al., 2010).

2. Family Sciuridae—squirrels, prairie dogs, and woodchucks

a Ground squirrels—*Urocitellus, Ictodomys,* and *Spermophilus* sp.

The most common species of ground squirrels used in research include *Urocitellus richardsonii* (Richardson's ground squirrel), *Ictidomys tridecemlineatus* (13-lined ground squirrel), *Spermophilus lateralis* (golden-mantled ground squirrel), and *Spermophilus beecheyi* (California ground squirrel; rock squirrel).

Manual restraint: Wild-caught ground squirrels are difficult to manually restrain. They may be transferred from a nest box to a sac by placing the nest box in a sac and opening the nest box. The squirrel is subsequently anesthetized using injectables through the sac or by isoflurane induction in a chamber (Sainsbury, 2003).

Chemical restraint: Induction using isoflurane in a chamber (3%–5%) requires minimal handling and reduces the likelihood of trauma from handling (Sainsbury, 2003). Anesthesia is maintained by administering isoflurane (0.5%–3%) via a mask or an endotracheal tube. A combination of ketamine (85 mg/kg) and xylazine (10 mg/kg) IM can be used for injectable anesthesia in ground squirrels (Hahn, 2019). Analgesic doses found in Table 22.6 can be used in this species as well.

b Black-tailed prairie dog—*Cynomys ludovicianus*

Manual restraint: Prairie dogs acquired at a young age may be acclimated to handling and restraint; however, wild-caught or stressed animals should not be restrained without the use of thick towels or leather gloves (Eshar and Gardhouse, 2020). Stressed prairie dogs will prolapse anal glands and may become dyspneic since they are obligate nasal breathers (Klaphake, 2006).

Chemical restraint: Isoflurane inhalation anesthesia via induction chamber (3%–5%), followed by face mask or endotracheal intubation to effect requires minimal handling of uncooperative animals (Hernandez-Divers, 2004; Johnson-Delaney, 2006; Sainsbury, 2003). Premedication with butorphanol (0.2 mg/kg SQ, IM) contributes to a smooth induction (Hernandez-Divers, 2004). Most prairie dogs develop respiratory acidosis and azotemia regardless of the length of time under isoflurane anesthesia, so hydration should be provided at the time of surgery in the form of a balanced crystalloid solution given subcutaneously or intravenously (80–100 mL/kg) (Eshar and Gardhouse, 2020). Atropine (0.05 mg/kg SQ, IM) or glycopyrrolate (0.01–0.02 mg/kg SQ, IM) can be given to decrease bronchial secretions during induction (Hahn, 2019). Injectable anesthetics, sedatives, and analgesics are provided in Tables 22.7 and 22.8.

Vascular access: 24-gauge catheters can be placed in the cephalic veins for intravascular access. The medial

TABLE 22.7 Injectable anesthetics and sedatives for prairie dogs.

Drug	Dosage and route	References
Acepromazine	0.5–2.5 mg/kg IM—sedation	Hahn (2019)
Diazepam	0.2–5 mg/kg PO, IM. IV—sedation	Morrisey and Carpenter, 2020
Etomidate	1 mg/kg IV	Hahn (2019)
Ketamine	20–40 mg/kg SQ, IM, IV—sedation	Morrisey and Carpenter, 2020
Ketamine plus dexmedetomidine plus midazolam	40 mg/kg SQ, IM; 0.25 mg/kg SQ, IM; 1.5 mg/kg SQ, IM	Morrisey and Carpenter, 2020
Ketamine plus diazepam	30 mg/kg IM; 0.5 mg/kg IM	Hahn (2019)
Ketamine plus midazolam	5–10 mg/kg IM; 0.5–1 mg/kg IM	Mayer and Mans (2018)
Lidocaine	1–4 mg/kg SQ—local	Morrisey and Carpenter, 2020
Midazolam	0.5 mg/kg SQ, IM—sedation	Morrisey and Carpenter, 2020
Propofol	3–5 mg/kg IV	Morrisey and Carpenter, 2020
Tiletamine/zolazepam (Telazol)	20 mg/kg IM	Hahn (2019)
Xylazine	5–10 mg/kg IP, SQ	Hahn (2019)

TABLE 22.8 Analgesics for prairie dogs.

Drug	Dosage and route	References
Buprenorphine	0.03–0.05 mg/kg SQ, IM, IV q 8–12 hours	Morrisey and Carpenter, 2020
Buprenorphine, sustained release (Buprenorphine SR, Zoo-Pharm)	1.2 mg/kg SQ q 72 hours	Mayer and Mans (2018)
Butorphanol	0.1–0.5 mg/kg SQ, IM q 6–8 hours	Morrisey and Carpenter, 2020
Carprofen	4 mg/kg SQ q 24 hours	Hahn (2019)
Flunixin meglumine	2.5 mg/kg SQ, IM q 12–24 hours	Hahn (2019)
Ketoprofen	2 mg/kg SQ, IM q 12 hours	Morrisey and Carpenter, 2020
Meloxicam	0.3–0.5 mg/kg PO, SQ, IM q 24 hours	Morrisey and Carpenter, 2020
Meloxicam, sustained release (Meloxicam SR, ZooPharm)	4 mg/kg SQ, q 72 hours	Mayer and Mans (2018)
Morphine	2–5 mg/kg SQ, IM q 4 hours	Hahn (2019)

saphenous veins may also be used for IV catheterization. Blood collection can be done through the jugular, cranial vena cava, cephalic, saphenous, and femoral veins, and is not complicated in this species. For the majority of sites, immobilization with general anesthesia is required for blood collection (Eshar and Gardhouse, 2020).

c Woodchuck—*Marmota monax*

The eastern woodchuck, a 2.5–5.0-kg Sciuridae rodent, is found throughout the midwestern and eastern United States and southern Canada (Bellezza et al., 2015). Woodchucks, as obligate hibernators, experience a doubling of body weight in the summer while preparing for hibernation and up to 50% weight loss during fall and winter hibernation (Bellezza et al., 2015). They are used in research programs to study viral hepatitis, obesity, energy balance, and hibernation (Bellezza et al., 2015; McKenzie et al., 2006).

Manual restraint: Elkhide elbow-length leather gloves are used to protect against serious bites from aggressive individuals. The woodchuck is pinned behind the neck with one hand while the opposite hand grasps the base of the tail for subsequent intramuscular injections (alternating gastrocnemius or quadriceps muscles for serial injections) or placement in an isoflurane anesthesia induction chamber

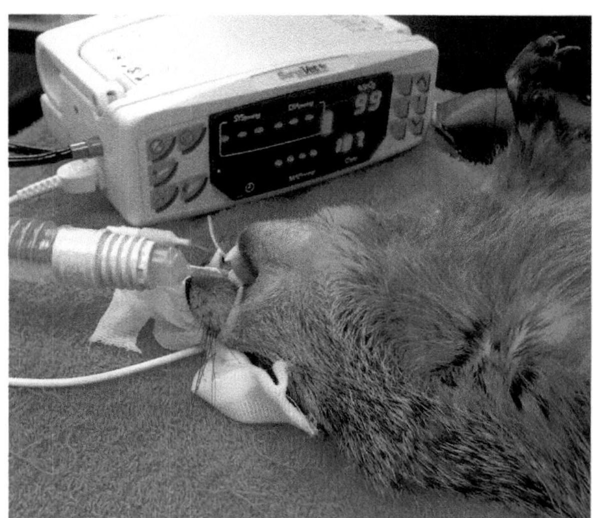

FIGURE 22.5 A woodchuck (*Marmota monax*) intubated for maintenance of isoflurane anesthesia. Courtesy of University of Calgary.

or face mask (Bellezza et al., 2015; McKenzie et al., 2006; Sainsbury, 2003).

Chemical restraint: Isoflurane may be administered via induction chamber or face mask (3%–5%) and given to effect via face mask (Fig. 22.5) or endotracheal intubation for maintenance (Bellezza et al., 2015; Sainsbury, 2003). Injectable anesthetics are listed in Table 22.9. Unlike many rodents, woodchucks can vomit, which necessitates a preanesthetic fasting period or careful monitoring during induction (Bellezza et al., 2015). Consideration must be given to seasonal body conditions (i.e., fat content) when anesthetizing wild or hibernating woodchucks (Beiglbock and Zenker, 2003). Analgesic doses found in Table 22.6 can be used in this species as well.

Vascular access: Blood collection is typically done under anesthesia, and can be performed using the cephalic, femoral, or jugular veins (Fig. 22.6). Indwelling catheterization of the peripheral veins is challenging in the woodchuck but has been done for single procedures using the

TABLE 22.9 Injectable anesthetics for woodchucks.

Drug	Dosage and route	Comments	References
Ketamine plus xylazine	50 mg/kg IM; 5 mg/kg IM	20 minutes anesthesia plus half dose for supplement	Bellezza et al. (2015)
Sodium pentobarbital	2–6 mg/kg IV	Sublingual vein or implanted catheter (20–40 minutes anesthesia)	Bellezza et al. (2015)
Fentanyl/droperidol (Innovar Vet)	0.35 mL/kg IM	Reversed with naloxone	Bellezza et al. (2015)
Ketamine plus xylazine	40 mg/kg IM; 3 mg/kg IM	Short-term surgery in Spring lean marmots	Beiglbock and Zenker (2003)[a]
Ketamine plus xylazine	60 mg/kg IM; 20 mg/kg IM	Short-term surgery in late Summer/Fall fat marmots	Beiglbock and Zenker (2003)[a]
Ketamine plus xylazine	80 mg/kg IM; 20 mg/kg IM	Long-term surgery in Spring lean marmots	Beiglbock and Zenker (2003)[a]
Ketamine plus medetomidine	35 mg/kg IM; 0.25 mg/kg IM	Short-term surgery in Spring lean marmots	Beiglbock and Zenker (2003)[a]
Ketamine plus medetomidine	60 mg/kg IM; 0.2 mg/kg IM	Short-term surgery in late Summer/Fall fat marmots	Beiglbock and Zenker (2003)[a]
Ketamine plus medetomidine	70 mg/kg IM; 0.5 mg/kg IM	Long-term surgery in Spring lean marmots	Beiglbock and Zenker (2003)[a]
Tiletamine/zolazepam (Telazol) plus xylazine	15 mg/kg IM; 3 mg/kg IM	Short-term surgery in Spring lean marmots	Beiglbock and Zenker (2003)[a]
Tiletamine/zolazepam (Telazol) plus xylazine	15 mg/kg IM; 10 mg/kg IM	Short-term surgery in late Summer/Fall fat marmots	Beiglbock and Zenker (2003)[a]
Tiletamine/zolazepam (Telazol) plus xylazine	20 mg/kg IM: 10 mg/kg IM	Long-term surgery in Spring lean marmots	Beiglbock and Zenker (2003)[a]

[a]*Free ranging* Marmota marmota.

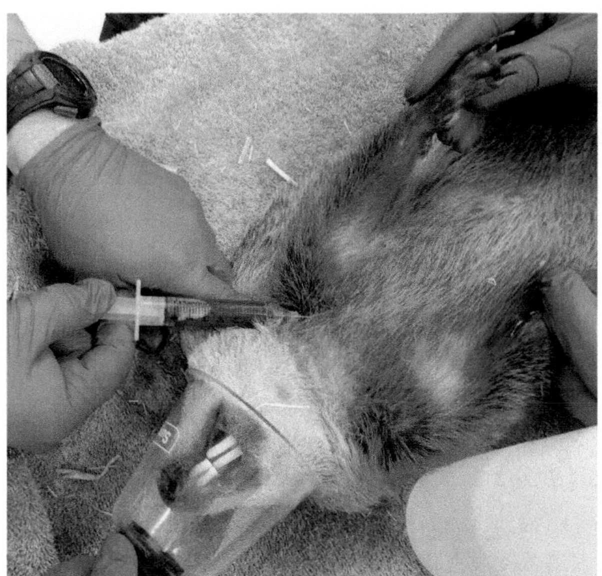

FIGURE 22.6 Blood is collected from the lower portion of the jugular vein in a woodchuck (*Marmota monax*) while under isoflurane anesthesia. Maintenance of anesthesia can be done with a well-fitted mask for simple procedures such as this. *Courtesy of University of Calgary.*

cephalic vein. For animals that may need repeat access to blood samples, central lines have been successfully placed with vascular access ports (personal communication with Dr. Kristie Brock, DVM, Case Western Reserve University).

C. Suborder Hystricomorpha

Suborder Hystricomorpha

Family Chinchillidae: chinchillas

Family Octodontidae: degu

Family Heterocephalidae: naked mole rats

1. *Family Chinchillidae—chinchillas (*Chinchilla laniger*)*

a Manual restraint

Chinchillas are relatively easy to handle and best restrained by firmly grasping the base of the tail with one hand and supporting the ventrum with the other hand, extending two fingers between the forelegs (Klaphake, 2006). Care should be taken to never pick up a chinchilla by the tail or grasp it by the fur alone, as they can experience fur slip as a defensive mechanism (Hsu et al., 2015; Mans and Donnelly, 2020).

b Chemical restraint

Isoflurane anesthesia may be induced by a chamber or mask (3%–5%) and maintained to effect by mask or endotracheal intubation (Sainsbury, 2003) or injectable anesthetics (Table 22.10). Similar to guinea pigs, chinchillas have a palatal ostium (a structure created by the fusion of the soft palate with the base of the tongue), which complicates endotracheal intubation. Use of an endoscope and stylet can

TABLE 22.10 Anesthetics and sedatives for chinchillas and degus.

Species	Drug	Dosage and route	References
Chinchilla	Bupivacaine	1–2 mg/kg SQ—local	Morrisey and Carpenter (2020)
	Diazepam	0.5–3 mg/kg IM, IV—sedation	Morrisey and Carpenter (2020)
	Ketamine	20–40 mg/kg IM—sedation	Mayer and Mans (2018)
	Ketamine plus dexmedetomidine	4 mg/kg IM; 0.015 mg/kg IM	Morrisey and Carpenter (2020)
	Ketamine plus diazepam	20–40 mg/kg IM; 1–2 mg/kg IM	Mayer and Mans (2018)
	Ketamine plus midazolam	5–10 mg/kg IM; 0.5–1 mg/kg IM	Morrisey and Carpenter (2020)
	Ketamine plus xylazine	40 mg/kg IM; 2 mg/kg IM	Mayer and Mans (2018)
	Lidocaine	1–4 mg/kg SQ—local	Morrisey and Carpenter (2020)
	Midazolam	1–2 mg/kg SQ, IM, IV—sedation	Morrisey and Carpenter (2020)
	Propofol	3–5 mg/kg IV	Mayer and Mans (2018)
	Tiletamine/zolazepam (Telazol)	20–40 mg/kg IM	Mayer and Mans (2018)
Degu	Ketamine plus medetomidine	5–10 mg/kg IM; 0.02–0.04 mg/kg IM	Mayer and Mans (2018)
	Ketamine plus midazolam	3–6 mg/kg IM; 0.2–0.4 mg/kg IM—sedation	Jekl (2020)
	Ketamine plus midazolam plus butorphanol	5–10 mg/kg IM; 0.2–0.4 mg/kg IM; 0.3–0.5 mg/kg IM	Mayer and Mans (2018)

TABLE 22.11 Analgesics for chinchillas and degus.

Species	Drug	Dosage and route	References
Chinchilla	Buprenorphine	0.1–0.2 mg/kg SQ, IM q 6 hours	Morrisey and Carpenter (2020)
	Butorphanol	0.2–2.0 mg/kg SQ, IM q 2–4 hours	Morrisey and Carpenter (2020)
	Carprofen	2–5 mg/kg PO, SQ q 12–24 hours	Morrisey and Carpenter (2020)
	Gabapentin	3–5 mg/kg PO q 12–24 hours	Morrisey and Carpenter (2020)
	Hydromorphone	1–2 mg/kg SQ q 4 hours	Morrisey and Carpenter (2020)
	Ketoprofen	1–2 mg/kg SQ, IM q 12–24 hours	Morrisey and Carpenter (2020)
	Meloxicam	≥0.5 mg/kg PO, SQ q 24 hours	Morrisey and Carpenter (2020)
	Morphine	2–5 mg/kg SQ, IM q 4 hours	Morrisey and Carpenter (2020)
Degu	Buprenorphine	0.05 mg/kg SQ q 8–12 hours	Johnson-Delaney (2006)
	Butorphanol	0.4–2.0 mg/kg SQ q 8–12 hours	Johnson-Delaney (2006)
	Carprofen	2–5 mg/kg PO, SQ q 12–24 hours	Mayer and Mans (2018)
	Morphine	2–5 mg/kg SQ q 4 hours	Johnson-Delaney (2006)

help avoid traumatizing this highly vascular structure during endotracheal intubation (Hawkins and Pascoe, 2020). Atropine (0.1–0.2 mg/kg IM, SQ) or glycopyrrolate (0.01–0.02 mg/kg SQ) reduces oral and respiratory mucus secretions (Mayer and Mans, 2018). Analgesics are listed in Table 22.11.

c Vascular access

The jugular veins are the preferred site of blood collection for any diagnostics that require larger blood samples in chinchillas. Collecting blood from the jugular veins can be done with manual restraint or under anesthesia. Smaller amounts of blood can be drawn from either the cephalic or lateral saphenous veins. The cephalic vein can also be used for the placement of a peripheral intravenous catheter (using a 24- to 26-gauge catheter) under anesthesia (Mans and Donnelly, 2020).

2. *Family Octodontidae—degus (*Octodon degus*)*

a Manual restraint

Degus are susceptible to tail slip and should not be picked up by the tail. Restraint is best performed by grasping the animal around the neck and shoulders. Scruffing the skin over the neck and shoulders is not an appropriate method of restraint for this species (Jekl, 2020).

b Chemical restraint

Isoflurane anesthesia may be induced by chamber or mask (3%–5%) and maintained in effect by mask or endotracheal intubation or injectable anesthetics (Table 22.10). Analgesics are listed in Table 22.11.

c Vascular access

Blood collection should only be performed under anesthesia in degus. Blood can be collected from the cranial vena cava, lateral saphenous veins, or femoral veins. Due to the small size of the peripheral veins and the risk of fatal hemorrhage in catheterizing the jugular vein, intraosseous catheterization of the proximal femur or humerus is the suggested method for intravascular access in this species (Jekl, 2020).

3. *Family Heterocephalidae—naked mole-rats (*Heterocephalus glaber*)*

The naked mole rat is one of only two eusocial mammal species currently known, with a single queen that is the only reproducing female in a colony (Raines, 2019). There has been ongoing debate on the taxonomy of the naked mole rat—at the time of this writing, it has been reclassified from its previous Bathyergidae family to the Heterocephalidae family (of which *Heterocephalus glaber* is the only member) (Patterson and Upham, 2014). Naked mole rats weigh approximately 35g, similar to a laboratory mouse, but live far longer, with a lifespan of up to 30 years in captivity. Due to their eusocial structure and longevity, they are interesting models of behavior and aging. Additionally, they have natural resistances to both cancer and hypoxia, which make them valuable models in those areas of research (Donnelly et al., 2015).

a Chemical restraint

When an animal is removed from the colony for a procedure, care must be taken to always have gloves on, as foreign odors can cause other members of the colony to attack the individual once reintroduced. Naked mole rats tolerate anesthesia with isoflurane or sevoflurane while maintained on a facemask, like other rodents (Raines, 2019). Due to the species' unique physiologic adaptations, it is not recommended to extrapolate injectable doses from other rodent species. Several recent publications have described injectable combinations that were safe and effective in naked mole rats, including alfaxalone plus ketamine (A: 4 mg/kg IM; K: 20 mg/kg IM) (Ambar et al., 2020) and dexmedetomidine plus ketamine plus midazolam (D: 0.06 mg/kg IM; K: 20 mg/kg IM; M: 1 mg/kg IM) (Huckins et al., 2020). Response to analgesics in these naked mole rats may be minimal as they lack several neurotransmitters, but analgesics should still be included in any procedural plan that may cause pain. Meloxicam has been successfully given to naked mole rats at 0.1–0.2 mg/kg PO q 24 hours (Raines, 2019).

V. Xenarthra: edentates (nine-banded armadillo—*Dasypus novemcinctus*)

A. Manual restraint

Armadillos do not usually attempt to bite, but they have powerful legs and sharp claws that may inflict injury. They may be picked up by their sides. Restraining by the tail alone can result in self-injury and should be avoided (Rojas Moreno, 2019). The handler must be careful not to get their fingers pinched under the carapace plates as they curl up when handled.

B. Chemical restraint

Armadillos may hold their breath for up to 10 minutes making induction with isoflurane in a chamber or face mask difficult (Gillespie, 1993). Premedication with injectable anesthetics followed by administration relaxes the armadillo and minimizes breath holding (Gillespie, 2003). Another technique that can be used is starting with 100% oxygen and slowly increasing the isoflurane dosage to promote continuous spontaneous breathing (Rojas Moreno, 2019). Once induced with 3%–5% isoflurane or by injectables, armadillos may be intubated with polyethylene tubing (0.6–1.3 cm) and maintained with 1%–2% isoflurane (Gillespie, 1993). Table 22.12 list injectable anesthetics. The thigh is the best site to administer an IM injection (Rojas Moreno, 2019). Atropine (0.02–0.04 mg/kg IM) controls salivation (Aguilar and Superina, 2015). Monitoring both body temperature and room temperature during surgical procedures with armadillos is recommended, as their body temperature is strongly influenced by environmental temperature and significant changes in body temperature should be controlled for during anesthesia (Rojas Moreno, 2019). There is a lack of published information on analgesic doses for this species, but one source states either flunixin meglumine (2.5 mg/kg SQ q 24 hours for 3 days) or tramadol (0.5 mg/kg IM q 12–24 hours) may be given (Aguilar and Superina, 2015).

C. Vascular access

Blood may be collected from the superficial femoral vein of an anesthetized armadillo, or the caudal tail vein located on the ventrum between the second, third, and fourth bony tail segments (Gillespie, 2003).

VI. Chiroptera: bats

Bats are one of the most widespread mammals on earth, second only to rodents (Heard, 2003). They are the only mammal with powered flight, with the term Chiroptera translating literally to "hand wing". Ecology and anatomy, not size, separate the two suborders Megachiroptera (fruit eaters) and Microchiroptera (insectivores/omnivores/carnivores) (Buckles, 2015). Three families of microchiropterans (Phyllostomidae, Vespertilionidae, and Mormoopidae) and one family of megachiropterans (Pteropodidae) have been studied in biomedical research (Tuval et al., 2018).

TABLE 22.12 Injectable anesthetics for armadillos.

Drug	Dosage and route
Ketamine plus butorphanol plus medetomidine	15 mg/kg IM; 0.1 mg/kg IM; 0.07 mg/kg IM
Ketamine plus dexmedetomidine plus midazolam	5 mg/kg IM; 0.015 mg/kg IM; 0.1 mg/kg IM
Ketamine plus medetomidine	7.5 mg/kg IM; 0.075 mg/kg IM
Ketamine plus midazolam	5–10 mg/kg IM; 0.2 mg/kg IM—short procedures
Ketamine plus xylazine	40 mg/kg IM; 1 mg/kg IM
Tiletamine/zolazepam (Telazol)	8.5 mg/kg IM—prolonged recovery

All dosages are from Rojas Moreno, 2019.

Family Phyllostomidae (new world leaf-nosed bats)

Phyllostomus discolor (lesser spear-nosed bat)

Glossophaga soricina (long-tongued bat)

Carollia perspicillata (short-tailed fruit bat)

Desmodus rotundus (common vampire bat)

Family Vespertilionidae (evening bats)

Eptesicus fuscus (big brown bat)

Family Mormoopidae (mustached bats)

Pteronotus parnellii (Parnell's mustached bat)

Family Pteropodidae (flying foxes)

Rousettus aegyptiacus (Egyptian fruit bat)

A. Manual restraint

Soft, pliable leather gloves and butterfly nets may be used for handling microchiropterans weighing 10–50 g. The body is palmed with wings gently folded, while the head is restrained between the thumb and the middle finger with the index finger placed on top of the head (Pye, 2001). Care should be taken to avoid bending wings in unnatural positions, traumatizing flapping wings, pulling locked toes, causing distal femoral epiphyseal fractures, and injuring teeth while biting gloves (Pye, 2001). Excessive pressure on the chest or neck can compromise respiratory function (Buckles, 2015). Manual restraint should be minimized to reduce stress and hyperthermia (Heard, 2003).

B. Chemical restraint

Inhalant anesthesia via face mask or induction chamber (5%) followed by maintenance (2%–3%) by face mask is recommended (Pye, 2001) (Figs. 22.7 and 22.8). Glycopyrrolate (0.01 mg/kg IM) or atropine (0.02 mg/kg SC) reduces pharyngeal secretions (Hahn, 2019). Bats should not be preoperatively fasted to prevent hypoglycemia. Under general anesthesia, wings should be folded, and the animal placed on a warm water–circulating heating pad. The wing patagium may be irritated and damaged by alcohol- and iodine-containing compounds (Heard, 2003). Injectable anesthetics and analgesics are listed in Tables 22.13 and 22.14. Lactated Ringer's Solution can be given subcutaneously to microchiropterans at a volume of 0.1–0.2 mL/5 g body weight for fluid support (Hahn, 2019).

C. Vascular access

Cephalic and saphenous (interfemoral) veins are options for safe and efficient blood collection in anesthetized or manually restrained bats of various sizes (Eshar and Weinberg, 2010). The external jugular vein may also be used for blood collection, but care should be taken to avoid fatal hematoma (Heard, 2003).

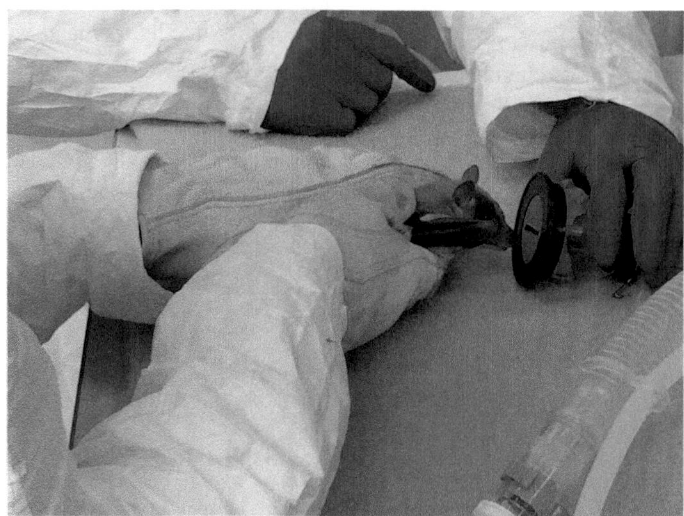

FIGURE 22.7 An Egyptian fruit bat (*Rousettus aegyptiacus*) is gently restrained with the wings folded back to be induced with isoflurane anesthesia through a face mask. Courtesy of Brown University.

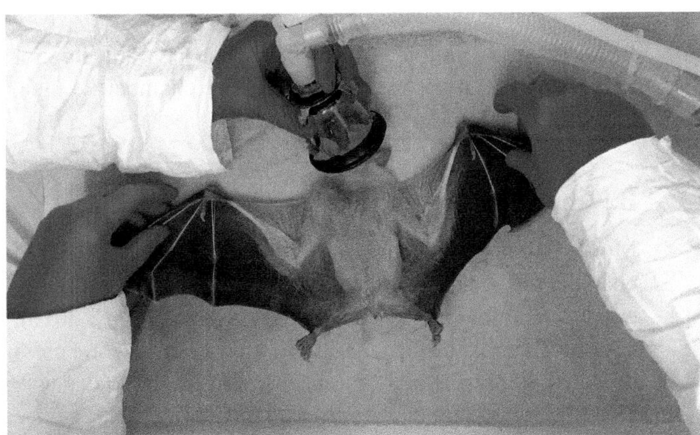

FIGURE 22.8 An Egyptian fruit bat (*Rousettus aegyptiacus*) being maintained on isoflurane anesthesia through used of a well-fitted face mask. Courtesy of Brown University.

TABLE 22.13 Injectable anesthetics for bats.

Species	Drug	Dosage and route	References
Microchiropterans	Ketamine plus acepromazine	10 mg/kg IM; 1 mg/kg IM	Hahn (2019)
	Ketamine plus xylazine	10 mg/kg IM; 2 mg/kg IM	Hahn (2019)
	Propofol	6–8 mg/kg IV	Hahn (2019)
	Tiletamine/zolazepam (Telazol)	10 mg/kg IM	Hahn (2019)
Egyptian fruit bat	Alfaxalone plus midazolam	15 mg/kg SQ; 2 mg/kg SQ—sedation	Tuval et al. (2021)
	Flumazenil	0.3 mg/kg SQ—reversal for midazolam	Tuval et al. (2021)
	Ketamine plus acepromazine	10 mg/kg IM; 1 mg/kg IM	Hahn (2019)
	Ketamine plus medetomidine	6 mg/kg IM; 0.06 mg/kg IM	Hahn (2019)
	Ketamine plus xylazine	10–20 mg/kg IM; 2–4 mg/kg IM	Hahn (2019)
	Medetomidine plus midazolam	0.15 mg/kg SQ; 1.5 mg/kg SQ	Tuval et al. (2018)
	Medetomidine plus midazolam plus fentanyl	0.15 mg/kg SQ; 1.5 mg/kg SQ; 0.015 mg/kg SQ	Tuval et al. (2018)
	Medetomidine plus midazolam plus ketamine	0.15 mg/kg SQ; 1.5 mg/kg SQ; 10 mg/kg SQ	Tuval et al. (2018)
	Medetomidine plus midazolam plus morphine	0.15 mg/kg SQ; 1.5 mg/kg SQ; 1.5 mg/kg SQ	Tuval et al. (2018)
	Propofol	8–10 mg/kg IV	Hahn (2019)
	Tiletamine/zolazepam (Telazol)	10 mg/kg IM	Hahn (2019)

TABLE 22.14 Injectable analgesics for bats.

Species	Drug	Dosage and route
Microchiropterans	Buprenorphine	0.05–0.0.1 mg/kg SQ or IM q 6–12 hours
	Butorphanol	0.2 mg/kg SQ or IM q 4 hours
	Carprofen	3–5 mg/kg SQ, IM, or PO q 12 hours
	Meloxicam	1–2 mg/kg SQ, IM, or PO q 12 hours
	Morphine	2–5 mg/kg SQ or IM q 4–6 hours
Egyptian fruit bat	Buprenorphine	0.03 mg/kg SQ or IM q 6–12 hours
	Butorphanol	0.4 mg/kg SQ or IM q 4 hours
	Carprofen	1–4 mg/kg SQ or IM q 24 hours; PO q 12 hours
	Meloxicam	0.1–0.3 mg/kg SQ, IM, or PO q 12 hours
	Morphine	0.5–1 mg/kg SQ or IM q 4–6 hours
	Tramadol	0.5–2 mg/kg PO q 24 hours

All dosages are from Hahn (2019).

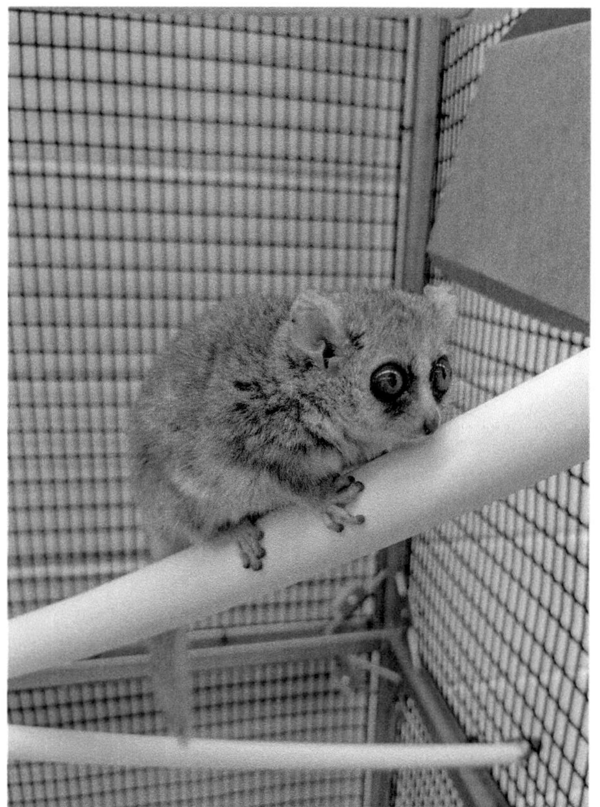

FIGURE 22.9 Gray mouse lemurs (*Microcebus murinus*) are small and quick, making them difficult to capture in the cage. Nest boxes can be used to help transport them to anesthesia induction boxes. *Courtesy of Megan Albertelli*

D. Recovery

Microchiropterans should be lightly wrapped in a drape to prevent erratic wing flapping until they are coordinated well enough to crawl out (Heard, 2003).

VIII. Prosimii: gray mouse lemur (*Microcebus murinus*)

Prosimians are ancestrally extant primates, including lemurs, pottos, lorises, and galagos. Several articles describe the anesthetic management of a variety of prosimians in wild, zoo, or primate center settings as part of behavioral or health assessment studies (Junge, 2003; Kästner et al., 2016; Williams, 2015). The gray mouse lemur is a small prosimian used as a model for cognitive and aging studies (Fritz et al., 2020).

A. Manual restraint

Cotton or thin leather gloves may be used to gently restrain mouse lemurs in a cupped hand. They may be transferred from a nest box into a cloth sac for subsequent injection or placement in an isoflurane induction chamber (Junge, 2003) (Fig. 22.9).

B. Chemical restraint

Mouse lemurs may be placed in an isoflurane induction chamber (3%–5%) and maintained to effect via face mask or endotracheal intubation (Junge, 2003; Kästner et al., 2016). Care must be taken when masking a mouse lemur to not press the mask up against the prominent eyes and cause damage. Standard masks and nose cones for laboratory rodents can be adapted to avoid ocular damage. A short fasting period (<6 hours) is indicated to prevent vomiting at induction (Kästner et al., 2016). Care must be taken to avoid hypothermia during anesthesia just as with any small laboratory animal. Atropine (0.1 mg/kg SC) or glycopyrrolate (0.02–0.04 mg/kg SC) can be used prior to induction to decrease salivation (Kästner et al., 2016). Table 22.15 lists anesthetic and analgesic doses for gray mouse lemurs.

C. Vascular access

No veins are accessible for catheterization, but subcutaneous fluids may be given as described for mice and rats. Blood collection from the saphenous vein has been described (Kästner et al., 2016). A small blood sample (<0.3 mL) may be collected by advancing a 25-gauge needle on a tuberculin syringe at a 45 degrees angle and accessing a coccygeal blood vessel located approximately one-third down the ventral midline of the tail (personal communication from E.E. Louis, DVM, Omaha Henry Doorly Zoo).

TABLE 22.15 Injectable anesthetics and analgesics for gray mouse lemurs.

Drug	Dosage and route
Diazepam	20–30 mg/kg IM—sedation
Ketamine	10 mg/kg SQ—sedation
Ketamine plus diazepam	100 mg/kg IM; 2 mg/100 g IM
Ketamine plus diazepam	100 mg/kg IP; 1 mg/100g SQ
Ketamine plus medetomidine	130–140 mg/kg IM; 0.25 mg/kg IM
Ketamine plus xylazine	65 mg/kg IM; 6 mg/kg IM
Meloxicam	0.2 mg/kg SQ
Tiletamine/zolazepam (Telazol)	10 mg/kg IM

All dosages are from Kästner et al. (2016).

Acknowledgments

This chapter builds upon the related chapter in the second edition of this text. Portions of text from the previous edition have been retained, updated, and added. The author of the present chapter is greatly indebted to Jeff Wyatt, the author of the previous edition, for the work he previously did on this text.

References

Aguilar, R.F., Superina, M., 2015. Xenarthra. In: Miller, R.E., Fowler, M.E. (Eds.), Fowler's Zoo and Wild Animal Medicine, vol. 8. Elsevier, St. Louis, pp. 355–369.

Ambar, N., Eshar, D., Shrader, T.C., Beaufrère, H., 2020. Anesthetic effects of intramuscular alfaxalone-ketamine in naked mole rats (*Heterocephalus glaber*). J. Am. Assoc. Lab. Anim. Sci. 59 (5), 539–545.

Barbiers, R., 2003. Insectivora (Hedgehogs, Tenrecs, Shrews, Moles). In: Fowler, M.E., Miller, R.E. (Eds.), Zoo and Wild Animal Medicine, fifth ed. W.B. Saunders, St. Louis, pp. 304–315.

Barnett, G.J., Barnett, I.J., Wilson, S.R., Smith, P.C., 2017. Comparison of 6 injectable anesthetic regimens and isoflurane in gray short-tailed opossums (*Monodelphis domestica*). J. Am. Assoc. Lab. Anim. Sci. 56 (5), 544–549.

Bathgate, R.A.D., Sernia, C., Gemmel, R.T., 1992. Plasma concentrations of arginine vasopressin in an Australian marsupial, the brushtail opossum, *Trichosurus vulpecula*. Gen. Comp. Endocrinol. 88 (2), 217–223.

Beiglbock, C., Zenker, W., 2003. Evaluation of three combinations of anesthetics for use in free-ranging alpine marmots (*Marmota marmota*). J. Wildl. Dis. 39 (3), 665–674.

Bellezza, C.A., Sexton, S., Curtain, L.I., Concannon, P.W., Baldwin, B.H., Graham, L.A., et al., 2015. The Laboratory Woodchuck (*Marmota monax*). In: Fox, J.G., Anderson, L.C., Otto, G., Pritchett-Corning, K.R., Whary, M.T. (Eds.), Laboratory Animal Medicine, third ed. Academic Press, San Diego, pp. 351–386.

Brust, D.M., Mans, C., 2018. Sugar gliders. In: Carpenter, J.W., Marion, C.J. (Eds.), Exotic Animal Formulary. Elsevier, St. Louis, pp. 432–442.

Buckles, E.L, 2015. In: Miller, R.E., Fowler, M.E. (Eds.), Fowler's Zoo and Wild Animal Medicine, 8. Elsevier, St. Louis, pp. 281–290.

Cantwell, S.L., 2001. Ferret, Rabbit, and Rodent Anesthesia. In: Heard, D.J. (Ed.), The Veterinary Clinics of North America, Exotic Animal Practice, Analgesia and Anesthesia. W.B. Saunders, Philadelphia, pp. 169–191.

D'Agostino, J., 2015. Insectivores (Insectivora, Macroscelidea, Scandentia). In: Miller, R.E., Fowler, M.E. (Eds.), Fowler's Zoo and Wild Animal Medicine, vol. 8. Elsevier, St. Louis, pp. 275–281.

Donnelly, T.M., Bergin, I., Ihrig, M., 2015. Biology and diseases of other rodents. In: Fox, J.G., Anderson, L.C., Otto, G., Pritchett-Corning, K.R., Whary, M.T. (Eds.), Laboratory Animal Medicine, third ed. Academic Press, San Diego, pp. 285–349.

Eshar, D., Gardhouse, S., 2020. Prairie dogs. In: Quesenberry, K.E., Orcutt, C.J., Mans, C., Carpenter, J.W. (Eds.), Ferrets, Rabbits, and Rodents Clinical Medicine and Surgery, fourth ed. Elsevier, St. Louis, pp. 334–344.

Eshar, D., Weinberg, M., 2010. Venipuncture in bats. Lab. Anim. (NY) 39 (6), 175–176.

Fritz, R.G., Zimmermann, E., Meier, M., Mestre-Francés, N., Radespiel, U., Schmidtke, D., 2020. Neurobiological substrates of animal personality and cognition in a nonhuman primate (*Microcebus murinus*). Brain Behav. 10 (9), e01752.

Geyer, B., Erickson, N.A., Müller, K., Grübel, S., Hueber, B., Hetz, S.K., Brecht, M., 2022. Establishing and maintaining an Etruscan shrew colony. J. Am. Assoc. Lab. Anim. Sci. 61 (1), 52–60.

Gillespie, D., 1993. Edentata: diseases. In: Fowler, M.E. (Ed.), Zoo and Wild Animal Medicine Current Therapy 3. W.B. Saunders, Philadelphia, pp. 304–321.

Gillespie, D., 2003. Xenarthra: Edentata (Anteaters, Armadillos, Sloths). In: Fowler, M.E., Miller, R.E. (Eds.), Zoo and Wild Animal Medicine and Surgery, fifth ed. W.B. Saunders, St. Louis, pp. 397–407.

Hahn, A., 2019. Zoo and Wild Mammal Formulary, first ed. John Wiley & Sons, Inc., Hoboken.

Heard, D.J., 2003. In: Fowler, M.E., Miller, R.E. (Eds.), Zoo and Wild Animal Medicine, fifth ed. W.B. Saunders, St. Louis, pp 315–333.

Hawkins, M.G., Pascoe, P.J., 2020. In: Quesenberry, K.E., Orcutt, C.J., Mans, C., Carpenter, J.W. (Eds.), Ferrets, Rabbits, and Rodents Clinical Medicine and Surgery, fourth ed. Elsevier, St. Louis, pp. 536–558.

Hernandez-Divers, S.M., 2004. Veterinary Clinics of North America, Exotic Animal Medicine, Wound Healing and Management. W.B. Saunders, Philadelphia, pp. 1–18.

Holz, P., 2003. Marsupialia (Marsupials). In: Fowler, M.E., Miller, R.E. (Eds.), Zoo and Wild Animal Medicine, fifth ed. W.B. Saunders, St. Louis, pp. 288–303.

Hsu, C.C., Chan, M.M., Wheler, C.L., 2015. Biology and diseases of Chinchillas. In: Fox, J.G., Anderson, L.C., Otto, G., Pritchett-Corning, K.R., Whary, M.T. (Eds.), Laboratory Animal Medicine, third ed. Academic Press, San Diego, pp. 387–409.

Huckins, G.L., Eshar, D., Shrader, T., Beaufrère, H., 2020. Anesthetic effect of dexmedetomidine-ketamine-midazolam combination administered intramuscularly to zoo-housed naked mole rats (*Heterocephalus glaber*). J. Zoo Wildl. Med. 51 (1), 59–66.

Isenbugel, E., Baumgartner, R., 1993. Insectivora. In: Fowler, M.E. (Ed.), Zoo & Wild Animal Medicine Current Therapy 3. W.B. Saunders, Philadelphia, pp. 294–302.

Jekl, V., 2020. Degus. In: Quesenberry, K.E., Orcutt, C.J., Mans, C., Carpenter, J.W. (Eds.), Ferrets, Rabbits, and Rodents Clinical Medicine and Surgery, fourth ed. Elsevier, St. Louis, pp. 323–333.

Johnson-Delaney, C.A., 2006. Common Procedures in Hedgehogs, Prairie Dogs, Exotic Rodents, and Companion Marsupials. In: Griffin, C. (Ed.), Veterinary Clinics of North America, Exotic Animal Practice, Common Procedures. W.B. Saunders, Philadelphia, pp. 415–435.

Johnson-Delaney, C., 2021. Sugar Gliders. In: Quesenberry, K.E., Orcutt, C.J., Mans, C., Carpenter, J.W. (Eds.), Ferrets, Rabbits, and Rodents Clinical Medicine and Surgery, fourth ed. Elsevier, St. Louis, pp. 385–400.

Junge, R.E., 2003. Prosimians. In: Fowler, M.E., Miller, R.E. (Eds.), Zoo and Wild Animal Medicine, fifth ed. W.B. Saunders, St. Louis, pp. 334–346.

Kastenmayer, R.J., Moak, H.B., Jeffress, E.J., Elkins, W.R., 2010. Management and care of African dormice (*Graphiurus kelleni*). J. Am. Assoc. Lab. Anim. Sci. 49 (2), 173–176.

Kästner, S.B.R., Tünsmeyer, J., Schütter, A.F., 2016. How to anesthetize mouse lemurs. In: Lehman, S.M., Radespiel, U., Zimmermann, E. (Eds.), The Dwarf and Mouse Lemurs of Madagascar: Biology, Behavior, and Conservation Biogeography of the Cheirogaleidae. Cambridge University Press, Cambridge, pp. 135–160.

Klaphake, E., 2006. Common rodent procedures. In: Griffin, C. (Ed.), Veterinary Clinics of North America, Exotic Animal Practice, Common Procedures. W.B. Saunders, Philadelphia, pp. 389–413.

Long, J.P., West, C.L., 2012. Dormouse. In: Suckow, M.A., Stevens, K.A., Wilson, R.P. (Eds.), The Laboratory Rabbit, Hamster, Guinea Pig, and Other Rodents, first ed. Elsevier, St. Louis, pp. 1089–1094.

Mans, C., Donnelly, T.M., 2020. Chinchillas. In: Quesenberry, K.E., Orcutt, C.J., Mans, C., Carpenter, J.W. (Eds.), Ferrets, Rabbits, and Rodents Clinical Medicine and Surgery, fourth ed. Elsevier, St. Louis, pp. 298–322.

Mayer, J., Mans, C., 2018. Rodents. In: Carpenter, J.W., Marion, C.J. (Eds.), Exotic Animal Formulary. Elsevier, St. Louis, pp. 459–493.

McKenzie, E.J., Jackson, M., Turner, A., Gregorash, L., Harapiak, L., 2006. Chronic care and monitoring of woodchucks (*Marmota monax*) during repeated magnetic resonance imaging of the liver. J. Am. Assoc. Lab. Anim. Sci. 45 (2), 26–30.

Ness, R.D., Johnson-Delaney, C., 2012. Sugar Gliders. In: Quesenberry, K.E., Carpenter, J.W. (Eds.), Ferrets, Rabbits, and Rodents Clinical Medicine and Surgery, third ed. Elsevier, St. Louis, pp. 393–410.

Morrisey, J.K., Carpenter, J.W., 2020. Appendix - Formulary. In: Quesenberry, K.E., Orcutt, C.J., Mans, C., Carpenter, J.W. (Eds.), Ferrets, Rabbits, and Rodents Clinical Medicine and Surgery, fourth ed. Elsevier, St. Louis, pp. 620–630.

Ohl, F., Michaelis, T., Fujimori, H., 1999. Volumetric MRI measurements of the tree shrew hippocampus. J. Neurosci. Methods 88 (2), 189–193.

Ostdiek, A. (2021). Personal communication.

Patterson, B.D., Upham, N.S., 2014. A newly recognized family from the Horn of Africa, the Heterocephalidae (Rodentia: Ctenohystrica). Zool. J. Linn. Soc. 172 (4), 942–963.

Pye, G.W., 2001. Marsupial, insectivore, and chiropteran anesthesia. In: Heard, D.J. (Ed.), The Veterinary Clinics of North America, Exotic Animal Practice, Anesthesia and Analgesia. W.B. Saunders, Philadelphia, pp. 211–237.

Raines, J., 2019. In: Miller, R.E., Lamberski, N., Calle, P.P. (Eds.), Fowler's Zoo and Wild Animal Medicine Current Therapy, 9. Elsevier, St. Louis, pp. 514–518.

Rojas Moreno, G., 2019. In: Miller, R.E., Lamberski, N., Calle, P.P. (Eds.), Fowler's Zoo and Wild Animal Medicine Current Therapy, 9. Elsevier, St. Louis, pp. 527–534.

Sainsbury, A.W., 2003. Rodentia (Rodents). In: Fowler, M.E., Miller, R.E. (Eds.), Zoo and Wild Animal Medicine, fifth ed. W.B. Saunders, St. Louis, pp. 420–442.

Schultz, D.A., Sagartz, J.E., Huso, D.L., Buller, R.M., 2009. Experimental infection of an African dormouse (*Graphiurus kelleni*) with monkeypox virus. Virology 383 (1), 86–92.

Shima, A.L., 1999. Sedation and anesthesia in marsupials. In: Fowler, M.E., Miller, R.E. (Eds.), Zoo & Wild Animal Medicine, fourth ed. W.B. Saunders, Philadelphia, pp. 333–336.

Tuval, A., Las, L., Shilo-Benjamini, Y., 2018. Evaluation of injectable anaesthesia with five medetomidine-midazolam based combinations in Egyptian fruit bats (*Rousettus aegyptiacus*). Lab. Anim. 52 (5), 515–525.

Tuval, A., Dror-Maman, I., Las, L., Bdolah-Abram, T., Shilo-Benjamini, Y., 2021. Evaluation of alfaxalone and midazolam with or without flumazenil reversal in Egyptian fruit bats (*Rousettus aegyptiacus*). Vet. Anaesth. Analg. 48 (2), 239–246.

Vogelnest, L., 2015. Marsupialia (marsupials). In: Miller, R.E., Fowler, M.E. (Eds.), Fowler's Zoo and Wild Animal Medicine, vol. 8. Elsevier, St. Louis, pp. 255–274.

Williams, C.V., 2015. Prosimians. In: Miller, R.E., Fowler, M.E. (Eds.), Fowler's Zoo and Wild Animal Medicine, vol. 8. Elsevier, St. Louis, pp. 291–301.

Yarto-Jaramillo, E., 2015. Rodentia. In: Miller, R.E., Fowler, M.E. (Eds.), Fowler's Zoo and Wild Animal Medicine, vol. 8. Elsevier, St. Louis, pp. 384–421.

Chapter 23

Anesthesia and analgesia in birds

Jeff Wyatt
School of Medicine & Dentistry, University of Rochester, Rochester, NY, United States

Chapter outline

Anesthesia and Analgesia in Laboratory Animals. https://doi.org/10.1016/B978-0-12-822215-7.00016-0

I. Avian physiology and anatomy relevant to anesthesia and analgesia

The limited, species-specific pharmacokinetic (PK), safety, and efficacy data for analgesic and anesthetic drugs potentially useful in the wide range of avian species enrolled in scientific studies challenges practitioners and researchers to move beyond a "trial and error" approach. Interspecies scaling of drugs has been attempted in zoo animals using three methods: (1) linear extrapolation from domestic species, (2) metabolic scaling, and (3) allometric scaling (Hunter and Isaza 2008). Linear extrapolation risks overdosing large animals and underdosing small animals (Hunter and Isaza 2008). The highly variable inter and intraspecies basal metabolic rates in birds driven by season, wild, or captive status, domestication, flight capability, and diet, hinder extrapolation of dosages within or across species (Houben et al., 2016; McKenchie et al., 2006). Allometric scaling of metabolic traits (bioavailability, absorption, distribution, and body clearance) theoretically correlated with body mass has been used to extrapolate drug dosages across mammals (Boxenbaum, 1982). For example, a more rapid body clearance of a drug like ketamine hydrochloride in a mouse with a higher metabolic rate requires a higher mg/kg body weight dosage to produce the same anesthetic effect in a great ape. Even though drugs are generally metabolized by the liver and excreted by the kidneys in both birds and mammals, the hepatic microenzyme activity is dictated differently for omnivorous, herbivorous, and carnivorous birds. Birds' lower, intermittent glomerular filtration rates make extrapolation from mammals problematic. Optimizing allometric scaling across bird species requires consideration of species-specific, physiological, pharmacological, toxicological, dosing, and environmental variables (Dorrestein 1991; Dorrestein and Miert 1988). The variation in avian species' pharmacokinetics and phenotypic flexibility in metabolic rates often makes anesthetic and analgesic dosing in birds largely empirical, based on clinical experience. Where possible, the analgesic and anesthetic regimens described in this chapter are supported by species-specific clinical efficacy and PK peer-reviewed, published studies.

The avian trachea lacks an epiglottis, posing a higher risk for aspiration in the nonintubated subject. All birds have complete tracheal rings, prohibiting the expansion required for the safe use of cuffed endotracheal tubes (ET) in mammals (Lierz and Korbel, 2012). The trachea splits at the syrinx, the structure responsible for bird vocalizations from melodious songs to raucous calls (Gunkel and Lafortune, 2005). Beyond the syrinx, primary bronchi branch into 11−15 secondary ventro-, dorso-, and latero-bronchi that communicate with the air sacs. The avian trachea is 2.7 times longer and 1.3 times wider compared with mammals with 4 times the amount of anatomical dead space produced by seven to nine air sacs unique to the bird respiratory tract (Duncker, 1972; Jaensch et al., 2002; James et al., 1976; Gunkel and Lafortune, 2005). The firm, dorsal attachment of each lung to the rigid rib cage above the intercostal juncture and absence of a diaphragm require a breathing technique very different from mammals. Hinge-like lifting and lowering of the sternum and lateral motion of the ribs caudal to the lungs move air in and out of the air sacs through the pulmonary parenchyma of each lung (Duncker, 1972; James et al., 1976). Lateral body positioning of an anesthetized bird promotes unrestricted sternal movement in contrast to dorsal or ventral recumbency, which compresses air sacs (Degernes, 2008; Gunkel and Lafortune, 2005; Guzman and Beaufrere, 2021) with the exception of red-tailed hawks, where neither dorsal nor lateral recumbency compromised ventilation or oxygen transport (Hawkins et al., 2013).

The three to four paired air sacs (cervical, cranial thoracic, caudal thoracic, and abdominal) and the single interclavicular air sac act as bellows, moving air in a unidirectional pattern through the primary, secondary, and tertiary bronchi termed parabronchi making up the bulk of the pulmonary parenchyma (Gill, 2007). Pulmonary parenchymal arterioles and parabronchi give rise to an interdigitating, dense, honeycomb-like network of microscopic, thin-walled blood and air capillaries, respectively. This aerated vascular structure provides on a unit volume basis more efficient gas exchange with a ten-fold higher vascular-respiratory interface than mammals (Duncker, 1972; James et al., 1976; West et al., 2006). For the first inhalation, fresh air enters through the nares and trachea primarily into the posterior (caudal thoracic and abdominal) air sacs and partially into the parabronchial gas exchange area, where oxygen diffuses from air capillaries into blood capillaries. Respirations are accomplished with two consecutive cycles each with an inhalation and exhalation phase. The first exhalation displaces deoxygenated air in the parabronchi with oxygenated air from posterior air sacs. The second inhalation displaces deoxygenated air from the parabronchi to the anterior air sacs as it pulls fresh air through the nares and trachea, mostly into the posterior air sacs with some air entering the parabronchi for oxygen diffusion. The second exhalation pushes deoxygenated air from the anterior air sacs through the trachea and nares in synchrony with pulling fresh air from the posterior air sacs into the parabronchi for gas exchange. These two consecutive respiratory cycles allow fresh, oxygenated air to pass over the parabronchial gas exchange areas of the lung during both inhalation and exhalation, producing a continuous state of oxygen diffusion from fresh air within the bird's lungs (Gill, 2007).

As a flight adaptation, select bones (femur, humerus, synsacrum, and thoracic vertebrae) are pneumatized with direct connections to the respiratory tract. Traumatic injury or infection in these pneumatized bones will affect the respiratory tract. Other bones, specifically the radius, ulna, and tibiotarsus, are relatively hollow with sinusoid connections to the venous system making them as useful as veins to cannulate for fluid therapy (Degernes, 2008; Duncker, 1972; Gunkel and Lafortune, 2005; Lierz and Korbel, 2012).

II. Preprocedural considerations

A. Planning and preparation

Given the deleterious effects of handling of birds, including elevated corticosteroids, heart rate, respiratory rate, core body temperature, apnea, cardiac arrhythmias, and risk of injury, the most valuable parts of an avian anesthetic procedure are planning and preparation (Gunkel and Lafortune, 2005; Lierz and Korbel, 2012). A written anesthetic plan should include the calculation of all anesthetics, analgesics, reversal agents, and emergency drugs. Anesthetics and analgesics should be drawn up, labeled, and readily accessible. All anesthetic induction, maintenance, monitoring, recovery, and support equipment should be assessed for readiness. Consumables, drugs, and tools necessary for the anesthetic procedure should be immediately within reach. The most prepared avian anesthetic team utilizes a checklist and talks through the procedure as a tabletop exercise, confirming all materials and equipment are present and that everyone knows their roles and responsibilities. This holds true for avian anesthetic protocols in the laboratory, classroom, and field. Preoperative observation of the research bird already acclimated to its housing enclosure, ideally at a time when animal care staff normally service the room, provides an opportunity to observe the bird in a setting where it is most likely not stressed so it may demonstrate, not hide, clinical signs of disease. When stressed, birds feign well-being even in the face of disabling disease, a natural adaptation retained as a prey species.

B. History and records

Birds raised as laboratory animals should have records detailing parentage, age, behaviors, social experience, enrichment, macroenvironment, microenvironment, and husbandry. Documentation of flock or individual bird health monitoring, a wholesome diet, potable water, and species-appropriate temperature, lighting, and humidity parameters should be available to the anesthetist. In contrast, field researchers consider the natural history of avian subjects, including the impact that the breeding, nesting and migratory season, weather, nutritional resources, and epizootics may have on a successful anesthetic outcome.

C. Patient evaluation, physical examination and diagnostic tests

Captive-bred, laboratory birds, like their mammal counterparts, living in a strictly controlled environment and characterized by a health monitoring program, generally do not require a comprehensive, preanesthetic health assessment including complete blood counts (CBC), serum chemistry panels, and imaging. Undefined, wild caught or farm-acquired poultry may, however, warrant such diagnostic health assessments. A preanesthetic CBC, serum chemistry panel, fecal Gram stain, cloacal culture, and radiography commonly performed for companion birds may inform the anesthetist of disease states and health risks likely to compromise anesthesia (Degernes, 2008). A scaled down, simpler blood assessment including packed cell volume, total protein, and glucose will rapidly rule out anemia, hypoproteinemia, dehydration, and hypoglycemia before proceeding with anesthesia (Guzman and Beaufrere, 2021). Blood samples, not exceeding 1% body weight, may be collected by the experienced phlebotomist from the hematoma-prone jugular, cutaneous ulnar/basilic, or metatarsal veins (Gunkel and Lafortune, 2005). Minimally, the anesthetist should evaluate the laboratory or wild bird's body condition, mucous membrane color for paleness or cyanosis, examine the eyes and nares for discharges, auscult the heart for arrhythmias and respiratory track for congestion and palpate the crop and lower coelomic cavity for masses (impaction, eggs, masses) when also being handled for anesthetic induction (Degernes, 2008).

III. Preoperative management

A. Fasting

Practices and recommendations vary widely regarding the need to fast birds prior to anesthesia. The author and others have found a risk of hypoglycemia in fasting birds less 200 g (Gunkel and Lafortune, 2005). Full crops of larger birds such as parrots, poultry, waterfowl, and raptors risk regurgitation and aspiration, as well as weigh down the sternum compromising ventilation (Lierz and Korbel, 2012). A full gastro-intestinal tract in an anesthetized, recumbent bird may also press on air sacs impairing ventilation of the lungs (Gunkel and Lafortune, 2005). Table 23.1 lists preanesthetic fasting recommendations based on body weight.

B. Premedication

Premedicant drugs, such as parasympatholytics (e.g., atropine and glycopyrrolate), used in mammals are not recommended for birds. These drugs thicken salivary and tracheal mucosal secretions increasing the risk of tracheal or ET plugging (Gunkel and Lafortune, 2005; Guzman and Beaufrere, 2021).

TABLE 23.1 Preanesthetic fasting.

Body weight	Fasting to empty crop and proventriculus	References
<200 g	1–2 hours	Lierz and Korbel (2012)
>200 g	2–4 hours but not >6 hours	Gunkel and Lafortune (2005)
<300 g	3–6 hours	Degernes (2008)
>300 g	8–12 hours	Degernes (2008)
200–400 g	2–4 hours	Lierz and Korbel (2012)
400–600 g	4–6 hours	Lierz and Korbel (2012)
0.6–1.0 kg	6–12 hours	Lierz and Korbel (2012)
>1 kg	12–48 hours	Lierz and Korbel (2012)

However, these drugs may be beneficial for intraoperatively treating anesthetic-related bradycardia or managing the oculocardiac reflex during ophthalmic surgery (Guzman and Beaufrere, 2021; Lierz and Korbel, 2012). While anxiolytics such as benzodiazepines may be beneficial in some fractious birds, the additional handling and delay in anesthetic induction should be balanced with increased risk of distress and physiological harm (Fair et al., 2010; Gunkel and Lafortune, 2005; Mans, 2014). Application of an ophthalmic lubricant prevents corneal drying caused by decreased tear production in anesthetized birds (Guzman and Beaufrere, 2021).

C. Preoperative sedatives, anxiolytics and local anesthetics

1. Sedation

Sedation is a state in which responses to external stimuli are depressed, but a response can be elicited with sufficient stimulation. In contrast, anesthesia is a state of amnesia, analgesia, loss of responsiveness, and skeletal muscle reflexes. The benefits of sedation may outweigh the risks of inducing deeper anesthesia, especially in fractious, distressed, or dehydrated birds simply requiring examinations, blood sample collection, catheterization, imaging, bandaging, rehydration, or stabilization before general anesthesia (Mans, 2014). A wide range of avian subjects have been sedated with butorphanol given at 1–3 mg/kg IM combined with midazolam given at 0.1–2.0 mg/kg IM. Alfaxalone, a neuroactive steroid anesthetic, has produced 30 minutes of mild to deep sedation in budgerigars (*Melopsittacus undulatus*) dosed at 15–20 mg/kg IM (Romano et al., 2020). Intranasal administration of select sedatives over 5–10 seconds (delivered by atomizer or directly from the syringe tip) rapidly sedates birds within 3–5 minutes while avoiding the need for keel access and the pain associated with intramuscular injections. Despite eliciting sneezing that may risk complete drug delivery, the 5–10 second, intranasal administration of midazolam (2 mg/kg), diazepam (0.2–2 mg/kg), butorphanol (1–3 mg/kg), or butorphanol combined with midazolam (each at 1–2 mg/kg) rapidly sedate birds within 3–5 minutes. Intramuscular or intranasal administration of flumazenil reverses the sedative effect of benzodiazepine within 10–15 minutes (Mans, 2014). In an experimental trial, intranasal dosing of diazepam (0.8 mg/kg) in propylene glycol produced standing chemical restraint within minutes. Midazolam (0.4–0.8 mg/kg) and xylazine (2–4 mg/kg) each alone produced mild-to-moderate sedation within 4 minutes of intranasal administration, producing standing chemical restraint and up to 20 minutes of sternal recumbency affording adequate analgesia for minor invasive procedures (Araghi et al., 2016).

2. Local anesthetics

Two local anesthetics, bupivacaine (2 mg/kg) or lidocaine (1–2.5 mg/kg) may safely be subcutaneously infiltrated as an adjunctive analgesic in sedated birds to mitigate pain associated with minor procedures such as intraosseous (IO) cannulation, digit amputation, or tendon repair (Lee and Lennox, 2016; Lennox, 2011; Strick et al., 2004). Bupivacaine has also been used as a local anesthetic in birds at skin incision sites and as a ring block at 2 mg/kg (Degernes, 2008). However, bupivacaine administered at slightly higher dosages of 2.7–3.3 mg/kg immediately caused self-limiting recumbency and drowsiness in chickens. Lidocaine hydrochloride administered at higher doses (2.7–4 mg/kg) has caused seizures and cardiac arrest in birds (Degernes, 2008; Gunkel and Lafortune, 2005; Machin, 2005a; Machin, 2005b). Therefore, local anesthetics should be used with caution and close attention for species-specific toxicity.

3. *Muscle relaxants*

The handling stress associated with dosing birds with a muscle relaxant such as benzodiazepine prior to anesthetic induction may outweigh the benefit (Fair et al., 2010; Gunkel and Lafortune, 2005). However, the alpha-2 agonists (medetomidine, dexmedetomidine, and xylazine) and benzodiazepines (diazepam, midazolam, and zolazepam) prevent muscle rigidity, tremors and opisthotonos seen when administered in conjunction with dissociative anesthetics such as ketamine and tiletamine (Gunkel and Lafortune, 2005; Lierz and Korbel, 2012).

IV. Anesthetic agents

Depending upon the dose, the following drugs may produce sedation to anesthesia. Table 23.1.

A. Intramuscular route

The pectoralis muscle located on either side of the keel makes for the largest and most accessible site for administering intramuscular injections. Subcutaneous injections may be made in the interscapular, inguinal, or axillary regions. The advantages of using injectable anesthetic agents outweigh the disadvantages, especially for relatively short (e.g., 45 minutes) procedures and for procedures requiring frequent manipulation or relocation of an anesthetized bird. The combination of ketamine with alpha-2 agonists or benzodiazepines may provide safe, dose-dependent, and reversible chemical restraint to a surgical plane of anesthesia. Given the dose-dependent cardiovascular and respiratory depressant effects of injectable agents, supplementation of any single component of the combination to maintain anesthesia beyond that initial dose is not recommended. Inhalation gas anesthesia or intravenous (IV) continuous rate infusion (CRI) may be used to extend the duration of anesthesia.

The injectable drugs ketamine, xylazine, medetomidine, acepromazine, diazepam, and tiletamine-zolazepam, commonly used in laboratory mammals may be administered alone or in combination for chemical restraint or surgical anesthesia of birds. Anesthetic induction should take place in a quiet, warm, and dimly lit room. Given the absence of a diaphragm, special attention must be given when restraining birds by hand so as not to compromise the requirement to lift the sternum and expand the caudal ribs for inhalation and exhalation (Duncker, 1972; West, 2009; James et al., 1976; Hawkins and Paul-Murphy, 2011). Dyspnea caused by over-restraint all too often rapidly leads to fatal cardiac arrest misleading the handler to overestimate the risk of ever again attempting to anesthetize birds.

Disadvantages of injectables compared with inhalation agents include the need to take an accurate body weight to deliver the safest dosage and the inability to adjust the dose once administered. An overdose of injectable agents will exaggerate their cardiopulmonary depressant effects (Lierz and Korbel, 2012). The higher tissue solubility of injectable drugs compared to gas anesthetics requires optimal hydration for liver metabolism and renal excretion. Injectable agents generally provide only 30–45 minutes of chemical restraint or anesthesia, making them most suitable for short procedures. While some of the injectable agents may be given intravenously, the handling stress to gain IV access poses physiological undesirable effects (doubling of respiratory rate, a 2.3°C spike in body temperature, tachycardia, and arrhythmias) within the first 4–15 minutes of manual restraint (Fair et al., 2010; Gunkel and Lafortune, 2005). The advantages of injectable agents include ease of administration without the need for specialized equipment like vaporizers, especially beneficial in field settings.

1. *Ketamine*

Ketamine, a phencyclidine dissociative anesthetic, alone provides insufficient analgesia for painful procedures, provides no muscle relaxation, and produces tremors, opisthotonos, and prolonged, excitable recovery with forceful body flailing and wing flapping. Ketamine should be used in combination with alpha-2 agonists or benzodiazepines for muscle relaxation and smooth inductions and recoveries (Gunkel and Lafortune, 2005; Lierz and Korbel, 2012). Ketamine should not be used alone in Coturnix quail (*Coturnix coturnix*), pigeons (*Columbia livia*), and most other species in the author's experience due to muscle rigidity, hyperthermia, and excitable recovery (Durrani et al., 2009, 2014).

2. *Alpha-2 adrenergic agonists*

Xylazine, dexmedetomidine, and medetomidine, each being an alpha-2 agonist, when combined with ketamine provide chemical restraint with excellent muscle relaxation and dose-dependent analgesia for painful procedures. Disadvantages of alpha-2 agonists include dose-dependent respiratory depression, hypotension, bradycardia, and partial atrioventricular block (Virtanen, 1989). The cardiopulmonary depression caused by xylazine and dexmedetomidine may be reversed by yohimbine and atipamezole, respectively. The smooth recovery associated with a ketamine and alpha-2 agonist combination may be maintained but shortened by administration of alpha-2 antagonists. Xylazine and medetomidine alone administered IM, do not reliably and safely provide chemical restraint or anesthesia (Gunkel and Lafortune, 2005; Lierz and Korbel, 2012).

However, a much higher, intranasal dosing of ostriches, an avian species used for orthopedic and joint research, with xylazine at 2–4 mg/kg produced 20 minutes of profound sedation in sternal recumbency within minutes of dosing (Araghi et al., 2016).

3. Benzodiazepines

Benzodiazepines (diazepam, midazolam) administered alone provide dose-dependent sedation and mild analgesia without the cardiovascular effects of alpha-2 agonists (Lierz and Korbel, 2012; Mahmud et al., 2014; Mans, 2014). Diazepam administered alone at 10 mg/kg IM provided 3 hours of deep sedation in zebra finches (*Taeniopygia guttata*) suitable for minor invasive procedures successfully reversed with flumazenil 0.3 mg/kg IM (Prather, 2012). Midazolam and midazolam/butorphanol provide dose-dependent sedation adequate for clinical procedures such as physical examination, blood collection, and imaging in most species (Guzman and Beaufrere, 2021). Diazepam administered intranasally (IN) at 0.8 mg/kg in ostriches (*Struthio camelus*) provided standing chemical restraint. Midazolam dosed 0.4–0.8 mg/kg IN produced 20 minutes of standing chemical restraint to sternal recumbency with deep sedation (Araghi et al., 2016). Being water soluble, midazolam may be administered intramuscularly or subcutaneously without irritating local tissue as seen with water-insoluble diazepam (Mans, 2014).

4. Ketamine and alpha-2 agonist combinations

A wide variety of intramuscularly administered ketamine and alpha-2 agonist sedative combinations providing dose-dependent effects from chemical restraint with analgesia to a surgical plane of anesthesia for research and clinical purposes in all taxa of birds from hummingbirds to ostriches have been published (Pytte et al., 2004; Jiang et al., 2015). The potent sedative, muscle relaxing, and analgesic benefits of xylazine (5 mg/kg IM) when combined with ketamine (35 mg/kg) provide 30–45 minutes surgical anesthesia in most birds suitable for major invasive surgery (Bhavsar et al., 2010; Durrani et al., 2009, 2014). Given the cardiopulmonary depression caused by alpha-2 agonists, risks must be considered when anesthetizing unhealthy birds (Virtanen, 1989). Yohimbine and atipamezole (Table 23.2) reverse the sedative as well as the cardiopulmonary depressant effects of xylazine and medetomidine or dexmedetomidine, respectively. Intramuscular supplementation of partial or full doses of either ketamine or xylazine is not recommended given dose-dependent cumulative adverse cardiopulmonary effects (Lierz and Korbel, 2012). Procedures requiring a longer duration of surgical anesthesia should be performed using more controllable and titratable inhalation or intravenous CRI anesthesia.

5. Ketamine and benzodiazepine combinations

Benzodiazepines such as diazepam and midazolam may be added to ketamine to provide excellent muscle relaxation without the cardiopulmonary depression seen with alpha-2 agonists. Diazepam causes tissue damage unless given intravenously due to its propylene glycol content. Midazolam, which is typically formulated as an aqueous solution not containing propylene glycol, may be administered intramuscularly or subcutaneously without irritating local tissue (Mans, 2014). While flumazenil (Table 23.2) may be administered intramuscularly or IN to antagonize the effects of either of the benzodiazepines to shorten recovery, the anxiolytic and muscle relaxation afforded by benzodiazepines may be desirable to promote a smooth anesthetic recovery (Gunkel and Lafortune, 2005; Lierz and Korbel, 2012; Mans, 2014). Benzodiazepines are minimum alveolar concentration (MAC) sparing drugs permitting the use of lower concentrations of isoflurane or sevoflurane (Gunkel and Lafortune, 2005). Flumazenil delivered IM or IN reverses the effects sedative effects of benzodiazepines.

6. Tiletamine-zolazepam

Tiletamine-zolazepam, or Telazol™, an anesthetic used commonly in zoo animals, combines all of the benefits of a phencyclidine and benzodiazepine in one product, providing muscle relaxation and longer duration of anesthesia than using ketamine alone. Telazol™ may in some cases produce prolonged, possibly stormy recoveries in birds, warranting gentle wrapping in a towel to prevent flapping of wings (Gunkel and Lafortune, 2005; Lierz and Korbel, 2012; Guzman and Beaufrere, 2021).

B. Subcutaneous route

Both intramuscular and subcutaneous routes have been shown to be equally effective for many of the analgesics and anesthetic agents used in birds (Tables 23.1 and 23.2). The subcutaneous tissue is preferred as an injection site to avoid local irritation of relatively large, space-occupying drug volumes, especially in small birds, as evidenced by elevated muscle enzymes in serum biochemistry panels (Mans, 2014).

A regimen of continuously infusing ketamine and dexmedetomidine subcutaneously safely anesthetized budgerigars throughout a 2–3 hours surgery implanting electrodes in the brain for postoperative, awake neurophysiological recording. Anesthesia was induced with subcutaneous administration of ketamine (3–5 mg/kg) and dexmedetomidine (0.08–0.1 mg/kg), followed by CRI by syringe pump of ketamine (6–10 mg/kg/hr) and dexmedetomidine (0.16–0.27 mg/kg/hr) in lactated ringers (30–50 mL/kg/hr). Upon completion of the surgery,

TABLE 23.2 Anesthetics, sedatives and reversal drugs.

Drug(s)	mg/kg	Route[a]	Species	Comments	References
Acepromazine + Propofol	A: 0.25 + P: 4.0	A: IM P: IV	ostrich	Recumbent for 9 minutes anesthesia, hooded	Ciboto et al. (2006)
Acepromazine + Ketamine + Diazepam	A: 0.25 K: 5 D: 0.25	A: IM K: IV D: IV	ostrich	Recumbent and nonresponsive for 9 minutes (hooded)	Ciboto et al. (2006)
Acepromazine + Telazol (tiletamine:zolazepam)	A: 0.25 T: 3	A: IM T: IV	ostrich	17 minutes recumbent (hooded)	Ciboto et al. (2006)
Alfaxalone	10–25 mg/kg	IM	budgerigar	Mild to deep sedation	Romano et al. (2020)
Alfaxalone + Butorphanol	A: 30 B: 0.7	A: SC B: SC	Bengalese finch	15 minutes moderate sedation with minimal analgesia	Perrin et al. (2017)
Alfaxalone + Midazolam	A: 30 Mz: 0.7	A: SC Mz: SC	Bengalese finch	15 minutes moderate sedation with analgesia	Perrin et al. (2017)
Alpha chloralose	20–30	PO	duck, goose	Baited in bread, Chemical immobilization for translocation	Woronecki et al. (1990)
Alpha chloralose	30–60	PO	urban pigeon	Baited in corn, Chemical immobilization	Woronecki et al. (1990)
Atipamezole (Antisedan™)	0.25–5 *or* 5 X medetomidine dose	IM, IV	most species	Alpha-2 antagonist reversal of medetomidine, dexmedetomidine	Lierz and Korbel (2012)
Bupivacaine	2–8	Local infiltration	chicken, duck	Local anesthetic	Malik and Valentine, 2018
Butorphanol	1–3	IM	psittacine	Sedation and preanesthetic	Lee and Lennox (2016) Mans (2014)
Butorphanol	1–4 mg/kg loading dose CRI: 1–4 mg/kg/hr	IV IV	cockatoo, guinea fowl, chicken	Isoflurane MAC sparing 21%–25%	Schnellbacher and Comolli (2020)
Butorphanol + Midazolam	B: 1–2 + Mz: 1–2	IM, IN	multiple	Deep sedation	Mans (2014)
Diazepam	0.2–2	IM, IV	multiple	Sedation, Anxiolytic, Tissue damage if given IM	Lierz and Korbel (2012) Mans (2014)
Diazepam	10	IM	zebra finch	Deep sedation for 3 hours reversed by flumazenil).3 mg/kg IM. No adverse effect or tissue damage reported	Prather (2012)
Diazepam	0.5	IM	chicken	Sedation	Mahmud et al. (2014)
Diazepam	0.4	IN	ostrich	20 minutes standing restraint, hooded	Araghi et al. (2016)
Fentanyl	0.02 bolus CRI: 0.007 –0.02 mg/kg/hr CRI: 0.1 –0.15 mg/kg/hr	IV IV IV	hawk, parrot, chicken	MAC Isoflurane sparing 31%–54%	Schnellbacher and Comolli (2020)

Continued

TABLE 23.2 Anesthetics, sedatives and reversal drugs.—cont'd

Drug(s)	mg/kg	Route[a]	Species	Comments	References
Flumazenil	0.01–0.1	IM IN	multiple	Reverses benzodiazepines within 15 minutes 2nd dose may be required	Mans (2014)
Isoflurane	3%–5% induction 1%–2.5% maintenance	INH	multiple, cockatoo, zebra finch	Endotracheal or Air Sac Intubation or Face Mask in 100% 02	Gunkel and Lafortune (2005), Jaensch et al. (2001) Korschgen et al. (1996) Lierz and Korbel (2012) Nilson et al. (2005)
Ketamine	20–50	SC, IM, IV	psittacine	Not a mono anesthetic: No muscle relaxation. Poor analgesia	Gunkel and Lafortune (2005) Lierz and Korbel (2012)
Ketamine + Diazepam	K: 10–50 + D: 0.5–2	IM	psittacine	Dose dependent restraint with analgesia and muscle relaxation to surgical anesthesia	Gunkel and Lafortune (2005)
Ketamine + Diazepam	K: 25 + D: 7.5	IM	multiple	Dose dependent short-term anesthesia	Lierz and Korbel (2012)
Ketamine + Diazepam	K: 10 D: 2	IM	chicken	Anesthesia depth sufficient for surgery	Mahmud et al. (2014)
Ketamine + Medetomidine	K: 3–7 M: 0.075–0.1	IM	psittacine	Dose dependent restraint with analgesia and muscle relaxation to anesthesia (sufficient for surgery)	Gunkel and Lafortune (2005)
Ketamine + medetomidine	K: 2–5 M: 0.05–0.2	IM	raptors, psittacine, ostrich	Short term anesthesia	Lierz and Korbel (2012)
Ketamine + Midazolam	K: 10–25 + Mz: 0.5–1	IM IM	psittacine	Dose dependent restraint with analgesia and muscle relaxation to anesthesia (sufficient for surgery)	Gunkel and Lafortune (2005)
Ketamine + Xylazine	K: 35 X: 5 ISO: 2%–4% maintenance	IM IM INH	white leghorn chicken	Anesthesia for flexor tendon adhesion model	Bhavsar et al. (2010)
Ketamine + Xylazine	K: 30 + X: 9	IM	coturnix quail, pigeon	Anesthesia depth sufficient for surgery	Durrani et al. (2014) Durrani et al. (2009)
Ketamine + Xylazine	K: 40 X: 10	IM	multiple	Short term anesthesia (sufficient for surgery)	Lierz and Korbel (2012)
Ketamine + Xylazine	K: 30 X: 8 CRI K; 1 mg/mL 4–6 drops per second	IM CRI	ostrich	Anesthesia (sufficient for surgery) for 2 hours	Jiang et al. (2015)

Continued

TABLE 23.2 Anesthetics, sedatives and reversal drugs.—cont'd

Drug(s)	mg/kg	Route[a]	Species	Comments	References
Ketamine + Xylazine	K: 24 X: 12	IM	blue throated humming-bird	Anesthesia for Auditory Brain-stem Recordings reversed by yohimbine 0.6 mg/kg IM	Pyette et al. (2004)
Ketamine + Xylazine + Midazolam	K: 15 + X:2.5 + Mz: 0.3	IM	guinea fowl	Short term anesthesia (sufficient for surgery)	Lierz and Korbel (2012)
Lidocaine hydrochloride without epinephrine	2	Infiltrated-ted IM, SC	chicken	Dilute 1:10, Local anesthetic at flexor tendon resection	Strick et al. (2004) Malik and Valentine, 2018
Midazolam	0.4–0.8	IN	ostrich	20 minutes standing chemical restraint with analgesia	Araghi et al. (2016)
Midazolam	0.5–3	IM	multiple	Sedation, anxiolytic wide margin of safety	Lee and Lennox (2016) Mans (2014)
Midazolam + Butorphanol + Isoflurane	Mz: 2 B: 1 ISO: 4% mask induction 2.5% ET maintenance	IM IM INH	Mallard duck	Anesthesia for cataract removal	Wilson and Pettifer (2004)
Propofol	5–15 induction CRI 0.5–1.0 mg/kg/min	IV	multiple, parrot, barn owl, mute swan	Short term anesthesia, apnea, assist ventilate	Gunkel and Lafortune (2005) Mama et al. (1996)
Propofol	2-8 loading dose 0.4–1.0 mg/kg/min	IV IV	hawk, owl, parrot, swans	Anesthesia sufficient for surgery (requires ventilatory support)	Schnellbacher and Comolli (2020)
Sevoflurane	5%–8% induction 3%–4% maintenance	INH	multiple	Endotracheal or Air Sac Intubation or Face Mask in 100% 02	Lierz and Korbel (2012)
Tiletamine-zolazepam	20–30	IM	multiple	Short term anesthesia	Lierz and Korbel (2012)
Yohimbine	0.2–2.0	IM, IV	most species	Alpha-2 antagonist reverses xylazine	Lierz and Korbel (2012)
Xylazine	2–4	IN	ostrich	Standing chemical restraint with analgesia	Araghi et al. (2016)
Xylazine	1–2	IM	multiple	Sedation, Cardiopulmonary depression	Lierz and Korbel (2012)
Xylazine	18	IM	coturnix quail, pigeon	Sedation	Durrani et al. (2009) Durrani et al. (2014)
Xylazine + Ketamine + Diazepam	X: 1.0 K: 5 D: 0.25	X: IM K: IV D: IV	ostrich	Recumbent, 12 minutes anesthesia, hooded	Ciboto et al. (2006)
Xylazine + tiletamine:zolazepam	X: 1.0 T: 3	X: IM T: IV	ostrich	Recumbent, 19 minutes anesthesia, hooded	Ciboto et al. (2006)

[a]*CRI, continuous rate infusion;* IN, *intranasal;* INH, *inhalation;* IM, *intramuscular;* IV, *intravenous;* SC, *subcutaneous;* PO, *oral.*

anesthesia was smoothly reversed with a subcutaneous injection of atipamezole (0.5 mg/kg), followed by carprofen (1 mg/kg/kg) SID (Henry et al., 2016; Henry et al., 2017; Wang et al., 2021). This regimen underscores the opportunity to explore the delivery of anesthetic agents subcutaneously in birds by CRI.

C. Intravenous route

Intravenous drug administration may be performed in manually restrained birds into the jugular vein (the right being larger in many species), the wing vein (cutaneous ulnar/basilic vein), or the tibiotarsal vein (most prominent in poultry, waterfowl, and cranes). Be aware that birds are prone to hematomas, and repeated IV access is best accomplished through a catheter. Agents may be given as a bolus or by CRI. CRI of anesthetics intravenously delivered by a syringe pump enhances operative and postoperative outcomes by providing a steady state and precisely adjustable plane of anesthesia replicating the advantages of inhalation gas anesthesia (Sayce et al., 2020; Schnellbacher and Comolli, 2020).

1. Propofol

Propofol, a short-acting, nonbarbiturate isopropyl phenol anesthetic and muscle relaxant, must be administered intravenously. The intravenous induction typically causes self-limiting apnea that may require assisted ventilation. The extent of apnea may be limited by slow administration of propofol to effect; one-quarter of the predicted dose delivered over 15 seconds. Because of breath-holding behavior when using inhalation gas anesthetics, waterfowl may best be induced by IV injection with propofol at 4−6 mg/kg IV (Guzman and Beaufrere, 2021). Propofol's ultrashort anesthetic duration of minutes requires either continuous infusion or a transition to another general anesthetic to maintain a surgical plane. Barn owls (*Tyto alba*) used in auditory brainstem response studies to localize auditory pathways may be anesthetized with a 4 mg/kg intravenous bolus of propofol slowly administered over 30 seconds, followed by 0.5 mg/kg/min by CRI (Mama et al., 1996). CRI of propofol at 0.2 mg/kg/min after a 3 mg/kg IV bolus in premedicated adult ostriches (ketamine 2 mg/kg and medetomidine 80 μg/kg IM) produced brief self-limiting bradycardia and normal PAO2 throughout 30 minutes of a light plane of anesthesia with negative palpebral and pedal but positive corneal reflexes (Langan et al., 2000). Oxygen should routinely be administered as a safeguard against hypoxia by face mask or endotracheal intubation (ET) throughout the CRI of propofol (Guzman and Beaufrere, 2021). The slower metabolism of propofol in birds compared with mammals may explain prolonged recovery times (Schnellbacher and Comolli, 2020).

2. Opioids

A loading dose of fentanyl (20 μg/kg) followed by CRI at 7−20 μg/kg/h in poultry and birds of prey and at 100−150 μg/kg/h in parrots reduced isoflurane MAC by 17.6%−42.6%, respectively (Schnellbacher and Comolli, 2020). Butorphanol dosed initially at 1−4 mg/kg followed by CRI at 1−4 mg/kg/hr spares MAC concentration across most bird species (Schnellbacher and Comolli, 2020).

D. Intraosseous route

The radius, ulna, and tibiotarsus are relatively hollow with sinusoid connections to the venous system, making them as useful as veins to cannulate for intra and postoperative drug administration and fluid therapy (Degernes, 2008; Duncker, 1972; Gunkel and Lafortune, 2005; Lierz and Korbel, 2012). IO catheterization is a valuable alternative to catheterizing birds with small or damaged veins. IO catheters, 3 cm long, 14−20 g with a metal stylet are commercially available (Global Veterinary Products, Inc). Spinal needles work well. A hypodermic needle may be used, but be aware of plugging of the cannula with bone. Before IO catheterization, pluck the feathers and aseptically prep the skin at the insertion site. The proximal and distal ulna and the proximal tibiotarsus are the most common IO cannulation sites. Correct placement of an IO catheter is well described in the literature (Gunkel and Lafortune, 2005). The IO catheter may be capped and secured in place under a figure-8 wing bandage for postop fluid and drug therapy.

E. Inhalation route

Inhalant anesthetic agents, the safest and most preferred of all choices, offer the advantage to titrate dosing throughout the procedure as delivered with a vaporizer and controlled oxygen flow (Lierz and Korbel, 2012). Due to the bird's greater lung surface area with a ten-fold higher vascular-respiratory interface, and more efficient gas exchange, induction with gas anesthesia is much more rapid than seen in mammals (Degernes, 2008; James et al., 1976; West et al., 2006; West, 2009). For this chapter, the more common and less expensive inhalation agent, isoflurane, will be described. Anesthetists may however prefer using sevoflurane given its slightly more rapid induction and recovery times; however, these advantages are reduced when sedative drugs are also administered. Unless the bird is accustomed to handling, the anesthetist may want to choose an induction chamber to avoid extended, manual restraint during mask induction. Nonrebreathing systems such as a Bain coaxial circuit or Ayre's T-piece with a 0.25−1.0 L reservoir bag work best for most birds weighing less than 7 kg. The high flow rate (e.g., 150−200 mL/oxygen/kg/min for a Bain system and 400 mL/kg/min for Ayre's T-piece) decreases resistance to breathing and eliminates the buildup of carbon dioxide. Manual ventilation "bagging" should not exceed 15–20 cm H20. The anesthetist may rely on capnography for monitoring CO2 levels to correctly make changes in respiratory rate and quality (Degernes, 2008; Gunkel and Lafortune, 2005; Guzman and Beaufrere, 2021).

The inhalation agents, isoflurane, and sevoflurane, may safely be administered using an induction chamber or a face mask with a vaporizer. The gently wrapped, handheld bird is induced via a face mask or is loosely wrapped inside a dimly lit, padded, chamber to a rapidly increasing gas concentration from 0% to 4% for isoflurane or to 6% for sevoflurane at high oxygen flow rates. This technique takes several minutes until the loss of righting reflex. Another technique gradually increases the gas concentration 0.5% increments per minute until the loss of righting reflex (Guzman and Beaufrere, 2021). The author prefers the more rapid induction minimizing the potential for the bird struggling during a prolonged excitement phase. Preoxygenation of chickens for 3 minutes before isoflurane anesthesia conferred no benefit after experimental induction of apnea compared with nonpreoxygenated birds (Pierre et al., 2021).

After induction by an injectable drug combination or inhaled gas, the bird is endotracheally intubated. The lack of an epiglottis and easy access at the base of the tongue make ET simple for even the novice anesthetist. After an assistant opens the mouth with gauze strips placed on the upper and lower beaks, followed by gentle retraction of the tongue with a cotton tip applicator gauze, the anesthetist inserts the ET through the glottis. Since all birds have closed cartilaginous tracheal rings, an uncuffed ET should be used to prevent ring fracture or mucosal necrosis (Degernes, 2008; Gunkel and Lafortune, 2005; James et al., 1976; Lierz and Korbel, 2012). Birds weighing less than 80 g may experience soft tissue trauma and lumen plugging when endotracheally intubated (Gunkel and Lafortune, 2005). However, an intravenous Teflon catheter sheath or urinary catheter has successfully been used in some small birds (Degernes, 2008). For birds weighing more than 100 g, a Cole pediatric ET with a narrower to progressively larger circumference allows advancement beyond the glottis until resistance is met to create a relatively airtight seal. Uncuffed avian ETs may be purchased from commercial sources (Portex Cole's Neonatal Tube, JorVet Jorgensen Labs, Bivona Inc) (Gunkel and Lafortune, 2005). For birds weighing greater than 300 g, an ET with a Murphy eye and uninflated cuff is preferred. The author and others prefer to use larger-cuffed ETs with slightly inflated cuffs in large waterfowl and ratites (Ciboto et al., 2006; Guzman and Beaufrere, 2021; Jiang et al., 2015; Langan et al., 2000; Troy et al., 2007). ET provides numerous important advantages, including consistent delivery of inhalant anesthetic agents carried in high concentrations of oxygen, reducing the risk of foreign material (e.g., secretions, blood) being aspirated into the trachea, the ability to assist ventilation (including preventing apnea from progressing to cardiac arrest), and reducing exposure to waste anesthetic gas (Degernes, 2008; Gunkel and Lafortune, 2005).

Air sac perfusion anesthesia or caudal thoracic air sac intubation or cannulation offers a novel method to deliver inhalation anesthetics when the head must be free of anesthetic equipment for maximum access for neurosurgery (Gunkel and Lafortune, 2005; Jaensch et al., 2001; Nilson et al., 2005). The avian veterinarian experienced with laparoscopic sexing of birds may use the same approach. The bird, already anesthetized with isoflurane delivered via a face mask or ET, is placed in right lateral recumbency with the wings taped upward above the body and the left leg secured caudally, exposing the left paralumbar fossa between the last two ribs, the cranial aspect of the thigh (femur), and the synsacrum (analogous to the mammal's pelvis). The anesthetist focally plucks feathers and aseptically prepares the site for a 0.5–1.0 cm skin incision. A small hemostat is used to bluntly dissect through the body wall so that a quick, controlled stab is made through the left caudal thoracic air sac, the largest of the air sacs in most birds (Gunkel and Lafortune, 2005). An air sac cannula about the same diameter of the trachea made from a red rubber feeding tube with two side ports is inserted about 2 cm into a 300-gram bird. Larger cannula may be adapted for more sizable birds. The correct placement is verified by checking air flow out of the catheter which is most easily accomplished by holding a downy feather over the end of the cannula lumen. The cannula is secured to the skin with a purse string or butterfly suture and a finger trap suture pattern. An ET adapter is used to connect the cannula to the anesthetic machine, delivering isoflurane at 1%–2.5% concentration at a flow rate of 0.3 L/kg/min for a 300-g bird instead of previously through the trachea. A CO2 washout from the respiratory tract may cause hypoventilation or apnea, requiring assisted ventilation and monitoring of PO2 by pulse oximetry. This technique may be used in birds the size of cockatoos (Jaensch et al., 2001) to finches (Nilson et al., 2005). At the end of the anesthetic procedure, administering 100% oxygen for a few minutes flushes the respiratory tract free of isoflurane, leading to spontaneous breathing within 4 minutes, followed by full recovery (Lierz and Korbel, 2012).

F. Intranasal route

Many of the injectable avian sedatives and anesthetics and antagonists, including butorphanol, midazolam, diazepam, xylazine, and flumazenil may effectively and easily be administered IN in birds (Mans, 2014). Given the high bioavailability and absorption of the drugs delivered IN, the onset of sedation is within three to 5 minutes (Mans, 2014). Disadvantages of the IN route include the risk of incomplete delivery with sneezing and limitations of larger volumes of less concentrated drugs for the more sizable birds. However, the IN route has proven as effective and easier to administer sedatives compared with IM or IV in unruly ratites often used in orthopedic research (Araghi et al., 2016).

V. Anesthetic monitoring, management and emergencies

"The proper use of anesthetics and analgesics in research animals is an ethical and scientific imperative. It should be considered that procedures that cause pain in humans may also cause pain in other animals" (National Research Council, 2010a). Mammals and birds share the same stages of anesthesia from induction (stage I) through excitatory (stage II), light (stage III), moderate (stage IV) to deep (stage V). Righting, pedal (toe pinch), and palpebral reflexes are lost, jaw (beak) tone is relaxed, and respiratory and heart rates decrease as the bird reaches a moderate depth of anesthesia (stage IV) suitable for performing surgery. Loss of corneal reflex and slow, shallow, and intermittent respirations accompanied by bradycardia indicate a dangerously deep level of anesthesia (stage IV) progressing to apnea and cardiac arrest (Lierz and Korbel, 2012). Table 23.3 lists the most commonly used and best studied emergency drugs used in birds.

A. Monitoring and management

Documenting anesthetic parameters in an anesthetic chart facilitates monitoring trends at 5-min intervals and assists with oversight body assessments of the program.

1. Heart rate and quality

It is important to monitor and record trends in rate from the baseline given the rapid rate at which birds may decompensate (Machin, 2005b). Heart rate may be auscultated over the keel, thoracic inlet, axilla, and over the back lateral to the vertebrae (Degernes, 2008). An esophageal stethoscope is useful when passed beyond the crop into the thoracic esophagus (Guzman and Beaufrere, 2021). As with mammals, heart rate will increase with nociception, light anesthesia, and blood loss. An 8 MHz ultrasonic Doppler transducer affixed over the cranial tibial artery (cranial aspect of the hock joint), superficial ulnar artery (ventral

TABLE 23.3 Emergency drugs.

Emergency drug	mg/kg	Route[a]	Species	Comments	References
Atropine	0.02–0.5	IM, IV, IO, IT	all	bradycardia	Gunkel and Lafortune (2005) Lierz and Korbel (2012)
Caffeine-sodium salicylate	Per drop	PO, IN	all	Cardiopulmonary arrest	Lierz and Korbel (2012)
Calcium gluconate	50–100	IM, IV	all	Hypocalcemia	Gunkel and Lafortune (2005)
Doxapram	5–20	IM, IV, IO, IT	all	Respiratory arrest, apnea, CPR	Lierz and Korbel (2012)
Dexamethasone	2–6	IM, IV	all	Shock	
Epinephrine (1:1000)	0.5–1.0	IM, IV, IO, IT		Cardiac arrest	Gunkel and Lafortune (2005) Lierz and Korbel (2012)
Dextrose 50%	500	Slow IV	all	Hypoglycemia, Never IM or SC	Gunkel and Lafortune (2005)
Glycopyrrolate	0.01–0.03	IM, IV	all	Bradycardia	Gunkel and Lafortune (2005) Lierz and Korbel (2012)
Sodium bicarbonate	1–5 mEq/kg	IV, IO	all	Metabolic acidosis, CPR	Gunkel and Lafortune (2005)
Prednisolone sodium succinate	10–30	Sublingual, IM, IV, IO	all	Shock, CPR	Lierz and Korbel (2012)

[a]*IM, intramuscular; IN, intranasal; IO, intraosseous; IT, intratracheal; IV, intravenous; PO, oral; SC, subcutaneous.*

surface of the elbow), and the deep radial artery (ventral surface of the radius near the carpus), or an esophageal stethoscope aid in monitoring heart rate (Degernes, 2008; Lierz and Korbel, 2012). A modified Lead II electrocardiogram measures electrical differences between the patagium, the wing skin web between the humerus and radius elbow joint, and the inguinal skin fold where the femur meets the body wall. As with mammals, each electrode may be connected directly to the skin with flattened alligator clips or more indirectly attached with alligator clips on a hypodermic needle advanced into the skin. While a typical Lead II reading is not produced, arrhythmias and rates may easily be identified. Heart rate decreases with dose-dependent cardio-depressant agents and deep anesthesia. The presence of arrhythmias is often evidence of poor oxygenation.

2. Respiratory rate and quality

As with heart rate, monitor, and document trends from the baseline given the propensity of avian species for rapid decompensation under anesthesia (Guzman and Beaufrere, 2021). Respiratory rates for larger species (10–25/min) and smaller birds (30–40/min) should be maintained spontaneously or with assistance, either manually or by a mechanical ventilator. The anesthetist should observe the keel lifting and dropping with each respiratory cycle. Optimal lateral body positioning avoids the restricted sternal movement and compression of air sacs posed by dorsal or ventral recumbency (Degernes, 2008; Gunkel and Lafortune, 2005; Guzman and Beaufrere, 2021). In contrast to other species, dorsal recumbency did not compromise ventilation and oxygen transport in red-tailed hawks when compared with lateral positioning (Hawkins et al., 2013). Apnea from any cause rapidly leads to cardiac arrest in birds. Diligently monitor and document respiratory rate and be prepared to provide respiratory support with oxygen supplementation and assisted ventilation via an ET while problem-solving with priority on assessment of a mucus-plugged airway.

3. Oxygenation

Pulse oximeters used in mammals may underestimate the PO2 values in birds, especially at lower levels due to differences in avian hemoglobin absorption characteristics (Degernes, 2008; Perrin et al., 2017). Absolute PaO2 values may not correlate exactly with blood gas values and motion results in discontinuous and fluctuating values. Regardless, documentation and tracking trends may be useful if a reliable location on the unpigmented toes, lower legs, skin webbing, or wattle is accessible (Guzman and Beaufrere, 2021; Schmitt et al., 1998). Pulse oximeters measuring heart rates up to and over 300 are valuable for use in birds. Oxygen supplementation is recommended by face mask or ET as a precaution when delivering propofol by CRI (Guzman and Beaufrere, 2021). Oxygen flow rates of 150 mL/kg/min for small birds and 1 L/min for birds greater than 300 g work well for an endotracheally intubated in a nonrebreathing system or face mask (Guzman and Beaufrere, 2021). Intermittent positive pressure ventilation prevents hypercapnia (Guzman and Beuafrere, 2021).

4. Carbon dioxide

Capnography may be accomplished in an endotracheally intubated with a side-stream monitor as used in mammals. Target maintaining an end-tidal carbon dioxide (ETCO2) range of 30–45 mmHg under anesthesia when spontaneously breathing or using positive pressure ventilation. A normal physiological ETCO2 range in awake birds is 25–40 mmHg (Degernes, 2008; Lierz and Korbel, 2012; Guzman and Beaufrere, 2021). Elevated CO2 values may indicate a plugged or kinked ET or hypoventilation, requiring assisted ventilation (e.g., bagging). Lower than preferred ETCO2 values may be caused by hyperventilation, warranting a reduction in manual or assisted ventilation. Even in spontaneously breathing, intubated subjects, the anesthetist should assist-ventilate or "sigh" the bird once per minute to avoid hypercapnia, hypoxia, and acidosis (Degernes, 2008).

5. Body temperature

Normothermia assists with intra and postoperative anesthetic drug metabolism and speeds recovery. Monitor and document body temperature with a cloacal or esophageal probe, and be prepared to intervene. The preferred body temperature to maintain ranges between 104 and 109°F (Lierz and Korbel, 2012). The same risks of hypothermia in small mammals apply more so for birds given their larger surface area relative to body mass and the large volume of anesthetic gas flow in the air sacs (Degernes, 2008). General anesthesia causes hypothermia as a result of depression of thermoregulation and, with many anesthetics, vasodilation. Keep anesthetic episodes as short as possible by using agents with low tissue absorption like isoflurane, sevoflurane, and propofol, or those drugs whose effects can be antagonized. Pluck as few feathers as necessary and sparingly apply liquid antiseptics at the surgical site. Monitor and document body temperature with a cloacal or esophageal probe and be prepared to intervene (Lierz and Korbel, 2012). Maintain a warm environment throughout the perioperative period from anesthetic induction through recovery. Warm the operating room. Surround the bird with radiant heat as accomplished with warm air or water pads followed by covering the bird with a transparent drape (Guzman and Beaufrere, 2021). Humidify and warm inhalation gas. Anesthetized birds may lose 2.8–3.3°C body temperature within 40 minutes. Active warming methods (e.g., forced air warmer [e.g., Bair Hugger™], conductive polymer blankets [e.g., HotDog™], or circulating water blankets) benefit birds as for small mammals. Note: circulating water blankets are no longer recommended unless their temperature output is checked as they have been associated with thermal burns. A continuous IV or IO infusion of warmed fluids at (10−20 mL/kg/hr) for prolonged procedures or a postoperative subcutaneous (30−40 mL/kg) bolus of warm (38−40°C) fluids may mitigate intraoperative risk or reverse hypothermia as the bird recovers from anesthesia (Degernes, 2008; Gunkel and Lafortune, 2005; Lierz and Korbel, 2012). Recover the loosely wrapped bird in a dimly lit incubator warmed to 25−30°C.

6. Fluid therapy

Place an IV (jugular vein, basilic/cutaneous ulnar vein, or medial metatarsal vein) or IO catheter for procedures greater than 30 minutes. Warmed IV or IO fluids, preferable lactated ringers, delivered at 10−20 mL/kg/hr or up to 40 mL/kg subcutaneous bolus will prevent or treat hypothermia or hypotension. Favored subcutaneous sites for fluid therapy include the inguinal web, interscapular, or paravertebral (Degernes, 2008; Lierz and Korbel, 2012). Be careful not to inject fluids into the cervical air sacs most prominent around the neck of select bird species such as cockatoos (Janesch et al., 2002). Fluids will readily be absorbed via an IO catheter, most placed in the distal ulna or proximal tibiotarsus. Sinusoids in these bones carry fluids into veins. The IO catheter may be capped and secured in place under a figure-8 wing bandage for postop fluid therapy. Fluids should never be injected into the femur or humerus, as these can be pneumatized bones, connecting directly to the respiratory tract (Gunkel and Lafortune, 2005).

7. Blood pressure

Indirect monitoring of blood pressure with a pressure cuff is not reliable. Direct monitoring of blood pressure via arterial cannulation is possible. Systolic blood pressure should be maintained above 90 mmHg (Lierz and Korbel, 2012).

B. Common anesthetic emergencies and drugs

The prepared team should have written emergency protocols for the following situations. A standardized approach to address emergencies under anesthesia should include reduction of the inhalation anesthetic concentration, assisted ventilation, and administration of an injectable antagonist to reverse the alpha-2 agonist or benzodiazepine component of a ketamine combination anesthetic regimen.

1. Apnea

Confirm a mucus plug is not blocking the trachea or ET (see Section 2, below). Turn off inhalation gas or intravenously inject relevant reversal agents (atipamezole, yohimbine, or flumazenil). Assist-ventilate "bag" 10−20 breaths per minute with 100% oxygen into the trachea by endotracheal tube not to exceed 15−20 cm H2O (Guzman and Beaufrere, 2021).

2. Endotracheal tube blockage

A plugged ET is evidenced by increased respiratory effort and compromised or prolonged exhalation despite air sacs filling with positive pressure ventilation (Guzman and Beaufrere, 2021). Remove and examine the ET and tracheal lumen for a mucous plug or obstruction. Suction trachea if feasible. Replace the ET, assist ventilation with 100% O2, and observe the respiratory cycle.

3. Hypothermia

If body temperature drops below 38°C, increase thermal support and begin IV or IO infusion with warm (38.3−40.5°C) isotonic fluids at 10−20 mL/kg/h (Degernes, 2008; Gunkel and Lafortune, 2005; Lierz and Korbel, 2012).

4. Regurgitation

Hold the head low to drain material away from the glottis. Suction or clean the oral cavity with cotton-tipped applicators or gauze. Suction the ET and trachea if feasible. Place a patent and clean ET in the trachea. Start on antibiotics.

5. Hypotension

First, correct hypothermia if present (Guzman and Beaufrere, 2021). Volume replacement with warm isotonic crystalloid fluids given slowly at 10−20 mL/kg/h until correction of rapid, thready, weak pulse and prolonged capillary refill time. Consider synthetic colloid (e.g., hetastarch at 10 mL/kg IV to effect; typically, over 10−15 minutes) (Degernes, 2008; Gunkel and Lafortune, 2005; Lierz and Korbel, 2012). Dobutamine (CRI at 5−15 μg/kg/min) and dopamine (CRI at 5−10 μg/kg/min) have corrected anesthetic-induced hypotension in Hispaniola parrots (Guzman and Beaufrere, 2021).

6. Cardiac arrest

Turn off the anesthetic vaporizer or administer relevant antagonists (atipamezole, yohimbine, or flumazenil). Endotracheally intubate and assist ventilation ("bag") with 100% oxygen at a frequency of 10−12 breaths per minute, not to exceed 15–20 cm H2O. Administer atropine 0.02–0.5 mg/kg IM, IV, IO, or intratracheally (IT) at 0.5–1 mg/kg and 1:1000 epinephrine IV, IO or IT at 0.5–1.0 mg/kg and attempt 60 lateral sternal compressions per minute (Degernes, 2008; Gunkel and Lafortune, 2005; Guzman and Beaufrere, 2021; Lierz and Korbel, 2012).

7. Hypoglycemia

Preoperative fasting and prolonged anesthetic procedures may contribute to hypoglycemia. While glucose is not routinely monitored intraoperatively, a hand held, human glucometer has been validated to provide rapid and reliable results in domestic pigeons (Mohsenzadeh et al., 2015). Lactated ringers with 2.5% dextrose infused IV or IO at 20 mL/kg/hr will prevent or treat hypoglycemia (Gunkel and Lafortune, 2005).

8. Bradycardia

Reduce anesthetic, if possible, administer 100% oxygen, treat with IV or IO fluids, anticholinergics (atropine 0.02–0.5 mg/kg IM, IV, IO, or IT or glycopyrrolate at 0.01–0.02 mg/kg IM or IV) (Degernes, 2008; Guzman and Beaufrere, 2021).

9. Subcutaneous crepitus

Subcutaneous crepitus is evidence of trauma caused by a ruptured air sac after forceful positive pressure ventilation or a misplaced caudal thoracic air sac cannula. The crepitus alone is usually not life-threatening. The source of sudden appearance of subcutaneous crepitus should be explored intraoperatively especially since it may require correction of placement of an air sac cannula or attention to forceful assisted ventilation greater than 20 cm pressure. The crepitus may resolve over days or require tapping with a needle and syringe (Lee et al., 2011).

VI. Anesthetic recovery

After the anesthetic procedure is completed, attention must be given to patient recovery. Extubate only in the presence of spontaneous breathing and head movement. The benefits and risks of reversing components of anesthetic combinations should carefully be considered. The analgesic, anxiolytic and muscle relaxant benefits of benzodiazepines, alpha-2 agonists and narcotics may be advantageous to retain for promoting a smooth recovery. In cases of prolonged recovery nonresponsive to reversal agents, hypothermia, hypotension, acid-base imbalance, hypoxemia and inadequate pain control should be ruled out (Degernes, 2008).

Birds recovering from anesthesia should be loosely wrapped in a towel or drape to prevent flailing, flapping and injury during recovery especially after use of ketamine. Be careful not to impair sternal and caudal rib cage movement necessary for respirations. Place in lateral recumbency to ease upward motion of the keel and visceral compression of air sacs. Place the bird in a dimly lighted, quiet and warm (25–30°C or 77–86°F) room or a heated incubator supplemented with oxygen especially in cases of hypoventilation.

Provide food and water as soon as fully conscious. Low perches provide safe choices for recovering birds to regain normal postures.

VII. Analgesia

Analgesia includes pharmacologic, physical, environmental, and behavioral management (Machin, 2005a). Birds perceive pain like mammals with nociceptors in the nidopallium, which is analogous to the mammalian pain center in the prefrontal cortex (Gill, 2007; Lierz and Korbel, 2012). The paucity of species-specific pharmacokinetic studies requires the clinician to implement a pharmacodynamic (PD) approach clinically observing for analgesic efficacy (Gill, 2007; Hawkins and Paul-Murphy, 2011; Machin, 2005b). As a prey species, most birds feign well-being even in the presence of pain and disease. Acute pain may be manifested by escape or defense behaviors, vocalization, crouching, closed eyelids, semi- to nonweight bearing, wing droop, immobility and increased blood pressure, heart and respiratory rates. When experiencing chronic pain, birds may have a decreased appetite, weight loss, and demonstrate lethargy, aggression, abnormal posture, guarding behavior, lameness, ruffled feathers and decreased grooming (Gill, 2007; Guzman and Beaufrere; 2021; Lierz and Korbel, 2012; Machin, 2005a). Table 23.4 lists the most commonly used and best studied analgesics used in birds.

A. Multimodal analgesia

Multimodal or balanced analgesia incorporates drugs from different classes to provide pain relief through different mechanisms. If drug synergism occurs, the required dose of individual drugs may be reduced (Guzman and Beaufrere, 2021). Multimodal analgesia is recommended across species, especially to manage moderate to high pain intensity (National Research Council 2010b).

B. Preventive analgesia

Preemptive analgesia using the agents listed below is the standard of care for birds. Birds should never preoperatively have water removed to avoid dehydration and renal toxicity posed especially by nonsteroidal antiinflammatory drugs (NSAID) analgesics (Degernes, 2008).

C. Pharmacologic options

1. Opioids

Opioid drugs mimic the effects of endogenous endorphins, enkephalins, and dynorphins on mu, kappa, and gamma receptors on cell membranes. A lack of published data on opioid receptor distribution in birds, mechanisms of action, and use of opioids beyond butorphanol impedes their informed use by clinicians (Hawkins and Murphy, 2011; Machin, 2015a). Opioids are used to manage moderate-to-severe pain and have minimal cardiopulmonary adverse effects (Guzman and Beaufrere, 2021). When given preemptively, they are MAC-sparing, so lower concentrations of inhalant anesthesia are required (Escobar et al., 2017; Lierz and Korbel, 2012; Guzman and Beaufrere, 2021). Butorphanol may be administered at 5 mg/kg IM with redosing every 2–4 hours. An investigation testing liposomal butorphanol in Hispaniolan parrots demonstrated analgesic efficacy for 3–5 days based on serum levels and thermal antinociceptive foot withdrawal (Gill, 2007; Guzman and Beaufrere, 2021; Sladky et al., 2006).

Carprofen and meloxicam, both cyclooxygenase (COX) inhibitors are the most studied and commonly used NSAIDs in many bird species for managing postsurgical pain. NASIDs prevent the biosynthesis of prostaglandin, decreasing inflammation as described in mammals (Gill, 2007; Guzman and Beaufrere, 2021; Lierz and Korbel, 2012; Machin, 2005a). After the preemptive injectable dose, either drug may easily be delivered postoperatively orally in treats eliminating handling stress associated with injections. Dehydration significantly increases risk of NSAID nephrotoxicity in birds (Hawkins and Paul-Murphy, 2011; Lierz and Korbel, 2012). Flunixin has been reported to be nephrotoxic in Coturnix quail (*Coturnix coturnix*) when given at 0.1 mg/kg for 7 days (Hawkins and Paul-Murphy, 2011). Large-scale mortality of wild vultures in India occurred after consuming diclofenac (NSAID) treated bovine carcasses (Hawkins and Paul-Murphy, 2011). Pharmacokinetic studies of meloxicam, flunixin, and sodium salicylate in chickens, ostriches, mallard ducks, turkeys, and pigeons identified rapid elimination from the body, resulting in highly variable pharmacodynamic results (Hawkins and Paul-Murphy, 2011). NSAIDs, including acetylsalicylic acid, celecoxib, carprofen, flunixin meglumine, ibuprofen, ketoprofen, meloxicam, piroxicam, and phenylbutazone, are listed in Table 23.3 with clinical or experimental evidence of analgesic efficacy in birds.

Tramadol is a synthetic with opioid, adrenergic, and serotonin receptor activity. PK and clinical investigations demonstrate analgesic promise and efficacy of tramadol across species from penguins to peafowl without adverse effect (Guzman et al., 2014; Kilburn et al., 2014; Malik and Valentine, 2018; Black et al., 2010). Tramadol, given orally at 30 mg/kg maintained therapeutic concentrations for 12 hours in Muscovy ducks (Bailey et al., 2019). A thermal antinociception experiment and PK serum levels in Hispaniola parrots demonstrated 6–8 hours of analgesic efficacy at 30 mg/kg PO (Sanchez et al., 2012; Souza et al., 2013).

2. Corticosteroids

Betamethasone (0.04 mg/kg), dexamethasone (0.06 mg/kg), and methylprednisolone (2 mg/kg) have reduced postoperative inflammation in turkeys and chickens. NSAIDs are preferred over corticosteroids in birds considering the potential reversal of analgesic efficacy of endogenous corticosteroids and the risk of immunosuppression (Machin, 2005b).

D. Nonpharmacologic supportive care

Postoperative recovery and animal well-being may be enhanced with supportive care in addition to analgesic drugs. Hydration of postoperative birds demonstrating a reduced interest in drinking and eating may be accomplished by subcutaneous administration of a 10–40 mL/kg body weight bolus of warmed (101–105°F) subcutaneous 2.5%–5% dextrose fluids over the scapula and in the inguinal skin web before the animal fully recovers from anesthesia (Degernes, 2008; Lierz and Korbel, 2012). This may need to be repeated daily depending upon food and water intake. Dehydration will increase the risk of NSAID analgesic toxicity. Maintain IV access via an IO or intravascular catheter protected under bandaging and/or by an Elizabethan collar to maintain hydration and normoglycemia in a debilitated postop patient. Administer 2.5%–5% dextrose-containing fluids delivered at 40–60 mL/kg/day (Miller and Buttrick, 1999).

Provide supplemental humidified and warmed oxygen inside an incubator or via caudal thoracic air sac cannula to enhance the oxygenation of a hypoventilating patient.

Provide fresh food and water daily within easy reach by the bird. Postoperative nursing care may include syringe feeding strained baby food meat or fruit baby food or pediatric cream of wheat to carnivorous, omnivorous, and granivorous birds in addition to electrolyte-balanced rehydration fluids such as Pedialyte. Avoid feeding mealworms or crickets with chitinous exoskeletons risking impaction, especially in a dehydrated bird.

Immobilization of wings with figure 8 bandages or legs with casting will minimize the pain associated with orthopedic or musculoskeletal procedures.

Oral analgesics should be mixed in a preferred treat (e.g., a grape or strawberry, or mouse pink) instead of handling for injection. If antibiotics are required, select palatable oral or sustained-release injectable forms to avoid frequent handling.

VIII. Anesthesia for specific situations

A. Celiotomy

The lack of a diaphragm creates one coelomic cavity, despite the frequent use of the terms thorax and abdomen in avian medicine. The most common reasons to surgically enter the coelomic cavity are to visualize gonads for sexing monomorphic species, biopsy an organ, or implant a radio transmitter. All of these brief (5−10 minutes) procedures may be accomplished via laparoscopy or a small incision on the lateral side of the bird immediately caudal to the ribs. Short-acting general anesthesia using inhalants or reversible chemical agents promotes a rapid recovery, which is especially useful for field work where animals must be returned to their habitat fully recovered to avoid predation and injury. Preoperative administration of an NSAID listed in Table 23.4 manages the potential pain associated with these procedures.

B. Craniotomy

Infiltration of the scalp incision site with bupivacaine or lidocaine as described in Table 23.2 should be considered. Stereotaxic neurosurgery requires the surgeon to have unobstructed access to the cranium. Preventive and postoperative treatment with an analgesic listed in Table 23.4 will manage the potential pain associated with craniotomies without compromising a rapid recovery.

C. Orthopedic

A deeper plane of anesthesia may be required for painful orthopedic surgeries, but appropriate analgesia (including regional anesthesia techniques) should always be provided. Sustained-release analgesics provide the advantage of infrequently handling the postoperative patient.

D. Minor invasive

Surgical procedures not invading the coelomic cavity such as laceration repair, and placement of an IO or caudal thoracic catheter or cannula may be accomplished in a lighter plane of surgical anesthesia enhanced by judicious use of local anesthetics. An NSAID analgesic is the first choice in a well-hydrated bird. Debilitated, potentially dehydrated birds will benefit most from the nonpharmacologic pain and distress-relieving techniques described below.

E. Imaging and sample collection

A light plane of anesthesia accomplished simply by inhalant anesthesia administered by face mask or ketamine and reversible alpha-2 agonists or benzodiazepines by one IM injection is preferred given the frequent repositioning required for blood sample collection, bandaging, and imaging.

F. Neuromuscular blocking agents

Topical application of saline-diluted vecuronium (0.8 mg/mL) without an additional corneal penetrating agent like saponin has been used safely in psittacines with few systemic effects to paralyze the skeletal muscles of the pupil to produce mydriasis to facilitate cataract surgery (Ramer et al., 1996). The combination of topically administered vecuronium (0.16 mg per eye) and 1% atropine and 2.5% phenylephrine produced maximal 6.2 mm pupil dilation with no systemic effects in cormorants (Loerzel et al., 2002). Intravenously dosing isoflurane-anesthetized chickens with atracurium at 0.46 mg/kg experimentally achieved 95% muscle twitch depression in 95% of the birds for up to an hour with small increases in heart rate and blood pressure. The muscle relaxation was reversed with 0.5 mg/kg IV edrophonium (Nicholson and Ilkiw, 1992). The use of neuromuscular blocking drugs in anesthetized birds requires close monitoring of anesthetic depth (i.e., heart rate and blood pressure) and preparedness for respiratory support (Guzman and Beaufrere, 2021). Please refer to Chapter 8 (Neuromuscular Blocking Agents) for a detailed description of monitoring.

G. Field work

Challenges faced with anesthetizing birds in the field include a lack of sophisticated anesthetic delivery and monitoring equipment as well as the requirement to select an anesthetic regimen with a rapid, full recovery. Continuous and attentive monitoring of respiratory rate, reflexes, and muscle relaxation abate the need for elaborate monitoring equipment. A portable pulse oximeter clipped on the wing or leg musculature may continuously display percent blood oxygenation and audibly track heart rate trends. Using either an inhalant anesthetic delivered in a chamber or beak/head mask or an injectable, reversible ketamine and sedative combination hasten a full recovery. A warm, dry, dimly lighted, padded container, such as a small Kritter Keeper™ or appropriately sized sky kennel large enough for

TABLE 23.4 Analgesics.[a]

Drug(s)	mg/kg	Route	Species	Comments	References
Acetylsalicylic acid	5–10	PO	multiple	Minimum 3 days	Machin et al. (2005a) Lierz and Korbel (2012)
Betamethasone	0.1	IM	turkey, chicken	Degenerative hip disorders in turkeys, Uric acid induced arthritis in chickens	Machin et al. (2005a)
Buprenorphine	0.01 –0.05	IM	most species	Effective for 8–12 hours for moderate to severe pain but variable duration of action by species No effect in African Grey parrots	Lierz and Korbel (2012) Machin et al. (2005a)
Buprenorphine	0.25–0.5	IM	pigeon, chicken	5–12 hours analgesia	Hawkins and Paul-Murphy (2011) Malik and Valentine (2018)
Buprenorphine	0.1–0.6	IM	falcon	QID	Guzman and Beaufrere (2021)
Butorphanol	1–3	IM	most species	Opioid drug of choice for moderate to severe pain	Guzman and Beaufrere (2021) Hawkins and Paul-Murphy (2011) Lierz and Korbel (2012) Machin et al. (2005a)
Carprofen	1–4	IM, SC, PO	most species	BID– TID	Hawkins and Paul-Murphy (2011) Lierz and Korbel (2012) Machin et al. (2005a)
Celecoxib	10	PO	most species	SID—treats psittacine proventricular disease for 6–24 weeks	Malik and Valentine (2018)
Fentanyl	0.01 –0.02	IV	African gray parrot	1.3 hours half life	Lierz and Korbel (2012)
Flunixin meglumine	1–5	IM	duck, chicken, pigeon, budgerigar	Muscle necrosis, severe renal toxicity	Hawkins and Paul-Murphy (2011)
Gabapentin	10–11		cockatoo, falcon	SID-BID	Malik and Valentine (2018)
Hydromorphone	0.1–0.3	IM	falcon	Every 3–6 hours	Guzman and Beaufrere (2021)
Ketoprofen	1–5	IM, SC	quail, chicken, duck, budgerigar	SID–TID Renal tubular necrosis in budgerigars dosed at 2.5 mg/kg SID x 7	Hawkins and Paul-Murphy (2011) Lierz and Korbel (2012) Machin et al. (2005a)
Ibuprofen	5–10	PO	not given	BID—TID, pediatric syrup	Machin et al. (2005a)
Meloxicam	1	PO	domestic duck	Analgesia for arthritis animal model	Bailey et al. (2019)
Meloxicam	2	IM, PO	pigeon	IM followed by PO BID analgesia for orthopedic- osteotomy research	Desmarchelier et al. (2012)

Continued

TABLE 23.4 Analgesics.[a]—cont'd

Drug(s)	mg/kg	Route	Species	Comments	References
Meloxicam	1−1.5	IM, PO	psittacine	BID	Guzman and Beaufrere (2021)
Meloxicam	0.3−0.5	IM, IV, PO	most species	SID− BID− NSAID of choice Renal glomerular congestion in budgerigars dosed SID at 0.1 mg/kg × 7 days	Hawkins and Paul-Murphy (2011) Lierz and Korbel (2012)
Nalbuphine	12.5	IM	Hispaniolan amazon parrot	3 hours analgesia	Hawkins and Paul-Murphy (2011)
Piroxicam	0.5−1.0	PO	psittacine	BID for chronic osteoarthritis	Machin et al. (2005a) Malik and Valentine (2018)
Prednisolone	7	PO	multiple	Antiinflammatory	Machin et al. (2005a)
Tramadol	5−30	PO	domestic duck, Hispaniolan parrot, peafowl, hawk, eagle	Analgesia for arthritis animal model 6 hours of analgesia for foot withdrawal in antinociception model	Bailey et al. (2019) Guzman and Beaufrere (2021) Black et al. (2010) Malik and Valentine (2018)
Tramadol	5	PO	American kestrel	Foot withdrawal in antinociception model	Guzman et al. (2014)

[a]*IM, intramuscular;* IV, *intravenous;* PO, *oral;* SC, *subcutaneous.*

the bird to stand with a visual access helps the anesthetist realize when a fully recovered bird may safely be released to the wild.

References

Araghi, M., Azizi, S., Vesal, N., Dalir-Naghade, B., 2016. Evaluation of the sedative effects of diazepam, midazolam, and xylazine after intranasal administration in juvenile ostriches (*Struthio camelus*). J. Avian Med. Surg. 30 (3), 221−226.

Bailey, R.S., Sheldon, J.D., Allender, M.C., Adkesson, M.J., Chinnadurai, S.K., 2019. Analgesic efficacy of tramadol compared with meloxicam in ducks (*Cairina moschata domestica*) evaluated by ground-reactive forces. J. Avian Med. Surg. 33 (2), 133−140.

Bhavsar, D., Shettko, D., Tenenhaus, M., 2010. Encircling the tendon repair site with collagen-GAG reduces the formation of postoperative tendon adhesions in a chicken flexor tendon model. J. Surg. Res. 159 (2), 765−771.

Black, P.A., Cox, S.K., Macek, M., Tieber, A., Junge, R.E., 2010. Pharmacokinetics of tramadol hydrochloride and its metabolite O-desmethyltramadol in peafowl (*Pavo cristatus*). J. Zoo Wildl. Med. 41 (4), 671−676.

Boxenbaum, H., 1982. Interspecies scaling, allometry, physiological time, and the ground plan of pharmacokinetics. J. Pharmacokinet. Biopharm. 10 (2), 201−227.

Ciboto, R., Cortopassi, S.R.G., Lopes, M.A.E., Carvalho, R.C., Baitelo, C.G., 2006. Comparison of chemical restraint techniques in ostrich (*Struthio camelus*). Braz. J. Poult. Sci. 8, 119−123.

Degernes, L., 2008. Anesthesia for companion birds. Compendium 30 (10), 1−11.

Desmarchelier, M., Troncy, E., Fitzgerald, G., Lair, S., 2012. Analgesic effects of meloxicam administration on postoperative orthopedic pain in domestic pigeons (*Columba livia*). Am. J. Vet. Res. 73 (3), 361−367.

Dorrestein, G.M., 1991. The pharmacokinetics of avian therapeutics. Vet. Clin. Small Anim. Pract. 21 (6), 1241−1264.

Dorrestein, G.M., Miert, A.V., 1988. Pharmacotherapeutic aspects of medication of birds. J. Vet. Pharmacol. Therapeut. 11 (1), 33−44.

Duncker, H.R., 1972. Structure of avian lungs. Respir. Physiol. 14 (1−2), 44−63.

Durrani, U.F., Ashraf, M., Khan, M.A., 2009. A comparison of the clinical effects associated with xylazine, ketamine, and a xylazine-ketamine cocktail in pigeons (*Columba livia*). Turk. J. Vet. Anim. Sci. 33 (5), 413−417.

Durrani, U.F., Mahmood, A.K., Shahid, A., Iqbal, Z., Waqas, M., Imran, S., Hussain, R., 2014. Comparative study on sedative and anesthetic effects of Xylazine, Ketamine and Xylazine-Ketamine Combination in quails (*Coturnix coturnix*). IOSR J. Agric. Vet. Sci. 7 (6), 29−33.

Escobar, A., da Rocha, R.W., Midon, M., de Almeida, R.M., Zangirolami Filho, D., Werther, K., 2017. Effects of tramadol on the minimum anesthetic concentration of isoflurane in white-eyed parakeets (Psittacara leucophthalmus). J. Zoo Wildl. Med. 48 (2), 380−387.

Fair, J.M., Paul, E., Jones, J., 2010. Guidelines to the Use of Wild Birds in Research.

Gill, F.B., 2007. Ornithology. W.H. Freeman and Company, New York.

Gunkel, C., Lafortune, M., October 2005. Current techniques in avian anesthesia. Seminars in Avian and Exotic Pet Medicine, Vol. 14, No. 4. WB Saunders, pp. 263–276.

Guzman, D.S.M., Beaufrère, H., 2021. Avian pain management and anesthesia. Exotic Anim. Emerg. Crit. Care Medicine 488–502.

Guzman, D.S.M., Drazenovich, T.L., Olsen, G.H., Willits, N.H., Paul-Murphy, J.R., 2014. Evaluation of thermal antinociceptive effects after oral administration of tramadol hydrochloride to American kestrels (*Falco sparverius*). Am. J. Vet. Res. 75 (2), 117–123.

Hawkins, M.G., Paul-Murphy, J., 2011. Avian analgesia. Vet. Clin. Exotic Anim. Pract. 14 (1), 61–80.

Hawkins, M.G., Malka, S., Pascoe, P.J., Solano, A.M., Kass, P.H., Ohmura, H., Jones, J.H., 2013. Evaluation of the effects of dorsal versus lateral recumbency on the cardiopulmonary system during anesthesia with isoflurane in red-tailed hawks (*Buteo jamaicensis*). Am. J. Vet. Res. 74 (1), 136–143.

Henry, K.S., Neilans, E.G., Abrams, K.S., Idrobo, F., Carney, L.H., 2016. Neural correlates of behavioral amplitude modulation sensitivity in the budgerigar midbrain. J. Neurophysiol. 115 (4), 1905–1916.

Henry, K.S., Abrams, K.S., Forst, J., Mender, M.J., Neilans, E.G., Idrobo, F., Carney, L.H., 2017. Midbrain synchrony to envelope structure supports behavioral sensitivity to single-formant vowel-like sounds in noise. J. Assoc. Res. Otolaryngol. 18 (1), 165–181.

Houben, R., Antonissen, G., Croubels, S., Backer, P.D., Devreese, M., 2016. Pharmacokinetics of drugs in avian species and the applications and limitations of dose extrapolation. Vlaams Diergeneeskundig Tijdschrift 85 (3), 124–132.

Hunter, R.P., Isaza, R., 2008. Concepts and issues with interspecies scaling in zoological pharmacology. J. Zoo Wildl. Med. 39 (4), 517–526.

Jaensch, S.M., Cullen, L., Raidal, S.R., 2001. Comparison of endotracheal, caudal thoracic air sac, and clavicular air sac administration of isoflurane in sulphur-crested cockatoos (*Cacatua galerita*). J. Avian Med. Surg. 15 (3), 170–177.

Jaensch, S.M., Cullen, L., Raidal, S.R., 2002. Air sac functional anatomy of the sulphur-crested cockatoo (*Cacatua galerita*) during isoflurane anesthesia. J. Avian Med. Surg. 16 (1), 2–9.

James Jr., A.E., Hutchins, G., Bush, R.M., Natarajan, T.K., Burns, B., 1976. How birds breathe: correlation of radiographic with anatomical and pathological studies. J. Am. Vet. Radiol. Soc. 17, 77–86.

Jiang, W., Wang, P., Wan, Y., Xin, D., Fan, M., 2015. A simple method for establishing an ostrich model of femoral head osteonecrosis and collapse. J. Orthop. Surg. Res. 10 (1), 1–10.

Kilburn, J.J., Cox, S.K., Kottyan, J., Wack, A.N., Bronson, E., 2014. Pharmacokinetics of tramadol and its primary metabolite O-desmethyltramadol in African penguins (*Spheniscus demersus*). J. Zoo Wildl. Med. 45 (1), 93–99.

Korschgen, C.E., Kenow, K.P., Gendron-Fitzpatrick, A., Green, W.L., Dein, F.J., 1996. Implanting intra-abdominal radiotransmitters with external whip antennas in ducks. J. Wildl. Manag. 132–137.

Langan, J.N., Ramsay, E.C., Blackford, J.T., Schumacher, J., 2000. Cardiopulmonary and sedative effects of intramuscular medetomidine-ketamine and intravenous propofol in ostriches (*Struthio camelus*). J. Avian Med. Surg. 14 (1), 2–7.

Lee, A., Lennox, A., 2016. Sedation and local anesthesia as an alternative to general anesthesia in 3 birds. J. Exot. Pet Med. 25 (2), 100–105.

Lee, S.Y., Kim, H.J., Kim, J.W., 2011. Deflation treatment for subcutaneous emphysema in a Goffin Cockatoo (Cacatua goffini). J. Vet. Clin. 28 (5), 519–521.

Lennox, A.M., 2011. Sedation as an alternative to general anesthesia in pet birds. In: Proc Annu Conf Assoc Avian Vet, pp. 289–292.

Lierz, M., Korbel, R., 2012. Anesthesia and analgesia in birds. J. Exot. Pet Med. 21 (1), 44–58.

Loerzel, S.M., Smith, P.J., Howe, A., Samuelson, D.A., 2002. Vecuronium bromide, phenylephrine and atropine combinations as mydriatics in juvenile double-crested cormorants (*Phalacrocorax auritus*). Vet. Ophthalmol. 5 (3), 149–154.

Machin, K.L., October 2005a. Avian analgesia. Seminars in Avian and Exotic Pet Medicine, Vol. 14, No. 4. WB Saunders, pp. 236–242.

Machin, K.L., 2005b. Controlling avian pain. Compendium April 27, 299–307.

Mahmud, M.A., Shaba, P., Yisa, H.Y., Gana, J., Ndagimba, R., Ndagi, S., 2014. Comparative efficacy of Diazepam, Ketamine, and Diazepam-Ketamine combination for sedation or anesthesia in cockerel chickens. J. Adv. Vet. Anim. Res. 1 (3), 107–113.

Malik, A., Valentine, A., 2018. Pain in birds: a review for veterinary nurses. Vet. Nurs. J. 33 (1), 11–25.

Mama, K.R., Phillips Jr., L.G., Pascoe, P.J., 1996. Use of propofol for induction and maintenance of anesthesia in a barn owl (*Tyto alba*) undergoing tracheal resection. J. Zoo Wildl. Med. 27, 397–401.

Mans, C., 2014. Sedation of pet birds. J. Exot. Pet Med. 23 (2), 152–157.

McKechnie, A.E., Freckleton, R.P., Jetz, W., 2006. Phenotypic plasticity in the scaling of avian basal metabolic rate. Proc. Biol. Sci. 273 (1589), 931–937.

Miller, W., Buttrick, M., 1999. Current anesthesia recommendations for companion birds. Iowa State University Veterinarian 61 (2), 3.

Mohsenzadeh, M.S., Zaeemi, M., Razmyar, J., Azizzadeh, M., 2015. Comparison of a point-of-care glucometer and a laboratory auto-analyzer for measurement of blood glucose concentrations in domestic pigeons (*Columba livia domestica*). J. Avian Med. Surg. 29 (3), 181–186.

National Research Council, 2010a. Guide for the Care and Use of Laboratory Animals.

National Research Council, 2010b. Recognition and Alleviation of Pain in Laboratory Animals.

Nicholson, A., Ilkiw, J.E., 1992. Neuromuscular and cardiovascular effects of atracurium in isoflurane-anesthetized chickens. Am. J. Vet. Res. 53 (12), 2337–2342.

Nilson, P.C., Teramitsu, I., White, S.A., 2005. Caudal thoracic air sac cannulation in zebra finches for isoflurane anesthesia. J. Neurosci. Methods 143 (2), 107–115.

Perrin, K.L., Nielsen, J.B., Thomsen, A.F., Bertelsen, M.F., 2017. Alfaxalone anesthesia in the Bengalese finch (Lonchura domestica). J. Zoo Wildl. Med. 48 (4), 1146–1153.

Pierre, C.L.S., Desprez, I., Chang, S., Machin, K., Ambros, B., 2021. Effect of preoxygenation before isoflurane induction and rocuronium-induced apnea on time until hemoglobin desaturation in domestic chickens (Gallus gallus domesticus). Vet. Anaesth. Analg. 48, 524–531.

Prather, J.F., 2012. Rapid and reliable sedation induced by diazepam and antagonized by flumazenil in zebra finches (*Taeniopygia guttata*). J. Avian Med. Surg. 26 (2), 76–84.

Pytte, C.L., Ficken, M.S., Moiseff, A., 2004. Ultrasonic singing by the blue-throated hummingbird: a comparison between production and perception. J. Comp. Physiol. 190 (8), 665–673.

Ramer, J.C., Paul-Murphy, J., Brunson, D., Murphy, C.J., 1996. Effects of mydriatic agents in cockatoos, African gray parrots, and blue-fronted Amazon parrots. J. Am. Vet. Med. Assoc. 208 (2), 227–230.

Romano, J., Hasse, K., Johnston, M., 2020. Sedative, cardiorespiratory, and thermoregulatory effects of alfaxalone on budgerigars (*Melopsittacus undulatus*). J. Zoo Wildl. Med. 51 (1), 96–101.

Sanchez-Migallon Guzman, D., Souza, M.J., Braun, J.M., Cox, S.K., Keuler, N.S., Paul-Murphy, J.R., 2012. Antinociceptive effects after oral administration of tramadol hydrochloride in Hispaniolan Amazon parrots (*Amazona ventralis*). Am. J. Vet. Res. 73 (8), 1148–1152.

Sayce, L.J., Powell, M.E., Kimball, E.E., Chen, P., Gartling, G.J., Rousseau, B., 2020. Continuous rate infusion of ketamine hydrochloride and dexmedetomidine for maintenance of anesthesia during laryngotracheal surgery in New Zealand white rabbits (*Oryctolagus cuniculus*). J. Am. Assoc. Lab. Anim. Sci. 59 (2), 176–185.

Schmitt, P.M., Göbel, T., Trautvetter, E., 1998. Evaluation of pulse oximetry as a monitoring method in avian anesthesia. J. Avian Med. Surg. 12, 91–99.

Schnellbacher, R., Comolli, J., 2020. Constant rate infusions in exotic animals. J. Exot. Pet Med. 35, 50–57.

Sladky, K.K., Krugner-Higby, L., Meek-Walker, E., Heath, T.D., Paul-Murphy, J., 2006. Serum concentrations and analgesic effects of liposome-encapsulated and standard butorphanol tartrate in parrots. Am. J. Vet. Res. 67 (5), 775–781.

Souza, M.J., Gerhardt, L., Cox, S., 2013. Pharmacokinetics of repeated oral administration of tramadol hydrochloride in Hispaniolan Amazon parrots (*Amazona ventralis*). Am. J. Vet. Res. 74 (7), 957–962.

Strick, M.J., Filan, S.L., Hile, M., McKenzie, C., Walsh, W.R., Tonkin, M.A., 2004. Adhesion formation after flexor tendon repair: a histologic and biomechanical comparison of 2-and 4-strand repairs in a chicken model. J. Hand Surg. 29 (1), 15–21.

Troy, K.L.R., Lundberg, H.J., Conzemius, M.G., Brown, T.D., 2007. Habitual hip joint activity level of the penned EMU (Dromaius novaehollandie). Iowa Orthop. J. 27, 17.

Virtanen, R., 1989. Pharmacological profiles of medetomidine and its antagonist, atipamezole. Acta Vet. Scand. Suppl. 85, 29–37.

Wang, Y., Abrams, K.S., Carney, L.H., Henry, K.S., 2021. Midbrain-level neural correlates of behavioral tone-in-noise detection: dependence on energy and envelope cues. J. Neurosci. 41 (34), 7206–7223.

West, J.B., 2009. Comparative physiology of the pulmonary blood-gas barrier: the unique avian solution. Am. J. Physiol. Regul. Integr. Comp. Physiol. 297 (6), R1625–R1634.

West, J.B., Watson, R.R., Fu, Z., 2006. The honeycomb-like structure of the bird lung allows a uniquely thin blood-gas barrier. Respir. Physiol. Neurobiol. 152 (1), 115–118.

Wilson, D., Pettifer, G.R., 2004. Anesthesia case of the month. Mallard undergoing phacoemulsification of a cataract. J. Am. Vet. Med. Assoc. 225 (5), 685–688.

Woronecki, P.P., Dolbeer, R.A., Seamans, T.W., 1990. Use of alpha-chloralose to remove waterfowl from nuisance and damage situations. Proceedings of the Vertebrate Pest Conference Vol. 14, No. 14.

Further reading

Bloomfield, T.C., Gentner, T.Q., Margoliash, D., 2011. What birds have to say about language. Nat. Neurosci. 14 (8), 947–948.

Graham, J.E., July 2004. Approach to the dyspneic avian patient. Seminars in Avian and Exotic Pet Medicine, Vol. 13, No. 3. WB Saunders, pp. 154–159.

Machin, K.L., Caulkett, N.A., 1999. Cardiopulmonary effects of propofol infusion in canvasback ducks (*Aythya valisineria*). J. Avian Med. Surg. 13, 167–172.

McKechnie, A.E., 2008. Phenotypic flexibility in basal metabolic rate and the changing view of avian physiological diversity: a review. J. Comp. Physiol. B 178 (3), 235–247.

Woronecki, P.P., Dolbeer, R.A., Seamans, T.W., Lance, W.R., 1992. Alpha-chloralose efficacy in capturing nuisance waterfowl and pigeons and current status of FDA registration. Proceedings of the Vertebrate Pest Conference Vol. 15, No. 15.

Yu, P.H., Hsiao, Y.T., 2019. Delayed evoked potentials in zebra finch (*Taeniopygia guttata*) under midazolam-butorphanol-isoflurane anesthesia. PeerJ 7, e7937.

Chapter 24

Anesthesia and analgesia in reptiles

Catherine J.A. Williams[1,2] **and Mads F. Bertelsen**[3]

[1]*Zoophysiology, Department of Biology, Aarhus University, Aarhus, Denmark;* [2]*Department of Biomedical Sciences, Ontario Veterinary College, University of Guelph, Guelph, ON, Canada;* [3]*Center for Zoo and Wild Animal Health, Copenhagen Zoo, Copenhagen, Denmark*

Chapter outline

Anesthesia and Analgesia in Laboratory Animals. https://doi.org/10.1016/B978-0-12-822215-7.00009-3

I. Introduction

This chapter is intended as a concise review of reptilian species in common laboratory use. For more detailed information and a wider species range, readers are directed to (Doss et al., 2021; Doss and Sladky, 2021; Schnellbacher et al., 2019) and for a wider formulary to (Klaphake et al., 2018).

A. Brief review of current species used in research

Reptiles (here read as nonavian reptiles) are an extremely diverse, speciose group of taxa that have evolved over a 300 million-year period from the sauropsid lineage, with birds diverging from crocodilians 240 million years ago (mya). The lineage that led to mammals (synapsids) diverged from sauropsids between 320 and 315 mya. Across extant reptile diversity, there are similarities: reptiles are (i) scaled amniotes, (ii) display primarily poikilothermy (reliance on external sources to set body temperature), (iii) possess a relatively low metabolic rate 5–10 times lower than that of a mammal at the same body temperature, and (iv) reproduce independent of water due to the formation of a resilient egg or live birth after internal fertilization. These features have relevance for their anesthesia—specifically considerations of metabolic rate and the cardio-respiratory system that supports it. Reptiles' long evolutionary trajectory and the diversity of extant species underline that despite these similarities there is likely to be a wide range of physiologies and anatomies that impact on their anesthesia in terms of drug pharmacokinetics and pharmacology.

Reptiles are usually divided (Fig. 24.1) into (i) Squamata: comprising the single extant Rhynchocephalian (*Sphenodon,* the tuatara), over 7000 species of extant lizards, and over 3900 species of snake (Tonini et al., 2016). (ii) Chelonia: 348–361 extant species comprising side-necked (Pleurodira) and soft shell, marine and freshwater turtles (collected under Cryptodira) (Thomson et al., 2021; Uetz, 2021). (iii) Crocodilia: 24–26 extant species (IUCN Crocodile Specialist Group, n.d.; Uetz, 2021).

B. Squamates

Squamates (lizards and snakes) have diversified to establish niches in all continents except Antarctica, including burrowing, semiaquatic, terrestrial, and arboreal forms. Their body size varies from the miniaturized chameleon *Brookesia nano* at 13–30 mm snout-vent length to 1.5 m in the Komodo dragon (*Varanus komodoensis*) or more than 6 m in the reticulated python (*Malayopython reticulatus*), and multiple species have evolved limb loss. Squamates form the vast majority of extant reptilians, and several species are common in laboratory science. These species have been historically amenable to laboratory management, available through the pet trade, or of specific interest due to their natural history. Specific charismatic species such as *Varanus* spp. and venomous species, which are not routinely managed in a laboratory setting, have also often been studied in the context of non-laboratory captive collections. In the field, ecological or ecophysiological studies of wild squamates have taken place in e.g., fence lizards, anoles, and garter snakes. Of the Iguania, the green anole (*Anolis carolinensis*) has been commonly used in laboratory studies of reproductive behavior and morphology and was the first reptile to have a reported genome sequence, and use of CRISPR technology (Alföldi et al., 2011; Lovern et al., 2004; Rasys et al., 2019b). The green iguana (*Iguana iguana*) has also been commonly studied historically, e.g., (Moberly, 1968; Wang et al., 1997). The feeding behavior of pythons (*Python* spp.) as well as their invasive status in some of their modern range for large species such as *Python bivittatus* (Card et al., 2018; Larsen, 2016; Wang and Rindom, 2021) and seasonal endothermy of tegus, *Salvator merianae* (Tattersall et al., 2016), have made them study species in comparative physiology (Burggren et al., 2014). Venomous snakes such as *Crotalus* spp. (rattlesnakes) are used in toxicology and physiology (Filogonio et al., 2020; Gracheva et al., 2010; Nielsen et al., 2019). The reproductive behavior of garter snakes (*Thamnophis* spp.) has made them important reptilian endocrinology study species (Friesen et al., 2016; Palacios et al., 2012). Rat snakes (*Pantherophis* spp.), e.g., the corn snake, are commonly used in herpetology teaching (O'Rourke et al., 2018), while the regenerative capacity of, e.g., leopard geckos (*Eublepharis macularius)* makes them of biomedical interest e.g., (Peacock et al., 2015; Vickaryous and Gilbert, 2019). The recent surge of genetic information available in squamates will have an increased impact in terms of a more diverse range of reptiles being amenable to genetic studies, and therefore their increased presence in research.

C. Chelonia

Turtles (Chelonia) inhabit freshwater and marine habitats over a wide range of latitudes, and are also one of the clades of vertebrates most vulnerable to extinction, with ¾ of species current listed as being at serious risk (Thomson et al., 2021). Chelonians have been widely studied in comparative in vivo physiology (e.g., the red-eared slider *Trachemys scripta*, the painted turtle *Chrysemys picta,* and the box turtle *Terrapene* spp.) for their hypoxia and temperature tolerance (Bickler and Buck, 2007; Overgaard et al., 2002; Warren and Jackson, 2008), with knock-on utility as durable ex vivo preparations for the study of basic neurophysiology (Wright and Wessel, 2017). Red-footed tortoises form a large part of the growing literature on reptilian cognition (Wilkinson and Huber, 2012), while marine species have usually been studied in the context of their conservation priority and ecology.

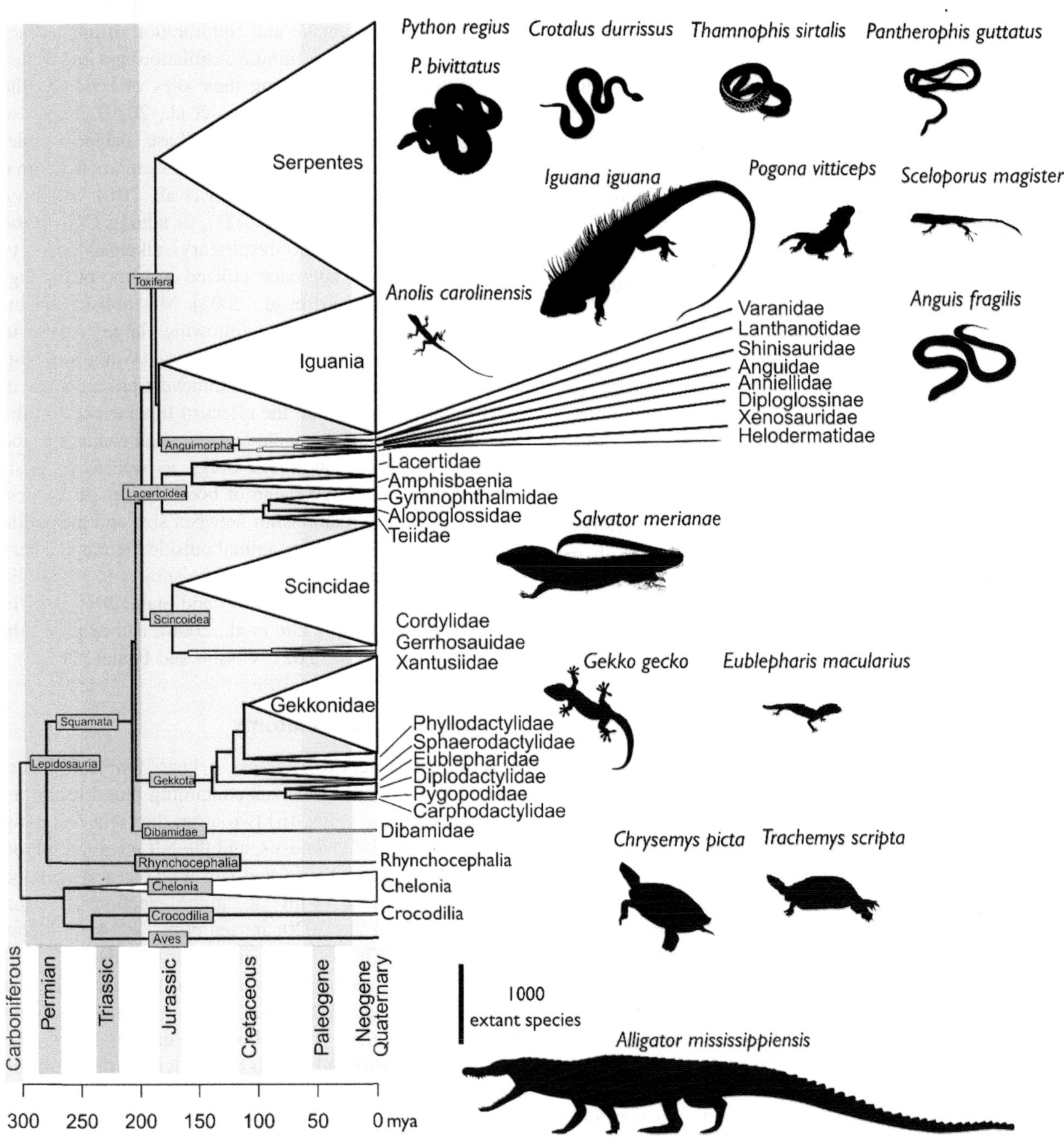

FIGURE 24.1 A phylogeny of extant reptiles (tree as per (Zheng and Wiens, 2016)) over geological time. Tip width is proportional to the number of extant species (Uetz, 2021), and silhouettes (not to scale) are provided for common laboratory species (source phylopic.com, or by CW from silhouettes from CC BY acknowledged photographers). Silhouettes from *top to bottom* and *left to right*, snakes: python species (ball and Burmese), rattlesnake species, garter snakes, rat snakes (here exemplified by the corn snake), lizards: green anole, green iguana, bearded dragon, fence lizard, slow worm, tegu, tokay gecko and leopard gecko, turtles: painted turtle and red eared slider, crocodilians: the American alligator. *Figure was created using R Studio Team (2015) and (Revell, 2012).*

D. Crocodylia

Crocodilians are apex predators usually with an ambush predatory strategy at the water/land transition over estuarine and freshwater habitats across the tropics, where half of the species are listed as vulnerable to extinction or critically endangered (IUCN Crocodile Specialist Group, n.d.). Historically, the most commonly used species in laboratory science is the American alligator (*Alligator mississippiensis*), due to their relatively good temperament, funding for research, and ease of access (Axelsson et al., 1989; Axelsson and Franklin, 2011; Conner et al., 2019; Seebacher and Franklin, 2004; Skovgaard et al., 2016). However, there is interest in comparative anatomy (Monticelli et al., 2019), ecology, physiology (Findsen et al., 2018; Gräns et al., 2010; Stegmann et al., 2017), and cognition (Reber et al., 2021; Tisdale et al., 2018) among a broader range of crocodilians, which leads to requirements for their safe handling, sedation, and anesthesia.

II. Reptilian anatomy and physiology of anesthetic and analgesic relevance

Readers are directed to the comparative anatomical and physiological literature for more comprehensive descriptions and general anatomy. Reptiles have resilient physiologies, which have historically been exploited by immobilization protocols that rely on their relative robustness to hypoxia and cold tolerance. However, in the last 30 years, protocols tailored to reptilian physiologies have been developed, optimizing anesthesia and analgesia, with the aim of not only improving the welfare of reptiles under laboratory care but also the quality of scientific data produced.

A. Ectothermy

All physiological processes are temperature dependent. Reptiles usually rely on behavioral responses and external conditions to provide internal body temperatures—they are ectothermic poikilotherms. Very large individual species are able to maintain higher body temperatures than their surroundings due to a lower surface area to volume ratio and therefore lower loss of metabolic heat production to the environment, e.g., in leatherback turtles and large crocodilians, while endothermy can be found seasonally in the tegu and some species of python can raise their body temperature through muscle action, e.g., when surrounding and incubating eggs (Alexander, 2018; Paladino et al., 1990; Tattersall et al., 2016). Reptilian ectothermy means that it is essential to know and maintain a species' normal/preferred body temperature (often referred to as the POTZ or preferred optimal temperature zone) under anesthesia and during recovery. The uptake, dose requirement, and elimination of anesthetics and analgesics as well as heart and respiratory rate and healing will be very sensitive to variations within normal "room temperature" or between laboratory or field habitat conditions and an unheated or uncooled anesthetic station (Kischinovsky et al., 2013; Preston et al., 2010; Stegmann et al., 2017; Williams et al., 2020). Reptiles also have metabolic rates that, even when held at the same temperature as an endotherm, are 5–10 times lower, mainly due to mitochondrial processes (Nagy, 2005; Ruben, 1995). As cardiac output and minute ventilation usually match metabolic needs, this will in particular slow the uptake and equilibration of inhaled anesthetics, which rely on minute ventilation and cardiovascular distribution for reaching their sites of action in the central nervous system (Williams et al., 2020). This also means that maintaining, e.g., acid-base balance under anesthesia relies on matching ectotherm ventilation (normal veterinary practice, e.g., (Bertelsen et al., 2014; Jakobsen et al., 2017; Williams et al., 2021), or adding CO_2 to the inhaled gas to prevent respiratory alkalosis due to overventilation—an approach utilized in some physiological studies (Overgaard et al., 2002). Metabolism can increase by up to 5 times following large meals in infrequently fed species such as pythons (Wang and Rindom, 2021), therefore fasting recommendations are made in order to take into account the effect of this increase on the animal under anesthesia, including potential changes to the pharmacokinetics of anesthetic drugs, as well as on postprandial data. The large range of body masses of reptiles, and the allometric relationship between size and metabolic rate means that dosages for animal outside the range where the dose has been reported should be subject to metabolic scaling e.g., for the theory (Divers and Stahl, 2019; Martin and Sedgwick, 1994; White et al., 2006), and examples in practice (Freitag et al., 2021; Olsson and Phalen, 2012a).

B. Cardiovascular anatomy

Noncrocodilian reptiles possess a heart that comprises: (i) a contractile sinus venosus containing blood returning from the systemic veins, (ii) two atria: the right receiving blood from the sinus venosus, and the left receiving blood from the pulmonary veins, and (iii) a single, trabeculated (spongy) ventricle with a high ejection fraction (Abramochkin et al., 2020; Jensen et al., 2014; Williams et al., 2019a). The ventricle is to varying degrees subdivided into the cavum pulmonale, on the right, and the cavum venosus and arteriosus, on the left. Blood leaving the ventricle enters the pulmonary arteries (from the cavum pulmonale) and the right and left aortas from the cavum arteriosus. However, because the barrier between these ventricular subchambers is incomplete, (i) pulmonary and systemic pressures are equal in most noncrocodilian reptiles (Joyce et al., 2016), and (ii) blood can shunt intraventricularly, depending on the relative resistance of the pulmonary arteries and the aortae. This cardiac shunt can be either one of, or a mixture of, a right-to-left shunt, where deoxygenated systemic venous blood recirculates into the systemic system, bypassing the lungs, or left-to-right shunt, where oxygenated blood returns to the pulmonary circuit, bypassing the body. The degree of this intraventricular shunt is regulated by the autonomic nervous system in the conscious reptile, e.g., a resting small degree of the right-to-left shunt, with decreased right-to-left shunt, or overt left-to-right shunt during breathing bouts or exercise (Burggren et al., 2020). Intraventricular shunting will vary under anesthesia with anesthetic depth, temperature, hypoxia, and the action of the anesthetic on the vascular resistance (e.g., systemic vasodilation under isoflurane leading to large right-to-left shunts (Greunz et al., 2018)). Pythons and varanid lizards have more complete functional systolic separation of the ventricle, allowing separation of systemic and pulmonary pressures (Jensen et al., 2010; Millard and Johansen, 1974). This intraspecific difference has implications for inhaled anesthesia, as right-to-left shunts delay the equilibration of inhaled anesthesia (Williams et al., 2020), and therefore the measured concentration of inhaled anesthetic required in a species may depend on its degree of ventricular separation (Kristensen et al., 2022; Larouche, 2019). This also means that modifying the extent of the right-to-left shunt can aid in the uptake and equilibration of the anesthetic. This can be done using atropine to reduce pulmonary constriction (Greunz et al., 2018; Kristensen et al., 2022), or by increasing sympathetic tone in recovery from nonsurgical anesthesia e.g., by adrenaline or acupuncture (Gatson et al., 2017; Goe et al., 2016).

1. Crocodilian cardiovascular anatomy

Crocodilian hearts have complete ventricular separation, and thus possess two atria and two ventricles with no *intraventricular* shunting. There are two aortae (the left emerging from the right ventricle and mainly serving the gut, and the right aorta from the left ventricle serving the caudal tissue mass as the dorsal aorta). The pulmonary trunk also emerges from the right ventricle via a complex valve system with passive and active (cog tooth) components (Axelsson and Franklin, 2011). The left aorta can be filled from the right aorta (and therefore from the left ventricle) via the foramen of Panizza (a small smooth-muscle-controlled opening between the two aortae). This produces a 'no shunt' condition as right ventricular flow fills the pulmonary trunk. This is the case when under high sympathetic tone, the systemic pressure is high and the pulmonary conus cog-tooth valve is open. However, under conditions of low sympathetic tone, e.g., at rest, there is low systemic blood pressure, and right ventricular pressure exceeds systemic arterial pressure, also there is increased pulmonary resistance due to the increased resistance at the cog-tooth valve. Then, the left aortic valve opens, and there is a right-to-left shunt (Axelsson et al., 1989). There is also communication between the two aortae at the anastomosis, a muscular vessel under vasoactive regulation, caudal to the heart and cranial to the gut. The relevance of this complex cardiovascular anatomy for the anesthetist is that, as with noncrocodilian reptiles, right-to-left shunting that bypasses the lungs, will slow uptake and equilibration of inhaled gas anesthetics and changes in shunting under anesthesia will change the pharmacokinetics of the anesthesia (Williams et al., 2020).

C. Respiratory anatomy and physiology

Moving from rostral to caudal in the respiratory system, the glottis is located immediately caudal to the tongue, and is easily visualized in most snakes and lizards (Fig. 24.2). In chelonians, it can be obscured by a broader fleshy tongue, but may usually be lifted by mild external pressure under the ventral gular region. In crocodilians, the palatal flap (*velum palati*) has to be moved aside from its normal position to visualize the glottis. Usually, the velum apposes the gular fold to form a water-tight seal during diving behavior. Visualizing the glottis and intubation usually requires deep sedation in both chelonians and crocodilians, as well as the use of gags to ensure the safety of the operator, and stress reduction for the animal. The trachea can possess incomplete rings of cartilage (snakes and lizards) or complete rings (turtles and crocodilians), and the tracheal mucosa is delicate and liable to scarring, so uncuffed ET tubes (or modified feeding tubes or iv catheters depending on animal size) are used, except when underwater experimentation is required (Harms et al., 2009). The tracheal length is also variable—bronchial division is high in many chelonian species and care and short e.g., Cole tubes, are used to minimize the chance of damage and subsequent tracheal fibrosis. Lung anatomy is variable among reptiles (Cieri and Farmer, 2016; Perry, 1989) from more 'simple' single compartment lungs in geckos to multi-cameral unidirectional flow lungs in, e.g., crocodilians. In general—the gas exchange surface is across shallow faveoli rather than alveoli, and the diffusive barrier of the faveoli to red blood cells in reptiles is wider than in mammals and birds. Reptilian lungs are more highly compliant than those of mammals or birds, i.e., a greater volume change per unit change in airway pressure (Perry and Duncker, 1980; Williams et al., 2021). The gas exchange surface is also often limited to areas within the respiratory tree, e.g., the cranial half of a snake lung, while one lung may be very reduced, e.g., loss or vestigial remains of the left lung in most snakes (Soldt et al., 2015), and loss of the right lung in amphisbaena lizards (Perry, 1983). In some species, there is proven unidirectional movement of air during normal breathing (Cieri and Farmer, 2016), which is not maintained under mechanical ventilation under anesthesia. The absence of a diaphragm is common to all noncrocodilian reptiles, and different taxa use different muscle groups to aid respiratory movements, e.g., extensive use of the rib musculature in snakes, limb and intracarapacial musculature in chelonians where the ribs are fused to the carapace, and the use of ribs and the hepato-pelvic ligament to draw visceral organs caudally, thus increasing pulmonary capacity in crocodilians (Lyson et al., 2014; Taylor et al., 2010). In most reptiles, at surgical depths of anesthesia, voluntary breathing is lost. Voluntary breathing is often a discontinuous pattern in reptiles, and due to the low metabolic rate, the effect of respiratory depression or the normal complete apnea under anesthesia is not as immediately threatening as it would be in a mammal. However, to maintain normal physiology, aid tissue oxygenation, and the removal of CO_2 (and thus acid-base status), assisted ventilation is normally recommended (Bertelsen, 2019; Sladky and Mans, 2012a). This should ideally match metabolic requirements, and normal guidance for species where acid-base status has been studied, indicate minute ventilation of 100–150 mL/minute/kg, with a maximum airway pressure of 10 cm H_2O. In practice, an airway pressure of 5 cm H_2O is a good starting point and can be gradually increased to where the inspiratory depth matches that of a voluntary breath, e.g., the start of cranial limb movement in chelonians, or a small excursion of the ribs over the lung in snakes (Bertelsen et al., 2014; Jakobsen et al., 2017; Williams et al., 2021). Respiratory frequency is usually set at 1–10 breaths per minute dependant usually either on the minimal setting of the ventilator, or whether manual ventilation is used. An inspiratory phase of 1/3 of the total respiratory period is common. Control of respiration in reptiles depends on central and peripheral chemoreceptors as well as pulmonary stretch receptors, and $PaCO_2$ provides the dominant drive to breathing, with a more minor role in response to oxygen content or delivery to the receptor (Milsom, 1991; Taylor et al., 2010). Thus, maintaining a physiological $PaCO_2$ via ventilation matched to metabolism is important for recovery of spontaneous breathing after anesthesia; moving to ventilation on room air in recovery with a lower respiratory frequency will aid this, although probably not through the lowering of PaO_2—as shown in the nonsignificant difference in recovery times on 21% or 100% oxygen (Churgin et al., 2014; Odette et al., 2015; Ratliff et al., 2019) (Figs. 24.2 and 24.3).

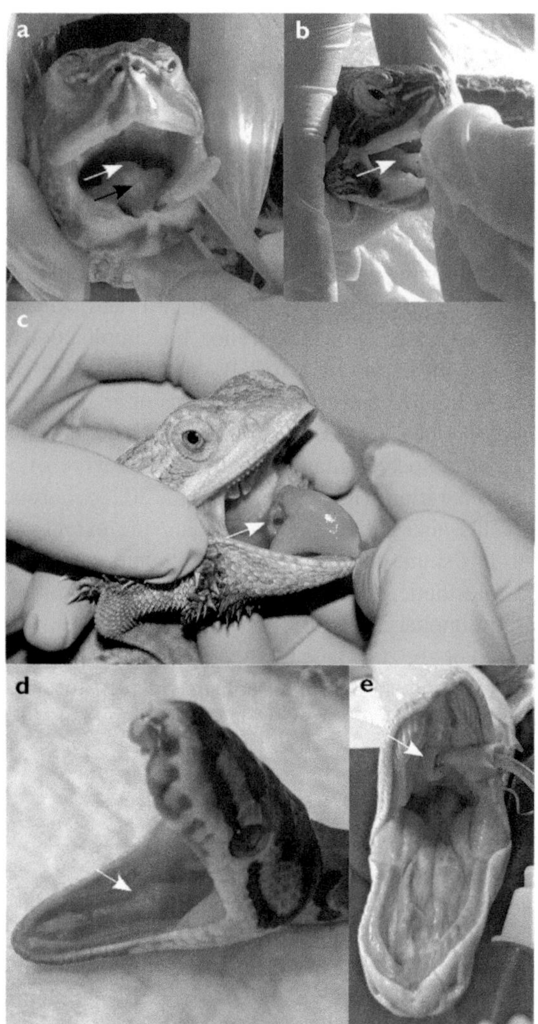

FIGURE 24.2 Glottal position in reptiles (A) Propofol sedated freshwater slider (*Trachemys scripta* spp.) with tongue (*black arrow*) and glottis (*closed white arrow*). (B) The same individual with uncuffed endotracheal tube in place within the glottis (*white arrow*). (C) Bearded dragon (*Pogona vitticeps*) with open glottis (*white arrow*) caudal to the tongue. (D) Conscious ball python (*Python regius*) with closed glottis (*white arrow*) caudal to a retracted tongue. (E) Isoflurane anesthetized python (*Python molurus bivittatus*) in dorsal recumbency showing in-place endotracheal tube at the glottis (*white arrow*).

D. Vascular beds—the influence of hepatic and renal portal systems

The connected renal and hepatic portal systems have been reported in reptiles for over 150 years (Jacquart, 1855); however, it is only recently that their effects on the pharmacodynamics of injectable anesthetics and analgesics in reptiles have come into focus. As a consequence of these portal systems, blood draining the caudal body including the hind legs and tail, first bathes the tubules of the renal system as a mixture with arterial blood from the renal artery, where the proportion of arterial blood is dependent on hydration status (Holz et al., 1997). Blood can then move from the renal portal system into the hepatic portal system or drain directly from the hindquarters into the hepatic portal system via the abdominal vein. Therefore, injections given subcutaneously or intramuscularly into the caudal body may be subject to excretion if filtered at the renal tubules or first-pass metabolism via the hepatic portal system. This does not necessarily apply to drugs given intravenously into the caudal ventral tail vein in squamates, as this drains directly into the caudal vena cava, but may also be relevant in turtles where blood drains into the ventral abdominal vein and thus the hepatic portal system and caudal vena cava

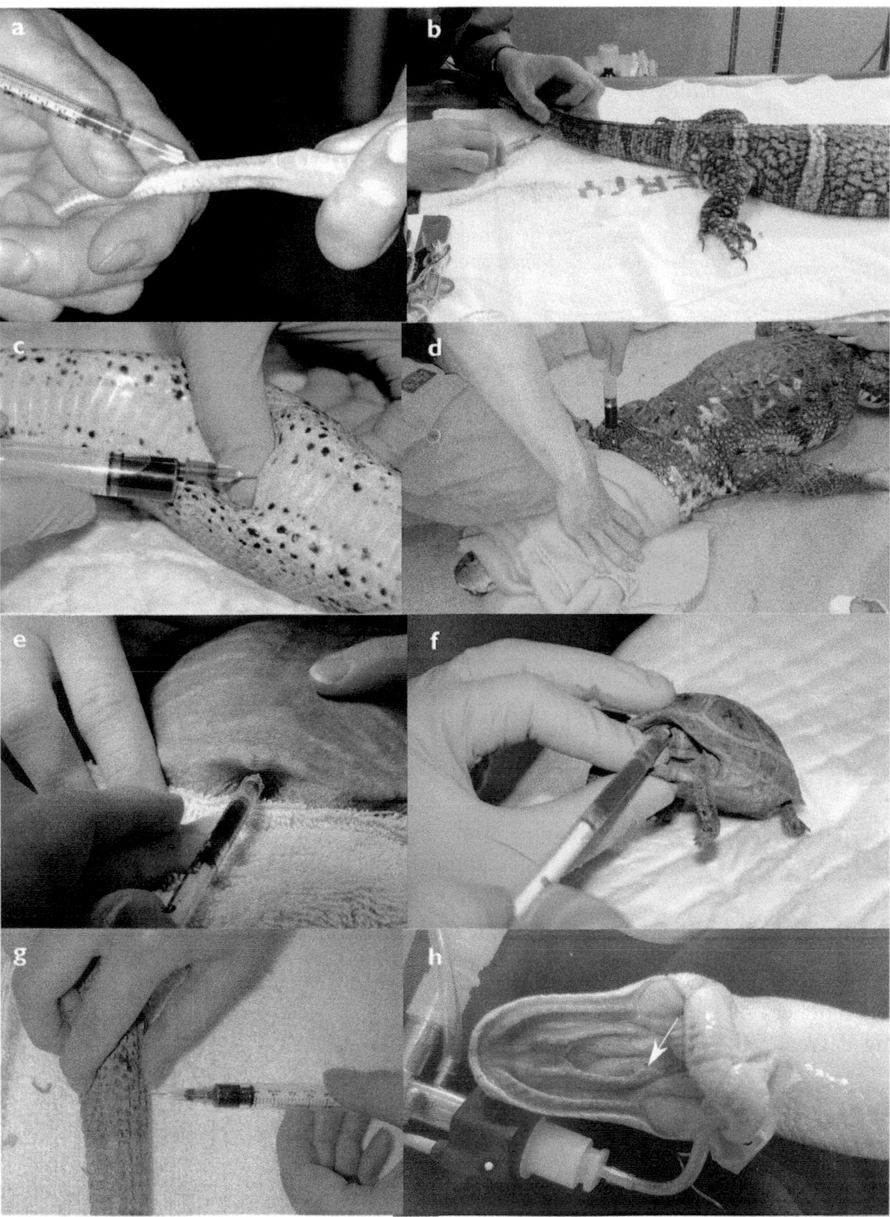

FIGURE 24.3 Vascular sampling and injection sites: (A) Ventral tail vein in a red-tailed green ratsnake (*Gonyosoma oxycephalum*), (B) lateral tail vein in a Dumeril's monitor (*Varanus dumerili*), (C) intraventricular puncture in an anesthetised Burmese python (*Python molurus bivittatus*) (D) occipital puncture in a Nile crocodile (*Crocodylus niloticus*), (E) subcarapacial plexus in Chinese softshell turtle (*Pelodiscus sinensis*) and (F) juvenile terrestrial chelonian (*Testudo horsfieldii*), (G) lateral tail (*Varanus niloticus*) and (H) right palatine vein (*white arrow*) in python (*Python molurus bivittatus*).

(Di Giuseppe et al., 2018; Morici et al., 2021). In terms of anesthetics, the effect of the hepatic portal system has been repeatedly demonstrated for the neuroactive steroid alfaxalone, where pythons injected caudally required 50% higher doses to attain a similar effect to a cranial injection (James et al., 2018; Yaw et al., 2018). This effect was not found significant in a similar study on corn snakes (Rockwell et al., 2021); however, cranial injection is still recommended by the authors. Similarly to alfaxalone, the action of medetomidine or dexmedetomidine and combinations containing them was found to be decreased when administered caudally in red-eared sliders, leopard geckos, and saltwater crocodiles (Fink et al., 2018; Lahner et al., 2011; Olsson and Phalen, 2012b). First-pass metabolism may also result in increased doses of effective metabolites, e.g., tramadol in terrapins (Giorgi et al., 2015). Variable efficacy of the injection site was also found between cranial body locations in the anole (Rasys et al., 2019a). Vascular access is illustrated in Fig. 24.3 and details provided in Table 24.1.

TABLE 24.1 Vascular beds—sites for blood sampling and access for injection.

Taxa	Vascular access site	Notes	References
Snakes	Ventral tail vein Palatine vein Intraventricular puncture Arterial access—surgical via vertebral artery catheter	Difficult in pythons and obese animals. Larger on right hand side, care with access in venomous species. Authors' preference is to use only under anesthesia. Mixed arterial/venous sample	Bertelsen et al. (2014) Isaza et al. (2004) Jakobsen et al. (2017)
Lizards	Ventral tail vein	Caution with species that shed tail, e.g., geckos.	
Terrapins (relatively shallow carapace)	Supravertebral/subcarapacial plexus, often referred as a sinus in the literature. Jugular vein, Dorsal tail vein	Mixed sample and lymph contamination possible.	Bonnet et al. (2016), Hernandez-Divers et al. (2002), Innis et al. (2010) and Ziolo and Bertelsen (2009)
Tortoises (relatively steep carapace)	Jugular vein, Supravertebral/subcarapacial plexus, Brachial plexus, Dorsal tail vein	Use for injection not recommended due to incidence of intrathecal penetration	Innis et al. (2010)
Crocodilians	Postoccipital sinus Ventral and lateral tail veins		Stegmann et al. (2017)

III. Preprocedural considerations

A. Planning

1. Health and safety

a. Venomous and predatory species

Large numbers of snakes and smaller numbers of lizards (e.g., *Heloderma* spp.) are to varying degrees venomous, including some species used in laboratory science. Specialist equipment such as handling tubes (Fig. 24.4), snake tongs, and snake hooks are vital to safely handling these species, and specialist training should be attained before experiments using these taxa and their anesthesia are planned (Antonio, 2014; Schnellbacher et al., 2019). Liaison with local healthcare facilities in terms of acute treatment in the case of envenomation is also required, as

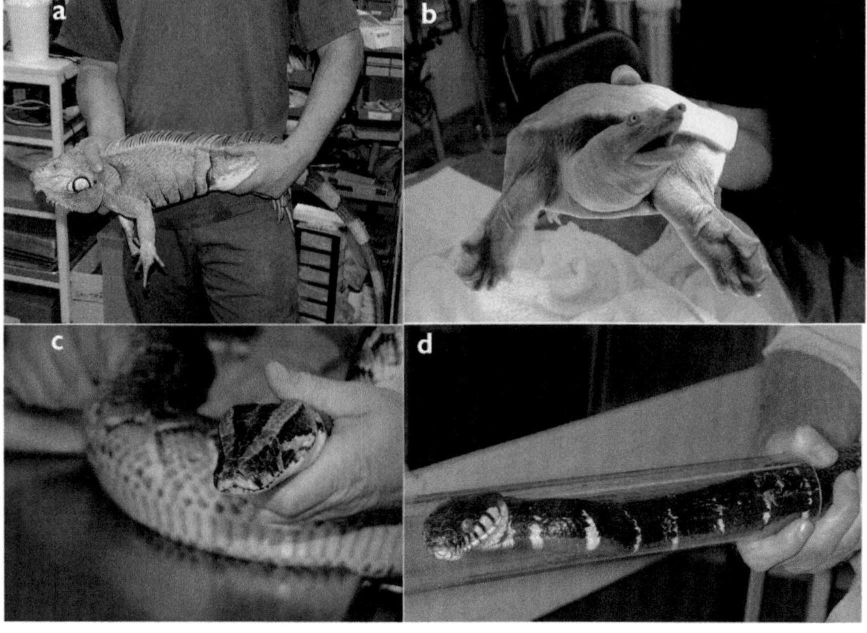

FIGURE 24.4 Handling practices for (A) a green iguana (*Iguana iguana*), (B) softshell turtle (*Pelodiscus sinensis*), (C) Burmese python (*Python molurus bivittatus*), (D) snake tube used on a venomous mangrove snake (*Boiga dendrophila*).

treatment protocols and availability will vary with the venom type and geographical region.

Large predatory species such as all crocodilians, large constrictor snakes, large chelonians e.g., snapping turtles, and large lizards (e.g., varanids) require specialist handling. The use of e.g., croc muzzles, snake bags, and training for handling and restraint can be used to aid handling and reduce the potential for injury and stress to staff and animals alike (Schnellbacher et al., 2019).

b. Zoonoses

Several zoonotic bacteria can be carried asymptomatically and be intermittently shed by reptiles. These include *Salmonella enteritidis, S. typhimurium*, etc., (McWhorter et al., 2021; Pedersen et al., 2009). Other potential zoonoses include *Pseudomonas*, *Mycobacterium*, *Cryptosporidium*, *Rickettsia* spp., and pentastomidas (arachnid lung parasites). Normal precautions, such as wearing disposable gloves and maintaining personal hygiene following the handling of reptiles, are recommended. Ectoparasites of imported reptiles can also carry zoonoses, so adequate quarantine and treatment are required (Andoh et al., 2015). Meanwhile, within laboratory collections, quarantine, care with handling, and disinfection are required to prevent cross infection with bacteria and viruses, within captive reptile populations, e.g., inclusion body disease in snakes, and amebic dysentery (Jensen et al., 2021; Pasmans et al., 2008).

c. Field versus laboratory anesthesia

Field anesthesia requires protocols that minimize equipment, achieve short recoveries, and allow reproducible anesthesia, often with lower staffing levels. Often, this has led to greater reliance on injectable protocols, including regional anesthesia (Preston et al., 2010; Rivera et al., 2011), or when using inhalants, on an open drop method, although the use of vaporizers has been reported (Hale et al., 2017). Modern fast-acting anesthetics such as alfaxalone that can be administered IM or SC may be useful in field situations in combination with local anesthesia, e.g., for telemeter placement. Other drug combinations that have been used include ketamine alpha-2 adrenergic agonist combinations. Due to the potential for risk of predation in the postoperative period, it is usually recommended to allow animals to fully recover prior to release back into the wild.

B. History and records

Knowing the origin of animals is of paramount importance. The use of wild-caught animals not only needs to be considered carefully from an ethical standpoint, but also should prompt consideration in terms of quarantine and isolation. Wild-caught animals should undergo a thorough physical examination in terms of body condition score and total protein prior to use. Given the large increases in metabolic demand during digestion in many reptiles, especially those with infrequent feeding patterns, a note of when the animal last fed will help with planning the anesthetic. Normal anesthetic record keeping is recommended with caveats on the accuracy of some monitoring equipment, see below.

1. *Patient evaluation*

Normal behavior of the species and e.g., feeding behavior, normal posture, and enclosure used by the individual, should ideally be established prior to the anesthetic event to enable postoperative monitoring for signs of pain. Respiratory rate may be estimated from coelomic movements e.g., over the ribs in lizards snakes and crocodilians, and movements of limbs and head in chelonians. Heart rate is usually assessed by Doppler positioned over the heart, e.g., in snakes 1/4 to 1/3 total body length from the rostrum, over the ventral pectoral girdle in lizards, midline and cranial of midpoint in small chelonians on the ventral plastron, or over a large vessel, e.g., brachial plexus or femoral artery. Both respiratory rate and heart rate are likely to increase markedly in handled reptilians (Bertelsen et al., 2021; Williams, 2019), in comparison with unobserved controls, but can serve as a handled baseline for that individual. Animals that are or recently were gravid may be expected to have longer recoveries, and may also warrant lower anesthetic doses (Preston et al., 2010).

Weight and body condition scores are important to assess as in animals in poor body condition, dose reduction of especially protein-bound drugs may be required, as the effective agent dose is higher when less of the drug is protein bound in the plasma (e.g., anesthetic induction agents, such as propofol and alfaxalone). Body condition is assessed in chelonians by weight to straight carapace length or body volume, while snout vent-to-weight ratios can be used in lizards and snakes, as well as visual analogue scales.

The animal's body temperature should be within its species' preferred optimal temperature zone.

2. *Laboratory investigation*

Especially in cases of poor condition or suspected dehydration, blood sampling to assess total protein and hematocrit is quick and may inform immediate anesthetic choices in terms of drug doses and fluids. More extensive hematology and biochemistry are useful in specific laboratory situations, e.g., to help assess health status prior to experimental inclusion, or in the case of clinical cases within a laboratory population, and species-specific reference ranges should be employed wherever possible (Divers and Stahl, 2019; Klaphake et al., 2018).

3. Fasting

Especially in infrequently feeding species, digestion is associated with a large increase in metabolism and oxygen consumption, liver activity, and heart rate with reductions in respiratory rate. As these are likely to impact the distribution and metabolism of injectable and inhaled anesthetics alike, fasting prior to anesthesia is preferred and will also remove a confounding factor from data collected during (and therefore including during terminal studies) and immediately after anesthesia. The physical effects of digesta, especially in animals with no diaphragm, may potentially reduce lung volume or obscure surgical sites. Fasting recommendations will depend on the species' normal gut clearance and feeding interval, but a general recommendation could be to miss one normal feeding period prior to anesthesia, e.g., 2–3 days in *T. scripta* and 2 weeks in *P. regius*.

IV. Chemical restraint versus anesthesia

A. Historical approaches and nonchemical strategies

Historically, there has been some use of neuromuscular junction (NMJ) blockers, e.g., gallamine for transportation or nonpainful procedures in crocodilians (Fleming, 2014), or the use of hypothermia for nonchemical restraint, or reliance on physical restraint methods only. This has been superseded by the use of combinations of reversible or short-acting sedatives and anesthetics, e.g., midazolam, medetomidine, and alfaxalone (Olsson et al., 2013; Olsson and Phalen, 2012a, 2012b, 2013). The sole use of NMJ blockers is not recommended by the authors, even for nonnociceptive procedures, due to the stress of immobility with retained sensory function (AVMA panel on euthanasia, 2020; West et al., 2014).

Hypothermia is variably tolerated by many reptiles in their natural environment with sufficient environmental cues (e.g., the gradual reduction in light, temperature, and feeding in the autumn priming for torpor in hypothermic, hypoxic conditions in *T. scripta*). This is dependent on their natural history, has profound effects on immune status, drug metabolism times, and return to normal behavior, and importantly, is not associated with analgesia. Hypothermia for immobilization is therefore not currently recommended clinically and will have an impact on scientific data collected from reptiles exposed to it.

Vaso-vagal responses after the application of slight eye pressure, and the vasovagal response to dorsal recumbency have been used to aid positioning, e.g., for imaging, but may be unreliable.

B. Requirement for analgesia

Reptiles have nociceptive apparatus, endogenous opioids, and changes to long-term behavior following experiences expected to be painful in other species (James et al., 2017; Williams et al., 2019b). The provision of analgesia in those circumstances is therefore not only legally mandated in laboratory species in some jurisdictions but also benefits postoperative welfare, return to normal function, and the collection of robust, representative scientific data.

C. Balanced anesthesia

The use of balanced anesthesia is becoming more common in clinical reptilian practice, and while the effect of multiple agents is often a matter for concern in laboratory studies, the use of multiple agents may allow lower doses of the agents used and therefore reduce unwanted side effects, e.g., MAC reduction in pythons via midazolam (Larouche et al., 2019a,b), and the use of local anesthesia and systemic analgesia (Sladky and Mans, 2012b, 2019). Examples of balanced anesthesia in a chelonian, snake, and crocodilian are now also appearing in the scientific literature, utilizing premedication, induction and maintenance agents, with local and systemic analgesia (Joyce et al., 2018; Larouche et al., 2019a,b; Monticelli et al., 2019).

D. Chemical restraint

Combinations of benzodiazepines, with an alpha-2 agonist, ketamine, or an opioid have also been utilized for providing some degree of chemical restraint. The need to proceed to full anesthesia from minimal chemical restraint can occur when procedures are invasive, e.g., any surgery, expected nociceptive stimulation, or if ventilation is required. Table 24.2 represents a summary of chemical restraint agents in current use.

E. Monitoring under chemical restraint

The commonly monitored reflexes under sedation include righting reflex, cranial and caudal muscle tone, and, where present, limb withdrawal, cloacal tone, jaw tone, palpebral and corneal reflexes (not possible in snakes), tongue withdrawal (in snakes), and nociceptive withdrawal. These are lost in approximately this order across species (Bertelsen, 2019; Kristensen et al., 2022), and chemical restraint will usually allow the maintenance of cloacal and some jaw tone, tongue withdrawal, and nociceptive responses to pinch or deep pain.

Respiratory depression or frank apnea is usually minimal under injectable chemical restraint, but as depth and duration are reported to vary widely with these injectable agents between individuals, it is always advisable to have equipment for intubation and provision of supplemental

TABLE 24.2 Table of chemical restraint agents in current use.

Drug(s)	Species	Dosage	Duration	Antagonist	Comments
Chemical restraint agents: sole agents					
Midazolam	Multiple; e.g., in snakes (*Python regius*), crocodilians (*C. porosus*), *lizard and chelonian species*	1–2 mg/kg IM 0.1–1 mg/kg IM with local anesthesia and opiate	Variable ~80 - minutes at 26°	Flumazenil 0.01 –0.05 mg/kg SC/IM	Light and variable sedation, MAC reduction in *Python regius* (Larouche et al., 2019a,b) as premedication e.g., in crocodilians (Olsson, 2013). Ineffective as sole agent (Arnett-Chinn et al., 2016; Lopes et al., 2017; Miller et al., 2018; Olsson, 2013; Oppenheim and Moon, 1995)
Alfaxalone	Multiple species including: Bearded dragon *P. vitticeps* Ball python (*P. regius*) Prairie rattlesnake (*Crotalus viridis*) Green anole (*A. carolensis*) Estuarine and Australian freshwater crocodiles (*C. porosus and johnstoni*)	5–10 mg/kg IV 5–20 mg/kg SC/IM (cranial injection)	Variable with dose and temperature. ~20 minutes at 30°	None	Immobilization and sedation (Ferreira and Mans, 2018; James et al., 2018; Yaw et al., 2018; Webb et al., 2021; Rasys et al., 2019a; Olsson et al., 2013)
Medetomidine	Crocodilians	0.5 mg/kg for 40 kg animals with metabolic scaling for larger individuals leading to doses of 0.15 mg/kg		Atipamezole 0.5 mg/kg IM	Olsson and Phalen (2012a)
Combinations					
Midazolam: medetomidine/ dexmedetomidine	Small to medium sized lizard species: central bearded dragon (*Pogona vitticeps*) Uromastyx (*Uromastyx* sp.) Chinese water dragon (*Physignathus cocincinus*) Veiled chameleon (*Chamaeleo calyptratus*) Panther chameleon (*Furcifer pardalis*) Oustalet's chameleon (*Furcifer oustaleti*) Green iguana (*Iguana iguana*) Blue iguana (*Cyclura lewisi*) Mojave black-collared lizard (*Crotaphytus bicinctores*) Black tree monitor (*Varanus beccarii*) Savannah monitor (*Varanus exanthematicus*) Leopard gecko (*Eublepharis macularius*) Argentine black and white tegu (*Salvator merianae*) Green basilisk (*Basiliscus plumifrons*) Mexican beaded lizard (*Heloderma horridum*) Scheltopusik (*Pseudopus apodus*)	0.5–2:0.2/0.1 mg/kg IM		Flumazenil 0.01 –0.05 mg/kg SC: atipamezole 0.5 mg/kg IM	Budden et al. (2018) and Doss et al. (2017)
Midazolam: ketamine	Lizard species as above, and Komodo dragon (*Varanus komodoensis*). Chelonians: Galapagos (*Chelonoidis nigra*), Aldabra (*Aldabrachelys gigantea*), and African Spurred Tortoises (*Centrochelys sulcata*). Leatherback turtles (*Dermochelys coriacea*), red eared slider (*T. scripta*)	2:5–40 mg/kg IM	Variable	Flumazenil 0.01 –0.05 mg/kg SC	Budden et al. (2018), Harms et al. (2014), Holz and Holz (1994), Spelman et al. (1996) and Turner et al. (2021)
Dexmedetomidine: midazolam: ketamine	Chelonians, lizard species as above	0.1:1:10 mg/kg IM	Max effect at 35 minutes, 20 minutes sedation duration	Atipamezole 0.5 mg/kg IM: flumazenil 0.05 mg/kg SC	Budden et al. (2018) and Eshar et al. (2021)

oxygenation available. Heart rate can be monitored visually, e.g., in small snakes in dorsal recumbency, or with transillumination with a cold light source in lizards. In most reptiles, heart rates can be monitored using a Doppler probe that is placed over the heart or a major artery.

Pulse oximetry providing SpO_2 may be available depending on the sedation level, and the pigmentation of the individual, e.g., over the tongue, cloacal muscosa, or a skin fold. However, while % tissue oxygenation may be valid, calculated pO_2 is calibrated to mammalian hemoglobin saturation curves, and is not validated for use in reptiles. Therefore, while trends over time in an individual may be useful, individual values are unlikely to be accurate or valuable. Cloacal or esophageal reflectance probe SpO_2 may be available in deeply sedated individuals.

Body temperature will determine the time span of drug action and recovery, so monitoring and maintaining temperature is essential. Cloacal temperature is the most common route for assessing body temperature; esophageal may also be used.

F. Support

Temperature maintenance is crucial and can be provided via covered heating pads and warm air blowers, with care to avoid local overheating. Fluids may be required for long sedations or in debilitated individuals (Minor et al., 2021). Balanced crystalline fluids such as combinations of 0.9% saline and ringers and dextrose-containing fluids are commonly used in practice, with an aim to be isosmotic with reptile plasma at 260−290 mOsm/L, with a wider range of species-specific figures reported in biological and clinical sources of 248−408 mOsm/L (Dessauer, 1970; Kanda and Brandão, 2021; Klaphake et al., 2018). Rates of maintenance fluids are usually lower than those in mammals as reptiles' lower metabolic rate is reflected in fluid turnover where liquid waste production (urate/urine/ammonia) is very variable between species: daily maintenance fluid recommendations are 5−15 mL/kg/24 hours (Kanda and Brandão, 2021). Providing lubrication is recommended both to eyes in species without a spectacle and to exposed tissues, e.g., the tongue extended for SpO_2 probe placement.

V. Anesthesia

A. Premedication

1. Sedation and MAC sparing

Midazolam has been shown to reduce the MAC of isoflurane in pythons, while alpha-2 agonists have antinociceptive action and can be administered intranasally in recalcitrant individuals (Cermakova et al., 2018; Lahner et al., 2011; Larouche et al 2019b; Schnellbacher et al., 2014).

2. Systemic analgesia

Mu opiates such as morphine (0.2−10 mg/kg), methadone 0.2−5 mg/kg, and hydromorphone 0.2−0.5 mg/kg have been shown to have antinociceptive effects in crocodilians, lizards, and chelonians in Hargreaves tests and surgical models, so they are good premedication for surgical procedures (Couture et al., 2017; Kinney et al., 2011; Leal et al., 2017; Mans et al., 2012; Rasys et al., 2019a; Turner et al., 2021; Williams et al., 2016). The respiratory depression that accompanies mu opiate use means supplemental oxygenation and the ability to intubate is essential for anesthetics following opiate administration (Kinney et al., 2011; Malte et al., 2018). Mu opiate use in snakes for analgesia is not validated in preclinical nociceptive models (Sladky et al., 2008; Williams et al., 2016), but appears to be clinically successful in chronically painful individuals. While butorphanol was previously used commonly in reptiles, it appears to have mainly sedative rather than antinociceptive effect and is no longer recommended (Fleming and Robertson, 2012; Kinney et al., 2011; Leal et al., 2017; Sladky and Miletic, 2007; Trnkova et al., 2007b; Trnková et al., 2008; Ward et al., 2012; Williams et al., 2016). Buprenorphine has not been shown to have antinociceptive activity in reptiles and therefore is not recommended as a premedication (Greenacre et al., 2006; Mans et al., 2012). Tramadol has less respiratory depression, good nociceptive activity, and a long duration in *T. scripta*, and therefore may also be a good option for premedication for surgery (Baker et al., 2011a; Giorgi et al., 2015).

3. Modification of cardiac shunting

Atropine is not used in reptiles to specifically prevent oral secretions or to increase heart rate, (although it will usally cause the latter, at least in conscious individuals (Greunz et al., 2018; Kristensen et al., 2022)). However, atropine has been shown to have an effective MAC-sparing effect, as it prevents pulmonary artery constriction and therefore acts to reduce right-to-left cardiac shunting. It may therefore aid in the uptake and control of inhaled anesthetic levels. However, published dosages (1−2 mg/kg) are currently drawn from the physiological literature and not optimized for clinical use (Greunz et al., 2018; Kristensen et al., 2022; Williams et al., 2020).

B. Induction

Table 24.3 presents options for induction of anesthesia, both injectable and inhaled.

C. Anesthetic maintenance

1. Inhalation anesthetics

Isoflurane and sevoflurane are commonly used for maintenance (Table 24.4), with MAC (minimum anesthetic concentration required to ensure no response to a

TABLE 24.3 Table of induction agents.

Drug(s)	Species	Dosage	Duration	Antagonist	Comments
Injectable single agent and combinations					
Propofol	Multiple species including snakes; South American rattle snake (*C. durissus*), lizards (*P. vitticeps*), crocodilians: American alligator and nile crocodile, and chelonians (e.g., *T. scripta*)	5–20 mg/kg IV	20–45 minutes dose and temperature dependant	None	Intravascular only. Plasma protein bound so effective dose increased in animals with reduced total protein (Bertelsen et al., 2014, 2021; Gorczak et al., 2017; Perrin and Bertelsen, 2017; Stegmann et al., 2017; Ziolo and Bertelsen, 2009)
Alfaxalone	Multiple species including snakes (*P. regius, C durissus, C. viridis, Pantherophis guttatus*), lizards (*I. iguana, A. carolinensis, Eublepharis macularis*) *Crocodilians (C. porosus), and chelonians (T. scripta* spp.)	5–15 mg/kg IV 10–30 mg/kg IM/SC	20–45 minutes dose and temperature dependent	None	Plasma protein bound so care in animals with reduced TP. SC and IM administration in cranial body to avoid hepatic portal circulation and first pass metabolism (Bertelsen et al., 2021; Ferreira et al., 2019; Ferreira and Mans, 2018; James et al., 2018; Kischinovsky et al., 2013; Knotek, 2014; Knotek et al., 2013, 2011; Morici et al., 2018; Rasys et al., 2019a; Shepard et al., 2013; Trnkova et al., 2007b; Webb et al., 2021; Yaw et al., 2020, 2018)
Ketamine: alpha-2 agonist (dexmedetomidine)	Multiple lizard, snake and chelonian species	30–60 mg/kg (100 for very extended anesthesia): 0.5–0.2 mg/kg	1–2, 16 hours for extended anesthesia. Individually variable duration	Atipamezole to reverse alpha-2 agonist (5 times dose of initial agent, administered IM)	Budden et al. (2018), Bunke et al. (2018), Christiansen et al. (2013), Cushing et al. (2020), Doss et al. (2017), Fink et al. (2018), Harms et al. (2014) and Rasys et al. (2019b)
Ketamine: alpha-2 agonist (medetomidine)	Multiple lizard, snake and chelonian species	30–60 mg/kg (100 for very extended anesthesia): 0.1–0.4 mg/kg	1–2, 16 hours for extended anesthesia. Individually variable duration	Atipamezole to reverse alpha-2 agonist (5 times dose of initial agent, administered IM)	Barrillot et al. (2018), Budden et al. (2018), Doss et al. (2017), Fink et al. (2018), Harms et al. (2007, 2009) and Monticelli et al. (2019)

Continued

TABLE 24.3 Table of induction agents.—cont'd

Drug(s)	Species	Dosage	Duration	Antagonist	Comments
Methohexital	Multiple in physiology studies including (*Thamnophis sirtalis parietalis*)	15 mg/kg	50–200 minutes	None	Preston et al. (2010)
Pentobarbital	Multiple species of snakes (e.g., *P regius, P. molurus*) lizards, chelonians (*T. scripta* spp.)	30–60 mg/kg IP, 30 mg/kg IV	Terminal anesthesia only.	None	Terminal anesthesia only, to be used in conjunction with local anesthesia to provide perioperative antinociception (Enok et al., 2016; Joyce et al., 2018; Williams et al., 2021)
Inhaled agents					
Isoflurane	Multiple (see Table 24.5 for MAC values)	4%–5% from vaporiser for inline chamber induction. 0.5–1 mL/L chamber volume for closed drop chamber induction	Variable dependent on open/closed drop and ventilation.	None	Uptake affected by minute ventilation of the reptile and extent of cardiac shunting. Therefore impractical for normal induction in aquatic chelonians (Williams et al., 2020) Keep liquid anesthetic out of direct contact with animal. Care with exposure of staff to anesthetic agent. Practical for small lizards and snakes in plastic chamber/robust plastic bag.
Sevoflurane	Multiple	6%–7% from vapouriser. 1 mL/L chamber volume for closed drop induction chamber	Variable dependant on open/closed drop and ventilation.	None	Uptake affected by minute ventilation of the reptile and extent of cardiac shunting. Therefore impractical for normal induction in aquatic chelonians (Williams et al., 2020)

TABLE 24.4 Table of maintenance anesthetic agents.

Drug(s)	Species	Dosage	Duration	Antagonist	Comments
Maintenance anesthetic agents					
Inhaled agents					
Isoflurane	Multiple	2.5% maintenance for surgical depth anesthesia. See Table 24.5 for MAC determinations where they have been made.		None	Long equilibration times, especially in breath holding individuals, dose reduction required over long anesthetics, elimination requires ventilation and the resumption of spontaneous ventilation. (Barter et al., 2006; Brosnan et al., 2006; Greunz et al., 2018; Kristensen et al., 2022; Larouche et al., 2019a,b; Williams et al., 2020)
Sevoflurane	Multiple	3.5% average maintenance	Variable dependant on open/closed drop and ventilation.	None	Uptake affected by minute ventilation of the reptile and extent of cardiac shunting. Therefore impractical for normal induction in aquatic chelonians (Williams et al., 2020)
Injectable agents					
Ketamine: alpha-2 agonist (dexmedetomidine)	Multiple lizard, snake and chelonian species	30–60 mg/kg (100 for very extended anesthesia): 0.5–0.2 mg/kg	1–2, 16 hours for extended anesthesia. Individually variable duration	Atipamezole to reverse alpha-2 agonist, (5 times dose of initial agent, administered IM)	Budden et al. (2018), Bunke et al. (2018), Christiansen et al. (2013), Cushing et al. (2020), Doss et al. (2017), Fink et al. (2018), Harms et al. (2014) and Rasys et al. (2019b)
Ketamine: alpha-2 agonist (medetomidine)	Multiple lizard, snake and chelonian species	30–60 mg/kg (100 for very extended anesthesia): 0.1–0.4 mg/kg	1–2, 16 hours for extended anesthesia. Individually variable duration	Atipamezole to reverse alpha-2 agonist (5 times dose of initial agent, administered IM)	Barrillot et al. (2018), Budden et al. (2018), Doss et al. (2017), Fink et al. (2018), Harms et al. (2007, 2009) and Monticelli et al. (2019)
Pentobarbital	multiple species including snakes (*P. regius and P. molurus bivittatus*), lizards, chelonians (*T. scripta*) and crocodilians	30–60 mg/kg IP	Terminal anesthesia only. Expected duration 1–3 hours.	None	Terminal anesthesia only, to be used in conjunction with local anesthesia to provide perioperative antinociception (Joyce et al., 2018). Low therapeutic index and reduction in cardiac output over time (Williams et al., 2021)
Propofol	Iguana iguana Multiple species	0.5 mg/kg/minute Intraosseous following 5 mg/kg induction 1–2 mg/kg boli given 10–30 minutes apart IV following 5 mg/kg induction	Cumulative effects unknown over long administration, 30 minutes duration in study and authors' experience dependent on feeding status	None	Bennett et al. (1998)

supramaximal nociceptive stimulus in 50% of a population) used to compare the potency of inhaled anesthetics. MAC, which is very consistent across mammalian species, is quite variable across the reptile species studied, likely mainly due to variation in intracardiac shunting (Table 24.5). MAC_{iso} is reported from 1.1% in pythons to 3.5% in red-footed tortoises and sliders with sole agent isoflurane, which can be reduced to 1.5% by the used of atropine and propofol for induction (Barter et al., 2006; Bertelsen et al., 2005b; Greunz et al., 2018; Kristensen et al., 2022; Larouche 2019b; Mosley et al., 2003). In practice, 1.3 x MAC is recommended for surgical anesthesia to account for individual variation, so a maintenance dose of 2.5% will account for most reptiles, either after isoflurane induction (e.g., small lizards and snakes) or an injectable induction with propofol or alfaxalone (e.g., in chelonians or larger animals) (Bertelsen, 2019). Maintenance doses should be lowered over time to account for the slow equilibration of the drugs in the arterial blood and CNS (Barter et al., 2006; Brosnan et al., 2006; Williams et al., 2020). MAC_{sevo} is higher, as in mammals, and maintenance doses of 3.5% will usually be sufficient. Reductions in the maintenance dose can be made if additional induction agents or premedication are employed, e.g., with opiates or midazolam (Table 24.4).

2. Injectable anesthetics

Long-duration anesthesia has been reported using high doses and repeated administrations of ketamine and medetomidine for specific experimental requirements in tegus (Barrillot et al., 2018). Repeated or continuous dosing of propofol or alfaxalone is feasible, and an intraosseous protocol has been described (Bennett et al., 1998).

D. Anesthetic management and monitoring

1. Peri-anesthetic support

Temperature maintenance is key to peri-anesthetic support. It is best maintained via cloacal feedback heat pads, especially if data is collected under the anesthetic, but Bair huggers or separate covered heating pads can be used. Care must be taken to minimise the potential for thermal burns (Kischinovsky et al., 2013; Williams et al., 2020).

Ventilation is usually required at a surgical depth of anesthesia in reptiles. While the comparative hypoxia tolerance of their tissues means that temporary apnea is not as deleterious as it would be in mammals, the provision of ventilation that matches metabolic needs helps ensure acid-base balance and gives a swifter recovery from, e.g., inhaled anesthetic (Bertelsen et al., 2014; Jakobsen et al., 2017; Williams et al., 2021). This is usually provided by mechanical ventilation with a maximum airway pressure of 10 cm H_2O, minute volumes of 50–150 mL/minute/kg, and frequencies of 0.5–5 breaths per minute at 20–30°C.

Evaporative losses in surgery are lower than those of endotherms, but the use of parenteral fluids is recommended to aid recover from preoperative dehydration, compensate for losses in excreta or blood over the surgical period, and ameliorate the potential for reduced fluid and food intake in the postsurgical period. Balanced crystalline fluids such as combinations of 0.9% saline and ringers and

TABLE 24.5 Table of published literature values for MAC (minimum anesthetic concentration) for isoflurane in reptiles.

Species	MAC isoflurane (%) (mean ± sd)	Temperature (°C) (mean ± sd)
Yellow-bellied slider (*Trachemys scripta*) Kristensen et al. (2022)	3.3 ± 0.8	29 ± 0.3
Ball pythons (Python regius) Larouche et al. (2019b)	1.11 ± 0.26	30.1 ± 0.4
Radiated rat snake (*Elaphe radiata*) Maas and Brunson (2002)	1.68 ± 0.3	NR
Dumeril's monitor (*Varanus dumerili*) Bertelsen et al. (2005a)	1.54 ± 0.17	32–33
Desert iguanas (*Dipsosaurus dorsalis*) Dohm and Brunson (1998)	3.14 3.10 2.83	35 30 20
Green iguanas (*Iguana iguana*) Barter et al. (2006) Mosley et al. (2003)	2.1 ± 0.5[a] 1.8 ± 0.3 2.0 ± 0.6 2.1 ± 0.6	35.5 ± 0.3 35.5 ± 0.4 30–32
Red-footed tortoise (*Chelonoidis carbonaria*) Greunz et al. (2018)	2.2 ± 0.3 (with atropine) 3.2 ± 0.4 (without atropine)	30 ± 1

[a]*Average over three time points, 1.8 value represents latest time point predicted to be closest to true MAC at equilibrium.*

dextrose-containing fluids are commonly used in practice with an aim to be isosmotic with reptile plasma, at 260–290 mOsm/L.

2. Anesthetic monitoring

Reflexes are monitored as with those for chemical restraint, but with an expected further progression to loss of nociceptive response. Loss of the combination of corneal, cloacal, and general deep pain responses should warrant caution as anesthetic depth may become excessive, although the loss of general deep pain is preferred for surgical depths of anesthesia.

Doppler ultrasound may be used to obtain heart rate through anesthetic procedures. Electrocardiogram (ECG) is useful and easy to obtain by connecting leads ending in crocodile clips to either electrolyte-saturated pads in thin-skinned species, or needles that are gently placed subcutaneously in heavily scaled species. However, the divorce of cardiac from CNS function may be seen especially in hypoxia-tolerant species, so continuing ECG activity should not be used as a proxy for continued life, and vice versa, loss of cardiac activity does not guarantee irrecoverable CNS function. Capnography, using minimal dead space mainstream models and low input sidestream models, is useful for assessing continued tissue metabolism and ventilation quality (Fig. 24.5). Given cardiac shunting, $etCO_2$ may not reflect arterial $PaCO_2$, thus trends should be given more weight than individual measurements. $EtCO_2$ tends to be lower than $PaCO_2$ in studies where both are measured, and maintenance of $etCO_2$ at 10–20 mmHg is acceptable.

Pulse oximetry (reflectance probe functions best and can be used at esophageal or cloacal locations) is best used for within patient trends only, as it is not calibrated to reptilian hemoglobin saturation curves, so while % saturation may be valid, internal calculated pO_2 will not, and equipment may have difficulty with pigmented skin and penetration.

Blood gases are feasible with the correct equipment, which needs to be calibrated to temperature, and ideally, to species hemoglobin saturations curves (Malte et al., 2014); however, arterial samples require surgical approaches, and there is a limited utility of venous samples, as they reflect not only tissue metabolism, but also any degree of cardiac shunting. For further details, please refer to Bertelsen (2019) and Mans (2018).

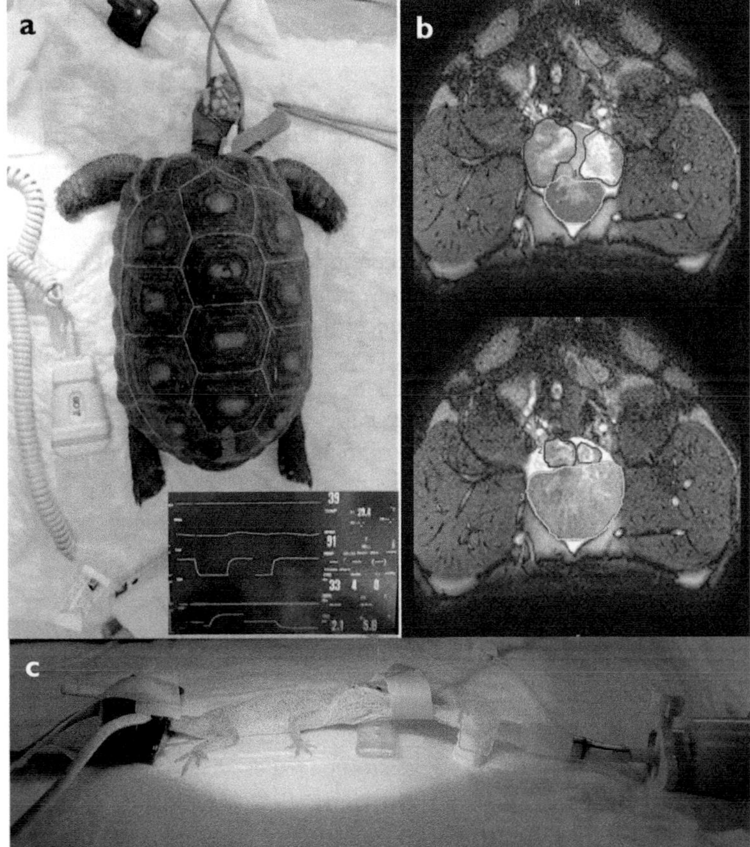

FIGURE 24.5 Anesthetic monitoring during experimentation on (from *top*) intubated 2 kg red footed tortoise (*Chelonoidis carbonaria*), showing esophageal temperature, Doppler for heart rate, tissue oxygenation, end tidal anesthetic gases. Insert: display of monitoring output. Cardiac silhouette on ECG gated MRI, showing ventricular outline (*green*) right atrium (*blue*) and left atrium (*red*) in systole (*top*) and diastole (*bottom*). Intubated 4 g green anole (*Anolis carolinensis*) with tissue oxygenation, cloacal temperature and end tidal gas analysis.

3. Anesthetic emergencies

Emergencies are relatively uncommon due to the robust nature of reptilian physiology but are best avoided by accurate dosing of injectable drugs, with dose reductions in animals with a low total protein and prompt recognition and resolution of problems.

Respiratory depression is ubiquitous at surgical depths of anesthesia. The provision of even minimal manual intermittent positive pressure ventilation (IPPV) will avoid respiratory acidosis, while IPPV provided by a low-RR ventilator can match physiological conditions and hasten recovery (Bertelsen et al., 2014; Jakobsen et al., 2017; Williams et al., 2021).

Rapid injection of high doses of propofol, or overdose of isoflurane (e.g., in a closed drop system, if the animal remains in contact with high partial pressures for an extended period) can lead to cardiac depression and asystole. External cardiac massage in snakes is possible by gently compressing the ventricle from caudal to cranial, and with the provision of ventilation and lowered concentrations of isoflurane or time after propofol injection, will usually result in the resumption of normal cardiac activity. In animals with less obvious cardiac anatomy, continued ventilatory support and withdrawal of anesthetic agents will usually suffice; however, cardiac support can also be given using relatively low doses of adrenaline (10 μg/kg) and atropine (e.g., 1 mg/kg) IV to prevent the right-to-left shunting and enable elimination of inhaled anesthetics (Gatson et al., 2017; Goe et al., 2016; Greunz et al., 2018; Kristensen et al., 2022).

4. Reversal agents

Where agents have been used that have specific reversal agents, e.g., flumazenil for benzodiazepines (flumazenil 0.01–0.05 mg/kg IM/SC) and atipamezole for alpha-2-agonists (5 times dose of original alpha-2, IM) the reversal should be given in the case of anesthetic emergencies, prior to the use of adrenaline or atropine, or when the procedure is completed to hasten recovery. The reversal of opiate analgesics to reverse respiratory depression is possible with naloxone, but will also reverse analgesic effects, and the half-life of the reversal agent may be less than that of the original drug, therefore care must be taken to monitor closely in recovery for any resumption of apnea.

VI. Anesthesia for specific situations

A. Field anesthesia

For short procedures where venous access (Fig. 24.3) is available then propofol or alfaxalone with local anesthesia is the authors' agent of choice. Alfaxalone can also be used intramuscularly in cases where venous access is not possible. A flow-over vaporizer or closed-drop method of isoflurane anesthesia is easy but requires more equipment and can be less finely controlled. Ventilation via intubation and manual bagging at 1–4 breaths per minute to coelomic expansion equivalent to a normal breath is recommended, whichever induction agent is used. Analgesia is recommended via local anesthetics (e.g., lidocaine <10 mg/kg, or bupivacaine, <4 mg/kg) and systemic analgesics (e.g., meloxicam, 0.3 mg/kg). Release while under the influence of any anesthetic, including opiate pain relief, is not recommended due to the potential for respiratory depression, and potential issues for predators if a released animal is consumed, given relative dosages in reptiles and therapeutic doses in mammals.

B. Laboratory anesthesia

As discussed throughout the chapter, this is likely to depend on species and study design. A first pilot protocol for most studies would consist of induction with propofol or alfaxalone with maintenance under inhaled anesthesia for large individuals or those that breath-hold, especially in aquatic chelonians. Induction and maintenance with inhaled anesthesia for small lizards or snakes where vaporizer equipment is available. Ventilation will be required at surgical depths of anesthesia.

C. Imaging

If prolonged imaging is required, then the use of inhaled anesthesia is practical and can be MRI-compatible (Greunz et al., 2018; Williams et al., 2019a), while injectable combinations have also been used for prolonged anesthesia where neurological recording precluded the use of inhaled anesthetics (Barrillot et al., 2018). For short-duration imaging, the use of chemical restraint +/− the vasovagal reflex can be considered, e.g., midazolam, dexmedetomidine combinations +/− ketamine depending on the degree of sedation required. Ventilation may be required based on the depth of sedation, positioning, and loss of spontaneous respiratory drive.

D. Laparoscopy

Induction with propofol/alfaxalone, with maintenance on inhaled anesthesia is recommended dependent on the procedure, as injectable induction agents such as propofol may allow sufficient time for e.g., sex determination, but not for sterilization, or other invasive procedures. Local anesthesia is recommended at laparoscopy sites (Alworth et al., 2011; Chatigny et al., 2017; Divers, 2019; MacLean et al., 2008; Schnellbacher et al., 2019).

E. Open coeliotomy

For snakes, lizards, and crocodilians, the incision is via soft tissue, but for chelonians, an open coeliotomy involves a bone incision through the plastron, therefore the necessary degree of analgesia should be carefully considered, and premedication with a mu-opioid +/− midazolam can be considered. In all cases, given the lack of diaphragm and dorsal position of the lungs, assisted ventilation, usually via IPPV, is required at approximately 100−150 mL/kg/minute, airway pressures of 5−10 cm H_2O, and respiratory frequencies 0.5−5 breaths per minute (Bertelsen et al., 2014; Jakobsen et al., 2017; Williams et al., 2021). Induction can be performed via injectable anesthesia, e.g., propofol or alfaxalone (especially in turtles, large lizards, and crocodilians) or inhalational anesthesia (small lizards and snakes), with maintenance of inhaled anesthesia using IPPV.

F. Long-term anesthesia

Prolonged anesthesia can be managed via inhalational means, remembering that the slow equilibration of inhaled anesthetics means that the dose provided at the vaporizers should be decreased over a long anesthetic to avoid overdose (Barter et al., 2006; Brosnan et al., 2006; Williams et al., 2020). Ketamine combinations have also been used for prolonged surgical/neurological experiments (Barrillot et al., 2018), but it should be noted that recoveries can be extremely slow, and using combinations where some of the agents may be reversed (e.g., midazolam, dexmedetomidine), may be beneficial. Providing thermal support is essential in all ectotherm anesthesia, especially so in long-term anesthesia, where the rate of metabolism of drugs is key to the maintenance of a steady plane of anesthesia and the ability of the animal to recover. Fluid support may be maintained via intravenous catheters, where placed, or via intracoelomic injection or subcutaneous administration (Minor et al., 2021). The requirement for fluid support will depend on whether the experimental animal is healthy versus for example, a dehydrated individual, the temperature of the species in comparison with environmental conditions in terms of the degree of evaporation. The requirement for fluid support can be assessed via preanesthetic check, interoperative tissue observation, PCV, and TP.

G. Brumation and torpor/hibernation

During periods of brumation/torpor/hibernation the dosages of anesthetics may require reduction, especially those interacting with receptors also involved in the maintenance of metabolic suppression and reduced neural activity during, e.g., hypoxic or hypothermic overwintering in *T. scripta* (Madsen et al., 2013; Nilsson and Lutz, 1993). Therefore, pilot dosages especially of injectable drugs should be tested, or inhalational agents, with IPPV matching metabolic requirements, should be used.

H. Terminal procedures

Commonly pentobarbital (30−50 mg/kg IP or IV, dose species dependent) has been used for terminal procedures e.g., in comparative physiology (Enok et al., 2016; Joyce et al., 2018; Williams et al., 2021). Inhaled anesthesia (isoflurane at 1.3X species MAC (Kristensen et al., 2022; Larouche et al., 2019b, b)) is another potential route to the good provision of long-anesthesia times. With both regimes, the use of local anesthesia at the surgical site, and for pentobarbital on injection IP will provide antinociception and prevent wind-up under anesthesia that may affect physiological parameters (e.g., blood pressure, heart rate, c-fos spinal activation (Khoo et al., 2018)).

VII. Postanesthetic recovery and care

A. Recovery period

Ventilation in recovery should be optimized to allow the elimination of inhaled anesthetic gases (Jakobsen et al., 2017; Williams et al., 2020), but also allow normal or slightly rising $PaCO_2$ to stimulate the return to spontaneous ventilation. In practice, after inhaled anesthesia, the authors maintain animals on IPPV until head withdrawal, with care for ET tube placement, and then monitor for spontaneous breathing, with supplementary manual bagging if required at 0.2−1 breath per minute. In some animals, once the ET tube is removed and sometimes after the end of anesthetic provision, the reptile can again become more sedated, presumably as cardiac shunting or movement of anesthetics from adipose tissue into circulation increases the CNS concentration. Therefore, animals should be monitored for the first few hours after inhalational anesthesia in case additional ventilation is required.

The temperature should be maintained within the POTZ for the species (Rossi, 2019) in recovery in order to optimize the metabolism of drugs, the resumption of normal behavior, and immune status. Adrenaline or stimulation has been used to shorten recovery time in nonsurgical procedures in reptiles anesthetized with inhaled anesthetics (Gatson et al., 2017; Goe et al., 2016). There may also be a place for atropine to change shunt patterns in recovery, but this has not yet been studied (Greunz et al., 2018).

Aquatic animals such as fresh water and marine turtles and crocodilians should be maintained in dry dock in recovery to avoid inhalation of water before full glottal and head and neck muscular control is resumed. Hydration should be maintained by the use of SC fluids during or after the procedure, and/or the provision of drinking water and normal humidity after recovery. Refeeding should only be attempted when the animal is fully recovered, with the knowledge that pain or the prior use of opiate drugs may reduce appetite (James et al., 2017; Kinney et al., 2011), and that digestion is a metabolically costly activity in infrequently feeding ectotherms.

Recoveries may be prolonged in animals at lower temperatures, for those animals with lower body condition scores, and in recently gravid females where longer monitoring and ventilation may be required.

B. Supportive care

Supportive care may include the provision of fluids (S/C or intracoelomically (Kanda and Brandão, 2021; Minor et al., 2021)) peri and postanesthesia, assisted feeding with species-appropriate processed foods in fully recovered animals (Kanda and Brandão, 2021) and careful provision of temperature gradients (Rossi, 2019) within areas with the provision of hides, etc.

C. Pain assessment

There are no verified pain scales in reptiles, but behavioral ethograms have been found to differ in animals following surgery and opiate administration (Kinney et al., 2011; Rasys et al., 2019a). Clinical and behavioral indications of pain include changes in posture (e.g., reluctance to touch the ventral to the substrate after Colectomy), decreased food intake, drop in body condition score, a change from normal escape behavior e.g., anoles, and/or a general inactivity, or loss of normal cage behavior (i.e., climbing and jumping on wall and roof surfaces).

D. Return to group housing

The timing and extent of a return to group housing will depend on species. Some reptiles may be housed singly due to behavioral constraints; group housing is not then recommended in recovery. Some species are prone to damaging surgical sites on conspecifics, e.g., *T. scripta*, and here return to group housing should only take place after the healing of any surgical sites. In groups with strong hierarchy, e.g., crocodilians, careful planning is needed to reduce the occurrence of conspecific aggression on the return of anesthetized animals to the group (Stegmann et al., 2017).

VIII. Analgesia

A. Approach to analgesia in the given species

While reptiles have historically been perceived as less susceptible to pain, or even unable to perceive it, it is the authors' opinion that the weight of modern evidence is that reptiles experience pain and that it should be treated. Lines of evidence include (i) the nociceptive apparatus in reptiles, including connections to the thalamus and forebrain (Williams et al., 2019b), (ii) the amelioration of abnormal behavior and posture following clinical analgesics in conditions considered painful in mammals (Sladky and Mans, 2019) (iii) the reduction in feeding (a behavioral tradeoff) following nociception under anesthesia if specific analgesia is not given (James et al., 2017), and (iv) the species-specific response to analgesics in nociceptive tests (Couture et al., 2017; Leal et al., 2017; Sladky and Miletic, 2007; Sladky et al., 2008; Williams et al., 2016).

Multimodal analgesia has had less history in reptiles used in laboratory science, due often to concerns over drug effects on data collection, and a lack of information on efficacy. The rapid expansion of the literature on reptilian analgesia in the last 10–20 years will hopefully spur greater uptake of analgesia in laboratory reptilian anesthesia (Table 24.6).

B. Preventative analgesia

Analgesia can be provided as part of the anesthetic protocol prior to the nociceptive stimulus, e.g., the use of alpha-2 agonists and ketamine agents as anesthetics, and the use of opiate premedication and local anesthesia prior to surgical incision. There is little direct evidence for antinociception from nonsteroidal antiinflammatory drugs, but there is expression of COX 1 and 2 in inflamed tissue (Sadler et al., 2016; Thompson et al., 2018), and clinically, meloxicam 0.3 mg/kg and ketoprofen 2–3 mg/kg have analgesic activity in postoperative cases, therefore their use as premedications is limited but possible (Hernandez-Divers, 2006; Sladky and Mans, 2012b; Spadola et al., 2016; Trnkova et al., 2007a).

Postoperative analgesia encompasses therapeutics given in the postoperative period, lengthening the provision of pain relief during tissue healing; and options are given below and in Table 24.6.

C. Pharmacologic options

1. Opioids

Mu opiates such as morphine and hydromorphone have proved effective in nociceptive tests in chelonians, crocodilians, and lizards (Kanui and Hole, 1992; Kinney et al., 2011; Leal et al., 2017; Makau et al., 2017; Sladky and Miletic, 2007; Sladky et al., 2008), and there is clinical empirical evidence in chronically painful snakes but not in healthy nonpainful snakes subjected to nociceptive testing (Bertelsen, 2019; Mans et al., 2019). Fentanyl has been shown to penetrate reptile skin from a transdermal system, and clinical effects have been noted in chronic reptile cases,

TABLE 24.6 Table of analgesia agents.

Drug(s)	Species	Dosage	Duration	Antagonist	Comments
Opiates					
Morphine	Multiple species including chelonians (*T. scripta*), lizards (*P. vitticeps, Salvator merianae*), crocodilians (*C. niloticus*). Not currently validated in snakes.	1–10 mg/kg IM	8–12 hours	Naloxone, naltrexone	Moderate sedation, respiratory depression and feeding behavior reduction (Kanui and Hole, 1992; Kinney et al., 2011; Leal et al., 2017; Malte et al., 2018; Sladky et al., 2008; Williams et al., 2016)
Hydromorphone	Multiple including chelonians (*T. scripta*) and lizards (*P. vitticeps*)	0.5–1 mg/kg IM/SC	12–24 hours *T. scripta*, 24 hours *P. vitticeps*	Naloxone, naltrexone	Immobilization, light to moderate sedation (Hawkins et al., 2019)
Tramadol	Chelonians	5–10 mg/kg PO	72 hours (Norton et al., 2015)	Naloxone, naltrexone	Baker et al. (2011b)
Methadone		3–5 mg/kg SC/IM	24 hours	Naloxone, naltrexone	Respiratory depression unknown
Fentanyl	Pharmacokinetics and some clinical efficacy for snakes e.g., *P. regius,* lizards e.g., *Corucia zebrata*	2.5–12.5 μg/hour transcutaneous	Dependant on exposure	Naloxone, naltrexone	Available as patches transdermal systems (Darrow et al., 2017; Gamble, 2008)
Nonsteroidal antiinflammatory					
Meloxicam	Multiple including pharmacokinetics in loggerhead turtles (*Caretta caretta*), sliders (*Trachemys scripta* spp.), green iguana, (*Iguana iguana*)	0.2–0.4 mg/kg IM	24 hours		Di Salvo et al. (2016), Divers et al. (2010), Hernandez-Divers (2006), Lai et al. (2015), Trnkova et al. (2007a,b) and Uney et al. (2016)
Ketoprofen	Multiple including pharmacokinetics in loggerhead turtles *Caretta caretta*	2–3 mg/kg	24 hours		Thompson et al. (2018)
Local anesthesia					
Lidocaine	Multiple species of snakes, lizards crocodilians and chelonians	1–10 mg/kg SC	Unknown in reptiles	None	Sladky and Mans (2012b)
Bupivacaine	Multiple, specific use in *P. regius.*	1–4 mg/kg SC	Unknown in reptiles	None	Sladky and Mans (2012b) and Williams (2019)
Mepivacaine	Multiple, specific use in crocodilians.	1 mg/kg SC	Unknown in reptiles	None	Wellehan et al. (2006)
Lidocaine/ prilocaine	Multiple chelonian species	Cream at a dose of 1 g/10 cm^2 mucosa of 25 mg/g formulation Patch at 25 mg/ 25 mg	Active 20–40 minutes after application		Joyce et al. (2018), Spadola et al. (2015) and Williams et al. (2021)
Alpha-2-adrenergic agonist					
Dexmedetomidine Medetomidine	Multiple including Argentinian tegu (*Salvator merianae*) and ball python (*Python regius*) Multiple including desert tortoise (*Gopherus agassizii*)	0.1–0.2 mg/kg 0.1–0.2 mg/kg	Over 8 hours at the doses given, when not reversed	Atipamezole (0.05 mg/kg IM)	Dose from nociceptive studies, no sedation reported at this dosage used as a sole agent in snakes, but respiratory depression noted, and sedation in chelonians (Bisetto et al., 2018; Bunke et al., 2018; Sleeman and Gaynor, 2000)

including snakes, but not in acute antinociception where tested in pythons (Darrow et al., 2017; Gamble, 2008; Kharbush et al., 2017; Savageau and Gamble, 2016). Tramadol has been associated with less respiratory depression than pure mu agonists such as morphine and hydromorphine. Care must be taken with the position of injection regarding hepatic metabolism, which will affect drugs travelling via the hepatic portal system which drains the caudal body. This may reduce the dose of some opiates, and increase the concentration of effective metabolites in others, e.g., tramadol (Baker et al., 2011b; Kinney et al., 2011; Leal et al., 2017; Sladky and Miletic, 2007; Sladky et al., 2008; Williams et al., 2016). Butorphanol has been used in reptiles, but it yields sedation rather than analgesia in most species. In those corn snakes where antinociception was reported in preclinical nociceptive trials, dosages with associated respiratory depression were too high for clinical use (Sladky et al., 2008; Williams et al., 2016).

2. Nonsteroidal antiinflammatories

There is current debate over the use of selective versus nonselective nonsteroidal drugs in reptiles, given the preference for selective COX-2 inhibitors in mammals but little evidence of selective expression of COX-2 at inflamed sites in reptiles (Royal et al., 2012; Thompson et al., 2018). The current clinical approach encompasses the use of meloxicam 0.2−0.3 mg/kg, versus ketoprofen 2 mg/kg, but there is little evidence of antinociception in preclinical trials (Olesen et al., 2008; Trnkova et al., 2007a). However, there is good clinical evidence of improvement in pain-related behavior (Hernandez-Divers, 2006).

3. Local and regional anesthesia

Local/regional blocks have been reported in the literature for caudal surgery in chelonians (Mans, 2014), neuraxial anesthesia (lidocaine with or without morphine) in bearded dragons (Ferreira and Mans, 2018; Fink et al., 2021), and nerve blocks especially in crocodilians (Wellehan et al., 2006). Regional anesthesia has been recently reviewed (d'Ovidio and Adami, 2019; Mans et al., 2019). Local preoperative injection, splash blocks, and the use of EMLA have also been reported (Bianchi et al., 2020; Ferreira and Mans, 2018; Joyce et al., 2018; Mans, 2014; Rivera et al., 2011; Spadola et al., 2015; Wellehan et al., 2006). As the mechanism of action applies across reptiles, the drugs are available, inexpensive, and effective, local analgesia should be routine across all situations where nociceptive stimulation is predicted. Current dosages in terms of toxicity and duration are drawn from the mammalian literature, i.e., 2−4 mg/kg lidocaine and 1−2 mg/kg bupivacaine, and standard formulations can be diluted. The authors would recommend local anesthesia use even in terminal preparations where physiological data is collected, as nociceptive sympathetic cascades can have effects on the data (Williams et al., 2019b).

4. Other agents

Dexmedetomidine has been recently shown to have antinociceptive effects, as well as moderate respiratory depression in pythons and tegus, and contribute to surgical analgesia in bull snakes (Bisetto et al., 2018; Bunke et al., 2018; Sadar and Ambros, 2019).

Anxiolytics and muscle relaxants, such as Midazolam have been reported to have MAC-sparing effects—thus supporting some analgesic action or inhalant potentiation at the spinal level in *Python regius* (Larouche et al., 2019b).

NO_2 has been shown to act as a MAC-sparing agent, and where it can be used safely may be integrated into anesthesia protocols as published in *Python regius* and *Iguana iguana* (Bertelsen et al., 2005b; Larouche et al., 2019b).

D. Nonpharmacological options

While nonpharmaceutical options for analgesia have not been widely reported in reptiles, the minimal and mandatory provision of a species-specific diet and husbandry as well as meeting behavioral needs will both enable pain behavior to be noticed and reduce stress in the animals, potentially improving healing times.

Clinically, acupuncture and electroacupuncture have been reported successfully in reptile patients (Mader and Divers, 2014).

IX. Euthanasia

The ectothermic metabolism and hypoxia tolerance of many reptilian species mean that neural tissue can recover or retain function in situations where mammalian nervous tissue would have become irrecoverably compromised. This robust nature of the CNS must be taken into account at euthanasia—protocols that stop cardiorespiratory function do not indicate that CNS function has been abolished, and therefore a two-stage euthanasia with physical destruction of the CNS is required in most circumstances (AVMA panel on Euthanasia, 2020; Doss and Sladky, 2021; Nevarez et al., 2014; Schnellbacher et al., 2019). This can be via pithing while under deep surgical anesthesia, e.g., after overdose of pentobarbital (300−400 mg/kg), or surgical depths of anesthesia with other chemical agents, via chemical destruction e.g., perfusion fixation with formalin under deep anesthesia if the structure of the CNS is to be retained for research, or fast freezing while under terminal surgical anesthesia. Pentobarbital 300−400 mg/kg IV or IP (with local anesthesia in the hub of the IP needle advised due to the high pH of the drug (Khoo et al., 2018)) is the most common chemical means of abolishing central nervous system function in laboratory species. In larger species: bolt guns have been used to concuss or in combination with pithing in crocodilian farming but require specialist equipment to be used safely. The use of high concentrations of MS222 IP has been used (Conroy et al., 2009), but the low pH of the solution requires buffering, which increases volume, so a two-stage process of an initial buffered injection, followed by an unbuffered further dose once fully anesthetised has been proposed. The use of chemicals to stop cardiac function, e.g., potassium chloride etc., should only be used under a surgical depth of anesthesia and when followed by a physical means to confirm CNS destruction.

While there is some renewed debate about the use of cold as an adjunct to anesthesia, or as a means of euthanasia (Keifer and Zheng, 2017; Lillywhite et al., 2017), this is not currently recommended due to i) the potential for reversal of function if then warmed, ii) effects on stress and immune status of previous hypothermia, iii) the potential for pain if ice crystals form before the loss of nociception, and iv) the range of cold tolerance in reptilian species. An exception is reptiles under 4 g where the use of fast freezing is considered an acceptable euthanasia method (AVMA panel on Euthanasia, 2020; European Council, 2010).

Acknowledgments

The authors gratefully acknowledge Lauren James and Dr. Christian Damsgaard for use of photographs of the ball python and anole in this chapter, and Professor Tobias Wang for discussion of the physiology sections. Silhouettes from phylopic.org used under Public Domain Dedication 1.0, from images by Blair Perry, Christoph Schomburg, Michael Scroggie, Jack Mayer Wood, Birgit Szabo, and CC 3.0 license by Scott Harman, or created by CW under CC 2.0 license from photos by Matt Reinbold, Judy Gallagher, Squamata55, Longitude Latitude and Brian Gratwicke.

References

Abramochkin, D.V., Matchkov, V., Wang, T., 2020. A characterization of the electrophysiological properties of the cardiomyocytes from ventricle, atrium and sinus venosus of the snake heart. J. Comp. Physiol. B. 190, 63–73. https://doi.org/10.1007/s00360-019-01253-5.

Alexander, G.J., 2018. Reproductive biology and maternal care of neonates in southern African python (*Python natalensis*). J. Zool. 305, 141–148.

Alföldi, J., Di Palma, F., Grabherr, M., Williams, C., Kong, L., Mauceli, E., et al., 2011. The genome of the green anole lizard and a comparative analysis with birds and mammals. Nature 477, 587–591.

Alworth, L.C., Hernandez, S.M., Divers, S.J., 2011. Laboratory reptile surgery: principles and techniques. J. Am. Assoc. Lab. Anim. Sci. 50, 11–26.

Andoh, M., Sakata, A., Takano, A., Kawabata, H., Fujita, H., Une, Y., et al., 2015. Detection of rickettsia and ehrlichia SPP. In ticks associated with exotic reptiles and amphibians imported into Japan. PLoS ONE 10, 1–14.

Antonio, F.B., 2014. Venomous reptile restraint and handling. In: Zoo Animal and Wildlife Immobilization and Anesthesia. Wiley, pp. 337–350.

Arnett-Chinn, E.R., Hadfield, C.A., Clayton, L.A., 2016. Review of intramuscular midazolam for sedation in reptiles at the National Aquarium, Baltimore. J. Herpetol. Med. Surg. 26, 59–63.

AVMA panel on Euthanasia, 2020. AVMA Guidelines for the Euthanasia of Animals: 2020 Edition.

Axelsson, M., Franklin, C.E., 2011. Elucidating the responses and role of the cardiovascular system in crocodilians during diving: fifty years on from the work of C.G. Wilber. Comp. Biochem. Physiol. A. Mol. Integr. Physiol. 160, 1–8.

Axelsson, M., Holm, S., Nilsson, S., 1989. Flow dynamics of the crocodilian heart. Am. J. Physiol. 256, R875–R879.

Baker, B.B., Sladky, K.K., Johnson, S.M., 2011a. Evaluation of the analgesic effects of oral and subcutaneous tramadol administration in red/eared slider turtles. J. Am. Vet. Med. Assoc. 238, 220–227.

Baker, B.B., Sladky, K.K., Johnson, S.M., 2011b. Evaluation of the analgesic effects of oral and subcutaneous tramadol administration in red-eared slider turtles. J. Am. Assoc. Lab. Anim. Sci. 238, 1356–1362.

Barrillot, B., Roux, J., Arthaud, S., Averty, L., Clair, A., Herrel, A., Libourel, P.-A., 2018. Intramuscular administration of ketamine-medetomidine assures stable anaesthesia needed for long term surgery in the argentine tegu *Salvator merianae*. J. Zoo Wildl. Med. 49, 291–296.

Barter, L.S., Hawkins, M.G., Brosnan, R.J., Antognini, J.F., Pypendop, B.H., 2006. Median effective dose of isoflurane, sevoflurane, and desflurane in green iguanas. Am. J. Vet. Res. 67, 392–397.

Bennett, R.A., Schumacher, J., Hedjazi-Haring, K., Newell, S.M., 1998. Cardiopulmonary and anesthetic effects of propofol administered intraosseously to green iguanas. J. Am. Vet. Med. Assoc. 212, 93–98.

Bertelsen, M.F., 2019. Anaesthesia and analgesia. In: BSAVA Manual of Reptiles. British Small Animal Veterinary Association, pp. 200–209.

Bertelsen, M.F., Buchanan, R., Jensen, H.M., Leite, C.A.C., Abe, A.S., Nielsen, S., Wang, T., 2014. Assessing the influence of mechanical ventilation on blood gases and blood pressure in rattlesnakes. Vet. Anaesth. Analg. 42, 1–8.

Bertelsen, M.F., Buchanan, R., Jensen, H.M., Leite, C.A.C., Abe, A.S., Wang, T., 2021. Comparative biochemistry and physiology, part A pharmacodynamics of propofol and alfaxalone in rattlesnakes (*Crotalus durissus*). Comp. Biochem. Physiol. Part A 256, 110935.

Bertelsen, M.F., Mosley, C.A.E., Crawshaw, G.J., Dyson, D., Smith, D.A., 2005a. Minimum alveolar concentration of isoflurane in mechanically ventilated Dumeril monitors. J. Am. Vet. Med. Assoc. 226, 1098–1101.

Bertelsen, M.F., Mosley, C.A.E., Crawshaw, G.J., Dyson, D.H., Smith, D.A., 2005b. Anesthetic potency of sevoflurane with and without nitrous oxide in mechanically ventilated Dumeril monitors. J. Am. Vet. Med. Assoc. 227, 575–578.

Bianchi, C., Adami, C., Dirrig, H., Cuff, A., d'Ovidio, D., Monticelli, P., 2020. Mandibular nerve block in juvenile Nile crocodile: a cadaveric study. Vet. Anaesth. Analg. 47, 835–842.

Bickler, P.E., Buck, L.T., 2007. Hypoxia tolerance in reptiles, amphibians, and fishes: life with variable oxygen availability. Annu. Rev. Physiol. 69, 145–170.

Bisetto, S.P., Melo, C.F., Carregaro, A.B., 2018. Evaluation of sedative and antinociceptive effects of dexmedetomidine, midazolam and dexmedetomidine-midazolam in tegus (*Salvator merianae*). Vet. Anaesth. Analg. 45, 320–328.

Bonnet, X., El Hassani, M.S., Lecq, S., Michel, C.L., El Mouden, E.H., Michaud, B., Slimani, T., 2016. Blood mixtures: impact of puncture site on blood parameters. J. Comp. Physiol. B Biochem. Syst. Environ. Physiol. 186, 787–800.

Brosnan, R.J., Pypendop, B.H., Barter, L.S., Hawkins, M.G., 2006. Pharmacokinetics of inhaled anesthetics in green iguanas (*Iguana iguana*). Am. J. Vet. Res. 67, 1670–1674.

Budden, L., Doss, G., CLyde, V., Mans, C., 2018. Retrospective evaluation of sedation in 16 lizard species with dexmedetomidine-midazolam with or without ketamine (2010–2016). J. Herpetol. Med. Surg. 28, 47–50.

Bunke, L.G., Sladky, K.K., Johnson, S.M., Bunke, 2018. Antinociceptive efficacy and respiratory effects of dexmedetomidine in ball pythons (*Python regius*). Am. J. Vet. Res. 79, 718–726.

Burggren, W., Filogonio, R., Wang, T., 2020. Cardiovascular shunting in vertebrates: a practical integration of competing hypotheses. Biol. Rev. 95, 449–471.

Burggren, W.W., Christoffels, V.M., Crossley, D.A., Enok, S., Farrell, A.P., Hedrick, M.S., et al., 2014. Comparative cardiovascular physiology: future trends, opportunities and challenges. Acta Physiol. 210, 257–276.

Card, D.C., Perry, B.W., Adams, R.H., Schield, D.R., Young, A.S., Andrew, A.L., et al., 2018. Novel ecological and climatic conditions drive rapid adaptation in invasive Florida Burmese pythons. Mol. Ecol. 27, 4744–4757.

Cermakova, E., Ceplecha, V., Knotek, Z., 2018. Efficacy of two methods of intranasal administration of anaesthetic drugs in red-eared terrapins (*Trachemys scripta elegans*). Vet. Med. (Praha). 63, 87–93.

Chatigny, F., Kamunde, C., Creighton, C.M., Stevens, E.D., 2017. Uses and doses of local anesthetics in fish, amphibians, and reptiles. J. Am. Assoc. Lab. Anim. Sci. 56, 244–253.

Christiansen, E.F., Piniak, W.E.D., Lester, L.A., Harms, C.A., 2013. Underwater anesthesia of diamondback terrapins (*Malaclemys terrapin*) for measurement of auditory evoked potentials. J. Am. Assoc. Lab. Anim. Sci. 52, 792–797.

Churgin, S.M., Sladky, K.K., Smith, L., 2014. Comparison of induction and recovery parameters between isoflurane in 100% oxygen and 21% oxygen in bearded dragons (*Pogona vitticeps*). In: Proceedings of the Association of Reptilian and Amphibian Veterinarians, p. 40.

Cieri, R.L., Farmer, C.G., 2016. Unidirectional pulmonary airflow in vertebrates: a review of structure, function, and evolution. J. Comp. Physiol. B Biochem. Syst. Environ. Physiol. 186, 541–552.

Conner, J.L., Crossley, J.L., Elsey, R., Nelson, D., Wang, T., Crossley, D.A., 2019. Does the left aorta provide proton-rich blood to the gut when crocodilians digest a meal? J. Exp. Biol. jeb201079.

Conroy, C., Papenfuss, T., Parker, J., Hahn, N., 2009. Use of tricaine methanesulfonate (MS222) for euthanasia of reptiles. J. Am. Assoc. Lab. Anim. Sci. 48, 28–32.

Couture, É.L., Monteiro, B.P., Aymen, J., Troncy, E., Steagall, P.V., Couture, E.L., et al., 2017. Validation of a thermal threshold nociceptive model in bearded dragons (*Pogona vitticeps*). Vet. Anaesth. Analg. 44, 676–683.

Cushing, A.C., Smith, C.K., Ramsay, E.C., Nelson, S., Giori, L., 2020. Transcutaneous oxygen monitoring in lousiana pine snakes (*Pitouphis ruthveni*). J. Zoo Wildl. Med. 50, 874–878.

d'Ovidio, D., Adami, C., 2019. Locoregional anesthesia in exotic pets. Vet. Clin. N. Am. Exot. Anim. Pract. 22, 301–314.

Darrow, B.G., Myers, G.E., KuKanich, B., Sladky, K.K., 2017. Fentanyl transdermal therapeutic system provides rapid systemic fentanyl absorption in two ball pythons (*Python regius*). J. Herpetol. Med. Surg. 26, 94–99.

Dessauer, H.C., 1970. Blood chemistry of reptiles: physiological and evolutionary aspects. In: Gans, C., Parsons, T.H. (Eds.), Biology of the Reptilia. Academic Press, New York, pp. 1–72.

Di Giuseppe, M., Morici, M., Nastasi, B., Spadola, F., 2018. Preliminary survey on influence of renal portal system during propofol anesthesia in yellow-bellied turtle (*Trachemys scripta scripta*). J. Vet. Med. Allied Sci. 2, 2–5.

Di Salvo, A., Giorgi, M., Catanzaro, A., Deli, G., della Rocca, G., 2016. Pharmacokinetic profiles of meloxicam in turtles (*Trachemys scripta scripta*) after single oral, intracoelomic and intramuscular administrations. J. Vet. Pharmacol. Ther. 39, 102–105.

Divers, S.J., 2019. Endoscope-assisted and endoscopic surgery. In: Mader's Reptile and Amphibian Medicine and Surgery, third ed.

Divers, S.J., Papich, M., McBride, M., Stedman, N.L., Perpinan, D., Koch, T.F., et al., 2010. Pharmacokinetics of meloxicam following intravenous and oral administration in green iguanas (*Iguana iguana*). Am. J. Vet. Res. 71, 1277–1283.

Divers, S.J., Stahl, S.J., 2019. Section 8: endoscopy. In: Divers, S., Stahl, S. (Eds.), Mader's Reptile and Amphibian Medicine and Surgery. Elsevier, Missouri, p. 1511.

Dohm, L., Brunson, D., 1998. Effective dose of isoflurane for the desert iguana (*Dipsosaurus dorsalis*) and the effect of hypothermia on effective dose. Proc. Am. Coll. Vet. Anesth. 543.

Doss, G.A., Fink, D.M., Sladky, K.K., Mans, C., 2017. Comparison of subcutaneous dexmedetomidine-midazolam versus alfaxalone-midazolam sedation in leopard geckos (*Eublepharis macularius*). Vet. Anaesth. Analg. 44, 1175–1183.

Doss, G.A., Mans, C., Sladky, K.K., 2021. Analgesia, anesthesia and monitoring. In: Graham, J.E., Doss, G.A., Beaufrere, H. (Eds.), Exotic Animal Emergency and Critical Care Medicine. Wiley-Blackwell, pp. 746–756.

Doss, G.A., Sladky, K.K., 2021. CPR and euthanasia. Exot. Anim. Emerg. Crit. Care Med. 738–745.

Enok, S., Leite, G.S.P.C., Leite, C.A.C., Gesser, H., Hedrick, M.S., Wang, T., 2016. Improved cardiac filling facilitates the postprandial elevation of stroke volume in *Python regius*. J. Exp. Biol. 219, 3009–3018.

Eshar, D., Rooney, T.A., Gardhouse, S., Beaufrère, H., 2021. Evaluation of the effects of a dexmedetomidine-midazolam-ketamine combination administered intramuscularly to captive red-footed tortoises (*Chelonoidis carbonaria*). Am. J. Vet. Res. 82, 858–864.

European Council, 2010. Directive 2010/63/EU of the European parliament and of the council on the protection of animals used for scientific purposes. Off. J. Eur. Union 1, 33–79.

Ferreira, T.H., Mans, C., 2018. Evaluation of neuraxial anesthesia in bearded dragons (*Pogona vitticeps*). Vet. Anaesth. Analg. 46, 126–134.

Ferreira, T.H., Mans, C., Di Girolamo, N., 2019. Evaluation of the sedative and physiological effects of intramuscular lidocaine in bearded dragons (*Pogona vitticeps*) sedated with alfaxalone. Vet. Anaesth. Analg. 46, 496–500.

Filogonio, R., Sartori, M.R., Morgensen, S., Tavares, D., Campos, R., Abe, A.S., et al., 2020. Cholinergic regulation along the pulmonary arterial tree of the South American rattlesnake: vascular reactivity, muscarinic receptors, and vagal innervation. Am. J. Physiol. 319, R156–R170.

Findsen, A., Crossley, D.A., Wang, T., 2018. Feeding alters blood flow patterns in the American alligator (*Alligator mississippiensis*). Comp. Biochem. Physiol. Part A Mol. Integr. Physiol. 215, 1–5.

Fink, D.M., Doss, G.A., Sladky, K.K., Mans, C., 2018. Effect of injection site on dexmedetomidine-ketamine induced sedation in leopard geckos (*Eublepharis macularius*). J. Am. Vet. Med. Assoc. 253, 1146–1150.

Fink, D.M., Ferreira, T.H., Mans, C., 2021. Neuraxial administration of morphine combined with lidocaine induces regional antinociception in inland bearded dragons (*Pogona vitticeps*). Am. J. Vet. Res. 83, 1–6.

Fleming, G.J., 2014. Crocodilians (crocodiles, alligators, caiman, and gharial). In: Zoo Animal and Wildlife Immobilization and Anesthesia, pp. 325–336.

Fleming, G.J., Robertson, S.A., 2012. Assessments of thermal antinociceptive effects of butorphanol and human observer effect on quantitative evaluation of analgesia in green iguanas (*Iguana iguana*). Am. J. Vet. Res. 73, 1507–1511.

Freitag, F.A., Barboza, T.K., Dutton, C., Buck, R.K., 2021. Alfaxalone for anesthesia of a giant snake. Vet. Anaesth. Analg. 9–10.

Friesen, C.R., Uhrig, E.J., Mason, R.T., Brennan, P.L.R., 2016. Female behaviour and the interaction of male and female genital traits mediate sperm transfer during mating. J. Evol. Biol. 29, 952–964.

Gamble, K., 2008. Plasma fentanyl concentrations achieved after transdermal fentanyl patch application in prehensile-tailed skinks, *Corucia zebrata*. J. Herpetol. Med. Surg. 18, 31–35.

Gatson, B.J., Goe, A., Granone, T.D., Wellehan, J.F.X., 2017. Intramuscular epinephrine results in reduced anesthetic recovery time in american alligators (*Alligator mississippiensis*) undergoing isoflurane anesthesia. J. Zoo Wildl. Med. 48, 55–61.

Giorgi, M., Salvadori, M., De Vito, V., Owen, H., Demontis, M.P., Varoni, M.V., 2015. Pharmacokinetic/pharmacodynamic assessments of 10 mg/kg tramadol intramuscular injection in yellow-bellied slider turtles (*Trachemys scripta scripta*). J. Vet. Pharmacol. Ther. 38, 488–496.

Goe, A., Shmalberg, J., Gatson, B., Bartolini, P., Curtiss, J., Wellehan, J.F.X., 2016. Epinephrine or Gv-26 electrical stimulation reduces inhalant anesthestic recovery time in common snapping turtles (*Chelydra serpentina*). J. Zoo Wildl. Med. 47, 501–507.

Gorczak, R., Chaves, R.O., Teixeira, M.L., de Freitas, I.B., Martins, R.C., Valandro, M.A., et al., 2017. Anesthesia in American alligator (*Alligator mississipiensis*) for a limb amputation. Acta Sci. Vet. 45, 1–5.

Gracheva, E.O., Ingolia, N.T., Kelly, Y.M., Cordero-Morales, J.F., Hollopeter, G., Chesler, A.T., et al., 2010. Molecular basis of infrared detection by snakes. Nature 464, 1006–1011.

Gräns, A., Olsson, C., Pitsillides, K., Nelson, H.E., Cech Jr., J.J., Axelsson, M., 2010. Effects of feeding on thermoregulatory behaviours and gut blood flow in white sturgeon (*Acipenser transmontanus*) using biotelemetry in combination with standard techniques. J. Exp. Biol. 213, 3198–3206.

Greenacre, C., Takle, G., Schumacher, J., Klaphake, E.K., Harvey, R.C., 2006. Comparative antinociception of morphine, butorphanol, and buprenorphine versus saline in the green iguana (*Iguana iguana*) using electrostimulation. J. Herpetol. Med. Surg. 16, 88–92.

Greunz, E.M., Williams, C.J., Ringgaard, S., Hansen, K., Wang, T., Bertelsen, M.F., 2018. Elimination of intracardiac shunting provides stable gas anesthesia in tortoises. Sci. Rep. 8, 1712.

Hale, V.L., MacGowan, B., Corriveau, L., Huse, D.C., Currylow, A.F.T., Thompson, S., 2017. Radio transmitter implantation and movement in the wild timber rattlesnake (*Crotalus horridus*). J. Wildl. Dis. 53, 591–595.

Harms, C.A., Eckert, S.A., Jones, T.T., Dow Piniak, W.E., Mann, D.A., 2009. A technique for underwater anesthesia compared with manual restraint of sea turtles undergoing auditory evoked potential measurements. J. Herpetol. Med. Surg. 19, 8–12.

Harms, C.A., Eckert, S.A., Kubis, S.A., Campbell, M., Levenson, D.H., Crognale, M.A., 2007. Field anaesthesia of leatherback sea turtles (*Dermochelys coriacea*). Vet. Rec. 161, 15–21.

Harms, C.A., Piniak, W.E.D., Eckert, S.A., Stringer, E.M., Harms, A.C.A., Piniak, W.E.D., et al., 2014. Sedation and anesthesia of hatchling leatherback sea turtles (*Dermochelys coriacea*) for auditory evoked potential measurement in air and in water. J. Zoo Wildl. Med. 45, 86–92.

Hawkins, S.J., Cox, S., Yaw, T.J., Sladky, K., 2019. Pharmacokinetics of subcutaneously administered hydromorphone in bearded dragons (*Pogona vitticeps*) and red-eared slider turtles (*Trachemys scripta elegans*). Vet. Anaesth. Analg. 46, 352–359.

Hernandez-Divers, S.J., 2006. Meloxicam and repiles, a practical approach to analgesia. Small Anim. Exot. Proc. N. Am. Vet. Conf. 1636–1637.

Hernandez-Divers, S.M., Hernandez-Divers, S.J., Wyneken, J., 2002. Angiographic, anatomic and clinical technique descriptions of a subcarapacial venipuncture site for chelonians. J. Herpetol. Med. Surg. 12, 32–37.

Holz, P., Barker, I.K., Burger, J.P., Crawshaw, G.J., Peter, D., 1997. The effect of the renal portal system on pharmacokinetic parameters in the red-eared slider (*Trachemys scripta elegans*). J. Zoo Wildl. Med. 28, 386–393.

Holz, P., Holz, R.M., 1994. Evaluation of ketamine, ketamine xylazine, and ketamine midazolam anesthesia in red-eared sliders (*Trachemys scripta elegans*). J. Zoo Wildl. Med. 25, 531–537.

Innis, C., DeVoe, R., Mylniczenko, N., Young, D., Garner, M., 2010. A call for additional study of the safety of subcarapacial venipuncture in chelonians. In: Proceedings of the Association of Reptilian and Amphibian Veterinarians, pp. 8–10.

Isaza, R., Andrews, G., Coke, R., Hunter, R., 2004. Assessment of multiple cardiocentesis in ball pythons (*Python regius*). Contemp. Top. Lab. Anim. Sci. 43, 35–38.

IUCN Crocodile Specialist Group, n.d. http://www.iucncsg.org/. (Accessed 20 October 2021).

Jacquart, H., 1855. Memoire sur les organes de la circulation chez le serpent python. Ann. Sci. Nat. 4, 321–364.

Jakobsen, S.L., Williams, C.J.A., Wang, T., Bertelsen, M.F., 2017. The influence of mechanical ventilation on physiological parameters in ball pythons (*Python regius*). Comp. Biochem. Physiol. Part A Mol. Integr. Physiol. 207, 30–35.

James, L.E., Williams, C.J.A., Bertelsen, M.F., Wang, T., 2017. Evaluation of feeding behavior as an indicator of pain in snakes. J. Zoo Wildl. Med. 48, 196–199.

James, L.E., Williams, C.J.A., Bertelsen, M.F., Wang, T., 2018. Anaesthetic induction with alfaxalone in the ball python (*Python regius*): dose response and effect of injection site. Vet. Anaesth. Analg. 45, 329–337.

Jensen, B., Moorman, A.F.M., Wang, T., 2014. Structure and function of the hearts of lizards and snakes. Biol. Rev. Camb. Philos. Soc. 89, 302–336.

Jensen, B., Nielsen, J.M., Axelsson, M., Pedersen, M., Löfman, C., Wang, T., 2010. How the python heart separates pulmonary and systemic blood pressures and blood flows. J. Exp. Biol. 213, 1611–1617.

Jensen, M.T., Jensen, U.T., Bertelsen, M.F., 2021. Assessing the effects of biosecurity measures in terrarium management. J. Zoo Aquar. Res. 9, 157–160.

Joyce, W., Axelsson, M., Altimiras, J., Wang, T., 2016. *In situ* cardiac perfusion reveals interspecific variation of intraventricular flow separation in reptiles. J. Exp. Biol. 219, 2220–2227.

Joyce, W., Williams, C.J.A., Crossley, D.A., Wang, T., Crossley II, D.A., Wang, T., 2018. Venous pressures and cardiac filling in turtles during apnoea and intermittent ventilation. J. Comp. Physiol. B Biochem. Syst. Environ. Physiol. 188, 481–490.

Kanda, I., Brandão, J., 2021. Nutrition and fluid therapy. In: Graham, J.E., Doss, G.A., Beaufrère, H. (Eds.), Exotic Animal Emergency and Critical Care Medicine. Wiley, pp. 764–767.

Kanui, T.I., Hole, K., 1992. Morphine and pethidine antinociception in the crocodile. J. Vet. Pharmacol. Ther. 15, 101–103.

Keifer, J., Zheng, Z., 2017. Cold block of in vitro eyeblink reflexes: evidence supporting the use of hypothermia as an anesthetic in pond turtles. J. Exp. Biol. 220, 4370–4373.

Kharbush, R., Gutwilling, A., Hartzler, K., Gardner, A., Abbott, A., Cox, S., et al., 2017. Antinociceptive and respiratory effects following application of transdermal fentanyl patches and assessment of brain μ-opioid receptor mRNA expression in ball pythons. Am. J. Vet. Res. 78, 785–795.

Khoo, S.Y.-S., Lay, B.P.P., Joya, J., McNally, G.P., 2018. Local anaesthetic refinement of pentobarbital euthanasia reduces abdominal writhing without affecting immunohistochemical endpoints in rats. Lab. Anim. 52, 152–162.

Kinney, M.E.M., Johnson, S.M., Sladky, K.K., 2011. Behavioral evaluation of red-eared slider turtles (*Trachemys scripta elegans*) administered either morphine or butorphanol following unilateral gonadectomy. J. Herpetol. Med. Surg. 21, 54–62.

Kischinovsky, M., Duse, A., Wang, T., Bertelsen, M.F., 2013. Intramuscular administration of alfaxalone in red-eared sliders (*Trachemys scripta elegans*)—effects of dose and body temperature. Vet. Anaesth. Analg. 40, 13–20.

Klaphake, E., Gibbons, P.M., Sladky, K.K., Carpenter, J.W., 2018. Reptiles. In: Exotic Animal Formulary, fifth ed., pp. 81–166.

Knotek, Z., 2014. Alfaxalone as an induction agent for anaesthesia in terrapins and tortoises. Vet. Rec. 175, 327.

Knotek, Z., Hrda, A., Kley, N., Knotkova, Z., 2011. Alfaxalon anaesthesia in veiled chameleon (*Chamaeleo calyptratus*). Proc. Arav 181.

Knotek, Z., Hrdá, A., Knotková, Z., Trnková, Š., Babák, V., 2013. Alfaxalone anaesthesia in the green iguana (*Iguana iguana*). Acta Vet. Brno 82, 109–114.

Kristensen, L., Zardo, J.Q., Hansen, S.M., Bertelsen, M.F., Alstrup, A.K.O., Wang, T., Williams, C.J.A., 2022. The effect of atropine and propofol on the minimum anaesthetic concentration of isoflurane in the freshwater turtle *Trachemys scripta scripta* (yellow-bellied slider). Vet. Anaesth. Analg. https://doi.org/10.1016/j.vaa.2021.10.008.

Lahner, L.L., Mans, C., Sladky, K.K., Aczm, D., 2011. Comparison of anesthetic induction and recovery times after intramuscular, subcutaneous or intranasal dexmedetomidine in red eared slider turtles (*Trachemys scripta*). Proc. Assoc. Reptil. Amphib. Vet. 136–137.

Lai, O.R., Di Bello, A., Soloperto, S., Freggi, D., Marzano, G., Cavaliere, L., Crescenzo, G., 2015. Pharmacokinetic behavior of meloxicam in loggerhead sea turtles (*Caretta caretta*) after intramuscular and intravenous administration. J. Wildl. Dis. 51, 509–512.

Larouche, C.B., 2019. The Use of Midazolam, Isoflurane, and Nitrous Oxide for Sedation and Anesthesia of Ball Pythons (*Python regius*). University of Guelph.

Larouche, C.B., Beaufrere, H., Mosley, C., Nemeth, N.M., Dutton, C., 2019a. Evaluation of the effects of midazolam and flumazenil in the ball python (*Python regius*). J. Zoo Wildl. Med. 50, 579–588.

Larouche, C.B., Mosley, C., Beaufrère, H., Dutton, C., 2019b. Effects of midazolam and nitrous oxide on the minimum anesthetic concentration of isoflurane in the ball python (*Python regius*). Vet. Anaesth. Analg. 46, 807–814.

Larsen, G.D., 2016. The peculiar physiology of the python. Lab Anim. (NY) 45, 205.

Leal, W.P., Carregaro, A.B., Bressan, T.F., Bisetto, S.P., Melo, C.F., Sladky, K.K., 2017. Antinociceptive efficacy of intramuscular administration of morphine sulfate and butorphanol tartrate in tegus. Am. J. Vet. Res. 78, 1019–1024.

Lillywhite, H.B., Shine, R., Jacobson, E., Denardo, D.F., Gordon, M.S., Navas, C.A., et al., 2017. Anesthesia and euthanasia of amphibians and reptiles used in scientific research: should hypothermia and freezing be prohibited? Bioscience 67, 53–61.

Lopes, I.G., Armelin, V.A., Braga, V.H. da S., Florindo, L.H., 2017. The influence of midazolam on heart rate arises from cardiac autonomic tones alterations in Burmese pythons, *Python molurus*. Auton. Neurosci. Basic Clin. 208, 103–112.

Lovern, M.B., Holmes, M.M., Wade, J., 2004. The green anole (*Anolis carolinensis*): a reptilian model for laboratory studies of reproductive morphology and behavior. Inst. Lab. Anim. Res. J. 45, 54–64.

Lyson, T.R., Schachner, E.R., Botha-Brink, J., Scheyer, T.M., Lambertz, M., Bever, G.S., Rubidge, B.S., de Queiroz, K., 2014. Origin of the unique ventilatory apparatus of turtles. Nat. Commun. 5, 5211.

Maas, A., Brunson, D.B., 2002. Comparison of anesthetic potency and cardiopulmonary effects of isoflurane and sevoflurane in colubrid snakes. In: Proceedings of the American Association of Zoo Veterinarians, pp. 306–308.

MacLean, R., Harms, C., Braun-McNeill, J., 2008. Propofol anesthesia in loggerhead (*Caretta caretta*) sea turtles. J. Wildl. Dis. 44, 143–150.

Mader, D.R., Divers, S.J., 2014. Current Therapy in Reptile Medicine and Surgery. Elsevier.

Madsen, J.G., Wang, T., Beedholm, K., Madsen, P.T., 2013. Detecting spring after a long winter: coma or slow vigilance in cold, hypoxic turtles? Biol. Lett. 9.

Makau, C.M., Towett, P.K., Abelson, K.S.P.P., Kanui, T.I., 2017. Modulation of formalin-induced pain-related behaviour by clonidine and yohimbine in the Speke's hinged tortoise (*Kiniskys spekii*). J. Vet. Pharmacol. Ther. 40, 439–446.

Malte, C.L., Bundgaard, J., Jensen, M.S., Bertelsen, M.F., Wang, T., 2018. The effects of morphine on gas exchange, ventilation pattern and ventilatory responses to hypercapnia and hypoxia in dwarf caiman

(*Paleosuchus palpebrosus*). Comp. Biochem. Physiol. Part A Mol. Integr. Physiol. 222, 60–65.

Malte, C.L., Jakobsen, S.L., Wang, T., 2014. A critical evaluation of automated blood gas measurements in comparative respiratory physiology. Comp. Biochem. Physiol. A. Mol. Integr. Physiol. 178C, 7–17.

Mans, C., 2014. Clinical technique: intrathecal drug administration in turtles and tortoises. J. Exot. Pet Med. 23, 67–70.

Mans, C., 2018. Unique species considerations: reptiles. In: Veterinary Anesthetic and Monitoring Equipment, pp. 489–495.

Mans, C., Lahner, L.L., Baker, B.B., Johnson, S.M., Sladky, K.K., 2012. Antinociceptive efficacy of buprenorphine and hydromorphone in red-eared slider turtles (*Trachemys scripta elegans*). J. Zoo Wildl. Med. 43, 662–665.

Mans, C., Steagall, P., Sladky, K.K., 2019. 51—regional anesthesia and analgesia. In: Divers, S.J., Stahl, S.J. (Eds.), Mader's Reptile and Amphibian Medicine and Surgery, third ed. W.B. Saunders, St. Louis (MO), pp. 475–479.e1.

Martin, J.C., Sedgwick, C.J., 1994. A review of allometric scaling with considerations for its application. Proc. Assoc. Reptil. Amphib. Vet. 55–58.

McWhorter, A., Owens, J., Valcanis, M., Olds, L., Myers, C., Smith, I., et al., 2021. In vitro invasiveness and antimicrobial resistance of *Salmonella enterica* subspecies isolated from wild and captive reptiles. Zoonoses Public Health 68, 402–412.

Millard, R.W., Johansen, K., 1974. Ventricular outflow dynamics in the lizard, *Varanus niloticus*: responses to hypoxia, hypercarbia and diving. J. Exp. Biol. 60, 871–880.

Miller, L.J., Fetterer, D.P., Garza, N.L., Lackemeyer, M.G., Donnelly, G.C., Steffens, J.T., et al., 2018. A fixed moderate-dose combination of tiletamine+zolazepam outperforms midazolam in induction of short-term immobilization of ball pythons (*Python regius*). PLoS ONE 13, 1–15.

Milsom, W.K., 1991. Intermittent breathing in vertebrates. Annu. Rev. Physiol. 53, 87–105.

Minor, R.L., Doss, G.A., Mans, C., 2021. Evaluation of glucose absorption rates following intracoelomic or subcutaneous administration in experimentally dehydrated inland bearded dragons (*Pogona vitticeps*). Am. J. Vet. Res. 82, 9–12.

Moberly, W.R., 1968. The metabolic responses of the common iguana, *Iguana iguana*, to walking and diving. Comp. Biochem. Physiol. 27, 21–32.

Monticelli, P., Ronaldson, H.L., Hutchinson, J.R., Cuff, A.R., D'Ovidio, D., Adami, C., 2019. Medetomidine-ketamine-sevoflurane anaesthesia in juvenile Nile crocodiles (*Crocodylus niloticus*) undergoing experimental surgery. Vet. Anaesth. Analg. 46, 84–89.

Morici, M., Di Giuseppe, M., Spadola, F., Oliveri, M., Knotkova, Z., Knotek, Z., 2018. Intravenous alfaxalone anaesthesia in leopard geckos (*Eublepharis macularis*). J. Exot. Pet Med. 27, 11–14.

Morici, M., Lubian, E., Costa, G.L., Spadola, F., 2021. Difference between cranial and caudal intravenous alfaxalone administration in yellow-bellied sliders (*Trachemys scripta scripta*). Acta Vet. Eurasia 47, 88–92.

Mosley, C.A.E., Dyson, D., Smith, D.A., 2003. Minimum alveolar concentration of isoflurane in green iguanas and the effect of butorphanol on minimum alveolar concentration. J. Am. Vet. Med. Assoc. 222, 1559–1564.

Nagy, K.A., 2005. Field metabolic rate and body size. J. Exp. Biol. 208, 1621–1625.

Nevarez, J.G., Strain, G.M., da Cunha, A.F., Beaufrere, H., Anderson, F., da Cunha, A.F., Beaufrere, H., 2014. Evaluation of four methods for inducing death during slaughter of American alligators. Am. J. Vet. Res. 75, 536–546.

Nielsen, V.G., Frank, N., Afshar, S., 2019. De novo assessment and review of pan-american pit viper anticoagulant and procoagulant venom activities via kinetomic analyses. Toxins (Basel) 11.

Nilsson, G.E., Lutz, P.L., 1993. Role of GABA in hypoxia tolerance, metabolic depression and hibernation-possible links to neurotransmitter evolution. Comp. Biochem. Physiol. Part C Comp. 105, 329–336.

Norton, T.M., Cox, S., Nelson Jr., S.E., Kaylor, M., Thomas, R., Hupp, A., et al., 2015. Pharmacokinetics of tramadol and o-desmethyltramadol in loggerhead sea turtles (*Caretta caretta*). J. Zoo Wildl. Med. 46, 262–265.

O'Rourke, D.P., Cox, J.D., Baumann, D.P., 2018. Non-traditional species. In: Management of Animal Care and Use Programs in Research, Education, and Testing. CRC Press, pp. 579–596.

Odette, O., Churgin, S.M., Sladky, K.K., Smith, L., 2015. Anesthetic induction and recovery parameters in bearded dragons (*Pogona vitticeps*): comparison of isoflurane delivered in 100% oxygen versus 21% oxygen. J. Zoo Wildl. Med. 46, 534–539.

Olesen, M.G., Bertelsen, M.F., Perry, S.F., Wang, T., 2008. Effects of preoperative administration of butorphanol or meloxicam on physiologic responses to surgery in ball pythons. J. Am. Vet. Med. Assoc. 232, 1183–1188.

Olsson, A., 2013. Investigation into Developing Reliable Immobilisation Protocol for Use Under Varying Environmental Temperatures in Estuarine and Australian Freshwater Crocodiles. University of Sydney.

Olsson, A., Phalen, D., 2012a. Medetomidine immobilisation and atipamezole reversal in large estuarine crocodiles (*Crocodylus porosus*) using metabolically scaled dosages. Aust. Vet. J. 90, 240–244.

Olsson, A., Phalen, D., 2012b. Preliminary studies of chemical immobilization of captive juvenile estuarine (*Crocodylus porosus*) and Australian freshwater (*C. johnstoni*) crocodiles with medetomidine and reversal with atipamezole. Vet. Anaesth. Analg. 39, 345–356.

Olsson, A., Phalen, D., 2013. The effects of decreased body temperature on the onset, duration and action of medetomidine and its antagonist atipamezole in juvenile farmed estuarine crocodiles (*Crocodylus porosus*). Vet. Anaesth. Analg. 40, 272–279.

Olsson, A., Phalen, D., Dart, C., 2013. Preliminary studies of alfaxalone for intravenous immobilization of juvenile captive estuarine crocodiles (*Crocodylus porosus*) and Australian freshwater crocodiles (*Crocodylus johnstoni*) at optimal and selected sub-optimal thermal zones. Vet. Anaesth. Analg. 40, 494–502.

Oppenheim, Y.C.C., Moon, P.F.F., 1995. Sedative effects of midazolam in red-eared slider turtles (*Trachemys scripta elegans*). J. Zoo Wildl. Med. 26, 409–413.

Overgaard, J., Stecyk, J.A.W., Farrell, A.P., Wang, T., 2002. Adrenergic control of the cardiovascular system in the turtle *Trachemys scripta*. J. Exp. Biol. 205, 3335–3345.

Palacios, M.G., Sparkman, A.M., Bronikowski, A.M., 2012. Corticosterone and pace of life in two life-history ecotypes of the garter snake thamnophis elegans. Gen. Comp. Endocrinol. 175, 443–448.

Paladino, F.V., O'Connor, M.P., Spotila, J.R., 1990. Metabolism of leatherback turtles, gigantothermy, and thermoregulation of dinosaurs. Nature 344, 858–860.

Pasmans, F., Blahak, S., Martel, A., Pantchev, N., 2008. Introducing reptiles into a captive collection: the role of the veterinarian. Vet. J. 175, 53–68.

Peacock, H.M., Gilbert, E.A.B.B., Vickaryous, M.K., 2015. Scar-free cutaneous wound healing in the leopard gecko, *Eublepharis macularius*. J. Anat. 227, 596–610.

Pedersen, K., Lassen-Nielsen, A.M., Nordentoft, S., Hammer, A.S., 2009. Serovars of salmonella from captive reptiles. Zoonoses Public Health 56, 238–242.

Perrin, K.L., Bertelsen, M.F., 2017. Intravenous alfaxalone and propofol anesthesia in the bearded dragon (*Pogona vitticeps*). J. Herpetol. Med. Surg. 27, 123–126.

Perry, S.F., 1983. Reptilian lungs. Functional anatomy and evolution. Adv. Anat. Embryol. Cell Biol. 79, 1–81.

Perry, S.F., 1989. Structure and function of the reptilian respiratory system. In: Lenfant, C., Wood, S. (Eds.), Lung Biology in Health and Disease. Comparative Pulmonary Physiology. Current Concepts. Marcel Dekker, New York, NY, pp. 193–236.

Perry, S.F., Duncker, H.R., 1980. Interrelationship of static mechanical factors and anatomical structure in lung evolution. J. Comp. Physiol. B 138, 321–334.

Preston, D.L., Mosley, C.A.E., Mason, R.T., 2010. Sources of variability in recovery time from methohexital sodium anesthesia in snakes. Copeia 2010, 496–501.

Rasys, A.M., Divers, S.J., Lauderdale, J.D., Menke, D.B., 2019a. A systematic study of injectable anesthetic agents in the brown anole lizard (*Anolis sagrei*). Lab. Anim. 00, 1–12.

Rasys, A.M., Park, S., Ball, R.E., Alcala, A.J., Lauderdale, J.D., Menke, D.B., 2019b. CRISPR-Cas9 gene editing in lizards through microinjection of unfertilized oocytes. Cell Rep. 28, 2288+.

Ratliff, C., Parkinson, L.A.B., Mans, C., 2019. Effects of the fraction of inspired oxygen on alfaxalone-sedated inland bearded dragons (*Pogona vitticeps*). Am. J. Vet. Res. 80, 129–134.

Reber, S.A., Oh, J., Janisch, J., Stevenson, C., Foggett, S., Wilkinson, A., 2021. Early life differences in behavioral predispositions in two Alligatoridae species. Anim. Cogn. 24, 753–764.

Revell, L.J., 2012. Phytools: An R package for phylogenetic comparative biology (and other things). Methods Ecol. Evol. 3, 217–223. https://doi.org/10.1111/j.2041-210X.2011.00169.x.

Rivera, S., Divers, S.J., Knafo, S.E., Martinez, P., Cayot, L.J., Tapia-Aguilera, W., Flanagan, J., 2011. Sterilisation of hybrid Galapagos tortoises (*Geochelone nigra*) for island restoration. Part 2: phallectomy of males under intrathecal anaesthesia with lidocaine. Vet. Rec. 168, 78.

Rockwell, K., Boykin, K., Padlo, J., Ford, C., Aschebrock, S., Mitchell, M., 2021. Evaluating the efficacy of alfaxalone in corn snakes (*Pantherophis guttatus*). Vet. Anaesth. Analg.

Rossi, J.V., 2019. General husbandry and management. In: Divers, S.J., Stahl, S.J. (Eds.), Mader's Reptile and Amphibian Medicine and Surgery, third ed. W.B. Saunders, St. Louis (MO), pp. 109–130.e1.

Royal, L.W., Lascelles, B.D.X., Lewbart, G.A., Correa, M.T., Jones, S.L., 2012. Evaluation of cyclooxygenase protein expression in traumatized versus normal tissues from eastern box turtles (*Terrapene carolina carolina*). J. Zoo Wildl. Med. 43, 289–295.

Ruben, J., 1995. Endothermy in birds and mammals: from physiology to fossils. Annu. Rev. Physiol. 57, 69–95.

Sadar, M.J., Ambros, B., 2019. Use of alfaxalone or midazolam–dexmedetomidine–ketamine for implantation of radiotransmitters in bullsnakes (*Pituophis catenifer sayi*). J. Herpetol. Med. Surg. 28, 93–98.

Sadler, R.A., Schumacher, J.P., Rathore, K., Newkirk, K.M., Cole, G., Seibert, R., Cekanova, M., 2016. Evaluation of the role of the cyclooxygenase signaling pathway during inflammation in skin and muscle tissues of ball pythons (*Python regius*). Am. J. Vet. Res. 77, 487–494.

Savageau, N.R., Gamble, K.C., 2016. Clinical challenge: renal adenocarcinoma in a beaded lizard (*Heloderma horridum horridum*). J. Zoo Wildl. Med. 47, 945–947.

Schnellbacher, R.W., Hernandez, S.M., Tuberville, T.D., Mayer, J., Alhamhoom, Y., Arnold, R.D., 2014. The efficacy of intranasal administration of dexmedetomidine and ketamine to yellow-bellied sliders (*Trachemys scripta scripta*). J. Herpetol. Med. Surg. 22, 91–98.

Schnellbacher, R.W., Shepard, M., Mans, C., Sladky, K., Schumacher, J., Steagall, P., et al., 2019. Section 6: anesthesia, chapters 48–53. In: Mader's Reptile and Amphibian Medicine and Surgery, pp. 444–483.

Seebacher, F., Franklin, C.E., 2004. Integration of autonomic and local mechanisms in regulating cardiovascular responses to heating and cooling in a reptile (*Crocodylus porosus*). J. Comp. Physiol. B. 174, 577–585.

Shepard, M.K., Divers, S., Braun, C., Hofmeister, E.H., 2013. Pharmacodynamics of alfaxalone after single-dose intramuscular administration in red-eared sliders (*Trachemys scripta elegans*): a comparison of two different doses at two different ambient temperatures. Vet. Anaesth. Analg. 40, 590–598.

Skovgaard, N., Crossley, D.A., Wang, T., 2016. Low cost of pulmonary ventilation in American alligators (*Alligator mississippiensis*) stimulated with doxapram. J. Exp. Biol. 219, 933–936.

Sladky, K., Miletic, V., 2007. Analgesic efficacy and respiratory effects of butorphanol and morphine in turtles. J. Am. Vet. Med. Assoc. 230, 1–7.

Sladky, K.K., Kinney, M.E., Johnson, S.M., 2008. Analgesic efficacy of butorphanol and morphine in bearded dragons and corn snakes. J. Am. Assoc. Lab. Anim. Sci. 233, 267–273.

Sladky, K.K., Mans, C., 2012a. Clinical anesthesia in reptiles. J. Exot. Pet Med. 21, 17–31.

Sladky, K.K., Mans, C., 2012b. Clinical analgesia in reptiles. J. Exot. Pet Med. 21, 158–167.

Sladky, K.K., Mans, C., 2019. 50—analgesia. In: Divers, S.J., Stahl, S.J. (Eds.), Mader's Reptile and Amphibian Medicine and Surgery, third ed. W.B. Saunders, St. Louis (MO), pp. 465–474.e3.

Sleeman, J., Gaynor, J., 2000. Sedative and cardiopulmonary effects of medetomidine and reversal with atipamezole in desert tortoises (*Gopherus agassizii*). J. Zoo Wildl. Med. 31, 28–35.

Soldt, B.J.V., Metscher, B.D., Poelmann, R.E., Vervust, B., 2015. Heterochrony and early left-right asymmetry in the development of the cardiorespiratory system of snakes. PLoS ONE 10, 1–28.

Spadola, F., Morici, M., Knotek, Z.Z., 2015. Combination of lidocaine/prilocaine with tramadol for short time anaesthesia-analgesia in chelonians: 18 cases. Acta Vet. Brno 84, 71–75.

Spadola, F., Morici, M., Oliveri, M., Knotek, Z., 2016. Description of cloacoscopy in the loggerhead sea turtle (*Caretta caretta*). Acta Vet. Brno 85, 367–370.

Spelman, L.H., Cambre, R.C., Walsh, T., Rosscoe, R., 1996. Anesthetic techniques in Komodo dragons (*Varanus komodoensis*). Proc. Am. Assoc. Zoo Vet. 247–250.

Stegmann, G.F., Williams, C.J.A., Franklin, C., Wang, T., Axelsson, M., 2017. Long-term surgical anaesthesia with isoflurane in human habituated Nile crocodiles. J. S. Afr. Vet. Assoc. 88, 1–6.

Tattersall, G.J., Leite, C.A.C., Sanders, C.E., Cadena, V., Andrade, D.V., Abe, A.S., Milsom, W.K., 2016. Seasonal reproductive endothermy in tegu lizards. Sci. Adv. 2, 1–8.

Taylor, E.W., Leite, C.A.C., McKenzie, D.J., Wang, T., 2010. Control of respiration in fish, amphibians and reptiles. Braz. J. Med. Biol. Res. 43, 409–424.

Thompson, K.A., Papich, M.G., Higgins, B., Flanagan, J., Christiansen, E.F., Harms, C.A., 2018. Ketoprofen pharmacokinetics of R- and S-isomers in juvenile loggerhead sea turtles (*Caretta caretta*) after single intravenous and single- and multidose intramuscular administration. J. Vet. Pharmacol. Ther. 41, 340–348.

Thomson, R.C., Spinks, P.Q., Bradley Shaffer, H., 2021. A global phylogeny of turtles reveals a burst of climate-associated diversification on continental margins. Proc. Natl. Acad. Sci. USA 118, 1–10.

Tisdale, R.K., Lesku, J.A., Beckers, G.J.L., Rattenborg, N.C., 2018. Bird-like propagating brain activity in anesthetized Nile crocodiles. Sleep 41.

Tonini, J.F.R., Beard, K.H., Ferreira, R.B., Jetz, W., Pyron, R.A., 2016. Fully-sampled phylogenies of squamates reveal evolutionary patterns in threat status. Biol. Conserv. 204, 23–31.

Trnkova, S., Knotkova, Z., Hrda, A., Knotek, Z., 2007a. Effect of non-steroidal anti-inflammatory drugs on the blood profile in the green iguana (*Iguana iguana*). Vet. Med. Czech J. Vet. Med. 52, 507–511.

Trnkova, S., Knotkova, Z., Knotek, Z., 2007b. Light anaesthesia in terrapins and lizards. In: British Veterinary Zoological Society Preceedings, pp. 28–29.

Trnková, Š., Knotková, Z., Knotek, Z., 2008. Effect of butorphanol on anaesthesia induction by isoflurane in the green iguana (*Iguana iguana*). Acta Vet. Brno 77, 245–249.

Turner, R.C., Gatson, B.J., Hernandez, J.A., Alexander, A.B., Aitken-palmer, C., Vigani, A., Heard, D.J., 2021. Sedation and Anesthesia of Galapagos (*Chelonoidis nigra*), Aldabra (*Aldabrachelys gigantea*), and African Spurred Tortoises (*Centrochelys sulcata*): A Retrospective Review (2009–2019).

Uetz, P., 2021. The Reptile Database (Accessed 20 October 2021). http://www.reptile-database.org.

Uney, K., Altan, F., Aboubakr, M., Cetin, G., Dik, B., 2016. Pharmacokinetics of meloxicam in red-eared slider turtles (*Trachemys scripta elegans*) after single intravenous and intramuscular injections. Am. J. Vet. Res. 77.

Vickaryous, M.K., Gilbert, E.A.B., 2019. Reptile embryology and regeneration. Methods Mol. Biol. 1920, 219–246.

Wang, T., Carrier, D.R., Hicks, J.W., 1997. Ventilation and gas exchange in lizards during treadmill exercise. J. Exp. Biol. 200, 2629–2639.

Wang, T., Rindom, E., 2021. The physiological response to digestion in snakes: a feast for the integrative physiologist. Comp. Biochem. Physiol. Part A Mol. Integr. Physiol. 254.

Ward, J.L., Mccartney, S.P., Chinnadurai, S.K., Posner, L.P., 2012. Development of a minimum-anesthetic-concentration depression model to study tion depression model to study the effects of. J. Zoo Wildl. Med. 43, 214–222.

Warren, D.E., Jackson, D.C., 2008. Lactate metabolism in anoxic turtles: an integrative review. J. Comp. Physiol. B Biochem. Syst. Environ. Physiol. 178, 133–148.

Webb, J.K., Keller, K.A., Chinnadurai, S.K., Kadotani, S., Allender, M.C., Fries, R., 2021. Optimizing the pharmacodynamics and evaluating cardiogenic effects of the injectable anesthetic alfaxalone in prairie rattlesnakes (*Crotalus viridis*). J. Zoo Wildl. Med. 52.

Wellehan, J.F.X., Gunkel, C.I., Kledzik, D., Robertson, S.A., Heard, D.J., 2006. Use of a nerve locator to facilitate administration of mandibular nerve blocks in crocodilians. J. Zoo Wildl. Med. 37, 405–408.

West, G., Heard, D., Caulkett, N., 2014. Zoo Animal and Wildlife Immobilization and Anesthesia, second ed.

White, C.R., Phillips, N.F., Seymour, R.S., 2006. The scaling and temperature dependence of vertebrate metabolism. Biol. Lett. 2, 125–127.

Wilkinson, A., Huber, L., 2012. Cold-blooded cognition: reptilian cognitive abilities. Oxford Handb. Comp. Evol. Psychol. 9780199738, 1–25.

Williams, C.J.A., 2019. Anaesthesia and Analgesia in Reptiles and Amphibians: Physiological Implications. Aarhus University.

Williams, C.J.A., Greunz, E.M., Ringgaard, S., Hansen, K., Bertelsen, M.F., Wang, T., 2019a. Magnetic resonance imaging (MRI) reveals high cardiac ejection fractions in red-footed tortoises (*Chelonoidis carbonarius*). J. Exp. Biol. 222.

Williams, C.J.A., Hansen, K., Williams, N., Jakobsen, S.R., Pedersen, C.C.E., Bertelsen, M.F., Wang, T., 2021. The influence of assisted ventilation and recumbency on cardiorespiratory physiology in the anesthetized freshwater turtle *Trachemys scripta scripta*. Comp. Biochem. Physiol. Part A Mol. Integr. Physiol. 260, 111036.

Williams, C.J.A., James, L.E., Bertelsen, M.F., Wang, T., 2016. Tachycardia in response to remote capsaicin injection as a model for nociception in the ball python (*Python regius*). Vet. Anaesth. Analg. 43, 429–434.

Williams, C.J.A., James, L.E., Bertelsen, M.F., Wang, T., 2019b. Analgesia for non-mammalian vertebrates. Curr. Opin. Physiol. 11, 75–84.

Williams, C.J.A., Malte, C.L., Malte, H., Bertelsen, M.F., Wang, T., 2020. Ectothermy and cardiac shunts profoundly slow the equilibration of inhaled anaesthetics in a multi-compartment model. Sci. Rep. 10.

Wright, N.C., Wessel, R., 2017. Network activity influences the subthreshold and spiking visual responses of pyramidal neurons in the three-layer turtle cortex. J. Neurophysiol. 118, 2142–2155.

Yaw, T.J., Mans, C., Johnson, S., Bunke, L., Doss, G.A., Sladky, K.K., 2020. Evaluation of subcutaneous administration of alfaxalone-midazolam and dexmedetomidine-midazolam for sedation of ball pythons (*Python regius*). J. Am. Vet. Med. Assoc. 256, 573–579.

Yaw, T.J., Mans, C., Johnson, S.M., Doss, G.A., Sladky, K.K., 2018. Effect of injection site on alfaxalone-induced sedation in ball pythons (*Python regius*). J. Small Anim. Pract. 59, 747–751.

Zheng, Y., Wiens, J.J., 2016. Combining phylogenomic and supermatrix approaches, and a time-calibrated phylogeny for squamate reptiles (lizards and snakes) based on 52 genes and 4162 species. Mol. Phylogenet. Evol. 94, 537–547. https://doi.org/10.1016/j.ympev.2015.10.009.

Ziolo, M.S., Bertelsen, M.F., 2009. Effects of propofol administered via the supravertebral sinus in red-eared sliders. J. Am. Vet. Med. Assoc. 234, 390–393.

Chapter 25

Anesthesia and analgesia in amphibians

Catherine J.A. Williams[1,2] and Mads F. Bertelsen[3]

[1]Zoophysiology, Department of Biology, Aarhus University, Aarhus, Denmark; [2]Department of Biomedical Sciences, Ontario Veterinary College, University of Guelph, Guelph, ON, Canada; [3]Center for Zoo and Wild Animal Health, Copenhagen Zoo, Copenhagen, Denmark

Chapter outline

I. Introduction

This short chapter is intended as a concise introduction to the anesthesia of laboratory-relevant species. For more in-depth perspective, readers are directed to (Baitchman and Stetter, 2014; Doss et al., 2021; Schnellbacher et al., 2019; Wright and Whitaker, 2001).

A. Brief review of current species used in research

Amphibians form a large, diverse, and acutely vulnerable range of over 8300 extant species, divided into frogs and toads (Anura, ~7394 species), salamanders (Caudata, ~765 species), and caecilians (Gymnophiona, ~215 species), with native ranges from the tropics to high latitudes, e.g., the freeze-tolerant wood frog of Northern America (California, 2021; Jetz and Pyron, 2018). Of these species, between 1/3 and 1/2 are considered threatened with extinction due to a combination of global environmental change, disease (particularly chytridiomycosis), and anthropogenic impacts. These interact catastrophically with amphibians' physiological and biological characteristics, such as semipermeable skin and common dependence on small microclimates (Amphibian Specialist Group, 2019; González-del-Pliego et al., 2019). This makes amphibians

Anesthesia and Analgesia in Laboratory Animals. https://doi.org/10.1016/B978-0-12-822215-7.00006-8

current subjects for increased research, and therefore safe and effective anesthetics and analgesics are of increased importance in veterinary medicine, conservation biology, and physiological sciences.

Of the vast species range, only a few distantly related species have been the subjects of the majority of biomedical and biological research (Fig. 25.1). These include the historic extensive use of the somewhat atypically aquatic anurans *Xenopus laevis* and *X. tropicalis,* especially in egg production for developmental research and pregnancy testing (Reed and Research Animals Department, 2005; Voss et al., 2009). Common species have been studied as subjects of physiological research, and are also often species that are known to be locally invasive, e.g., the cane toad *Rhinella marina*, the American bullfrog *Rana catesbeiana*, and the Northern leopard frog *Rana pipiens.* Among salamanders, the axolotl *Ambystoma mexicanum,* while endangered in the wild, has an extensive presence in regenerative medicine laboratories. *Notophthalmus viridescens, Necturus maculosus, and Ambystoma tigrinum*, and the Plethodontidae lungless salamanders have also been much studied (Burggren and Warburton, 2007). Rare species may be more likely to be subject to anesthesia and/or analgesia in the future in the context of conservation and research into amphibian population health and global change. The diversity of amphibia should be borne in mind, as it may affect the ability to extrapolate drugs, dosages, and ventilation requirements, e.g., between more and less aquatic taxa (Brod et al., 2019; Burggren and Warburton, 2007; Martinelli et al., 2021; O'Rourke, 2007; Taylor et al., 2021). Therefore, performing pilot trials of anesthetic protocols on species where they have not been previously optimized is recommended.

II. Anatomy and physiology relevant to anesthesia

A. Ectothermy

Amphibians, being ectothermic, have physiologies that are highly dependent on external temperature, and this will have direct effects on their metabolism, oxygen requirements, and drug pharmacokinetics. This is vital to remember in the context of anesthesia induction, maintenance, and recovery. Even when kept at the same temperature, ectotherm metabolism is only approximately 1/5th to 1/10th that of endotherms (Nagy, 2005), so oxygen requirements and CO_2 production are much lower, and drug metabolism is predicted to be much slower than that in endotherms (White et al., 2006).

B. Semipermeable skin

With variable but characteristically glandular semipermeable skin, both desired (e.g., cutaneous/immersion anesthetic administration, electrolytes) and unwanted (e.g., intoxication from cleaning agents) chemicals can easily become systemically circulated (Campbell et al., 2012; Quaranta et al., 2009). Multiple respiratory modes provide gas exchange: cutaneous, lung/pulmonary (where present), gill/brachial (where present), and buccopharyngeal, where the extent of each mode depends greatly on

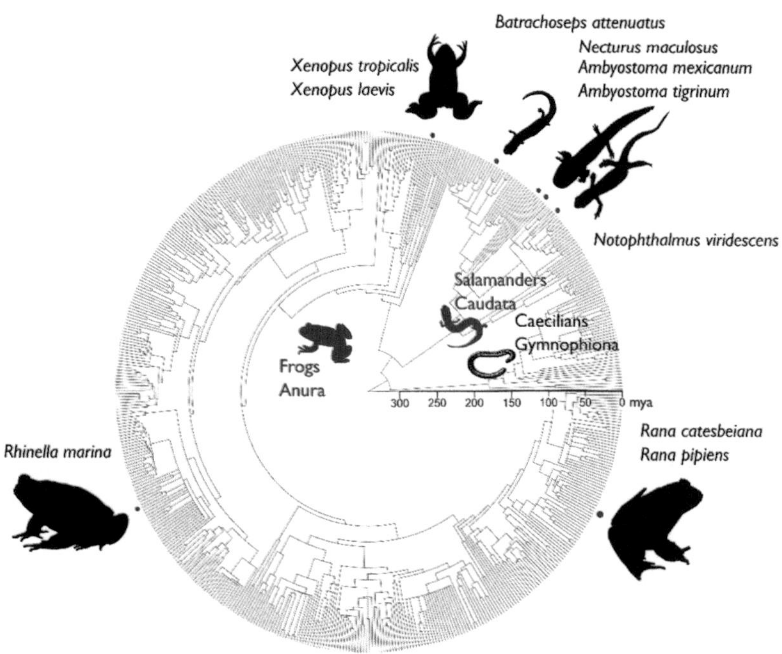

FIGURE 25.1 A genus level phylogeny of Amphibia, showing caecilians (black), salamanders (dark blue) and frogs (blue). Silhouettes of species commonly anesthetized in research are highlighted. Tree created in phytools (Revell, 2012) using data from (Jetz and Pyron, 2018), silhouettes phylopic.com see acknowledgments.

the taxa and developmental stage; larval stages are more dependent on gill and cutaneous respiration, and adults more on pulmonary respiration in those species where lungs develop during metamorphosis (Milsom et al., 2022; Taylor et al., 2010).

C. Metamorphosis

The characteristic natural metamorphosis of amphibians (except notable neotenous species such as the axolotl where metamorphosis can still be artificially induced) has relevance to anesthesia, especially as the primary means of gas exchange shifts from gill/cutaneous to lung in those species which possess them—this changing the risks for, e.g., drowning in recovery for adult anurans, but also as the changing metabolism and cutaneous permeability makes earlier life stages at greater risk of intoxication, and requiring lower immersion anesthesia doses (Mitchell, 2009).

D. Cardiovascular

The characteristic adult amphibian heart possesses two atria and an undivided, spongy-walled ventricle. Atrial septation occurs late in developing larval amphibia and is variable between species and classes of amphibia (Jensen et al., 2019; Lewis and Hanken, 2017). Oxygen-poor systemic blood enters the right atrium, and oxygen-rich blood from the lungs enters the left atrium, from where they both enter the single ventricle. Leaving the ventricle, blood is ejected via the contractile conus arteriosus, containing a spiral valve that aids the separation of the blood streams such that the oxygen-poor blood primarily enters the pulmocutaneous artery, while the oxygenated blood travels into the carotid and systemic arteries. The oxygen-rich blood that returns from the skin enters the venous system, raising right atrial oxygenation above that of mixed venous blood (Wang et al., 1999). The lack of anatomical ventricular separation means that pulmonary and systemic arterial blood pressures are equal, but also allows intraventricular shunting of blood to take place. Hence, oxygen-poor blood can recirculate to the systemic system, or oxygen-rich blood to the lungs and skin, depending on the passive physical resistance of the receiving vessels, and any regulated constriction of these vessels (Andersen and Wang, 2003; Hillman et al., 2014). A net right-to-left shunt (where deoxygenated blood recirculates) usually prevails at rest, but under conditions especially of increased cardiac output, such as digestion, exercise, increased temperature, or hypoxia, the right-to-left shunt can be reduced or even reversed. Heart rate and cardiac output are usually depressed under deep anesthesia, but not always in the initial or lighter planes: e.g., the common amphibian immersion anesthetic MS222 usually results in a stable or elevated heart rate until very deep anesthesia where heart rate will fall.

There is considerable lymph volume and flux in amphibian species (Hedrick et al., 2013, 2014), and lymph hearts (from 6 in anurans to 200 in caecilians) provide secondary circulatory propulsion, which may affect the pharmacokinetics of injected drugs, especially if close to lymph sacs (Williams et al., 2017).

The pharmacokinetics of drugs injected in the caudal half of the animal may be affected by the venous drainage of these areas into the renal and hepatic portal systems, as well as the hydration status of the amphibian (Killorn and Toews, 2001). Therefore, administration in the forelimb or cranially to the hind limbs is recommended to increase predictability (Fig. 25.2).

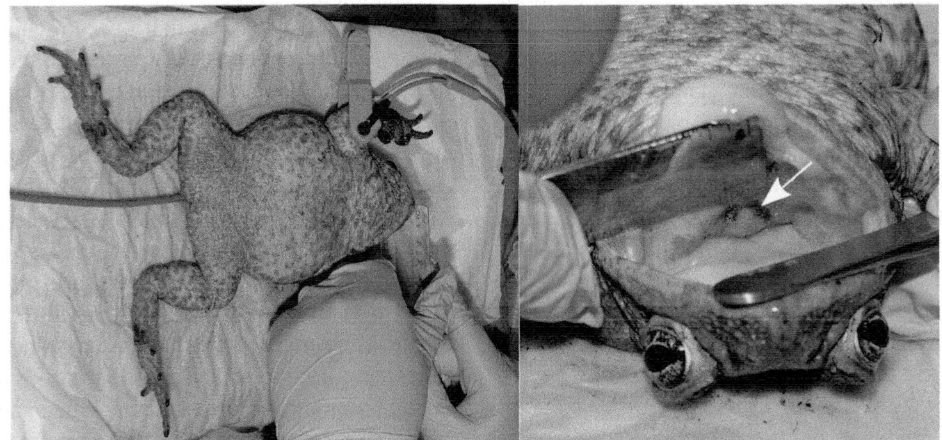

FIGURE 25.2 Anesthetized (1 g/L buffered MS222) Rhinella marina showing positioning of cloacal temperature probe, forelimb spO_2 probe, and characteristic ventral erythema under anesthesia as well as semiextended forelimb posture. If intubation is required, the (closed) glottis is highlighted (right, white arrow).

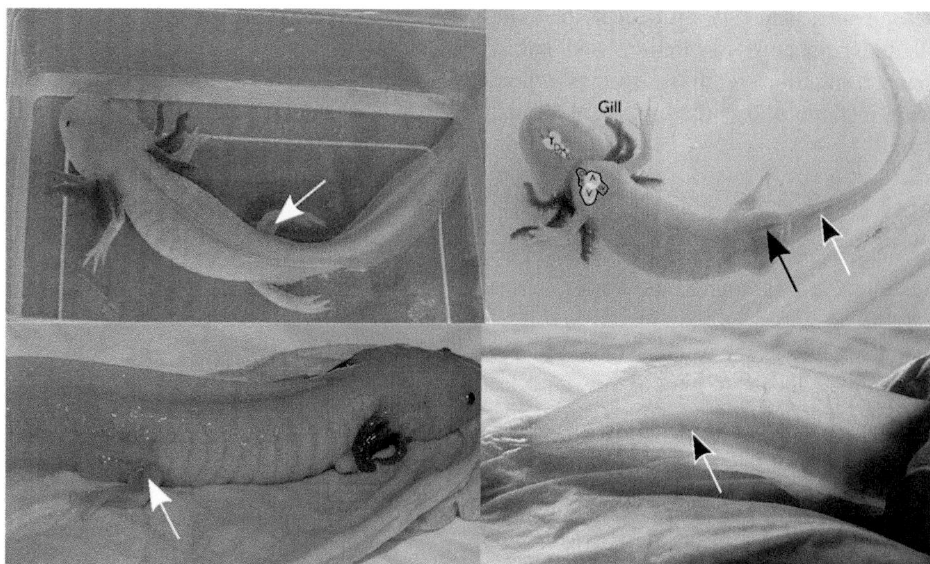

FIGURE 25.3 Anesthesia of the axolotl. Clockwise from top left: (A) A male leucistic axolotl (*A. mexicanum*) in home tank water for observation in a round sided clear plastic container. The location of the right femoral vein is highlighted with a white arrow. (B) The same individual in a ventral view while anesthetized with buffered 200 mg/L MS222, showing position of gills, and cloaca (black arrow), ventral tail vein (white/black arrow), and overlay showing diagrams of the position of the heart (ventricle (V), atria (A), sinus venosus (SV) and outflow tract (OT), and brain (telencephalon (T), diencephalon (D), mesencephalon (M) and rhombencephalon (R)). (C) Transillumination of the tail, high-lighting the position of the ventral tail vein (D) Anesthetized (200 mg/L, buffered MS222) axolotl maintained on wet towel moistened with buffered anesthetic for blood sampling, femoral vein highlighted by the white arrow.

Vascular access, although limited by animal body mass, can be provided by the ventral midline abdominal vein, femoral vein behind the stifle (Fig. 25.3), axillary venous plexus, sublingual plexus (Fig. 25.5), and the ventral tail vein (in Caudata, see Fig. 25.3). Vessel pathways can be highlighted by transillumination (Fig. 25.3). Cardiac puncture should be reserved for surgically anesthetized animals and ideally, terminal procedures. The position of the heart in axolotls is illustrated in Fig. 25.3. While amphibians are variably capable of cardiac regeneration, from low potential in adult *Xenopus* to high capacity in, e.g., axolotls (Marshall et al., 2019; Voss et al., 2009), cardiac access is likely to cause nociception, pain, and stress. Regeneration is also likely to be time and energy-consuming for the animal. Cardiac samples are likely to be of mixed oxygenated/deoxygenated blood. For arterial samples, an indwelling catheter is used for research purposes, commonly in the femoral artery in anurans. Venous samples from the plexus may be diluted with lymph. Sampling from the tail vein may result in a tail autotomy in species that can shed their tails in response to handling (certain salamanders).

E. Ventilation

While juvenile individuals of all species rely on cutaneous and brachial gas exchange, ventilation of the usually saccular lungs is developed by adult anurans and lunged adult salamanders. Exceptions are the gill retention in paedomorphic/neotenic axolotls (*Ambystoma mexicanum),* and lack of lung development (and the lack of atrial septation) in the lungless salamanders. Lung ventilation is via a positive pressure buccal pump in anurans and Caudata, and different rates of gular and abdominal breathing are often noted. Surgical levels of anesthesia are usually accompanied by marked hypopnea or apnea, making cutaneous/branchial respiration the sole means of gas exchange. Cutaneous vessels often dilate under anesthesia (Fig. 25.2), and cutaneous gas exchange is usually relied upon for oxygenation and CO_2 elimination under anesthesia in most species. Arterial PO_2 may fall over the anesthesia period, especially in more terrestrial species, and a mixed respiratory and metabolic acidosis can result from CO_2 retention and lactate production (Andersen and Wang, 2002), typically resolving over 24 hours, while tissue spO_2 in the more aquatic *Xenopus laevis* was stable over 2 hours of MS222 anesthesia in unbubbled water (Lalonde-Robert et al., 2012a). Both hypercapnia and hypoxia are respiratory stimuli, while hyperoxia may reduce respiratory drive (e.g., gill ventilation in conscious larval *Rana catesbeiana* (Jia and Burggren, 1997)), but ensure cutaneous oxygenation. Therefore, a practical solution is to bubble the water with an air or air/oxygen mix, e.g., with an aquarium pump. Maintaining skin hydration throughout anesthesia is essential for animal health and surgical recovery. Some terrestrial species have a particularly well-vascularized and permeable ventral pelvic patch, while other species have more generalized high permeability and are at greater risk of dehydration.

III. Preprocedural considerations

A. Planning

1. Health and safety

The glandular skin of amphibians has often developed toxic secretions that necessitate care with handling, e.g., those of the parotid glands of the cane toad, *Rhinella marina* located on the dorsal cranium caudal to the eyes (Fig. 25.2), and those dependent on toxic food consumption, e.g., poison dart frogs, *Dendrobates* spp. Therefore, the use of disposable gloves premoistened in the amphibians' home water, bottled water, or amphibian ringers is recommended (Mitchell, 2009; Mylniczenko, 2009; Pasmans and Martel, 2019). Eye protection when handling large species with parotid glands (e.g., *Rhinella marina*) is recommended. Some Caecilians may also have a proteolytic venom associated with very small dental structures (Mailho-Fontana et al., 2020).

Zoonotic risks are mainly of bacterial origin, such as Salmonella and atypical Mycobacteria (e.g., *M. marinum*), *Chlamydophila pneumoniae* and *C. psittaci*, and *Aeromonas* spp., which are carried asymptomatically or mildly symptomatically by the animal (Alworth and Harvey, 2007). Fecal material or contaminated water is also a source of waterborne bacteria such as *E. coli* and other common enteric pathogens. The use of disposable gloves, good hand hygiene, and lab clothing are common sense mitigations of risk.

Some larger species, such as hellbenders, African bullfrogs, and horned frogs, can deliver serious bites and should be handled with care.

There is a serious risk of cross-contamination with, e.g., chytrid fungus (*Batrachochytrium dendrobatidis* (Bd) and *Batrachochytrium salamandrivorans* (Bsal)) and iridoviruses when species of amphibians handling equipment or their surrounding environment are brought together (Lips, 2016). Therefore adequate quarantine, testing of animals (PCR), cleaning of shared equipment, and use of disposable gloves are vital to prevent transmission (Thomas et al., 2020; Jensen et al., 2021; Van Rooij et al., 2017).

2. History and records

For risk assessment and quarantine assessment, wild-caught versus captive-bred status should be known. Body mass, body condition, and the staging of metamorphosis are important for calculating anesthetic doses.

Sex determination may be difficult to assess in many species, especially in juvenile individuals or those outside of the breeding season. The larger size and rounder body type of females, the appearance of nuptial pads in male anurans and salamanders, as well as the appearance of eggs in the abdomen of females visible via transillumination, are common strategies for sexing amphibians. For species-specific guides, please refer to general amphibian literature.

Housing temperature, water temperature and pH should be noted and replicated in the anesthesia setting if species appropriate (Pasmans and Martel, 2019). Laboratory records on the quality of a home tank water sample may be used to determine if suitable for use during anesthesia.

B. Patient evaluation

1. Physical examination

The use of prewetted single-use, powder-free gloves, e.g., **rinsed** nitrile is highly recommended both for personal protection, and also to avoid damage to the fragile and chemically porous amphibian skin, which mandates minimal handling where possible (Cashins et al., 2008; Thomas et al., 2020). The use of clear plastic bags partially filled with home water and the animal can aid in examination and any imaging. Aquatic species should be retrieved directly into home tank water using nonknotted aquarium nets or a plastic bag to minimize skin trauma.

Body condition score (BCS) is important as emaciated animals may have low total protein, which will unpredictably increase the effect of normally protein-bound drugs such as propofol. BCSs have been developed for several species in captivity or field conditions based on visual aids such as diagrams of species anatomy at varying scores or the individuals' residual from a species regression of body mass against snout-vent length (Jayson et al., 2018, James Abraham in Divers and Stahl, 2019).

External examination of body posture and mentation, skin condition, heart rate HR (via doppler ultrasound), and respiratory RR (gular rate) may be made. Manual restraint focuses on preventing escape motions in anurans by holding the hind legs extended in one hand in small specimens, and supporting the body on the top of the hand, or by grasping large anurans behind the forelimbs and then gripping the hindlimbs with the other hand. Examination in a cup or plastic bag is often optimal for getting a full external physical examination. In salamanders, manual restraint may be via grip behind the head, in front of the forelimbs, or in front of the hind limbs. Some species will autotomize their tails if pressure is placed caudally. Aquatic salamanders should be examined in the water to maintain skin integrity and water balance and minimize handling (Fig. 25.3). Caecilians are usually examined in a clear container.

2. Laboratory testing

The use of preanesthetic laboratory testing in amphibians is limited, but may include preintroduction chytrid or ranavirus screening, and measurement of total protein to aid dosage calculation for protein-bound anesthetics (e.g., propofol, alfaxalone).

Chambers and surfaces for handling amphibians, especially in their early life stages, must be carefully cleaned and rinsed so as to minimize residues of chemicals from cleaning, disinfection, or e.g., nitrile glove coatings, which can negatively affect amphibians, as well as any secretions from animals previously held in the container (Cashins et al., 2008; Thomas et al., 2020). In the field, it is important to avoid releasing this rinse water with chemical residues into the environment.

3. *Fasting*

Fasting recommendations vary in the literature, as the amphibian glottis usually remains closed under anesthesia (Fig. 25.2). However, due to the pressure of a full gut on other organs and the possibility of peri/postanesthetic regurgitation with some agents (especially clove oil), the authors recommend 24 hours of gut emptying prior to anesthesia, with larger insectivorous amphibians fasting for 48 hours (Alworth et al., 2011; Baitchman and Stetter, 2014). Large rodent-eating species may be fasted for up to a week to reduce gut fill and potential for ileus (Gentz, 2007). It should also be noted that digestive status will markedly affect metabolism, acid-base status, and heart rate, with a postprandial increase in metabolism and heart rate, especially in those species where large infrequent meals are normal (Andersen et al., 2003; Andersen and Wang, 2003).

IV. Chemical restraint versus anesthesia

The same agents are often used for chemical restraint and full anesthesia in amphibians, where the dose and duration of exposure to the induction dose, and the dose used for maintenance are changed to allow differing depths to be attained. Therefore, agents are here considered in parallel for both purposes. Historically and currently, a single immersion agent (usually buffered MS222 or benzocaine) has been the most common anesthetic regime in amphibians; however, there is increased and due attention on balanced anesthesia, if supplementary agents can improve postoperative analgesia or produce better experimental results. A separate provision of analgesia in amphibians had previously not been considered necessary, as they were studied as models for nociception (the sensation of harmful stimuli) without being considered able to experience pain (Stevens, 1992). This is no longer supported by clinical opinion and by many legislative bodies or mandated approval committees for laboratory research (Alworth and Harvey, 2007; Canadian Council on Animal Care, 2021; European Council, 2010; Gebhart et al., 2009; University Federation of Animal Welfare, 2010), where there is a general requirement to consider analgesia where the pain would be anticipated in a similar situation in a mammal. In the case of the United States, despite amphibians not being covered under the Animal Welfare Act, permits for publicly funded research use of amphibians are covered by IACUCs, which have to follow guidance, including the use of analgesia in amphibians (Alworth and Harvey, 2007; University Federation of Animal Welfare, 2010). Specific analgesia, based on antinociceptive research and clinical experience is now recommended; however, this area also requires further study (Coble et al., 2011; Hausmann et al., 2021; Martinelli et al., 2021; Stevens, 2011).

A. Premedication

Preemptive analgesia may be considered for animals undergoing surgical procedures; however, the common use of immersion anesthesia, and the need to minimize handling mean that injectable premedication is rarely used in amphibians. Ketamine at 20−40 mg/kg intramuscularly to the forelimb has been historically used clinically (Mitchell, 2009), but not by the present authors in laboratory species. Combinations including ketamine with others agents have been used for chemical restraint (Yaw et al., 2020).

V. Chemical restraint

Agents and doses are summarized in Table 25.1.

A. Immersion agents

Immersion agents are the most commonly used, comprising MS222 benzocaine, propofol, alfaxalone, etomidate, and eugenol (Adami et al., 2016a,b; d'Ovidio et al., 2015; Sladakovic et al., 2014; Stathopoulou et al., 2022; Thygesen et al., 2017). An initial induction bath of the anesthetic agent in neutral pH, unchlorinated, deionized (no nitrate, nitrate, or ammonia) fresh water (or, if of appropriate quality, home tank water) is used. After a common initial excitatory phase, where the use of a closed container with soft sides such as a plastic bag with round corners (available from fish shops) is useful to prevent damage, the animal will sequentially lose spontaneous movement and other responses until an anesthetic plane is reached, usually judged as the loss of righting reflex. The animal is then removed from the induction solution, rinsed and placed on a moist towel or in shallow water (maximum to the level of the humero-scapular joint to prevent drowning), either with no or a lower concentration of the active drug. Figs. 25.4 and 25.5 depict anesthesia and positioning of aquatic amphibians (axolotl and *Xenopus*, respectively). The anesthetic plane will often then deepen further (probably by recirculation of the drug in the extensive lymph system) and can attain a surgical plane, assessed by lack of

TABLE 25.1 Anesthetic and sedative agents in common amphibian use.

Drug(s)	Species	Dose	Duration	Antagonist**	Comments
Immersion agents					
MS222	Multiple Axolotl, *Plethodon* spp, *Xenopus, Rhinella marina* (Andersen and Wang, 2002; Lalonde-Robert et al., 2012a; Novarro et al., 2017; Smith et al., 2018; Zullian et al., 2016)	0.1–2 g/L induction to effect, lower end doses in larval stages, small species and aquatic species. Up to 3 g/L have been used for *Rhinella*.	Species dependant but usually 30–60 minutes from inductive bathing, high doses give a longer duration of activity. Maintenance via moist paper towel in induction dose, or 1/3 dose for maintenance.	None, clearance via metabolism and cutaneous elimination.	Requires active buffering to pH 7–7.4. Stock solution to be kept in darkened glass. Care with handling as can absorbed over human skin. Species variability in dose, e.g., higher dose requirement (2 g/L) *Plethodon cinereus* than other salamanders (Novarro et al., 2017)
Benzocaine	Multiple	0.05–0.5 g/L lower doses for larval stages, small and aquatic species e.g., 0.2 g/L in axolotls for surgery. (Dittrich and Lauridsen, 2021)	30 minutes of 0.2 g/L immersion gives 150 minutes of anesthesia in axolotls when animals maintained in 0.2 g/L anesthetic-soaked tissue		For dissolution requires small volume of ethanol or acetone, followed by dilution in home tank water or distilled water
Alfaxalone	Axolotl, small anuran (e.g., publications on *Bombina orientalis*)	5–200 mg/L in freshwater bath. Top ups over gills required at low doses for surgical anesthesia plane. 2 g/L ineffective in bullfrogs.		None, hepatic metabolism.	Requires buffering to pH 7 at high doses. Little to no analgesia provision. May be combined with morphine for analgesia (50 mg/L morphine concentration) (Adami et al., 2015; McMillan and Leece, 2011; Posner et al., 2013)
Propofol	Axolotl, small anuran.	2–4 mg/L		None, hepatic metabolism	No analgesia provision. Maintained regenerative and improved nerve responses in research in comparison with MS222 (Thygesen et al., 2017)
Eugenol	Xenopus	350 mg/L for 15 minutes immersion		None, proposed hepatic metabolism	Respiratory depression, short duration of surgical depth after immersion (15–30 minutes) dependent on frog size. Vomiting and abdominal contraction on contact and recovery. Variable toxicity across species, high mortality reported in cane toads (Guénette et al., 2007; Hernández et al., 2012)

Continued

TABLE 25.1 Anesthetic and sedative agents in common amphibian use.—cont'd

Drug(s)	Species	Dose	Duration	Antagonist**	Comments
Etomidate	Xenopus	15–30 mg/L			Longer duration with higher induction dose (Smith et al., 2018)
Inhalation agents					
Isoflurane	Multiple, exact data for *Rhinella marina* (Morrison et al., 2016)	3%–5% for swift induction in oxygen 2%–3% for induction within 15 minutes, In *Rhinella marina*	2–5 hours to return of righting reflex		Preparation of gel for cutaneous absorption also possible
Sevoflurane	Multiple, data for *Rhinella marina* (Morrison et al., 2016)	3%–5% for swift induction in oxygen, 2%–3% for induction within 15 minutes	2–7 hours to return of righting reflex		Preparation of gel for cutaneous absorption also possible
Desflurane	Multiple, data for *Rhinella marina* (Morrison et al., 2016)	6% for induction within 15 minutes	1–4 hours to return of righting reflex		Preparation of gel for cutaneous absorption also possible
Injectable agents					
MS222	Multiple	200 mg/kg IC			Used mainly for euthanasia, requires aseptic preparation and buffering to pH 7–7.4 for injectable use.
Propofol	Multiple, data for *Pelodryas caerulea, Rana catesbeiana*	9–30 mg/kg IC 10 mg/kg IV			Higher doses caused mortality in *P caerulea* (Von Esse and Wright, 1999; Williams et al., 2018; Wojick et al., 2010)
Alfaxalone	Multiple, specific data for *Rana catesbeiana Litoria* spp. *Dendrobates* in combination	10 mg/kg IV and 10–20 mg/kg IM 20–30 mg/kg IM, 40 mg/kg SC with midazolam 40 mg/kg and dexmedetomidine (5 mg/kg) in *Dendrobates*	Loss of righting 5 minutes, loss of muscle tone 10 minutes, recovery of muscle tone at 60 (50–70) min (mean [range]) after 10 mg/kg and 120 minutes after 20 mg/kg in Rana, and 1 hour in *Litoria* spp, after 20–30 mg/kg IM		(Posner et al., 2013; Sladakovic et al., 2014; Williams et al., 2018; Yaw et al., 2020)
Ketamine	Majority of species, *Rhinella marina, Dendrobates* in combination	70–100 mg/kg sole agent 100 mg/kg with 40 mg/kg midazolam, 5mg/kg dexmedetomidine in *Dendrobates tinctorius azureus* 200 mg/kg with 0.2 mg/kg diazepam in *Rhinella marina*	Recovery within 12 hours, but species diverse 60 minutes to induction, 8 hours to recovery		Wright and Whitaker (2001) Hernández et al. (2012); Yaw et al. (2020)

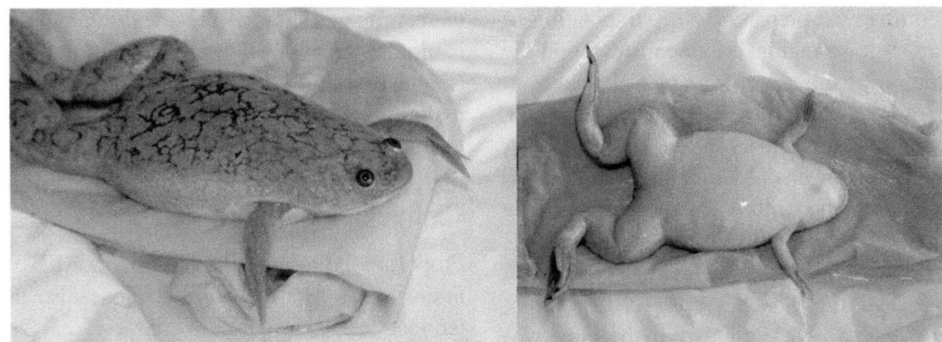

FIGURE 25.4 Anesthesia of *Xenopus*. A female *Xenopus laevis*, anesthetized with 1 g/L buffered MS222 by immersion, placed on a moistened tissue pad, over a covered heat pad, to maintain body temperature. Ventral view of the same animal.

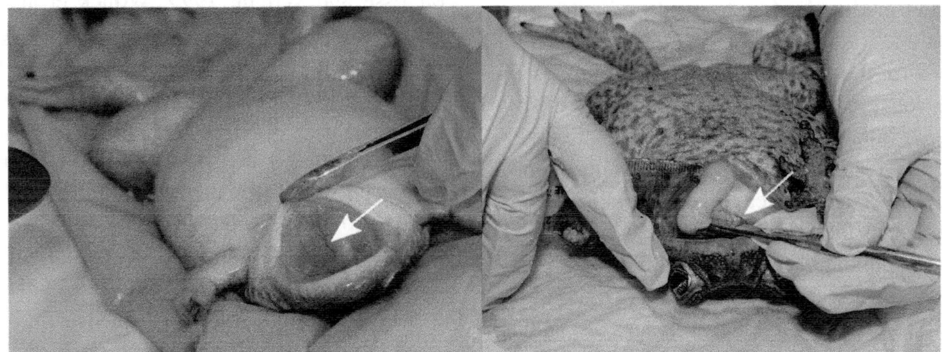

FIGURE 25.5 Ventral tongue plexus location. Anesthesia of (1 g/L buffered MS222) *Xenopus laevis* (left) and *Rhinella marina* (right), showing position of ventral tongue venous plexus as blood sampling site.

withdrawal and nociceptive response. The animal is recovered by exposure to fresh water, at temperatures in the preferred temperature zone for the species.

MS222 (otherwise named tricaine methanesulfonate, ethyl 3-aminobenzoate methanesulfonate—a voltage-gated sodium channel blocker) is the most commonly used immersion anesthesia drug. Stock solutions should be maintained in light-proof containers. MS222 requires buffering, as without it in soft water conditions, its low pH can cause extensive skin irritation, and also hinder the uptake of the drug (Torreilles et al., 2009). Common procedure is to use an equal dry mass of sodium bicarbonate to MS222, or where possible to measure pH to titrate to pH 7.0–7.4 with sodium hydroxide, sodium bicarbonate, or EDTA (Gentz, 2007; Mitchell, 2009; Sladakovic and Divers, 2019; Stathopoulou et al., 2022). EDTA will also have effects on dissolved calcium and magnesium levels and is therefore not preferred.

Benzocaine is another sodium channel blocker commonly used, which requires predissolving in ethanol or acetone prior to dilution in water. For both of these agents, loss of righting and corneal reflexes occurs earliest, with spontaneous movement, gular respiration, and withdrawal response lost sequentially afterward as depth increases. Bradycardia and loss of cardiac impulse indicate excessive anesthetic depth. The mechanism of action via sodium channels makes it likely that the use of these anesthetics will affect measurements dependent on sensory neuronal function such as the auditory brainstem response, or on neural control, e.g., of respiration or motor responses (Cui et al., 2017; Hedrick and Winmill, 2003; Medler, 2019). Both MS222 and benzocaine provide general hypnosis but also have been shown to decrease sensory and motor neuron activity and MS222 appears to impact antinociception for some hours after exposure (Ramlochansingh et al., 2014; Smith et al., 2018).

Eugenol is the active ingredient in clove oil and has been marketed commercially as AQUI-S. It has actions at sodium and transient receptor potential channels. Its dose response appears to be variable between species. Doses are reported for *Xenopus, Litoria ewingii anurans, Amphiuma, and Ambystoma tigrinum* salamanders (Baitchman and Stetter, 2014; Goulet et al., 2010; Guénette et al., 2007; Mitchell et al., 2009; Pojman and Fonteno, 2014; Speare et al., 2014; Weber et al., 2019). Its use has been associated with abdominal contraction and vomiting and regurgitation on contact and recovery (Mitchell et al., 2009). Renal tubular necrosis which progressed with repeated dosing has been reported in *Xenopus laevis* (Goulet et al., 2011). Eugenol is available in pharmaceutical grade for dilution in ethanol and via commercial preparations. Extrapolation of doses from the literature should take into consideration the variable concentration of the active ingredient in the noncommercial preparations which have previously been used.

Etomidate, propofol, and alfaxalone all act at GABA channels, and have all been less commonly used as amphibian immersion agents, with a sedative to anesthetic effects dependent on the dose utilized and exposure time, but have no specific analgesic effects (Adami et al., 2015; McMillan and Leece, 2011; Sanches et al., 2018; Smith et al., 2018; Thygesen et al., 2017). Dexmedetomidine was found to increase antinociception under alfaxalone immersion but decrease the anesthetic plane. This was hypothesized by the authors to be due to the vasoconstrictive effects of dexmedetomidine leading to a reduced cutaneous uptake of alfaxalone (Adami et al., 2016b). Cutaneous uptake is also used for the administration of gels to the skin, either containing local anesthetic agents, which are absorbed systemically, or inhalation agents as liquids mixed with aqueous gels (e.g., 1 mL isoflurane, 1 mL water, 3 mL water-soluble gel; however, clinical reports of skin lesions with isoflurane suggests that sevoflurane may be preferred). Isoflurane has been bubbled through water baths, as compounded gel, or administered directly to the skin as a liquid. Care is required to prevent human exposure to agents evaporating from the bath or degassing from the gel, while direct exposure to isoflurane has been associated with skin irritation.

B. Inhaled anesthesia

Amphibians can be chamber-induced with inhaled anesthetics, and large specimens maintained on an inhaled anesthetic via intubation with short noncuffed endotracheal tubes. However, controlling depth may be complicated by cutaneous gas diffusion and intraventricular shunting. Due to these processes, there is a long time for CNS equilibration (approximately 4 hours), so higher anesthetic doses that give a practical time for induction are used (2%–3% isoflurane). These are higher than the presumed mean anesthetic concentration for immobility ($MAC_{immobility}$ 1.15%–1.12% isoflurane in *Rana pipiens,* $MAC_{loss\ of\ righting\ reflex\ <15\ minutes}$ 1.4 in *Rhinella marina*). Anesthetists should be aware that any change in the provided anesthetic level will take hours to reach equivalent levels in the brain and spinal cord, so the animal is always in a nonequilibrium state. Thus, in practice, animals are induced at 2%–3% isoflurane or 5%–8% sevoflurane, left in the chamber for 5–15 minutes following the loss of righting reflex, and then, if necessary, intubated (Baitchman and Stetter, 2014; Barter et al., 2006, 2007; Barter and Antognini, 2008; Morrison et al., 2016; Williams et al., 2020). After 15 minutes in a 1.5 $MAC_{loss\ righting\ reflex}$ induction chamber postloss of righting reflex in cane toads, recovery times were around 3 hours for sevoflurane (range 2–6 hours), isoflurane (range 2–4 hours), and 80 minutes for desflurane (range 1–4 hours) (Morrison et al., 2016). This variability makes inhaled anesthesia a secondary choice in amphibians to immersion anesthesia.

C. Injectable anesthesia

Propofol and alfaxalone (10 mg/kg) have been used as intravascular agents, with alfaxalone also used intramuscularly at the same dose (Williams et al., 2018), and intracoelomic (IC) use of MS222 and propofol (early high doses of 35 mg/kg reported IC) although IC high doses were associated with high variability (Lalonde-Robert et al., 2012b; Von Esse and Wright, 1999; Wojick et al., 2010). Neither propofol nor alfaxalone possess specific analgesic effects, so they are less useful as sole agents for painful procedures, but can be combined with analgesia or other injectable sedatives (Yaw et al., 2020). For terminal use, pentobarbital (30–60 mg/kg IC) has been widely used in physiological research but has a low therapeutic index and little analgesic potential, so it may lead to nociceptive changes with resulting physiological effects on the collected data, if not combined with an analgesic. Ketamine has been used as a sole agent, but with highly variable interspecific dose-response (20–200 mg/kg), variable time to induction, very delayed recovery (up to 12 hours), and large volumes required to provide the average surgical dose range of 75–100 mg/kg. Therefore ketamine's sole use for research purposes is limited, and clinical recommendations have been as a premedication of 20–40 mg/kg (Mitchell, 2009). A combination of ketamine (50 mg/kg) with medetomidine (0.5 mg/kg), meloxicam (0.2 mg/kg), and butorphanol (25 mg/kg) intramuscularly has been reported in *Xenopus*, with the medetomidine reversible with an equal volume of atipamezole has been reported (Chai, 2015), and in combination with midazolam and dexemedetomidine in *Dendrobates* (Yaw et al., 2020), but medetomidine was not advised as a sole agent in *Rana pipiens* (Lafortune et al., 2001).

VI. Monitoring

A. Reflexes

The usual course of events as the plane of anesthesia deepens is as follows: loss of spontaneous movement, loss of righting reflex, loss of corneal reflex, and loss of deep pain to toe pinch.

B. Cardiovascular and respiratory monitoring

Doppler can be used to determine HR over the thoracic girdle, or over a femoral artery. Respiratory rate is usually determined via observation of the gular movements, nares, or abdomen. Electrocardiography (ECG) can be applied via moist gel patches on limbs or subcutaneous placement of sterile hypodermic needles attached to the crocodile clips of an ECG to minimize tissue trauma. Capnography is rare as only large terrestrial species are commonly intubated, and the relatively large intake to side-stream capnography in comparison with the tidal volume of the animal and dead space of mainstream analyzers, make capnography less well supported. Also, the potential for intraventricular shunts means that end-tidal CO_2 will not exactly reflect arterial levels. However, where used, a trend in data may be useful for individuals, rather than single data points reflecting an arterial level. Similarly, pulse oximeters are not calibrated for amphibian hemoglobin oxygen saturation curves, but may provide an indication of heart rate and a trend for oxygenation status (Fig. 25.2 and Stathopoulou et al., 2022).

C. Support

Temperature is vital to maintaining physiological processes and providing less variable induction and recovery. The temperature of induction chambers, recovery, and the animal during surgery should be maintained in the preferred temperature zone for the species, usually considered as 18–22°C (65–72°F) for temperate species and 24–27°C (75–80°F) for tropical species.

Hydration, especially of the skin, must be maintained for cutaneous drug uptake and elimination, and the longer-term immune and electrolyte balance of the animal. Aerated, deionized unchlorinated tap water may be used, but it will be hypotonic to the animal (amphibian plasma is 230 mOsm/L). For clinically dehydrated, or longer-term maintenance cases, bathing in a solution isotonic with amphibian plasma will reduce the potential for edema, and energy use associated with maintaining electrolyte balance. 0.6% saline may be appropriate or a combination with Holtfreter's Solution (NaCl 3.46 g/L, KCl 0.05 g/L, $CaCl_2$ 0.1 g/L, $NaHCO_3$ 0.2 g/L) or amphibian ringers (6.6 g/L NaCl, 0.15 g/L KCl, 0.15 g/L $CaCl_2$, 0.2 g/L $NaHCO_3$ in distilled water).

Oxygenation can be maintained using aeration or oxygenation of the induction and maintenance water. With larger species, there is the potential for tracheal intubation for long procedures and to maintain PCO_2 (Fig. 25.2). If intubated, the very short trachea of, e.g., anurans should be noted to prevent intubating one bronchus and tissue damage. Uncuffed tubes (e.g., Cole, modified feeding tubes, or IV catheters) and airway pressures of 5 cmH_2O are recommended to avoid damage to the tracheal mucosa and saccular lungs. Humidification of the inhaled gases is recommended to prevent drying of the lung surface.

D. Common anesthetic emergencies

Hypoxia, bradycardia, and hypothermia are the most common anesthetic emergencies, and the provision of clean flowing water at the species preferred body temperature will be the most efficient means of reducing anesthetic concentrations for the immersion anesthetics and speeding recovery. Where injectable agents with specific antidotes are used (uncommon use of alpha-2-agonists or benzodiazepines), the reversal agent should be given (usually for alpha-2-agonists at a 5:1 dose of, e.g., atipamezole to medetomidine previously administered). Otherwise, treatment to support cardiac function (adrenaline, 10 μg/kg; atropine, dose 1–2 mg/kg (Herman and Sandoval, 1983; Williams et al., 2020) may also speed the reduction in inhaled and possibly immersion anesthetic concentrations by decreasing the right-to-left shunt and increasing pulmonary perfusion and cardiac output, but may also increase cardiac oxygen requirements.

VII. Analgesia

A. Approach to analgesia in the given species

Nociceptive pathways are present in amphibians, and the potential for analgesia to act to reduce their sensation of tissue damage and pain has been reviewed elsewhere (Guénette et al., 2013; Machin, 1999; Stevens, 2011). Analgesia, where tissue damage has taken place, and pain is inferred, is mandated in European jurisdictions (European Council, 2010; Keifer and Zheng, 2017) and recommended in mandatory guidelines for publicly funded research in North America (Alworth and Harvey, 2007; Gebhart et al., 2009); however, information is limited as to effective modalities, dosages, and potential side effects across species. Information here is taken from physiological research using the acetic acid wiping test to determine antinociceptive doses of drugs, surgical studies, and some clinical reports. The acetic acid wiping test (AAT) is where serial dilutions of acetic acid are applied to the dorsal femoral area. An effective analgesic is one where the animal does not show a wiping response that is demonstrated in a control situation and is dependent on C-fiber nociceptive transmission (Stevens, 2004). This technique has been applied successfully with opiates, alpha-2 agonists, and nonsteroidal anti-inflammatory drugs. More research is required into the use of multimodal analgesia, in *Rana* and particularly in other genera. The use of thermal nociceptive methods for determining analgesia efficacy has not been well supported (Coble et al., 2011; Hausmann et al., 2021; Martinelli et al., 2021; Vachon, 2014).

B. Pharmacologic options (see Table 25.2)

Local anesthetics (such as 1–50 mg/kg lidocaine) have been used in amphibians, in addition to the similar compounds (MS222/benzocaine) employed as general anesthetics. However, care should be taken as regional/general spread of subcutaneously injected local anesthetics via the lymph is reported, leading to a loss of, or lack of, a local antinociceptive effect and systemic sedation at higher doses (Chatigny et al., 2017; Williams et al., 2017).

Opiates have been used as immersive and injected adjuncts to anesthesia and as analgesics (Adami et al., 2016a; Chai, 2015; Stevens, 2011). In frogs, this use as analgesia has been based on results from the acetic acid test (AAT) in *Rana pipiens*, with morphine, fentanyl, and buprenorphine via injection, and butorphanol and morphine via immersion being the most commonly used agents (Adami et al., 2016a; Stevens, 2004; Stevens et al., 1994). There is still comparatively little species-specific analgesic information on amphibians (Martinelli et al., 2021). In salamanders, the use of opiates has been assessed and validated via their postoperative behavior (Koeller, 2009); however, this efficacy has not yet been replicated in axolotls, where morbidity occurred following buprenorphine use (Llaniguez et al., 2020).

Among nonsteroidal agents, flunixin and ketorolac 25 mg/kg have been advocated based on their efficacy in the AAT (Stevens, 2011). Meloxicam 0.1 mg/kg reduced the change in circulating PGE2 in bullfrogs and is clinically recommended (Archibald et al., 2015; Minter et al., 2011). This dose did not, however, provide long-lasting plasma concentrations in the smoky jungle frog *Leptodactylus pentadactylus,* again highlighting the need for greater species-specific information on nonsteroidal utility, pharmacokinetics, and pharmacodynamics in normal and inflamed tissue (Balko et al., 2019).

Dexmedetomidine (0.06–0.12 mg/kg) and other alpha-2-agonists have had positive analgesic action in the AAT over 30 minutes to 9 hours, at doses that did not provide a delay in reflexes (and thus are argued to not show sedative effect) in *Rana pipiens*. An equipotent solution of medetomidine also did not lead to sedation, although it was associated with a reduction in respiratory rate (Brenner et al., 1994; Lafortune et al., 2001).

C. Nonpharmacological options

There have, to the authors' knowledge, not been studies on the effect of acupuncture, nutrition, housing, or conspecifics on amphibian pain, above the general relation between increased stress and the release of endogenous opiates, which is not considered a clinical aim.

While regional hypothermia has been shown to reduce reaction to the AAT in *Rana pipiens* in an opiate-dependent manner, this should not be used clinically, as the effects of hypothermia are likely to be effective via the effects of stress-released endogenous opiates, as well as via a reduction in the function of nociceptive nerves (Stevens, 2011). General hypothermia will have effects on anesthetic recovery, tissue healing, and immune function, so while it has been used for immobilization postsurgically (Dittrich and Lauridsen, 2021), this is not generally recommended.

VIII. Anesthesia and analgesia for specific situations

A. Sedation, noninvasive procedure

Examples include use to provide sedation to swab for disease status and swift imaging procedures. Alfaxalone 5 mg/L immersion, propofol 3–4 mg/L, and buffered MS222 200 mg/L (Fig. 25.3).

B. Anesthesia for physiological data collection

For situations such as sensory physiology data collection or cardiovascular echocardiographic imaging, common approaches include use of immersive use of buffered MS222 or benzocaine (prediluted in ethanol or acetone) at 200 mg/L-1 g/L species dependent or immersion in propofol 3–4 mg/L or alfaxalone 5 mg/L for noninvasive study. Induction time is approximately 20–50 minutes dependent on the species (Adami et al., 2015; Hernández et al., 2012; Thygesen et al., 2017). Recovery time in freshwater is approximately 60 minutes. Analgesia can be provided by buprenorphine, pure mu opiates, or meloxicam (See Table 25.2). Where invasive procedures are included but Na+ channel blockers must be avoided for experimental reasons, then a combination of opiate, ketamine, and alpha-2 agonists may be used e.g., ketamine (50 mg/kg) with medetomidine (0.5 mg/kg), meloxicam (0.2 mg/kg), and butorphanol (25 mg/kg) intramuscularly in *Xenopus* (Chai, 2015). In physiological data collection, e.g., sensory and cardiovascular physiology and after transmitter placement, meloxicam 0.1–0.2 mg/kg has been employed (Chai, 2015) injectably at induction, and separately, 0.4 mg/kg every 24 hours orally postoperatively (Yaw et al., 2017).

C. Surgery

Common procedures supported by anesthesia include reproductive surgery: for egg harvesting in *Xenopus laevis* (Fig. 25.4), usually performed as a partial ovariectomy, induction using 1–2 g/L solution of MS222 buffered to pH 7.0 by sodium bicarbonate in a home tank or unchlorinated, deionized water is commonly used. The MS222 dose should be based on expected surgical time, 30 minutes - 1 g/L, 60 minutes 2 g/L (Lalonde-Robert et al., 2012a).

TABLE 25.2 Table of Analgesic agents in current use.

Drug(s)	Species	Dose	Duration	Antagonist**	Comments
Analgesia					
Local anesthesia					
Lidocaine	Multiple	5–50 mg/kg			Systemic circulation of the drug may result in deepening general anesthetic plane, with loss of local anesthetic effect (Williams et al., 2017)
Benzocaine	Multiple	20 mg/L by immersion (Dittrich and Lauridsen, 2021)	For duration of immersion	None	For dissolution requires small volume of ethanol or acetone, followed by dilution in home tank water or distilled water
Nonsteroidal anti-inflammatories (NSAIDs)					
Meloxicam	*Rana catesbeiana*	0.1–0.2 mg/kg		None	Reduction in PGE synthesis reported (*R. catesbeiana* (Minter et al., 2011)) and clinical reports of efficacy, no effect in antinociceptive testing performed in *Xenopus* (Coble et al., 2011).
Flunixin	*Xenopus laevis*, *Rana pipiens*	25 mg/kg	To 24 hours	none	Leads to long lasting antinociception in AAT in *Xenopus* and *R. pipiens* (Coble et al., 2011; Smith et al., 2018; Terril-Robb et al., 1996). Higher doses cause toxicity, some local reaction in xenopus at this dose.
Opiates					
Morphine	*Rana pipiens*	ED_{50} 33 mg/kg,	>4 hours	Naloxone, not clinically used.	AAT tested (Stevens, 2011)
Fentanyl	*Rana pipiens*	ED_{50} 0.8 mg/kg	>4 hours	Naloxone, not clinically used.	AAT tested (Stevens, 2011)
Butorphanol	*Rana pipiens* *Notophthalmus viridescens*	AAT tested dose 33 mg/kg SC 0.5 mg/L immersion for 72 hours		Naloxone, not clinically used.	Stevens (2011) Shortened time to normal behavior (Koeller, 2009), no significant effect in axolotls (Llaniguez et al., 2020)
Buprenorphine	*Rana pipiens* *Notophthalmus viridescens*	ED_{50} 45 mg/kg SCin dorsal lymph sac 50 mg/kg IC q24 h		Naloxone, not clinically used.	AAT tested(Stevens, 2011) Shortened time to normal behavior (Koeller, 2009), this dose caused ileus and prompted euthanasia in axolotl (Llaniguez et al., 2020)
Alpha-2-agonists					
Dexmedetomidine	*Rana pipiens* *Bombina orientalis*	0.1–0.2 mg/kg SC into dorsal lymph sac 3 mg/L by immersion	>8 hours	Atipamezole at 2:1 volume used in research or 5:1 mg/mg dose (clinical norm)	AAT tested (Brenner et al., 1994) Withdrawal and von Frey and (Adami et al., 2016b)
Xylazine	*Rana pipiens*	10 mg/kg			AAT test (Terril-Robb et al., 1996)

Time to induction is approximately 20 minutes to loss of righting reflex and withdrawal. Rinse the animal from the induction solution with clean water and place it on a moist towel with nares in the air. Intraoperative analgesia is inconsistently used currently, but 0.1–0.2 mg/kg meloxicam to the dorsal lymph sac may be recommended, or 25 mg/kg flunixin (care with potential tissue irritation) (Coble et al., 2011; Kalpravidh et al., 1984; Smith et al., 2018). Opiates such as buprenorphine at 30–40 mg/kg could also be considered based on studies in *Rana pipiens*, however, use prior to removal of oocytes is not recommended due to potential effects on the oocytes, therefore injection postsurgically, but prerecovery may be more supported, but clinical studies are lacking. Similarly, nonsteroidal injection may be delayed to prerecovery if there are surgical concerns about a theoretical contribution to increased intraoperative bleeding. Postoperative analgesia is also potentially available via low (25 mg/L) concentrations of benzocaine as immersive analgesia (Dittrich and Lauridsen, 2021). For invasive surgery or fracture management—mu opioids such as morphine 10–100 mg/kg (Stevens, 2011) and *Xenopus spp.* dose of 40 mg/kg (Coble et al., 2011) are appropriate, and doses are drawn from the experimental literature.

D. Regenerative medicine research

Regenerative medicine is an area of increasing research interest. Common examples are limb amputation, cardiac puncture/injury, and neural injury, e.g., in axolotl. For cardiac cryoinjury, a protocol could include induction in 250 mg/L benzocaine (prediluted in 3 mL acetone, then into a home tank or deionized water), followed by maintenance on moist towels. Postoperative analgesia is possible via low (25 mg/L) concentrations of benzocaine as immersive analgesia (Dittrich and Lauridsen, 2021). The use of nonsteroidal or opiate analgesics is currently debated due to unknown effects on the regenerative process being studied; however, some early support exists for opiate use from a zebrafish model (Lelek et al., 2020). MS222 anesthesia is also commonly used. Morphine 10–100 mg/kg or buprenorphine 50 mg/kg intracelomically (Koeller, 2009) are potential options; however, buprenorphine cannot currently be recommended in axolotls, where gastrointestinal side effects have been noted at this dose (Llaniguez et al., 2020). The known interaction of inflammation and regeneration means that nonsteroidal drugs have not found favor in the regeneration research community; however, the specific effects of NSAIDs on regeneration have not been studied.

IX. Postprocedural recovery and care

Normal posture of the animal should be maintained in recovery so that the nares and mouth are in the air to prevent drowning in adult anurans. Provision of clean aerated water or electrolyte solution matching home tank conditions is the ideal recovery environment, with water changes being required if extended anesthesia times are experienced, to remove residual anesthetic being equilibrated with the recovery water.

Supportive care: Maintenance of temperature and hydration is key, while aeration of the tank water is recommended to allow a return to normal oxygenation and acid-base balance.

Pain assessment: The resumption of normal posture, behavior, and feeding are used for amphibian pain assessment; however, validated pain scales are currently lacking in amphibian species. In their absence, the experience of the care staff with the normal behavior of the species and individuals in question is essential. Behaviors to monitor for normal recovery can include resumption of normal feeding, posture in the tank, e.g., position on the substrate or aerial tank features for arboreal anurans, and normal reaction to observation and startle behaviors while those that could indicate pain include anorexia, repeated wiping at surgical sites, and immobility.

Return to group housing: activity following anesthesia and surgery is often not encouraged due to the fragility of sutures placed in amphibian skin. Therefore, individual housing may be required following surgery.

X. Euthanasia

As with anesthesia, immersion in MS222 (buffered, 1–5 g/L dependent on species, for >1 hour) is the mainstay of laboratory euthanasia in amphibians to provide CNS depression and loss of respiratory and cardiac function (AVMA Panel on Euthanasia, 2020; European Council, 2010). Intracoelomic injection of buffered MS222 (200–300 mg/kg) has also been used but is unreliable in some species (e.g., *Xenopus*) (Torreilles et al., 2009). Overdose of pentobarbital (>1000 mg/kg IP) and benzocaine 20% gel (>180 mg/kg topically) was also found to be effective over hours of exposure in *Xenopus*, while lower doses are used in other species.

Note that the loss of respiratory or even cardiac rhythm is not sufficient to guarantee **irreversible** loss of CNS function in these low-metabolism, hypoxia, and hypercarbia tolerant, cutaneous respiration-capable animals (Lalonde-Robert et al., 2012b; Torreilles et al., 2009; Woodbury, 2014). Therefore, the overdose of chemical anesthesia to give a deep anesthetic plane, which occurs much faster than the cessation of cardiac activity, should be followed up with a physical means of CNS destruction, such as a double pithing, concussion, or fast freezing (AVMA Panel on Euthanasia, 2020; Leary et al., 2016; Medler, 2019). Double pithing in practice means the insertion of a blunt probe into the brain via the caudal occiput, and destroying it by moving laterally, then reversing the direction of the probe into the proximal spinal cord, with physical disruption of the nerves. If the CNS is the subject of study and cannot be physically disrupted, then longer exposure (over 3 hours) to the chemical means described above is possible, or removal and functional destruction by fixation are possible under the deep anesthetic plane created.

The science, ethics, and practicalities of euthanasia of large numbers of specimens in field situations/teaching/for invasive species are a matter of current scientific and regulatory debate (Kay and Mawson, 2021; Leary et al., 2013, 2016; Lillywhite et al., 2017; Woodbury, 2014). The variable species-specific tolerances to cold and hypercarbia mean that neither cooling followed by freezing, nor prolonged 4% CO_2 exposure are recommended by the authors for general use in laboratory settings.

Acknowledgments

The authors thank Per Henriksen for the photographs used in this chapter, and Professor Tobias Wang for the discussion of the physiology sections. Silhouettes from phylopic.com are used under Public Domain Dedication 1.0 license from images by Beth Reinke, Dennis C. Murphy, Jake Warner, and Yan Wong from illustration by Charles Orbigny and Creative Commons license 3.0 from C. Camilo Julián-Caballero.

References

Adami, C., D'Ovidio, D., Casoni, D., 2016a. Alfaxalone-butorphanol versus alfaxalone-morphine combination for immersion anaesthesia in oriental fire-bellied toads (*Bombina orientalis*). Lab. Anim. 50, 204–211.

Adami, C., D'Ovidio, D., Casoni, D., 2016b. Alfaxalone versus alfaxalone-dexmedetomidine anaesthesia by immersion in oriental fire-bellied toads (*Bombina orientalis*). Vet. Anaesth. Analg. 43, 326–332.

Adami, C., Spadavecchia, C., Angeli, G., d'Ovidio, D., 2015. Alfaxalone anesthesia by immersion in oriental fire-bellied toads (*Bombina orientalis*). Vet. Anaesth. Analg. 42, 547–551.

Alworth, L.C., Harvey, S.B., 2007. IACUC issues associated with amphibian research. ILAR J. 48, 278–289.

Alworth, L.C., Hernandez, S.M., Divers, S.J., 2011. Laboratory reptile surgery: principles and techniques. J. Am. Assoc. Lab. Anim. Sci. 50, 11–26.

Amphibian Specialist Group, 2019. IUCN SSC Amphibian Specialist Group. https://www.iucn-amphibians.org/. (Accessed 20 August 2021).

Andersen, J.B., Andrade, D.V., Wang, T., 2003. Effects of inhibition gastric acid secretion on arterial acid-base status during digestion in the toad *Bufo marinus*. Comp. Biochem. Physiol. A. Mol. Integr. Physiol. 135, 425–433.

Andersen, J.B., Wang, T., 2002. Effects of anaesthesia on blood gases, acid-base status and ions in the toad *Bufo marinus*. Comp. Biochem. Physiol. Mol. Integr. Physiol. 131, 639–646.

Andersen, J.B., Wang, T., 2003. Cardiorespiratory effects of forced activity and digestion in toads. Physiol. Biochem. Zool. 76, 459–470.

Archibald, K.E., Minter, L.J., Dombrowski, D.S., O'Brien, J.L., Lewbart, G.A., 2015. Cystic urolithiasis in captive waxy monkey frogs (*Phyllomedusa sauvagii*). J. Zoo Wildl. Med. 46, 105–112.

AVMA panel on Euthanasia, 2020. AVMA Guidelines for the Euthanasia of Animals, 2020 Edition.

Baitchman, E., Stetter, M., 2014. Amphibians. In: West, G., Heard, D.J., Caulkett, N. (Eds.), Zoo Animal and Wildlife Immobilization and Anesthesia. John Wiley & Sons, Inc., pp. 303–311.

Balko, J.A., Watson, M.K., Papich, M.G., Posner, L.P., Chinnadurai, S.K., 2019. Plasma concentrations of ketoprofen and meloxicam after subcutaneous and topical administration in the smoky jungle frog (*Leptodactylus pentadactylus*). J. Herpetol. Med. Surg. 28, 89–92.

Barter, L.S., Antognini, J.F., 2008. Kinetics and potency of halothane, isoflurane, and desflurane in the Northern Leopard frog *Rana pipiens*. Vet. Res. Commun. 32, 357–365.

Barter, L.S., Hawkins, M.G., Brosnan, R.J., Antognini, J.F., Pypendop, B.H., 2006. Median effective dose of isoflurane, sevoflurane, and desflurane in green iguanas. Am. J. Vet. Res. 67, 392–397.

Barter, L.S., Mark, L.O., Smith, A.C., Antognini, J.F., 2007. Isoflurane potency in the northern leopard frog *Rana pipiens* is similar to that in mammalian species and is unaffected by decerebration. Vet. Res. Commun. 31, 757–763.

Brenner, G.M., Klopp, A.J., Deason, L.L., Stevens, C.W., 1994. Analgesic potency of alpha adrenergic agents after systemic administration in amphibians. J. Pharmacol. Exp. Therapeut. 270, 540–545.

Brod, S., Brookes, L., Garner, T.W.J., 2019. Discussing the future of amphibians in research. Lab. Anim. (NY) 48, 16–18.

Burggren, W.W., Warburton, S., 2007. Amphibians as animal models for laboratory research in physiology. ILAR J. 48, 260–269.

California, U. of, 2021. AmphibaWeb. https://amphibiaweb.org. (Accessed 20 August 2021).

Campbell, C.R., Voyles, J., Cook, D.I., Dinudom, A., 2012. Frog skin epithelium: electrolyte transport and chytridiomycosis. Int. J. Biochem. Cell Biol. 44, 431–434.

Canadian Council on Animal Care, 2021. CCAC Guidelines: Amphibians.

Cashins, S.D., Alford, R.A., Skerratt, L.F., 2008. Lethal effect of latex, nitrile, and vinyl gloves on tadpoles. Herpetol. Rev. 39, 298–301.

Chai, N., 2015. Endoscopy in Amphibians. Vet. Clin. N. Am. Exot. Anim. Pract. 18, 479–491.

Chatigny, F., Kamunde, C., Creighton, C.M., Stevens, E.D., 2017. Uses and doses of local anesthetics in fish, Amphibians, and reptiles. J. Am. Assoc. Lab. Anim. Sci. 56, 244–253.

Coble, D.J., Taylor, D.K., Mook, D.M., 2011. Analgesic effects of meloxicam, morphine sulfate, flunixin meglumine, and xylazine hydrochloride in African-clawed frogs (*Xenopus laevis*). J. Am. Assoc. Lab. Anim. Sci. 50, 355–360.

Cui, J., Zhu, B., Fang, G., Smith, E., Brauth, S.E., Tang, Y., 2017. Effect of the level of anesthesia on the auditory brainstem response in the emei music frog (*Babina daunchina*). PLoS One 12, e0169449.

d'Ovidio, D., Spadavecchia, C., Angeli, G., Adami, C., 2015. Etomidate anaesthesia by immersion in oriental fire-bellied toads (*Bombina orientalis*). Lab. Anim. 49, 319–326.

Dittrich, A., Lauridsen, H., 2021. Cryo-injury induced heart regeneration in the axolotl and echocardiography and unbiased quantitative histology to evaluate regenerative progression. J. Vis. Exp. 2021, 1–13.

Divers, S.J., Stahl, S.S. (Eds.), 2019. Mader's Reptile and Amphibian Medicine and Surgery, third ed. Elsevier.

Doss, G.A., Mans, C., Sladky, K.K., 2021. Analgesia, anesthesia and monitoring. In: Graham, J.E., Doss, G.A., Beaufrere, H. (Eds.), Exotic Animal Emergency and Critical Care Medicine. Wiley-Blackwell, pp. 746–756.

European Council, 2010. Directive 2010/63/EU of the european parliament and of the council on the protection of animals used for scientific purposes. Off. J. Eur. Union 1, 33–79.

Gebhart, G.F., Basbaum, A.I., Bird, S.J., Flecknell, P., Goodly, L., Karas, A.Z., Kelley, S.T., Lacher, J., Mason, G., Sneddon, L.U., Soriano, S.G., Shafford, H.L., 2009. Recognition and alleviation of pain in laboratory animals. In: Laboratory Animals. The National Academies Press, p. 380.

Gentz, E.J., 2007. Medicine and surgery of amphibians. ILAR J. 48, 255–259.

González-del-Pliego, P., Freckleton, R.P., Edwards, D.P., Koo, M.S., Scheffers, B.R., Pyron, R.A., Jetz, W., 2019. Phylogenetic and trait-based prediction of extinction risk for data-deficient Amphibians. Curr. Biol. 29, 1557–1563.e3.

Goulet, F., Hélie, P., Vachon, P., 2010. Eugenol anesthesia in African clawed frogs (*Xenopus laevis*) of different body weights. J. Am. Assoc. Lab. Anim. Sci. 49, 460–463.

Goulet, F., Vachon, P., Hélie, P., 2011. Evaluation of the toxicity of eugenol at anesthetic doses in African clawed frogs (*Xenopus laevis*). Toxicol. Pathol. 39, 471–477.

Guénette, S.A., Hélie, P., Beaudry, F., Vachon, P., 2007. Eugenol for anesthesia of African clawed frogs (*Xenopus laevis*). Vet. Anaesth. Analg. 34, 164–170.

Guénette, S.A., Giroux, M.-C., Vachon, P., 2013. Pain perception and anaesthesia in research frogs. Exp. Anim. 62, 87–92.

Hausmann, J.C., Krisp, A.R., Mans, C., Johnson, S.M., Sladky, K.K., 2021. Analgesic efficacy of tramadol and morphine in white's tree frogs (*Litoria caerulea*). J. Am. Assoc. Lab. Anim. Sci. 60, 681–686.

Hedrick, M.S., Hansen, K., Wang, T., Lauridsen, H., Thygesen, J., Pedersen, M., 2014. Visualising lymph movement in anuran amphibians with computed tomography. J. Exp. Biol. 217 (17), 2990–2993. https://doi.org/10.1242/jeb.106906.

Hedrick, M.S., Hillman, S.S., Drewes, R.C., Withers, P.C., 2013. Lymphatic regulation in nonmammalian vertebrates. J. Appl. Physiol. 115 (3), 297–308. https://doi.org/10.1152/japplphysiol.00201.2013.

Hedrick, M.S., Winmill, R.E., 2003. Excitatory and inhibitory effects of tricaine (MS-222) on fictive breathing in isolated bullfrog brain stem. Am. J. Physiol. Regul. Integr. Comp. Physiol. 284, R405–R412.

Herman, C.A., Sandoval, E.J., 1983. Catecholamine effects on blood pressure and heart rate in the American bullfrog, *Rana catesbeiana*. Gen. Comp. Endocrinol. 52, 142–148.

Hernández, S.E., Sernia, C., Bradley, A.J., 2012. The effect of three anaesthetic protocols on the stress response in cane toads (Rhinella marina). Vet. Anaesth. Analg. 39, 584–590.

Hillman, S.S., Hedrick, M.S., Kohl, Z.F., 2014. Net cardiac shunts in anuran amphibians: physiology or physics? J. Exp. Biol. 217, 2844–2847.

Jayson, S., Harding, L., Michaels, C.J., Tapley, B., Hedley, J., Goetz, M., Barbon, A., Garcia, G., Lopez, J., Flach, E., 2018. Development of a body condition score for the mountain chicken frog (*Leptodactylus fallax*). Zoo Anim. Wildl. Immobil. Anesth. 37, 196–205.

Jensen, M.T., Jensen, U.T., Bertelsen, M.F., 2021. Assessing the effects of biosecurity measures in terrarium management. J. Zoo Aquarium Res. 9, 157–160.

Jensen, B., Wang, T., Moorman, A.F.M., 2019. Evolution and development of the atrial septum. Anat. Rec. 302, 32–48.

Jetz, W., Pyron, R.A., 2018. The interplay of past diversification and evolutionary isolation with present imperilment across the amphibian tree of life. Nat. Ecol. Evol. 2, 850–858.

Jia, X., Burggren, W., 1997. Developmental changes in chemoreceptive control of gill ventilation in larval bullfrogs (*Rana catesbeiana*). I. Reflex ventilatory responses to ambient hyperoxia, hypoxia and NaCN. J. Exp. Biol. 200, 2229–2236.

Kalpravidh, M., Lumb, W.V., Wright, M., Heath, R.B., 1984. Effects of butorphanol, flunixin, levorphanol, morphine, and xylazine in ponies. Am. J. Vet. Res. 45, 217–223.

Kay, W., Mawson, P., 2021. An efficient method for the euthanasia of cane toads (*Rhinella marina*) under northern Australian field conditions. Animals 11, 2239.

Keifer, J., Zheng, Z., 2017. Cold block of in vitro eyewink reflexes: evidence supporting the use of hypothermia as an anesthetic in pond turtles. J. Exp. Biol. 220, 4370–4373.

Killorn, E.E., Toews, D.P., 2001. The dynamics of venous return and response to hypervolemia in the toad, *Bufo marinus* (L.). BMC Physiol. 1, 1–6.

Koeller, C.A., 2009. Comparison of buprenorphine and butorphanol analgesia in the eastern red-spotted newt (*Notophthalmus viridescens*). J. Am. Assoc. Lab. Anim. Sci. 48, 171–175.

Lafortune, M., Mitchell, M.A., Smith, J.A., 2001. Evaluation of medetomidine, clove oil and propofol for anesthesia of leopard frogs, *Rana pipiens*. J. Herpetol. Med. Surg. 11, 13–18.

Lalonde-Robert, V., Beaudry, F., Vachon, P., 2012a. Pharmacologic parameters of MS222 and physiologic changes in frogs (*Xenopus laevis*) after immersion at anesthetic doses. J. Am. Assoc. Lab. Anim. Sci. 51, 464–468.

Lalonde-Robert, V., Desgent, S., Duss, S., Vachon, P., 2012b. Electroencephalographic and physiologic changes after tricaine methanesulfonate immersion of African clawed frogs (*Xenopus laevis*). J. Am. Assoc. Lab. Anim. Sci. 51, 622–627.

Leary, S., Regenstein, J., Shearer, J., Smith, S.A., Golab, G.C., 2016. AVMA Guidelines for the Humane Slaughter of Animals, 2016 Edition.

Leary, S., Underwood, W., Anthony, R., Cartner, S., Corey, D., Walla, W., Grandin, T., Greenacre, C., Gwaltney-Brant, S., McCrackin, M.A., Meyer, R., Miller, D., Shearer, J., Yanong, R., Golab, G.C., Patterson-kane, E., 2013. AVMA Guidelines for the Euthanasia of Animals: 2013 Edition. American Veterinary Medical Association.

Lelek, S., Simoes, M., Hu, B., Alameldeen, A., Czajkowski, M., Meyer, A., Ferrara, F., Junker, J., Panakova, D., 2020. Morphine alleviates pain after heart cryoinjury in zebrafish without impeding regeneration. bioRxiv.

Lewis, Z.R., Hanken, J., 2017. Convergent evolutionary reduction of atrial septation in lungless salamanders. J. Anat. 230, 16–29.

Lillywhite, H.B., Shine, R., Jacobson, E., Denardo, D.F., Gordon, M.S., Navas, C.A., Wang, T., Seymour, R.S., Storey, K.B., Heatwole, H., Heard, D., Brattstrom, B., Burghardt, G.M., 2017. Anesthesia and euthanasia of Amphibians and reptiles used in scientific research: should hypothermia and freezing be prohibited? Bioscience 67, 53–61.

Lips, K.R., 2016. Overview of chytrid emergence and impacts on amphibians. Philos. Trans. R. Soc. B Biol. Sci. 371, 20150465.

Llaniguez, J.T., Szczepaniak, M.A., Rickman, B.H., Gelovani, J.G., Hish, G.A., Cotroneo, T.M., 2020. Quantitative and qualitative behavioral measurements to assess pain in axolotls (*Ambystoma mexicanum*). J. Am. Assoc. Lab. Anim. Sci. 59, 186–196.

Machin, K., 1999. Amphibian pain and analgesia. J. Zoo Wildl. Med. 30, 2–10.

Mailho-Fontana, P.L., Antoniazzi, M.M., Alexandre, C., Pimenta, D.C., Sciani, J.M., Brodie, E.D., Jared, C., 2020. Morphological evidence for an oral venom system in caecilian amphibians. iScience 23, 101234.

Marshall, L.N., Vivien, C.J., Girardot, F., Péricard, L., Scerbo, P., Palmier, K., Demeneix, B.A., Coen, L., 2019. Stage-dependent cardiac regeneration in Xenopus is regulated by thyroid hormone availability. Proc. Natl. Acad. Sci. U. S. A. 116, 3614–3623.

Martinelli, L.M., Johnson, S.M., Sladky, K.K., 2021. Comparison of thermal and mechanical noxious stimuli for testing analgesics in white's tree frogs (*Litoria caerulea*) and northern leopard frogs (*lithobates pipiens*). J. Am. Assoc. Lab. Anim. Sci. 60, 687–691.

McMillan, M.W., Leece, E.A., 2011. Immersion and branchial/transcutaneous irrigation anaesthesia with alfaxalone in a Mexican axolotl. Vet. Anaesth. Analg. 38, 619–623.

Medler, S., 2019. Anesthetic MS-222 eliminates nerve and muscle activity in frogs used for physiology teaching laboratories. Adv. Physiol. Educ. 43, 69–75.

Milsom, W.K., Kinkead, R., Hedrick, M.S., Gilmour, K., Perry, S., Gargaglioni, L., Wang, T., 2022. Evolution of vertebrate respiratory central rhythm generators. Respir. Physiol. Neurobiol. 295, 103781.

Minter, L.J., Clarke, E.O., Gjeltema, J.L., Archibald, K.E., Posner, L.P., Lewbart, G.A., 2011. Effects of intramuscular meloxicam administration on prostaglandin E2 synthesis in the north American bullfrog (*Rana catesbeiana*). Zoo Biol. 42, 680–685.

Mitchell, M.A., 2009. Anesthetic considerations for amphibians. J. Exot. Pet Med. 18, 40–49.

Mitchell, M.A., Riggs, S.M., Singleton, C.B., Diaz-Figueroa, O., Hale, L.K., 2009. Evaluating the clinical and cardiopulmonary effects of clove oil and propofol in tiger salamanders (*Ambystoma tigrinum*). J. Exot. Pet Med. 18, 50–56.

Morrison, K.E., Strahl-Heldreth, D., Clark-Price, S.C., 2016. Isoflurane, sevoflurane and desflurane use in cane toads (*Rhinella marina*). Vet. Rec. Open 3, 1–6.

Mylniczenko, N., 2009. Amphibians. In: Mitchell, M., Tully, T. (Eds.), Manual of Exotic Pet Practice. Elsevier, p. 160.

Nagy, K. a, 2005. Field metabolic rate and body size. J. Exp. Biol. 208, 1621–1625.

Novarro, A.J., Blackman, A., Bailey, S.D., 2017. Tricaine methanesulfonate (MS-222) as a short-term anesthetic for the eastern red-backed salamander, *Plethodon cinereus*. Herpetol. Rev. 48, 320–322.

O'Rourke, D.P., 2007. Amphibians used in research and teaching. ILAR J. 48, 183–187.

Pasmans, F., Martel, A., 2019. 28 - Amphibians. In: Divers, S.J., Stahl, S.J. (Eds.), Mader's Reptile and Amphibian Medicine and Surgery, third ed. W.B. Saunders, St. Louis (MO), pp. 224–234.e1.

Pojman, J.A., Fonteno, C.L., 2014. Use of clove oil as an anesthetic for PIT tagging and surgery with the three-Toed Amphiuma (*Amphiuma tridactylum*) and determination of recovery time as a function of body mass. Herpetol. Rev. 45, 25–27.

Posner, L.P., Bailey, K.M., Richardson, E.Y., Motsinger-Reif, A.A., Harms, C.A., 2013. Alfaxalone anaesthesia in Bullfrogs (*Lithobates catesbeiana*) by injection or immersion. J. Zoo Wildl. Med. 44, 965–971.

Quaranta, A., Bellantuono, V., Cassano, G., Lippe, C., 2009. Why amphibians are more sensitive than mammals to xenobiotics. PLoS One 4, 2–5.

Ramlochansingh, C., Branoner, F., Chagnaud, B.P., Straka, H., 2014. Efficacy of tricaine methanesulfonate (MS-222) as an anesthetic agent for blocking sensory-motor responses in *Xenopus laevis* tadpoles. PLoS One 9, e101606.

Reed, B.T., Research Animals Department, R., 2005. Guidance on the Housing and Care of the African Clawed Frog *X. laevis*.

Revell, L.J., 2012. phytools: An R package for phylogenetic comparative biology (and other things). Methods Ecol. Evol. 3, 217–223.

Sanches, P.G., Op't Veld, R.C., de Graaf, W., Strijkers, G.J., Grull, H., 2018. Novel axolotl cardiac function analysis method using magnetic resonance imaging. PLoS One 12, 1–15.

Schnellbacher, R.W., Shepard, M., Mans, C., Sladky, K., Schumacher, J., Steagall, P., Sladakovic, I., Divers, S.J., 2019. Section 6: Anesthesia, Chapters 48–53. In: Mader's Reptile and Amphibian Medicine and Surgery, pp. 444–483.

Sladakovic, I., Divers, S.J., 2019. 52 - Amphibian Anesthesia. In: Divers, S.J., Stahl, S.J. (Eds.), Mader's Reptile and Amphibian Medicine and Surgery, third ed. W.B. Saunders, St. Louis (MO), pp. 480–485.e1.

Sladakovic, I., Johnson, R.S., Vogelnest, L., 2014. Evaluation of intramuscular alfaxalone in three Australian frog species (*Litoria caerulea, Litoria aurea, Litoria booroolongensis*). J. Herpetol. Med. Surg. 24, 36–42.

Smith, B.D., Vail, K.J., Carroll, G.L., Taylor, M.C., Jeffery, N.D., Vemulapalli, T.H., Elliott, J.J., 2018. Comparison of etomidate, benzocaine, and MS222 anesthesia with and without subsequent flunixin meglumine analgesia in african clawed frogs (*Xenopus laevis*). J. Am. Assoc. Lab. Anim. Sci. 57, 202–209.

Speare, R., Speare, B., Muller, R., Bishop, P., 2014. Anesthesia of tadpoles of the southern brown tree frog (*Litoria ewingii*) with isoeugenol (Aqui-S). J. Zoo Wildl. Med. 45, 492–496.

Stathopoulou, T., Light, J., Lamas, L.P., Pierce, S.E., Pelligand, L., 2022. A Protocol for Prolonged Surgical Anaesthesia with Recovery in Fire Salamanders Using Tricaine Mesylate (MS-222): A Case Series. Lab. Anim. 56 (6), 540–549.

Stevens, C., 1992. Alternatives to the use of mammals for pain research. Life Sci. 50, 901–912.

Stevens, C., 2011. Analgesia in amphibians: preclinical studies and clinical applications. Vet. Clin. N. Am. Exot. Anim. Pract. 14, 33–44.

Stevens, C.W., 2004. Opioid research in amphibians: an alternative pain model yielding insights on the evolution of opioid receptors. Brain Res. Brain Res. Rev. 46, 204–215.

Stevens, C.W., Klopp, A.J., Facello, J.A., 1994. Analgesic potency of mu and kappa opioids after systemic administration in Amphibians. J. Pharmacol. Exp. Therapeut. 200, 1086–1093.

Taylor, E.N., Diele-Viegas, L.M., Gangloff, E.J., Hall, J.M., Halpern, B., Massey, M.D., Rödder, D., Rollinson, N., Spears, S., Sun, B.J., Telemeco, R.S., 2021. The thermal ecology and physiology of reptiles and amphibians: a user's guide. J. Exp. Zool. Part A Ecol. Integr. Physiol. 335, 13–44.

Taylor, E.W., Leite, C.A.C., McKenzie, D.J., Wang, T., 2010. Control of respiration in fish, amphibians and reptiles. Braz. J. Med. Biol. Res. 43, 409–424.

Terril-Robb, L.A., Suckow, M.A., Grigdesby, C.F., 1996. Evaluation of the analgesic effects of butorphanol tartrate, xylazine hydrochloride, and flunixin meglumine in leopard frogs (*Rana pipiens*). Contemp. Top. Lab. Anim. Sci. 35, 54–56.

Thomas, V., van Rooij, P., Meerpoel, C., Stegen, G., Wauters, J., Vanhaecke, L., Martel, A., Pasmans, F., 2020. Instant killing of pathogenic chytrid fungi by disposable nitrile gloves prevents disease transmission between amphibians. PLoS One 15, 1–16.

Thygesen, M.M., Rasmussen, M.M., Madsen, J.G., Pedersen, M., Lauridsen, H., 2017. Propofol (2,6-diisopropylphenol) is an applicable immersion anesthetic in the axolotl with potential uses in hemodynamic and neurophysiological experiments. Regeneration 4, 121–131.

Torreilles, S.L., McClure, D.E., Green, S.L., 2009. Evaluation and refinement of euthanasia methods for *Xenopus laevis*. J. Am. Assoc. Lab. Anim. Sci. 48, 512–516.

University Federation of Animal Welfare, 2010. The care and management of laboratory and other research animals. J. Chem. Inf. Model. (Wiley-Blackwell).

Vachon, P., 2014. Hargreaves does not evaluate nociception following a surgical laparotomy in *Xenopus leavis* frogs. Res. Vet. Sci. 97, 470–473.

Van Rooij, P., Pasmans, F., Coen, Y., Martel, A., 2017. Efficacy of chemical disinfectants for the containment of the salamander chytrid fungus *Batrachochytrium salamandrivorans*. PLoS One 12, 1–10.

Von Esse, F.V., Wright, K.M., 1999. Effect of intracoelomic propofol in white's tree frogs, *Pelodryas caerulea*. Bull. Assoc. Reptil. Amphib. Vet. 9, 7–8.

Voss, S.R., Epperlein, H.H., Tanaka, E.M., 2009. *Ambystoma mexicanum*, the axolotl: a versatile amphibian model for regeneration, development, and evolution studies. Cold Spring Harb. Protoc. 4, 1–9.

Wang, T., Hedrick, M.S., Ihmied, Y.M., Taylor, E.W., 1999. Control and interaction of the cardiovascular and respiratory systems in anuran amphibians. Comp. Biochem. Physiol. Mol. Integr. Physiol. 124, 393–406.

Weber, L., Šmejkal, M., Bartoň, D., Rulík, M., 2019. Testing the applicability of tagging the Great crested newt (*Triturus cristatus*) using passive integrated transponders. PLoS One 14, 1–14.

White, C.R., Phillips, N.F., Seymour, R.S., 2006. The scaling and temperature dependence of vertebrate metabolism. Biol. Lett. 2, 125–127.

Williams, C.J., Alstrup, A.K., Bertelsen, M.F., Jensen, H.M., Leite, C.A., Wang, T., 2018. Cardiovascular effects of alfaxalone and propofol in the bullfrog, *Lithobates catesbeianus*. J. Zoo Wildl. Med. 49, 92–98.

Williams, C.J., Malte, C.L., Malte, H., Bertelsen, M.F., Wang, T., 2020. Ectothermy and cardiac shunts profoundly slow the equilibration of inhaled anaesthetics in a multi-compartment model. Sci. Rep. 10, 1–11.

Williams, C.J.A., Alstrup, A.K.O., Bertelsen, M.F., Jensen, H.M., Leite, C.A.C., Wang, T., 2017. When local anesthesia becomes universal: pronounced systemic effects of subcutaneous lidocaine in bullfrogs (*Lithobates catesbeianus*). Comp. Biochem. Physiol. Part A Mol. Integr. Physiol. 209, 41–46.

Wojick, K.B., Langan, J.N., Mitchell, M.A., 2010. Evaluation of MS-222 (tricaine methanesulfonate) and propofol as anesthetic agents in sonoran desert toads (*Bufo alvarius*). J. Herpetol. Med. Surg. 20, 79–83.

Woodbury, M., 2014. Euthanasia. In: West, G., Heard, D., Caulkett, N.J. (Eds.), Zoo Animal and Wildlife Immobilization and Anesthesia. Wiley-Blackwell, pp. 149–154.

Wright, K.M., Whitaker, B.R., 2001. Amphibian Medicine and Captive Husbandry. Krieger Publishing Company.

Yaw, T.J., Mans, C, Martinelli, L., Sladky, K.K., 2020. Comparison of subcutaneous administration of alfaxalone-midazolam-dexmedetomidine with ketamine-midazolam-dexmedetomidine for chemical restraint in juvenile blue poison dart frogs (Dendrobates tinctorius azureus). J. Zoo Wildl. Med. 50, 868–873.

Yaw, T.J., Swanson, J.E., Pierce, C.L., Muths, E., Smalling, K.L., Vandever, M.W., Zaffarano, B.A., 2017. Placement of intracoelomic radiotransmitters and silicone passive sampling devices in northern leopard frogs (*Lithobates pipiens*). J. Herpetol. Med. Surg. 27, 111–115.

Zullian, C., Dodolet-Devillers, A., Roy, S., Vachon, P., Dodelet-Devillers, A., Roy, S., Vachon, P., 2016. Evaluation of the anesthetic effects of MS222 in the adult Mexican axolotl (*Ambystoma mexicanum*). Vet. Med. Reports 7, 1–7.

Chapter 26

Anesthesia and analgesia in invertebrates

Sarah J. Wahltinez[1], Craig A. Harms[2] and Gregory A. Lewbart[3]

[1]College of Veterinary Medicine, University of Florida, Gainesville, FL, United States; [2]College of Veterinary Medicine and Center for Marine Sciences and Technology, North Carolina State University, Morehead City, NC, United States; [3]College of Veterinary Medicine, North Carolina State University, Raleigh, NC, United States

Chapter outline

I. Introduction

Some invertebrate species like the octopus, horseshoe crab, and various species of insects, have been used in research laboratories for decades. Their contribution has led to knowledge about pesticide and heavy metal toxicity, vision and color perception, embryology, and a long list of diseases, including multiple sclerosis and Parkinson's disease.

Invertebrates are playing an ever-increasing and important role in research. The elevated awareness and influence of animal welfare and the attempts and efforts to replace, reduce, and refine the use of vertebrate species in laboratory studies have had some impact on the invertebrate animal model. The overall public perception that invertebrates are more acceptable than vertebrates in research settings, is mainly present because of the commonly held belief that invertebrates do not experience pain. This has led to invertebrates being offered as a major "alternative" in any IACUC and animal welfare and research constitution. Much research is supported when animal models (microorganisms or invertebrates) can be used in place of vertebrates (NIH, n.d.). Selecting invertebrate species as an alternative to vertebrates for research makes the process of IACUC regulations and oversight very easy because there are no regulations or restrictions in the U.S. on invertebrate use. Despite some concerns from different sources, the Animal Welfare Act and PHS Policy do not require coverage for invertebrates. Some organizations, including some zoos and aquariums, do require a protocol for invertebrates used in research protocols. The United States Department of Agriculture has an "Information Resource on the Care and Use of Invertebrates" (AWIC Resource Series No. 8, 2000), which has an extensive number of references for invertebrates in research.

The controversial discussion about animal welfare and pain recognition in invertebrates is slowly moving and many changes are initiated from the U.K. and other European countries (Berry et al., 2015; Cooke et al., 2019; ; Cooper, 2022; Diggles, 2019; Elwood, 2019). It is hoped that the increased veterinary interest in invertebrate medicine will result in more research and scientific findings leading to appropriate care for invertebrate species in clinical and laboratory settings. Some invertebrates may eventually be included in US animal welfare regulations,

Anesthesia and Analgesia in Laboratory Animals. https://doi.org/10.1016/B978-0-12-822215-7.00022-6

leading to regulatory oversight for living invertebrate species in research. Cephalopod mollusks are protected in the European Union under EU Directive 2010/63/EU and in the United Kingdom, Canada, and Australia. Decapod crustaceans are protected in addition to cephalopod mollusks in Switzerland, Norway, and New Zealand (Smith et al., 2013). Evidence for sentience in some cephalopod mollusks and decapod crustaceans was recently reviewed with implications for animal welfare regulations in mind (Birch et al., 2021). Criteria evaluated included (1) possession of nociceptors, (2) possession of integrative brain regions, (3) connections between nociceptors and integrative brain regions, (4) responses affected by potential local anesthetics or analgesics, (5) motivational trade-offs demonstrating balancing of threat vs. opportunity for reward, (6) flexible self-protective behaviors in response to injury and threat, (7) associative learning beyond habituation and sensitization, and (8) behavior demonstrating the animal values local anesthetics or analgesics when injured. On the basis of these criteria, Birch et al. (2021) concluded that there is very strong evidence of sentience in octopods and strong evidence for true crabs (infraorder Brachyura).

Animal welfare considerations aside, adequate anesthesia can facilitate the successful completion of planned procedures more efficiently, and often with less physical and physiologic disruption than physical restraint alone, leading to more representative research results. The UFAW Handbook on the Care and Management of Laboratory Animals has in its eighth edition a section on cephalopods with references (Hubrecht and Kirkwood, 2010). Several reviews, references, and recommendations have recently been published on behaviors and husbandry of different invertebrate species (Anderson and Wood, 2001; Fiorito et al., 2015; Smith and Berkson, 2005; Wood and Anderson, 2004). This may reflect the interest in animal welfare for invertebrates and may lead to a change in perception about these animals and their needs.

This chapter reviews common anesthetic techniques for invertebrates with a focus on these species that are frequently seen in laboratory facilities, as well as a brief review of acceptable euthanasia methods.

II. Anesthesia

A. General considerations

It is important to note that hypothermia, despite its popularity in the literature, is not an anesthetic and does not provide analgesia or muscle relaxation. Hypothermia itself is considered to be painful and should therefore not be used as an anesthetic, especially during surgical procedures. Mortalities and distress have been reported from hypothermia in squid (Bower et al., 1999). The underestimation of cardiovascular and respiratory system compromise during hypothermia, as well as in the phase of warming, maybe one of the leading causes of adverse outcomes.

There is a lack of research on anesthetic monitoring for invertebrate species. Knowledge of the species' respiratory and cardiovascular systems, where applicable, should inform anesthetic monitoring. For most invertebrate taxa, Ruppert et al. (2004) contain relevant information on life history and physiology that can be helpful in determining anesthetic depth and monitoring invertebrate animals under anesthesia.

1. Aquatic invertebrates

For any aquatic species, the water being used for anesthesia should match the water quality of the animal's tank or environmental water as closely as possible (e.g., temperature, salinity, osmolality, hardness, and pH). Induction, maintenance, and recovery water should be well aerated. Immersion anesthetic agents may be delivered as a static bath treatment for short-term procedures, or via a recirculating system for longer- duration procedures (Fig. 26.1).

Magnesium salts ($MgCl_2 \bullet 6H_2O$ and $MgSO_4 \bullet 7H_2O$) are commonly used as immersion agents for restraint, sedation, anesthesia, and euthanasia of marine invertebrates, and they work well for most taxa, with the exception of crustaceans. The hexahydrate magnesium chloride and heptahydrate magnesium sulfate (Epsom salts) are the forms most commonly available, and typically what is meant when $MgCl_2$ and $MgSO_4$ are referred to in invertebrate anesthesia literature, although often not specified. For the purposes of this chapter, $MgCl_2$ and $MgSO_4$ will refer to $MgCl_2 \bullet 6H_2O$ and $MgSO_4 \bullet 7H_2O$, respectively. Anhydrous and other hydrated forms of these magnesium salts occur and can be procured, however, which would affect the molar

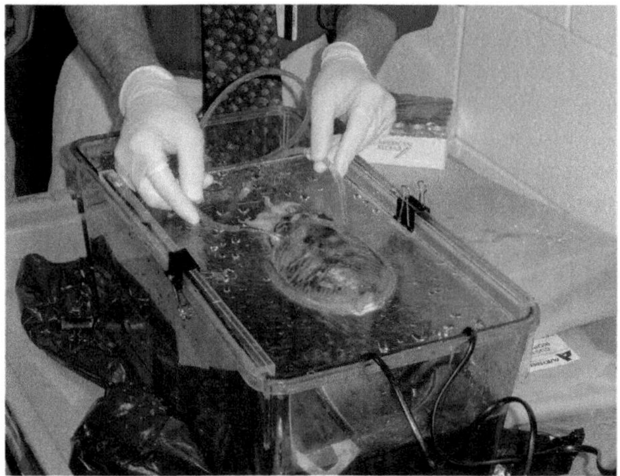

FIGURE 26.1 Cuttlefish (*Sepia officinalis*) on a recirculating anesthetic system for removal of a granuloma. Anesthesia was induced with 3% ethanol and maintained on 1.5% ethanol for the procedure. *Image by C. Harms.*

concentration of the active Mg^{++} ion considerably if dosed identically on a weight-per-volume basis. $MgCl_2{\bullet}6H_2O$ at a 7.5% concentration (75 g/L) in distilled water is nearly isosmotic with seawater. Therefore, 7.5% stock solution can be added in increasing proportions to seawater without altering osmotic pressure, whereas adding $MgCl_2{\bullet}6H_2O$ directly to seawater can increase osmolarity markedly, an important consideration for anesthetizing marine invertebrates for survival procedures.

Differing opinions have been expressed about the ability of $MgCl_2$ to produce adequate sedation and analgesia via blocking nerve transmission and neurotransmitter release or acting only as a neuromuscular blocking agent (Clark et al., 1996). Differences in vertebrate versus invertebrate anatomy/physiology, as well as routes of administration seem to play a role in the effects, but the issue remains unresolved for all taxa (Clark et al., 1996). There is evidence that the magnesium ion acts centrally in suppressing neural activity in cephalopods (Messenger et al., 1985), and cephalopods have further been found to lose both afferent and efferent nerve transmission, indicating true anesthesia (Butler-Struben et al., 2018), but further research is needed to evaluate $MgCl_2$ as an anesthetic across other invertebrate taxa.

Ethanol is another commonly used immersion agent for aquatic invertebrates. Depressive effects on the CNS have been well described, and include inhibition of neuronal sodium and calcium channels in mollusks (Deitrich et al., 1989). Note that the concentrations of ethanol used for anesthesia (up to 10%) are far lower than those used as a tissue preservative (70% and greater), and the latter high concentrations are unsuitable for use for anesthesia or as a single-step euthanasia procedure.

Tricaine methanesulfonate (MS-222), an immersion anesthetic agent for fish, is often assumed to be a logical choice to try on aquatic invertebrates, simply because of their common aquatic environment. In practice, with the exception of some echinoderms, jellyfish (Fig. 26.2), and anemones, MS-222 is generally less effective for aquatic invertebrates (Butler-Struben et al., 2018; Gorges et al., 2022), or requires substantially higher concentrations for effect (Applegate et al., 2016).

Other agents used for aquatic invertebrate anesthesia include eugenol/clove oil, menthol, 2-phenoxyethanol (2-PE), propylene phenoxetol, urethane, benzocaine, ketamine, xylazine, lidocaine, tiletamine-zolazepam, and pentobarbital. See specific taxa below for further details on their use and caveats.

2. *Terrestrial invertebrates*

Terrestrial invertebrates can be anesthetized or immobilized with various gaseous and volatile agents, including isoflurane, sevoflurane, desflurane, chloroform, and CO_2.

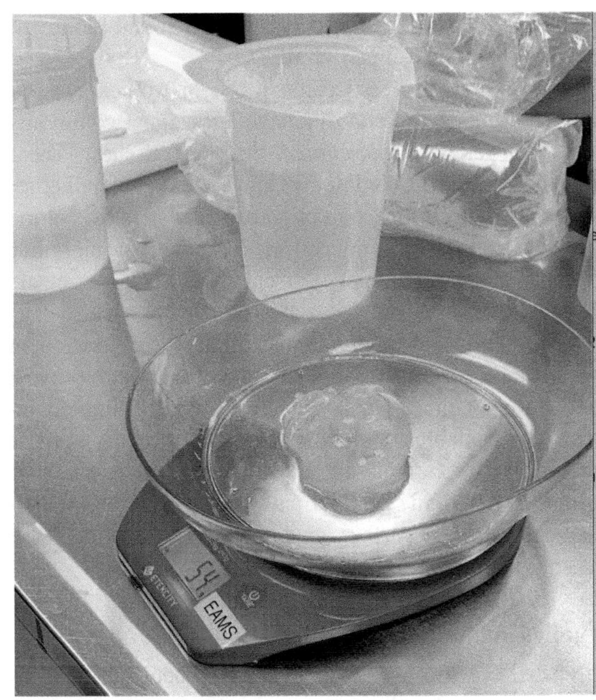

FIGURE 26.2 This moon jelly (*Aurelia aurita*) has been euthanized with an overdose of magnesium chloride (142 g/L for 15 min) and is being weighed prior to fixation in Davidson's fixative. *Image by G. Lewbart.*

These are administered in an exposure chamber, either commercially designed for invertebrates, adapted from small mammal chambers, or custom-made. Anesthetics may be administered via precision vaporizer into the chamber, or by adding liquid anesthetic to a fibrous matrix (e.g., cotton ball, rayon ball, and filter paper) within the chamber, ensuring no direct contact with the invertebrate to be anesthetized. This latter method is simpler, but less controlled, and can result in high anesthetic concentrations with a greater risk of mortality. See the arachnid section below for additional details on anesthetic chambers for terrestrial invertebrates.

B. Considerations for anesthesia by taxa

1. *Cnidaria*

Cnidarians have a radially symmetric body with a single opening surrounded by tentacles and are well known for their cnidocytes or stinging cells. Cnidarians are found in two basic body forms called polyps and medusae, which may occur at different life stages in the same individual. Polyps are tube-shaped and attached to the benthos, while medusae are bell-shaped and free-swimming. There are over 11,000 species of cnidarians, including corals, jellyfish, and anemones. The nervous system of cnidarians is composed of a pair of nerve nets comprised of interconnected neurons. In the medusae form, the nervous system also has nerve rings and ganglia found along the edges of the bell (Ruppert et al., 2004).

Many cnidarians, especially those in tropical waters, may have endosymbiotic dinoflagellates, most commonly from the genus *Symbiodinium* in their tissues. These intracellular algae, commonly known as zooxanthellae, allow cnidarians to thrive in oligotrophic waters by sharing products from photosynthesis in exchange for inorganic nutrients from the animal host cnidarian (Ruppert et al., 2004).

Most reports of cnidarian anesthesia are relaxation or narcotization in preparation for terminal fixation to prevent contraction of the animal. Therefore, there is limited information available about the recovery and impacts of these narcotization solutions on animals. Further research is needed to determine optimal anesthetic protocols for survival procedures in this phylum. Doses for cnidarian anesthesia are reported in Table 26.1.

a. Jellyfishes

Jellyfish have a polyp stage in development but exist as medusae as adults (Ruppert et al., 2004). Jellyfish have been anesthetized using a menthol solution (Fuentes et al., 2011) and MS-222. Moon jellyfish immersed in MS-222 at 0.3 and 0.6 g/L had a reduced response to stimuli and decreased movement, with no mortality observed (Gorges et al., 2022). They have also been relaxed with $MgSO_4$ isoosmotic to seawater (Colley and Trench, 1985), isotonic $MgCl_2$ (Kikinger, 1992), and menthol (Park, 1998); however, these animals were then fixed and dehydrated for histology. Adjustments may need to be made for anesthesia.

To evaluate anesthetic depth a rocking stimulus test, probe stimulus test, bell contraction quality, and body tone have been used (Gorges et al., 2022).

b. Sea anemones

Sea anemones are most commonly found as large solitary polyps and lack a medusa stage (Ruppert et al., 2004). Sea anemones have been anesthetized by immersion in sea water with menthol crystals titrated until the animals were nonresponsive. This method did not appear to impact their regeneration (Bossert et al., 2013). Juvenile and adult anemones have also been relaxed in $MgCl_2$ (71.4 g/L) diluted 1:6 with 1/3-strength artificial seawater for 10−15 min (Amiel and Rottinger, 2021). Another reported anesthetic dose is 7 g of $MgCl_2$ dissolved in 100 mL of 1/3-strength artificial seawater (Stefanik et al., 2013).

Prior to fixation, anemones have been relaxed using immersion in menthol crystals (50 g of crystals in 100 mL of water), $MgCl_2$ (19 or 35−75 g/L), $MgSO_4$ (35−75 g/L), and tricaine methanesulfonate (MS-222, 200−500 mg/L) (England, 1987; Haussermann, 2004; Moore, 1989; Morrall et al., 2000; Sebens and Paine, 1978; Spano and Flores, 2013). The time required for the immersion may depend on the size of the animal. Menthol or a combination of menthol and $MgSO_4$ may be more effective in larger sea anemones (England, 1987). $MgCl_2$ (60 g/L) has also been administered directly into the gastrovascular cavity of anemones immediately before immersion in fixative (Spano and Flores, 2013). Since these animals did not recover, doses may need to be adjusted for anesthesia.

c. Corals

Corals are a diverse group that includes two main types: stony corals (Scleractinia), which create a calcium carbonate exoskeleton, such as staghorn and elkhorn corals, and soft corals (Octocorallia), which lack a stony skeleton, such as sea plumes, sea fans, and sea pens. Corals may be colonial or solitary (Ruppert et al., 2004).

Corals have been anesthetized using menthol crystals and recovered quickly (Agostini et al., 2008). Prior to fixation, corals were relaxed in calcium-free seawater (Chen et al., 2008). This method is not recommended for anesthesia due to potential physiological derangements. Corals have also been relaxed using $MgSO_4$ prior to dissection for electron microscopy (Kawaguti, 1964). To relax soft corals, a $MgSO_4$ solution (110 g/L) was added to the coral in seawater in 5 mL increments every 15−20 min prior to fixation (Janes, 2008).

2. Mollusks

The mollusks are a diverse and large group of animals that occupy terrestrial, freshwater, and marine environments. There are probably about 100,000 described species in this extensive phylum, with high environmental importance and as a source of food, animals for pets, display, and research, and as jewelry, artwork, and the lucrative shell-collecting hobby. Details of molluscan natural history, anatomy, and physiology can be found in a number of references, including Ruppert et al. (2004), Lewbart (2022), and any general invertebrate zoology text. Presented here are three major groups of mollusks (gastropods, cephalopods, and bivalves), with the most economically important classes discussed regarding anesthesia and analgesia. Doses for anesthesia in mollusks are reported in Table 26.2.

a. Gastropods

The gastropods are a large, important, and easily recognized group that includes abalone, snails, slugs, nudibranchs, and sea hares, among others. Most are aquatic and have a well-developed head with eyes and other sensory organs, an external shell, a muscular foot, and gills within a chamber for respiration. Many aquatic gastropods have an operculum that can close and seal the shell aperture, which closure can impede anesthetic induction.

TABLE 26.1 Doses for anesthesia of cnidarians.

Cnidaria					
Order	Agent	Dose	Method of administration	Species	Source
Rhizostomeae (Jellyfish)	Magnesium Chloride ($MgCl_2•6H_2O$)	Iso-osmotic to seawater[a]	Immersion	*Cotylorhiza tuberculata*	Kikinger (1992)
	Magnesium Sulfate ($MgSO_4•7H_2O$)	Iso-osmotic to seawater[a]	Immersion	*Cassiopeia xamachana*	Colley and Trench (1985)
	Menthol	Titrated to nonresponse	Immersion	*Rhizostoma pulmo*	Fuentes et al. (2011)
	MS-222	0.3 and 0.6 g/L	Immersion	*Aurelia aurita*	Gorges et al. (2022)
Limnomedusae (Freshwater Jellyfish)	Menthol	Titrated to nonresponse[a]	Immersion	*Craspedacusta sowerbii*	Park (1998)
Actiniaria (Anemones)	Magnesium Chloride ($MgCl_2•6H_2O$)	60 g/L[a]	Directly administered to gastrovascular cavity	*Anthopleura hermaphroditica, Bunodactis hermafroditica*	Spano and Flores (2013)
		70 g/L	Immersion	*Nematostella vectensis*	Stefanik et al. (2013)
		41 g/L[a]	Immersion	*Aiptasia pallida*	Morrall et al. (2000)
		35 g/L[a]	Immersion	South American sea anemones	Sebens and Paine (1978)
		18.75 g/L[a]	Immersion	British sea anemones	Moore (1989)
		14.3 g/L	Immersion	*Nematostella vectensis*	Amiel and Rottinger (2021)
	Magnesium Sulfate ($MgSO_4•7H_2O$)	35–40 g/L[a]	Immersion	Sea anemones from the tropical Red Sea and Indo-Pacific Ocean	England (1987)
	Menthol	Titrated to nonresponse	Immersion	*Nematostella vectensis*	Bossert et al. (2013)
				Chilean shallow-water sea anemones	Haussermann (2004)
				British sea anemones	Moore (1989)
		500 g/L[a]	Immersion	*Anthopleura hermaphroditica, Bunodactis hermafroditica*	Spano and Flores (2013)
	MS-222	200–500 mg/L[a]	Immersion	British sea anemones	Moore (1989)
Scleractinia (Stony Corals)	Magnesium Sulfate ($MgSO_4•7H_2O$)	Not given	Immersion	*Oulastrea crispata*	Kawaguti (1964)
	Menthol	Titrate to nonresponse	Immersion	*Galaxea fascicularis*	Agostini et al. (2008)
Octocorallia (Soft Corals)	Magnesium Sulfate ($MgSO_4•7H_2O$)	Titrated to nonresponse[a]	Immersion	Octocorals	Janes (2008)

[a]*Not all animals were recovered, dose may need to be adjusted for anesthesia.*

TABLE 26.2 Doses for anesthesia of mollusks.

Mollusca					
Class	**Agent**	**Dose**	**Method of administration**	**Species**	**Source**
Gastropoda	Benzocaine	100 mg/L	Immersion	*Haliotis iris*	Aquilina and Roberts (2000)
				Haliotis laevigata, Haliotis rubra	Edwards et al. (2000)
	Ethanol	3%	Immersion	*Haliotis laevigata, Haliotis rubra*	Edwards et al. (2000)
		5%	Immersion	*Cryptomphalus aspersa*	Flores et al. (1983)
	Isoflurane	MAC 1.09%	Inhalation	*Lymnaea stagnalis*	Girdlestone et al. (1989)
	Listerine® (ethanol 21.9%, menthol 0.042%)	10%	Immersion	*Lymnaea stagnalis*	Woodall et al. (2003)
	Magnesium Chloride ($MgCl_2 \bullet 6H_2O$)	50 g/L	Immersion	*Aplysia californica*	Anderson et al. (2010)
		200 g/L[a]	Intracoelomic injection (30 mL)	*Aplysia californica*	Junge and Ortiz (1978)
		Isotonic	Injection into foot (25% body weight)	*Aplysia californica*	Kanz et al. (1979)
	Magnesium Sulfate ($MgSO_4 \bullet 7H_2O$)	40–220 g/L	Immersion	*Haliotis midae*	White et al. (1996)
	2-Phenoxyethanol	1 mL/L	Immersion	*Haliotis laevigata, Haliotis rubra*	Edwards et al. (2000)
		0.5–3 mL/L	Immersion	*Haliotis midae*	White et al. (1996)
	Sodium Pentobarbital	50 mg/L	Immersion	*Haliotis iris*	Aquilina and Roberts (2000)
		400 mg/L	Immersion	*Biomphalaria* spp.	Martins-Sousa et al. (2001)
	Sodium Pentobarbital and MS-222	80 mg/L and 3 g/L	Immersion	*Lymnaea stagnalis*	Joose and Lever (1958)
				Bulinus spp., *Lymnaea* spp., *Gyraulus* spp., *Anisus* spp.	Mutani (1982)
		120 mg/L and 3 g/L	Immersion	*Biomphalaria* spp., *Helisoma* spp.	Mutani (1982)

Continued

TABLE 26.2 Doses for anesthesia of mollusks.—cont'd

Mollusca					
Class	Agent	Dose	Method of administration	Species	Source
Cephalopoda	Ethanol	1.5%–3%	Immersion	*Sepia officinalis*	Harms et al. (2006)
		2%	Immersion	*Octopus vulgaris*	Andrews and Tansey (1981)
	Magnesium Chloride ($MgCl_2•6H_2O$)	6.8 g/L	Immersion	*Sepia officinalis*	Gore et al. (2005)
		37.5 g/L	Immersion	*Sepia officinalis, Loligo forbesi, Allo-teuthis subulata, Octopus vulgaris, Ele-done cirrhosa*	Messenger et al. (1985)
Bivalvia	Chloral Hydrate	4 g/L	Immersion	*Ostrea edulis*	Heasman et al. (1995)
	Magnesium Chloride ($MgCl_2•6H_2O$)	35 g/L	Immersion	*Ostrea edulis*	Culloty and Mulcahy (1992)
		30–50 g/L	Immersion	*Pecten fumatus*	Heasman et al. (1995)
	Propylene Phenoxetol	1–3 mL/L	Immersion	*Pinctada maxima*	Mills et al. (1997)
		2–3 mL/L	Immersion	*Pinctada albina, Pinctada margaritifera*	Norton et al. (1996)

[a]*Not all animals were recovered, dose may need to be adjusted for anesthesia.*

Gastropods are generally slow-moving and easy to restrain manually or with a protective container. While most gastropods are harmless to humans, members of the tropical genus *Conus* can inflict serious injury or even death with small toxic "harpoons," which are modified teeth from the radula.

Snails can be anesthetized using menthol, 5% ethanol (Flores et al., 1983), or inhalant agents like isoflurane (Girdlestone et al., 1989). Anesthesia in snails is defined when the body and tentacle withdrawal response to gentle stimulation is absent. Tentacle withdrawal reflex remaining under inhalant anesthesia may suggest an insufficient depth for surgery (Girdlestone et al., 1989). A commercial 10% Listerine solution (ethanol 21.9%, menthol 0.042%) in normal *Lymnaea* saline is commonly used to anesthetize snails in research settings (Woodall et al., 2003). Sodium pentobarbital at 400 mg/L in water has been reported with a very slow onset (8 h) but good effects and a low mortality rate (Martins-Sousa et al., 2001). A combination of sodium pentobarbital and MS-222 has been described as a useful method of relaxation and anesthetizing various species of snails (Joosse and Lever, 1958; Mutani, 1982) with an onset time of 60 min and a long-lasting effect.

Anesthesia via isoflurane for terrestrial snails requires an anesthetic chamber with the ability for fresh gas inflow and waste gas scavenging (Girdlestone et al., 1989). The minimum alveolar concentration (MAC) of isoflurane in the pond snail is reported at 1.09% (Girdlestone et al., 1989). Induction is relatively fast (<10 min), but an excitatory period is common. One disadvantage is the need to take the animal out of the chamber for a procedure, which results in fluctuation of anesthetic depth and increased pollution of the work area. Furthermore, the depth of anesthesia may not be adequate for surgical procedures.

Ketamine and propofol do not induce anesthesia and might even have an excitatory effect (Woodall and McCrohan, 2000). Ketamine in combination with xylazine may have toxic effects (Martins-Sousa et al., 2001).

Aplysia spp. sea snails are commonly anesthetized with intracoelomic or intramuscular administration of $MgCl_2$ (Junge and Ortiz, 1978; Kanz et al., 1979). Induction is fast (2–5 min) and smooth, leading to good muscle relaxation.

Immersion in $MgCl_2$ at 50 g/L (0.246 M) resulted in an initial increase in activity followed by progressive sedation (loss of attachment to tanks and righting reflex) and anesthesia (immobile and nonresponsive) over the course of 35 min, with rapid recovery (seconds to 1.5 min) following rinsing in and return to anesthesia-free water (Anderson et al., 2010). Halothane and MS-222 appear to be ineffective (administered as immersion or intracoelomic) anesthetic agents in these species (Clark et al., 1996).

Abalones are commercially farmed and frequently require physical examination and sizing, pearl seeding, and removal from the tanks for maintenance and harvesting (White et al., 1996). Research in abalone involves furthering knowledge of its ecological role, reproduction, and genetics. Removal of abalones is often only possible with mechanical assistance due to their ability to tightly adhere to the substratum. This forced removal may result in injury with slow recovery or even death. Therefore, a muscle-relaxing or anesthetic agent may be necessary to avoid stress and mechanical injuries related to dislodging. Protocols used in abalones for removal and research include ethanol (3%), 2-phenoxyethanol (1 mL/L), benzocaine (100 mg/L), $MgSO_4$ (40−220 g/L), and sodium pentobarbital (1 mL/L) (Aquilina and Roberts, 2000; Edwards et al., 2000; White et al., 1996). $MgSO_4$ is administered in water (4−22 g/100 mL) with dose ranges depending on the size of the abalone (higher doses for larger animals) (White et al., 1996). Induction time is fast (5−8 min), and recovery is uneventful (3−35 min, depending on dose and anesthesia time). Phenoxyethanol is administered at 0.5−3.0 mL/L and also shows a fast induction period (1−3 min) and good recovery time (5−20 min) (White et al., 1996). Nembutal (sodium pentobarbital, 1 mL/L) produces good muscle relaxation with an induction time of 15 min and complete recovery (Aquilina and Roberts, 2000). Clove oil (0.5−1.5 mL/L) and propylene phenoxetol (2.5 mL/L) are not recommended since both agents can cause unacceptable high mortalities (Aquilina and Roberts, 2000; Edwards et al., 2000). MS-222 (1 g/L) and benzocaine (0.1 g/L) are ineffective as muscle relaxants in this species (Aquilina and Roberts, 2000). Both MS-222 and propylene phenoxetol cause significant excitation at induction, resulting in copious mucus production and loss of pigment (Aquilina and Roberts, 2000).

Recovery from any anesthetic includes thorough washing of the abalone and exposure to fresh flowing seawater at its optimal temperature (18°C) until muscle strength returns.

b. Cephalopods

This group of predatory and specialized mollusks includes such familiar forms as the squid, cuttlefish, octopus, and chambered nautilus, which have been extensively studied in various research projects. Cephalopods are exclusively marine and have the ability for fast locomotion. They have closed circulatory systems, high metabolic rates, and advanced nervous systems that include excellent vision and tactile senses. Most have an internal skeleton (shell), with the exceptions being the octopuses (no shell) and the nautilus (external shell).

Cephalopods are generally easily stressed, which often results in "inking." They can be difficult to handle, other than for a quick move or relocation, without sedation. Wearing cloth gloves by the handler prevents cephalopod suckers from gaining purchase on hands and wrists, and allows a somewhat greater degree of control for brief manual restraint. Buckets, plastic nets, or other objects may be used to capture or restrain cephalopods, but it should be considered that these species are "specialized escape artists" (Wood and Anderson, 2004). Artificial turf lining the upper reaches of aquatic containers discourages climbing by octopuses.

The two most commonly used anesthetic agents in these marine invertebrate species are $MgCl_2$ and ethanol. $MgCl_2$ is the preferred anesthetic agent for use in cephalopods. It is used by preparing an isotonic solution of 7.5% (75 g/L) $MgCl_2$ (in distilled water) mixed with an equal volume of seawater (Messenger et al., 1985). Induction time lies between 1.5 and 13 min, with a short period of hyperventilation, then a gradual increase in arm flaccidity and righting reflexes; it is considered to be very smooth (Messenger et al., 1985). Respiration decreases and even ceases if the anesthetic concentration is not reduced. The gills should be intermittently or constantly perfused with anesthetic seawater. Time of recovery from $MgCl_2$ is fairly quick (1−10 min), but dependent on the length and type of procedure (up to 20 min after longer procedures).

Cuttlefish have been successfully anesthetized with 1.5%−3% ethanol (15−30 mL/L) diluted in seawater (Harms et al., 2006). Inductions are rapid (1 min), especially at higher doses, and dilution to a lower concentration (10−15 mL/L) to decrease the risk of overdosing should be considered. During inductions with lower concentrations of ethanol occasional transient excitement has been noticed (Harms et al., 2006). If the procedure cannot be performed in the water, anesthesia is maintained with a recirculating anesthesia system (Lewbart and Harms, 1999). The anesthetic concentration of the water is adjusted over time to the depth of anesthesia desired.

If $MgCl_2$ is used as an anesthetic agent in cuttlefish, a 7.5% (75 g/L) $MgCl_2$ stock solution is prepared with distilled water (Gore et al., 2005). This stock solution is mixed with a known amount of seawater to prepare an anesthetic concentration suitable for induction. A final concentration of 6.8 g/L (100 mL of the stock solution mixed with 1 L of seawater) has been reported to have an induction time of 6−12 min without side effects (Gore et al., 2005). Due to the size of the cuttlefish, a total water volume of 6−8 L is commonly needed. Induction is usually smooth and without a period of excitation. Decreases in concentration via dilution may be necessary over time to adjust the depth of anesthesia.

Octopuses are anesthetized in a similar manner. Two commonly employed anesthetic agents are ethanol and $MgCl_2$. Ethanol (2% v/v in seawater) can produce excitement during the short induction time [increased respiratory rate, attempts to climb out of the solution, and ink ejection (Andrews and Tansey, 1981)]. Induction time has been reported to be 4 min and time to full recovery as 2.5 min (Andrews and Tansey, 1981). Ethanol (2%) is not effective in cold-water species (below 15°C) (Gleadall, 2013).

The use of urethane has been reported (Andrews and Tansey, 1981; Messenger et al., 1985; Gleadall, 1991) and was routinely used in the 1970s and 80s, but despite its good anesthetic effects, the traumatic effects on the animals from an excitement phase during induction could be severe, and there are human exposure concerns. Chloroform, chloral hydrate, and CO_2 are unsuitable anesthetic agents in cephalopods as they can cause high mortality (Garcia-Franco, 1992; Gleadall, 1991).

For recovery or resuscitation, the cephalopod is placed into a container with anesthesia-free seawater. Ideally, the water in this container is circulated and aerated. Anesthesia-free water should be directed over the gills for a washout effect. If spontaneous respiration is not present, gentle and slow mantle massage of the whole mantle/body can be used to provide a combination of circulatory and respiratory support until normal respiration is restored. The tentacles remain extended and flaccid in the first phase of recovery and will retract in response to light pinching with progressive awakening (Harms et al., 2006).

Cephalopods are commonly monitored with visualization of respiratory rate and pattern. Normal awake values for *Octopus vulgaris* in a weight range from 100 to 800 g are 26–30 breaths/min (Andrews and Tansey, 1981). The cardiovascular system is assessed by placing a Doppler probe on the dorsal area (above the aorta) or behind the gills (above either branchial heart) to monitor heart rate and blood flow. In transparent species (esp. with $MgCl_2$), the pallial organs can be observed. The depth of anesthesia is difficult to assess in cephalopods. One guideline is that the level of anesthesia seems adequate when no response to tactile and surgical stimuli is present (withdrawal of appendices or movement, contraction of the skin around the eye in response to pressure on the eyeball, withdrawal of the animal in response to a pinch of the skin over the eye (Andrews and Tansey, 1981)). Further indicators of anesthetic depth are the flaccidity of the arms, the loss of normal posture, and the inability to regain normal posture after disturbance (Andrews and Tansey, 1981). Respiration usually remains spontaneous; a depression or cessation is a sign of a critically deep level of anesthesia.

c. Bivalves

This large and economically important group of highly adapted aquatic mollusks includes clams, mussels, oysters, and scallops. They lack a well-developed head, are generally nonvisual (the scallops are an exception), feed by filtration utilizing the gills for food transport, and utilize a muscular and sometimes large foot for locomotion. Research on these species primarily focuses on fishery and ecology projects.

Most bivalves are easy to handle and restrain safely. Nearly all will tightly close their calcareous valves when handled or disturbed and may require sedation or physical manipulation (prying) to open the valves, which are held fast by strong adductor muscles. This behavioral response can greatly impede anesthetic induction, particularly if the anesthetic is irritating to any degree.

Propylene phenoxetol is used as a 1% solution to anesthetize oysters in a dose range from 1 to 3 mL/L. Higher doses induce a rapid and relatively deep level of anesthesia (Mills et al., 1997) and may need diluting throughout the procedure to decrease the recovery time (Norton et al., 1996). Generally, concentrations of 1–2 mL/L are safe and effective. The oyster should be placed hinge-down in the solution, leaning against the walls of the aerated container to facilitate monitoring. Induction time is reported to be between 6 and 15 min. Adequate anesthesia is reached when the oyster gapes wide enough to part the gill curtain and shows no responsiveness to handling (Mills et al., 1997) or contraction of the tissue to a stimulus (Norton et al., 1996). A decrease in stress from handling before placing oysters into the anesthesia container will improve the anesthetic effects and opening. Recovery time is short (less than 30 min), although it depends on the length of the procedure, the concentration of anesthetic, and temperature (Norton et al., 1996).

$MgCl_2$ seems to have variable effects on oysters. Some workers describe the little effect of $MgCl_2$ in pearl oysters (Mills et al., 1997; Norton et al., 1996), mainly due to long induction times (1–2 h). Culloty and Mulcahy (1992) reported good anesthetic effects, but also long induction and recovery times (90 min) at 3.5%. The effect of $MgCl_2$ seems dependent on species and concentration. MS-222 and chloral hydrate are not effective in oysters (slow induction and recovery) and are associated with complications (death; some of it may be related to the low pH of unbuffered MS-222) (Norton et al., 1996).

Anesthesia in scallops may be required for muscle relaxation and opening of the valves. In general, the depth of anesthesia/relaxation is adequate when handling and stimulating the mantle tissue fails to produce shell closure. Recovery is often defined as the regained ability for shell closure in response to handling (Heasman et al., 1995).

$MgCl_2$ is the drug of choice in scallops due to its rapid and consistent induction and recovery. The agent is pre-dissolved in seawater and then added to the aerated induction container to reach a concentration of 30–50 g/L. Induction times at these concentrations are quick and in the range of 2–6 min. Recovery time in scallops anesthetized with $MgCl_2$ seems to be consistently short (10 min) regardless of concentration used or temperature (Heasman et al., 1995).

Chloral hydrate seems to have variable effects in scallops, with significant changes in induction and recovery at different concentrations and temperatures (Heasman et al., 1995). A concentration of 4 g/L produces anesthesia in about 10–25 min if the temperature is held at 24°C. Lower temperatures significantly slow the induction period. Higher concentrations shorten the induction time but can result in high mortality. Recovery time at 4 g/L is between 20 and 30 min but varies widely depending on temperature (and concentration). Aerated seawater recovery tanks and continuous flushing with seawater facilitate recovery.

Other drugs have been examined for scallop anesthesia with little success. MS-222 causes hyperactivity and hyperextension, benzocaine causes initial hyperactivity, metomidate results in shell closure, ethanol does not seem to have any effect, and $MgSO_4$ leads to high mortality (Heasman et al., 1995).

Giant clams (*Tridacna* sp.) have been anesthetized with propylene phenoxetol (Mills et al., 1997).

3. Annelids

The annelids are a large and diverse group of segmented worm-like animals that are divided into three main classes: the polychaetes, oligochaetes, and hirudineans. All are characterized by regular segmentation of the coelomic cavity as well as the circulatory, excretory, and nervous systems. This segmentation probably evolved as a means of burrowing via peristaltic contractions (Ruppert et al., 2004). A cuticle covers the animal, and segmented setae occur in nearly all annelids. A more or less straight gut tube lies between the anterior mouth and posterior anus (Ruppert et al., 2004). Doses for anesthesia of annelids are reported in Table 26.3.

a. Polychaetes

Like many marine invertebrates, polychaetes can be sedated with $MgCl_2$ in the water. While it is possible, if not likely, that some species are more sensitive than others, a concentration of between 7.5% and 8.0% seems to work well for relaxation (Lewbart and Riser, 1996; Müller et al., 2003). A 2016 study determined that a product called Dentol (Khoraman laboratory, Iran), which contains 10% carvacrol, was very safe and effective for the relaxation of nereid polychaetes prior to the study. Worms were placed

TABLE 26.3 Doses for anesthesia of annelids.

Annelida					
Class	**Agent**	**Dose**	**Method of administration**	**Species**	**Source**
Polychaeta	Dentol	8%[a]	Immersion	Nereididae worms from Persian Gulf	Bonyadi-Naeini et al. (2016)
	Magnesium Chloride ($MgCl_2 \bullet 6H_2O$)	75 g/L	Immersion	*Parapionosyllis manca*	Lewbart and Riser (1996)
		80 g/L[a]	Immersion	*Eurythoe complanata*	Müller et al. (2003)
Oligochaeta	Alcohol (presumably Ethanol)	5%	Immersion	*Lumbricus terrestris*	Cooper et al. (1986)
	Ethanol	5%	Immersion	*Lumbricus terrestris, Eisenia foetida*	Cooper (1968); Marks and Cooper (1977)
		5%	Immersion	*Lumbricus terrestris*	Salgado et al. (2014)
Hirudinea	Benzocaine	400 mg/L	Immersion	*Hirudo medicinalis*	Cooper et al. (1986)
	Mephenesin	Saturated	Immersion	*Hirudo medicinalis, Glossiphonia complanata*	Tettamanti et al. (2003)
	Soda Water (50%)	500 mL/L	Immersion	*Hirudo medicinalis*	Cooper et al. (1986)

[a]*Not all animals were recovered, dose may need to be adjusted for anesthesia.*

in an 8% Dentol solution in seawater and relaxed in less than 1 min. Carvacrol is an aromatic oil found in many different plants (Bonyadi-Naeini et al., 2016). Unfortunately, Dentol may be hard to find outside of Iran.

b. Oligochaetes

Cooper and Roch (1986) anesthetized *Lumbricus terrestris* with a 5% alcohol (presumably ethanol) solution for a period of 1 h prior to tissue grafting experiments. In some earlier experiments, Cooper (1968) used 5% ethanol in Rushton's Ringers solution until the worms (*L. terrestris and E. foetida*) were immobilized. Marks and Cooper (1977) used 5% ethanol at a temperature of 23°C for *L. terrestris* and *E. foetida*, and Salgado et al. (2014) reported success using 5% ethanol for anesthetizing *L. terrestris*.

c. Hirudineans

The literature on leech anesthesia is minimal. One study found that immersion of *Hirudinaria medicinalis* in 400 mg/L benzocaine adequately immobilized the animals with a recovery time of approximately 3 h (Cooper et al., 1986). The same study found that 50% soda water, at a concentration of 500 mL/L, was effective following a 2 min excitatory period. This protocol resulted in a variable recovery period of up to 4.5 h. An article describes the use of saturated mephenesin (3-(*o*-toloxy)-1,2-propanediol) to anesthetize leeches for grafting research (Tettamanti et al., 2003).

4. *Arachnida*

Doses for anesthesia of arachnids are reported in Table 26.4.

a. Spiders and scorpions

Physical restraint is commonly used to handle and transport spiders, but it is advisable to wear latex or nitrile gloves because some tarantula species are capable of shedding urticating hairs that can be quite irritating, especially to individuals allergic to these structures. Direct handling of scorpions on the other hand should be kept to a minimum for both the safety of the handler and the animal. Clear plastic containers and in some cases, utensils like long forceps can be employed for moving an animal from one place to another (Frye, 2022). The primary drawbacks to manual restraint of spiders or scorpions are stress and injury to the animal and the potential envenomation of the handler. Caution should be taken not to drop the spider or have it leap or fall to the ground.

Spiders and scorpions are most commonly and successfully anesthetized with inhalant anesthetic agents. All agents (isoflurane, sevoflurane, and desflurane) can be used, depending on cost and availability, although most commonly isoflurane and sevoflurane are used for spiders and scorpions (Cooper, 2001; Melidone and Mayer, 2005; Pizzi and Kennedy, 2022; Sheldon et al., 2019; Zachariah et al., 2009, 2014).

Several different induction chambers have been described (Cooper, 2001; Melidone and Mayer, 2005; Pizzi and Kennedy, 2022) and used successfully for delivering inhalant anesthesia primarily to spiders but also scorpions. These chambers are ideally commercially available invertebrate-specific induction chambers with appropriate fresh gas inflow and scavenging outflow, regular small mammal induction chambers, or simple self-made clear plastic containers.

TABLE 26.4 Doses for anesthesia of arachnids.

Arachnida					
Group	Agent	Dose	Method of administration	Species	Source
Spiders and Scorpions	CO_2	98%	Inhalant	*Nephila edulis*	Madsen and Vollrath (2000)
	Isoflurane	5%	Inhalant	*Heterometrus longimanus, Pandinus dictator*	Sheldon et al. (2019)
				Theraphosa blondi, Grammostola rosea	Zachariah et al. (2009)
	Sevoflurane	5%	Inhalant	*Grammostola rosea*	Zachariah et al. (2014)
Horseshoe Crabs	MS-222	1 g/L	Immersion	*Limulus polyphemus*	Archibald et al. (2019)
	2-Phenoxyethanol	2 mL/L	Immersion		

If plastic containers without the use of an inflow and outflow system are used, a cotton wool swab soaked with a small amount of inhalant agent is placed into the box. The animal itself should be placed in a separate smaller container with small pores. The smaller container holding the spider or scorpion is placed into the larger box allowing the inhalant to diffuse into the box with the animal while ensuring that no direct contact with the inhalant-soaked cotton swab will occur. This method is not ideal because of the higher exposure risk to the personnel of the anesthetic agent, less control of the amount of anesthetic given to the animal, and higher risk of overdose (e.g., up to 32% isoflurane in the air).

An induction chamber using anesthetic gas given via a precision vaporizer is much preferred. The animal is placed into the chamber and the chamber is filled with the anesthetic gas (about 3%–5% for isoflurane and 4%–6% for sevoflurane). To increase the filling time in larger chambers the oxygen flow rate is high at the beginning (1–3 L/min), but can be decreased to a minimum if there are no major leaks in the system (300–1000 mL/min). Oxygen flow lower than 200 mL/min decreases the accuracy of the vaporizer and may decrease the amount of anesthetic agent in the chamber due to the uptake of the animal; the amount of carbon dioxide built up in the chamber may also be increased using low fresh gas flows. An appropriate scavenging system is necessary to decrease pollution and exposure of the staff to anesthetic gases. With increasing depth of anesthesia, the vaporizer can be adjusted (decreased over time). The MAC of the different anesthetic agents in spiders or scorpions has not been determined.

The advantages of the chamber technique are the convenience of use, low cost, and safety to the patient associated with the setup. The disadvantage associated with this type of system is that the animal can only be temporarily sedated or anesthetized. For any physical examination or surgery, the animal is removed from the chamber, which limits the time for any procedure before the animal recovers. This may require repeated inductions, but it also increases the exposure of the clinician and staff to the anesthetic gases. A surgery chamber has been developed (Melidone and Mayer, 2005) that allows the clinician to perform the surgery or other manipulations on the animal without taking the animal out of the chamber.

Another interesting technique is to induce the spider in an anesthetic chamber and then place its abdomen (with the associated book lungs/tracheae) into a smaller chamber "sealed" with a latex glove. This technique appears to have some merit when a procedure must be performed on the cephalothorax or limbs (Dombrowski, 2006a; Cooper, 2022).

Other agents like carbon dioxide and nitrogen, as well as hypothermia, have been used to immobilize spiders (Madsen and Vollrath, 2000; Pizzi and Kennedy, 2022). No reports about the amount of nitrogen used or the quality of nitrogen anesthesia could be found. Carbon dioxide is administered as a gas in a chamber, often producing 98% saturation. Dilution with air or oxygen is hard to achieve, resulting in an increased risk for mortalities (Pizzi and Kennedy, 2022). Side effects of CO_2 anesthesia are well recognized in vertebrates (e.g., respiratory acidosis, and behavioral signs of distress) and should be considered when used in invertebrate species.

Observing the spider or scorpion for righting reflexes and leg movements assists in monitoring the depth of anesthesia. During induction, it may take 10–15 min, with several attempts of the animal to move and reposition itself until full immobilization has occurred. During the procedure, leg movements in response to stimuli are an obvious sign of the insufficient depth of anesthesia. An increase in heart rate and respiratory rate may be seen, but it is often unrecognized. A deep level of anesthesia is more difficult to evaluate, and slow respiratory rates and low heart rates are often the only ways to assess a patient for excessive depth of anesthesia. An analgesic administered for painful stimulations may make it easier for the clinician to maintain a consistent level of anesthesia.

Respiratory rate is observed at the cranial lateral side of the animal. The heart rate can often only be monitored in larger spiders or scorpions. The spider's heart lies under the dorsal surface of the body. With a Doppler (pinpoint–crystal head) placed over the heart area, a rate can be obtained. Normal heart rates are considered to be 30–70 beats/min in large spiders and up to 200 beats per minute in smaller species.

After turning off the inhalant and maintaining the animal on fresh oxygen flow or room air, the recovery from anesthesia is gradual and can take between 3 and 20 min depending on ambient room temperature and the depth of anesthesia during the procedure. Slow leg movements and righting attempts occur and increase over time. When fully awake, the animal should be returned to its enclosure and maintained at its preferred ambient temperature. Feeding after anesthesia should be withheld for 48 h (Pizzi and Kennedy, 2022).

b. Horseshoe crabs

The American horseshoe crab (*Limulus polyphemus*) is the most common one of four different species and is frequently used as a laboratory animal model to study its eye, and nervous system and to represent marine invertebrate embryology (Smith and Berkson, 2005; Smith, 2022). Most extensive might be the research on the blue blood of the horseshoe crab as the pharmaceutical compound limulus amebocyte lysate (LAL).

Horseshoe crabs can easily be handled and restrained, although strong locomotion and righting reflexes can make examinations difficult (Smith and Berkson, 2005).

The holder is cautioned not to pinch their fingers between the lateral edge of the opisthosoma and the genal angle of the prosoma (Smith, 2022).

The tubular heart of the horseshoe crab is located dorsally over the entire length of the body (Spotswood and Smith, 2007). The blood/hemolymph collection site has been extensively reported (Smith and Berkson, 2005; Smith, 2022) and is easy to perform. Trends in hemolymph pH and blood gases may be measured for monitoring anesthesia (Archibald et al., 2019). ECG patches placed on the cephalothorax detect a heart rate, and normal awake heart rates in horseshoe crabs are reportedly 30 beats per minute depending on temperature (23°C) (Redmond et al., 1982). Ultrasonography may also be used to measure heart rate, as well as cardiac contractility and respiratory rate through the carapace without having to invert the animal to view the book gill excursions (Archibald et al., 2019). Resting heart rate, cardiac fractional shortening, and respiratory rate in that study at 22.8–28°C were ~22–50/min, ~32–50%, and ~35–53/min, respectively (Archibald et al., 2019). Immersion in MS-222 at 1 g/L buffered with sodium carbonate, and 2-phenoxyethanol at 2 mL/L, provided effective anesthesia with clinically useful induction and recovery times (Archibald et al., 2019). Effective buffering of MS-222 at that high concentration required the use of sodium carbonate rather than sodium bicarbonate in order to avoid simultaneously markedly increasing the salinity of the anesthesia water. Both anesthetics reduced cardiac contractility and respiratory rate, with minimal effect on heart rate. 2-phenoxyethanol subjectively provided smoother and more reliable anesthesia than MS-222.

5. Crustaceans

The crustaceans are a large and diverse group of arthropods that are all aquatic at some stage of their life histories. The majority of the most conspicuous and economically important crustaceans belong to the order Decapoda, which includes crabs, crayfish, hermit crabs, lobsters, and shrimp. Research in this order involves genetics, morphology, reproduction, ecology, behavior, and fisheries.

Some species can be manually restrained with gloved hands or, in some cases, with the help of utensils such as nets or tongs. Since some crustaceans, like lobsters and large crabs, can cause serious injury to handlers, care should be taken when manipulating or restraining these animals.

Crustaceans can be anesthetized with various agents. Doses for the anesthesia of crustaceans are reported in Table 26.5. Depending on the animal's size and procedure, immersion in isobutyl alcohol or clove oil, and injections of lidocaine, ketamine, xylazine, tiletamine-zolazepam, and alfaxalone have been reported (Brown et al., 1996; Ferraro and Pressacco, 1996; Foley et al., 1966; Gardner 1997; Minter et al., 2013; Oswald, 1977; Quesada et al., 2011). An intravascular injection can be performed in adult giant crabs through the coxal arthrodial membrane of a cheliped (Oswald, 1977; Gardner, 1997) using a small needle (25 gauge). Anesthetic immersions commonly used in other aquatic invertebrate taxa, such as MS-222, 2-phenoxyethanol, and magnesium salts ($MgCl_2$ and $MgSO_4$), are generally accepted as not effective to produce anesthesia in decapod crustaceans (Coyle et al., 2005; Foley et al., 1966; Fregin and Bickmeyer, 2016; Gardner, 1997; Oswald, 1977). Immersion in isobutyl alcohol (1.5–7.0 mL/L) results in sedation at low doses and anesthesia at high doses. The induction time and duration of effect are dose-dependent (Foley et al., 1966).

Lidocaine (0.4–1 mg/g) can be injected intramuscularly into the tail and lasts for about 5–30 min in crayfish, depending on the dose administered, with an average induction time of 1.5 min (Brown et al., 1996). Lidocaine (0.2 mg/g) injected intravascularly lasted approximately 3 min in blue crabs (*Callinectes sapidus*) (Quesada et al., 2011).

Ketamine has been used in crayfish (40–90 mg/kg [mcg/g]) (Brown et al., 1996), Australian giant crab (*Pseudocarcinus gigas*) (0.025–0.1 mg/kg IV) (Gardner, 1997), and blue crabs (*C. sapidus*) (Quesada et al., 2011) with variable responses. Ketamine given intramuscularly to crayfish provides consistent anesthesia (induction time: 1 min) for over 10 min (40 mcg/g) to almost 2 h (>90 mcg/g) without excitatory side effects during induction or recovery (Brown et al., 1996). When ketamine alone was given to the giant crab *(P. gigas)* intravascularly, a short period of excitement occurred, but induction time was fast (15–45 s). The duration of anesthesia was dose-dependent and lasted between 8 and 40 min (Gardner, 1997). Intravascular injections of ketamine (20 mg/kg) in blue crabs (*C. sapidus*) resulted in a smooth and fast induction (<60 s), but the duration of anesthesia was only between 3 and 12 min. The majority of crabs were categorized as having light anesthesia. Intracardiac injections of ketamine (20 mg/kg) resulted in death in four out of five crabs (Quesada et al., 2011).

Xylazine has shown good anesthetic effects in adult giant crabs when used at doses between 16 and 22 mg/kg IV (Gardner, 1997) or in common shore crabs (*Carcinus maenas*) at 70 mg/kg IV (Oswald, 1977). Induction seems to be smooth and fairly fast (3–5 min), and immobilization lasts 25–45 min (depending on the dose administered). Side effects like bradycardia, extrasystoles, and dysrhythmias have been reported with high doses (70 mg/kg) (Oswald, 1977). A similar fast induction (30–60 s) was seen in blue crabs administered xylazine (20 mg/kg) IV, with a duration lasting 5–30 min (Quesada et al., 2011). Higher doses of xylazine (70 mg/kg) resulted in death in blood-spotted crabs *(Portunus sanguinolentus)*

TABLE 26.5 Doses for the anesthesia of crustaceans.

Crustacea					
Order	Agent	Dose	Method of administration	Species	Source
Decapoda	Alfaxalone	15 mg/kg[a], 100 mg/kg	Intravascular injection	*Callinectes sapidus*	Minter et al. (2013)
	AQUI-S	100 mg/L	Immersion	*Macrobrachium rosenbergii*	Coyle et al. (2005)
		40–200 mg/L[a]	Immersion	*Jasus edwardsii*	Roberston et al. (2018)
	Clove Oil	>0.125 mL/L (induction)	Immersion	*Pseudocarcinus gigas*	Gardner (1997)
	Eugenol	>0.2 mL/L	Immersion	*Macrobrachium rosenbergii*	Saydmohammed and Pal (2009)
	Isobutyl Alcohol	1.5–7.0 mL/L[a]	Immersion	*Homarus americanus*	Foley et al. (1966)
	Ketamine	40–90 mg/kg	Intramuscular injection	*Orconectes virilis*	Brown et al. (1996)
		0.025–0.1 mg/kg	Intravascular injection	*Pseudocarcinus gigas*	Gardner (1997)
		20 mg/kg	Intravascular injection	*Callinectes sapidus*	Quesada et al. (2011)
	Ketamine-Xylazine	20 mg/kg each	Intravascular injection	*Callinectes sapidus*	Quesada et al. (2011)
	Lidocaine	0.4–1 mg/g	Intramuscular injection	*Orconectes virilis*	Brown et al. (1996)
		0.2 mg/g	Intravascular injection	*Callinectes sapidus*	Quesada et al. (2011)
	Procaine	25 mg/kg	Intravascular injection	*Carcinus maenas*	Oswald (1977)
	Tiletamine-Zolazepam	30 mg/kg	Injection	*Callinectes sapidus*	Quesada et al. (2011)
	Xylazine	16–22 mg/kg	Intravascular injection	*Pseudocarcinus gigas*	Gardner (1997)
		20 mg/kg	Intravascular injection	*Callinectes sapidus*	Quesada et al. (2011)
		70 mg/kg	Intravascular injection	*Carcinus maenas*	Oswald (1977)

[a]*Sedation at lower doses, anesthesia at higher doses.*

(Premarathna et al., 2016). Care should be taken when using doses of xylazine at the high end of the reported range.

Ketamine combined with xylazine (20 mg/kg each) IV resulted in a quick induction (30–40 s) and lasted 5–10 min in blue crabs (*C. sapidus*). Tiletamine-zolazepam (30 mg/kg) IV also had a quick induction (20–60 s) and lasted 5–7 min (Quesada et al., 2011). Intravascular injections of alfaxalone provide sedation (15 mg/kg) and anesthesia (100 mg/kg). Induction is rapid (<1 min) but prolonged recoveries have been observed with higher doses (Minter et al., 2013). Intravascular injections of etomidate (16 mg/kg) were ineffective, and propofol (20 mg/kg) is not recommended for use as it resulted in limb autotomies in blue crabs (*C. sapidus*). Pentobarbital (20 mg/kg) IV produced inadequate sedation in five out of six blue crabs, and light sedation in the remaining crab (Quesada et al., 2011).

Procaine (25 mg/kg IV) has also been used in crabs and provides good anesthesia with a very short induction time (20–30 s). This included a 10-second-long excitatory phenomenon that led to tonic contraction before paralysis. Duration was very long (2–3 h) with slow recoveries (Oswald, 1977), and it may be reserved for long-term experimental anesthesia.

For smaller crabs, in which an IV or IM injection is impractical, clove oil can be used as a bath treatment and has shown a 16 min onset of anesthesia at a dose of >0.125 mL/L and a long recovery phase (2.5 h). Once the animal is anesthetized, a reduction of concentration is necessary because clove oil at 0.125 mL/L over a longer period of time is also used for the euthanasia of these animals (Gardner, 1997). Freshwater prawns (*Macrobrachium rosenbergii*) were anesthetized with immersion in eugenol and experienced a lower oxygen consumption rate at doses higher than 0.2 mL/L. Induction and recovery times were similar with immersion in eugenol alone and a mixture of eugenol and menthol (Saydmohammed and Pal, 2009). Immersion in AQUI-S (100 mg/L) has been reported for anesthesia of the freshwater prawn (*M. rosenbergii*) (Coyle et al., 2005). Southern rock lobsters (*Jasus edwardsii*) immersed in AQUI-S (40–200 mg/L) exhibited sedation at the lower end of the dose range and anesthesia at the higher end of the dose range (Robertson et al., 2018).

Crustacean heart rates can be assessed by applying ECG pads with ample gel on the shell above the heart, or by Doppler flow probe (Fig. 26.3). The normal heart rate for lobsters is between 5 and 20 beats per minute with a circadian influence (higher at night) (Aguzzi et al., 2004) and 30–70 beats per minute for the shore crab (Styrishave et al., 2003), depending on pH and temperature. Anesthetic depth is evaluated in crustaceans by the relaxation of the body and the ability to withdraw extremities, and the very slow withdrawal of their antennae (Fig. 26.4).

More research is needed to determine effective analgesic agents in crustaceans. Morphine has been shown to decrease the response of crabs (100 mg/kg) and shrimp (91 mg/kg) to noxious stimuli, and this effect is reversible with naloxone administration (Lozada et al., 1988; Maldonado and Miralto, 1982; Tomsic and Maldonado, 1990). However, this decreased response appears to be due to sedation rather than analgesia (Barr and Elwood, 2011). Ketorolac administered intracardiac was fatal to blue crabs (*C. sapidus*); consistent concentrations were observed when administered to crabs intramuscularly (0.25–0.75 mg/kg); however, more data is needed on the safety of this drug (Souza et al., 2020).

6. Insects

The insects are an incredibly diverse and numerous group with nearly a million described species that some taxonomists term the Hexapoda. Insects are arthropods with three major body segments (head, thorax, and abdomen) and three pairs of legs. Most have keen eyesight, well-developed mouthparts, sensory antennae, and wings. They have an open circulatory system that contains hemolymph and gases are exchanged through spiracles that open into a system of tracheae. Insects have been used for years in a variety of research. *Drosophila* may be its most known representative for genetic research studies, but other species are important contributors of information on pathogen-vector interaction in various diseases, metamorphosis and anatomy/physiology (facet eye, senses),

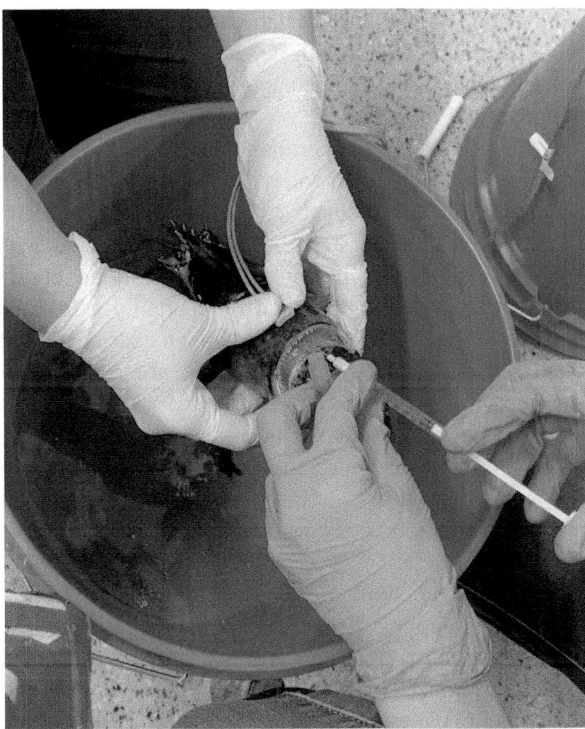

FIGURE 26.3 This American lobster (*Homarus americanus*) has been anesthetized with eugenol immersion and is being euthanized with injectable intracardiac potassium chloride. A Doppler is being used to monitor heart rate. Within seconds of the potassium chloride administration the heart stopped beating. *Image by G. Lewbart.*

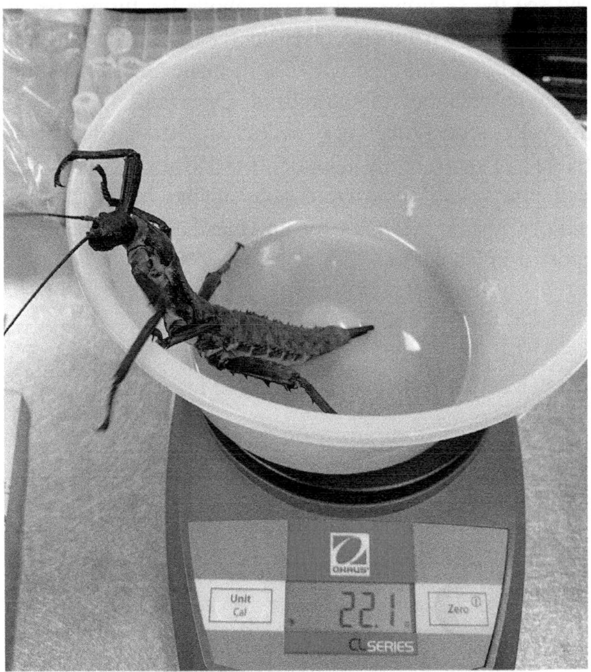

FIGURE 26.4 This fully awake Australian thorny devil stick bug (*Eurycantha calcarata*) is being weighed prior to a study. Insects and other terrestrial invertebrates can frequently be examined and weighed without the need for anesthesia. In cases where anesthesia is required a number of inhalant agents have been successfully used. *Image by G. Lewbart.*

ecology, and agriculture, pharmaceutical control, etc. Several recent works investigate the effects of isoflurane (Troup et al., 2019), sevoflurane (Chen et al., 2019), and isoflurane and sevoflurane on *Drosophila* (MacMillan et al., 2017). This latter paper found that both gas inhalants were superior to cold and carbon dioxide with regards to side effects such as reproductive compromise and mortality of juvenile flies. Not a single side effect was noted with sevoflurane anesthesia in fruit flies (MacMillan et al., 2017). Chen et al. (2019) found no mortality associated with sevoflurane, but the gas did lead to an exacerbation of the eye phenotype in the offspring of anesthetized flies.

In most cases, depending on size and species, insects can be handled and restrained manually without risk to the animal or handler. In some cases, gloves are recommended as a protective measure, and various utensils can be employed to immobilize or restrain insects (Cooper et al., 2022).

Carbon dioxide remains a popular agent to immobilize insects in entomological research, although multiple side effects, including convulsions and excitation at induction, are well recognized and mortality is high (Nicolas and Sillans, 1989; Valles and Koehler, 1994; MacMillan et al., 2017). Its use remains controversial, and a more progressive approach would be the use of a volatile anesthetic agent like isoflurane or sevoflurane. This requires a chamber apparatus to allow for appropriate delivery and scavenging of the inhalant agent (Walcourt and Ide, 1998) (and see the section on arachnids above for further details on anesthetic chambers). Transient exposure to airborne chloroform or desflurane in custom-made small glass tube induction chambers immobilized *Drosophila* larvae for survival confocal imaging (Cevik et al., 2019). Chloroform resulted in more rapid induction but slower recovery than desflurane, with less depression of the heart rate and auditory response. Doses for the anesthesia of insects are reported in Table 26.6.

Hypothermia also has been reported for immobilization of insects, but its use is discouraged for surgical or otherwise stressful/painful procedures (Cooper et al., 2022; MacMillan et al., 2017).

7. Nematodes

Nematodes are one of the largest groups of invertebrates, with around 500,000 known species (Bodri, 2022). Numerous species have been extensively used in research for plant-parasite effects, diseases, and genetics.

Caenorhabditis elegans is probably the most researched nematode, as it is commonly used as an animal model due to its size, small and consistent number of somatic cells, and easily accessible nervous system. Research on *C. elegans* has led to scientific information about meiosis, nicotine dependence, volatile anesthetics, and genetics. Due to its popularity, most anesthetic agents reported for nematodes are based on their use in *C. elegans*, and their anesthetic effects on the animal are well described (Bodri, 2022). *C. elegans* has been anesthetized with CO_2 (Bodri, 2022), 4.5% ethanol (Morgan and Sedensky, 1995), propylene phenoxetol (Nelson and Riddle, 1984), and several inhalants, including chloroform, flurothyl, fluorxene, halothane, and isoflurane (Crowder et al., 1996; Morgan and Cascorbi, 1985; Morgan et al., 1990). Much higher concentrations of inhalant anesthetics are required for *C. elegans* compared to vertebrates, as reviewed by Zalucki and van Swinderen (2016). Crowder et al. (1996) recommend 6.5% isoflurane. The effective dose $(ED)_{50}$ (the concentration where half of the animals tested were immobile for longer than 10 s) values for the nine different inhalant agents were established in Morgan's studies, and the anesthetic chamber for these species is described (Morgan and Cascorbi, 1985; Bodri, 2022). This included isoflurane with a concentration range of 5.6%−7.18%, consistent with the findings of Crowder et al. (1996). Doses for the anesthesia of nematodes are reported in Table 26.7.

TABLE 26.6 Doses for anesthesia of insects.

Insecta					
Order	**Agent**	**Dose**	**Method of administration**	**Species**	**Source**
Diptera	Chloroform	30s × 2	Inhalant	*Drosophila melanogaster*	Cevik et al. (2019)
	Desflurane	10 m × 2			Cevik et al. (2019)
	Isoflurane	$ED_{50} = 0.3\%$[a]			Troup et al. (2019)
		4.6%			MacMillan et al. (2017)
	Sevoflurane	2.1%, 3%			Chen et al. (2019)
		6.7%			MacMillan et al. (2017)

[a]*The effective dose $(ED)_{50}$ is the concentration where half of the animals tested were immobile for longer than 10 s.*

TABLE 26.7 Doses for anesthesia of nematodes.

Nematoda					
Order	Agent	Dose	Method of administration	Species	Source
Rhabditida	Chloroform	$ED_{50} = 0.52\%$[a]	Inhalant	*Caenorhabditis elegans*	Morgan and Cascorbi (1985)
		$ED_{50} = 1.47\%$[a]	Inhalant		Morgan et al. (1990)
	Ethanol	4.5%	Immersion		Morgan and Sedensky (1995)
	Flurothyl	$ED_{50} = 8.1\%$[a]	Inhalant		Morgan and Cascorbi (1985)
		$ED_{50} = 14.3\%$[a]	Inhalant		Morgan et al. (1990)
	Fluroxene	$ED_{50} = 10.9\%$[a]	Inhalant		Morgan and Cascorbi (1985)
		$ED_{50} = 10.8\%$[a]	Inhalant		Morgan et al. (1990)
	Halothane	$ED_{50} = 0.85\%$[a]	Inhalant		Morgan and Cascorbi (1985)
		$ED_{50} = 3.18\%$[a]	Inhalant		Morgan et al. (1990)
		$ED_{50} = 3.6\%$[a]	Inhalant		Crowder et al. (1996)
	Isoflurane	$ED_{50} = 4.9\%$[a]	Inhalant		Morgan and Cascorbi (1985)
		$ED_{50} = 6.5\%$[a]	Inhalant		Crowder et al. (1996)
		$ED_{50} = 7.18\%$[a]	Inhalant		Morgan et al. (1990)
	Propylene Phenoxetol	0.5 μL/mL for L1 larvae, 1.5 μL/mL for L2 larvae, 2.0 μL/mL for L3 larvae, 4.0 μL/mL for dauer larvae, 2.5 μL/mL for L4 larvae, and 3.0 μL/mL for adults	Agar Pad		Nelson and Riddle (1984)

[a] *The effective dose $(ED)_{50}$ is the concentration where half of the animals tested were immobile for longer than 10 s.*

8. Echinoderms

Echinoderms have pentaradial symmetry as adults, a calcium carbonate endoskeleton, and deuterostome development. There are approximately 7000 species divided into five classes, including brittle and basket stars (Ophiuroidea), feather stars and sea lilies (Crinoidea), sea cucumbers (Holothuroidea), sea stars (Asteroidea), and sea urchins, sea biscuits, and sand dollars (Echinoidea) (Ruppert et al., 2004). The echinoderm nervous system is composed of a circumoral nerve ring and radial nerves that extend from the circumoral nerve ring. While the circumoral nerve ring is centrally located in the echinoderm body, it does not appear to have a coordinating function and is not a true central nervous system (Cobb, 1995).

Most species of the echinoderm phylum can be handled safely and effectively without anesthesia or sedation. They tend to be slow-moving and quite hardy (one exception being the brittle stars). Certain species of sea urchins can inflict a painful "sting" with movable, sharp spines. Nets, tongs, and gloves can aid in the safe handling of many species for physical restraint. Anesthesia and analgesia should be used for invasive and potentially painful procedures. If echinoderms need to be anesthetized/immobilized, immersion in $MgCl_2$ or MS-222 is commonly used (Harms, 2022). Doses for the anesthesia of echinoderms are reported in Table 26.8.

a. Brittle and basket stars

Brittle stars have thin arms, while basket stars have branched arms (Ruppert et al., 2004). They must be handled gently to prevent arm autotomies.

MS-222 (1 g/L), $MgCl_2$ (1:1 ratio of iso-osmotic $MgCl_2$ to seawater), menthol (1/2 saturation), and 2-phenoxyethanol (5%) have been shown to reduce or prevent arm autotomy in brittle stars (Dobson, 1985). Details pertaining to the anesthetic plane are not reported, but the brittle stars recovered. A 2.5%–5% solution of menthol in seawater has been reported for anesthesia of *Amphipholis squamata* (Costello and Henley, 1971). Prior to fixation, brittle stars have been anesthetized by immersion in propylene phenoxetol (1 g/L) (Wilkie, 1992).

b. Feather stars and sea lilies

Feather stars and sea lilies are the most ancient of the echinoderms. They are typically sessile or semisessile, feather stars are free swimming, while sea lilies are attached to the substrate with a stalk. They are suspension feeders, collecting food using their branched arms (Ruppert et al., 2004).

There are a few reports of anesthetizing feather stars and sea lilies. They reportedly do not respond to magnesium salts; MS-222 (1 g/L) (Hendler, 2004) and propylene phenoxetol titrated to effect (Nichols, 1960) may be more effective. Bubbling nitrogen gas in seawater for 10–15 min has also been reported to reversibly anesthetize feather stars (Zmarzly, 1984).

c. Sea cucumbers

Sea cucumbers have an elongated cylindrical body shape with a soft and leathery body wall, characterized by a thick dermis. Their mouth and anus are found at opposite ends of their oblong bodies (Ruppert et al., 2004).

Some sea cucumbers may respond less to magnesium salts and better to propylene phenoxetol (Hendler et al., 1995). When exposed to seawater saturated with propylene phenoxetol, sea cucumbers exhibited increased activity for the first 30 min, began to relax after 1 h, and were fully relaxed after 2 h. These animals recovered in running seawater. Sea cucumbers left in the same solution for 13 h did not survive (Hill and Reinschmidt, 1976). Another reported dose for propylene phenoxetol is 2 g/L (VandenSpiegel and Jangoux, 1987), however, these sea cucumbers were dissected and did not recover. Menthol crystals have also been used to anesthetize sea cucumbers (Costelloe and Keegan, 1984).

d. Sea stars

Most sea star species have 5 rays, or arms, which extend from their central disc, but some species can have more than 40 (Ruppert et al., 2004).

A common anesthetic for sea stars is $MgCl_2$. A 75 g/L $MgCl_2$ solution (75 g $MgCl_2$ in 1 L of dechlorinated freshwater) is isotonic to natural seawater (Wahltinez et al., 2021). Immersion in an 80 g/L $MgCl_2$ solution (Anderson, 1965) or a 1:1 mixture of a 7.5% stock solution with seawater has been reported (McCurley and Kier, 1995). Higher concentrations may be necessary for induction (note that higher concentrations may be hyperosmotic), but adjustments over time during maintenance of anesthesia may be required by gradually administering more seawater. A wide range of MS-222 doses have been reported, and it can be used in a concentrated form (1–10 g/L in seawater) (O'Neill, 1989, 1994). Other reported anesthetic agents are menthol (10 g/L) (Pinn et al., 2014; Saha et al., 2006) and propylene phenoxetol (1 g/L in seawater) (Santos et al., 2005).

e. Sea urchins

Sea urchins have roughly spherical bodies with long spines, except the flattened "irregular" urchins which bury themselves in the sand or mud, such as sea biscuits and sand dollars (Ruppert et al., 2004).

Anesthesia in sea urchins is primarily geared toward preventing spawning, thus preserving the commercial value of the gonad. $MgCl_2$ doses may vary by species and age of urchins. A low dose of $MgCl_2$ (1.0 g/L) prevented spawning and decreased mortality in adult purple urchins (*Paracentrotus lividus*), while higher doses of 8.1–20.3 g/L were associated with increased mortality (Arafa et al., 2007). However, no mortality was observed in juvenile green sea urchins (*Strongylocentrotus droebachiensis*) immersed in 100 g/L $MgCl_2$ (Hagen, 2003). MS-222 buffered with sodium bicarbonate was an effective sedative (0.4 g/L) and anesthetic (0.8 g/L) for sea urchins (Applegate et al., 2016). Criteria for evaluating anesthetic effects included drooping spines, loss of adhesion to a vertical surface, response to tactile stimuli, and righting response (Applegate et al., 2016). Other anesthetics reported for use in sea urchins are KCl (2.5–50 g/L) and 2-phenoxyethanol (30 g/L). Benzocaine (20 g/L) has been deemed to be unsuitable (Hagen, 2003).

TABLE 26.8 Doses for anesthesia of echinoderms.

Echinodermata					
Class	**Agent**	**Dose**	**Method of administration**	**Species**	**Source**
Ophiuroidea	MS-222	1 g/L	Immersion	*Ophiophragmus filograneus*	Dobson (1985)
	Magnesium Chloride ($MgCl_2•6H_2O$)	1:1 ratio iso-osmotic $MgCl_2$ to seawater	Immersion	*Ophiophragmus filograneus*	Dobson (1985)
	Menthol	2.5%–5%[a]	Immersion	*Amphipholis squamata*	Costello and Henley (1971)
		½ saturation	Immersion	*Ophiophragmus filograneus*	Dobson (1985)
	2-Phenoxyethanol	5%	Immersion	*Ophiophragmus filograneus*	Dobson (1985)
	Propylene Phenoxetol	1 g/L[a]	Immersion	*Ophiophragmus filograneus*	Wilkie (1992)
Crinoidea	MS-222	1 g/L	Immersion	Not specified	Hendler (2004)
	Nitrogen	Bubbled for 10–15 min	Immersion	6 species of crinoids from the Marshall Islands	Zmarzly (1984)
	Propylene Phenoxetol	Titrated to effect[a]	Immersion	*Antedon bifida*	Nichols (1960)
Holothuroidea	Menthol	Not given[a]	Immersion	*Aslia lefevrei*	Costelloe and Keegan (1984)
	Propylene Phenoxetol	2 g/L[a]	Immersion	*Holothuria forskali*	VandenSpiegel and Jangoux (1987)
		Saturated[a]	Immersion	*Stichopus badionotus*	Hill and Reinschmidt (1976)
Asteroidea	Magnesium Chloride ($MgCl_2•6H_2O$)	37.5 g/L[a]	Immersion	*Luidia clathrate, Astropecten articulatus*	McCurley and Kier (1995)
		80 g/L	Immersion	*Asterias forbesi*	Anderson (1965)
	Menthol	10 g/L[a]	Immersion	*Asterina pectinifera*	Saha et al. (2006)
		Not given	Immersion	5 species of asteroids from Malaysia	Pinn et al. (2014)
	MS-222	1 g/L[a]	Immersion	*Echinaster spinulosus*	O'Neill (1989)
		10 g/L[a]	Immersion	*Coscinasterias calamaria*	O'Neill (1994)
	Propylene Phenoxetol	1 g/L[a]	Immersion	*Marthasterias glacialis*	Santos et al. (2005)
Echinoidea	Magnesium Chloride ($MgCl_2•6H_2O$)	100 g/L	Immersion	*Strongylocentrotus droebachiensis*	Hagen (2003)
	MS-222	0.4 g/L[b], 0.8 g/L	Immersion	*Arbacia punctulata*	Applegate et al. (2016)
	2-Phenoxyethanol	30 g/L	Immersion	*Strongylocentrotus droebachiensis*	Hagen (2003)
	Potassium Chloride (KCl)	2.5–50 g/L	Immersion	*Strongylocentrotus droebachiensis*	Hagen (2003)

[a]*Not all animals were recovered, dose may need to be adjusted for anesthesia.*
[b]*Sedation at low dose, anesthesia at high dose.*

III. Pain and analgesia in invertebrates

More research will likely occur to answer questions about pain perception by invertebrates. To date, the concept that invertebrates "feel pain" is a topic of debate. The crux of the debate may lie in the differentiation between nociception and pain. Nociception describes the neurophysiologic components leading to the sensation of pain but excludes the central perception of nociceptive input that ultimately leads to the sensation of pain. Strictly defined pain is "an unpleasant sensory and emotional experience associated with, or resembling that associated with, actual or potential tissue damage" (IASP, 2020). In humans, pain is modulated by various parts of the cerebral cortex (Xie et al., 2009). Although invertebrates do not possess a central nervous system with a well-described cortex or similar structure, it has been shown that a nociceptive response is present in invertebrates (Tobin and Bargmann, 2004), that nociceptor cells are present (Nicholls and Baylor, 1968), and that opioid systems have a functional role in invertebrate nociception (Kavaliers et al., 1983; Kavaliers, 1988; Fiorito, 1986; Saksida et al., 1993; Smith, 1991; Thomas et al., 1997). However, no definitive answer exists as to whether invertebrates perceive pain and would suffer emotional distress from it. The animals' response to a mechanical, chemical, and electrical stimulus is seen by withdrawal and escape behaviors. This response is decreased or slowed when an analgesic is used (Kavalier and Hirst, 1983; Kavaliers et al., 1983). It is not yet clear if this decreased response is due to a sedative effect or an analgesic effect of the drug. With the general trend of pain research and animal welfare recognition our knowledge on this delicate topic will expand and these questions can be answered.

Until more information is available regarding pain perception by invertebrates, an anesthetic should be given to any animal that is subjected to a painful procedure, and the amount of stress and pain induced should be reduced by decreasing awareness via appropriate choices of anesthetic agents.

The use of analgesic agents in invertebrate species has its own limitations due to the fact that very few reports can be found in the literature documenting the administration and dosing of analgesic agents, especially in the very small species, or, more importantly, evaluating the effects and impacts of the different analgesics on the patient, receptors, the anesthesia, and the recovery.

Assessment of pain or discomfort in invertebrates is very difficult, despite the fact that some avoidance behavior has been described (Mather, 2001; Tobin and Bargmann, 2004). The effect of analgesia is even harder to evaluate.

Obviously, more research is required in this area, but in the meantime, if possible, drugs with analgesic properties should be used to anesthetize invertebrates when invasive procedures are performed to decrease the nociceptive pathway. Hypothermia and CO_2 do not possess analgesic properties and may even show hyperalgesia characteristics. Generally, an inhalant agent is preferred over the latter methods. Although inhalant agents do not possess true analgesic properties, they do render mammalian patients insensible to painful stimuli when administered at sufficient anesthetizing doses. Unfortunately, the insensibility to painful stimuli only lasts as long as the animal is anesthetized; if the procedure is expected to be associated with significant postoperative pain, the administration of an analgesic would be advisable. Knowledge concerning analgesic receptors in invertebrate taxa, and if or how commonly used analgesics of vertebrates would apply is sparse. Lidocaine injections have been shown to block afferent signals to the CNS and prevent behavioral responses to noxious stimuli in cephalopods, which would indicate analgesic properties (Butler-Struben et al., 2018; Crook, 2021). Morphine does not appear to have analgesic properties in decapod crustaceans (Bar and Elwood, 2011).

IV. Euthanasia

A section on invertebrates was included in the AVMA Guidelines for the Euthanasia of Animals for the first time in the 2013 Edition and was expanded upon in the 2020 Edition. Further guidance can be found in other sources (Cooper, 2022a; Murray, 2022; Reilly, 2001; Poole, 1999).

Due to challenges in confirming death in many invertebrate species, a two-step euthanasia protocol is recommended, where the first step renders the animal nonresponsive and the second step ensures death. Acceptable first-step methods for aquatic invertebrates include immersion in magnesium salts, clove oil or eugenol, and ethanol (up to 10%). Acceptable first-step methods for terrestrial invertebrates include inhalant gas anesthetics delivered via a suitably sized induction chamber, and injection of pentobarbital-containing euthanasia solution into the circulating hemolymph. Acceptable second-step methods include immersion in fixatives such as 70% alcohol and 10% formalin and physical methods such as pithing, freezing, and boiling. Methods that do not cause rapid death or cause stress and trauma prior to loss of response cannot be considered euthanasia. Unacceptable methods as a solo or first step for euthanasia of invertebrates include removal of aquatic animals from water or immersion of terrestrial animals in water to die by hypoxia, leaving animals in a container without aeration to die by anoxia, freezing, or immersion in caustic chemical such as tissue fixative (Leary et al., 2020).

Despite the ongoing debate on the capacity of invertebrates to perceive pain, it is well-recognized that different species of invertebrates show various types of stress responses and react to noxious stimuli. Even if the perception of pain is not fully understood, it is our responsibility to treat every living creature with respect, assure the well-being of these animals, and decrease any stress we put on the individual animal in the best way possible (Murray, 2022). Euthanasia should be performed in an effective, fast, pain-free, and stress-free manner.

The most commonly used methods for euthanasia are terminal anesthesia followed by physical destruction of the nervous system. The physical destruction of the nervous system/primary ganglia may be added to the chemical method because death is often difficult to verify in invertebrates (Hackendahl and Mashima, 2002). It is important to keep in mind that the nervous system varies in the different invertebrate species and that decapitation alone may not always be a suitable method (Hackendahl and Mashima, 2002). Other destructive methods may have to be implemented when doubts about the confirmation of the death from an anesthetic overdose are present. More information about ideal species-specific methods of euthanasia is needed due to the large variety of invertebrate species.

Some recommendations have been made regarding acceptable or recommended euthanasia in specific invertebrate species. Emphasis is placed on methods that reduce stress for the animal until more is known about the effects of stress and pain on these species. Special consideration and adjustments may be necessary for research that relies on the preservation of specific tissues or interference of anesthetic agents with the research purpose.

Specific euthanasia methods and techniques can be adjusted based on planned sample analyses and research goals. Horseshoe crabs can be euthanized with an injection of 1–2 mL of pentobarbital-containing euthanasia solution directly into the cardiac sinus (Smith and Berkson, 2005). Sea stars have been euthanized by immersion in $MgCl_2$ (75 g/L) until they are nonresponsive followed by a physical method of quick dissection. This method allowed for the isolation of high-quality RNA (Wahltinez et al., 2021). Jellyfish euthanized in an immersion of $MgCl_2$ (142 g/L) were suitable for NMR-spectroscopy-based metabolomics analysis (Doerr and Stoskopf, 2019). The recommendations for cephalopods are an overdose of ethanol or $MgCl_2$, followed by brain destruction (Murray, 2022; Reilly, 2001; Scimeca et al., 2022). Recommended euthanasia methods for crustaceans are an overdose of ethanol or clove oil followed by brain destruction (Reilly, 2001). Eugenol immersion at 500 mg/L followed by intracardiac KCl at 10 mmol/kg or ivermectin at 5 mg/kg were effective, rapid methods of euthanasia in blue crabs (*Callinectes sapidus*) (Mones et al., 2022). Injection of KCl at 13 mmol/kg at the base of the second walking leg to flood the hemolymph sinus containing the ventral nerve cord has been recommended as an effective method for euthanasia of American lobsters (*Homarus americanus*) (Battison et al., 2000), but despite presumed rapid effects on the central nervous system, this method may be better applied as the second step of a 2-step protocol. This method has also been applied to terrestrial arthropods and termed "targeted hyperkalosis" to describe terminal depolarization of the thoracic ganglia leading to death (Bennie et al., 2012). Pizzi and Kennedy describe the immersion in 70% ethanol after general anesthesia as an acceptable method for euthanasia in spiders (Pizzi & Kennedy, 2022).

References

Agostini, S., Suzuki, Y., Casareto, B.E., Nakano, Y., Fairoz, M.F.M., Shiroma, K., Irikawa, A., Daigo, K., 2008. New approach to study the coral symbiotic complex: application to vitamin B12. Proc. 11th Int. Coral Reef Symp. 2, 917–921.

Aguzzi, J., Abello, P., Depledge, M.H., 2004. Endogenous cardiac activity rhythms of continental slope *Nephrops norvegicus* (Decapoda: nephropidea). Mar. Freshw. Behav. Physiol. 37 (1), 55–64.

Amiel, A.R., Rottinger, E., 2021. Experimental tools to study regeneration in the sea anemone Nematosella vectensis. In: Developmental Biology of the Sea Urchin and Other Marine Invertebrates: Methods and Protocols. Humana, New York, NY, pp. 69–80.

Anderson, E.T., Davis, A.S., Law, J.M., Lewbart, G.A., Christian, L.S., Harms, C.A., 2010. Gross and histologic evaluation of 5 suture materials in the skin and subcutaneous tissue of the California sea hare (*Aplysia californica*). J. Am. Assoc. Lab Anim. Sci. 49, 64–68.

Anderson, J.M., 1965. Studies on visceral regeneration in sea stars. III. Regeneration of the cardiac stomach in *Asterias forbesi*. Biol. Bull. 129, 454–470.

Anderson, R.C., Wood, J.B., 2001. Enrichment for giant pacific octopuses: happy as a clam? J. Appl. Anim. Welfare Sci. 4 (2), 157–168.

Andrews, P.L.R., Tansey, E.M., 1981. The effects of some anesthetic agents in *Octopus vulgaris*. Comp. Biochem. Physiol. 70C, 241–247.

Applegate, J.R., Dombrowski, D.S., Christian, L.S., Bayer, M.P., Harms, C.A., Lewbart, G.A., 2016. Tricaine methanesulfonate (MS-222) sedation and anesthesia in the purple-spined sea urchin (*Arbacia punctulata*). J. Zoo Wildl. Med. 47, 1025–1033.

Aquilina, B., Roberts, R., 2000. A method for inducing muscle relaxation in the abalone, *Haliotis iris*. Aquaculture 190, 403–408.

Arafa, S., Sadok, S., Abed, A.E., 2007. Assessment of magnesium chloride as an anaesthetic for adult sea urchins (*Paracentrotus lividus*): incidence on mortality and spawning. Aquacult. Res. 38, 1673–1678.

Archibald, K.E., Scott, G.N., Bailey, K.M., Harms, C.A., 2019. 2-Phenoxyethanol (2-PE) and tricaine methanesulfonate (MS-222) immersion anesthesia of American horseshoe crabs (*Limulus polyphemus*). J. Zoo Wildl. Med. 50, 96–106.

AWIC Resource Series No 8 (May 2000; Slightly Revised October 2000, edited by M.D. Kreger, M.S.

Barr, S., Elwood, R.W., 2011. No evidence of morphine analgesia to noxious shock in the shore crab, *Carcinus maenas*. Behav. Process. 86, 340–344.

Battison, A., MacMilan, R., MacKenzie, A., Rose, P., Cawthorn, R., Horney, B., 2000. Use of injectable potassium chloride for euthanasia of American lobsters (*Homarus americanus*). Comp. Med. 50, 545–550.

Bennie, N.A.C., Loaring, C.D., Bennie, M.M.G., Trim, S.A., 2012. An effective method for terrestrial arthropod euthanasia. J. Exp. Biol. 215, 4237–4241.

Berry, A., Vitale, A., Carere, C., Alleva, E., 2015. EU guidelines for the care and welfare of an "exceptional invertebrate class" in scientific research. Ann. Istituto Super. Sanita 51 (4), 267–269.

Birch, J., Burn, C., Schnell, A., Browning, H., Crump, A., 2021. Review of the evidence of sentience in cephalopod molluscs and decapod Crustaceans. In: LSE Consulting, London School of Economics and Political Science, London, p. 107.

Bodri, M.S., 2022. Nematodes. In: Lewbart, G.A. (Ed.), Invertebrate Medicine, *third ed.* Wiley-Blackwell Publishing, Ames, IA, pp. 537–561.

Bonyadi-Naeini, A., Hassan, R., Glasby, C.J., 2016. A new substance to relax polychaete worms (Annelida) prior to morphological study. ZooKeys 594, 1.

Bossert, P.E., Dunn, M.P., Thomsen, G.H., 2013. A staging system for the regeneration of a polyp from the aboral physa of the anthozoan cnidarian *Nematostella vectensis*. Dev. Dynam. 242, 1320–1331.

Bower, J.R., Sakurai, Y., Yamamoto, J., Ishii, H., 1999. Transport of the ommastrephid squid *Todarodes pacificus* under cold-water anesthesia. Aquaculture 170, 127–130.

Brown, P.B., White, M.R., Chaille, J., Russell, M., Oseto, C., 1996. Evaluation of three anesthetic agents for crayfish (*Orconectes virilis*). J. Shellfish Res. 15 (2), 433–435.

Butler-Struben, H.M., Brophy, S.M., Johnson, N.A., Crook, R.J., 2018. *In vivo* recording of neural and behavioral correlates of anesthesia induction, reversal, and euthanasia in cephalopod molluscs. Front. Physiol. 9, 109.

Cevik, D., Acker, M., Arefi, P., Ghaemi, R., Zhang, J., Selvaganapathy, P.R., Dworking, I., Jacobs, J.R., 2019. Chloroform and desflurane immobilization with recovery of viable *Drosophila* larvae for confocal imaging. J. Insect Physiol. 17, 103900.

Chen, C., Dai, C.F., Plathong, S., Chiou, C.Y., Chen, C.A., 2008. The complete mitochondrial genomes of needle corals, *Seriatopora* spp. (Scleractinia: pocilloporidae): an idiosyncratic atp8, duplicated trnW gene, and hypervariable regions used to determine species phylogenies and recently diverged populations. Mol. Phylogenet. Evol. 46, 19–33.

Chen, C.W., Lin, W.Y., Cheng, J., Chen, K.B., Kuo, Y.C., Li, C.Y., Hsin-Ping, L., 2019. Inhalational Aesthetic Sevoflurane Exacerbates Eye Phenotype of SCA3 Transgenic Drosophila Model.

Clark, T.R., Nossov, P.C., Apland, J.P., Filbert, M.G., 1996. Anesthetic agents for use in the invertebrate sea snail, *Aplysia californica*. Contemp. Top. Lab. Anim. Sci. 35 (5), 75–79.

Cobb, J.L.S., 1995. The nervous systems of Echinodermata: recent results and new approaches. In: Breidbach, O., Kutsch, W. (Eds.), The Nervous Systems of Invertebrates: An Evolutionary and Comparative Approach, pp. 407–424.

Colley, N.J., Trench, R.K., 1985. Cellular events in the reestablishment of a symbiosis between a marine dinoflagellate and a coelenterate. Cell Tissue Res. 239, 93–103.

Cooke, G.M., Tonkins, B.M., Mather, J.A., 2019. Care and enrich- ment for captive cephalopods. In: Carere, C., Mather, J. (Eds.), The Welfare of Invertebrate Animals. Springer, Cham, Switzerland, pp. 179–208.

Cooper, E.L., 1968. Transplantation immunity in annelids. Transplantation 6 (3), 322–337.

Cooper, E.L., Roch, P., 1986. Second-set allograft responses in the earthworm *Lumbricus terrestris*. Transplantation 41 (4), 514–520.

Cooper, J.E., 2001. Invertebrate anesthesia. In: Heard, D. (Ed.), Exotic Anesthesia and Analgesia, pp. 57–67.

Cooper, J.E., Pellett, S., O'Brien, M., 2022a. Insects. In: Lewbart, G.A. (Ed.), Invertebrate Medicine, third ed. Wiley-Blackwell Publishing, Ames, IA, pp. 413–437.

Cooper, M.E., 2022. Laws and regulations. In: Lewbart, G.A. (Ed.), Invertebrate Medicine, 3rd Ed. Wiley-Blackwell Publishing, Oxford, UK, pp. 651–668.

Cooper, J.E., Mahaffey, P., Applebee, K., 1986. Anaesthesia of the medicinal leech (*Hirudo medicinalis*). Vet. Rec. 118, 589–590.

Costello, D.P., Henley, C., 1971. Methods of Obtaining and Handling Marine Eggs and Embryos, second ed. Marine Biological Laboratory, Woods Hole, MA, pp. 247–250.

Costelloe, J., Keegan, B.F., 1984. Feeding and related morphological structures in the dendrochirote *Aslia lefevrei* (Holothuroidea: echinodermata). Mar. Biol. 84, 135–142.

Coyle, S.D., Dasgupta, S., Tidwell, J.H., Beavers, T., Bright, L.A., Yasharian, D.K., 2005. Comparative efficacy of anesthetics for the freshwater prawn *Macrobrachium rosenbergii*. J. World Aquacult. Soc. 36, 282–290.

Crook, R.J., 2021. Behavioral and neurophysiological evidence suggests affective pain experience in octopus. iScience 24, 102229.

Crowder, C.M., Shebester, L.D., Schedl, T., 1996. Behavioral effects of volatile anesthetics in *Caenorhabditis elegans*. Anesthesiology 85, 901–912.

Culloty, S.C., Mulcahy, M.F., 1992. An evaluation of anesthetics for *Ostrea edulis* (L.). Aquaculture 107 (2–3), 249–252.

Deitrich, R.A., Dunwiddie, T.V., Harris, R.A., Erwin, V.G., 1989. Mechanism of action of ethanol: initial central nervous system actions. Pharmacol. Rev. 41, 489–537.

Diggles, B.K., 2019. Review of some scientific issues related to crustacean welfare. ICES (Int. Counc. Explor. Sea) J. Mar. Sci. 76 (1), 66–81.

Dobson, W.E., 1985. A pharmacological study of neural mediation of disc autotomy in *Ophiophragmus filograneus* (Lyman) (Echinodermata: ophiuroidea). J. Exp. Mar. Biol. Ecol. 94, 223–232.

Doerr, M., Stoskopf, M.K., 2019. Evaluation of euthanasia of moon jellyfish (*Aurelia aurita*) using simple salt solutions. J. Zoo Wildl. Med. 50, 123–126.

Dombrowski, D., 2006a. Personal Communication/unpublished Data.

Edwards, S., Burke, C., Hindrum, S., Johns, D., 2000. Recovery and growth effects of anaesthetic and mechanical removal on greenlips (*Haliotis laevigata*) and blacklip (*Haliotis rubra*) abalone. J. Shellfish Res. 19 (1), 510.

Elwood, R.W., 2019. Assessing the potential for pain in crustaceans and other invertebrates. In: Carere, C., Mather, J. (Eds.), The Welfare of Invertebrate Animals. Springer, Cham, Switzerland, pp. 147–177.

England, K.W., 1987. Certain actiniaria (Cnidaria, anthozoa) from the red sea and tropical indo-pacific ocean. Bull. Br. Museum (Natural Hist. Zool. Ser.) 53, 205–292.

Ferraro, E.A., Pressacco, L., 1996. Anesthetic procedures for crustaceans. An assessment of isobutanol and xylazine as general anaesthetics for *Squilla mantis* (Stomapoda). Mem. Biol. Mar. Oceanogr. 12, 471–475.

Fiorito, G., 1986. Is there "pain" in invertebrates? Behav. Process. 12, 383–388.

Fiorito, G., Affuso, A., Basil, J., et al., 2015. Guidelines for the care and welfare of cephalopods in research – a consensus based on an initiative by CephRes, FELASA and the Boyd Group. Lab. Anim. 49 (S2), 1–90.

Flores, D.V., Salas, P.J.I., Vedra, J.P.S., 1983. Electroretinography and ultrastructural study of the regenerated eye of the snail *Cryptomphallus aspera*. J. Neurobiol. 14 (3), 167–176.

Foley, D.M., Stewart, J.E., Holley, R.A., 1966. Isobutyl alcohol and methyl pentynol as general anesthetics for the lobster, *Homarus americanus* Milne-Edwards. Can. J. Zool. 44, 141–143.

Fregin, T., Bickmeyer, U., 2016. Electrophysiological investigation of different methods of anesthesia in lobster and crayfish. PLoS One 11, 1–19.

Frye, F., 2022. Scorpions. In: Lewbart, G.A. (Ed.), Invertebrate Medicine, *third ed.* Wiley-Blackwell Publishing, Ames, IA, pp. 349–365.

Fuentes, V., Straehler-Pohl, I., Atienza, D., Franco, I., Tilves, U., Gentile, M., Acevedo, M., Olariaga, A., Gili, J.M., 2011. Life cycle of the jellyfish *Rhizostoma pulmo* (Scyphozoa: rhizostomeae) and its distribution, seasonality and inter-annual variability along the Catalan coast and the Mar Menor (Spain, NW Mediterranean). Mar. Biol. 158, 2247–2266.

Garcia-Franco, M., 1992. Anaesthetics for the squid *Sepioteuthis sepioidea* (Mollusca: cephalopoda). Comp. Biochem. Physiol. 103C (1), 121–123.

Gardner, C., 1997. Options for immobilization and killing crabs. J. Shellfish Res. 16 (1), 219–224.

Girdlestone, D., Cruickshank, S.G.H., Winlow, W., 1989. The actions of 3 volatile anaesthetics on the withdrawal response of the pond snail *Lymnaea stagnalis*. Comp. Biochem. Physiol. 92C (1), 39–43.

Gleadall, I.G., 1991. Comparison of anaesthetics for octopuses. Bull. Mar. Sci. 49 (1–2), 663.

Gleadall, I.G., 2013. The effects of prospective anaesthetic substances on cephalopods: a summary of original data and a brief review of studies over the past two decades. J. Exp. Mar. Biol. Ecol. 447, 23–30.

Gore, S.R., Harms, C.A., Kukanich, B., Forsythe, J., Lewbart, G.A., Papich, M.G., 2005. Enrofloxacin pharmacokinetics in the European cuttlefish, *Sepia officinalis*, after a single i.v. injection and bath administration. J. Vet. Pharmacol. Therapeut. 28, 433–439.

Gorges, M.A., Martinez, K.M., Labriola, N.F., Phillips, B.E., Christian, L.S., Chen, E.P., Posner, L.P., Lewbart, G.A., Dombrowski, D.S., 2022. Effects of tricaine methanesulfonate (MS-222) in a managed collection of moon jellyfish (*Aurelia aurita*). J. Zoo Wildl. Med. 53 (1), 100–107.

Hackendahl, N., Mashima, T.Y., 2002. Considerations in aquatic invertebrate euthanasia. In: Proceedings of the American Association of Zoo Veterinarians, pp. 324–329.

Hagen, N.T., 2003. KCl induced paralysis facilitates detachment of hatchery reared juvenile green sea urchins, Strongylocentrotus droebachiensis. Aquaculture 216, 155–164.

Harms, C.A., 2022. Echinoderms. In: Lewbart, G.A. (Ed.), Invertebrate Medicine. Blackwell Publishing, Ames, IA, pp. 579–598.

Harms, C.A., Lewbart, G.A., McAlarney, R., Christian, L.S., Geissler, K., Lemons, C., 2006. Surgical excision of mycotic (*Cladosporium* sp.) granulomas from the mantle of a cuttlefish (*Sepia officinalis*). J. Zoo Wildl. Med. 37, 524–530.

Hausserman, V., 2004. Identification and taxonomy of soft-bodied hexacorals exemplified by Chilean sea anemones; including guidelines for sampling, preservation and examination. J. Mar. Biol. Assoc. U. K. 84, 931–936.

Heasman, M.P., O'Connor, W.A., Frazer, A.W.J., 1995. Induction of anesthesia in the commercial scallop, Pecten fumatus reeve. Aquaculture 131, 231–238.

Hendler, G., Miller, J.E., Pawson, D.L., Kier, P.M., 1995. Sea Stars, Sea Urchins and Allies: Echinoderms of Florida and the Caribbean. Smithsonian Institution Press, Washington, DC, pp. 21–27.

Hendler, G., 2004. Collecting, Preserving and Archiving Echinoderms. Natural History Museum of Los Angeles County.

Hill, R.B., Reinschmidt, D., 1976. Relative importance of the antioxidant and anesthetic properties of propylene phenoxetol in its action as a "preservative" for living holothurians. J. Invertebr. Pathol. 28, 131–135.

Hubrecht, R.C., Kirkwood, J. (Eds.), 2010. The UFAW Handbook on the Care and Management of Laboratory and Other Research Animals. John Wiley & Sons.

International Association for the Study of Pain IASP Announces Revised Definition of Pain. 2020. Available online: www.iasp-pain.org. Accessed 18 January 2023.

Janes, M.P., 2008. Laboratory methods for the identification of soft corals (octocorallia: alcyonacea). In: Leewis, J.M., Janes, M.P. (Eds.), Advances in Coral Husbandry in Public Aquariums. Public Aquarium Husbandry Species 2, pp. 413–426.

Joosse, J., Lever, J., 1958. Techniques for narkotization and operation for experiments with *Lymnaea stagnalis* (Gastropoda Pulmonata). Proc. Kon. Ned. Akad. Wetensch. C 62, 145–149.

Junge, D., Ortiz, C.L., 1978. Measurement of electrogenic-pump current in *Aplysia* neurones with constant-current and constant-voltage techniques. J. Exp. Biol. 72, 141–151.

Kanz, J.E., Eberly, L.B., Cobbs, J.S., Pinsker, H.M., 1979. Neuronal correlates of siphon withdrawal in freely behaving *Aplysia*. J. Neurophysiol. 42, 1538–1556.

Kavaliers, M., 1988. Evolutionary and comparative aspects in nociception. Brain Res. Bull. 21, 923–931.

Kavaliers, M., Hirst, M., 1983. Tolerance to morphine-induced thermal response in terrestrial snail, *Cepaea nemoralis*. Neuropharmaology 22, 1321–1326.

Kavaliers, M., Hirst, M., Teskey, G.C., 1983. A functional role for an opiate system in snail thermal behavior. Science 220 (4592), 99–101.

Kawaguti, S., 1964. Electron microscopic study of the nerve plexus in the polyp of a reef coral. Proc. Jpn. Acad. 40, 121–124.

Kikinger, R., 1992. *Cotylorhiza tuberculata* (Cnidaria: scyphozoa) - life history of a stationary population. Mar. Ecol. 13, 333–362.

Leary, S., Underwood, W., Anthony, R. Cartner, S., Grandin, T., Greenacre, C., Gwaltney-Brant, S. McCrackin, M.A., Meyer, R., Miller, D, Shearer, J., Turner, T., Yanong, R., 2020. AVMA Guidelines for the euthanasia of animals: 2020 edition. https://www.avma.org/sites/default/files/2020-02/Guidelines-on-Euthanasia-2020.p df (Accessed 18 January 2023).

Lewbart, G., Riser, N., 1996. Nuchal organs of the polychaete *Parapionosyllis manca*. (Syllidae). Invertebr. Biol. 115 (4), 286–298.

Lewbart, G.A., Harms, C.A., 1999. Building a fish anesthesia delivery system. Exot. DVM 1 (2), 25–28.

Lewbart, G.A., 2022. In: Lewbart, G.A. (Ed.), In: Invertebrate Medicine, third ed. Wiley-Blackwell Publishing, Oxford. 752 pp.

Lozada, M., Romano, A., Maldonado, H., 1988. Effect of morphine and naloxone on a defensive response of the crab *Chasmagnathus granulatus*. Pharmacol. Biochem. Behav. 30, 635–640.

MacMillan, H.A., Nørgård, M., MacLean, H.J., Overgaard, J., Williams, C.J., 2017. A critical test of *Drosophila* anaesthetics: isoflurane and sevoflurane are benign alternatives to cold and CO2. J. Insect Physiol. 101, 97–106.

Madsen, B., Vollrath, F., 2000. Mechanism and morphology of silk dawn from anesthetized spiders. Naturwissenschaften 87, 149–153.

Maldonado, H., Miralto, A., 1982. Effect of morphine and naloxone on a defensive response of the mantis shrimp (*Squilla mantis*). J. Comp. Physiol. 147, 455–459.

Marks, D.H., Cooper, E.L., 1977. *Aeromonas hydrophila* in the coelomic cavity of the earthworms *Lumbricus terrestris* and *Eisenia foetida*. J. Invertebr. Pathol. 29, 382–383.

Martins-Sousa, R.L., Negrao-Correa, D., Bezerra, F.S.M., Coelho, P.M.Z., 2001. Anesthesia of *Biomphalaria* spp. (Mollusca, Gastropoda): sodium pentobarbital is the drug of choice. Mem. Inst. Oswaldo Cruz 96 (3), 391–392.

Mather, J.A., 2001. Animal suffering: an invertebrate perspective. J. Appl. Anim. Welfare Sci. 4 (2), 151–156.

McCurley, R.S., Kier, W.M., 1995. The functional morphology of starfish tube feet: the role of a crossed-fiber helical array in movement. Biol. Bull. 188, 197–209.

Melidone, R., Mayer, J., 2005. How to build an invertebrate surgery chamber. Exot. Dvm 7 (5), 8–10.

Messenger, J.B., Nixon, M., Ryan, K.P., 1985. Magnesium chloride as an anesthetic for cephalopods. Comp. Biochem. Physiol. 82C (1), 203–205.

Mills, D., Tlili, A., Norton, J., 1997. Large-scale anesthesia of the silver-lip pearl oyster, *Pinctada maxima* Jameson. J. Shellfish Res. 16 (2), 573–574.

Minter, L.J., Harms, C.A., Archibald, K.E., Broadhurst, H., Bailey, K.M., Christiansen, E.F., Lewbart, G.A., Posner, L.P., 2013. Efficacy of alfaxalone for intravascular anesthesia and euthanasia in blue crabs (*Callinectes sapidus*). J. Zoo Wildl. Med. 44, 694–699.

Mones, A.B., Harms, C.A., Balko, J.A., 2022. Evaluation of intracardiac administration of potassium chloride, ivermectin, and lidocaine hydrochloride for euthanasia of anesthetized blue crabs (*Callinectes sapidus*). In: Proceedings of the International Association for Aquatic Animal Medicine, 2022.

Moore, S.J., 1989. Narcotising sea anemones. J. Mar. Biol. Assoc. United Kingdom. 69, 803–811.

Morgan, P.G., Cascorbi, H.F., 1985. Effect of anesthetics and a convulsant on normal and mutant *Caenorhabditis elegans*. Anesthesiology 62, 738–744.

Morgan, P.G., Sedensky, M.M., 1995. Mutations affecting sensitivity to ethanol in the nematode, *Caenorhabditis elegans*. Alcohol Clin. Exp. Res. 19, 1423–1429.

Morgan, P.G., Sedensky, M., Meneely, P.M., 1990. Multiple site of action of volatile anesthetics in *Caenorhabditis elegans*. Proc. Natl. Acad. Sci. U.S.A. 87, 2965–2985.

Morrall, C.E., Galloway, T.S., Trapido-Rosenthal, H.G., Depledge, M.H., 2000. Characterisation of nitric oxide synthase activity in the tropical sea anemone *Aiptasia pallida*. Comp. Biochem. Physiol. B Biochem. Mol. Biol. 125, 483–491.

Murray, M.J., 2022. Euthanasia. In: Lewbart, G.A. (Ed.), Invertebrate Medicine, 3rd Ed. Wiley-Blackwell Publishing, Oxford, UK, pp. 645–650.

Müller, M.C.M., Berenzen, A., Westheide, W., 2003. Experiments on anterior regeneration in *Eurythoe complanata* (Polychaeta: Amphinomidae): reconfiguration of the nervous system and its function for regeneration. Zoomorphology 122 (2), 95–103.

Mutani, A., 1982. A technique for anaesthetizing pulmonate snails of medical and veterinary importance. Z. Parasitenkd. 68, 117–119.

Nelson, F.K., Riddle, D.L., 1984. Functional study of the *Caenorhabditis elegans* secretory-excretory system using laser microsurgery. J. Exp. Zool. 231 (1), 45–56.

Nicholls, J.G., Baylor, D.A., 1968. Specific modalities and receptive fields of sensory neurons in the C leech. J. Neurophysiol. 31, 740–756.

Nichols, D., 1960. The histology and activities of the tube-feet of *Antedon bifida*. J. Cell. Sci. 101, 105–117.

Nicolas, G., Sillans, D., 1989. Immediate and latent effects of carbon dioxide on insects. Annu. Rev. Entomol. 34, 97–116.

NIH. (n.d.) Research Using Vertebrate Animals. https://www.niaid.nih.gov/grants-contracts/research-vertebrate-animals.

Norton, J.H., Dashorst, M., Lansky, T.M., Mayer, R.J., 1996. An evaluation of some relaxants for use with pearl oysters. Aquaculture 144, 39–52.

O'Neill, P.L., 1989. Structure and mechanics of starfish body wall. J. Exp. Biol. 147, 53–89.

O'Neill, P.L., 1994. The effect of anesthesia on spontaneous contraction of the body wall musculature in the asteroid Coscinasterias calamaria. Mar. Behav. Physiol. 24, 137–150.

Oswald, R.L., 1977. Immobilization of decapod crustaceans for experimental purposes. J. Mar. Biol. Assoc. U. K. 57, 715–721.

Park, J.H., 1998. First record of a freshwater jellyfish, *Craspedacusta sowerbii* lankester, 1880 (Limnomedusae, Olindiidae) from reservoirs in Korea. Kor. J. Biol. Sci. 2, 303–308.

Pinn, W.S., Fang, A.N.P., Razalli, N.M., Nilamani, N., Peng, T.C., Yasin, Z., Tan, S.W., Fujita, T., 2014. New records of sea stars (Echinodermata Asteroidea) from Malaysia with notes on their association with seagrass beds. Biodivers. J. 5, 453–458.

Pizzi, R., Kennedy, B., 2022. Spiders. In: Lewbart, G.A. (Ed.), Invertebrate Medicine, *third ed.* Wiley-Blackwell Publishing, Ames, IA, pp. 301–347.

Poole, T., 1999. UFAW Handbook on the Care and Management of Laboratory Animals, seventh ed., Vol 2. Part 3. Blackwell Publishing.

Premarathna, A.D., Pathirana, I., Rajapakse, R.P.V.J., Pathirana, E., 2016. Evaluation of efficacy of selected anesthetic agents on blood-spotted crab (*Portunus sanguinolentus*). J. Shellfish Res. 35, 237–240.

Quesada, R.J., Smith, C.D., Heard, D.J., 2011. Evaluation of parenteral drugs for anesthesia in the blue crab (*Callinectes sapidus*). J. Zoo Wildl. Med. 42, 295–299.

Redmond, J.R., Jorgensen, D.D., Bourne, G.B., 1982. Circulatory physiology of *limulus*. Prog. Clin. Biol. Res. 81, 133–146.

Reilly, R.S., 2001. Euthanasia of animals used for scientific purposes. ANZCCART (2), 98–99.

Robertson, J.D., Delorme, N.J., Hickey, A., Jeffs, A.G., 2018. Assessment of the potential of the anesthetic AQUI-S for live transportation of the southern rock lobster, *Jasus edwardsii*. Bull. Mar. Sci. 94, 1137–1151.

Ruppert, E.E., Fox, R.S., Barnes, R.D., 2004. Invertebrate Zoology: A Functional Evolutionary Approach, seventh ed. Thompson-Brooks/Cole, Belmont, California. 963 pp.

Saksida, L.M., Galea, L.A., Kavaliers, M., 1993. Antinociceptive effects of the enkephalinase inhibitor, SCH 34826, in the snail, *Cepaea nemoralis*. Peptides 14 (4), 763–765.

Saha, A.K., Tamori, M., Inoue, M., Nakajima, Y., Motokawa, T., 2006. NGIWYamide-induced contraction of tube feet and distribution of NGIWYamide-like immunoreactivity in nerves of the starfish *Asterina pectinifera*. Zool. Sci. (Tokyo) 23, 627–632.

Salgado, M.A., Lewbart, G.A., Christian, L.S., Griffith, E.H., Law, J.M., 2014. Evaluation of five different suture materials in the skin of the earthworm (*Lumbricus terrestris*). SpringerPlus 3 (1), 1–7.

Santos, R., Haesaerts, D., Jangoux, M., Flammang, P., 2005. The tube feet of sea urchins and sea stars contain functionally different mutable collagenous tissues. J. Exp. Biol. 208, 2277–2288.

Saydmohammed, M., Pal, A.K., 2009. Anesthetic effect of eugenol and menthol on handling stress in *Macrobrachium rosenbergii*. Aquaculture 298, 162–167.

Scimeca, J.M., Barord, G.J., Lewbart, G.A., 2022. Cephalopods. In: Lewbart, G.A. (Ed.), Invertebrate Medicine, *third ed.* Wiley- Blackwell Publishing, Ames, IA, pp. 177–201.

Sebens, K., Paine, R., 1978. Biogeography of anthozoans along the west coast of South America: habitat, disturbance, and prey availability. Proc. Int. Symp. Mar. Biogeogr. Evol. South Hemisph. 137, 219–237.

Sheldon, J.D., Adamovicz, L., Burvenich, P., Chinnadurai, S.K., Allender, M.C., 2019. Effects of oxygen and isoflurane anesthesia on hemolymph gas analysis and righting reflex of asian forest (*Heterometrus longimanus*) and dictator scorpions (*Pandinus dictator*). J. Zoo Wildl. Med. 50 (1), 111–122.

Smith, J., 1991. A question of pain in invertebrates. ILAR J. 33 (1–2), 25–31.

Smith, S.A., 2022. Horseshoe crabs. In: Lewbart, G.A. (Ed.), Invertebrate Medicine, *third ed.* Wiley-Blackwell Publishing, Ames, IA, pp. 283–300.

Smith, S.A., Berkson, J., 2005. Laboratory culture and maintenance of the horseshoe crab (*Limulus polyphemus*). Lab. Anim. 34 (7), 27–34.

Smith, J.A., Andrews, P.L.R., Hawkins, P., Louhimies, S., Ponte, G., Dickel, L., 2013. Cephalopod research and EU Directive 2010/63/EU: requirements, impacts and ethical review. Elsevier B.V. J. Exp. Mar. Biol. Ecol. 447, 31–45.

Souza, A.R., Lewbart, G.A., Papich, M.G., 2020. Pilot pharmacokinetic study of ketorolac in the blue crab, *Callinectes sapidus*. J. Surv. Fish Sci. 6, 93–97.

Spano, C., Flores, V., 2013. Staining protocol for the histological study of sea anemones (Anthozoa: actiniaria) with recommendations for anesthesia and fixation of specimens. Lat. Am. J. Aquat. Res. 41, 1019–1024.

Spotswood, T., Smith, S.A., 2007. Cardiovascular and gastrointestinal radiographic contrast studies in the horseshoe crab (*Limulus polyphemus*). Vet. Radiol. Ultrasound 48 (1), 14–20.

Stefanik, D.J., Friedman, L.E., Finnerty, J.R., 2013. Collecting, rearing, spawning and inducing regeneration of the starlet sea anemone, *Nematostella vectensis*. Nat. Protoc. 8, 916–923.

Styrishave, B., Andersen, O., Depledge, M.H., 2003. In situ monitoring of heart rates in shore crabs *Carcinus maenas* in two tidal estuaries: effects of physico-chemical parameters on tidal and diel rhythms. Mar. Freshw. Behav. Physiol. 36 (3), 161–175.

Tettamanti, G., Grimaldi, A., Ferrarese, R., Palazzi, M., Perletti, G., Valvassori, R., Cooper, E.L., Lanzavecchia, G., de Eguileor, M., 2003. Leech responses to tissue transplantation. Tissue Cell 35, 199–212.

Thomas, A.W., Kavaliers, M., Prato, F.S., Ossenkopp, K.P., 1997. Antinociceptive effects of a pulsed magnetic field in the land snail, Cepaea nemoralis. Neurosci. Lett. 31 (2), 107–110, 222.

Tobin, D.M., Bargmann, C.I., 2004. Invertebrate nociception: behaviors, neurons and molecules. J. Neurobiol. 61, 161–174.

Tomsic, D., Maldonado, H., 1990. Central effect of morphine pretreatment on short- and long-term habituation to a danger stimulus in the crab *Chasmagnathus*. Pharmacol. Biochem. Behav. 36, 787–793.

Troup, M., Zalucki, O.H., Kottler, B.D., Karunanithi, S., Anggono, V., van Swinderen, B., 2019. Syntaxin1A neomorphic mutations promote rapid recovery from isoflurane anesthesia in *Drosophila melanogaster*. Anesthesiology 131 (3), 555–568.

Valles, S.M., Koehler, P.G., 1994. Influence of carbon dioxide anesthesia on chlorpyrifos toxicity in the German cockroach (*Dictyoptera: Blattellidae*). J. Econ. Entomol. 87 (3), 709–713.

Van den Spiegel, D., Jangoux, M., 1987. Cuvierian tubules of the holothuroid *Holothuria forskali* (Echinodermata): a morphofunctional study. Mar. Biol. 96, 263–275.

Wahltinez, S.J., Kroll, K.J., Nunamaker, E.A., Denslow, N.D., Stacy, N.I., 2021. Practical euthanasia method for common sea stars (*Asterias rubens*) that allows for high-quality RNA sampling. Animals 11, 1–12.

Walcourt, A., Ide, D., 1998. A system for the delivery of general anesthetics and other volatile agents to the fruit-fly *Drosophila melanogaster*. J. Neurosci. Methods 84, 115–119.

White, H.I., Hecht, T., Potgieter, B., 1996. The effect of four anaesthetics on *Haliotis midae* and their suitability for application in commercial abalone culture. Aquaculture 140, 145–151.

Wilkie, I.C., 1992. Variable tensility of the oral arm plate ligaments of the brittlestar *Ophiura ophiura* (Echinodermata: ophiuroidea). J. Zool. 228, 5–26.

Wood, J.B., Anderson, R.C., 2004. Interspecific evaluation of Octopus escape behavior. J. Appl. Anim. Welfare Sci. 7 (2), 95–106.

Woodall, A.J., McCrohan, C.R., 2000. Excitatory actions of propofol and ketamine in the snail *Lymnaea stagnalis*. Comp. Biochem. Physiol. 127C, 297–305.

Woodall, A.J., Naruo, H., Prince, D.J., Feng, Z.P., Winlow, W., Takasaki, M., Syed, N.I., 2003. Anesthetic treatment blocks synaptogenesis but not neuronal regeneration of cultured *Lymnaea* neurons. J. Neurophysiol. 90, 2232–2239.

Xie, Y.F., Huo, F.Q., Tang, J., 2009. Cerebral cortex modulation of pain. Acta Pharmacol. Sin. 30, 31–41.

Zachariah, T.T., Mitchell, M.A., Guichard, C.M., Singh, R.S., 2009. Isoflurane anesthesia of wild-caught goliath birdeater spiders (*Theraphosa blondi*) and Chilean rose spiders (*Grammostola rosea*). J. Zoo Wildl. Med. 40, 347–349. https://doi.org/10.1638/2007-0060.1.

Zachariah, T.T., Mitchell, M.A., Watson, M.K., et al., 2014. Effects of sevoflurane anesthesia on righting reflex and hemolymph gas analysis variables for Chilean rose tarantulas (*Grammostola rosea*). Am. J. Vet. Res. 75, 521–526. https://doi.org/10.2460/ajvr.75.6.521.

Zalucki, O., van Swinderen, B., 2016. What is unconsciousness in a fly or worm? A review of general anesthesia in different animal models. Conscious. Cognit. 44, 72–88.

Zmarzly, D.L., 1984. Distribution and ecology of shallow-water crinoids at Enewetak Atoll, Marshall Islands, with an annotated checklist of their symbionts. Pac. Sci. 38, 105–122.

Further reading

AAZV, 2006. Guidelines for Euthanasia of Non-domestic Animals.

Hancock-Ronemus, A., Buote, M., Lewbart, G.A., 2022. Crustaceans. In: Lewbart, G.A. (Ed.), Invertebrate Medicine, 3rd Ed. Wiley-Blackwell Publishing, Oxford, UK, pp. 367–398.

Walls, E.A., Berkson, J., Smith, S.A., 2002. The horseshoe crab, *Limulus polyphemus*: 200 million years of existence, 100 years of study. Rev. Fish. Sci. 10, 39–73.

Section VI

Special topics

Chapter 27

Management of chronic pain

Klas Abelson[1] and Carsten Grøndahl[2]

[1]*Department of Experimental Medicine, University of Copenhagen, Copenhagen, Denmark;* [2]*Veterinarian Department, Copenhagen Zoo, Copenhagen, Denmark*

Chapter outline

I. Introduction

Chronic pain is a significant problem in many aspects, not only causing suffering among humans and animals but also being a potential confounding factor and source of variation in animal experimentation. Thus, in order to minimize any suffering as well as a potential adverse impact on experimental results, the recognition, assessment, and alleviation of chronic pain in laboratory animals are highly important.

Detection and treatment of chronic pain conditions in animals are far from easy, though, since chronic pain may have many different causes related to different animal species, different background diseases, and a diversity of underlying mechanisms. Due to the complexity of chronic pain conditions, they are in general very difficult to treat and alleviate satisfactorily.

The aim of the present chapter is to present an overview of different types of chronic pain conditions based on their mechanisms of action, and to provide guidance on how to recognize, assess, and—where possible—alleviate such conditions.

A. Definition and prevalence of chronic pain

In human medicine, chronic pain is most often referred to as "pain which persists past the normal time of healing" (Bonica, 1953). More specifically, the International Association for the Study of Pain (IASP) has defined chronic pain as pain that persists or recurs for longer than 3 months (Treede et al., 2019). IASP has also published a range of articles on the classification and details of various conditions of chronic pain. These involve neuropathic pain (Scholz et al., 2019), cancer-related pain (Bennett et al., 2019), postsurgical and posttraumatic pain (Schug et al., 2019), orofacial pain and headache (Benoliel et al., 2019), visceral pain (Aziz et al., 2019), and musculoskeletal pain (hereunder inflammatory pain including rheumatoid arthritis and osteoarthritis (Perrot et al., 2019).

The IASP definition of pain includes pain in both humans and animals. The inclusion of nonhuman species in the definition was not explicit in the original definition from 1979, but in the revised definition published in 2020, it is emphasized that "verbal description is only one of several

Anesthesia and Analgesia in Laboratory Animals. https://doi.org/10.1016/B978-0-12-822215-7.00015-9

behaviors to express pain; inability to communicate does not negate the possibility that a human or a nonhuman animal experiences pain" (Raja et al., 2020). Chronic pain in animals, however, is not as well studied and understood within veterinary medicine as it is in human medicine. To understand chronic pain, it is important to be aware that chronic pain constitutes enduring syndromes characterized by unpleasant sensations or distress. Most important is that chronic pain is a pathological function of the nervous system and not simply persistent acute pain (Breen, 2002; Grachev et al., 2000). Therefore, the terms "adaptive" and "maladaptive" pain have been suggested to better distinguish between pain conditions, rather than acute or chronic pain (Adrian et al., 2017; Woolf, 2010). However, the term "chronic" is most commonly used and will be used in this chapter.

When it comes to laboratory animals, chronic pain can arise both intentionally, where the pain is part of the model, and unintentionally, due to unwanted effects from the invasive procedure used to induce the disease or phenomenon of interest. The chronic pain could also possibly arise from a naturally occurring disease in the animal, such as osteoarthritis or cancer. Although the precise mechanisms underlying the development of chronic pain are not yet fully known, neuroplasticity is likely critical to the transformation of acute to chronic pain (Jabbur and Saadé, 1999; Ji and Woolf, 2001). In neuropathic, inflammatory, and cancer models, neuroplastic changes proposed to be involved with chronic pain developed 2–3 weeks after pain induction or lesioning (Cain et al., 2001; Calzà et al., 1998; Hains et al., 2003; Schwei et al., 1999; Sharif Naeini et al., 2005; Shimoyama et al., 2005; Wang et al., 2002; Yen et al., 2006). Some of these changes peak at 4–6 weeks (Brenowitz, 1983; Yen et al., 2006), and sometimes between 3 and 11 weeks (Calzà et al., 2000) postpain initiation. Consequently, the IASP definition of chronic pain as a condition lasting more than 3 months is not fully applicable in the context of animal models. Thus, the above-mentioned data—as well as clinical experience—(Muir et al., 2004) support considering pain persisting for 1 month or more, rather than three, as a practical point for defining a transition from acute to chronic pain in animals.

The prevalence of chronic pain in laboratory animals is for the most part unknown, and it is most unlikely that such information will be forthcoming. A huge number of animals—especially mice and rats—are used for experimentation every year, and many of these experiments last for several weeks or months. Given the difficulties of detecting chronic pain in animals under these circumstances, it is practically impossible to determine any relevant figure of prevalence. However, by utilizing existing data or screening for chronic pain in selected models, it could be possible to draw conclusions that could help institutions judge the potential for chronic pain within a given establishment. For example, a study of outpatients at a veterinary teaching hospital demonstrated that the prevalence of chronic pain is higher in older populations (Muir et al., 2004). Naturally occurring hyperalgesia, allodynia (Kitagawa et al., 2005; Lovell et al., 2000; Novak et al., 1999), and chronic pain-related neuroplasticity (Iwata et al., 2002; Ramer and Bisby, 1998) occur in aged rats. The prevalence of osteoarthritis, a known etiology for chronic pain, is significantly greater in older macaques (Carlson et al., 1996; Lim et al., 1996; Rothschild et al., 1999), baboons (reviewed in (Black and Lane, 2002), cats, rats, mice, and guinea pigs (Bendele, 2001; Clarke and Bennett, 2006). Thus, the prevalence of chronic pain is likely high in populations of aged animals.

Conversely, data with respect to gender and chronic pain paints a different picture. In humans, the prevalence of chronic pain is considerably influenced by gender and found to be greater in female populations (Bartley and Fillingim, 2013; Marcus, 2003; Meana et al., 2004; Orfila et al., 2006; Rustøen et al., 2004). Sexual dimorphism relevant to chronic pain has also been demonstrated in rodent models. When compared to male rats, female rats have more persistent induced thermal hyperalgesia (Tall et al., 2001), greater induced mechanical allodynia (DeLeo and Rutkowski, 2000; LaCroix-Fralish et al., 2005), and reduced antinociception (Gaumond et al., 2005). The experimental data in this case points to sex as a factor in the development of induced chronic pain.

In addition to age- and sex-related differences, the strain of the mouse or rat has also been shown to influence the development of pain and response to analgesic treatment, which also should be considered when attempting to survey the prevalence of chronic pain (Hestehave et al., 2020; Smith, 2019).

B. Impact on experimental readouts

Numerous studies have demonstrated that chronic pain exerts both physiologic and behavioral effects, which may introduce confounding variables or bias experimental data. The following section will discuss some of the effects on the immune system, the endocrine system, the nervous system, and behavior related to anxiety and depression, as have been observed in models of chronic pain. These systems are closely integrated with each other and thus affect several physiologic and behavioral processes, and there is therefore great potential for chronic pain to confound experimental data in many research fields.

The section is not intended to provide a comprehensive review of the field, but to exemplify what systems may be affected and the potential consequences. The list and variety of consequences are likely to increase over time, given that more attention is paid to the consequences of chronic pain by researchers.

1. Immune system

Peripheral immunomodulation has been shown in rat models of chronic neuropathic pain. Chronic constriction injury (CCI) of the sciatic nerve in the rat causes a neuron-dependent increase in delayed-type hypersensitivity (DTH) and decreased antigen-specific IgG (Herzberg et al., 1994, 1996b). The neuropathic enhancement of DTH was ascribed to an increase in substance P release in CCI rats and activation of NK-1 receptors (Herzberg et al., 1996a). Upregulation of mRNA for the potent immune-modulating bradykinin receptor in lumbar dorsal horn ganglia (Levy and Zochodne, 2000) and increased levels of IL-1β, IL-2, IL-6, and IL-10 in sciatic nerve (Romero-Sandoval and Eisenach, 2006) have also been demonstrated in neuropathic rat models.

Neuroimmune activation (NA) is defined as the production of substances and the expression of surface antigens from endothelial and glial cells that enhance CNS immune cascades (DeLeo and Yezierski, 2001). In chronic pain, NA-mediated effects are likely due to activated astrocytes (DeLeo et al., 2004; Gordh et al., 2006). Astrocyte activation has been demonstrated in neuropathic and inflammatory models of chronic pain (Garrison et al., 1994; Herzberg and Sagen, 2001; Raghavendra et al., 2004; Tanga et al., 2004) and shown to persist for 150 days in a neuropathic model (Zhang and De Koninck, 2006). Once activated, astrocytes release proinflammatory and neuroexcitatory chemicals such as cytokines, reactive nitrogen species, prostaglandins, and glutamate (Liu et al., 2004; Wieseler-Frank et al., 2004, 2005). Astrocytes also regulate numerous aspects of neuronal physiology, including modulation of synaptic activity (Araque et al., 1999b). As such, the potential exists for chronic pain-activated astrocytes to influence a wide range of neuronal functions (Araque, 2006; Araque et al., 1999a; Eddleston and Mucke, 1993; Mucke and Eddleston, 1993).

2. Endocrine system

The hypothalamic–pituitary–adrenal (HPA) axis plays a central role in neuroendocrine responses to chronic pain. In humans, chronic pain can result in altered HPA function and stress-related syndromes, such as elevated cortisol levels, lower levels of cortisol due to enhanced negative feedback, or a delayed cortisol response from a stressor. These phenomena are associated with functional disturbances in the HPA (Gaab et al., 2005; McBeth et al., 2005). The relationship between pain and the endocrine system appears to be the same in animals. Pain, in general, affects the HPA axis since activation of the nociceptive system is a significant stressor. This may—besides being a welfare issue—have an impact on the experimental data, since HPA axis activation affects metabolism and thus introduces confounding variables (Abelson, 2017; Abelson et al., 2021). The effects on HPA function by chronic pain have been demonstrated in rats and appear to be model dependent. Changes in HPA function have been well documented in a rat model of induced inflammatory chronic pain but not in neuropathic models, for yet unknown reasons (Berke et al., 2022; Bomholt et al., 2005; Hestehave et al., 2020; Ulrich-Lai et al., 2006). Most data on the relationship between HPA function and chronic pain has been demonstrated in the rat adjuvant-induced inflammatory arthritis (AA) model. HPA alterations noted in the AA model include increased basal plasma ACTH and corticosterone, increased excretion of fecal corticosterone metabolites, increased hypothalamic vasopressin, induction of arginine vasopressin mRNA in the paraventricular nucleus (PVN), and proopiomelanocortin mRNA expression in the anterior pituitary, decreased portal (brain) corticotropin-releasing hormone (CRH) concentrations, and decreased expression of PVN CRH, and hippocampal mineralocorticoid and glucocorticoid receptor (GR) mRNA (Berke et al., 2022; Blackburn-Munro, 2004; Blackburn-Munro and Blackburn-Munro, 2001; Bomholt et al., 2005). In addition, AA has been shown to blunt acute physical and psychological stress-induced increases in plasma ACTH and cortisone (Aguilera et al., 1997; Harbuz et al., 1997; Windle et al., 2001) and their normal circadian fluctuations (Persellin et al., 1972; Sarlis et al., 1992).

3. Receptor systems and synaptic transmission

Chronic inflammation as well as nerve damage cause alterations in both the peripheral and central nervous systems and are significant causes of chronic pain conditions.

Inflammation initiates a cascade of events in the periphery, often referred to as the "inflammatory soup" with the production and release of prostaglandins, bradykinin, serotonin, and histamine, among others, in the injured tissue, which causes peripheral sensitization and activation of afferent nerve fibers. Subsequent synaptic transmission in the spinal cord dorsal horn involves activation of excitatory receptor systems such as N-methyl-D-aspartate (NMDA)- and alfa-amino-3-hydroxy-5-methyl-4-isoxazolepropionic acid (AMPA)-receptors, neuropeptide substance P (SP), and calcitonin gene-related peptide (CGRP), as well as inhibitory systems such as the gamma-aminobutyric acid (GABA), neuropeptide Y (NPY), opioid, serotoninergic, noradrenergic, and cholinergic systems. In addition, non-neuronal cell types such as astrocytes and microglia also regulate nociceptive transmission in the dorsal horn. Sensitization at the spinal cord level is primarily mediated through "wind-up" mechanisms involving NMDA and AMPA receptors (reviewed in (Abelson, 2005; D'Mello and Dickenson, 2008). The mentioned mechanisms are most beneficial to the organism during inflammation under normal circumstances. However, if the inflammation remains and becomes chronic, the risk of alterations in the systems described being prolonged is increased, resulting in chronic pain (Abelson, 2017).

Nerve damage in the peripheral nervous system is often caused by trauma, such as surgical procedures, but can also result from various neurological diseases. A common consequence of peripheral nerve damage is the formation of traumatic neuromas, i.e., small bundles forming tumors along the nerve at the injured site that cause intense pain arising from a simple touch or without external stimulation. Such formations are not uncommon after surgery in humans and are also known to be present in common laboratory species like rats and pigs (Alant et al., 2012; Sandercock et al., 2016). Another consequence is damage to the myelin sheaths surrounding Aβ- or Aδ-fibres, which may cause ephaptic transmission (communication that does not involve synapses) between Aβ- and C-fibres or between damaged Aβ- and Aδ-fibres, giving rise to pain from nonnoxious stimuli similar to that arising from neuromas (D'Mello and Dickenson, 2008).

Peripheral nerve damage, similar to persistent nociceptive input from chronic inflammation, will result in plasticity changes both in the spinal cord and in the somatosensory cortex, involving several of the above-mentioned receptor systems as well as microglia (Basbaum et al., 2009; Hiraga et al., 2022).

These alterations are often the target of interest in animal models of chronic pain, where the objective is to seek an understanding of the etiology of pain. However, when chronic pain occurs through natural processes, unintentionally after surgery or other interventions in animal models, where the pain is not a part of the model, the alterations and their potential treatments may have a negative and confounding impact on the experimental data. Hence, both animal welfare and validity of research outcomes should be considered when an experimental animal is experiencing chronic pain.

4. Behavior

Chronic pain is known to cause depression, anxiety, and impaired emotional decision-making in humans (Apkarian et al., 2004; Bair et al., 2003; Dworkin and Gitlin, 1991; Wilson et al., 2001), and this pain-depression comorbidity is also present in animals (Li, 2015). Chronic inflammatory and neuropathic pain in mice causes anxiety-like behaviors in the light-dark and elevated plus-maze tests (Narita et al., 2006a,b). Chronic pain has also been shown to alter gene expression (neurokinin (NK)-1 receptor, brain-derived neurotrophic factor (BDNF), CRH, and GR mRNA) and neurogenesis in limbic brain areas of rats, changes associated with anxiety and depression (Dranovsky and Hen, 2006; Duric and McCarson, 2006; Ulrich-Lai et al., 2006). Furthermore, the effects of induced inflammatory and neuropathic pain on animal performance in sucrose preference tests and forced swim tests have been recognized (Li, 2015).

II. Recognition and assessment of chronic pain

In experiments lasting for a month or more, any pain present should be classified as chronic, since pain persisting beyond the time when wound or lesion healing should be complete is to be considered chronic pain. Pain present in experiments where animal models are studied as models for human chronic pain conditions should also be classified as chronic, since they are mimicking chronic pain conditions even if the duration of the study does not exceed a month. When studying animal models for chronic pain conditions such as arthritis or neuropathy, specific parameters relevant to that specific model are studied as part of the investigation. How these models are established and what parameters are relevant are discussed in detail in other publications focusing on animal models of pain (Abelson et al., 2021) and will not be discussed further in the present chapter. Instead, particular attention is paid to the recognition and assessment of potential chronic pain that may arise unintentionally in animals used in prolonged studies, as it is in these situations where animal welfare may be compromised along with the risk of confounding experimental data.

Recognizing and assessing pain in many animals is generally a difficult task, especially when attempting to detect pain at a stage before it becomes severe, reaching a humane endpoint. Chronic pain is particularly difficult to recognize since obvious signs of pain may occur spontaneously and irregularly, or be of a character causing apparently subtle signs of pain. A comprehensive monitoring protocol should therefore always be established with several parameters, since this increases the likelihood of detecting less obvious signs of pain. The following section will discuss in general terms what possible parameters are present and how a monitoring protocol should be applied. We consider these applicable to both acute and chronic pains, and rather related to the experimental conditions and other circumstances than to the precise definition of the pain condition. Further, many of the parameters listed below are the result of nociception-induced stress or reflex responses, rather than an actual painful experience. Hence, it may not be possible to actually recognize and assess pain in itself. However, stress reactions or reflex responses elicited by a nociceptive event serve as a proxy measurement of pain, and are therefore considered valid parameters (Abelson, 2017; National Research Council Committee on and Alleviation of Pain in Laboratory, 2009).

There are different ways to recognize pain, and different methods may have different objectives. The objective of the assessment can either be to investigate whether, and to what extent, a certain procedure will cause pain and stress in the animal, and how this can be minimized or eliminated using different treatments. This is of utmost importance to establish relevant pain treatment protocols for a certain experimental procedure. Or the objective could be to assess any ongoing pain in the animal at a certain time point to determine whether there is a need for additional pain treatment or whether a humane endpoint has been reached. Regardless of the objective, methods for recognizing and assessing pain can be categorized into physiological parameters, biomarkers, and behavioral and clinical signs.

Physiologic parameters such as blood pressure, pulse, and body temperature tend to increase during pain and stress, and quantification of these can indicate if an animal is experiencing pain or stress. These parameters are fairly easily monitored in larger animals, but for rodents and other smaller animals, it may require radio telemetry for accurate measurement, which involves major surgery. Hence, physiological parameters in smaller animals are not used for routine welfare assessments, but mainly for determining effect of procedures and analgesic protocols, and often only in connection with studies where telemetry is applied for other purposes. One should also be aware that physiologic parameters can be rather insensitive and nonspecific, and influenced by other parameters (National Research Council Committee on and Alleviation of Pain in Laboratory, 2009). In addition, physiological parameters may not be applicable for chronic pain conditions, as animals may adapt their allostatic functions to the chronic pain condition.

There are several biomarkers for pain and stress. The most commonly applied biomarker for stress is probably increased levels of the glucocorticoid cortisol (in large animals such as pigs) or corticosterone (in small animals such as rodents) (Morton and Hau, 2021). These can be quantified in blood, plasma, serum, and urine, and their metabolites can be extracted from feces (Abelson et al., 2009; Kalliokoski et al., 2010; Siswanto et al., 2008). Quantification from the blood for chronic pain monitoring would call for repeated sampling, which is impractical unless automated blood sampling is possible. Therefore, quantification of fecal corticosteroid metabolites is preferable since it is noninvasive and can be done without any restriction in the duration of sampling. Limitations related to measuring chronic pain and stress are the facts that the response may be blunted in adjuvant-induced arthritic models (discussed above) and that long-term pain and stress may cause neuroendocrine dysfunction with depletion of the adrenal glands (Husebye et al., 2021; Smith and Vale, 2006). Other biomarkers are, for instance, secretory IgA quantified from saliva in larger animals to assess immune suppression due to long-term stress (Staley et al., 2018) or urinary excretion of 8-Oxo-2′-deoxyguanosine (8-oxo-dG) or isoprostanes (biologically active lipids) that are produced as a result of DNA damage after oxidative stress (Montuschi et al., 2004; Valavanidis et al., 2009). The peptide c-Fos can be quantified in the spinal cord, since c-fos expression is upregulated during nociceptive activation (Harris, 1998). Similar to physiological parameters, biomarkers are used for determining the effects of experimental procedures and analgesic protocols, since their quantification requires laboratory analysis or, in the case of c-Fos, only after the animal has been culled, and can thus only be used retrospectively.

Assessment of behavior and clinical signs can either be done subjectively or objectively. A subjective assessment can be performed by mere observation of the animal for a certain period of time and by subsequently giving a score on, for instance, a visual analog scale. The score is based on the observer's previous experiences, knowledge, and interpretation of the situation to assess the animal's condition. Although an easy and not particularly time-consuming method, it has the disadvantage that there may be considerable differences in the assessment between different observers (Roughan and Flecknell, 2006). An objective assessment is where a welfare monitoring protocol including a number of quantifiable or strictly defined behavioral parameters and clinical signs (and physiological parameters and biomarkers if relevant) is applied.

Behavioral monitoring requires an extensive knowledge of the animals' normal species-specific behavior, and knowledge of what can be expected during a certain experimental condition or from treatment with anesthetic and analgesic drugs or a certain substance being investigated as a drug candidate. Based on such knowledge, deviations from normal behavioral patterns can be assessed, for instance, increased or reduced activity, changed body posture or gait, licking or biting, abnormal sounds, or grooming behavior. Similarly, clinical signs such as reduced body weight gain, loss of body weight, reduced appetite, diarrhea, piloerection, and chromodacryorrhea (in rats) are closely related to pain and stress and should be included in a welfare monitoring scheme (Abelson, 2017; Morton and Hau, 2021).

Abdominal pain, such as after abdominal surgery, causes twitches of the skin of the back, abdominal press, writhing of the abdomen, staggering, back arching, and loss of balance with subsequent falling in rats and mice. These parameters are easily recognized with relatively little training needed by the observer and correlate well with pain from the abdomen (Jacobsen et al., 2012; Roughan and Flecknell, 2003, 2004), but their application in chronic pain conditions has not been studied in detail, as far as the authors are aware.

Typical symptoms associated with inflammatory and neuropathic pain are hyperalgesia, allodynia, and spontaneous pain. Hyperalgesia and allodynia can be assessed with numerous tests for evoked pain, which are those used in studies of animal models of these pain conditions, as described in (Abelson et al., 2021). Examples of such tests are von Frey filament testing and paw pressure for mechanical allodynia or hyperalgesia, or various thermal tests for heat or cold allodynia or hyperalgesia. Behaviors associated with spontaneous pain include licking/directed grooming (Grelik et al., 2005), biting, autotomy, scratching, lameness, paw lifting or shaking (Santos Tde et al., 1999), and guarding the affected area (Kingery and Vallin, 1989; Xu et al., 1997). Another method for assessing spontaneous pain, in general, is scoring facial expressions. Several research groups have established grimace scales with defined action units in facial expression in several animal species, including mice, rats, rabbits, sheep, goats, and horses. Examples of action units in small rodents are orbital tightening and altered position of ears, whiskers, noses, and cheeks. Although grimace scales were originally thought to only appear with acute spontaneous pain, recent studies have shown that these scales may also be applied to some chronic pain conditions, although more research is needed (Mogil et al., 2020; Mota-Rojas et al., 2020).

Apart from behaviors discussed above, analysis of the animal's gait or weight-bearing pattern can contribute significantly to the assessment of the pain, although this may require special equipment to provide accurate measurements and can be exhaustively time-consuming (Abelson et al., 2021; Tappe-Theodor et al., 2019), but it should be considered if available and feasible. The same goes for the assessment of nest building and burrowing behavior in small rodents, which can provide important information about the overall well-being of the animal (Deacon et al., 2001; Deacon, 2006; Gallo et al., 2020; Oliver et al., 2018).

In summary, recognition and assessment of pain, and pain-related stress, and welfare impairment is a task requiring time, motivation, and resources. There is no one-for-all solution, and thus a proper monitoring protocol needs to be established for each specific experimental situation, and this involves a thorough literature review of expected effects on pain and welfare discussion with and consultation from colleagues involved in similar experiments and experienced veterinary staff, and—not to forget—pilot studies to evaluate any risk of development of chronic pain or other welfare issues in the specific experiment.

III. Treatment

The key elements of the treatment of chronic pain are that the development of chronic pain should be prevented if possible and that the ultimate goal of the treatment should be to return pathological neurologic-endocrine-immune systems responsible for chronic pain to normal function. Unfortunately, it is painfully evident from human medicine that neither has had tremendous success. Once chronic pain develops, treatment involves a management endeavor, likely for the life of the afflicted. Chronic pain causes both substantial changes to pain signal transmission (wind-up) and perception, and radical changes in receptor density and location. Both peripheral and central sensitization increases pain impulses reaching supraspinal structures and are reducing the quality of life. Attempts to treat chronic pain are thus very challenging and often frustrating. In the situation of experimental animals, chronic pain naturally affects the animals' welfare. In addition, it could also be a significant confounder of experimental data, as could any treatment. This must therefore be carefully considered when designing monitoring and treatment options.

In people, the prevalence of chronic pain associated with surgical procedures is about 10%−50%. Postsurgical chronic pain can arise from inflammation or more likely from iatrogenic nerve damage (Kehlet et al., 2006). Although risk factors for the development of postsurgical chronic pain in animals have not been identified, good tissue handling, avoiding damage to major nerves, and using minimally invasive techniques (e.g., laparoscopic, thoracoscopic) during surgical procedures may help reduce the potential for developing chronic pain (Kehlet et al., 2006). It is also noteworthy that intense, acute, postoperative pain is a risk factor for the development of chronic pain (Perkins and Kehlet, 2000).

Although probably efficacious for preventing chronic inflammatory pain, preemptive and aggressive multimodal analgesia have not proven to be prophylactic "magic-bullets" for the development of postsurgical neuropathic pain (reviewed in (Brennan and Kehlet, 2005). Experimental and clinical evidence suggest that extended duration of complete nerve blockade combined with drugs to prevent glial activation may be needed to prevent postsurgical neuropathic pain. Clearly, novel strategies targeting neuronal and nonneuronal mechanisms need to be explored to better manage postsurgical pain. Considering the complexity of the laboratory animal environment, and the fact that there are few clinically tested regimes for managing chronic pain in animals, making specific treatment recommendations would not be productive. Therefore, the following section and references (Amir et al., 2006; Backonja et al., 2006; Chevlen et al., 2005; Leo, 2006; Schnitzer, 2006) are intended to serve as guidelines for treatment. Veterinary specific options for treating chronic pain (osteoarthritis, cancer, oral) may be found in (Beckman, 2006; Flecknell, 2001; Lester and Gaynor, 2000; McLaughlin, 2000). Doses and additional information for many of the drugs described may be found in (Grimm et al., 2015).

A. Ion channel modulation

1. *Sodium channel blockers*

a Lidocaine, mexiletine

Na channel blockers suppress spontaneous ectopic discharges at drug concentrations that do not inhibit normal impulse generation and propagation. As a result, these drugs can relieve chronic neuropathic pain with a high therapeutic index. Intravenous lidocaine and 5% lidocaine patches (the first drug FDA approved for postherpetic neuralgia) have both been shown efficacious for the treatment of neuropathic pain in people. Intravenous lidocaine has been shown to relieve neuropathic pain in rats (infusion) and people (bolus, infusion, and bolus plus infusion) for 3−21 days (Chaplan et al., 1995; Mao and Chen, 2000). Using published doses and infusion rates, lidocaine may prove effective in other species as well. Although the pharmacokinetics of a 5% lidocaine patch have been reported in dogs (Weiland et al., 2006) and appear to be well tolerated, no clinical studies have been performed. Mexiletine is an oral congener of lidocaine demonstrating, variable success in human clinical trials (Duby et al., 2004; Kingery, 1997). Some evidence suggests that a positive test with IV lidocaine predicts pain relief with mexiletine (Galer et al., 1996). Although used as an antiarrhythmic in veterinary medicine, mexiletine's efficacy for neuropathic pain in animals is unknown.

b Phenytoin

The anticonvulsant phenytoin is a classic neuroactive drug, reportedly effective in treating neuropathic pain in humans (reviewed in (Markman and Dworkin, 2006)) but with variable efficacy in experimental rat models (Hunter et al., 1997; Ko et al., 2006). Phenytoin's mechanism of action appears to be Na-channel blockade and inhibition of presynaptic glutamate release (Yaari et al., 1986). Although used as an anticonvulsant, its utility for managing chronic pain in animals is unexplored. Excessive sedation, ataxia, hepatocellular toxicity, and potential drug interactions may be limiting factors for its use. A potent analgesic impact of phenytoin on oxaliplatin-induced mechanical and cold hypersensitivity, and a modest effect on altered voluntary/spontaneous behavior have also been shown (Draxler et al., 2021).

2. *Calcium channel blockers*

Gabapentin and pregabalin are GABA analogs that bind to the $\alpha2\beta$ subunit of N-type calcium channels, a subunit upregulated by tissue inflammation and nerve injury. Although their definitive mechanism of action is unknown, gabapentin and pregabalin are postulated to inhibit pronociceptive neurotransmitter release from sensory nerve terminals (reviewed in (McGivern, 2006)). Gabapentin (and likely pregabalin) does not have any intrinsic analgesic activity and can be pronociceptive in the absence of clinical or pathologic pain (Gaynor and Muir, 2015). Both drugs are labeled for the treatment of a variety of neuropathic pain syndromes in people with pregabalin having improved potency and superior bioavailability. Experimental studies in rats and mice demonstrate that gabapentin and pregabalin may be viable drugs for treating neuropathic pain in animals (Draxler et al., 2021; Field et al., 1999; Laughlin et al., 2002; Peters et al., 2005; Walczak and Beaulieu, 2006; Walczak et al., 2006) and may be able to prevent the development of neuropathic pain if administered before nerve injury (Yasuda et al., 2005). Both drugs may be used for monotherapy or combined with other medications (Gilron et al., 2006), and some evidence suggests that gabapentin may be more effective when combined with morphine (Baillie and Power, 2005).

B. Tricyclic antidepressants

Tricyclic antidepressants (TCAs) are considered first-line drugs for the treatment of neuropathic pain and are used to treat a wide variety of chronic pain syndromes. Both experimental and clinical evidence indicates that these drugs have analgesic activity independent of their mood-altering properties (Fishbain et al., 2000; Max et al., 1987). Amitriptyline is the gold standard for analgesic antidepressants. Together with its metabolite nortriptyline, this drug has the best-documented efficacy in the treatment of neuropathic and many nonneuropathic pain syndromes (Bryson and Wilde, 1996; Saarto and Wiffen, 2007). Amitriptyline's analgesic mechanism of action has been ascribed to enhancing the activity of antinociceptive bulbospinal pathways by decreasing the reuptake of serotonin and norepinephrine at either spinal terminals or the brain stem (reviewed in (Esser and Sawynok, 1999)). Additional central and peripheral mechanisms for amitriptyline analgesia have been proposed. These include modulating central cytokine release and function (Obuchowicz et al., 2006; Reynolds et al., 2004), peripheral analgesia through blockade of tetrodotoxin-resistant Na channels (Bräu et al., 2001), and reduced adenosine reuptake (Lynch et al., 2005; Sawynok et al., 1999, 2005). Amitriptyline is used to treat idiopathic feline lower urinary tract disease (Chew et al., 1998) and may be effective for other chronic pain syndromes in animals. Experimentally, amitriptyline has been shown to be pro and antinociceptive or nonefficacious depending on the model used, route of administration, and behavioral endpoint (Beyreuther et al., 2006; Esser et al., 2001; LaBuda and Little, 2005; Walczak et al., 2005, 2006). Duloxetine, a serotonin-norepinephrine reuptake inhibitor (SNRI), significantly reduced oxaliplatin-induced chemotherapy-induced painful neuropathy in rats (Balayssac et al., 2014).

C. Opioids

As a class, opioids are some of the most potent and controversial drugs available for the treatment of chronic pain, regardless of etiology. Opioids have both central and peripheral effects that are mediated by complex interactions with mu, kappa, and delta receptors. Requisite dosing intervals (q 2–6 hours) make most current opioid formulations impractical for the management of chronic pain in laboratory animals. Patch, implant, or sustained-release formulations (fentanyl and buprenorphine) (Clemensen et al., 2018; Kleppner et al., 2010) may be useful, and the development of liposome-encapsulated oxymorphone holds great promise as well (Smith et al., 2003). Oral sustained-release preparations (morphine oxycodone, buprenorphine, and dihydrocodeine) are available and useful (Abelson et al., 2012), but may be poorly and erratically absorbed (KuKanich et al., 2005). Opioids are most effective in treating inflammatory and malignancy-related chronic pain, but questions persist about their use in the treatment of neuropathic pain. Although effective in many neuropathic conditions, their usefulness in central pain is still equivocal (reviewed in (Katz and Benoit, 2005)). Rodent studies indicate that buprenorphine (Christoph et al., 2005; Kouya et al., 2002), morphine (Decosterd et al., 2004; Walczak et al., 2005; Yasuda et al., 2005), and fentanyl (Stewart and Martin, 2003; Womer and Shannon, 2000; Zurek et al., 2001) are effective in the treatment of neuropathic pain. As with TCAs, opioid efficacy varies in experimental studies by drug, model, route of administration, and dependent measure (reviewed in (Martin and Eisenach, 2001)). In human medicine, transdermal fentanyl is recommended for, and shown to be efficacious in, the management of osteoarthritis and other conditions that do not respond well to nonopioid analgesics (Babić-Naglić et al., 2002; Langford et al., 2006; Le Loët et al., 2005). Transdermal fentanyl has demonstrated use for acute pain in cats, dogs, and pigs (Harvey-Clark et al., 2000; Hofmeister and Egger, 2004; Lafuente et al., 2005; Malavasi et al., 2006; Romans et al., 2005), and with some success also in rats (Clemensen et al., 2018).

Combination of mu opioids with cannabinoid receptor two-agonists has a strong opioid-sparing effect and a significant synergistic inhibition of preclinical pain while significantly reducing opioid-induced unwanted side effects (Grenald et al., 2017). Codeine has a dose-dependent effect on postsurgical pain-induced hypersensitivities (Draxler et al., 2021).

D. Corticosteroids

Corticosteroids as a group may be used as a primary or adjunctive treatment for chronic pain. In people, corticosteroids are used as adjuncts in the management of cancer-related chronic pain (Lussier et al., 2004) and may be a primary treatment for some neuropathic pain syndromes (Dabby et al., 2006; Kingery, 1997). Experimental models show dichotomous results with respect to glucocorticoids and neuropathic pain. Several studies suggest that glucocorticoids can inhibit and reverse neuropathic pain, possibly by inhibiting glial activation (Takeda et al., 2004) or central cytokine production (Xie et al., 2006). Others show upregulation of glucocorticoid receptors in response to induced neuropathic pain and a role for GR antagonists as treatment (Takasaki et al., 2005; Wang et al., 2004). When used judiciously, an experimental study in southern pig-tailed macaques (Leverenz et al., 1999) and clinical use in cats and dogs demonstrate that corticosteroids can be used for months with mild adverse effects (Cizinauskas et al., 2000; Preziosi et al., 2003).

E. Nonsteroidal anti-inflammatory drugs

Nonsteroidal antiinflammatory drugs (NSAIDs) are the most commonly used analgesic drugs in veterinary medicine. They also have the distinction of being the only medications with documented clinical efficacy and safety in the treatment of chronic pain (osteoarthritis). NSAIDs are primarily indicated for the treatment of pain arising from inflammatory musculoskeletal disease and osteoarthritis. Although not universally effective, NSAIDs can have a place in the management of chronic neuropathic or cancer pain (Robertson, 2008; Suyama et al., 2004) and can be synergistic with opioids. Other advantages of NSAIDs include the commercial availability of a wide variety of drugs in enteral and parenteral forms, which are useful in numerous species. Initial drug selection is usually based on clinical experience and is not always effective. For reasons unknown, animals (including people) may respond to one NSAID but not another, necessitating empirical trials to find an effective drug. To avoid toxicity or potentially fatal effects with long-term NSAID use, it is critical to use the lowest effective dose and, unless experimentally justified, never exceed approved or published dosage and never initiate the use of another NSAID or corticosteroid without an appropriate washout time (5–10 days) between drugs (Boston et al., 2003; KuKanich et al., 2005; Lascelles et al., 2005a,b; Nakagawa et al., 2005; Reed, 2002).

Periodic monitoring for fecal occult blood and evaluation of complete blood count (CBC) and serum chemistry are prudent during chronic NSAID treatment as well. For chronic use (weeks to years), a COX-2-selective NSAID may afford a greater margin of safety over a nonselective drug with respect to gastrointestinal and renal toxicity. However, all NSAIDs have ulcerogenic and nephrotoxic potential, and COX-2 selective inhibitors have been postulated to be prothrombotic, atherogenic, and hypertensive (Bolten, 2006; Krotz et al., 2005; Wang et al., 2005; Weir et al., 2003).

High doses of meloxicam (≥3.75 mg/kg) and ibuprofen (≥25 mg/kg) are predictably ulcerogenic in several rodent models (Bonabello et al., 2003; Khan and Akhter, 2005). Caution should also be taken when combining NSAID use with high doses of buprenorphine, due to a demonstrated risk of peritonitis development in rats (Hestehave et al., 2017). Some experimental evidence suggests that COX-2 selective agents have reduced ulcerogenic potential in rodents and may be safe for long-term use at recommended doses (Brown et al., 2000; Rainsford, 1987). A wide variety of NSAIDs are used acutely in ruminants, swine, lagomorphs, birds, and rodents.

Naproxen reduces most behavioral manifestations of carrageenan-induced inflammatory pain in a rat study (Draxler et al., 2021). The results show a behavioral impact of carrageenan-induced inflammatory pain on nonevoked behavioral parameters and distress beyond mechanical and thermal hypersensitivities. The behavioral test battery captured the clinically well-established potency of naproxen as an analgesic for inflammatory pain.

F. NMDA receptor antagonists

Ketamine, dextromethorphan, and amantadine are NMDA receptor (NMDAR) antagonists used in veterinary medicine that appear to have a role in the management of chronic pain (Fisher et al., 2000). NMDAR antagonists can inhibit the development and maintenance of central sensitization and are synergistic with opioids and NSAIDs (Petrenko et al., 2003; Visser and Schug, 2006). Thus, the primary indication for the use of NMDAR antagonists appears to be adjunctive or part of multimodal therapy with the goal of controlling central sensitization. Regrettably, their use is often limited by difficulty in administration or unacceptable adverse effects. Ketamine is one of the most potent NMDAR antagonists available, and one case report describes its use in the management of postamputation clinical signs in a cat (O'Hagan, 2006). Unfortunately, ketamine is rather difficult to use in the management of chronic pain since this application generally requires intravenous infusion protocols. Dextromethorphan has been used for years as an antitussive, and doses of 2 mg/kg BID PO appear to be well tolerated in dogs over 2 weeks of age (Dodman et al., 2004). However, the pharmacokinetic profile and adverse effects of dextromethorphan may limit its utility in the management of chronic pain (Kukanich and Papich, 2004). Amantadine is another oral form of NMDAR antagonist suggested for treating chronic pain in dogs and cats (Gaynor and Muir, 2015). None of the NMDAR antagonists have been evaluated in veterinary clinical trials for the management of chronic pain. For a review of NMDAR antagonists, including referenced doses, see Pozzi et al. (Pozzi et al., 2006).

G. Novel α^2A-agonists

PT-31 (a novel alpha2A-adrenoceptor agonist) shows promise as an oral analgesic for both acute and chronic pain without locomotor or hemodynamic impairments (Sudo et al., 2017). It is suggested that several pathways are responsible for this effect due to the attenuation of the analgesia by yohimbine, atropine, L-NAME, and naloxone.

H. Nerve growth factor antibodies (NGF-abs)

NGF-abs have now been shown to reduce chronic pain in rats and mice (Wild et al., 2007). In several neuropathic pain models, such as complete Freund's adjuvant-induced hind-paw inflammation, spinal nerve ligation, and streptozotocin-induced neuropathic pain models, a single treatment by an intraperitoneal injection of a polyclonal antiNGF antibody reversed tactile allodynia 3–7 days posttreatment, while the effects of thermal hyperalgesia were less prominent. In the mouse CCI model, a mouse monoclonal antiNGF antibody could reverse tactile allodynia 2 weeks postsurgery. Repeated administration during 3 weeks produced a sustained reversal (days 4–21) of tactile allodynia that returned 5 days after the end of dosing in the CCI mice. Hence, NGF seems to play an important role in models of neuropathic and inflammatory pain in rodents, with no observed tolerance or antagonism. NGF-Abs are marketed for use in both dogs and cats with monthly injections.

I. Substance P/neurokinin 1 (NK1) receptor antagonist

Aprepitant has been shown to have a significant impact on CCI-induced behavioral responses in rats, with the improvement of general locomotion and overall activity. Aprepitant administration induced a significant increase in grooming behavior in the splash test after sucrose application, and in the tests for affective behavior, aprepitant reduced the reduction of exploratory behavior and improved the nest-building behavior (Draxler et al., 2021).

J. Hyperbaric oxygen

Hyperbaric oxygen treatment appears to be successful in relieving neuropathic pain for an extended period of time. In two common models of neuropathic pain, L5 ligation and cCCI of the sciatic nerve, hyperbaric oxygen demonstrated significant relief of neuropathic pain during a 2-week period, with CCI animals recovering more quickly with a maintained recovery throughout the posttreatment period (Thompson et al., 2010).

Acknowledgments

This chapter is a revision of the chapter "Management of Chronic Pain" by George J. DeMarco, published in the previous (2nd) edition of Anesthesia and Analgesia in Laboratory Animals. The authors would like to express their sincere gratitude to Dr. DeMarco for his invaluable contribution to the field through that chapter and acknowledge the importance of his previous work has had for our authoring of the present chapter. We would also like to stress that parts of Dr. DeMarco's original chapter have been reused in the revised version—either rephrased and supplemented or in its original form.

References

Abelson, K., 2005. Acetylcholine in Spinal Pain Modulation: An in Vivo Study in the Rat. Acta Universitatis Upsaliensis, Uppsala.

Abelson, K.S., Fard, S.S., Nyman, J., Goldkuhl, R., Hau, J., 2009. Distribution of [3H]-corticosterone in urine, feces and blood of male Sprague-Dawley rats after tail vein and jugular vein injections. In Vivo 23, 381–386.

Abelson, K.S.P., 2017. Anaesthesia, analgesia, and euthanasia. In: Sørensen, D.B. (Ed.), Laboratory Animal Science: A Handbook on Experimental Animals and Animal Experimentation. Saxo, Copenhagen.

Abelson, K.S.P., Heegaard, A.M., Roughan, J., 2021. Animal models in pain research. In: Hau, J., Schapiro, S.J. (Eds.), Handbook of Laboratory Animal Science: Essential Principles and Practices, fourth ed. CRC Press, Bocar Raton.

Abelson, K.S.P., Jacobsen, K.R., Sundbom, R., Kalliokoski, O., Hau, J., 2012. Voluntary ingestion of nut paste for administration of buprenorphine in rats and mice. Lab. Anim. 46, 349–351.

Adrian, D., Papich, M., Baynes, R., Murrell, J., Lascelles, B.D.X., 2017. Chronic maladaptive pain in cats: a review of current and future drug treatment options. Vet. J. 230, 52–61.

Aguilera, G., Jessop, D.S., Harbuz, M.S., Kiss, A., Lightman, S.L., 1997. Differential regulation of hypothalamic pituitary corticotropin releasing hormone receptors during development of adjuvant-induced arthritis in the rat. J. Endocrinol. 153, 185–191.

Alant, J.D., Kemp, S.W., Khu, K.J., Kumar, R., Webb, A.A., Midha, R., 2012. Traumatic neuroma in continuity injury model in rodents. J. Neurotrauma 29, 1691–1703.

Amir, R., Argoff, C.E., Bennett, G.J., Cummins, T.R., Durieux, M.E., Gerner, P., Gold, M.S., Porreca, F., Strichartz, G.R., 2006. The role of sodium channels in chronic inflammatory and neuropathic pain. J. Pain 7, S1–S29.

Apkarian, A.V., Sosa, Y., Krauss, B.R., Thomas, P.S., Fredrickson, B.E., Levy, R.E., Harden, R.N., Chialvo, D.R., 2004. Chronic pain patients are impaired on an emotional decision-making task. Pain 108, 129–136.

Araque, A., 2006. Astrocyte-neuron signaling in the brain–implications for disease. Curr. Opin. Invest. Drugs 7, 619–624.

Araque, A., Parpura, V., Sanzgiri, R.P., Haydon, P.G., 1999a. Tripartite synapses: glia, the unacknowledged partner. Trends Neurosci. 22, 208–215.

Araque, A., Sanzgiri, R.P., Parpura, V., Haydon, P.G., 1999b. Astrocyte-induced modulation of synaptic transmission. Can. J. Physiol. Pharmacol. 77, 699–706.

Aziz, Q., Giamberardino, M.A., Barke, A., Korwisi, B., Baranowski, A.P., Wesselmann, U., Rief, W., Treede, R.-D., Pain, T.I.T.F.T.C.O.C., 2019. The IASP classification of chronic pain for ICD-11: chronic secondary visceral pain. Pain 160, 69–76.

Babić-Naglić, D., Jajić, Z., Gnjidić, Z., Stambuk, B., 2002. Treatment of chronic pain–use of transdermal fentanyl (Durogesic TTS). Reumatizam 49, 33–37.

Backonja, M.M., Irving, G., Argoff, C., 2006. Rational multidrug therapy in the treatment of neuropathic pain. Curr. Pain Headache Rep. 10, 34–38.

Baillie, J.K., Power, I., 2005. Morphine, gabapentin, or their combination for neuropathic pain. N. Engl. J. Med. 352, 2650–2651.

Bair, M.J., Robinson, R.L., Katon, W., Kroenke, K., 2003. Depression and pain comorbidity: a literature review. Arch. Intern. Med. 163, 2433–2445.

Balayssac, D., Ling, B., Ferrier, J., Pereira, B., Eschalier, A., Authier, N., 2014. Assessment of thermal sensitivity in rats using the thermal place preference test: description and application in the study of oxaliplatin-induced acute thermal hypersensitivity and inflammatory pain models. Behav. Pharmacol. 25, 99–111.

Bartley, E.J., Fillingim, R.B., 2013. Sex differences in pain: a brief review of clinical and experimental findings. Br. J. Anaesth. 111, 52–58.

Basbaum, A.I., Bautista, D.M., Scherrer, G., Julius, D., 2009. Cellular and molecular mechanisms of pain. Cell 139, 267–284.

Beckman, B.W., 2006. Pathophysiology and management of surgical and chronic oral pain in dogs and cats. J. Vet. Dent. 23, 50–60.

Bendele, A.M., 2001. Animal models of osteoarthritis. J. Musculoskelet. Neuronal Interact. 1, 363–376.

Bennett, M.I., Kaasa, S., Barke, A., Korwisi, B., Rief, W., Treede, R.-D., Pain, T.I.T.F.T.C.O.C., 2019. The IASP classification of chronic pain for ICD-11: chronic cancer-related pain. Pain 160, 38–44.

Benoliel, R., Svensson, P., Evers, S., Wang, S.-J., Barke, A., Korwisi, B., Rief, W., Treede, R.-D., Pain, T.I.T.F.T.C.O.C., 2019. The IASP classification of chronic pain for ICD-11: chronic secondary headache or orofacial pain. Pain 160, 60–68.

Berke, M.S., Fensholdt, L.K.D., Hestehave, S., Kalliokoski, O., Abelson, K.S.P., 2022. Effects of buprenorphine on model development in an adjuvant-induced monoarthritis rat model. PLoS One 17, e0260356.

Beyreuther, B., Callizot, N., Stöhr, T., 2006. Antinociceptive efficacy of lacosamide in a rat model for painful diabetic neuropathy. Eur. J. Pharmacol. 539, 64–70.

Black, A., Lane, M.A., 2002. Nonhuman primate models of skeletal and reproductive aging. Gerontology 48, 72–80.

Blackburn-Munro, G., 2004. Hypothalamo-pituitary-adrenal axis dysfunction as a contributory factor to chronic pain and depression. Curr. Pain Headache Rep. 8, 116–124.

Blackburn-Munro, G., Blackburn-Munro, R.E., 2001. Chronic pain, chronic stress and depression: coincidence or consequence? J. Neuroendocrinol. 13, 1009–1023.

Bolten, W.W., 2006. Problem of the atherothrombotic potential of non-steroidal anti-inflammatory drugs. Ann. Rheum. Dis. 65, 7–13.

Bomholt, S.F., Mikkelsen, J.D., Blackburn-Munro, G., 2005. Normal hypothalamo-pituitary-adrenal axis function in a rat model of peripheral neuropathic pain. Brain Res. 1044, 216–226.

Bonabello, A., Galmozzi, M.R., Canaparo, R., Isaia, G.C., Serpe, L., Muntoni, E., Zara, G.P., 2003. Dexibuprofen (S+-isomer ibuprofen)

reduces gastric damage and improves analgesic and antiinflammatory effects in rodents. Anesth. Analg. 97, 402–408.
Bonica, J., 1953. The Management of Pain. Lea and Febiger, Philadelphia.
Boston, S.E., Moens, N.M., Kruth, S.A., Southorn, E.P., 2003. Endoscopic evaluation of the gastroduodenal mucosa to determine the safety of short-term concurrent administration of meloxicam and dexamethasone in healthy dogs. Am. J. Vet. Res. 64, 1369–1375.
Bräu, M.E., Dreimann, M., Olschewski, A., Vogel, W., Hempelmann, G., 2001. Effect of drugs used for neuropathic pain management on tetrodotoxin-resistant Na(+) currents in rat sensory neurons. Anesthesiology 94, 137–144.
Breen, J., 2002. Transitions in the concept of chronic pain. ANS Adv. Nurs. Sci. 24, 48–59.
Brennan, T.J., Kehlet, H., 2005. Preventive analgesia to reduce wound hyperalgesia and persistent postsurgical pain: not an easy path. Anesthesiology 103, 681–683.
Brenowitz, G.L., 1983. Timecourse for receptive field plasticity following spinal cord hemisection. Brain Res. 279, 250–253.
Brown, W.A., Skinner, S.A., Malcontenti-Wilson, C., Misajon, A., Dejong, T., Vogiagis, D., O'brien, P.E., 2000. Non-steroidal anti-inflammatory drugs with different cyclooxygenase inhibitory profiles that prevent aberrant crypt foci formation but vary in acute gastrotoxicity in a rat model. J. Gastroenterol. Hepatol. 15, 1386–1392.
Bryson, H.M., Wilde, M.I., 1996. Amitriptyline. A review of its pharmacological properties and therapeutic use in chronic pain states. Drugs Aging 8, 459–476.
Cain, D.M., Wacnik, P.W., Turner, M., Wendelschafer-Crabb, G., Kennedy, W.R., Wilcox, G.L., Simone, D.A., 2001. Functional interactions between tumor and peripheral nerve: changes in excitability and morphology of primary afferent fibers in a murine model of cancer pain. J. Neurosci. 21, 9367–9376.
Calzà, L., Pozza, M., Arletti, R., Manzini, E., Hökfelt, T., 2000. Long-lasting regulation of galanin, opioid, and other peptides in dorsal root ganglia and spinal cord during experimental polyarthritis. Exp. Neurol. 164, 333–343.
Calzà, L., Pozza, M., Zanni, M., Manzini, C.U., Manzini, E., Hökfelt, T., 1998. Peptide plasticity in primary sensory neurons and spinal cord during adjuvant-induced arthritis in the rat: an immunocytochemical and in situ hybridization study. Neuroscience 82, 575–589.
Carlson, C.S., Loeser, R.F., Purser, C.B., Gardin, J.F., Jerome, C.P., 1996. Osteoarthritis in cynomolgus macaques. III: effects of age, gender, and subchondral bone thickness on the severity of disease. J. Bone Miner. Res. 11, 1209–1217.
Chaplan, S.R., Bach, F.W., Shafer, S.L., Yaksh, T.L., 1995. Prolonged alleviation of tactile allodynia by intravenous lidocaine in neuropathic rats. Anesthesiology 83, 775–785.
Chevlen, E., Davis, P.S., Rhiner, M., 2005. From mechanisms to management: translating the neuropathic pain consensus recommendations into clinical practice. J. Am. Acad. Nurse Pract. 17, 3–17 quiz 18.
Chew, D.J., Buffington, C.A., Kendall, M.S., Dibartola, S.P., Woodworth, B.E., 1998. Amitriptyline treatment for severe recurrent idiopathic cystitis in cats. J. Am. Vet. Med. Assoc. 213, 1282–1286.
Christoph, T., Kögel, B., Schiene, K., Méen, M., De Vry, J., Friderichs, E., 2005. Broad analgesic profile of buprenorphine in rodent models of acute and chronic pain. Eur. J. Pharmacol. 507, 87–98.
Cizinauskas, S., Jaggy, A., Tipold, A., 2000. Long-term treatment of dogs with steroid-responsive meningitis-arteritis: clinical, laboratory and therapeutic results. J. Small Anim. Pract. 41, 295–301.
Clarke, S.P., Bennett, D., 2006. Feline osteoarthritis: a prospective study of 28 cases. J. Small Anim. Pract. 47, 439–445.
Clemensen, J., Rasmussen, L.V., Abelson, K.S.P., 2018. Transdermal fentanyl solution provides long-term analgesia in the hind-paw incisional model of postoperative pain in male rats. In Vivo 32, 713–719.
D'mello, R., Dickenson, A.H., 2008. Spinal cord mechanisms of pain. Br. J. Anaesth. 101, 8–16.
Dabby, R., Gilad, R., Sadeh, M., Lampl, Y., Watemberg, N., 2006. Acute steroid responsive small-fiber sensory neuropathy: a new entity? J. Peripher. Nerv. Syst. 11, 47–52.
Deacon, R.M., Raley, J.M., Perry, V.H., Rawlins, J.N., 2001. Burrowing into prion disease. Neuroreport 12, 2053–2057.
Deacon, R.M.J., 2006. Assessing nest building in mice. Nat. Protoc. 1, 1117–1119.
Decosterd, I., Allchorne, A., Woolf, C.J., 2004. Differential analgesic sensitivity of two distinct neuropathic pain models. Anesth. Analg. 99, 457–463 (table of contents).
Deleo, J.A., Rutkowski, M.D., 2000. Gender differences in rat neuropathic pain sensitivity is dependent on strain. Neurosci. Lett. 282, 197–199.
Deleo, J.A., Tanga, F.Y., Tawfik, V.L., 2004. Neuroimmune activation and neuroinflammation in chronic pain and opioid tolerance/hyperalgesia. Neuroscientist 10, 40–52.
Deleo, J.A., Yezierski, R.P., 2001. The role of neuroinflammation and neuroimmune activation in persistent pain. Pain 90, 1–6.
Dodman, N.H., Shuster, L., Nesbitt, G., Weissman, A., Lo, W.Y., Chang, W.W., Cottam, N., 2004. The use of dextromethorphan to treat repetitive self-directed scratching, biting, or chewing in dogs with allergic dermatitis. J. Vet. Pharmacol. Therapeut. 27, 99–104.
Dranovsky, A., Hen, R., 2006. Hippocampal neurogenesis: regulation by stress and antidepressants. Biol. Psychiatr. 59, 1136–1143.
Draxler, P., Moen, A., Galek, K., Boghos, A., Ramazanova, D., Sandkühler, J., 2021. Spontaneous, voluntary, and affective behaviours in rat models of pathological pain. Front. Pain Res. 2, 672711.
Duby, J.J., Campbell, R.K., Setter, S.M., White, J.R., Rasmussen, K.A., 2004. Diabetic neuropathy: an intensive review. Am. J. Health Syst. Pharm. 61, 160–173 quiz 175-6.
Duric, V., Mccarson, K.E., 2006. Persistent pain produces stress-like alterations in hippocampal neurogenesis and gene expression. J. Pain 7, 544–555.
Dworkin, R.H., Gitlin, M.J., 1991. Clinical aspects of depression in chronic pain patients. Clin. J. Pain 7, 79–94.
Eddleston, M., Mucke, L., 1993. Molecular profile of reactive astrocytes–implications for their role in neurologic disease. Neuroscience 54, 15–36.
Esser, M.J., Chase, T., Allen, G.V., Sawynok, J., 2001. Chronic administration of amitriptyline and caffeine in a rat model of neuropathic pain: multiple interactions. Eur. J. Pharmacol. 430, 211–218.
Esser, M.J., Sawynok, J., 1999. Acute amitriptyline in a rat model of neuropathic pain: differential symptom and route effects. Pain 80, 643–653.
Field, M.J., Mccleary, S., Hughes, J., Singh, L., 1999. Gabapentin and pregabalin, but not morphine and amitriptyline, block both static and dynamic components of mechanical allodynia induced by streptozocin in the rat. Pain 80, 391–398.
Fishbain, D.A., Cutler, R., Rosomoff, H.L., Rosomoff, R.S., 2000. Evidence-based data from animal and human experimental studies on pain relief with antidepressants: a structured review. Pain Med. 1, 310–316.

Fisher, K., Coderre, T.J., Hagen, N.A., 2000. Targeting the N-methyl-D-aspartate receptor for chronic pain management. Preclinical animal studies, recent clinical experience and future research directions. J. Pain Symptom Manag. 20, 358–373.

Flecknell, P.A., 2001. Analgesia of small mammals. Vet. Clin. N. Am. Exot. Anim. Pract. 4, 47–56 vi.

Gaab, J., Baumann, S., Budnoik, A., Gmünder, H., Hottinger, N., Ehlert, U., 2005. Reduced reactivity and enhanced negative feedback sensitivity of the hypothalamus-pituitary-adrenal axis in chronic whiplash-associated disorder. Pain 119, 219–224.

Galer, B.S., Harle, J., Rowbotham, M.C., 1996. Response to intravenous lidocaine infusion predicts subsequent response to oral mexiletine: a prospective study. J. Pain Symptom Manag. 12, 161–167.

Gallo, M.S., Karas, A.Z., Pritchett-Corning, K., Garner Guy Mulder, J.P., Gaskill, B.N., 2020. Tell-tale TINT: does the time to incorporate into nest test evaluate postsurgical pain or welfare in mice? J. Am. Assoc. Lab. Anim. Sci. 59, 37–45.

Garrison, C.J., Dougherty, P.M., Carlton, S.M., 1994. GFAP expression in lumbar spinal cord of naive and neuropathic rats treated with MK-801. Exp. Neurol. 129, 237–243.

Gaumond, I., Arsenault, P., Marchand, S., 2005. Specificity of female and male sex hormones on excitatory and inhibitory phases of formalin-induced nociceptive responses. Brain Res. 1052, 105–111.

Gaynor, J.S., Muir, W.W., 2015. Handbook of Veterinary Pain Management. Elsevier, St. Louis, Missouri.

Gilron, I., Watson, C.P., Cahill, C.M., Moulin, D.E., 2006. Neuropathic pain: a practical guide for the clinician. CMAJ 175, 265–275.

Gordh, T., Chu, H., Sharma, H.S., 2006. Spinal nerve lesion alters blood-spinal cord barrier function and activates astrocytes in the rat. Pain 124, 211–221.

Grachev, I.D., Fredrickson, B.E., Apkarian, V.A., 2000. Abnormal brain chemistry in chronic back pain: an in vivo proton magnetic resonance spectroscopy study. Pain 89, 7–18.

Grelik, C., Bennett, G.J., Ribeiro-Da-Silva, A., 2005. Autonomic fibre sprouting and changes in nociceptive sensory innervation in the rat lower lip skin following chronic constriction injury. Eur. J. Neurosci. 21, 2475–2487.

Grenald, S.A., Young, M.A., Wang, Y., Ossipov, M.H., Ibrahim, M.M., Largent-Milnes, T.M., Vanderah, T.W., 2017. Synergistic attenuation of chronic pain using mu opioid and cannabinoid receptor 2 agonists. Neuropharmacology 116, 59–70.

Grimm, K.A., Lamont, L.A., Tranquilli, W.J., Greene, S.A., Robertson, S.A., 2015. Veterinary Anesthesia and Analgesia. Wiley Blackwell, Ames, Iowa.

Hains, B.C., Willis, W.D., Hulsebosch, C.E., 2003. Temporal plasticity of dorsal horn somatosensory neurons after acute and chronic spinal cord hemisection in rat. Brain Res. 970, 238–241.

Harbuz, M.S., Conde, G.L., Marti, O., Lightman, S.L., Jessop, D.S., 1997. The hypothalamic-pituitary-adrenal axis in autoimmunity. Ann. N. Y. Acad. Sci. 823, 214–224.

Harris, J.A., 1998. Using c-fos as a neural marker of pain. Brain Res. Bull. 45, 1–8.

Harvey-Clark, C.J., Gilespie, K., Riggs, K.W., 2000. Transdermal fentanyl compared with parenteral buprenorphine in post-surgical pain in swine: a case study. Lab. Anim. 34, 386–398.

Herzberg, U., Brown, D.R., Mullett, M.A., Beitz, A.J., 1996a. Increased delayed type hypersensitivity in rats subjected to unilateral mononeuropathy is mediated by neurokinin-1 receptors. J. Neuroimmunol. 65, 119–124.

Herzberg, U., Murtaugh, M., Beitz, A.J., 1994. Chronic pain and immunity: mononeuropathy alters immune responses in rats. Pain 59, 219–225.

Herzberg, U., Murtaugh, M.P., Carroll, D., Beitz, A.J., 1996b. Spinal cord NMDA receptors modulate peripheral immune responses and spinal cord c-fos expression after immune challenge in rats subjected to unilateral mononeuropathy. J. Neurosci. 16, 730–743.

Herzberg, U., Sagen, J., 2001. Peripheral nerve exposure to HIV viral envelope protein gp120 induces neuropathic pain and spinal gliosis. J. Neuroimmunol. 116, 29–39.

Hestehave, S., Abelson, K.S.P., Brønnum Pedersen, T., Finn, D.P., Andersson, D.R., Munro, G., 2020. The influence of rat strain on the development of neuropathic pain and comorbid anxio-depressive behaviour after nerve injury. Sci. Rep. 10, 20981.

Hestehave, S., Munro, G., Christensen, R., Bronnum Pedersen, T., Arvastson, L., Hougaard, P., Abelson, K.S.P., 2017. Is there a reasonable excuse for not providing post-operative analgesia when using animal models of peripheral neuropathic pain for research purposes? PLoS One 12, e0188113.

Hiraga, S.-I., Itokazu, T., Nishibe, M., Yamashita, T., 2022. Neuroplasticity related to chronic pain and its modulation by microglia. Inflamm. Regen. 42, 15.

Hofmeister, E.H., Egger, C.M., 2004. Transdermal fentanyl patches in small animals. J. Am. Anim. Hosp. Assoc. 40, 468–478.

Hunter, J.C., Gogas, K.R., Hedley, L.R., Jacobson, L.O., Kassotakis, L., Thompson, J., Fontana, D.J., 1997. The effect of novel anti-epileptic drugs in rat experimental models of acute and chronic pain. Eur. J. Pharmacol. 324, 153–160.

Husebye, E.S., Pearce, S.H., Krone, N.P., Kämpe, O., 2021. Adrenal insufficiency. Lancet 397, 613–629.

Iwata, K., Fukuoka, T., Kondo, E., Tsuboi, Y., Tashiro, A., Noguchi, K., Masuda, Y., Morimoto, T., Kanda, K., 2002. Plastic changes in nociceptive transmission of the rat spinal cord with advancing age. J. Neurophysiol. 87, 1086–1093.

Jabbur, S.J., Saadé, N.E., 1999. From electrical wiring to plastic neurons: evolving approaches to the study of pain. Pain Suppl. 6, S87–s92.

Jacobsen, K.R., Kalliokoski, O., Teilmann, A.C., Hau, J., Abelson, K.S.P., 2012. Postsurgical food and water consumption, fecal corticosterone metabolites, and behavior assessment as noninvasive measures of pain in vasectomized BALB/c mice. J. Am. Assoc. Lab. Anim. Sci. 51, 69–75.

Ji, R.R., Woolf, C.J., 2001. Neuronal plasticity and signal transduction in nociceptive neurons: implications for the initiation and maintenance of pathological pain. Neurobiol. Dis. 8, 1–10.

Kalliokoski, O., Hau, J., Jacobsen, K.R., Schumacher-Petersen, C., Abelson, K.S., 2010. Distribution and time course of corticosterone excretion in faeces and urine of female mice with varying systemic concentrations. Gen. Comp. Endocrinol. 168, 450–454.

Katz, N., Benoit, C., 2005. Opioids for neuropathic pain. Curr. Pain Headache Rep. 9, 153–160.

Kehlet, H., Jensen, T.S., Woolf, C.J., 2006. Persistent postsurgical pain: risk factors and prevention. Lancet (London, England) 367, 1618–1625.

Khan, M.S., Akhter, M., 2005. Synthesis, pharmacological activity and hydrolytic behavior of glyceride prodrugs of ibuprofen. Eur. J. Med. Chem. 40, 371–376.

Kingery, W.S., 1997. A critical review of controlled clinical trials for peripheral neuropathic pain and complex regional pain syndromes. Pain 73, 123–139.

Kingery, W.S., Vallin, J.A., 1989. The development of chronic mechanical hyperalgesia, autotomy and collateral sprouting following sciatic nerve section in rat. Pain 38, 321–332.

Kitagawa, J., Kanda, K., Sugiura, M., Tsuboi, Y., Ogawa, A., Shimizu, K., Koyama, N., Kamo, H., Watanabe, T., Ren, K., Iwata, K., 2005. Effect of chronic inflammation on dorsal horn nociceptive neurons in aged rats. J. Neurophysiol. 93, 3594–3604.

Kleppner, S.R., Patel, R., Costantini, L.C., Mcdonough, J., 2010. In-vitro and in-vivo characterization of a buprenorphine delivery system. J. Pharm. Pharmacol. 58, 295–302.

Ko, S.H., Jochnowitz, N., Lenkowski, P.W., Batts, T.W., Davis, G.C., Martin, W.J., Brown, M.L., Patel, M.K., 2006. Reversal of neuropathic pain by alpha-hydroxyphenylamide: a novel sodium channel antagonist. Neuropharmacology 50, 865–873.

Kouya, P.F., Hao, J.X., Xu, X.J., 2002. Buprenorphine alleviates neuropathic pain-like behaviors in rats after spinal cord and peripheral nerve injury. Eur. J. Pharmacol. 450, 49–53.

Krotz, F., Schiele, T.M., Klauss, V., Sohn, H.Y., 2005. Selective COX-2 inhibitors and risk of myocardial infarction. J. Vasc. Res. 42, 312–324.

Kukanich, B., Lascelles, B.D., Papich, M.G., 2005. Pharmacokinetics of morphine and plasma concentrations of morphine-6-glucuronide following morphine administration to dogs. J. Vet. Pharmacol. Therapeut. 28, 371–376.

Kukanich, B., Papich, M.G., 2004. Plasma profile and pharmacokinetics of dextromethorphan after intravenous and oral administration in healthy dogs. J. Vet. Pharmacol. Therapeut. 27, 337–341.

Labuda, C.J., Little, P.J., 2005. Pharmacological evaluation of the selective spinal nerve ligation model of neuropathic pain in the rat. J. Neurosci. Methods 144, 175–181.

Lacroix-Fralish, M.L., Rutkowski, M.D., Weinstein, J.N., Mogil, J.S., Deleo, J.A., 2005. The magnitude of mechanical allodynia in a rodent model of lumbar radiculopathy is dependent on strain and sex. Spine (Phila Pa 1976) 30, 1821–1827.

Lafuente, M.P., Franch, J., Durall, I., Díaz-Bertrana, M.C., Márquez, R.M., 2005. Comparison between meloxicam and transdermally administered fentanyl for treatment of postoperative pain in dogs undergoing osteotomy of the tibia and fibula and placement of a uniplanar external distraction device. J. Am. Vet. Med. Assoc. 227, 1768–1774.

Langford, R., Mckenna, F., Ratcliffe, S., Vojtassák, J., Richarz, U., 2006. Transdermal fentanyl for improvement of pain and functioning in osteoarthritis: a randomized, placebo-controlled trial. Arthritis Rheum. 54, 1829–1837.

Lascelles, B.D., Blikslager, A.T., Fox, S.M., Reece, D., 2005a. Gastrointestinal tract perforation in dogs treated with a selective cyclooxygenase-2 inhibitor: 29 cases (2002–2003). J. Am. Vet. Med. Assoc. 227, 1112–1117.

Lascelles, B.D., Mcfarland, J.M., Swann, H., 2005b. Guidelines for safe and effective use of NSAIDs in dogs. Vet. Therapeut. 6, 237–251.

Laughlin, T.M., Tram, K.V., Wilcox, G.L., Birnbaum, A.K., 2002. Comparison of antiepileptic drugs tiagabine, lamotrigine, and gabapentin in mouse models of acute, prolonged, and chronic nociception. J. Pharmacol. Exp. Therapeut. 302, 1168–1175.

Le Loët, X., Pavelka, K., Richarz, U., 2005. Transdermal fentanyl for the treatment of pain caused by osteoarthritis of the knee or hip: an open, multicentre study. BMC Muscoskel. Disord. 6, 31.

Leo, R.J., 2006. Treatment considerations in neuropathic pain. Curr. Treat. Options Neurol. 8, 389–400.

Lester, P., Gaynor, J.S., 2000. Management of cancer pain. Vet Clin North Am Small Anim Pract 30, 951–966 ix.

Leverenz, J.B., Wilkinson, C.W., Wamble, M., Corbin, S., Grabber, J.E., Raskind, M.A., Peskind, E.R., 1999. Effect of chronic high-dose exogenous cortisol on hippocampal neuronal number in aged nonhuman primates. J. Neurosci. 19, 2356–2361.

Levy, D., Zochodne, D.W., 2000. Increased mRNA expression of the B1 and B2 bradykinin receptors and antinociceptive effects of their antagonists in an animal model of neuropathic pain. Pain 86, 265–271.

Li, J.X., 2015. Pain and depression comorbidity: a preclinical perspective. Behav. Brain Res. 276, 92–98.

Lim, K.K., Kessler, M.J., Pritzker, K.P., Turnquist, J.E., Dieppe, P.A., 1996. Osteoarthritis of the hand in nonhuman primates: a clinical, radiographic, and skeletal survey of Cayo Santiago rhesus macaques. J. Med. Primatol. 25, 301–308.

Liu, Q.S., Xu, Q., Arcuino, G., Kang, J., Nedergaard, M., 2004. Astrocyte-mediated activation of neuronal kainate receptors. Proc. Natl. Acad. Sci. U. S. A. 101, 3172–3177.

Lovell, J.A., Novak, J.C., Stuesse, S.L., Cruce, W.L., Crisp, T., 2000. Changes in spinal serotonin turnover mediate age-related differences in the behavioral manifestations of peripheral nerve injury. Pharmacol. Biochem. Behav. 66, 873–878.

Lussier, D., Huskey, A.G., Portenoy, R.K., 2004. Adjuvant analgesics in cancer pain management. Oncol. 9, 571–591.

Lynch, M.E., Clark, A.J., Sawynok, J., Sullivan, M.J., 2005. Topical amitriptyline and ketamine in neuropathic pain syndromes: an open-label study. J. Pain 6, 644–649.

Malavasi, L.M., Nyman, G., Augustsson, H., Jacobson, M., Jensen-Waern, M., 2006. Effects of epidural morphine and transdermal fentanyl analgesia on physiology and behaviour after abdominal surgery in pigs. Lab. Anim. 40, 16–27.

Mao, J., Chen, L.L., 2000. Systemic lidocaine for neuropathic pain relief. Pain 87, 7–17.

Marcus, D.A., 2003. Gender differences in chronic pain in a treatment-seeking population. J. Gend. Specif. Med. 6, 19–24.

Markman, J.D., Dworkin, R.H., 2006. Ion channel targets and treatment efficacy in neuropathic pain. J. Pain 7, S38–S47.

Martin, T.J., Eisenach, J.C., 2001. Pharmacology of opioid and nonopioid analgesics in chronic pain states. J. Pharmacol. Exp. Therapeut. 299, 811–817.

Max, M.B., Culnane, M., Schafer, S.C., Gracely, R.H., Walther, D.J., Smoller, B., Dubner, R., 1987. Amitriptyline relieves diabetic neuropathy pain in patients with normal or depressed mood. Neurology 37, 589–596.

Mcbeth, J., Chiu, Y.H., Silman, A.J., Ray, D., Morriss, R., Dickens, C., Gupta, A., Macfarlane, G.J., 2005. Hypothalamic-pituitary-adrenal stress axis function and the relationship with chronic widespread pain and its antecedents. Arthritis Res. Ther. 7, R992–r1000.

Mcgivern, J.G., 2006. Targeting N-type and T-type calcium channels for the treatment of pain. Drug Discov. Today 11, 245–253.

Mclaughlin, R., 2000. Management of chronic osteoarthritic pain. Vet Clin North Am Small Anim Pract 30, 933–949 ix.

Meana, M., Cho, R., Desmeules, M., 2004. Chronic pain: the extra burden on Canadian women. BMC Wom. Health 4 (Suppl. 1), S17.

Mogil, J.S., Pang, D.S.J., Silva Dutra, G.G., Chambers, C.T., 2020. The development and use of facial grimace scales for pain measurement in animals. Neurosci. Biobehav. Rev. 116, 480–493.

Montuschi, P., Barnes, P.J., Roberts 2ND, L.J., 2004. Isoprostanes: markers and mediators of oxidative stress. FASEB J. 18, 1791–1800.

Morton, D.B., Hau, J., 2021. Welfare assessment and humane endpoints. In: Hau, J., Schapiro, S.J. (Eds.), Handbook of Laboratory Animal Science: Essential Principles and Practices, fourth ed. CRC Press, Boca Raton.

Mota-Rojas, D., Olmos-Hernández, A., Verduzco-Mendoza, A., Hernández, E., Martínez-Burnes, J., Whittaker, A.L., 2020. The utility of grimace scales for practical pain assessment in laboratory animals. Animals (Basel) 10, 1838.

Mucke, L., Eddleston, M., 1993. Astrocytes in infectious and immune-mediated diseases of the central nervous system. FASEB. J. 7, 1226–1232.

Muir 3rd, W.W., Wiese, A.J., Wittum, T.E., 2004. Prevalence and characteristics of pain in dogs and cats examined as outpatients at a veterinary teaching hospital. J. Am. Vet. Med. Assoc. 224, 1459–1463.

Nakagawa, K., Yamagami, T., Takemura, N., 2005. Hepatocellular toxicosis associated with the alternate administration of carprofen and meloxicam in a siberian husky. J. Vet. Med. Sci. 67, 1051–1053.

Narita, M., Kaneko, C., Miyoshi, K., Nagumo, Y., Kuzumaki, N., Nakajima, M., Nanjo, K., Matsuzawa, K., Yamazaki, M., Suzuki, T., 2006a. Chronic pain induces anxiety with concomitant changes in opioidergic function in the amygdala. Neuropsychopharmacology 31, 739–750.

Narita, M., Kuzumaki, N., Narita, M., Kaneko, C., Hareyama, N., Miyatake, M., Shindo, K., Miyoshi, K., Nakajima, M., Nagumo, Y., Sato, F., Wachi, H., Seyama, Y., Suzuki, T., 2006b. Chronic pain-induced emotional dysfunction is associated with astrogliosis due to cortical delta-opioid receptor dysfunction. J. Neurochem. 97, 1369–1378.

National Research Council Committee on, R. & Alleviation of Pain in Laboratory, A, 2009. The National Academies Collection: Reports Funded by National Institutes of Health. Recognition and Alleviation of Pain in Laboratory Animals. National Academies Press (US) Copyright © 2009, National Academy of Sciences, Washington (DC).

Novak, J.C., Lovell, J.A., Stuesse, S.L., Cruce, W.L., Mcburney, D.L., Crisp, T., 1999. Aging and neuropathic pain. Brain Res. 833, 308–310.

O'hagan, B.J., 2006. Neuropathic pain in a cat post-amputation. Aust. Vet. J. 84, 83–86.

Obuchowicz, E., Kowalski, J., Labuzek, K., Krysiak, R., Pendzich, J., Herman, Z.S., 2006. Amitriptyline and nortriptyline inhibit interleukin-1 release by rat mixed glial and microglial cell cultures. Int. J. Neuropsychopharmacol. 9, 27–35.

Oliver, V.L., Thurston, S.E., Lofgren, J.L., 2018. Using cageside measures to evaluate analgesic efficacy in mice (Mus musculus) after surgery. J. Am. Assoc. Lab. Anim. Sci. 57, 186–201.

Orfila, F., Ferrer, M., Lamarca, R., Tebe, C., Domingo-Salvany, A., Alonso, J., 2006. Gender differences in health-related quality of life among the elderly: the role of objective functional capacity and chronic conditions. Soc. Sci. Med. 63, 2367–2380.

Perkins, F.M., Kehlet, H., 2000. Chronic pain as an outcome of surgery. A review of predictive factors. Anesthesiology 93, 1123–1133.

Perrot, S., Cohen, M., Barke, A., Korwisi, B., Rief, W., Treede, R.-D., Pain, T.I.T.F.T.C.O.C., 2019. The IASP classification of chronic pain for ICD-11: chronic secondary musculoskeletal pain. Pain 160, 77–82.

Persellin, R.H., Kittinger, G.W., Kendall, J.W., 1972. Adrenal response to experimental arthritis in the rat. Am. J. Physiol. 222, 1545–1549.

Peters, C.M., Ghilardi, J.R., Keyser, C.P., Kubota, K., Lindsay, T.H., Luger, N.M., Mach, D.B., Schwei, M.J., Sevcik, M.A., Mantyh, P.W., 2005. Tumor-induced injury of primary afferent sensory nerve fibers in bone cancer pain. Exp. Neurol. 193, 85–100.

Petrenko, A.B., Yamakura, T., Baba, H., Shimoji, K., 2003. The role of N-methyl-D-aspartate (NMDA) receptors in pain: a review. Anesth. Analg. 97, 1108–1116.

Pozzi, A., Muir, W.W., Traverso, F., 2006. Prevention of central sensitization and pain by N-methyl-D-aspartate receptor antagonists. J. Am. Vet. Med. Assoc. 228, 53–60.

Preziosi, D.E., Goldschmidt, M.H., Greek, J.S., Jeffers, J.G., Shanley, K.S., Drobatz, K., Mauldin, E.A., 2003. Feline pemphigus foliaceus: a retrospective analysis of 57 cases. Vet. Dermatol. 14, 313–321.

Raghavendra, V., Tanga, F.Y., Deleo, J.A., 2004. Complete Freunds adjuvant-induced peripheral inflammation evokes glial activation and proinflammatory cytokine expression in the CNS. Eur. J. Neurosci. 20, 467–473.

Rainsford, K.D., 1987. Gastric ulcerogenicity of non-steroidal anti-inflammatory drugs in mice with mucosa sensitized by cholinomimetic treatment. J. Pharm. Pharmacol. 39, 669–672.

Raja, S.N., Carr, D.B., Cohen, M., Finnerup, N.B., Flor, H., Gibson, S., Keefe, F.J., Mogil, J.S., Ringkamp, M., Sluka, K.A., Song, X.-J., Stevens, B., Sullivan, M.D., Tutelman, P.R., Ushida, T., Vader, K., 2020. The revised International Association for the Study of Pain definition of pain: concepts, challenges, and compromises. Pain 161, 1976–1982.

Ramer, M.S., Bisby, M.A., 1998. Normal and injury-induced sympathetic innervation of rat dorsal root ganglia increases with age. J. Comp. Neurol. 394, 38–47.

Reed, S., 2002. Nonsteroidal anti-inflammatory drug-induced duodenal ulceration and perforation in a mature rottweiler. Can. Vet. J. 43, 971–972.

Reynolds, J.L., Ignatowski, T.A., Gallant, S., Spengler, R.N., 2004. Amitriptyline administration transforms tumor necrosis factor-alpha regulation of norepinephrine release in the brain. Brain Res. 1023, 112–120.

Robertson, S.A., 2008. Managing pain in feline patients. Vet Clin North Am Small Anim Pract 38, 1267–1290 vi.

Romans, C.W., Gordon, W.J., Robinson, D.A., Evans, R., Conzemius, M.G., 2005. Effect of postoperative analgesic protocol on limb function following onychectomy in cats. J. Am. Vet. Med. Assoc. 227, 89–93.

Romero-Sandoval, A., Eisenach, J.C., 2006. Perineural clonidine reduces mechanical hypersensitivity and cytokine production in established nerve injury. Anesthesiology 104, 351–355.

Rothschild, B.M., Hong, N., Turnquist, J.E., 1999. Skeletal survey of Cayo Santiago rhesus macaques: osteoarthritis and articular plate excrescences. Semin. Arthritis Rheum. 29, 100–111.

Roughan, J.V., Flecknell, P.A., 2003. Evaluation of a short duration behaviour-based post-operative pain scoring system in rats. Eur. J. Pain 7, 397–406.

Roughan, J.V., Flecknell, P.A., 2006. Training in behaviour-based post-operative pain scoring in rats—an evaluation based on improved recognition of analgesic requirements. Appl. Anim. Behav. Sci. 96, 327–342.

Roughan, J.V., Flecknell, R.A., 2004. Behaviour-based assessment of the duration of laparotomy-induced abdominal pain and the analgesic effects of carprofen and buprenorphine in rats. Behav. Pharmacol. 15, 461–472.

Rustøen, T., Wahl, A.K., Hanestad, B.R., Lerdal, A., Paul, S., Miaskowski, C., 2004. Gender differences in chronic pain–findings from a population-based study of Norwegian adults. Pain Manag. Nurs. 5, 105–117.

Saarto, T., Wiffen, P.J., 2007. Antidepressants for neuropathic pain. Cochrane Database Syst. Rev. Cd005454.

Sandercock, D.A., Smith, S.H., DI Giminiani, P., Edwards, S.A., 2016. Histopathological characterization of tail injury and traumatic neuroma development after tail docking in piglets. J. Comp. Pathol. 155, 40–49.

Santos Tde, J., De Castro-Costa, C.M., Giffoni, S.D., Santos, F.J., Ramos, R.S., Gifoni, M.A., 1999. The effect of baclofen on spontaneous and evoked behavioural expression of experimental neuropathic chronic pain. Arq. Neuropsiquiatr. 57, 753–760.

Sarlis, N.J., Chowdrey, H.S., Stephanou, A., Lightman, S.L., 1992. Chronic activation of the hypothalamo-pituitary-adrenal axis and loss of circadian rhythm during adjuvant-induced arthritis in the rat. Endocrinology 130, 1775–1779.

Sawynok, J., Reid, A.R., Esser, M.J., 1999. Peripheral antinociceptive action of amitriptyline in the rat formalin test: involvement of adenosine. Pain 80, 45–55.

Sawynok, J., Reid, A.R., Xue Jun, L., Parkinson, F.E., 2005. Amitriptyline enhances extracellular tissue levels of adenosine in the rat hindpaw and inhibits adenosine uptake. Eur. J. Pharmacol. 518, 116–122.

Schnitzer, T.J., 2006. Update on guidelines for the treatment of chronic musculoskeletal pain. Clin. Rheumatol. 25 (Suppl. 1), S22–S29.

Scholz, J., Finnerup, N.B., Attal, N., Aziz, Q., Baron, R., Bennett, M.I., Benoliel, R., Cohen, M., Cruccu, G., Davis, K.D., Evers, S., First, M., Giamberardino, M.A., Hansson, P., Kaasa, S., Korwisi, B., Kosek, E., Lavand'homme, P., Nicholas, M., Nurmikko, T., Perrot, S., Raja, S.N., Rice, A.S.C., Rowbotham, M.C., Schug, S., Simpson, D.M., Smith, B.H., Svensson, P., Vlaeyen, J.W.S., Wang, S.-J., Barke, A., Rief, W., Treede, R.-D., Group, C.C.O.T.N.P.S.I., 2019. The IASP classification of chronic pain for ICD-11: chronic neuropathic pain. Pain 160, 53–59.

Schug, S.A., Lavand'homme, P., Barke, A., Korwisi, B., Rief, W., Treede, R.-D., Pain, T.I.T.F.T.C.O.C., 2019. The IASP classification of chronic pain for ICD-11: chronic postsurgical or posttraumatic pain. Pain 160, 45–52.

Schwei, M.J., Honore, P., Rogers, S.D., Salak-Johnson, J.L., Finke, M.P., Ramnaraine, M.L., Clohisy, D.R., Mantyh, P.W., 1999. Neurochemical and cellular reorganization of the spinal cord in a murine model of bone cancer pain. J. Neurosci. 19, 10886–10897.

Sharif Naeini, R., Cahill, C.M., Ribeiro-DA-Silva, A., Ménard, H.A., Henry, J.L., 2005. Remodelling of spinal nociceptive mechanisms in an animal model of monoarthritis. Eur. J. Neurosci. 22, 2005–2015.

Shimoyama, M., Tatsuoka, H., Ohtori, S., Tanaka, K., Shimoyama, N., 2005. Change of dorsal horn neurochemistry in a mouse model of neuropathic cancer pain. Pain 114, 221–230.

Siswanto, H., Hau, J., Carlsson, H.E., Goldkuhl, R., Abelson, K.S.P., 2008. Corticosterone concentrations in blood and excretion in faeces after ACTH administration in male Sprague-Dawley rats. In Vivo 22, 435–440.

Smith, J.C., 2019. A review of strain and sex differences in response to pain and analgesia in mice. Comp. Med. 69, 490–500.

Smith, L.J., Krugner-Higby, L., Clark, M., Wendland, A., Heath, T.D., 2003. A single dose of liposome-encapsulated oxymorphone or morphine provides long-term analgesia in an animal model of neuropathic pain. Comp. Med. 53, 280–287.

Smith, S.M., Vale, W.W., 2006. The role of the hypothalamic-pituitary-adrenal axis in neuroendocrine responses to stress. Dialogues Clin. Neurosci. 8, 383–395.

Staley, M., Conners, M.G., Hall, K., Miller, L.J., 2018. Linking stress and immunity: immunoglobulin A as a non-invasive physiological biomarker in animal welfare studies. Horm. Behav. 102, 55–68.

Stewart, L.S., Martin, W.J., 2003. Influence of postoperative analgesics on the development of neuropathic pain in rats. Comp. Med. 53, 29–36.

Sudo, R.T., Do Amaral, R.V., Monteiro, C., Pitta, I.D.R., Lima, M.D.C., Montes, G.C., Ririe, D.G., Hayashida, K., Zapata-Sudo, G., 2017. Antinociception induced by a novel α(2A) adrenergic receptor agonist in rodents acute and chronic pain models. Eur. J. Pharmacol. 815, 210–218.

Suyama, H., Kawamoto, M., Gaus, S., Yuge, O., 2004. Effect of etodolac, a COX-2 inhibitor, on neuropathic pain in a rat model. Brain Res. 1010, 144–150.

Takasaki, I., Kurihara, T., Saegusa, H., Zong, S., Tanabe, T., 2005. Effects of glucocorticoid receptor antagonists on allodynia and hyperalgesia in mouse model of neuropathic pain. Eur. J. Pharmacol. 524, 80–83.

Takeda, K., Sawamura, S., Sekiyama, H., Tamai, H., Hanaoka, K., 2004. Effect of methylprednisolone on neuropathic pain and spinal glial activation in rats. Anesthesiology 100, 1249–1257.

Tall, J.M., Stuesse, S.L., Cruce, W.L., Crisp, T., 2001. Gender and the behavioral manifestations of neuropathic pain. Pharmacol. Biochem. Behav. 68, 99–104.

Tanga, F.Y., Raghavendra, V., Deleo, J.A., 2004. Quantitative real-time RT-PCR assessment of spinal microglial and astrocytic activation markers in a rat model of neuropathic pain. Neurochem. Int. 45, 397–407.

Tappe-Theodor, A., King, T., Morgan, M.M., 2019. Pros and cons of clinically relevant methods to assess pain in rodents. Neurosci. Biobehav. Rev. 100, 335–343.

Thompson, C.D., Uhelski, M.L., Wilson, J.R., Fuchs, P.N., 2010. Hyperbaric oxygen treatment decreases pain in two nerve injury models. Neurosci. Res. 66, 279–283.

Treede, R.-D., Rief, W., Barke, A., Aziz, Q., Bennett, M.I., Benoliel, R., Cohen, M., Evers, S., Finnerup, N.B., First, M.B., Giamberardino, M.A., Kaasa, S., Korwisi, B., Kosek, E., Lavand'homme, P., Nicholas, M., Perrot, S., Scholz, J., Schug, S., Smith, B.H., Svensson, P., Vlaeyen, J.W.S., Wang, S.-J., 2019. Chronic pain as a symptom or a disease: the IASP classification of chronic pain for the international classification of diseases (ICD-11). Pain 160, 19–27.

Ulrich-Lai, Y.M., Xie, W., Meij, J.T., Dolgas, C.M., Yu, L., Herman, J.P., 2006. Limbic and HPA axis function in an animal model of chronic neuropathic pain. Physiol. Behav. 88, 67–76.

Valavanidis, A., Vlachogianni, T., Fiotakis, C., 2009. 8-hydroxy-2'-deoxyguanosine (8-OHdG): a critical biomarker of oxidative stress and carcinogenesis. J. Environ. Sci. Health C Environ. Carcinog. Ecotoxicol. Rev. 27, 120–139.

Visser, E., Schug, S.A., 2006. The role of ketamine in pain management. Biomed. Pharmacother. 60, 341–348.

Walczak, J.S., Beaulieu, P., 2006. Comparison of three models of neuropathic pain in mice using a new method to assess cold allodynia: the double plate technique. Neurosci. Lett. 399, 240–244.

Walczak, J.S., Pichette, V., Leblond, F., Desbiens, K., Beaulieu, P., 2005. Behavioral, pharmacological and molecular characterization of the saphenous nerve partial ligation: a new model of neuropathic pain. Neuroscience 132, 1093–1102.

Walczak, J.S., Pichette, V., Leblond, F., Desbiens, K., Beaulieu, P., 2006. Characterization of chronic constriction of the saphenous nerve, a model of neuropathic pain in mice showing rapid molecular and electrophysiological changes. J. Neurosci. Res. 83, 1310–1322.

Wang, D., Wang, M., Cheng, Y., Fitzgerald, G.A., 2005. Cardiovascular hazard and non-steroidal anti-inflammatory drugs. Curr. Opin. Pharmacol. 5, 204–210.

Wang, H., Sun, H., Della Penna, K., Benz, R.J., Xu, J., Gerhold, D.L., Holder, D.J., Koblan, K.S., 2002. Chronic neuropathic pain is accompanied by global changes in gene expression and shares pathobiology with neurodegenerative diseases. Neuroscience 114, 529–546.

Wang, S., Lim, G., Zeng, Q., Sung, B., Ai, Y., Guo, G., Yang, L., Mao, J., 2004. Expression of central glucocorticoid receptors after peripheral nerve injury contributes to neuropathic pain behaviors in rats. J. Neurosci. 24, 8595–8605.

Weiland, L., Croubels, S., Baert, K., Polis, I., De Backer, P., Gasthuys, F., 2006. Pharmacokinetics of a lidocaine patch 5% in dogs. J. Vet. Med. A Physiol. Pathol. Clin. Med. 53, 34–39.

Weir, M.R., Sperling, R.S., Reicin, A., Gertz, B.J., 2003. Selective COX-2 inhibition and cardiovascular effects: a review of the rofecoxib development program. Am. Heart J. 146, 591–604.

Wieseler-Frank, J., Maier, S.F., Watkins, L.R., 2004. Glial activation and pathological pain. Neurochem. Int. 45, 389–395.

Wieseler-Frank, J., Maier, S.F., Watkins, L.R., 2005. Immune-to-brain communication dynamically modulates pain: physiological and pathological consequences. Brain Behav. Immun. 19, 104–111.

Wild, K.D., Bian, D., Zhu, D., Davis, J., Bannon, A.W., Zhang, T.J., Louis, J.C., 2007. Antibodies to nerve growth factor reverse established tactile allodynia in rodent models of neuropathic pain without tolerance. J. Pharmacol. Exp. Therapeut. 322, 282–287.

Wilson, K.G., Mikail, S.F., D'eon, J.L., Minns, J.E., 2001. Alternative diagnostic criteria for major depressive disorder in patients with chronic pain. Pain 91, 227–234.

Windle, R.J., Wood, S.A., Kershaw, Y.M., Lightman, S.L., Ingram, C.D., Harbuz, M.S., 2001. Increased corticosterone pulse frequency during adjuvant-induced arthritis and its relationship to alterations in stress responsiveness. J. Neuroendocrinol. 13, 905–911.

Womer, D.E., Shannon, H.E., 2000. Pharmacologic reversal of pertussis toxin-induced thermal allodynia in mice. Neuropharmacology 39, 1732–1739.

Woolf, C.J., 2010. What is this thing called pain? J. Clin. Investig. 120, 3742–3744.

Xie, W., Liu, X., Xuan, H., Luo, S., Zhao, X., Zhou, Z., Xu, J., 2006. Effect of betamethasone on neuropathic pain and cerebral expression of NF-kappaB and cytokines. Neurosci. Lett. 393, 255–259.

Xu, X.J., Hao, J.X., Andell-Jonsson, S., Poli, V., Bartfai, T., Wiesenfeld-Hallin, Z., 1997. Nociceptive responses in interleukin-6-deficient mice to peripheral inflammation and peripheral nerve section. Cytokine 9, 1028–1033.

Yaari, Y., Selzer, M.E., Pincus, J.H., 1986. Phenytoin: mechanisms of its anticonvulsant action. Ann. Neurol. 20, 171–184.

Yasuda, T., Miki, S., Yoshinaga, N., Senba, E., 2005. Effects of amitriptyline and gabapentin on bilateral hyperalgesia observed in an animal model of unilateral axotomy. Pain 115, 161–170.

Yen, L.D., Bennett, G.J., Ribeiro-Da-Silva, A., 2006. Sympathetic sprouting and changes in nociceptive sensory innervation in the glabrous skin of the rat hind paw following partial peripheral nerve injury. J. Comp. Neurol. 495, 679–690.

Zhang, J., De Koninck, Y., 2006. Spatial and temporal relationship between monocyte chemoattractant protein-1 expression and spinal glial activation following peripheral nerve injury. J. Neurochem. 97, 772–783.

Zurek, J.R., Nadeson, R., Goodchild, C.S., 2001. Spinal and supraspinal components of opioid antinociception in streptozotocin induced diabetic neuropathy in rats. Pain 90, 57–63.

Chapter 28

Anesthesia and analgesia in the fetus and neonate

Gerry Hish

Unit for Laboratory Animal Medicine, University of Michigan, Ann Arbor, MI, United States

Chapter outline

I. Introduction

Increasing attention is currently being given to fetal and neonatal anesthesia and analgesia by members of the medical and veterinary professions and animal research community. In contrast to human medicine, in veterinary clinical practice, interventions are rarely carried out on the fetus prior to labor. However, surgical or other invasive procedures in animals have been an integral part of fetal and neonatal research for many decades. For instance, animal models are commonly used to advance the clinical management of human infants before, during, and after birth (Mellor and Gregory, 2003) and to refine surgical techniques and therapies for in-utero procedures in human fetuses, such as intrauterine treatments for spina bifida (Eggink et al., 2005; Herrera et al., 2012; Watanabe et al., 2015), intrauterine growth restriction (Lopez-Tello et al., 2019) and fetal cardiopulmonary bypass (Ikai et al., 2005; Liu et al., 2011). Favored models for this work have frequently employed fetal sheep and nonhuman primates, in part because they are neurologically mature at birth, as is the human fetus. While large animal species represent the majority of the published maternal:fetal surgical models, intracranial injection and electroporation of fetuses are increasingly used for gene transfer during surgical exposure of the gravid uterus and have been described in rodents (Huang and Carcagno, 2018; Pacary and Guillemot, 2020; Sato et al., 2020) and ferrets (Kawasaki et al., 2012).

The findings of such work and its experimental approach have direct relevance in the veterinary context as

Anesthesia and Analgesia in Laboratory Animals. https://doi.org/10.1016/B978-0-12-822215-7.00024-X

well. Thus, fetal and neonatal instrumentation techniques employing surgery have also been directed at, for example, the causes and prevention of perinatal mortality and morbidity in farm livestock (Mellor, 1988; Mellor and Gregory, 2003; Mellor and Stafford, 2004), the clinical management of dystocia (Mellor and Gregory, 2003), and humane slaughter techniques for pregnant ruminants (Mellor and Gregory, 2003; van der Valk et al., 2004). Such research has employed anesthesia of the pregnant dam and newborn, but, until relatively recently, the use of intra or postoperative analgesia has rarely been considered.

The need for fetal anesthesia or analgesia is an area of current debate in human medicine. It is uncertain at what age a human fetus may be capable of experiencing or perceiving pain, or indeed whether a fetus can ever *experience* pain in utero (Lee et al., 2005; Mellor et al., 2005). The answer to this question will have a huge impact on attitudes toward the need for anesthesia or analgesia in fetuses undergoing surgery or invasive procedures. Further, the longer-term consequences arising from invasive procedures on the fetus, regardless of whether the stimuli so generated are perceived as painful or not, are unknown. Such stimuli can cause activation of the stress response and may potentially have a long-term influence on the processing of noxious stimuli (Mellor et al., 2005). These sequelae may justify the use of anesthesia and/or analgesia, even if the fetus is unconscious and unable to experience pain at the time of the intervention.

In the veterinary context, however, an additional factor needs to be considered. It is the neurological maturity of the fetus at birth because the implications for fetal and neonatal anesthesia and analgesia differ depending on whether the young are mature (precocial), as in cattle, deer, goats, sheep, horses, pigs, and guinea pigs (Ellingson and Rose, 1970; Mellor and Diesch, 2006; Mellor and Gregory, 2003; Mellor and Stafford, 2004), or relatively immature (altricial), as in cats, dogs, mice, rats, and rabbits (Ellingson and Rose, 1970).

In this chapter, 'fetus' refers to the antenatal individual during approximately the last two-thirds of pregnancy, including birth, and 'neonate' or 'newborn' to mammalian young within the first few days to weeks after birth, depending upon the species.

II. Anesthesia of the dam for fetal surgery

Pregnancy causes many physiological changes in the dam that will influence the pharmacokinetics and pharmacodynamics of administered anesthetic and analgesic drugs. While many of the general principles of anesthetic management can be applied to pregnant animals, there are unique physiologic and anatomic differences that must be considered during the planning and performance of obstetric anesthesia. Despite differences in reproductive characteristics such as gestation length and placental anatomy, pregnancy is associated with several changes common to both human and veterinary patients. Maternal adaptations are well-characterized and occur throughout pregnancy, initially associated with hormonal activity and later due to increasing fetal needs and the physical impacts of an enlarging uterus.

In response to increases in gestational hormones, a variety of circulatory adaptations occur during pregnancy. Blood volume increases significantly over the course of pregnancy, though the rise in red blood cell mass is modestly outpaced by increased plasma production, resulting in a relative hemodilution and reduction in hematocrit. Concurrent increases in cardiac output and heart rate are observed while mean arterial pressures (MAP) are maintained by vasodilation and reduced peripheral resistance. These changes ensure adequate uterine blood flow (UBF) and fetal support but can become compromised when using anesthetics that reduce cardiac output or during procedures that reduce blood volume. Maternal hypotension can lead to marked decreases in uterine and placental blood flow resulting in reduced oxygen delivery and fetal acidosis. In pregnant women, during the third trimester, there is a risk of compression of the great vessels by the gravid uterus, which can lead to reduced venous return and cardiac output as well as increased risk for deep vein thrombosis. These complications are uncommon in quadrupedal species under normal circumstances but can occur when animals, especially larger species, are placed in dorsal recumbency for ventral midline surgical approaches.

Hormonal actions also produce a number of changes in the respiratory system that can complicate anesthetic management during pregnancy. Higher oxygen consumption is facilitated by heightened sensitivity of the brain to carbon dioxide levels, and total ventilatory volume is increased secondary to bronchial relaxation and reduced total pulmonary resistance, leading to more rapid uptake of inhalant anesthetics. As pregnancy progresses, uterine enlargement may produce cranial displacement of the diaphragm and reduce the residual functional capacity of the lungs. As a result, pregnant patients are less able to compensate and are more likely to become hypoxic during periods of apnea or reduced ventilation that can occur during anesthetic induction or as side effects of some analgesics (Musk and Kemp, 2018). Allowing animals to breathe 100% oxygen for 3–5 minutes prior to anesthetic induction can reduce this hypoxic risk.

The need for dose adjustments for several drugs commonly administered to pregnant women has been established (Ansari et al., 2016); however, the clinical impact of these changes on anesthetic drug selection and dose in many animal species is still poorly characterized in the literature. Given the limited data describing the pharmacokinetics and pharmacodynamics of anesthetic drugs in pregnant animals, anesthetic drugs should be given 'to effect' to avoid inadvertent drug over- or underdosing. This key principle of anesthetic titration is best achieved with inhalant or rapidly metabolized intravenously administered anesthetics. Additionally, a balanced anesthetic approach that utilizes the synergism of several drugs while reducing the adverse effects seen with high doses of any single agent will generally provide improved stability for both the mother and the fetus.

As their circulation is intimately tied to that of the dam, the impacts on the fetus of any agents administered during pregnancy must be considered. There are several sources of variability in determining the effect of maternally given drugs on the fetus, including drug pharmacology and gestational age. The placental barrier is a lipoprotein, so drugs with higher lipid solubility will cross the placenta to exert an anesthetic action on the fetus. The thickness of the placenta decreases throughout gestation, which facilitates the diffusion of drugs across the placenta in older fetuses. However, the stage of gestation may also affect fetal drug metabolism. In the maturing human fetus, the liver is able to metabolize drugs, which influences fetal drug metabolism (Wunsch et al., 2003). The fetal liver in dogs has little capability to metabolize drugs, whereas the situation in other animal species is unknown.

The choice of anesthetic protocol for the individual patient will be determined by the species, the invasiveness of the procedure to be carried out on the fetus, and the stage of gestation. The fetal lamb is widely used for biomedical and veterinary studies of fetal and neonatal physiology, such that most experimental data describing the effects of anesthetics on fetal circulation have been obtained from experiments carried out in a sheep model. Therefore, general recommendations pertaining to maternal anesthesia for fetal surgery are usually derived from studies in sheep and extrapolated across species. In general, the same principles of anesthesia apply to pregnant animals as they do to any individual, particularly with regard to monitoring and maintenance of cardiovascular and respiratory function and with supportive measures such as fluid therapy. Animal users should always review recent literature and general veterinary anesthetic texts when formulating an anesthetic plan for a study.

A. Inhalational agents

The halogenated anesthetics are the most common inhalational agents utilized in veterinary medicine, and their use during pregnancy has multiple advantages when fetal manipulation is required, including producing uterine relaxation that can facilitate conditions for fetal surgery (Yoo et al., 2006). The low solubility of these anesthetics leads to relatively rapid changes in blood concentration and the ability to quickly change anesthetic depth during induction, maintenance, and recovery. Although halothane was historically widely used in human and veterinary medicine, it has been replaced by newer agents, including isoflurane and sevoflurane, which also have the added benefit of undergoing minimal hepatic metabolism. Inhalant agents administered to the mother cross the placenta and rapidly establish lower but proportional concentrations in the fetus (Biehl et al., 1983; Satoh et al., 1995). Work in sheep suggests that the fetus requires a lower concentration of inhalant agent to achieve the same level of anesthesia as the adult (Gregory et al., 1983), so that anesthetic concentrations sufficient to anesthetize the dam will also anesthetize the fetus.

While inhalant anesthetics offer multiple advantages for general anesthesia, their dose-dependent depression of both the respiratory and cardiovascular systems is well established, and a number of studies have investigated the effects of maternally administered inhalant agents on the fetal circulation. The placenta lacks the capacity to autoregulate blood flow, and perfusion is largely dependent upon maternal blood pressure. Palahniuk and Shnider (1974) found that the administration of isoflurane to sheep at twice the minimum alveolar concentration (MAC) resulted in the development of fetal acidosis and significant reductions in maternal cardiac output, MAP and UBF within 15 minutes of induction. A lower concentration of isoflurane (1 MAC) in the same study had no impact on UBF or fetal blood pH. Administration of isoflurane to sheep at ~1.5 MAC for 4 hours resulted in fetal bradycardia and hypotension but not a reduction in fetal brain oxygenation (McClaine et al., 2007). Higher doses of desflurane (Ngamprasertwong et al., 2013) and sevoflurane (Okutomi et al., 2009) induced similar changes in pregnant sheep that were absent at lower concentrations of the anesthetic.

The advantages of inhalant anesthetics, especially when administered at 1.5 MAC or below, make them excellent choices for procedures that require a surgical plane of anesthesia. Combination with other injectable anesthetics and some analgesics can serve to further reduce MAC and the adverse impacts that are seen with higher inhalant concentrations.

B. Propofol

Propofol is routinely used as both an induction agent and for continuous intravenous sedation and anesthesia. When administered to pregnant ewes, propofol rapidly crosses the placenta; however, fetal blood concentrations remain low relative to maternal levels (Andaluz et al., 2003; Ngamprasertwong et al., 2016). Though fetal uptake was lower, Andaluz et al. (2003) found that the half-life of propofol was 2–3 times longer in the fetus than in the ewe. Although survival was not affected, puppies delivered by cesarean section had lower APGAR scores in the first 60 minutes when propofol, versus alfaxalone, was used for induction (Doebeli et al., 2013). When utilized as a sole agent at sedative doses (2.5 mg/kg IV bolus, 0.3 mg/kg/minute CRI) in pregnant ewes, propofol was not associated with negative impacts on maternal or placental hemodynamics (Gaynor et al., 1998); however, at the higher doses (6 mg/kg IV bolus, 0.4 mg/kg/minute CRI) required to perform noxious procedures, propofol produced maternal and fetal acidosis and reduced maternal MAP in the first 15 minutes of induction (Andaluz et al., 2005). Propofol can also be associated with respiratory depression, and ventilatory support is frequently required at higher doses. Though potentially useful as an adjunct to other anesthetics, when used alone for anesthetic maintenance, propofol is probably best utilized for minimally invasive procedures and with careful monitoring.

C. Dissociative anesthetics

Ketamine is widely used in veterinary medicine either as a single agent for anesthesia/restraint or, more commonly, in combination with a sedative/hypnotic or an α_2 agonist. Its use in pregnant, nonrodent species in the laboratory is most often limited to anesthetic induction prior to acquiring venous access and transitioning to inhalant anesthesia. Ketamine readily crosses the placenta in sheep, and blood concentrations in the fetus approximate that of the ewe (Craft et al., 1983; Musk et al., 2012). Stümper et al. (2004) noted minimal hemodynamic and acid:base changes in late-gestation ewes and their fetuses following infusion of ketamine at clinically relevant doses. Most studies reporting the effects of ketamine anesthesia during pregnancy have evaluated it in combination with another agent, and it is difficult to draw conclusions about its impacts on the fetus; however, it appears to be well tolerated clinically in several species, whether used in combination or alone (Kinoshita et al., 2021; Sims et al., 1997). A combination injectable anesthetic containing tiletamine (a dissociative anesthetic) and zolazepam (a benzodiazepine) is available for use in cats and dogs, but its primary application in the research setting is in swine. Evaluation of distribution in pregnant swine showed that zolazepam, but not tiletamine, crossed the placenta (Li et al., 2017). This combination has been used successfully in pigs for anesthetic induction for fetal surgery (Boettcher et al., 2019).

In mice and rats, ketamine combinations are routinely administered to provide general anesthesia for invasive surgical manipulations. Numerous studies have reported the impacts of anesthetics, including ketamine, on fetal development as potential experimental confounders; however, few have evaluated the specific impacts on fetal or maternal physiology. Thaete et al. (2013) found that ketamine/xylazine anesthesia reduced fetal growth when administered at multiple timepoints during pregnancy but had no impact on litter size or pup survival. They further speculated that xylazine, not ketamine, was the cause of restricted fetal growth at E15 based upon preliminary work administering each individually at that timepoint.

D. α_2 adrenoreceptor agonists

Dexmedetomidine and xylazine are the most commonly utilized α_2 adrenergic receptor agonists in veterinary patients. Though largely supplanted by dexmedetomidine in companion animal practice due to its improved safety profile, xylazine is still widely used in farm animals and laboratory species.

At doses utilized to induce heavy sedation, xylazine has been well-documented to increase the contractility of the pregnant and nonpregnant uterus in several species (Jansen et al., 1984; Piccinno et al., 2016; Wheaton et al., 1989), resulting in an increase in intrauterine pressure. Xylazine can reduce UBF (Sakamoto et al., 1996; Waldvogel and Bleul, 2014) and has been associated with abortion when administered in the last third of pregnancy to cattle, presumably due to uterine contraction following drug administration (Hodgson et al., 2002). Xylazine rapidly crosses the placenta, and several effects associated with general fetal depression have been observed, including sedation, fetal acidosis (Sakamoto et al., 1996), a reduced fetal heart rate, the cessation of fetal breathing (Jansen et al., 1984).

Medetomidine and its dextrorotary enantiomer, dexmedetomidine, have an α_2:α_1 receptor specificity of 1620:1, making them approximately 10 times more selective than xylazine. Despite the higher selectivity, both have been associated with adverse impacts when used at the doses required to induce anesthesia in animals. A single intramuscular dose of medetomidine (40 μg/kg) in pregnant goats increased contractions and intrauterine pressure, reduced UBF, and produced fetal acidosis (Sakamoto et al., 1997). Kimizuka et al. (2021) demonstrated that dexmedetomidine increased oxytocin-induced myometrial contraction force in pregnant Wistar rats when infused at 30 μg/kg/hour but not at 6 μg/kg/hour.

Notably, both of these α_2-agonists produce strong somatic and visceral analgesia at doses considerably lower than those needed for anesthesia and with less cardiovascular depression. Placental transfer of dexmedetomidine is low in human infants (Yu et al., 2015) and absent in the amniotic fluid of puppies (Groppetti et al., 2019) following cesarean delivery; however, medetomidine levels were present in the same concentration in the umbilical and uterine vessels of sheep following maternal administration (Musk et al., 2012). Conscious pregnant sheep had reductions in maternal heart rate but a minimal reduction in

MAP and no changes in UBF, or fetal heart rate, or MAP when dexmedetomidine was infused intravenously at 1 μg/kg/hour for 3 hours (Uemura et al., 2012). At a higher dose of 2 μg/kg/hour, sheep anesthetized with sevoflurane had reductions in maternal HR, MAP, and UBF but maintained normal acid:base status (Lépiz et al., 2017). Fetal HR and MAP were unaffected in the same study, though fetal blood glucose and lactate levels did rise during anesthesia, suggesting the possibility of poor fetal perfusion. Low doses of medetomidine (equivalent to 1.5 μg/kg/hour of dexmedetomidine) provided effective analgesia without sedation in sheep when administered via an osmotic pump placed at the time of surgery.

While the α_2-agonists are still utilized in some species of pregnant animals, most notably rodents, the general effects of these drugs on uterine activity and fetal hemodynamics suggest that their use at anesthetic doses should be avoided. Those more selective for the α_2 receptor may have some advantages at lower doses for postoperative pain management or as inhalant-sparing adjuncts as part of a balanced anesthetic protocol.

E. Opioids

Opioids readily move across the placental barrier and can be detected in the fetus, though the rate and degree of fetal transfer from the maternal circulation are dependent upon the pharmacology of the specific agent and the placental characteristics of the individual species. In routine veterinary obstetric practice, where opioids are most often administered maternally during cesarean delivery, uptake fetal transfer can be problematic as the resulting sedation and respiratory depression complicate recovery without benefitting the normal, unoperated neonates. In contrast, except for minimally invasive procedures or those restricted to manipulation of placental and umbilical tissues that are devoid of pain receptors, opioid administration directly to the fetus is often recommended in human open uterine surgery to reduce movement and the fetal stress response (Chatterjee et al., 2021). As most animals exposed to open fetal surgery are under general inhalant anesthesia, fetal uptake is likely to be sufficient to provide a surgical plane and eliminate movement. In animal models involving fetal surgery, opioid analgesia is more commonly provided to the dam, either during surgery to reduce the dose requirement for inhalant agents or to ensure analgesia in the postoperative period.

Several opioids have shown to be useful in providing titratable, peri-operative analgesia using a continuous rate infusion with or without a loading bolus. Fentanyl and sufentanil are both rapidly transferred across the placenta to the fetal circulation, although rapid maternal reuptake of sufentanil limits fetal exposure compared to fentanyl (Loftus et al., 1995). Heikkinen et al. (2017) also observed fetal exposure to fentanyl when administered in several different ways, including by infusion, but found no significant fetal accumulation over the course of administration. Remifentanil, an ultrashort-acting μ-selective opioid, is of particular interest for use during pregnancy as it crosses the placental barrier rapidly but is hydrolyzed by plasma and tissue esterases. While fetal plasma levels in sheep are ~10% of the maternal levels during infusion and drop rapidly following discontinuation (Coonen et al., 2010), the lack of reliance upon mature renal or hepatic function for metabolism is a clear advantage for fetal elimination. Remifentanil infusions during surgery in ewes have been demonstrated to significantly reduce the MAC for halothane (Sato et al., 2017; Webster et al., 2005) and have been combined with propofol to deliver supplemental intravenous anesthesia (SIVA), reducing desflurane needs and improving maternal and fetal physiologic parameters (Ngamprasertwong et al., 2013).

The judicious use of opioids during the postoperative period plays a significant role in not only ensuring humane care but also safeguarding against premature labor and abortion. Compared to intermittent boluses, a continuous IV infusion of morphine administered in the postoperative period improved the tocolytic effect of indomethacin in a baboon model of open fetal surgery (Santolaya-Forgas et al., 2006). Oxytocin levels, which are correlated with uterine activity, were lower in animals receiving the infusion, suggesting that consistent pain control in the postoperative period is an important factor in fetal survival. Buprenorphine infused intraarterially for 48 hours following laparotomy in late-term baboons produced a similar, dose-dependent reduction in myometrial activity (Tame et al., 1999). Buprenorphine is a partial μ-agonist that is commonly used to provide analgesia in a number of species due to its efficacy, duration of the activity, and safety associated with its respiratory depression "ceiling effect" relative to the pure μ-agonists. Buprenorphine is also associated with relatively low fetal exposure following maternal administration in sheep (Hakomäki et al., 2021) and rats (Kongstorp et al., 2019). Both intramuscular buprenorphine and transdermal fentanyl provided good postoperative analgesia in pregnant ewes, and neither produced changes in fetal heart rate, arterial pressure, or blood:gas parameters (Padgett et al., 2020). In contrast, placental transfer was high in ewes receiving either IV or epidural administration of oxycodone, with fetal accumulation that exceeded maternal levels (Kinnunen et al., 2018).

F. Nonsteroidal anti-inflammatory drugs

Unlike opioids, nonsteroidal anti-inflammatory drugs (NSAIDs) lack significant depressant effects on the respiratory, cardiovascular, and central nervous systems and are commonly used for postoperative analgesia in both animals and humans due to their effectiveness and relative safety. NSAIDs inhibit cyclooxygenase (COX) production with a subsequent reduction in prostaglandin synthesis and are associated with a number of adverse effects on the human fetus, including premature closure of the ductus arteriosus and foramen ovale; nephrotoxicity; abnormalities of fetal hemostasis; and reductions in amniotic fluid production by the fetal kidney (Black et al., 2019). While animal models have been utilized to investigate many of these impacts, and Thaete et al. (2013) observed no negative effects on fetal or placental growth in pregnant mice receiving intramuscular meloxicam after embryonic day 4, there is scant data in the literature regarding the impact of NSAIDs on fetal development in animals at clinically relevant analgesic doses. There is some evidence that suggests meloxicam, a COX-2 selective NSAID, may be associated with fewer adverse effects than less selective alternatives in fetal sheep, rats, and rabbits. However, these studies evaluated infusions intended to reduce preterm labor (Rac et al., 2006, 2007) or assessed toxic effects following the administration of high, maximum-tolerated doses to dams (Cappon et al., 2003). Prostaglandins also play an important role in the maintenance of uterine and umbilical blood flow. The clinical impact of commonly used NSAIDs on the maintenance of adequate placental blood flow, particularly during maternal systemic hypotension, is unknown; however, an IV infusion of meloxicam to pregnant ewes with RU486-induced preterm labor resulted in no reductions in regional fetal blood flow and no abnormal maternal or fetal blood:gas values. While the prolonged administration of NSAIDs during pregnancy is currently not recommended (Boubred et al., 2006), careful use in the postoperative period appears unlikely to have a significant impact on the developing fetus and helps reduce maternal pain and stress that could lead to premature delivery and pregnancy loss.

G. Vasopressors and anticholinergics

Inhalant and neuraxial (epidural or spinal) anesthesia are two of the most commonly utilized techniques for obstetric surgery in human and veterinary medicine, and both can be associated with the development of maternal hypotension. As previously discussed, due to the absence of significant placental vascular autoregulation, this can have adverse impacts on the fetus, and the use of a vasopressor is common in human patients to prevent reductions in uteroplacental perfusion (Kinsella et al., 2018). Ephedrine and dopamine are among the more commonly used vasopressors in veterinary patients; however, their application in clinical practice is generally in emergent settings or as anesthetic support of nonpregnant animals. Dopamine has been demonstrated to reduce UBF (Rolbin et al., 1979) and increase uterine tone (Fishburne et al., 1980) in gravid sheep. Ephedrine is associated with more favorable responses in ewes, restoring maternal blood pressure and UBF (Strümper et al., 2005) and correcting fetal hypoxemia and placental hemodynamics (Erkinaro et al., 2006, 2007) in epidural-induced models of hypotension. Information regarding the use of vasopressors during pregnancy in rodents is limited, but ephedrine had similar positive effects on maternal blood pressure and UBF in pregnant guinea pigs (Chestnut et al., 1987, 1988).

The routine inclusion of anticholinergics in veterinary premedication protocols is not without some risk and has fallen out of common practice among many practitioners, reserving them instead for correction of bradycardias that develop during the anesthetic event or when high doses of opioids are utilized. Irrespective of how they are applied, glycopyrrolate may be preferred as it does not cross the placenta and will not increase the fetal heart rate, unlike atropine.

III. Neuraxial analgesia/anesthesia

Neuraxial anesthesia involves the epidural or intrathecal delivery of a combination of local anesthetics with an opioid and is routinely utilized in human medicine to provide regional anesthesia and analgesia in conscious patients during labor or cesarean section. While effective for pain control in the mother, little transfer occurs to the fetus or uterus, and surgery on unanesthetized fetuses of ewes given epidural anesthesia alone elicits strong leg, trunk, and/or neck movements in the fetus, especially after 120 days of gestation (Mellor and Gregory, 2003). These movements can make it difficult to carry out surgery on the fetus; therefore, epidural anesthesia alone is rarely used to provide maternal anesthesia and analgesia in more invasive experimental models. Uterine and fetal relaxation are critically important in human fetal surgery as well, and reliance upon neuraxial anesthetic techniques is reserved for minimally invasive procedures (Hoagland and Chatterjee, 2017).

While limited as a primary method of anesthesia, epidural or intrathecal drug administration can still be a useful tool in surgery during pregnancy. Peri-operative use may allow reductions in the amount of general anesthetics and provide analgesia after recovery from anesthesia, depending upon the agents utilized. Epidural catheters are also relatively easily placed during surgery and can be used to extend the duration of titratable postoperative analgesia beyond 24 hours. In humans, low doses of intrathecal or epidural opioids and local anesthetics administered during delivery are not generally associated with adverse neonatal effects (Capogna and Camorcia, 2004); however, practitioners should be aware of several considerations when using neuraxial techniques.

Epidural administration of local anesthetics can be associated with the development of maternal hypotension secondary to sympathetic blockade and has been reported in a variety of species, including dogs (Jones, 2001), swine (Vagts et al., 2003), and primates (Schäffer et al., 2017). Surgical teams should monitor blood pressure closely and be prepared to address reduced MAP with the judicious use of crystalloid fluids or the administration of pressors. Reducing the dose (Martin-Flores et al., 2019) or eliminating the local anesthetic component from the drug combination (Craft et al., 1982, 1984) may avoid the risk of hypotension while still providing a level of regional analgesia, especially when neuraxial administration is an adjunct to general anesthesia. While epidural administration of an anesthetic or analgesic agent often avoids the more significant systemic effects of the drug, it does not completely restrict it to the epidural space. Opioids have been found in the maternal circulation and the fetal blood of sheep (Kinnunen et al., 2018) and puppies (Romagnoli et al., 2019) following maternal epidural administration. While this should not preclude the use of regional anesthesia in pregnant animals, investigators should be aware that neuraxial techniques do not completely protect the fetus from anesthetic exposure.

IV. Prevention of post-operative preterm labor

Preterm labor is the most common and potentially most serious complication of fetal surgery. No single anesthetic agent has been implicated as a causative factor, and it is more likely that the stress response of the dam and fetus to surgery results in physiological changes that can trigger preterm labor. There are also significant differences among species in the sensitivity to uterine manipulation and hysterotomy. Sheep are notably tolerant, and preterm labor is relatively infrequent in this species following open fetal surgery, provided appropriate analgesia is provided. Nonhuman primates are more prone to develop postoperative uterine contractions and, like humans, may require additional interventions including, the administration of tocolytic drugs.

Optimizing the anesthetic regimen by moderating maternal-fetal stress and prioritizing the control of postoperative pain in the dam, as described previously in this chapter, can contribute to a reduced likelihood of abortion (Goodman, 2002). Though there is an increased risk of NSAID-associated fetal effects, the administration of indomethacin has been demonstrated to reduce uterine contractions following fetal surgery (Harrison et al., 1982) and in an interleukin 1β-induced model of preterm labor (Sadowsky et al., 2000) in pregnant macaques. Meloxicam is another NSAID that has demonstrated tocolytic effects in rat uterine tissue (Yousif and Thulesius, 1998) and in sheep models of preterm labor (Rac et al., 2006, 2007).

Continued progesterone secretion is essential for the maintenance of pregnancy in mammals, but there are differences in the principal site of progesterone secretion between species. In sheep, similar to humans, after approximately the first 55 days of pregnancy, the placenta produces sufficient progesterone to maintain pregnancy, whereas the corpus luteum is essential for progesterone secretion and maintenance of pregnancy in, for example, swine, cattle, goats, and horses. Supplementation with exogenous progestins before and after fetal surgery may be useful in some species if postoperative labor occurs. Altrenogest (Boettcher et al., 2019; Sims et al., 1997) and medroxyprogesterone (Swindle et al., 1996) have been used successfully in swine models to reduce fetal loss. Additional tocolytic agents that have been utilized in veterinary patients include terbutaline and nitroglycerin.

V. Functional maturity of key organ systems in newborn animals

While hormonal and mechanical changes in the pregnant female drive the need for anesthetic modifications, the primary considerations in most neonates undergoing anesthesia are the result of immature cardiovascular, respiratory, hepatic, and renal systems relative to adult animals.

Across species, there are huge differences in the stage of maturation of the animal at birth. In marsupial species, the young are born very immature and complete their embryonic development in the maternal pouch (marsupium). Relative to marsupial species, rats are more mature at birth, but they are still neurologically immature, hairless, and blind, and therefore completely dependent on their mother to feed and protect them. In contrast, lambs and other domesticated herbivores are neurologically precocious at birth. They are born with wool or hair covering their bodies, open eyes, and are able to stand shortly after birth. These differences have an impact on the approaches to anesthesia for the newborn animal.

Profound changes in physiology occur in every animal at birth. In particular, the cardiovascular and respiratory systems must rapidly adapt to the environment outside the uterus and to gas exchange occurring in the lungs rather than the placenta. Although physiological changes continue after birth over the following days and weeks, the magnitude and speed of these changes slow with increasing age. Anesthesia of neonatal animals in the first 24 hours after birth is uncommon in clinical or research practice. However, it is important to be aware of differences between neonatal and adult physiology in order to make informed decisions about the anesthetic management of neonatal patients. Species differences in neonatal physiology are evident and, to a certain extent are influenced by the maturity or precociousness of the neonate at birth.

A. Cardiovascular system

The neonate has a low-pressure, low-volume, and low peripheral resistance circulatory system compared to the adult animal (Adelman and Wright, 1985). Consequently, in order to maintain adequate peripheral perfusion in the face of these physiological changes, the neonate has a higher heart rate, plasma volume, and central venous pressure compared to the adult. Neonates demonstrate reduced myocardial contractility and are therefore largely dependent upon heart rate to maintain cardiac output. Because of this, bradycardia in neonates can rapidly result in hypotension and tissue hypoxia. Sympathetic innervation of the heart is incomplete in some neonates (Mace and Levy, 1983). Although there is evidence for structural maturity of the parasympathetic nervous system, the reduced responsiveness of neonatal heart rate to atropine suggests that vagal tone is reduced compared to adults (Fox, 1966; Mace and Levy, 1983). Hypoxia also causes bradycardia in neonates (Stowe et al., 1985; Swann et al., 1954), which is in direct contrast to the effect of hypoxia in adults.

B. Respiratory system

The mechanisms that control physiological function in the newborn develop before birth but require maturation in the postnatal period (Haddad and Mellins, 1984). Neonates show a biphasic response to hypoxia: initially, hypoxia causes an increase in minute ventilation, which is followed by a return to baseline levels if hypoxia persists (Haddad and Mellins, 1984; Nock et al., 2004). The early excitatory phase of the hypoxic ventilatory response is caused by peripheral chemoreceptor stimulation (Miller and Martin, 2011). The decline in ventilation is thought to be secondary to hypoxemia-induced central depression of respiration overriding the initial peripheral chemoreceptor stimulation (Hanson and Kumar, 1994). This may make neonates more vulnerable to apnea, due to hypoxic respiratory depression impairing the ventilatory response to apneic periods. The neonatal response to CO_2 follows a similar developmental pattern with the ventilatory response to hypercarbia increasing gradually after birth. Rat pups may be unique in demonstrating a triphasic response with a nadir of CO_2 sensitivity occurring at the end of the first week of life (Putnam et al., 2005).

The compliance of the chest wall is higher in neonates compared to adults and decreases during development (Papastamelos et al., 1995). Neonatal differences between chest wall and lung compliance predispose the neonate to alveolar collapse because of difficulties in passively maintaining residual lung volume (Papastamelos et al., 1995). In order to maintain functional residual capacity, neonates adopt an augmented breathing pattern with a high frequency of respiration combined with a relatively long expiratory time (Frappell and MacFarlane, 2005). Anesthesia may negatively influence gas exchange in neonates due to the respiratory depressant effects of most anesthetic agents. Pulmonary reserves may also be reduced in animals in the early postnatal period. The timing of lung maturation differs between altricial and precocial species, and while alveolar and bronchial development occurs during normal fetal growth in many larger laboratory animal species, formation does not occur until several days or weeks after birth in mice and rats (Szdzuy and Zeller, 2009).

The higher metabolic rate and oxygen requirements of neonates relative to mature animals can further complicate hypoxia during periods of apnea or airway obstruction, especially during induction. In addition, the expiratory resistance imposed by rebreathing anesthetic circuits may further impair ventilation, and the use of a nonrebreathing circuit or high flow rates should be applied when providing anesthesia to spontaneously breathing neonates.

C. Urinary system

There is significant variation in the degree of renal maturation at birth across species, and multiple developmental milestones of the kidney, including completion of nephrogenesis, maximal concentrating ability, and control of acid/base status, are reached only in the weeks after birth (Frazier, 2017), frustrating maintenance of fluid balance during anesthesia. Renal function reaches maturity in the first 2 weeks after birth in ruminants and pigs (Baggot and Short, 1984), whereas in other domestic species such as horses and dogs renal function matures over the first 4 weeks (Baggot and Short, 1984). Generally, renal blood flow in neonates is directly correlated with arterial blood pressure, and adult control of renal blood flow by angiotensin secretion is not fully developed at birth (Kleinman and Reuter, 1973). The functional immaturity of the kidney observed in neonates is associated with reduced glomerular filtration rate (GFR) and tubular secretory capacity (Bueters et al., 2020) and can decrease the renal excretion of some drugs and drug metabolites, potentially altering the pharmacokinetics of anesthetic and analgesic drugs.

D. Hepatobiliary system

During pregnancy, the placenta carries out many of the functions performed by the liver in the adult animal. During the first week after birth, dramatic changes in hepatic physiology occur, coupled with the loss of umbilical blood flow, increasing hepatic portal vein flow, and closure of the ductus venosus (Gow et al., 2001). The hepatic expression of P_{450} cytochromes matures and changes during the early neonatal period (Gow et al., 2001), and the glucuronide metabolic pathway is not fully developed for at least 6 weeks. The liver is therefore functionally immature at birth, and functionality increases over the subsequent weeks, although the rate of maturation varies between species (Baggot and Short, 1984). Clinically, this results in decreased hepatic metabolism of many anesthetic and analgesic drugs, and drug doses should be adjusted accordingly. The proportionally larger blood volume of neonatal animals compared to adults will also increase the volume of distribution and may impact the pharmacokinetics of some drugs.

VI. Anesthesia of neonatal animals

The specific approach to anesthesia for the neonate will be determined by the age, species, and size of the animal, coupled with a consideration of the invasiveness and duration of the procedure to be carried out. Smaller animals, such as neonatal mice and rats, pose challenges to anesthesia based on their size alone, resulting in practical difficulties such as establishing IV access and airway management. Specific to laboratory animals, investigators must also consider the impacts of anesthetics and analgesics on the disease or process that is ultimately being studied. Of particular concern in humans is the impact of N-methyl-D-aspartate (NMDA) antagonists and gamma aminobutyric acid (GABA) agonists on the development of the central nervous system (Houck and Vinson, 2017). Laboratory mice and rats, as altricial species in which considerable brain maturation may occur in the early postnatal period, may be especially prone to the effects of these agents. There is a growing body of data collected in animal models that has demonstrated anesthetic-induced apoptosis in the nervous system (Sanders et al., 2013), which has informed recent recommendations from the FDA regarding the clinical use of these drugs in human neonatal and pediatric patients (US FDA, 2017). It should be noted that many of these studies are designed to identify anesthetic neurotoxicity and often involve prolonged periods (>4 hours) or repeated episodes of anesthetic administration. While this may accurately model the exposure of human neonates undergoing surgical or diagnostic procedures, the shorter periods of anesthesia commonly used to facilitate experimental manipulations in neonatal animals do not necessarily induce the same apoptotic changes (Yahalom et al., 2011).

As a comprehensive guide to anesthesia for every neonatal model is beyond the scope of this chapter, it will instead focus on general principles that can be applied across species to all neonates. Investigators and practitioners should utilize these principles, in conjunction with a careful review of the current literature, to determine an optimal anesthetic approach for a given neonatal model.

A. Injectable general anesthetics

As previously discussed, immaturity of the hepatic and renal systems can have significant impacts on the rate of metabolism and elimination of anesthetic drugs. Additional physiologic characteristics unique to the neonate, including increased permeability of the blood-brain barrier and reduced plasma albumin, further contribute to the potential for increased or prolonged anesthetic effects relative to adults, especially with injectable drugs. Because of these differences and the difficulty predicting drug elimination in neonatal animals, parenterally administered sedatives and anesthetics should be given to effect to avoid overdosage. This approach has been successfully utilized with a variety of injectable anesthetics in swine (Gasthuys et al., 2017) and rabbits (Mooney et al., 2018), most often as single boluses for sedation or to facilitate rapid sequence induction and intubation. Even when vascular access permits controlled administration, unpredictable drug kinetics in neonatal animals require that repeated dosing or continuous rate infusions be utilized with caution as they may result in unexpected drug accumulation, though fentanyl, ketamine, and propofol infusions have been utilized to supplement or maintain anesthesia in neonatal animals (Clutton et al., 2014; Graham et al., 1998). Due to the potential for the development of apnea with fentanyl and propofol infusions, ventilation should be carefully monitored and support should be provided if needed.

While feasible for larger species, injectable anesthetic titration is frustrated by the technical challenges associated with securing venous access in small, altricial animals. Combinations of ketamine and xylazine are widely utilized in adult rodents to provide general anesthesia; however, these can be unpredictable in neonatal rats (Danneman and Mandrell, 1997; Tsukamoto et al., 2017) and are not recommended. Tsukamoto et al. (2017) found a combination of medetomidine, midazolam, and butorphanol to be effective at inducing anesthesia in neonatal rats, and a similar combination utilizing fentanyl in place of butorphanol provided 30 minutes of anesthesia in 2-day-old mice for intracranial viral injection (Tang et al., 2020). An advantage of these combinations is the ability to rapidly reverse one or more of the component drugs at the conclusion of the surgical procedure, though the use of naloxone for fentanyl reversal will abolish its analgesic effect in the recovering animal. Investigators may consider administering buprenorphine in place of naloxone to reduce residual respiratory depression while preserving some analgesia.

B. Inhalant general anesthetics

One of the primary characteristics of inhalant anesthetics, and the reason that they are so widely used in veterinary clinical practice, is their ability to rapidly titrate their effect to maintain an optimal anesthetic depth. Of particular relevance to neonatal animals, inhalant agents are largely eliminated by the lungs and undergo minimal hepatic metabolism facilitating more rapid recovery and effectively eliminating accumulation concerns. Isoflurane and sevoflurane are the most commonly used inhalant anesthetics in veterinary patients, and, despite minor differences in solubility and degree of hepatic metabolism, both are relatively safe for use in neonatal patients. In general, neonates have a higher MAC than adults of the same species and may require a higher inhaled concentration to achieve a surgical plane of anesthesia (Loepke et al., 2006). In general, the pharmacologic effects of inhalant anesthetics in neonates are similar to those in adults. Several studies have demonstrated stable physiologic parameters in neonatal rodents receiving volatile anesthetics, including heart rate, respiratory rate, and oxygen saturation (Huss et al., 2016; Mayer et al., 2018), though respiratory acidosis has been reported in otherwise stable mice (Loepke et al., 2006) and rats (Mayer et al., 2018) receiving isoflurane for anesthetic events of longer duration (60–90 minutes). A dose-dependent reduction in blood pressure may occur (Lerman et al., 1990; Loepke et al., 2006), consistent with the well-described vasodilatory effects of these anesthetics. Inhalant anesthetics have the potential to induce hypoglycemia in neonatal mice, independent of fasting, when administered for periods in excess of 1–2 hours and this can be successfully attenuated with intraperitoneal administration of 5% dextrose solution (Loepke et al., 2006, 2009; Yu et al., 2020).

Administration of gas anesthesia, while generally safe and effective for the patient, does pose a potential risk of exposure to personnel unless waste anesthetic gases are appropriately contained and scavenged. Placement of an endotracheal tube for delivery of gases and airway maintenance is ideal but can be difficult in some species. The potential for traumatic intubation can cause permanent damage to the trachea or larynx, and narrow-diameter endotracheal tubes can pose a high resistance to respiration and are at risk of obstruction from bronchial secretions, especially when animals are breathing spontaneously. Though tracheostomy may be a suitable alternative in some circumstances, orotracheal intubation is often possible using blind (Benito et al., 2021) or direct visualization techniques (Miranda et al., 2017), even in very small neonates. Inhalant agents can also be delivered via a nose cone or face mask, though these methods do not provide airway protection or assure respiratory delivery of anesthetic gases during positive pressure ventilation and leakage can increase the risk of occupational exposure. As obligate nasal breathers, tight-fitting nose cones have been used successfully to ventilate adult rodents in lieu of endotracheal intubation (Krutrök et al., 2021; Rindfield and McBrian, 2012). However, these are secured on the maxillary incisors, making them less practical in altricial species. Irrespective of whether delivery is accomplished by intubation or a mask, nonrebreathing circuits and high flow rates should be used for spontaneously breathing neonatal animals given their small size and reduced pulmonary reserve. This reduces the resistance of airflow in the circuit and prevents accumulation and rebreathing of carbon dioxide, but it can also exacerbate heat loss, a primary concern when anesthetizing newborn animals.

C. Cryoanesthesia/hypothermia

The induction of deep hypothermia in neonatal rodents has been described as a method of producing general anesthesia with relatively low mortality (Phifer and Terry, 1986). Cooling to 9°C halts nerve conduction and produces immobilization, respiratory arrest, and a marked reduction in heart rate and oxygen saturation compared to inhalant anesthetics (Huss et al., 2016). Though it seems unlikely that animals are capable of experiencing pain during the period of profound hypothermia, concerns regarding the potential for pain associated with rewarming (Herrmann and Flecknell, 2019) and the availability of safer and more easily titrated options make hypothermia a less desirable alternative, and the author prefers the use of inhalant anesthetics for most applications.

The acceptability of hypothermia for altricial rodent anesthesia and the ages at which it is permissible vary among institutions; however, there are several general principles that should be followed when using this method. Induction is usually accomplished by immersing the rodent pup in a slurry of water and crushed ice for approximately 5 minutes. To prevent injury to the skin, the animal must not directly contact the ice, and a finger from an exam glove makes a readily available sleeve for this purpose. After induction, the pup is placed onto an ice pack for the duration of the procedure. A glove filled with crushed ice can be molded to help maintain the position of the pup during the surgical procedure. Fiberoptic or LED lighting should be used to avoid heating the animal and premature recovery from anesthesia, and the total duration of hypothermia should be minimized to the shortest possible duration, not to exceed 30 minutes. Recovery can be prolonged (>30 minutes) and should occur gradually by placing the pup into an incubator or cage on a recirculating warm water pad.

VII. Supportive measures during neonatal anesthesia

A. Monitoring during anesthesia

Monitoring during anesthesia of neonates of all species is vital to warn of impending complications and allow early intervention. Manual monitoring of pulse rate and quality, observation of respiration, and assessment of the color and perfusion quality of the mucous membranes should be evaluated before and throughout the anesthetic event.

Additional monitoring of parameters such as electrocardiography, blood pressure, oxygen saturation, capnometry, and body temperature provides more detailed and precise information about the physiological status of the patient during anesthesia and are useful techniques for smaller animals where the manual monitoring of parameters is more challenging. Anesthetic monitoring equipment that is suitable for companion animal clinical practice will generally be suitable for neonates of most large animal species. Apparatus used in adult cats and dogs is usually suitable for use in neonates of these species, as well as some foals, calves, and pigs (depending on size). Specialized equipment is readily available for monitoring physiologic parameters in mice and rats, and sensors are available for neonates of these species.

B. Body temperature

Neonatal animals are generally at a higher risk of developing hypothermia than adults due to several anatomic and physiologic characteristics. Due to their relatively larger surface area to volume ratio and minimal subcutaneous fat accumulations, neonates are more susceptible to rapid cooling during anesthetic events. In the first few days after birth, the physiological adaptations to cold, such as vasoconstriction and shivering, are poorly developed (Lyon et al., 1997). Altricial young, both rodent and nonrodent, are most at risk, and while some degree of thermogenesis begins in the first 24 hours after birth, full control of body temperature is not achieved for 1–2 weeks in some species (Szdzuy and Zeller, 2009). Due to these factors, hypothermia can progress very quickly in newborn animals undergoing anesthetic events, even those of relatively short duration, and can lead to rapid deterioration if not addressed proactively.

Specific supportive measures are similar to those used in more mature animals and include regular monitoring, taking steps to reduce heat loss, and providing heat support through the anesthetic and recovery periods. Reducing heat loss by increasing the ambient environmental temperature and ensuring the animal does not lie on cold surfaces are vital to prevent heat loss. Two studies evaluating the impact of presurgical skin preparation on whole-body cooling in adult mice (Skorupski et al., 2017) and pediatric cats and dogs (Isaza et al., 2021) found no difference between the use of sterile water or saline compared to alcohol. There is probably no significant advantage to avoiding alcohol-based rinses or using warmed fluids in precocial neonates. However, care should still be taken to prevent excessive wetting of the body with cold fluids, especially with altricial species.

Measures to maintain normothermia during anesthesia include the use of forced air-warming devices (for example, a Bair Hugger®), isothermal heating pads, circulating warm water blankets, and heat lamps. Most of these devices can be easily modified for use in small animals such as rodents. Hyperthermia and skin burns can occur due to overzealous heating, and lack of attention to body temperature monitoring, particularly because the animal is immobile and unable to move away from direct heat sources. Measures to prevent skin burns (particularly when using heating devices on hairless animals) must be adopted.

C. Blood glucose

Blood glucose concentration is under tight metabolic control and is maintained within normal limits by glycogenolysis, gluconeogenesis, glycolysis, and insulin/glucagon secretion. In the first few hours after birth, neonates are at high risk of hypoglycemia because of limited glycogen stores at birth combined with the cessation of placental glucose supply (Mellor and Cockburn, 1986). This is especially so when colostrum or milk intake is inadequate. Anesthesia can further increase the risk of hypoglycemia in neonates because feeding is suspended during the period of anesthesia, though the development and severity of hypoglycemia may depend upon the species, the anesthetic used and the age of the animal (Yu et al., 2020). As mentioned previously in this chapter, inhalant anesthetics may induce hypoglycemia in rodents when administered for long-duration events.

When possible, monitoring blood glucose concentration during anesthesia can be a useful tool to guide supportive care. In addition to veterinary-specific point-of-care analyzers, commercially available, portable handheld glucometers for use by human patients are widely available, and require very little blood, but may need to be validated for the species of interest (Katsoulos et al., 2011; Morley et al., 2018). The frequency of testing and intervention can be adjusted depending on the stability of the measured blood glucose concentration. Alternatively, dextrose can be added to the intravenous fluids for administration during the anesthetic event or as intraperitoneal boluses in rodents. As the risk of hypoglycemia remains until the animal is able to resume normal feeding from the dam, monitoring of blood glucose should continue through the immediate postoperative period. Additional nutritional support can be provided to larger neonates by tube feeding maternal milk or colostrum via the mouth into the distal esophagus. This should not be undertaken until the neonate is able to swallow in order to reduce the risk of aspiration associated with this intervention.

VIII. Postanesthetic period

The recovery period is recognized to be a relatively high-risk period in veterinary anesthesia. The cardiovascular and respiratory side effects of anesthetic drugs remain until the animal is fully conscious, necessitating active support and continuous monitoring during the recovery period to prevent hypothermia, hypovolemia, and hypoxia. Derangements in fluid and energy balance may persist until the animal is able to maintain normal fluid and electrolyte balance and food intake. Oxygen should be supplemented using a face mask or oxygen tent until the animal is fully awake. An incubator can be a good environment in which to recover small neonatal animals. The environmental temperature can be controlled to prevent hypothermia, and the air in the incubator can easily be enriched with oxygen. Pain should also be frequently assessed during the postoperative period using behavioral indicators appropriate for that species.

Maternal acceptance of the neonate in the postoperative period is critically important for both altricial and precocial species. In the clinical setting, the introduction of infant nonhuman primates to their dams following cesarean delivery can be challenging, and several strategies have been reported to improve the chance of successful pairing (Bellanca et al., 2006; Ruggiero et al., 2009). Similarly, when sedating nonhuman primates for minor procedures it may be possible to keep their infants with them, avoiding neonatal stress. In contrast, when neonates undergo surgical procedures, separation from the dam is necessary, and manipulations that result in the introduction of new odors or physical changes to the neonate, such as incision sites or hair removal, can result in maternal inattention in some species. Reducing the period of time that offspring are separated from their mother during induction and recovery prevented maternal rejection and improved postoperative nursing and recovery in a scoliosis model in lambs (Clutton et al., 2014). Park et al. (1992), performing ocular surgery in day-old rat pups, minimized time away from the dam by removing pups individually from the litter and returning them as soon as they had recovered. They also described frequent, gentle handling of the pregnant rats and olfactory acclimation to materials like the tissue glue used for incisional closure in the days prior to parturition. Careful attention to the removal of blood and residual antiseptics from the skin followed by contact with bedding from the home cage has also been recommended to help reduce the introduction of novel odors following surgery in mice (Mahmoud et al., 2014).

IX. Neonatal analgesia

Historically, the use of analgesics in human neonates has not matched that of adults due to several factors, including concerns about altered drug pharmacokinetics, questions about the degree of pain perception, and difficulty assessing pain levels in nonverbal patients. The importance of adequate pain management in neonates is now recognized, and the routine use of analgesics in human infants has been facilitated by the development of pain scoring systems, a better understanding of neonatal physiology, and adherence to a balanced, multimodal approach (De Lima and Carmo, 2010; Haidon and Cunliffe, 2010). The potential for early pain experiences to alter the developing nervous system and produce functional changes that persist into adulthood has been demonstrated in both human (Taddio et al., 1997; Walker, 2019) and veterinary neonates (Carmo et al., 2016; Ranger et al., 2019; Victoria et al., 2014). Significantly, long-term changes in nociceptive sensitivity can be attenuated when analgesics are administered during the initial painful stimulus (van den Hoogen et al., 2021, 2016), though there may be variability between different analgesics and routes of delivery (Moriarty et al., 2018).

The assessment of pain is difficult in adult animals and is even more so in neonates, especially in altricial species due to their small size and lack of active behaviors (Henare et al., 2008). Ethograms have been developed to catalog behaviors observed in response to routine husbandry procedures in agricultural species (Hay et al., 2003; Molony et al., 1995, 2002). More recently, facial grimace scoring systems have been developed and validated specifically for piglets (Di Giminiani et al., 2016; Viscardi et al., 2017), lambs (Guesgen et al., 2016), and foals (van Loon et al., 2020). These systems can be utilized separately or in combination to aid in the assessment of pain in these species. In the absence of published behavioral criteria, animal users should consult the literature regarding analgesics with demonstrated impacts on analgesiometric assays in neonates. In general, it is useful to apply the same principles utilized in adults, namely multi-modal analgesia, preemptive administration, and regular assessment and treatment of pain-related behavior.

A. Nonsteroidal anti-inflammatory drugs

NSAIDs form a valuable component of peri-operative pain control in adult animals; however, recommendations for NSAID administration to neonates vary between species. NSAIDs are utilized for a variety of indications in human neonatology, including analgesia, antipyresis, and to induce closure of patent ductus arteriosus in premature infants (Aranda et al., 2017). Despite the utility of these drugs, NSAIDs are known to reduce the GFR, decreasing elimination and potentially resulting in acute renal failure (Donato et al., 2019). The intravenous administration of aspirin, indomethacin, and ibuprofen to neonatal rabbits resulted in reductions in renal blood flow and GFR (Guignard, 2002). These concerns have also limited their use in companion animal species, and NSAIDs are not advised in puppies and kittens less than 6 weeks of age (Mathews, 2008). Due to these concerns, careful consideration should be given to the use of NSAIDs in altricial young, and alternatives such as opioids and local anesthetics may be preferable options in these species.

In contrast, cattle and horses appear to be at a reduced risk of renal and gastrointestinal side effects from NSAIDs, and this class of drugs is commonly administered to horses and calves less than 1 month old (Crisman et al., 1996; Semrad, 1993). While this suggests that there may be fewer concerns in precocial young, the efficacy of these NSAIDs as analgesics can be both species and procedure specific. Using a grimace scale to assess foals with a variety of painful clinical conditions, van Loon et al. (2020) observed a significant reduction in pain scores in foals receiving intravenous flunixin meglumine or meloxicam. Growing interest in the treatment of pain resulting from routine husbandry practices in the agricultural setting has led to the evaluation of several NSAIDs in swine and sheep. Studies evaluating the effectiveness of NSAIDs in piglets following castration using routine management techniques have reported conflicting results. Several authors have reported effective postcastration analgesia with the preemptive use of meloxicam (Keita et al., 2010; Kluivers-Poodt et al., 2013), and a study by Nixon et al. (2021) suggested that flunixin and ketoprofen provided effective analgesia when administered to piglets 2 hours before castration and tail docking. In contrast, neither meloxicam (Burkemper et al., 2020; Viscardi et al., 2017) nor ketoprofen (Viscardi and Turner, 2018a) reduced pain-related behaviors or grimace scores in piglets when administered up to 20 minutes before surgery.

Similar variability in NSAID efficacy has been reported in lambs following mulesing, the surgical removal of perineal skin to prevent fly-strike in a wool production setting. Meloxicam with a topical anesthetic did not reduce pain behaviors in lambs when administered after mulesing and tail docking at 6–8 weeks of age (Grant et al., 2020), while carprofen and flunixin were both efficacious at reducing pain behaviors in 5-week-old lambs when given 90 minutes before mulesing (Paull et al., 2007). While this variability must be considered by practitioners, especially when using an NSAID as a sole analgesic in neonatal swine or sheep, it should also be noted that these studies evaluated the administration of NSAIDs shortly before the performance of noxious surgical procedures in nonsedated animals. In most instances, in a laboratory setting, piglets and lambs undergoing surgical procedures benefit from additional anesthesia, which could impact postoperative effects of these analgesics.

B. Opioids

Opioids lack the adverse impacts on renal function posed by the NSAIDs and provide more predictable and potent analgesia; however, as with adults, they can result in depression of the cardiovascular and respiratory systems. Neonates are generally more sensitive to opioids than older animals. Puppies required lower doses of morphine and fentanyl than older animals to induce analgesia (Luks et al., 1998) and respiratory depression (Bragg et al., 1995), and morphine, fentanyl, meperidine, and buprenorphine were all more potent in 3-day-old rat pups than in adult rats (McLaughlin and Dewey, 1994). Because the rate of maturational change in sensitivity is difficult to predict it is advisable to initially give low doses of opioids (e.g., half of the adult dose) and increase the dose as needed based upon the level of analgesia achieved. This is a safer way to achieve effective analgesia without excessive side effects. As a partial agonist, buprenorphine has the advantage of being less likely than pure μ-agonists to produce severe respiratory depression. Buprenorphine also has demonstrated efficacy in producing analgesia in neonatal animals. Thermal sensitivity in a neonatal rat model of incisional pain was reduced by buprenorphine HCl (Katz et al., 2021) and a sustained-release buprenorphine product (Blaney et al., 2021). Buprenorphine HCl was also effective in reducing facial grimace scores and pain behaviors in 5-day-old piglets following castration (Viscardi and Turner, 2018b). Reversal of excessive opioid side effects can be achieved with naloxone, although this may reverse opioid analgesia and expose the neonate to pain.

C. Local and neuraxial anesthesia

In order to avoid the potential for adverse effects associated with systemic NSAIDs or opioids, local and regional anesthetic techniques are commonly employed in human neonatal patients as an alternative or adjunct to other analgesics (Squillaro et al., 2019). The use of these techniques is also possible in many veterinary species and includes local or incisional application, perineural blockade, and neuraxial administration (e.g., epidural or intrathecal), each differing in technical difficulty and the extent and duration of effect.

The use of local infiltration, preferably before incision, is the simplest technique and can provide some analgesia but is limited by a relatively short duration of action. Lidocaine has shown minimal efficacy in the immediate postoperative period in neonatal rats (Katz et al., 2021) and piglets (Kluivers-Poodt et al., 2013), while bupivacaine has shown more promise in neonates. When applied for 30 seconds immediately following tail biopsy in neonatal mice, 0.5% bupivacaine prevented increases in corticosterone and blood glucose, a measure of hypothalamic/pituitary axis (HPA) activation and stress (Dudley et al., 2016). In contrast, application of a topical lidocaine (2.5%) or prilocaine (2.5%) cream up to 60 minutes prior to biopsy failed to prevent HPA activation in the same study, despite the accepted use of this product in human medicine as a topical anesthetic. Topical products containing mixtures of bupivacaine, lidocaine, and epinephrine have proven an effective means of reducing pain in piglets for up to 4 hours after castration when applied intraoperatively (Lomax et al., 2017; Sheil et al., 2021).

The perineural injection of local anesthetics has been described for several neonatal species and, while more challenging, offers an improved duration of effect relative to tissue infiltration alone. Blockade of the sciatic nerve with bupivacaine in 5-day-old rat pups reduced thermal nociception in the hindlimb for more than 2 hours (Kohane et al., 1998). Sciatic blockade with bupivacaine in 3-day-old rat pups before surgical incision of the paw prevented changcs in spinal nociceptive sensitivity in later life, suggesting a complete analgesic effect (Moriarty et al., 2018; Walker et al., 2015). Regional blockade in larger species is also possible and can be aided by the use of a peripheral nerve stimulator to ensure correct placement. Ghadirian et al. (2016) compared the duration of several local anesthetic combinations in a brachial plexus block in fat-tailed lambs and observed that sensory and motor blockade was significantly prolonged with bupivacaine (~5 hours) compared to lidocaine (~1.5 hours).

Epidural or intrathecal anesthesia, while technically demanding, has been described for both rodent and large animal neonates and can provide analgesia to a larger area (e.g., bilateral vs. unilateral) with a single administration. Evaluating intrathecal bupivacaine in rat pups, several authors (Hamurtekin et al., 2013; Yahalom et al., 2011) have demonstrated motor and sensory blockade without long-term impacts on gait or evidence of spinal cord toxicity. Intrathecal ketamine, in comparison, provides good anesthesia but is also neurotoxic, inducing histologic injury and prolonged motor alterations into adulthood (Walker et al., 2010). Epidural techniques are well described in the literature for larger species and lidocaine administered to lambs rapidly produced effective analgesia of the skin caudal to the flanks of approximately 1 hour duration (Habibian et al., 2011). The addition or substitution of tramadol as the epidural agent resulted in a slower onset but significantly longer duration of action compared to lidocaine alone.

Acknowledgments

This chapter builds upon the related chapter in the second edition of this text. Portions of text from the previous edition have been retained, updated, and added to. The author of the current chapter is indebted to the previous authors: Joanna C. Murrell, David J. Mellor, and Craig B. Johnson.

References

Adelman, R.D., Wright, J., 1985. Systolic blood pressure and heart rate in the growing beagle puppy. Dev. Pharmacol. Ther. 8, 396–401. https://doi.org/10.1159/000457064.

Andaluz, A., Trasserras, O., García, F., 2005. Maternal and fetal effects of propofol anaesthesia in the pregnant ewe. Vet. J. 170, 77–83. https://doi.org/10.1016/j.tvjl.2004.02.006.

Andaluz, A., Tusell, J., Trasserres, O., Cristòfol, C., Capece, B.P.S.C., Arboix, M., Garcia, F., 2003. Transplacental transfer of propofol in pregnant ewes. Vet. J. 166, 198–204. https://doi.org/10.1016/s1090-0233(02)00259-9.

Ansari, J., Carvalho, B., Shafer, S.L., Flood, P., 2016. Pharmacokinetics and pharmacodynamics of drugs commonly used in pregnancy and parturition. Anesth. Analg. 122, 786–804. https://doi.org/10.1213/ANE.0000000000001143.

Aranda, J.V., Salomone, F., Valencia, G.B., Beharry, K.D., 2017. Non-steroidal anti-inflammatory drugs in newborns and infants. Pediatr. Clin. N. Am. 64, 1327–1340. https://doi.org/10.1016/j.pcl.2017.08.009.

Baggot, J.D., Short, C.R., 1984. Drug disposition in the neonatal animal, with particular reference to the foal. Equine Vet. J. 16, 364–367. https://doi.org/10.1111/j.2042-3306.1984.tb01945.x.

Bellanca, R.U., Koberstein, D.R., Delio, P.J., Kelley, S.T., Crockett, C.M., 2006. Successful introduction of *Macaca nemestrina* infants to their mothers after cesarean delivery. J. Am. Assoc. Lab. Anim. Sci. 45, 27–32.

Benito, S., Hadley, S., Camprubí-Camprubí, M., Sanchez-de-Toledo, J., 2021. Blind endotracheal intubation in neonatal rabbits. J. Vis. Exp. https://doi.org/10.3791/61874.

Biehl, D.R., Yarnell, R., Wade, J.G., Sitar, D., 1983. The uptake of isoflurane by the foetal lamb in utero: effect on regional blood flow. Can. Anaesth. Soc. J. 30, 581–586. https://doi.org/10.1007/BF03015226.

Black, E., Khor, K.E., Kennedy, D., Chutatape, A., Sharma, S., Vancaillie, T., Demirkol, A., 2019. Medication use and pain management in pregnancy: a critical review. Pain Pract. 19, 875–899. https://doi.org/10.1111/papr.12814.

Blaney, A., Jampachaisri, K., Huss, M.K., Pacharinsak, C., 2021. Sustained release buprenorphine effectively attenuates postoperative hypersensitivity in an incisional pain model in neonatal rats (*Rattus norvegicus*). PLoS One 16. https://doi.org/10.1371/journal.pone.0246213.

Boettcher, A.N., Ahrens, A.P., Charley, S.E., Tuggle, C.K., 2019. A comprehensive protocol for laparotomy in swine to facilitate ultrasound-guided injection into the fetal intraperitoneal space. Comp. Med. 69, 123–129. https://doi.org/10.30802/AALAS-CM-18-000098.

Boubred, F., Vendemmia, M., Garcia-Meric, P., Buffat, C., Millet, V., Simeoni, U., 2006. Effects of maternally administered drugs on the fetal and neonatal kidney. Drug Saf. 29, 397–419. https://doi.org/10.2165/00002018-200629050-00004.

Bragg, P., Zwass, M.S., Lau, M., Fisher, D.M., 1995. Opioid pharmacodynamics in neonatal dogs: differences between morphine and fentanyl. J. Appl. Physiol. 79, 1519–1524. https://doi.org/10.1152/jappl.1995.79.5.1519.

Bueters, R., Bael, A., Gasthuys, E., Chen, C., Schreuder, M.F., Frazier, K.S., 2020. Ontogeny and cross-species comparison of pathways involved in drug absorption, distribution, metabolism, and excretion in neonates (review): kidney. Drug Metab. Dispos. 48, 353–367. https://doi.org/10.1124/dmd.119.089755.

Burkemper, M.C., Pairis-Garcia, M.D., Moraes, L.E., Park, R.M., Moeller, S.J., 2020. Effects of oral meloxicam and topical lidocaine on pain associated behaviors of piglets undergoing surgical castration. J. Appl. Anim. Welf. Sci. 23, 209–218. https://doi.org/10.1080/10888705.2019.1590717.

Capogna, G., Camorcia, M., 2004. Epidural analgesia for childbirth: effects of newer techniques on neonatal outcome. Paediatr. Drugs 6, 375–386. https://doi.org/10.2165/00148581-200406060-00005.

Cappon, G.D., Cook, J.C., Hurtt, M.E., 2003. Relationship between cyclooxygenase 1 and 2 selective inhibitors and fetal development when administered to rats and rabbits during the sensitive periods for heart development and midline closure. Birth Defects Res. B Dev. Reprod. Toxicol. 68, 47–56. https://doi.org/10.1002/bdrb.10008.

Carmo, E.D.C.D., Sanada, L.S., Machado, N.L.B., Fazan, V.P.S., 2016. Does pain in the neonatal period influence motor and sensory functions in a similar way for males and females during post-natal development in rats? Pain Med. 17, 1520–1529. https://doi.org/10.1093/pm/pnv117.

Chatterjee, D., Arendt, K.W., Moldenhauer, J.S., Olutoye, O.A., Parikh, J.M., Tran, K.M., et al., 2021. Anesthesia for maternal–fetal interventions: a consensus statement from the American Society of Anesthesiologists Committees on Obstetric and Pediatric Anesthesiology and the North American Fetal Therapy Network. Anesth. Analg. 132, 1164–1173. https://doi.org/10.1213/ANE.0000000000005177.

Chestnut, D.H., Ostman, L.G., Weiner, C.P., Hdez, M.J., Wang, J.P., 1988. The effect of vasopressor agents upon uterine artery blood flow velocity in the gravid guinea pig subjected to ritodrine infusion. Anesthesiology 68, 363–366.

Chestnut, D.H., Weiner, C.P., Wang, J.P., Herrig, J.E., Martin, J.G., 1987. The effect of ephedrine upon uterine artery blood flow velocity in the pregnant guinea pig subjected to terbutaline infusion and acute hemorrhage. Anesthesiology 66, 508–512. https://doi.org/10.1097/00000542-198704000-00010.

Clutton, R.E., Vettoratto, E., Schoeffman, G., Docherty, J., Burke, J., Gibson, A.J.N., 2014. The perioperative care of lambs and ewes when the former undergo major experimental (scoliotic) surgery. Lab. Anim. 48, 27–35. https://doi.org/10.1177/0023677213498718.

Coonen, J.B., Marcus, M.A.E., Joosten, E.A.J., van Kleef, M., Neef, C., van Aken, H., Gogarten, W., 2010. Transplacental transfer of remifentanil in the pregnant ewe. Br. J. Pharmacol. 161, 1472–1476. https://doi.org/10.1111/j.1476-5381.2010.00783.x.

Craft, J.B., Bolan, J.C., Coaldrake, L.A., Mondino, M., Mazel, P., Gilman, R.M., et al., 1982. The maternal and fetal cardiovascular effects of epidural morphine in the sheep model. Am. J. Obstet. Gynecol. 142, 835–839. https://doi.org/10.1016/S0002-9378(16)32528-5.

Craft, J.B., Coaldrake, L.A., Yonekura, M.L., Dao, S.D., Co, E.G., Roizen, M.F., et al., 1983. Ketamine, catecholamines, and uterine tone in pregnant ewes. Am. J. Obstet. Gynecol. 146, 429–434. https://doi.org/10.1016/0002-9378(83)90823-2.

Craft, J.B., Robichaux, A.G., Kim, H., Thorpe, D.H., Mazel, P., Woolf, W.A., Stolte, A., 1984. The maternal and fetal cardiovascular effects of epidural fentanyl in the sheep model. Am. J. Obstet. Gynecol. 148, 1098–1104. https://doi.org/10.1016/0002-9378(84)90635-5.

Crisman, M.V., Wilcke, J.R., Sams, R.A., 1996. Pharmacokinetics of flunixin meglumine in healthy foals less than twenty-four hours old. Am. J. Vet. Res. 57, 1759–1761.

Danneman, P.J., Mandrell, T.D., 1997. Evaluation of five agents/methods for anesthesia of neonatal rats. Lab. Anim. Sci. 47, 386–395.

De Lima, J., Carmo, K.B., 2010. Practical pain management in the neonate. Best Pract. Res. Clin. Anaesthesiol. 24, 291–307. https://doi.org/10.1016/j.bpa.2010.04.001.

Di Giminiani, P., Brierley, V.L.M.H., Scollo, A., Gottardo, F., Malcolm, E.M., Edwards, S.A., Leach, M.C., 2016. The assessment of facial expressions in piglets undergoing tail docking and castration: toward the development of the piglet grimace scale. Front. Vet. Sci. 3, 100. https://doi.org/10.3389/fvets.2016.00100.

Doebeli, A., Michel, E., Bettschart, R., Hartnack, S., Reichler, I.M., 2013. Apgar score after induction of anesthesia for canine cesarean section with alfaxalone versus propofol. Theriogenology 80, 850–854. https://doi.org/10.1016/j.theriogenology.2013.07.006.

Donato, J., Rao, K., Lewis, T., 2019. Pharmacology of common analgesic and sedative drugs used in the neonatal intensive care unit. Clin. Perinatol. 46, 673–692. https://doi.org/10.1016/j.clp.2019.08.004.

Dudley, E.S., Johnson, R.A., French, D.C., Boivin, G.P., 2016. Effects of topical anesthetics on behavior, plasma corticosterone, and blood glucose levels after tail biopsy of C57BL/6NHSD mice (*Mus musculus*). J. Am. Assoc. Lab. Anim. Sci. 55, 443–450.

Eggink, A.J., Roelofs, L.A.J., Feitz, W.F.J., Wijnen, R.M.H., Mullaart, R.A., Grotenhuis, J.A., et al., 2005. In utero repair of an experimental neural tube defect in a chronic sheep model using biomatrices. Fetal Diagn. Ther. 20, 335–340. https://doi.org/10.1159/000086808.

Ellingson, R., Rose, G., 1970. Ontogenesis of the electroencephalogram. In: Himwich, W.A., Williamina, A. (Eds.), Developmental Neurobiology. Thomas, Springfield, Ill, pp. 441–474.

Erkinaro, T., Kavasmaa, T., Päkkilä, M., Acharya, G., Mäkikallio, K., Alahuhta, S., Räsänen, J., 2006. Ephedrine and phenylephrine for the treatment of maternal hypotension in a chronic sheep model of increased placental vascular resistance. Br. J. Anaesth. 96, 231–237. https://doi.org/10.1093/bja/aei305.

Erkinaro, T., Mäkikallio, K., Acharya, G., Päkkilä, M., Kavasmaa, T., Huhta, J.C., et al., 2007. Divergent effects of ephedrine and phenylephrine on cardiovascular hemodynamics of near-term fetal sheep exposed to hypoxemia and maternal hypotension. Acta Anaesthesiol. Scand. 51, 922–928. https://doi.org/10.1111/j.1399-6576.2007.01327.x.

Fishburne, J.I., Meis, P.J., Urban, R.B., Greiss, F.C., Wheeler, A.S., James, F.M., et al., 1980. Vascular and uterine responses to dobutamine and dopamine in the gravid ewe. Am. J. Obstet. Gynecol. 137, 944–952. https://doi.org/10.1016/s0002-9378(16)32836-8.

Fox, M.W., 1966. Developmental physiology and behaviour. In: Himwich, W. (Ed.), Canine Pediatrics; Development, Neonatal, and Congenital Diseases. C. C. Thomas, Springfield, Ill., pp. 22–25

Frappell, P.B., MacFarlane, P.M., 2005. Development of mechanics and pulmonary reflexes. Respir. Physiol. Neurobiol. 149, 143–154. https://doi.org/10.1016/j.resp.2005.05.028.

Frazier, K.S., 2017. Species differences in renal development and associated developmental nephrotoxicity. Birth Defects Res. 109, 1243–1256. https://doi.org/10.1002/bdr2.1088.

Gasthuys, E., Schauvliege, S., van Bergen, T., Millecam, J., Cerasoli, I., Martens, A., et al., 2017. Repetitive urine and blood sampling in neonatal and weaned piglets for pharmacokinetic and pharmacodynamic modelling in drug discovery: a pilot study. Lab. Anim. 51, 498–508. https://doi.org/10.1177/0023677217692372.

Gaynor, J.S., Wertz, E.M., Alvis, M., Turner, A.S., 1998. A comparison of the haemodynamic effects of propofol and isoflurane in pregnant ewes. J. Vet. Pharmacol. Ther. 21, 69–73. https://doi.org/10.1046/j.1365-2885.1998.00110.x.

Ghadirian, S., Vesal, N., Maghsoudi, B., Akhlagh, S.H., 2016. Comparison of lidocaine, lidocaine-morphine, lidocaine-tramadol or bupivacaine for neural blockade of the brachial plexus in fat-tailed lambs. Vet. Anaesth. Analg. 43, 109–116. https://doi.org/10.1111/vaa.12280.

Goodman, S., 2002. Anesthesia for nonobstetric surgery in the pregnant patient. Semin. Perinatol. 26, 136–145. https://doi.org/10.1053/sper.2002.32203.

Gow, P.J., Ghabrial, H., Smallwood, R.A., Morgan, D.J., Ching, M.S., 2001. Neonatal hepatic drug elimination. Pharmacol. Toxicol. 88, 3–15. https://doi.org/10.1034/j.1600-0773.2001.088001003.x.

Graham, M.R., Thiessen, D.B., Mutch, W.A.C., 1998. Left ventricular systolic and diastolic function is unaltered during propofol infusion in newborn swine. Anesth. Analg. 86, 717–723. https://doi.org/10.1213/00000539-199804000-00008.

Grant, E.P., Wickham, S.L., Anderson, F., Barnes, A.L., Fleming, P.A., Miller, D.W., 2020. Preliminary findings on a novel behavioural approach for the assessment of pain and analgesia in lambs subject to routine husbandry procedures. Animals 10, E1148. https://doi.org/10.3390/ani10071148.

Gregory, G.A., Wade, J.G., Beihl, D.R., Ong, B.Y., Sitar, D.S., 1983. Fetal anesthetic requirement (MAC) for halothane. Anesth. Analg. 62, 9–14.

Groppetti, D., Di Cesare, F., Pecile, A., Cagnardi, P., Merlanti, R., D'Urso, E.S., et al., 2019. Maternal and neonatal wellbeing during elective C-section induced with a combination of propofol and dexmedetomidine: how effective is the placental barrier in dogs? Theriogenology 129, 90–98. https://doi.org/10.1016/j.theriogenology.2019.02.019.

Guesgen, M.J., Beausoleil, N.J., Leach, M., Minot, E.O., Stewart, M., Stafford, K.J., 2016. Coding and quantification of a facial expression for pain in lambs. Behav. Processes 132, 49–56. https://doi.org/10.1016/j.beproc.2016.09.010.

Guignard, J.-P., 2002. The adverse renal effects of prostaglandin-synthesis inhibitors in the newborn rabbit. Semin. Perinatol. 26, 398–405. https://doi.org/10.1053/sper.2002.37310.

Habibian, S., Bigham, A.S., Aali, E., 2011. Comparison of lidocaine, tramadol, and lidocaine-tramadol for epidural analgesia in lambs. Res. Vet. Sci. 91, 434–438. https://doi.org/10.1016/j.rvsc.2010.09.023.

Haddad, G.G., Mellins, R.B., 1984. Hypoxia and respiratory control in early life. Annu. Rev. Physiol. 46, 629–643. https://doi.org/10.1146/annurev.ph.46.030184.003213.

Haidon, J., Cunliffe, M., 2010. Analgesia for neonates. Contin. Educ. Anaesth. Crit. Care Pain 10, 123–127. https://doi.org/10.1093/bjaceaccp/mkq016.

Hakomäki, H., Kokki, H., Lehtonen, M., Räsänen, J., Voipio, H.-M., Ranta, V.-P., Kokki, M., 2021. Maternal and fetal buprenorphine pharmacokinetics in pregnant sheep during transdermal patch dosing: buprenorphine pharmacokinetics in pregnant sheep. Eur. J. Pharm. Sci. 165, 105936. https://doi.org/10.1016/j.ejps.2021.105936.

Hamurtekin, E., Fitzsimmons, B.L., Shubayev, V.I., Grafe, M.R., Deumens, R., Yaksh, T.L., Walker, S.M., 2013. Evaluation of spinal toxicity and long-term spinal reflex function following intrathecal levobupivacaine in the neonatal rat. Anesthesiology 119, 142–155. https://doi.org/10.1097/ALN.0b013e31828fc7e7.

Hanson, M., Kumar, P., 1994. Chemoreceptor function in the fetus and neonate. Adv. Exp. Med. Biol. 360, 99–108. https://doi.org/10.1007/978-1-4615-2572-1_9.

Harrison, M.R., Anderson, J., Rosen, M.A., Ross, N.A., Hendrickx, A.G., 1982. Fetal surgery in the primate I. Anesthetic, surgical, and tocolytic management to maximize fetal-neonatal survival. J. Pediatr. Surg. 17, 115–122. https://doi.org/10.1016/s0022-3468(82)80193-0.

Hay, M., Vulin, A., Génin, S., Sales, P., Prunier, A., 2003. Assessment of pain induced by castration in piglets: behavioral and physiological responses over the subsequent 5 days. Appl. Anim. Behav. Sci. 82, 201–218. https://doi.org/10.1016/S0168-1591(03)00059-5.

Heikkinen, E.M., Kokki, H., Heikkinen, A., Ranta, V.-P., Räsänen, J., Voipio, H.-M., Kokki, M., 2017. Foetal fentanyl exposure and ion trapping after intravenous and transdermal administration to the ewe. Basic Clin. Pharmacol. Toxicol. 120, 195–198. https://doi.org/10.1111/bcpt.12665.

Henare, S.J., Mellor, D.J., Lentle, R.G., Moughan, P.J., 2008. An appraisal of the strengths and weaknesses of newborn and juvenile rat models for researching gastrointestinal development. Lab. Anim. 42, 231–245. https://doi.org/10.1258/la.2007.007034.

Herrera, S.R.F., Leme, R.J.D.A., Valente, P.R., Caldini, É.G., Saldiva, P.H.N., Pedreira, D.A.L., 2012. Comparison between two surgical techniques for prenatal correction of meningomyelocele in sheep. Einstein São Paulo 10, 455–461. https://doi.org/10.1590/S1679-45082012000400011.

Herrmann, K., Flecknell, P., 2019. Retrospective review of anesthetic and analgesic regimens used in animal research proposals. Altex 36, 65–80. https://doi.org/10.14573/altex.1804011.

Hoagland, M.A., Chatterjee, D., 2017. Anesthesia for fetal surgery. Paediatr. Anaesth. 27, 346–357. https://doi.org/10.1111/pan.13109.

Hodgson, D.S., Dunlop, C.I., Chapman, P.L., Smith, J.A., 2002. Cardiopulmonary effects of xylazine and acepromazine in pregnant cows in late gestation. Am. J. Vet. Res. 63, 1695–1699. https://doi.org/10.2460/ajvr.2002.63.1695.

Houck, C.S., Vinson, A.E., 2017. Anaesthetic considerations for surgery in newborns. Arch. Dis. Child. Fetal Neonatal Ed. 102, F359–F363. https://doi.org/10.1136/archdischild-2016-311800.

Huang, C.-C., Carcagno, A., 2018. Electroporation of postimplantation mouse embryos in utero. Cold Spring Harb. Protoc. 2018. https://doi.org/10.1101/pdb.prot094060.

Huss, M.K., Chum, H.H., Chang, A.G., Jampachairsi, K., Pacharinsak, C., 2016. The physiologic effects of isoflurane, sevoflurane, and hypothermia used for anesthesia in neonatal rats (*Rattus norvegicus*). J. Am. Assoc. Lab. Anim. Sci. 55, 83–88.

Ikai, A., Riemer, R.K., Ramamoorthy, C., Malhatra, S., Cassorla, L., Amir, G., et al., 2005. Preliminary results of fetal cardiac bypass in nonhuman primates. J. Thorac. Cardiovasc. Surg. 129, 175–181. https://doi.org/10.1016/j.jtcvs.2004.09.003.

Isaza, D., DiGangi, B.A., Isaza, N., Isaza, R., 2021. Impact of surgical preparatory rinses with isopropyl alcohol or water on perioperative body temperature in pediatric female dogs and cats. Vet. Anaesth. Analg. 48, 198–204. https://doi.org/10.1016/j.vaa.2020.11.006.

Jansen, C.A.M., Lowe, K.C., Nathanielsz, P.W., 1984. The effects of xylazine on uterine activity, fetal and maternal oxygenation, cardiovascular function, and fetal breathing. Am. J. Obstet. Gynecol. 148, 386–390. https://doi.org/10.1016/0002-9378(84)90712-9.

Jones, R.S., 2001. Epidural analgesia in the dog and cat. Vet. J. 161, 123–131. https://doi.org/10.1053/tvjl.2000.0528.

Katsoulos, P.D., Minas, A., Karatzia, M.A., Pourliotis, K., Christodoulopoulos, G., 2011. Evaluation of a portable glucose meter for use in cattle and sheep. Vet. Clin. Pathol. 40, 245–247. https://doi.org/10.1111/j.1939-165X.2011.00309.x.

Katz, E.M., Huss, M.K., Jampachaisri, K., Pacharinsak, C., 2021. Buprenorphine, but not lidocaine, effectively attenuates post-operative thermal hypersensitivity in an incisional model in neonatal rats (*Rattus norvegicus*). Scand. J. Lab. Anim. Sci. 47. https://doi.org/10.23675/sjlas.v47i1.1057.

Kawasaki, H., Iwai, L., Tanno, K., 2012. Rapid and efficient genetic manipulation of gyrencephalic carnivores using in utero electroporation. Mol. Brain 5, 24. https://doi.org/10.1186/1756-6606-5-24.

Keita, A., Pagot, E., Prunier, A., Guidarini, C., 2010. Pre-emptive meloxicam for postoperative analgesia in piglets undergoing surgical castration. Vet. Anaesth. Analg. 37, 367–374. https://doi.org/10.1111/j.1467-2995.2010.00546.x.

Kimizuka, M., Tokinaga, Y., Azumaguchi, R., Hamada, K., Kazuma, S., Yamakage, M., 2021. Effects of anesthetic agents on contractions of the pregnant rat myometrium in vivo and in vitro. J. Anesth. 35, 68–80. https://doi.org/10.1007/s00540-020-02866-9.

Kinnunen, M., Kokki, H., Hautajärvi, H., Huhta, H., Ranta, V.-P., Räsänen, J., et al., 2018. Oxycodone pharmacokinetics and fetal exposure after intravenous or epidural administration to the ewe. Acta Obstet. Gynecol. Scand. 97, 1200–1205. https://doi.org/10.1111/aogs.13378.

Kinoshita, M., Crispi, F., Loreiro, C., Gratacós, E., Illa, M., Zamora, M., 2021. Strategies for intra-amniotic administration of fetal therapy in a rabbit model of intrauterine growth restriction. Exp. Biol. Med. 246, 1668–1679. https://doi.org/10.1177/15353702211003508.

Kinsella, S.M., Carvalho, B., Dyer, R.A., Fernando, R., McDonnell, N., Mercier, F.J., et al., Consensus Statement Collaborators, 2018. International consensus statement on the management of hypotension with vasopressors during caesarean section under spinal anaesthesia. Anaesthesia 73, 71–92. https://doi.org/10.1111/anae.14080.

Kleinman, L.I., Reuter, J.H., 1973. Maturation of glomerular blood flow distribution in the new-born dog. J. Physiol. 228, 91–103. https://doi.org/10.1113/jphysiol.1973.sp010074.

Kluivers-Poodt, M., Zonderland, J.J., Verbraak, J., Lambooij, E., Hellebrekers, L.J., 2013. Pain behaviour after castration of piglets; effect of pain relief with lidocaine and/or meloxicam. Anim. Int. J. Anim. Biosci. 7, 1158–1162. https://doi.org/10.1017/S1751731113000086.

Kohane, D.S., Sankar, W.N., Shubina, M., Hu, D., Nader, R., Berde, C.B., 1998. Sciatic nerve blockade in infant, adolescent, and adult rats: a comparison of ropivacaine with bupivacaine. Anesthesiology 89, 1199–1208. https://doi.org/10.1097/00000542-199811000-00021.

Kongstorp, M., Bogen, I.L., Stiris, T., Andersen, J.M., 2019. High accumulation of methadone compared with buprenorphine in fetal rat brain after maternal exposure. J. Pharmacol. Exp. Ther. 371, 130–137. https://doi.org/10.1124/jpet.119.259531.

Krutrök, N., Pehrsson, S., Van Zuydam, N., Jennbacken, K., Wikström, J., 2021. Ventilation via nose cone results in similar hemodynamic parameters and blood gas levels as endotracheal intubation during open chest surgery in rats. Lab. Anim. https://doi.org/10.1177/00236772211031039, 00236772211031039.

Lee, S.J., Ralston, H.J.P., Drey, E.A., Partridge, J.C., Rosen, M.A., 2005. Fetal pain: a systematic multidisciplinary review of the evidence. JAMA 294, 947–954. https://doi.org/10.1001/jama.294.8.947.

Lépiz, M.L., Sayre, R., Sawant, O., Barr, J., Pashmakova, M., Washburn, K., Washburn, S., 2017. Maternal and fetal effects of dexmedetomidine infusion in pregnant ewes anesthetized with sevoflurane. Am. J. Vet. Res. 78, 1255–1263. https://doi.org/10.2460/ajvr.78.11.1255.

Lerman, J., Oyston, J.P., Gallagher, T.M., Miyasaka, K., Volgyesi, G.A., Burrows, F.A., 1990. The minimum alveolar concentration (MAC) and hemodynamic effects of halothane, isoflurane, and sevoflurane in newborn swine. Anesthesiology 73, 717–721. https://doi.org/10.1097/00000542-199010000-00018.

Li, W., Li, G., Zhong, Z., Xie, B., Zhou, Z., Gu, W., et al., 2017. Validation of an HPLC assay for determination of Telazol in pregnant pigs: application to placental transfer study. J. Vet. Med. Sci. 79, 801–806. https://doi.org/10.1292/jvms.16-0300.

Liu, X., Zhou, C., Chen, J., Cen, J., Xu, G., Zhuang, J., 2011. A fetal goat model of cardiopulmonary bypass with cardioplegic arrest and hemodynamic assessment. J. Thorac. Cardiovasc. Surg. 142, 1562–1566. https://doi.org/10.1016/j.jtcvs.2011.06.022.

Loepke, A.W., Istaphanous, G.K., McAuliffe, J.J.I., Miles, L., Hughes, E.A., McCann, J.C., et al., 2009. The effects of neonatal isoflurane exposure in mice on brain cell viability, adult behavior, learning, and memory. Anesth. Analg. 108, 90–104. https://doi.org/10.1213/ane.0b013e31818cdb29.

Loepke, A.W., McCann, J.C., Kurth, C.D., McAuliffe, J.J., 2006. The physiologic effects of isoflurane anesthesia in neonatal mice. Anesth. Analg. 102, 75–80. https://doi.org/10.1213/01.ANE.0000181102.92729.B8.

Loftus, J.R., Hill, H., Cohen, S.E., 1995. Placental transfer and neonatal effects of epidural sufentanil and fentanyl administered with bupivacaine during labor. Anesthesiology 83, 300–308. https://doi.org/10.1097/00000542-199508000-00010.

Lomax, S., Harris, C., Windsor, P.A., White, P.J., 2017. Topical anaesthesia reduces sensitivity of castration wounds in neonatal piglets. PLoS One 12, e0187988. https://doi.org/10.1371/journal.pone.0187988.

Lopez-Tello, J., Arias-Alvarez, M., Gonzalez-Bulnes, A., Sferuzzi-Perri, A.N., 2019. Models of Intrauterine growth restriction and fetal programming in rabbits. Mol. Reprod. Dev. 86, 1781–1809. https://doi.org/10.1002/mrd.23271.

Luks, A.M., Zwass, M.S., Brown, R.C., Lau, M., Chari, G., Fisher, D.M., 1998. Opioid-induced analgesia in neonatal dogs: pharmacodynamic differences between morphine and fentanyl. J. Pharmacol. Exp. Ther. 284, 136–141.

Lyon, A.J., Pikaar, M.E., Badger, P., McIntosh, N., 1997. Temperature control in very low birthweight infants during first five days of life. Arch. Dis. Child. Fetal Neonatal Ed. 76, F47–F50. https://doi.org/10.1136/fn.76.1.f47.

Mace, S.E., Levy, M.N., 1983. Neural control of heart rate: a comparison between puppies and adult animals. Pediatr. Res. 17, 491–495. https://doi.org/10.1203/00006450-198306000-00014.

Mahmoud, A.I., Porrello, E.R., Kimura, W., Olson, E.N., Sadek, H.A., 2014. Surgical models for cardiac regeneration in neonatal mice. Nat. Protoc. 9, 305–311. https://doi.org/10.1038/nprot.2014.021.

Martin-Flores, M., Anderson, J.C., Sakai, D.M., Campoy, L., Cheong, S.H., Romano, M., Gleed, R.D., 2019. A retrospective analysis of the epidural use of bupivacaine 0.0625–0.125% with opioids in bitches undergoing cesarean section. Can. Vet. J. 60, 1349–1352.

Mathews, K.A., 2008. Pain management for the pregnant, lactating, and neonatal to pediatric cat and dog. Vet. Clin. N. Am. Small Anim. Pract. 38, 1291–1308. https://doi.org/10.1016/j.cvsm.2008.07.001 vi–vii.

Mayer, S., Peukert, N., Gnatzy, R., Gosemann, J.-H., Lacher, M., Suttkus, A., 2018. Physiologic changes in a small animal model for neonatal minimally invasive surgery. J. Laparoendosc. Adv. Surg. Tech. 28, 912–917. https://doi.org/10.1089/lap.2018.0075.

McClaine, R.J., Uemura, K., McClaine, D.J., Shimazutsu, K., de la Fuente, S.G., Manson, R.J., et al., 2007. A description of the preterm fetal sheep systemic and central responses to maternal general anesthesia. Anesth. Analg. 104, 397–406. https://doi.org/10.1213/01.ane.0000252459.43933.59.

McLaughlin, C.R., Dewey, W.L., 1994. A comparison of the antinociceptive effects of opioid agonists in neonatal and adult rats in phasic and tonic nociceptive tests. Pharmacol. Biochem. Behav. 49, 1017–1023. https://doi.org/10.1016/0091-3057(94)90258-5.

Mellor, D.J., 1988. Integration of perinatal events, pathophysiological changes and consequences for the newborn lamb. Br. Vet. J. 144, 552–569. https://doi.org/10.1016/0007-1935(88)90025-5.

Mellor, D.J., Cockburn, F., 1986. A comparison of energy metabolism in the new-born infant, piglet and lamb. Q. J. Exp. Physiol. 71, 361–379. https://doi.org/10.1113/expphysiol.1986.sp002995.

Mellor, D.J., Diesch, T.J., 2006. Onset of sentience: the potential for suffering in fetal and newborn farm animals. Appl. Anim. Behav. Sci. 100, 48–57. https://doi.org/10.1016/j.applanim.2006.04.012.

Mellor, D.J., Diesch, T.J., Gunn, A.J., Bennet, L., 2005. The importance of "awareness" for understanding fetal pain. Brain Res. Rev. 49, 455–471. https://doi.org/10.1016/j.brainresrev.2005.01.006.

Mellor, D.J., Gregory, N.G., 2003. Responsiveness, behavioural arousal and awareness in fetal and newborn lambs: experimental, practical and therapeutic implications. N. Z. Vet. J. 51, 2–13. https://doi.org/10.1080/00480169.2003.36323.

Mellor, D.J., Stafford, K.J., 2004. Animal welfare implications of neonatal mortality and morbidity in farm animals. Vet. J. 168, 118–133. https://doi.org/10.1016/j.tvjl.2003.08.004.

Miller, M.J., Martin, R.J., 2011. 91—pathophysiology of apnea of prematurity. In: Polin, R.A., Fox, W.W., Abman, S.H. (Eds.), Fetal and Neonatal Physiology, fourth ed. W.B. Saunders, Philadelphia, pp. 998–1011.

Miranda, A., Pêgo, J.M., Correia-Pinto, J., 2017. Animal facility videoendoscopic intubation station: tips and tricks from mice to rabbits. Lab. Anim. 51, 204–207. https://doi.org/10.1177/0023677216652342.

Molony, V., Kent, J.E., McKendrick, I.J., 2002. Validation of a method for assessment of an acute pain in lambs. Appl. Anim. Behav. Sci. 76, 215–238. https://doi.org/10.1016/S0168-1591(02)00014-X.

Molony, V., Kent, J.E., Robertson, I.S., 1995. Assessment of acute and chronic pain after different methods of castration of calves. Appl. Anim. Behav. Sci. 46, 33–48. https://doi.org/10.1016/0168-1591(95)00635-4.

Mooney, M.P., Shand, J.M., Burrows, A., Smith, T.D., Caccamese, J.F., Cooper, G.M., et al., 2018. Rescue of premature coronal suture fusion with TGF-β2 neutralizing antibody in rabbits with delayed-onset synostosis. Cleft Palate Craniofac. J. 55, 844–855. https://doi.org/10.1597/16-065.

Moriarty, O., Harrington, L., Beggs, S., Walker, S.M., 2018. Opioid analgesia and the somatosensory memory of neonatal surgical injury in the adult rat. Br. J. Anaesth. 121, 314–324. https://doi.org/10.1016/j.bja.2017.11.111.

Morley, L.A., Gomez, T.H., Goldman, J.L., Flores, R., Robinson, M.A., 2018. Accuracy of 5 point-of-care glucometers in C57BL/6J mice. J. Am. Assoc. Lab. Anim. Sci. 57, 44–50.

Musk, G.C., Kemp, M.W., 2018. Pregnant sheep develop hypoxaemia during short-term anaesthesia for caesarean delivery. Lab. Anim. 52, 497–503. https://doi.org/10.1177/0023677218764024.

Musk, G.C., Netto, J.D., Maker, G.L., Trengove, R.D., 2012. Transplacental transfer of medetomidine and ketamine in pregnant ewes. Lab. Anim. 46, 46–50. https://doi.org/10.1258/la.2011.010179.

Ngamprasertwong, P., Dong, M., Niu, J., Venkatasubramanian, R., Vinks, A.A., Sadhasivam, S., 2016. Propofol pharmacokinetics and estimation of fetal propofol exposure during mid-gestational fetal surgery: a maternal-fetal sheep model. PLoS One 11, e0146563. https://doi.org/10.1371/journal.pone.0146563.

Ngamprasertwong, P., Michelfelder, E.C., Arbabi, S., Choi, Y.S., Statile, C., Ding, L., et al., 2013. Anesthetic techniques for fetal surgery. Anesthesiology 118, 796–808. https://doi.org/10.1097/ALN.0b013e318283c954.

Nixon, E., Carlson, A.R., Routh, P.A., Hernandez, L., Almond, G.W., Baynes, R.E., Messenger, K.M., 2021. Comparative effects of nonsteroidal anti-inflammatory drugs at castration and tail-docking in neonatal piglets. PLoS One 16, e0254409. https://doi.org/10.1371/journal.pone.0254409.

Nock, M.L., Difiore, J.M., Arko, M.K., Martin, R.J., 2004. Relationship of the ventilatory response to hypoxia with neonatal apnea in preterm infants. J. Pediatr. 144, 291–295. https://doi.org/10.1016/j.jpeds.2003.11.035.

Okutomi, T., Whittington, R.A., Stein, D.J., Morishima, H.O., 2009. Comparison of the effects of sevoflurane and isoflurane anesthesia on the maternal-fetal unit in sheep. J. Anesth. 23, 392–398. https://doi.org/10.1007/s00540-009-0763-2.

Pacary, E., Guillemot, F., 2020. In utero electroporation to study mouse brain development. In: Sprecher, S.G. (Ed.), Brain Development: Methods and Protocols. Springer, New York, NY, pp. 513–523.

Padgett, A.L., Lepiz, M.L., Mackay, E.E., Driskill, A.J., Ivanov, I.V., Fajt, V.R., et al., 2020. Comparison of analgesic efficacy and fetal effects between transdermal administration of fentanyl and intramuscular administration of buprenorphine in pregnant sheep. Am. J. Vet. Res. 81, 581–593. https://doi.org/10.2460/ajvr.81.7.581.

Palahniuk, R.J., Shnider, S.M., 1974. Maternal and fetal cardiovascular and acid-base changes during halothane and isoflurane anesthesia in the pregnant ewe. Anesthesiology 41, 462–472. https://doi.org/10.1097/00000542-197411000-00010.

Papastamelos, C., Panitch, H.B., England, S.E., Allen, J.L., 1995. Developmental changes in chest wall compliance in infancy and early childhood. J. Appl. Physiol. 78, 179–184. https://doi.org/10.1152/jappl.1995.78.1.179.

Park, C.M., Clegg, K.E., Harvey-Clark, C.J., Hollenberg, M.J., 1992. Improved techniques for successful neonatal rat surgery. Lab. Anim. Sci. 42, 508–513.

Paull, D., Lee, C., Colditz, I., Atkinson, S., Fisher, A., 2007. The effect of a topical anaesthetic formulation, systemic flunixin and carprofen, singly or in combination, on cortisol and behavioural responses of Merino lambs to mulesing. Aust. Vet. J. 85, 98–106. https://doi.org/10.1111/j.1751-0813.2007.00115.x.

Phifer, C.B., Terry, L.M., 1986. Use of hypothermia for general anesthesia in preweanling rodents. Physiol. Behav. 38, 887–890. https://doi.org/10.1016/0031-9384(86)90058-2.

Piccinno, M., Rizzo, A., Mutinati, M., D'Onghia, G., Sciorsci, R.L., 2016. Lidocaine decreases the xylazine-evoked contractility in pregnant cows. Res. Vet. Sci. 107, 267–272. https://doi.org/10.1016/j.rvsc.2016.07.002.

Putnam, R.W., Conrad, S.C., Gdovin, M.J., Erlichman, J.S., Leiter, J.C., 2005. Neonatal maturation of the hypercapnic ventilatory response and central neural CO_2 chemosensitivity. Respir. Physiol. Neurobiol. 149, 165–179. https://doi.org/10.1016/j.resp.2005.03.004.

Rac, V.E., Scott, C.A., Small, C., Adamson, S.L., Rurak, D., Challis, J.R., Lye, S.J., 2007. Dose-dependent effects of meloxicam administration on cyclooxygenase-1 and cyclooxygenase-2 protein expression in intrauterine tissues and fetal tissues of a sheep model of preterm labor. Reprod. Sci. 14, 750–764. https://doi.org/10.1177/1933719107309042.

Rac, V.E., Small, C., Scott, C.A., Adamson, S.L., Rurak, D., Challis, J.R., Lye, S.J., 2006. Meloxicam effectively inhibits preterm labor uterine contractions in a chronically catheterized pregnant sheep model: impact on fetal blood flow and fetal-maternal physiologic parameters. Am. J. Obstet. Gynecol. 195, 528–534. https://doi.org/10.1016/j.ajog.2006.02.011.

Ranger, M., Tremblay, S., Chau, C.M.Y., Holsti, L., Grunau, R.E., Goldowitz, D., 2019. Adverse behavioral changes in adult mice following neonatal repeated exposure to pain and sucrose. Front. Psychol. 9, 2394. https://doi.org/10.3389/fpsyg.2018.02394.

Rindfield, T., McBrian, S., 2012. Assisted ventilation without endotracheal intubation in rats. J. Invest. Surg. 25, 197–199. https://doi.org/10.3109/08941939.2011.616257.

Rolbin, S.H., Levinson, G., Shnider, S.M., Biehl, D.R., Wright, R.G., 1979. Dopamine treatment of spinal hypotension decreases uterine blood flow in the pregnant ewe. Anesthesiology 51, 37–40.

Romagnoli, N., Barbarossa, A., Cunto, M., Ballotta, G., Zambelli, D., Armorini, S., et al., 2019. Evaluation of methadone concentrations in bitches and in umbilical cords after epidural or systemic administration for caesarean section: a randomized trial. Vet. Anaesth. Analg. 46, 375–383. https://doi.org/10.1016/j.vaa.2018.10.005.

Ruggiero, A.M., Novak, M.F.S.X., Woodward, R.A., Suomi, S.J., 2009. Successful behavioral strategy to unite mother and infant rhesus monkeys (*Macaca mulatta*) after cesarean delivery. Am. J. Primatol. 71, 510–522. https://doi.org/10.1002/ajp.20681.

Sadowsky, D.W., Haluska, G.J., Gravett, M.G., Witkin, S.S., Novy, M.J., 2000. Indomethacin blocks interleukin 1beta-induced myometrial contractions in pregnant rhesus monkeys. Am. J. Obstet. Gynecol. 183, 173–180. https://doi.org/10.1067/mob.2000.105968.

Sakamoto, H., Kirihara, H., Fujiki, M., Miura, N., Misumi, K., 1997. The effects of medetomidine on maternal and fetal cardiovascular and pulmonary function, intrauterine pressure and uterine blood flow in pregnant goats. Exp. Anim. 46, 67–73. https://doi.org/10.1538/expanim.46.67.

Sakamoto, H., Misumi, K., Nakama, M., Aoki, Y., 1996. The effects of xylazine on intrauterine pressure, uterine blood flow, maternal and fetal cardiovascular and pulmonary function in pregnant goats. J. Vet. Med. Sci. 58, 211–217. https://doi.org/10.1292/jvms.58.211.

Sanders, R.D., Hassell, J., Davidson, A.J., Robertson, N.J., Ma, D., 2013. Impact of anaesthetics and surgery on neurodevelopment: an update. Br. J. Anaesth. 110, i53–i72. https://doi.org/10.1093/bja/aet054.

Santolaya-Forgas, J., Romero, R., Mehendale, R., 2006. The effect of continuous morphine administration on maternal plasma oxytocin concentration and uterine contractions after open fetal surgery. J. Matern. Fetal Neonatal Med. 19, 231–238. https://doi.org/10.1080/14767050600593387.

Sato, M., Masui, K., Sarentonglaga, B., Yamaguchi, M., Fukumori, R., Nagao, Y., Sago, H., Sumikura, H., 2017. Influence of maternal remifentanil concentration on fetal-to-maternal ratio in pregnant ewes. J. Anesth. 31, 517–522. https://doi.org/10.1007/s00540-017-2332-4.

Sato, M., Takabayashi, S., Akasaka, E., Nakamura, S., 2020. Recent advances and future perspectives of in vivo targeted delivery of genome-editing reagents to germ cells, embryos, and fetuses in mice. Cells 9, 799. https://doi.org/10.3390/cells9040799.

Satoh, D., Iwatsuki, N., Naito, M., Sato, M., Hashimoto, Y., 1995. Comparison of the placental transfer of halothane, enflurane, sevoflurane, and isoflurane during cesarean section. J. Anesth. 9, 220–223. https://doi.org/10.1007/BF02479867.

Schäffer, D.P.H., de Araujo, N.L.L.C., Otero, A.R., Dórea Neto, F.D.A., Barbosa, V.F., Martins Filho, E.F., Oriá, A.P., 2017. Cardiorespiratory effects of epidural anesthesia using lidocaine with morphine or dexmedetomidine in capuchin monkeys (*Sapajus* sp.) undergoing bilateral tubal ligation surgery, anesthetized with isoflurane. J. Med. Primatol. 46, 311–319. https://doi.org/10.1111/jmp.12304.

Semrad, S.D., 1993. Comparison of flunixin, prednisolone, dimethyl sulfoxide, and a lazaroid (U74389F) for treating endotoxemic neonatal calves. Am. J. Vet. Res. 54, 1517–1522.

Sheil, M., De Benedictis, G.M., Scollo, A., Metcalfe, S., Innocent, G., Polkinghorne, A., Gottardo, F., 2021. Efficacy of intra-operative topical wound anaesthesia to mitigate piglet castration pain—a large, multi-centred field trial. Animals 11, 2763. https://doi.org/10.3390/ani11102763.

Sims, C.D., Butler, P.E., Casanova, R., Randolph, M.A., Yaremchuk, M.J., 1997. Prolonged general anesthesia for experimental craniofacial surgery in fetal swine. J. Invest. Surg. 10, 53–57. https://doi.org/10.3109/08941939709032126.

Skorupski, A.M., Zhang, J., Ferguson, D., Lawrence, F., Hankenson, F.C., 2017. Quantification of induced hypothermia from aseptic scrub applications during rodent surgery preparation. J. Am. Assoc. Lab. Anim. Sci. 56, 562–569.

Squillaro, A., Mahdi, E.M., Tran, N., Lakshmanan, A., Kim, E., Kelley-Quon, L.I., 2019. Managing procedural pain in the neonate using an opioid-sparing approach. Clin. Ther. 41, 1701–1713. https://doi.org/10.1016/j.clinthera.2019.07.014.

Stowe, D.F., Bosnjak, Z.J., Kampine, J.P., 1985. Effects of hypoxia on adult and neonatal pacemaker rates. Obstet. Gynecol. 66, 649–656.

Strümper, D., Gogarten, W., Durieux, M.E., Hartleb, K., Van Aken, H., Marcus, M.A.E., 2005. Effects of cafedrine/theodrenaline, etilefrine and ephedrine on uterine blood flow during epidural-induced hypotension in pregnant sheep. Fetal Diagn. Ther. 20, 377–382. https://doi.org/10.1159/000086816.

Strümper, D., Gogarten, W., Durieux, M.E., Hartleb, K., Van Aken, H., Marcus, M.A.E., 2004. The effects of S+-ketamine and racemic ketamine on uterine blood flow in chronically instrumented pregnant sheep. Anesth. Analg. 98, 497–502. https://doi.org/10.1213/01.ane.0000096243.74182.5e (table of contents).

Swann, H.G., Christian, J.J., Hamilton, C., 1954. The process of anoxic death in newborn pups. Surg. Gynecol. Obstet. 99, 5–8.

Swindle, M.M., Wiest, D.B., Smith, A.C., Garner, S.S., Case, C.C., Thompson, R.P., et al., 1996. Fetal surgical protocols in Yucatan miniature swine. Lab. Anim. Sci. 46, 90–95.

Szdzuy, K., Zeller, U., 2009. Lung and metabolic development in mammals: contribution to the reconstruction of the marsupial and eutherian morphotype. J. Exp. Zool. B Mol. Dev. Evol. 312B, 555–578. https://doi.org/10.1002/jez.b.21228.

Taddio, A., Katz, J., Ilersich, A.L., Koren, G., 1997. Effect of neonatal circumcision on pain response during subsequent routine vaccination. Lancet 349, 599–603. https://doi.org/10.1016/S0140-6736(96)10316-0.

Tame, J.D., Abrams, L.M., Ding, X.-Y., Yen, A., Giussani, D.A., Nathanielsz, P.W., 1999. Level of postoperative analgesia is a critical factor in regulation of myometrial contractility after laparotomy in the pregnant baboon: implications for human fetal surgery. Am. J. Obstet. Gynecol. 180, 1196–1201. https://doi.org/10.1016/S0002-9378(99)70616-2.

Tang, W., Zillmann, U., Sprengel, R., 2020. Alternative anesthesia of neonatal mice for global rAAV delivery in the brain with non-detectable behavioral interference in adults. Front. Behav. Neurosci. 14. https://doi.org/10.3389/fnbeh.2020.00115.

Thaete, L.G., Levin, S.I., Dudley, A.T., 2013. Impact of anaesthetics and analgesics on fetal growth in the mouse. Lab. Anim. 47, 175–183. https://doi.org/10.1177/0023677213480769.

Tsukamoto, A., Konishi, Y., Kawakami, T., Koibuchi, C., Sato, R., Kanai, E., Inomata, T., 2017. Pharmacological properties of various anesthetic protocols in 10-day-old neonatal rats. Exp. Anim. 66, 397–404. https://doi.org/10.1538/expanim.17-0037.

Uemura, K., Shimazutsu, K., McClaine, R.J., McClaine, D.J., Manson, R.J., White, W.D., et al., 2012. Maternal and preterm fetal sheep responses to dexmedetomidine. Int. J. Obstet. Anesth. 21, 339–347. https://doi.org/10.1016/j.ijoa.2012.06.010.

US FDA, 2017. FDA Drug Safety Communication: FDA approves label changes for use of general anesthetic and sedation drugs in young children. https://www.fda.gov/media/104705/download. (Accessed 22 August 2021).

Vagts, D.A., Iber, T., Puccini, M., Szabo, B., Haberstroh, J., Villinger, F., et al., 2003. The effects of thoracic epidural anesthesia on hepatic perfusion and oxygenation in healthy pigs during general anesthesia and surgical stress. Anesth. Analg. 97, 1824–1832. https://doi.org/10.1213/01.ANE.0000087062.94268.C5.

van den Hoogen, N.J., de Geus, T.J., Patijn, J., Tibboel, D., Joosten, E.A., 2021. Methadone effectively attenuates acute and long-term consequences of neonatal repetitive procedural pain in a rat model. Pediatr. Res. 89, 1681–1686. https://doi.org/10.1038/s41390-020-01353-x.

van den Hoogen, N.J., Tibboel, D., Honig, W.M.M., Hermes, D., Patijn, J., Joosten, E.A., 2016. Neonatal paracetamol treatment reduces long-term nociceptive behaviour after neonatal procedural pain in rats. Eur. J. Pain 20, 1309–1318. https://doi.org/10.1002/ejp.855.

van der Valk, J., Mellor, D., Brands, R., Fischer, R., Gruber, F., Gstraunthaler, G., et al., 2004. The humane collection of fetal bovine serum and possibilities for serum-free cell and tissue culture. Toxicol. Vitro 18, 1–12. https://doi.org/10.1016/j.tiv.2003.08.009.

van Loon, J., Verhaar, N., van den Berg, E., Ross, S., de Grauw, J., 2020. Objective assessment of acute pain in foals using a facial expression-based pain scale. Animals 10, 1610. https://doi.org/10.3390/ani10091610.

Victoria, N.C., Karom, M.C., Eichenbaum, H., Murphy, A.Z., 2014. Neonatal injury rapidly alters markers of pain and stress in rat pups. Dev. Neurobiol. 74, 42–51. https://doi.org/10.1002/dneu.22129.

Viscardi, A.V., Hunniford, M., Lawlis, P., Leach, M., Turner, P.V., 2017. Development of a piglet grimace scale to evaluate piglet pain using facial expressions following castration and tail docking: a pilot study. Front. Vet. Sci. 4. https://doi.org/10.3389/fvets.2017.00051.

Viscardi, A.V., Turner, P.V., 2018a. Use of meloxicam or ketoprofen for piglet pain control following surgical castration. Front. Vet. Sci. 5, 299. https://doi.org/10.3389/fvets.2018.00299.

Viscardi, A.V., Turner, P.V., 2018b. Efficacy of buprenorphine for management of surgical castration pain in piglets. BMC Vet. Res. 14, 318. https://doi.org/10.1186/s12917-018-1643-5.

Waldvogel, D., Bleul, U., 2014. Effect of xylazine, isoxsuprine, and lidocaine on Doppler sonographic uterine and umbilical blood flow measurements in cows during the last month of pregnancy. Theriogenology 81, 993–1003. https://doi.org/10.1016/j.theriogenology.2014.01.031.

Walker, S.M., 2019. Long-term effects of neonatal pain. Semin. Fetal Neonatal Med. 24, 101005. https://doi.org/10.1016/j.siny.2019.04.005.

Walker, S.M., Fitzgerald, M., Hathway, G.J., 2015. Surgical injury in the neonatal rat alters the adult pattern of descending modulation from the rostroventral medulla. Anesthesiology 122, 1391–1400. https://doi.org/10.1097/ALN.0000000000000658.

Walker, S.M., Westin, B.D., Deumens, R., Grafe, M., Yaksh, T.L., 2010. Effects of intrathecal ketamine in the neonatal rat: evaluation of apoptosis and long-term functional outcome. Anesthesiology 113, 147–159. https://doi.org/10.1097/ALN.0b013e3181dcd71c.

Watanabe, M., Kim, A.G., Flake, A.W., 2015. Tissue engineering strategies for fetal myelomeningocele repair in animal models. Fetal Diagn. Ther. 37, 197–205. https://doi.org/10.1159/000362931.

Webster, V.L., Cara, D.M., Walker, R.M., Ramsay, M.M., Aitkenhead, A.R., 2005. Description of a technique for anaesthetizing pregnant ewes for fetal surgery. Lab. Anim. 39, 94–99. https://doi.org/10.1258/0023677052886600.

Wheaton, L.G., Benson, G.J., Tranquilli, W.J., Thurmon, J.C., 1989. The oxytocic effect of xylazine on the canine uterus. Theriogenology 31, 911–915. https://doi.org/10.1016/0093-691x(89)90036-8.

Wunsch, M.J., Stanard, V., Schnoll, S.H., 2003. Treatment of pain in pregnancy. Clin. J. Pain 19, 148–155. https://doi.org/10.1097/00002508-200305000-00002.

Yahalom, B., Athiraman, U., Soriano, S.G., Zurakowski, D., Carpino, E., Corfas, G., Berde, C.B., 2011. Spinal anesthesia in infant rats: development of a model and assessment of neurological outcomes. Anesthesiology 114, 1325–1335. https://doi.org/10.1097/ALN.0b013e31821b5729.

Yoo, K.Y., Lee, J.C., Yoon, M.H., Shin, M.-H., Kim, S.J., Kim, Y.H., et al., 2006. The effects of volatile anesthetics on spontaneous contractility of isolated human pregnant uterine muscle: a comparison among sevoflurane, desflurane, isoflurane, and halothane. Anesth. Analg. 103, 443–447. https://doi.org/10.1213/01.ane.0000236785.17606.58.

Yousif, M.H., Thulesius, O., 1998. Tocolytic effect of the cyclooxygenase-2 inhibitor, meloxicam: studies on uterine contractions in the rat. J. Pharm. Pharmacol. 50, 681–685. https://doi.org/10.1111/j.2042-7158.1998.tb06905.x.

Yu, M., Han, C., Jiang, X., Wu, X., Yu, L., Ding, Z., 2015. Effect and placental transfer of dexmedetomidine during caesarean section under general anaesthesia. Basic Clin. Pharmacol. Toxicol. 117, 204–208. https://doi.org/10.1111/bcpt.12389.

Yu, Q., Li, J., Dai, C.-L., Li, H., Iqbal, K., Liu, F., Gong, C.-X., 2020. Anesthesia with sevoflurane or isoflurane induces severe hypoglycemia in neonatal mice. PLoS One 15. https://doi.org/10.1371/journal.pone.0231090.

Chapter 29

Anesthesia for in vivo imaging studies: practical considerations for experimental outcomes and animal welfare

Jordi L. Tremoleda[1] and Christoph W. Blau[2]

[1]*Queen Mary University of London, London, England, United Kingdom;* [2]*Charles River Laboratories Edinburgh Ltd., Tranent, Scotland, United Kingdom*

Chapter outline

I. Introduction

Imaging technologies are extensively used in biomedical research due to their remarkable scope for noninvasively studying biological processes in the living animal, providing a useful set of translational tools for studying disease models. Furthermore, they directly impact the 3Rs principles by enabling longitudinal studies with the acquisition of comprehensive anatomical, physiological, and functional parameters in real-time, thus reducing the number of animals used in serial studies. Furthermore, the acquisition of such clinically translatable readouts, in turn, also facilitates the care and welfare assessment of experimental animals and impacts the statistical power of the research acquired, representing a very valuable experimental refinement.

In contrast to human studies, imaging of animals generally requires anesthesia, which provides immobility therefore preventing movement that would adversely affect image quality (Tremoleda et al., 2012; Vesce et al., 2017; Gargiulo et al., 2012). During anesthesia, there is an inevitable autonomic nervous system depression that induces cardiovascular depression, respiratory depression, and hypothermia (see Chapters 6 and 10). These changes disrupt homeostasis, leading to potential health risks. In addition, there are other procedures performed along with imaging, such as the potential exposure to ionizing radiation, temporary fasting, serial blood sampling, gating,

Anesthesia and Analgesia in Laboratory Animals. https://doi.org/10.1016/B978-0-12-822215-7.00012-3

and/or the administration of contrast agents or imaging biomarkers that will also affect animal physiology and well-being, particularly when imaging animals used in disease models. These experimental interventions will influence animal physiology, which may confound the image quality and interpretation, or statistically speaking, lead to bias and increased variability, particularly when assessing functional parameters such as blood flow or tissue perfusion. Furthermore, repeated imaging sessions, while decreasing the number of animals required, will negatively impact the overall cumulative effects on the individual animals that are used. Therefore, it is important that researchers are well-familiarized with the imaging technologies available for laboratory animals and plan accordingly the appropriate handling and monitoring protocols to ensure the best animal welfare and quality data.

The modalities generally used for laboratory animal imaging include magnetic resonance imaging (MRI), computed tomography (CT), positron emission tomography (PET), single photon emission computed tomography (SPECT), high-frequency ultrasound (HFUS), optical imaging techniques such as bioluminescence imaging (BLI) and fluorescence imaging (FI), and photoacoustic imaging (PhAc) technologies. While all these modalities are implemented for in vivo imaging of laboratory animals, there are certain differences in terms of animal handling, monitoring, and follow-up on the recovery, particularly for serial imaging, which need to be considered. The aim of this chapter is to briefly describe how the most commonly used imaging modalities impact animal physiology and to discuss practical considerations to support appropriate anesthesia during imaging. In particular, recommendations will be made associated with setting up and carrying out the monitoring of the animals during imaging under anesthesia, including specific and unique considerations associated with each modality where appropriate. Specifics on anesthesia and drug protocols and doses are discussed in other chapters of this book and will not be discussed in detail here unless directly relevant. In particular, we will discuss how general procedures such as animal handling, induction, and maintenance of anesthesia, and physiological monitoring can be critical during imaging to promote appropriate animal care and minimize potential confounding effects during imaging studies. We will also discuss the impact of anesthesia on the experimental outcome, particularly its influence on normal physiology. The discussions in this chapter will aim to cover the species used most frequently for imaging studies, including mice, rats, nonhuman primates (NHP), and fish.

II. Imaging modalities

Similar to clinical practice, several imaging technologies are available for preclinical research, with different capabilities to acquire anatomical (e.g., μCT, MRI) and/or functional data (e.g., SPECT, PET) with different degrees of sensitivity and acquisition times. Moreover, some modalities, such as optical and photoacoustic imaging, have been specifically developed for research approaches based on the anatomical size and biological properties of some laboratory animal models (Kiessling and Pichler, 2016). Imaging technologies for laboratory animals have been extensively reviewed (Koba et al., 2011; Kagadis et al., 2010); but it is important to remind us of their key particularities and how they may affect animal physiology and how we can minimize any harms associated with the use of anesthesia (summary listed in Fig 29.1).

A. X-ray-based technologies

These include systems for imaging animals with standard X-rays, dual-energy X-ray absorptiometry (DEXA) for body composition analysis, and microcomputed tomography (μCT or microCT). These modalities rely on X-rays traveling through the body with the energy being absorbed at different rates by different parts of the body, which will be picked up by an X-ray detector.

1. Radiography and dual-energy X-ray absorptiometry

These systems provide two-dimensional radiography. The most widely available are the Faxitron systems, which provide ultrahigh-resolution imaging and are generally integrated with a dual-energy X-ray absorptiometry (DXA) system. This technology uses X-rays of two different energy levels that are absorbed differentially by various body tissue types. It is used primarily to provide information about body composition (differentiating mostly between mineralized tissue-bone, fat, and lean tissue). Most systems are self-contained X-ray units and workstations (Brommage, 2003).

2. Microcomputed tomography

Microcomputed tomography (MicroCT/μCT) involves the acquisition of a number of axial radiographic projections of the subject, which are subsequently reconstructed to enable three-dimensional visualization of the region(s) of interest (Bouxsein et al., 2010). It is the method of choice for imaging bones. Soft tissue assessment can be further enhanced with the use of iodine- or barium-based contrast agents (Hallouard et al., 2010). The duration of data acquisition will depend on the number of projections and the final image resolution. Depending on the particular system used, most in vivo μCT systems are capable of a resolution of 10–25 μm, although some systems provide a resolution of a few micrometers in isotropic voxel size (<5 μm). Higher resolutions will significantly prolong acquisition time and

Modality	Considerations for animal welfare during imaging
X-Ray-Based Technologies (Micro/uCT)	• Radiation exposure (particularly for repetitive studies and/or high resolution imaging requiring long acquisitions): acquisition time <> time under anaesthesia <> exposure to radiation • Gating during acquisition may be required to minimise movement artefacts • Account for the position of the animals as crucial for anatomical assessment and co-registration • Poor soft tissue contrast-may require the dosing of contrast agents: check guidelines for best route, volume, frequency and flow rate for dosing substances, particularly when imaging small lab rodents and aquatics
MRI/S	• No exposure to radiation • Excellent imaging contrast for soft tissue = Highly versatile for anatomical and functional data • Gating during acquisition may be required to minimise movement artefacts • Ensure non-magnetic monitoring equipment and set up for a remote monitoring • Capabilities for long term imaging (appropriate temperature, respiration and pulse monitoring) • High 3D resolution >> Long acquisition time >> long term anaesthesia
Nuclear Imaging techniques (SPECT/PET)	• Exposure to gamma radiation • Require dosing of radiotracers = good vascular line to avoid spillage and extravasation • Physiological stability critical for functional imaging with radiotracers • Co-registration with CT or MRI for data attenuation correction and identification of anatomical areas = multimodality imaging • Animals may require monitoring during decay period–account for housing shielded area and radiation exposure safety for all equipment and staff • Batched imaging >> management of anaesthesia
Optical Imaging (BLI/FLI)	• BLI requires genetic modification and injection of substrate • No exposure to radiation • High sensitivity and fast acquisition • Autofluorescence background (diet, fur) = consider the use of an alfalfa-free diet (at least a week prior to imaging) • Minimise animal hair (shave or depilate) and skin interference (when possible use hairless or albino animal strains) • Consider the position of the animal to avoid tissue signal attenuation
Ultrasound	• Thermoregulation is critical (immediate impact on cardiovascular function) • No exposure to radiation • Shaving required–cautious skin care and/or washing out of any depilatory cream • Handler require training (user dependent based on expertise)

FIGURE 29.1 Here commonly observed physiological effects and health risks during imaging and considerations for the management of anesthetized animals are listed.

anesthetic duration (Cherry, 2004). Additionally, longer acquisition times result in the animal receiving a higher dose of ionizing radiation, which must be balanced against the need for high-resolution images against the effect of radiation on the disease model (e.g., in studies of tumor biology and therapeutics).

The speed of acquisition is also important when using contrast agents since these agents can be rapidly cleared from the bloodstream. This is particularly relevant in laboratory rodents, which have high heart rates (mice; 400–600 bpm, rats; 250–400 bpm, compared to 60–80 bpm for adult humans) and very short circulation times ($\sim$10 seconds in mice compared to $\sim$30 seconds in humans). Another challenge for acquiring a good signal-to-noise ratio (SNR) relates to the interference effects of physiological movement created by the cardiac and respiratory cycle. The use of gating-based acquisition systems, allowing for images to be acquired simultaneously with, or triggered by a predetermined physiological point (e.g., maximum systole for heart imaging; Li et al., 2020), has greatly improved the quality of the images acquired.

B. Magnetic resonance imaging and spectroscopy

Magnetic resonance imaging (MRI) is a nonionizing 3D imaging technique that uses the magnetic properties of tissues and their interactions with both a large external magnetic field and radio frequency waves to create images. The proton 1H is the nucleus mostly used for anatomical imaging because of its abundance in tissues (water in the body; Driehuys et al., 2008). Preclinical systems can achieve high anatomical detail down to a 100-μm isotropic pixel size in living animals. Most MRI systems used for laboratory animal imaging have significantly higher magnetic field strengths than clinical MRI systems. This provides a higher image SNR, which can be used to increase imaging resolution alongside the use of specifically designed RF coils (Pautler, 2004).

As a highly versatile imaging approach, it provides anatomical, functional, and physiological data for studying a variety of organs, and it is very valuable for examining the central nervous system. The use of contrast agents or endogenous tissue properties can provide further functional information, such as changes in blood flow or oxygenation.

Magnetic resonance spectroscopy (MRS) confines the image acquisition to the spectral information of a particular nuclide. This is useful for imaging the tissue distribution of a particular drug or metabolite; however, the nuclide of interest is often present in low concentrations, limiting the spatial and temporal resolution (Driehuys et al., 2008; McConville et al., 2005).

The main challenges for preclinical MRI also relatc to the size of the region of interest and the final image resolution, particularly for 3D acquisitions. Considering the relatively small anatomical size of rodents compared to humans; for a mouse image to retain the same anatomical definition as that achieved in human images, the acquisition must be with a voxel volume approximately 3000 times smaller than that of a human, negatively impacting the entire scan time. This can be overcome by optimizing the radiofrequency (RF) coils and, as mentioned above, the use of stronger magnetic fields. Long imaging times represent one of the main MRI challenges, thus it is important that adequate physiological monitoring is used to maintain the physiological homeostasis of the anesthetized animal (critical for assisted ventilated animals, e.g., fMRI acquisitions). Specialized nonferrous monitoring equipment has to be used due to the presence of a magnetic field.

C. Nuclear imaging techniques (SPECT and PET)

Single photon emission computerized tomography (SPECT) and positron emission tomography (PET) rely on the detection of photons emitted from radiolabeled tracers in the body. SPECT systems record gamma rays directly after radionuclide emission via detectors that rotate around the animal. The photons pass through collimators (mostly multi-pinhole collimators) that "filter" them according to their direction, and impinge on the detector to provide a signal (Riemann et al., 2008; Peterson and Furenlid, 2011). PET systems also detect gamma rays, but the radionuclides emit positrons, which almost immediately come into contact with an electron in the tissue of interest. These two particles annihilate and emit two gamma photons in opposite directions. These dual emissions provide high signal intensities, providing high signal sensitivity.

SPECT radiopharmaceuticals generally have a medium half-life, are widely used in clinics, and are more readily available and cost-effective than PET tracers, which have a very short half-life and most require a cyclotron for their production (Khalil et al., 2011).

This highly specialized technology provides functional and metabolic information according to the type of isotope and radiochemistry used. Although these techniques are very sensitive, they provide poor spatial resolution and consequently are often used in conjunction with other modalities such as μCT or MRI that provide anatomical landmarks and support signal attenuation-correction. This multimodality acquisition is generally done consecutively, but preferably simultaneously, which may increase the anesthesia time. PET imaging dynamic study where the time distribution of a tracer is studied will also require longer anesthesia (Cherry, 2004; Cherry and Gambhir, 2001).

Adequate physiological monitoring to maintain good homeostasis is crucial for the assessment of functional/metabolic parameters measured through the radiotracers. Temperature monitoring remains critical during PET/SPECT acquisitions, as body temperature strongly confounds metabolic functions. There are important health and safety aspects related to the work with radioactive tracers and their waste, so handling anesthetized animals must address all the appropriate recommendations to minimize radiation exposure to researchers and other animals. Good patent vascular access is required to inject the tracer to ensure its distribution through the tissues/organs during the uptake period.

D. Optical

An increasing variety of optical imaging technologies is available for preclinical imaging. Many of these require genetic manipulation of either cells in vitro, which are subsequently implanted into the test animals, or the animal's genome, to express labeled proteins or enzymes (Wang et al., 2006; Hickson, 2009).

1. *Fluorescence*

Fluorescence imaging uses external dyes or fluorophores that can emit photons after excitation. An increasing number of genetic constructs with fluorophores incorporated into the genome of mice are extensively used as reporter proteins for genes or as cell labeling tools (Cherry, 2004). These fluorescent biomarkers can be used not only for tracking cells but can be engineered to signal a specific cell function (Ballou et al., 2005). Fluorescence imaging requires an external excitation source and multiple filters to obtain a spectrum of the light emitted, which can compromise the sensitivity. There is a relatively high level of background fluorescence (autofluorescence) and low transmission of light through tissues containing high levels of oxy- and deoxyhemoglobin. This can be minimized by using near-infrared spectrum fluorophores, which allow acquisition with lower background autofluorescence and greater sensitivity.

2. *Bioluminescence*

Bioluminescence results from the production of light by a biochemical reaction, requiring the presence of an active enzyme called luciferase and its substrate luciferin to produce light. The most commonly used luciferase is from fireflies, which produces light in yellow-green wavelengths. This technique allows the direct emission of photons in the targeted tissue with low background emission (tissues do not have endogenous bioluminescence; Sato et al., 2004). However, it requires the genetic integration of an exogenous transcript for luciferase into cells, or as a reporter gene in transgenic animals (Contag and Bachmann, 2002). Animals will need to be injected with the luciferin substrate to trigger the specific light-emitting enzymatic response.

Image acquisition requires placing the anesthetized animal into a light-proof chamber to enable signal detection by a sensitive camera, i.e., a charge-coupled device. Typically, the optical image is superimposed on another image, such as a low-resolution radiograph or photograph for anatomical reference. The advantage of these technologies is that they use low energy, nonionizing radiation with high sensitivity (μM-pM depending on the depth), and acquisition times are short, thus minimizing the time that animals are maintained under anesthesia. The main challenges are drop-off in signal with depth and low resolution (Leblond et al., 2010), background autofluorescence remains a major challenge for fluorescence imaging. This is generally reduced by a modified diet, minimizing skin fluorescence using nude animals and/or avoiding black-fur rodents, shaving the fur around the area of interest, as well as using techniques such as spectral unmixing to remove the unwanted autofluorescence signal from the image.

E. Ultrasound and photoacoustic modalities

This imaging modality is based on the propagation of sound waves created by a transducer through the soft tissues that are being imaged. These sound waves are reflected back from the tissues to the transducer and converted into a 3D image. Clinical systems that use relatively low-frequency probes (up to 15 MHz) are commonly used for imaging larger animals (e.g., dogs, cats, pigs, and horses), whereas high-frequency systems with probes ranging from 20 to 55 MHz are used for imaging small laboratory animals such as mouse, rat or zebrafish (Foster et al., 2002; Wang et al., 2018). These high-frequency systems provide good spatial resolution and adequate penetration for anatomical, functional, and hemodynamic real-time information in smaller animals. The images are acquired and visualized in real-time, delivering readily available data. Most systems also support techniques such as color flow Doppler, which is useful for functional vascular examinations. This technique is extensively used in cardiovascular research (Zhou et al., 2004), prenatal development, and for monitoring tumor growth and metastasis progression.

This modality has minimal impact on the animals; the hair must be removed to ensure the transducer has smooth contact with the skin via a gel. While most ultrasound examinations are done with animals under general anesthesia; it is possible to perform short examinations in conscious animals, being trained to accept a short and temporary manual restraint (Semeniuk et al., 2002).

Photoacoustic tomography is an emerging technology in which light absorption from either endogenous molecules (oxy-hemoglobin, deoxy-hemoglobin) or exogenous contrast agents creates thermally induced ultrasonic wave signals that are received to form images based on the acoustic detection of the optical absorption. It enables real-time anatomical, functional, and molecular imaging (Wang and Hu, 2012). Current technology requires hair removal and the animals may need to be immersed in a water bath under controlled anesthesia conditions, but there are promising ongoing developments with hand-held imaging probes.

III. Animal preparation and experimental planning

A. Regulatory requirements

Prior to planning for any imaging studies, it is critical to carefully evaluate the logistics for carrying out the imaging procedures and the need for anesthesia.

Animals can be conditioned to sufficient restraint to allow nonpainful, noninvasive imaging. For example, MRI in nonhuman primates can be performed without general anesthesia (Slater et al., 2016; Sandiego et al., 2013). Recent advances, such as 3D-printed restraint kits, have allowed conscious imaging of rats (Stenroos et al., 2018) and mice (Han et al., 2019) for fMRI and two-photon imaging (Villette et al., 2019). In particular, where the output is a functional measure of brain activity (e.g., fMRI), the quality of data obtained by avoiding anesthesia must form part of the cost-benefit analysis in deciding whether conscious imaging is an ethically acceptable choice. It may not be possible to avoid anesthesia completely (e.g., where a higher resolution image, for image registration, is required than can be obtained in the awake animal), but functional data may then be obtained in subsequent imaging sessions without anesthesia.

Where anesthesia is required, researchers need to carefully evaluate the health status and condition of the animals before imaging, recording essential parameters such as the animal's body weight, body condition (including an estimate of hydration), production of urine and feces, respiratory, and behavior patterns. This is particularly relevant when imaging disease models and/or genetically modified animals, which are likely to respond differently to anesthesia and thus might affect some of the functional imaging outcomes as well as having an increased risk of anesthetic complications. Special attention may be required when imaging neonates/pups, pregnant, and aged animals, taking extra care to support their recovery following anesthesia (e.g., enriched food, thermoregulation support).

Imaging is considered a regulated procedure as there is a recognized minimal threshold of pain and/or distress associated with the induction of anesthesia and if required, dosing of imaging agents. Therefore, even though imaging may be considered a minimally invasive procedure, researchers must ensure that these research activities are fully approved by their ethical and regulatory institutional frameworks (e.g., IACUC, AWB, or AWERB). As such, the frequency and timing of imaging, induction, and monitoring of anesthesia, and dosing protocols must be all included in the approved experimental procedures, even if imaging is done as a nonrecovery procedure.

B. Diet modification/fasting

Some studies may require some dietary restrictions. For example, alfalfa-free diets may be used in animals undergoing fluorescent imaging to minimize autofluorescence and improve imaging clarity (Bhaumik et al., 2007). Background autofluorescence generated via the ingested food (e.g., chlorophyll) poses a major setback for fluorescence imaging in mice. Compounds such as sodium perchlorate may be given in the food/drinking water to reduce the uptake of iodinated tracers into the thyroid and liver during SPECT imaging (Concilo et al., 2021). It is important to understand the impact that any of these modifications may have when anesthetizing animals during imaging.

Fasting before anesthesia is recommended in many laboratory animal species (dogs, cats, primates, and ferrets) to reduce the risk of regurgitation and the potential for aspiration pneumonia. In larger species (ruminants), fasting is also required to reduce the risk of bloat and consequent cardiorespiratory depression. Rodents and rabbits do not require fasting prior to anesthesia as they cannot vomit. However, fasting may be required for some metabolic/functional imaging procedures to achieve better uniformity of the tracer uptake during PET, minimizing background uptake in the GI tract linked to food ingestion. Researchers may generally apply up to ~12 hours fasting. However, one must consider that food consumption in most laboratory rodents is tied to the animals' circadian cycle, and thus the removal of food overnight (dark period) will have a stronger impact on their caloric intake as compared to withdrawal during the light period. In rodents, a fasting time of ~6 hours is effective to clear the stomach of food, and a longer fasting period may affect metabolism (e.g., a decrease of blood glucose and fatty acid levels) (Vermeulen et al., 1997). Food withdrawal should be carefully evaluated when working with neonates, pregnant, or aged animals. Water removal should be avoided due to the adverse effects of dehydration on the anesthetized animal. If withholding of water is required, it should be minimized, preferably not exceeding 1−2 hours before induction of anesthesia to avoid dehydration. In such cases, parenteral fluid support (ideally intravenously) during anesthesia should be provided.

C. Animal handling and preparation for imaging

Depending on the study, animals may require specific preparations like fur removal, placement of a superficial vascular port (e.g., tail, jugular vein), or specific handling acclimatization (e.g., imaging neonates). All these procedures will influence the animal's physiological homeostasis and thus must be carefully carried out to minimize stress.

When using chemical agents for fur removal, these must be carefully applied and appropriately washed off using a warm sterile solution to avoid skin inflammation.

Furthermore, the use of vascular access (rodents; tail, rabbits; ear or cephalic vein; larger species; cephalic, jugular, femoral, tail, or saphenous vein depending on species) is crucial to inject imaging tracers (e.g., PET/SPECT imaging) or contrast agents. For these procedures, sedatives/tranquillizers may be used to relieve anxiety (e.g., to reduce maternal distress when separating neonates for imaging), produce calmness, aid restraint (which can be critical for larger animals), smooth the induction of anesthesia, and reduce the dose of anesthetic needed. Other agents, like anticholinergic drugs, may be used to decrease oral and respiratory secretions, support cardiac output, and decrease gut motility.

If sampling before or during imaging/anesthesia is required, the access routes and volumes are to be considered to minimize potential adverse physiological effects from the procedure. This is particularly relevant for small laboratory animals with low blood volumes (e.g., mouse blood volume is only ~7% of body weight); sampling frequencies must follow recommended guidelines (Turner et al., 2011). Sampling frequency may be critical for some metabolic/tracer kinetics analysis and compartmental modeling during PET imaging, which requires frequent arterial blood sampling, so microsampling approaches may be required (Powles-Glover et al., 2014).

IV. Management of anesthesia in imaging studies

A. Anesthesia regimes

Anesthesia is generally required to ensure immobility without the stress associated with conscious restraint. However, most anesthetic agents induce a certain degree of autonomic nervous system depression, resulting in cardiovascular depression (e.g., reduction in cardiac output, blood pressure), respiratory depression (e.g., hypoxia, hypercapnia), and hypothermia (depression of thermoregulation and vasodilation). Ensuring the appropriate depth of anesthesia while maintaining animals in a stable physiological state during imaging is critical to minimize confounding effects on functional/metabolic outcomes (for further information, see Chapter 11). Animals have a poor ability to thermoregulate under anesthesia; this is particularly important in mice due to their high body surface-to-weight ratio and high metabolic rate. Mice undergoing long-term imaging procedures without adequate thermal support are at risk of developing hypoxia, respiratory depression, hypercapnia, and acidosis.

Inhalational anesthesia is most suitable and recommended for imaging due to its rapid onset and recovery times, and minimal requirement for metabolism. Furthermore, it allows for the management of the depth of anesthesia via a precision vaporizer, which, in combination with medical air or medical oxygen as a carrier gas, facilitates a better control of dosing, and consequently, anesthetic depth. Most imaging modalities are fitted with gas anesthesia circuits mounted to the imaging bed; generally via a nonrebreathing system to ensure minimum dead space and resistance to breathing. The anesthetic circuit is fitted with a nose cone that delivers the anesthetic gas directly to the animal and a scavenger port that removes waste/excess exhaled gas (see Chapter 9 for further information). Isoflurane remains the most commonly used agent, but other agents like, sevoflurane or desflurane may be used depending on specific institutional practices or for specific studies such as cardiac metabolic imaging (Flores et al., 2008).

Injectable agents continue to be used, possibly due to the large variety of anesthetic agents available and to avoid the use of an anesthesia rig (see Chapter 4 for further details on drugs and protocols). The choice of injectable agents will depend on the imaging experimental outcomes, thus it is important to assess their side effects and to consider the time required for imaging acquisition and recovery. The choice of commonly used agents, e.g., ketamine with xylazine, medetomidine, or dexmedetomidine, may be challenging as: 1. they often induce a prolonged recovery time, 2. it can be difficult to maintain a stable plane of anesthesia over longer periods, 3. additional (top-up) dosing can lead to overdose or a period of deep anesthesia. Some injectables can be administered via intravenous infusion (e.g., propofol), which may allow a more stable plasma concentration to be achieved over the course of imaging. Regardless of technique, the anesthetist must have experience and familiarity with the method chosen for an imaging protocol. When choosing an injectable agent, it is important to consider the expected physiologic adverse effects, particularly when planning to image genetically altered animals or models of disease, as these may respond differently or less predictably to anesthetic protocols. During the initial period of using a new drug protocol or when working with novel animals (species or models), it is important to monitor animals closely and make any adjustments necessary to the protocol for subsequent experiments.

For **larger species**, such as NHP, swine, and dogs, multimodal anesthesia regimes (typically combining injectable premedication and induction with maintenance using gas anesthetics $\pm$ intravenous anesthetic infusions) should be used where practicable. These allow for smooth induction, tight control of the anesthetic plane (via vaporizer), and decreased doses of each individual drug due to the synergistic actions of agents. Yet the same challenges on long-term dosing and metabolic effects of some drugs such as cardiovascular and respiratory depression, reduced perfusion and oxygenation, and higher acidosis, will still negatively impact imaging outcomes. Therefore, it is important for the researcher to consult with the imaging experts and the veterinarian to understand the drug effects and assess their influence on the imaging parameters.

Inhalant anesthesia provides the simplest and safest method for the maintenance of anesthesia and allows for ready and swift control of anesthetic depth. Multiple physiological systems should be monitored, at least including respiration rate and body temperature monitoring to enable the anesthetist to maintain the animal in a stable anesthetic depth with minimal perturbation of normal physiology. Hypothermia can develop very rapidly in anesthetized small animals, so the temperature should not only be measured but tightly controlled, for example by using feedback-controlled heating systems. Pulse oximetry measurements of blood oxygen levels are critically important to monitor cardiovascular function during imaging.

B. Adjuncts to anesthesia

Respiratory access is usually maintained simply via face mask, or by orotracheal intubation with an endotracheal tube. The latter has the following benefits: 1. provides a sealed airway, allowing for positive pressure ventilation, 2. the sealed airway also greatly reduces the risk of aspirating regurgitated material, and 3. minimizes pollution of the workplace (and subsequent personnel exposure) with anesthetic gases. Laryngeal 'masks' (supraglottic airway devices) are also available for certain species, such as rabbits and cats. Terminal studies may include tracheostomy surgery, which, while causing more surgical trauma, will decrease physiological dead space and can be secured in place surgically. Where the animal is positioned for imaging in such a way that airway patency may be compromised (e.g., hyperflexion of the neck for spinal imaging), an armored endotracheal tube should be used. Even when using injectable anesthetic regimes, it is advisable to provide oxygen to the animal, as injectable agents can also cause considerable respiratory depression.

Arterial access for serial blood gas sampling to determine physiological state may require further surgical preparation, and can provide reassurance that physiological homeostasis is maintained during data acquisition. In rodents, careful consideration must be taken of the volumes that may be removed for sampling, as discussed elsewhere.

Assisted ventilation may be used to manually or mechanically support the animal's respiratory function to support the maintenance of normal hemodynamic and pulmonary parameters during general anesthesia, as discussed in more detail in other chapters of this book. Ventilation can be required when tight control of physiology is required (e.g., brain blood flow, which is heavily altered by abnormal arterial carbon dioxide values), when hypoventilation is present (e.g., as an adverse effect of anesthesia), or when normal ventilation is unlikely to be achieved in the spontaneously breathing animal due to, for example, when imaging animals with specific thoracic interventions, during prolonged imaging sessions, or when close management of respiratory function may be required (e.g., fMRI). The use of assisted ventilation systems may also simplify the use of gating systems, as the imaging equipment can be gated to the automatically controlled ventilator cycles rather than to the spontaneous respiratory cycles of the animal.

C. Physiological monitoring: body temperature, cardiovascular, and respiratory function

Most anesthetic drugs will depress respiration, the cardiovascular system, and/or thermoregulation. Therefore, major consideration must be taken when setting up the anesthesia protocols and monitoring the animals during the imaging protocols. Confounding physiological effects can be most profound in those studies that are designed to assess some aspect of physiological function, like PET/SPECT, functional MRI, or echocardiography, and similarly for longer imaging procedures (Colby and Morenko, 2004).

While many preclinical imaging systems are increasingly integrating physiological monitoring devices, assessing respiratory function and supporting thermoregulation should be the minimum standard applicable to control the depth of anesthesia for any imaging study.

Direct visualization of the animals is generally not possible, so adapted monitoring equipment for each species has to be considered. Furthermore, laboratory rodents, with small body size and fast cardiac rates, are likely to require high-resolution acquisition, with longer imaging times and thus a greater need for accurate monitoring. It is crucial to consider the physical properties of the imaging devices and how the monitoring systems can be adapted with minimal interference in the imaging acquisition. In the case of MRI, devices must be nonferromagnetic to avoid any interference with the magnetized field, mostly using fiber-optic or carbon fiber equipment and power sources or batteries that are adequately filtered/isolated to avoid magnetic interference (Peden et al., 1992). For CT imaging, most temperature probes will provide a strong attenuation signal, thus it is important to assess the impact of any artifact effects on the region of interest to be imaged.

When multiple animals are imaged, for example during a high-throughput optical or PET system monitoring of individual animals must be provided (Greenwood et al., 2020; Gomes et al., 2018). Likewise, it is important to ensure that the position of the animal/animal does not restrict breathing, or circulation to the body and extremities to avoid any bruising, strains, or avulsions in the body structures.

Temperature: Maintenance of normal body temperature is instrumental during anesthesia to minimize the risk of hypothermia and prolonged recovery. Most anesthetic agents profoundly depress thermoregulation (Colby and Morenko, 2004). Rodents are highly susceptible to hypothermia due to their large surface area-to-body mass ratio and rapid metabolism. This is particularly critical when imaging nude or hairless mice. Hypothermia will have confounding effects on glucose metabolism and heart rate, which can significantly affect, e.g., FDG-PET studies and echocardiography outcomes. Therefore, monitoring and management of body temperature are crucial. This is mostly done using rectal thermometers that, ideally, will interface with an external heat source such as circulating hot water blankets or blowing air systems that help to maintain the animal's body temperature during imaging. It is highly recommendable to use a closed-loop system to ensure the appropriate regulation and monitoring of the temperature supplied by the warming systems. Hyperthermia is as dangerous as hypothermia, thus using a heat source that is "thermostatically controlled" and linked to the animal's core temperature measurements remains the most suitable approach. Importantly, heat loss must also be minimized during the animal preparation before imaging (e.g., hair removal, alcohol application), ensuring that active warming is initiated as early as possible and that any fluid replacement, if required, is prewarmed to 37°C.

Respiration: Most anesthetics are known to cause respiratory depression, thus it is important to reduce variability, due to poor ventilation including hypoxia, hypercapnia, and acidosis (Hauber et al., 2010; Pecchiari et al., 2014). Respiratory monitoring via direct visualization of chest movement is generally not possible when the animals are placed in the imaging device. Monitoring is generally carried out via detecting the breathing motion registered as compressions of a pneumatic respiratory sensor placed in contact with the animal's chest. Non kink plastic, nonelectrical sensors are recommended as they do not interfere with most imaging modalities (e.g., Baby Respiration Sensor, Viomedex, UK).

Other respiratory monitoring systems include digitized systems such as the capnograph, which measures the CO_2 level in the inhaled and exhaled gas between inspiration and expiration at the endotracheal tube connector or face masks (Beck et al., 2014).

It provides an estimate of the partial pressure of CO_2 in arterial blood, which is used to measure ventilation and alert the anesthetist during apnea. There are capnography specialized for small laboratory animals that provide real-time information on end-tidal CO_2 ($ETCO_2$). High $ETCO_2$ (hypercapnia) indicates hypoventilation associated with a deep anesthetic plane, respiratory depression, or animal's position. Low $ETCO_2$ (hypocapnia) indicates hyperventilation associated with reduced cardiac output, blood pressure, or pulmonary perfusion. Mice have rapid respiration and small tidal volume and the capnograph signal can be difficult to interrupt, but the changes in the $ETCO_2$ remain a valuable approach to monitoring respiratory function and alerting to problems with the equipment or the animal.

Other more specialized approaches include the use of arterial blood gas analysis to assess the level of oxygenation in circulating blood, which is very valuable during long-term procedures and/or functional imaging. Impaired gas exchange, or hyper- or hypoventilation, which remains important side effect of anesthesia is can be corrected by changing the anesthetic regime, including anesthetic agents and/or carrier gases of physiological support. It is particularly useful for studies that require the animal to be mechanically ventilated as the ventilation settings can then be adjusted to try to maintain physiological levels of O_2/CO_2, to ensure the animal does not develop hypercapnia or hypoxia (see other chapters of this book for more details on gas analysis.

Cardiovascular function: Assessment of blood perfusion and oxygenation remains a crucial parameter during anesthesia, which can be clinically evaluated through the color of the mucous membrane and capillary refill time. However, these approaches may not be easily accessible, as animals may be enclosed in the imaging devices and are not sensitive indicators of poor perfusion or hypoxia. Yet basic cardiovascular monitoring, including heart rate and pulse, is highly recommended for functional imaging. Pulse oximeters are highly recommended to monitor the pulse and arterial oxygenation, as systems provide real-time continuous measurements of arterial O_2, saturation, pulse strength, breathing rate, blood flow, and effort to breathe, to indicate any risk for hypoxemia. Electrocardiograms are also used to monitor heart rate and rhythm and can be used to synchronize the heart rate to the image acquisition during gated imaging. Blood pressure measurements are also used during imaging, with most methods requiring invasive access to an arterial line (Kramer and Remie, 2005), and are particularly relevant for functional MRI (addressed below) or when assessing the perfusion of contrast agents through specific tissues/organs during contrast-enhanced MRI (Thal and Plesnila, 2007).

Hydration/metabolic status: To support fluid homeostasis and systemic perfusion, physiological fluids such as normal saline or other balanced electrolyte solutions (e.g., Hartmann's) may be infused continuously or via SC dosing either pre and/or postprocedure, particularly during long imaging studies. Ensure osmolality, sterility, and preheating of the administered fluid. The stress of anesthesia itself may raise blood glucose levels (Vera et al., 2002), which may require specific supplemental fluid support. Eye protection by regular application of ophthalmic ointment is required to protect eyes from drying and the risk of exposure to keratitis and/or retinal damage caused by exposure to excessive light intensity in albino strains.

D. Relevance of anesthesia for functional magnetic resonance imaging

Functional magnetic resonance imaging (fMRI) is commonly used in preclinical models to detect changes in brain activity and the mechanism of pathology. As it relies on detecting changes in blood oxygen by measuring localized changes in oxyhemoglobin and deoxyhemoglobin levels caused by neuronal activity (the blood oxygen-level-dependent response, or BOLD; Crofts et al., 2020). Therefore it is critical to provide a stable and fully monitored anesthesia during imaging, as any alterations in the depth of anesthetics and their effects on physiological parameters will directly impact blood perfusion, cerebral blood flow, and cerebral metabolic rate of oxygen, thus affecting the BOLD signals and fMRI measurements. Consequently, addressing the anesthetic protocols used and how they may change physiological parameters remains critical for fMRI in laboratory animals. In fact, most anesthetic agents, doses, and timing will have an effect on fMRI results (Steiner et al., 2021). For example, animals under isoflurane anesthesia will have an increased CBF and vasodilation, thus affecting the fMRI signal. Hypercapnia also leads to vasodilation and increased CBF, and the use of mechanical ventilation helps avoid the increased $paCO_2$ improving the fMRI reproducibility. The impact of anesthesia on other physiological parameters, such as body temperature and peripheral cardiovascular activity, can modulate the quality of the measured functional measurements acquired during fMRI; thus, it is of the utmost importance to monitor these parameters and kept stable to assure normal physiological conditions during the acquisition. Anesthesia also affects CBF autoregulation in response to peripheral blood pressure changes; thus blood pressure measurements are of critical importance for fMRI. While technically challenging and invasive, blood pressure recordings can be carried out via arterial cannulation. Furthermore, it is important to understand the targets of different anesthetics used for laboratory animal studies; for example, isoflurane, propofol, and barbiturates are $GABA_A$ receptor agonists, and each drug may have subtle, unique characteristics on regional brain activity and cerebral blood volume across different brain areas. For further details on the impact of anesthetics on the cerebral networks of laboratory rodents and NHP and their effects during fMRI (Mandino et al., 2020).

E. Gating

Motion artifacts due to breathing, cardiac contraction, and/or chest movement can be eliminated from the images by employing gated imaging. Timing of image acquisition with specific stages of the respiratory or cardiac cycles is generally carried out during expiration to avoid the most prominent motion of the diaphragm and abdomen that occurs during inspiration. Most preclinical systems should be fitted with monitoring systems to trigger acquisition at some predefined physiological points (prospective gating) or to process postacquisition (retrospective gating). This allows controlling for the interference effects due to the physiological movement created through the cardiac and respiratory cycles and has greatly improved the quality of the images acquired. Respiratory and cardiac gating is extensively employed in CT and MRI imaging, being particularly relevant for the visualization and quantification of cardiac function (Li et al., 2020; Bartling et al., 2010). Inhalation anesthesia is highly recommended during gating since it allows for convenient adjustments and maintenance during scanning. Body temperature control is also critical to avoid the deterioration of the derived functional parameters due to cooling out of the animal, which will also alter the gating adjustments.

F. Repeated and long-term anesthesia

Some imaging protocols may require long acquisition times and/or high-frequency imaging with considerable impact on the cumulative effects of anesthesia. In these circumstances, it is recommended to use inhalational anesthesia, which generally allows for a quick induction, good control of the depth of anesthesia, and fast recovery. If specific studies require the use of injectable anesthetics, ideally this may be dosed via a continuous intravenous infusion with rapidly metabolized and eliminated agents such as propofol (or alfaxalone). Giving intermittent doses is likely to cause considerable variability of response, affecting physiological stability and functional imaging parameters. In any case, it is of utmost importance that appropriate physiological monitoring systems are in place and users are familiar with the anesthetic agent used. If a vascular line is in place, it is important to maintain good patency across the imaging acquisition; this is critical to avoid extravasation when irritant agents may be used (e.g., for the use of agents like α-chloralose in specifically regulated studies in which its use cannot be replaced by alternative agents and any extravasation would be highly irritable and critical to animal welfare; https://www.gv-solas.de/wp-content/uploads/2021/08/Chloralhydrat_Maerz_2016_EN_Sept_2019.pdf. When planning long-term imaging anesthesia, it is critical to minimize systemic accumulation of anesthetic metabolites, using an anesthetic circuit with minimal dead space and circuit resistance to support gas exchanges (avoid using small bore tubing for exhalation route), minimizing rebreathing, and providing an efficient scavenging of the exhaled gas. Monitoring with capnography can confirm rebreathing is not occurring. This may be particularly critical for long MRI studies, with animals being ventilated using long circuit hoses. Similarly, animals subjected to intravital microscopy procedures which enable high-resolution cellular imaging with generally long acquisition times will require well-controlled and monitored anesthesia to provide physiological stability.

In addition to the choice of anesthetic protocol, other considerations of particular importance during lengthy procedures include preventing dehydration by providing supporting fluids if necessary, maintenance of normothermia using an appropriate closed loop system, supporting organ perfusion and arterial blood pressure ensuring appropriate cardiovascular and respiratory functions during the lengthy anesthesia, and providing ocular protection (e.g., Lacri-lube) and relief from dry eyes. Particular attention will be needed to ensure supportive thermoregulation during recovery, as this may be slower, particularly in older animals and/or obese animals.

One of the major advantages of in vivo imaging is that it enables reimaging the same animal over time. However, frequent exposure to anesthesia is likely to cause increased stress and anxiety levels predominantly in the immediate postanesthetic recovery period (Hohlbaum et al., 2017). Similarly, other studies highlighted the variable response in anesthesia depth in rats, reduction of sleeping time, and weight loss as other significant adverse effects of repeated anesthesia, particularly when using injectable agents (Albrecht et al., 2014). The development of an aversion to reexposure to isoflurane has also been reported in laboratory rodents (Makowska and Weary, 2009). Therefore, an important consideration for studies with repeated imaging of animals is the frequency and time interval between imaging sessions. When planning such studies, it is important to address the number of imaging sessions that will be required in a specific time period in order to provide a prospective assessment of the expected cumulative severity across the study. Planning for the choice of anesthetic that is less likely to negatively impact the animals and ensuring a good recovery between imaging sessions will be valuable refinements.

G. Species-specific considerations

In vivo imaging of ***zebrafish*** has become a standard approach for studying developmental biology and disease modeling. The exceptional optical accessibility of zebrafish embryos, larvae, and/or GA nonpigmented strains, coupled with the new developments for cell labeling/reporting biological tools, allows for unique opportunities for high-resolution live imaging to study cell gene/cell functions in diseases. Despite all these advantages, it remains critically important to consider the impact of handling and anesthesia during these procedures, particularly accounting for their small size and the limited availability of physiological monitoring approaches (mostly focusing on environmental assessments).

Specific considerations for anesthesia regimes in fish are discussed in Chapter 16. As zebrafish are commonly used for assessing gene/cellular function, there are important factors to consider. First, account for the exposure to specific light wavelengths, as lengthy exposures can affect the optical properties of the yolk sack when imaging embryos (e.g., changes in opacity and viscosity); similarly, account for the transparent optical properties of mounting media such as low melt agarose if used. Consider the specific properties of the imaging chamber (round vs. flat-bottom plates, depending on the imaging targets), and avoid the use of damaging pressure from a coverslip. Controlling the environment during live imaging is critical, and systems should be equipped with a precise, controlled heating system to keep the animal relatively isolated from the laboratory's ambient temperature. Temperature will directly impact physiological processes (e.g., immune response), thus experimental conditions must be carefully monitored (Zhang et al., 2018). Some enclosures may also allow for the management of atmospheric gases—especially CO_2 and O_2, which may overcome some major challenges on oxygenation and the risk of anoxia, particularly for long-term imaging (Kamei and Weinstein, 2005). If requiring imaging modulators/contrast agents, routes of administration will have to be considered, as oral routes via simple addition to the water may be easier than other invasive routes (IV, IP).

In vivo imaging of **larger species** under anesthesia will largely follow established anesthetic protocols in that species, but consideration must still be taken of the imaging modality requirements and limitations. Firstly, any need for anesthesia must be carefully evaluated, as many species can readily be conditioned to tolerate certain imaging modalities (e.g., ultrasonography of the horse; fMRI of conscious primates; X-ray of the dog) with no chemical restraint or only mild sedation. Secondly, imaging equipment may prevent visualization of the animal, thus requiring additional monitoring equipment (e.g., cameras, pressure-sensitive respiratory sensors). Access to the animal may be limited, reducing the number of monitoring devices and supportive treatments that can be provided. In general, considerations discussed in Chapters 17 (Swine), 18 (Primates), etc. will dictate the regimes used. Due to the combination of the specific challenges of anesthesia in swine with the general imaging-related challenges already listed, this can be a particularly challenging species. In particular, there should be careful consideration of the need for assisted ventilation when designing protocols. Some primate imaging setups designed for use in awake animals, notably vertical bore MRI scanners, provide extra challenges when used on anesthetized animals, as keeping a patent airway is likely to require substantial physical supports for the animal, padding, and an MR-compatible IPPV system with adjunct monitoring capabilities, as discussed above. It is important to consider these requirements at the facility planning stage, as few facilities will have the resources to have both horizontal and vertical bore scanners that can accommodate primates.

V. Conclusions

The use of imaging has instrumentally revolutionized preclinical modeling by refining our animal studies, allowing for longitudinal in vivo cellular/organ anatomical and/or functional assessments. Yet, most imaging studies in laboratory animals will require anesthesia, which will directly impact animal physiology and, importantly, the imaging procedures and the data acquired. In this chapter, we have discussed the importance of undertaking comprehensive planning when addressing the anesthesia and monitoring protocols during imaging studies. Even though most imaging devices are reasonably user-friendly and provide relatively quick acquisitions, the impact on animal handling and anesthesia must always be taken into consideration. Their effects on animal physiology will modify imaging parameters such as those related to temperature and metabolic changes, blood perfusion, cardiovascular, or respiratory function (particularly related to functional imaging). Understanding the impact of the different modalities on animal physiology and how the use of anesthesia may affect this is crucial. Therefore, we encourage all researchers working in preclinical imaging to take into account all the considerations discussed in this chapter when planning their choice of anesthetics and monitoring approaches.

References

Albrecht, M., Henke, J., Tacke, S., Markert, M., Guth, B., 2014. Influence of repeated anaesthesia on physiological parameters in male Wistar rats: a telemetric study about isoflurane, ketamine-xylazine and a combination of medetomidine, midazolam and fentanyl. BMC Vet. Res. 10, 310. https://doi.org/10.1186/s12917-014-0310-8.

Ballou, B., Ernst, L.A., Waggoner, A.S., 2005. Fluorescence imaging of tumors in vivo. Curr. Med. Chem. 12 (7), 795–805. https://doi.org/10.2174/0929867053507324. PMID: 15853712.

Bartling, S.H., Kuntz, J., Semmler, W., 2010. Gating in small-animal cardio-thoracic CT. Methods 50 (1), 42–49. https://doi.org/10.1016/j.ymeth.2009.07.006. PMID: 19651213.

Beck, C., Barthel, F., Hahn, A.M., Vollmer, C., Bauer, I., Picker, O., 2014. Evaluation of a new side-stream, low dead space, end-tidal carbon dioxide monitoring system in rats. Lab. Anim. 48 (1), 1–5. https://doi.org/10.1177/0023677213501657. PMID: 24072488.

Bhaumik, S., DePuy, J., Klimash, J., 2007. Strategies to minimize background autofluorescence in live mice during noninvasive fluorescence optical imaging. Lab. Anim. (NY) 36 (8), 40–43. https://doi.org/10.1038/laban0907-40. PMID: 17721532.

Bouxsein, M.L., Boyd, S.K., Christiansen, B.A., Guldberg, R.E., Jepsen, K.J., Müller, R., 2010. Guidelines for assessment of bone microstructure in rodents using micro-computed tomography. J. Bone Miner. Res. 25 (7), 1468–1486. https://doi.org/10.1002/jbmr.141. PMID: 20533309.

Brommage, R., September 2003. Validation and calibration of DEXA body composition in mice. Am. J. Physiol. Endocrinol. Metab. 285 (3), E454–E459. https://doi.org/10.1152/ajpendo.00470.2002. PMID: 12759224.

Cherry, S.R., 2004. In vivo molecular and genomic imaging: new challenges for imaging physics. Phys. Med. Biol. 49 (3), R13–R48. https://doi.org/10.1088/0031-9155/49/3/r01. PMID: 15012005.

Cherry, S.R., Gambhir, S.S., 2001. Use of positron emission tomography in animal research. ILAR J. 42 (3), 219–232. https://doi.org/10.1093/ilar.42.3.219. PMID: 11406721.

Colby, L.A., Morenko, B.J., 2004. Clinical considerations in rodent bioimaging. Comp. Med. 54 (6), 623–630. PMID: 15679259.

Concilio, S.C., Suksanpaisan,L., Pham, L., Peng, K.W., Russell, S.J., 2021 Improved noninvasive in vivo tracking of AAV-9 gene therapy using the perchlorate-resistant sodium iodide symporter from Minke Whale. Mol. Ther. 29 (1), 236-243. https://doi.org/10.1016/j.ymthe.2020.09.036. PMID: 33038323; PMCID: PMC7791078.

Contag, C.H., Bachmann, M.H., 2002. Advances in in vivo bioluminescence imaging of gene expression. Annu. Rev. Biomed. Eng. 4, 235–260.

Crofts, A., Kelly, M.E., Gibson, C.L., 2020. Imaging functional recovery following ischemic stroke: clinical and preclinical fMRI studies. J. Neuroimaging 30 (1), 5–14. https://doi.org/10.1111/jon.12668.

Driehuys, B., Nouls, J., Badea, A., Bucholz, E., Ghaghada, K., Petiet, A., Hedlund, L.W., 2008. Small animal imaging with magnetic resonance microscope. ILAR J. 49 (1), 35–53. https://doi.org/10.1093/ilar.49.1.35. PMID: 18172332; PMCID: PMC2770253.

Flores, J.E., McFarland, L.M., Vanderbilt, A., Ogasawara, A.K., Williams, S.P., 2008. The effects of anesthetic agent and carrier gas on blood glucose and tissue uptake in mice undergoing dynamic FDG-PET imaging: sevoflurane and isoflurane compared in air and in oxygen. Mol. Imaging Biol. 10 (4), 192–200. https://doi.org/10.1007/s11307-008-0137-4. PMID: 18516648.

Foster, F.S., Zhang, M.Y., Zhou, Y.Q., Liu, G., Mehi, J., Cherin, E., et al., 2002. A new ultrasound instrument for in vivo microimaging of mice. Ultrasound Med. Biol. 28 (9), 1165–1172. https://doi.org/10.1016/s0301-5629(02)00567-7. PMID: 12401387.

Gargiulo, S., Greco, A., Gramanzini, M., Esposito, S., Affuso, A., Brunetti, A., Vesce, G., 2012. Mice anesthesia, analgesia, and care, part II: anesthetic considerations in preclinical imaging studies. ILAR J. 53 (1), E70–E81. https://doi.org/10.1093/ilar.53.1.70. PMID: 23382272.

Gomes, A.L., Gilchrist, S., Kersemans, V., Westcott, M., Smart, S., 2018. Refinement of in vivo optical imaging: development of a real-time respiration monitoring system. Lab. Anim. 52 (5), 531–535. https://doi.org/10.1177/0023677218757273. PMID: 29451416.

Greenwood, H.E., Nyitrai, Z., Mocsai, G., Hobor, S., Witney, T.H., 2020. High-throughput PET/CT imaging using a multiple-mouse imaging system. J. Nucl. Med. 61 (2), 292–297. https://doi.org/10.2967/jnumed.119.228692. PMID: 31519806; PMCID: PMC7002164.

Hallouard, F., Anton, N., Choquet, P., Constantinesco, A., Vandamme, T., 2010. Iodinated blood pool contrast media for preclinical X-ray imaging applications—a review. Biomaterials 31 (24), 6249–6268. https://doi.org/10.1016/j.biomaterials.2010.04.066. PMID: 20510444.

Han, Z., Chen, W., Chen, X., Zhang, K., Tong, C., Zhang, X., Li, C.T., Liang, Z., 2019. Awake and behaving mouse fMRI during Go/No-Go task. Neuroimage 188, 733–742. https://doi.org/10.1016/j.neuroimage.2019.01.002.

Hauber, H.P., Karp, D., Goldmann, T., Vollmer, E., Zabel, P., 2010. Effect of low tidal volume ventilation on lung function and inflammation in mice. BMC Pulm. Med. 10, 21. https://doi.org/10.1186/1471-2466-10-21. Erratum in: BMC Pulm Med. 2012;12:7. PMID: 20409304; PMCID: PMC2864238.

Hickson, J., 2009. In vivo optical imaging: preclinical applications and considerations. Urol. Oncol. 27 (3), 295–297. https://doi.org/10.1016/j.urolonc.2008.10.030. PMID: 19414115.

Hohlbaum, K., Bert, B., Dietze, S., Palme, R., Fink, H., Thöne-Reineke, C., 2017. Severity classification of repeated isoflurane anesthesia in C57BL/6JRj mice-assessing the degree of distress. PLoS One 12 (6), e0179588. https://doi.org/10.1371/journal.pone.0179588. PMID: 28617851; PMCID: PMC5472303.

https://www.gv-solas.de/wp-content/uploads/2021/08/Chloralhydrat_Maerz_2016_EN_Sept_2019.pdf (Accessed January 2023).

Kagadis, G.C., Loudos, G., Katsanos, K., Langer, S.G., Nikiforidis, G.C., 2010. In vivo small animal imaging: current status and future prospects. Med. Phys. 37 (12), 6421–6442. https://doi.org/10.1118/1.3515456. PMID: 21302799.

Kamei, M., Weinstein, B.M., 2005. Long-term time-lapse fluorescence imaging of developing zebrafish. Zebrafish 2, 113–123. https://doi.org/10.1089/zeb.2005.2.113. PMID: 18248171.

Khalil, M.M., Tremoleda, J.L., Bayomy, T.B., Gsell, W., 2011. Molecular SPECT imaging: an overview. Int. J. Mol. Imaging 2011, 796025. https://doi.org/10.1155/2011/796025. Epub 2011 Apr 5. PMID: 21603240; PMCID: PMC3094893.

Kiessling, F., Pichler, B.J., 2016. Small Animal Imaging: Basics and Practical Guide. Springer Science & Business Media.

Koba, W., Kim, K., Lipton, M.L., Jelicks, L., Das, B., Herbst, L., Fine, E., 2011. Imaging devices for use in small animals. Semin. Nucl. Med. 41 (3), 151–165. https://doi.org/10.1053/j.semnuclmed.2010.12.003. PMID: 21440693.

Kramer, K., Remie, R., 2005. Measuring blood pressure in small laboratory animals. Methods Mol. Med. 108, 51–62. https://doi.org/10.1385/1-59259-850-1:051. PMID: 16028675.

Leblond, F., Davis, S.C., Valdes, P.A., Pogue, B.W., 2010. Pre-clinical whole-body fluorescence imaging: review of instruments, methods and applications. J. Photochem. Photobiol. B Biol. 98, 77–94. https://doi.org/10.1016/j.jphotobiol.2009.11.007. Epub 2009 Nov 26. PMID: 20031443; PMCID: PMC3678966.

Li, H., Abaei, A., Metze, P., Just, S., Lu, Q., Rasche, V., 2020. Technical aspects of in vivo small animal CMR imaging. Front. Phys. https://doi.org/10.3389/fphy.2020.00183.

Makowska, I.J., Weary, D.M., 2009. Rat aversion to induction with inhalant anaesthetics. Appl. Anim. Behav. Sci. 119, 229–235.

Mandino, F., Cerri, D.H., Garin, C.M., Straathof, M., van Tilborg, G.A.F., Chakravarty, M.M., et al., 2020. Animal functional magnetic resonance imaging: trends and path toward standardization. Front. Neuroinform. 13, 78. https://doi.org/10.3389/fninf.2019.00078. PMID: 32038217; PMCID: PMC6987455.

McConville, P., Moody, J.B., Moffat, B.A., 2005. High-throughput magnetic resonance imaging in mice for phenotyping and therapeutic evaluation. Curr. Opin. Chem. Biol. 9 (4), 413–420. https://doi.org/10.1016/j.cbpa.2005.06.004. PMID: 16002325.

Pautler, R.G., 2004. Mouse MRI: concepts and applications in physiology. Physiology (Bethesda) 19, 168–175. https://doi.org/10.1152/physiol.00016.2004. PMID: 15304630.

Pecchiari, M., Monaco, A., Koutsoukou, A., Della Valle, P., Gentile, G., D'Angelo, E., 2014. Effects of various modes of mechanical ventilation in normal rats. Anesthesiology 120 (4), 943–950. https://doi.org/10.1097/ALN.0000000000000075. PMID: 24270126.

Peden, C.J., Menon, D.K., Hall, A.S., Sargentoni, J., Whitwam, J.G., 1992. Magnetic resonance for the anaesthetist. Part II: anaesthesia and monitoring in MR units. Anaesthesia 47, 508–517. https://doi.org/10.1111/j.1365-2044.1992.tb02278.x. PMID: 1616091.

Peterson, T.E., Furenlid, L.R., 2011. SPECT detectors: the anger camera and beyond. Phys. Med. Biol. 56 (17), R145–R182. https://doi.org/10.1088/0031-9155/56/17/R01. PMID: 21828904; PMCID: PMC3178269.

Powles-Glover, N., Kirk, S., Wilkinson, C., Robinson, S., Stewart, J., 2014. Assessment of toxicological effects of blood microsampling in the vehicle dosed adult rat. Regul. Toxicol. Pharmacol. 68 (3), 325–331. https://doi.org/10.1016/j.yrtph.2014.01.001. PMID: 24434616.

Riemann, B., Schäfers, K.P., Schober, O., Schäfers, M., 2008. Small animal PET in preclinical studies: opportunities and challenges. Q. J. Nucl. Med. Mol. Imaging 52 (3), 215–221. PMID: 18551093.

Sandiego, C.M., Jin, X., Mulnix, T., Fowles, K., Labaree, D., Ropchan, J., et al., 2013. Awake nonhuman primate brain PET imaging with minimal head restraint: evaluation of GABAA-benzodiazepine binding with 11C-flumazenil in awake and anesthetized animals. J. Nucl. Med. 54 (11), 1962–1968. https://doi.org/10.2967/jnumed.113.122077.

Sato, A., Klaunberg, B., Tolwani, R., 2004. In vivo bioluminescence imaging. Comp. Med. 54 (6), 631–634. PMID: 15679260.

Semeniuk, L.M., Kryski, A.J., Severson, D.L., 2002. Echocardiographic assessment of cardiac function in diabetic db/db and transgenic db/db-hGLUT4 mice. Am. J. Physiol. Heart Circ. Physiol. 283 (3), H976–H982. https://doi.org/10.1152/ajpheart.00088.2002. PMID: 12181126.

Slater, H., Milne, A.E., Wilson, B., Muers, R.S., Balezeau, F., Hunter, D., et al., 2016. Individually customisable non-invasive head immobilisation system for non-human primates with an option for voluntary engagement. J. Neurosci. Methods 269, 46–60. https://doi.org/10.1016/j.jneumeth.2016.05.009. PMID: 27189889.

Steiner, A.R., Rousseau-Blass, F., Schroeter, A., Hartnack, S., Bettschart-Wolfensberger, R., 2021. Systematic review: anesthetic protocols and management as confounders in rodent blood oxygen level dependent functional magnetic resonance imaging (BOLD fMRI)-part B: effects of anesthetic agents, doses and timing. Animals (Basel) 11 (1), 199. https://doi.org/10.3390/ani11010199.

Stenroos, P., Paasonen, J., Salo, R.A., Jokivarsi, K., Shatillo, A., Tanila, H., Gröhn, O., 2018. Awake rat brain functional magnetic resonance imaging using standard radio frequency coils and a 3D printed restraint kit. Front. Neurosci. 12, 548. https://doi.org/10.3389/fnins.2018.00548 eCollection 2018.

Thal, S.C., Plesnila, N., 2007. Non-invasive intraoperative monitoring of blood pressure and arterial pCO_2 during surgical anesthesia in mice. Neurosci. Methods 159 (2), 261–267. https://doi.org/10.1016/j.jneumeth.2006.07.016. Epub 2006 Sep 1. PMID: 16945419.

Tremoleda, J.L., Kerton, A., Gsell, W., 2012. Anaesthesia and physiological monitoring during in vivo imaging of laboratory rodents: considerations on experimental outcomes and animal welfare. EJNMMI Res. 2 (1), 44. https://doi.org/10.1186/2191-219X-2-44. PMID: 22877315; PMCID: PMC3467189.

Turner, P.V., Brabb, T., Pekow, C., Vasbinder, M.A., 2011. Administration of substances to laboratory animals: routes of administration and factors to consider. J. Am. Assoc. Lab. Anim. Sci. 50 (5), 600–613. PMID: 22330705; PMCID: PMC3189662.

Vera, E.R., Battell, M.L., Bhanot, S., McNeill, J.H., 2002. Effects of age and anesthetic on plasma glucose and insulin levels and insulin sensitivity in spontaneously hypertensive and Wistar rats. Can. J. Physiol. Pharmacol. 80 (10), 962. https://doi.org/10.1139/y02-124. PMID: 12450062.

Vermeulen, J.K., De Vries, A., Schlingmann, F., Remie, R., 1997. Food deprivation: common sense or nonsense? Anim. Technol. 48 (2), 45–54.

Vesce, G., Micieli, F., Chiavaccini, L., 2017. Preclinical imaging anesthesia in rodents. Q. J. Nucl. Med. Mol. Imaging 61 (1), 1–18. https://doi.org/10.23736/S1824-4785.16.02951-4. PMID: 27858407.

Villette, V., Chavarha, M., Dimov, I.K., Bradley, J., Pradhan, L., Mathieu, B., et al., 2019. Ultrafast two-photon imaging of a high-gain voltage indicator in awake behaving mice. Cell 179 (7), 1590–1608.e23. https://doi.org/10.1016/j.cell.2019.11.004.

Wang, L.V., Hu, S., 2012. Photoacoustic tomography: in vivo imaging from organelles to organs. Science 335 (6075), 1458–1462. https://doi.org/10.1126/science.1216210. PMID: 22442475; PMCID: PMC3322413.

Wang, D.S., Dake, M.D., Park, J.M., Kuo, M.D., 2006. Molecular imaging: a primer for interventionalists and imagers. J. Vasc. Interv. Radiol. 17 (9), 1405–1423. https://doi.org/10.1097/01.RVI.0000235746.86332.DF. PMID: 16990461.

Wang, L.W., Kesteven, S.H., Huttner, I.G., Feneley, M.P., Fatkin, D., 2018. High-frequency echocardiography-transformative clinical and research applications in humans, mice, and zebrafish. Circ. J. 82 (3), 620–628. https://doi.org/10.1253/circj.CJ-18-0027. PMID: 29415914.

Zhang, Q., Kopp, M., Babiak, I., Fernandes, J.M., 2018. Low incubation temperature during early development negatively affects survival and related innate immune processes in zebrafish larvae exposed to lipopolysaccharide. Sci. Rep. 8, 4142. https://doi.org/10.1038/s41598-018-22288-.

Zhou, Y.Q., Foster, F.S., Nieman, B.J., Davidson, L., Chen, X.J., Henkelman, R.M., 2004. Comprehensive transthoracic cardiac imaging in mice using ultrasound biomicroscopy with anatomical confirmation by magnetic resonance imaging. Physiol. Genom. 18 (2), 232–244. https://doi.org/10.1152/physiolgenomics.00026.2004. PMID: 15114000.

Chapter 30

Preclinical pain testing: a short guide to where we are and where we are going

Nick Andrews[1] and Jeffrey S. Mogil[2]

[1]*Behavior Testing Core, Salk Institute for Biological Studies, La Jolla, CA, United States;* [2]*Departments of Psychology and Anesthesia, Alan Edwards Centre for Research on Pain, McGill University, Montreal, QC, Canada*

Chapter outline

I. Why the need for animal use in pain research?

In a review published in 2010 (Mogil, Davis, and Derbyshire, 2010), we argued for the advantages and continuing value of the use of animal models in pain research. Animal models allow for detailed characterization of neurochemistry and anatomy, and the temporal and spatial resolution afforded by electrophysiology and now optogenetics. The use of animals allows high levels of environmental control and standardization, human safety, and controlled investigation into causal mechanisms that are simply impossible using human subjects. Over the last few decades, however, the failure to bring novel analgesics to market convinced many pharma companies to replace animal model data with human genetic data as such targets could yield greater translational success, having been identified from actual pain patients (Hayes et al., 2014). Additionally, neuroimaging technologies in human volunteers and patients have continued to develop, and many have advocated their use in analgesic development (Langley et al., 2008).

As a component of the 3Rs of animal research, replacement can be either *complete* (i.e., no animals used at all; that is, in silico, in vitro, or human clinical methods and technologies) or *partial*, which involves the use of invertebrates (not including octopuses, squid, or cephalopods) or immature vertebrates. Partial replacement also includes the in vitro use of animal cells or tissues taken from animals that were euthanized for that purpose only and did not undergo experimentation while alive. In vitro approaches over the last decade have gained some traction in the pain field with the development of nociceptor-like cells (partial replacement) from embryonic stem cells or induced pluripotent stem cells (iPSCs) generated by reprogramming fibroblasts from animals or (full replacement) healthy human volunteers (Boisvert et al., 2015; Chambers et al., 2012; Clark et al., 2017; Wainger et al., 2015; Wilson et al., 2018; Young et al., 2014) or even patients (e.g., Meents et al., 2019; Saito-Diaz et al., 2021). Reduced systems (tissue models such as spheroids, organoids, and "organs-on-chips") are just now beginning to be used to study conditions that are known to be associated with pain, such as chemotherapy-induced peripheral

Anesthesia and Analgesia in Laboratory Animals. https://doi.org/10.1016/B978-0-12-822215-7.00018-4

neuropathy (Pollard et al., 2021), osteoarthritis (He et al., 2020) and gastrointestinal inflammatory diseases (see Hartman et al., 2014 for review). However, such approaches do not yet model a sufficiently integrated system to fully represent the whole organism. Furthermore, they do not address pain as a whole, since they only offer the possibility to study nociception, whereas pain involves higher-level perception generated within the brain, and as yet only limited types of brain cells can be grown as organoids. A further limitation is that chronic pain can last for years, and maintenance of such microphysiological or cellular systems for such lengths of time is not possible at present. So, until such time as in vitro systems can model the full pain experience, including the complexity of responses by the brain, and over timeframes measured in months and years, animal models will be required.

If in vitro systems are still not advanced sufficiently to replace live animal studies, what about the promise of biomarkers? A biomarker is a characteristic that can be objectively measured and evaluated as an indicator of a normal or pathological process or a response to a therapeutic intervention. At present, there are no clinical biomarkers for pain approved by either the U.S. Food and Drug Administration (FDA) or the European Medicines Agency (EMA) for use in analgesic drug development trials. Areas that have received extensive attention in recent years as potential clinical biomarkers include tissue biopsies (typically skin) to measure transduction, microneurography to measure transmission, and use of quantitative sensory testing (QST) and electroencephalography/neuroimaging to measure perception (Coulombe et al., 2017; Gasparotti et al., 2017; Smith et al., 2017). In general, they have disappointed; a recent large study of patients with neuropathic pain, for example, reported no significant association whatsoever between QST measures and pain (Forstenpointner et al., 2021). As proposed by Tracey et al. (2019), it is highly likely that a composite of such biomarkers, alongside a self-report, will be required to accurately describe a painful condition. Others doubt that any biomarker(s) can ever replace human pain self-report, which of course is replete with its own limitations related to sensitivity, reliability, and validity (Smith et al., 2017).

With the availability of alternatives to live animals not yet specific and sensitive enough, there is still a clear need for live animal research in pain if progress is to be made in our understanding and treatment of pain in both humans and animals. Although rare genetic diseases have identified compelling analgesic drug targets, most notably *SCN9A* coding for the sodium channel subtype $Na_V1.7$ (Cox et al., 2006), this strategy has also failed thus far to produce a successful novel analgesic (Eagles et al., 2020). Neuroimaging has proven very useful in elucidating the cortical anatomy of pain but is much less able to reveal the kind of neurochemistry that leads to the pharmacology-based therapies that have been the mainstay of pain treatment. In fact, one thing that neuroimaging studies have clearly demonstrated is the importance of cortical processing and social, emotional, and cognitive context in pain, suggesting the limitations of any partial replacement strategy as discussed above.

At the same time, there have been major developments in the implementation of animal models of pain. There is now almost universal support for the idea that an exclusive reliance on the *status quo*—the measurement of reflexive withdrawal behavior from experimenter-delivered mechanical and thermal noxious stimuli to the plantar surface of a hind paw—is a poor way to measure pain in preclinical models. Recent years have seen the development of more realistic assays and measures of pain in animal models, and there are many excellent recent reviews of these developments (Abboud et al., 2021; Coderre and Laferriere, 2020; Cunha et al., 2020; Deuis et al., 2017; Mogil, 2019a; Negus, 2019; Tappe-Theodor et al., 2019; Sadler et al., 2022).

II. Animal models (assays) of pain

Having made the case that we do still need live animal models of pain in order to study the fundamental mechanisms that produce acute and chronic pain, what assays and measures are available for the pain scientist to use, and what are the issues to consider? Pain often begins as an acute sensation in response to a noxious stimulus that warns the organism to withdraw itself from that stimulus to avoid further injury and harm. Under normal circumstances, that is the end of the experience for the organism, as the sensation declines to below levels considered painful and, while remembering the incident to avoid it in the future, things return to normal. If the stimulus causes an injury (e.g., skin lesion leading to inflammation), an area of hypersensitivity develops, causing peripheral sensitization, which is again protective to the organism as it signals to avoid the use of the limb or area of the body until such time as the inflammation has resolved (Gold and Gebhart, 2010; Hucho and Levine, 2007). When the injury is more serious (e.g., directly to sensory nerves), the injury initially may (or may not) cause a painful stimulus that is incessant, activating nociceptors for a sustained period, leading to central sensitization (Latremoliere and Woolf, 2009), which may itself be protective by leading to hypervigilance (Crook et al., 2014; Lister et al., 2020).

Chronic pain assays can be broadly divided into neuropathic and inflammatory (see Table 30.1), based loosely on the dominant etiology, though there is considerable overlap in almost all cases as the relationship between the neuronal and immune systems is now recognized to be highly integrated and bidirectional. In terms of conceptualizing models of pain, it was suggested over 20 years ago (Woolf et al., 1998) that the field move away

TABLE 30.1 Assays of neuropathic and inflammatory pain in animals.

Category	Assay	Species[a]	Key references
Neuropathic pain			
Traumatic nerve injury	Spared nerve injury (SNI)	M, R	Decosterd and Woolf (2000), Shields et al. (2003)
	Spinal nerve ligation (SNL)	M, R	Kim and Chung (1992), Vilceanu et al. (2010)
	Spinal nerve transection (SNT)	M, R	Calvo et al. (2011), Mabuchi et al. (2003)
	Chronic constriction injury (CCI)	M, R	Bennett and Xie (1988), Ruscheweyh et al. (2007)
	Tibial nerve transection (TNT)	R	Lee et al. (2000)
	Partial sciatic nerve ligation (PSNL)	M, R	Malmberg and Basbaum (1998), Seltzer et al. (1990)
	Orofacial nerve transection	R	Vos et al. (1994)
Drug-induced	Chemotherapy-induced peripheral neuropathy (CIPN)	M, R	Hoke and Ray (2014) for review
	Antiretroviral drug induced peripheral neuropathy	M, R	Sanna et al. (2020), Wallace et al. (2007)
	Type 1 diabetic peripheral neuropathy (DPN)	M, R	Courteix et al. (1993), O'Brien et al. (2014) review;
Inflammatory pain			
Joint-related	Intra-articular CFA	M, R	Alvarado-Vazquez et al. (2015), Staton et al. (2007)
	Intra-articular mono-iodoacetate (MIA)	M, R	Liu et al. (2011), Moilanen et al. (2015)
	Intra-articular carrageenan	R, C, P	Dougherty et al. (1992), Sluka and Westlund (1993), Schaible et al. (1987)
	Intra-articular uric acid	M, R, C	Coderre and Wall (1987), Moilanen et al. (2015) Okuda et al. (1984)
	Collagen antibody-induced arthritis (CAIA)	M	Khachigian, (2006)
	Serum (K/BxN) transfer	M	Monach et al. (2008)
	Medial meniscal tear	M, R, D	McCoy (2015) for review
	Anterior cruciate ligament transection	M, R, D	McCoy (2015) for review
Nonjoint related	Intraplantar complete Freund's adjuvant (CFA)	M, R	Larson et al. (1986)
	Intraplantar carrageenan	M, R	Iadarola et al. (1988) Rocha et al. (2006)
	Intraplantar zymosan	M, R	Meller and Gebhart (1997), Staniland et al. (2010)
	Intraplantar formalin	M, R, C	Dubuisson and Dennis, (1977), McNamara et al. (2007), Tjolsen et al. (1992)
	Intra-dermal capsaicin	M, R, P	Gilchrist et al. (1996), Shimada and LaMotte (2008), Simone et al. (1991)
	Intraplantar mustard oil	M, R	Weng et al. (2012)
Visceral	Intracolonic mustard oil	M, R	Gonzalez-Cano et al. (2020), Ji et al. (2012)
	Irritant-induced (e.g., acetic acid) writhing	M, R	Feng et al. (2003), Stevenson et al. (2006), van der Wende and Margolin (1956)
	Intracolonic dextran sulfate sodium (DSS)	M, R	Gaudio et al. (1999), Okayasu et al. (1990)
Postsurgical	Plantar incision	M, R	Brennan et al. (1996), Pogatzki and Raja (2003)
	Laparotomy	M, R	Roughan and Flecknell (2001), Wolfe et al. (2015)

Continued

TABLE 30.1 Assays of neuropathic and inflammatory pain in animals.—cont'd

Category	Assay	Species[a]	Key references
Disease associated			
	Endometriosis	M	Fattori et al. (2020)
	Sickle cell anemia	M	Sadler et al. (2019)
	Parkinson's disease	M, R	Valek et al., (2019) for review
	Postherpetic neuralgia (PHN)	M, R	Dalziel et al. (2004), Silva et al. (2020)
	Vulvodynia	M	Farmer et al. (2011)
	Type 2 DPN	M, R	O'Brien et al. (2014) review

[a]*Species abbreviations: C, cat; D, dog; M, mouse; P, primate; R, rat.*

from defining the models according to etiology and instead in terms of underlying pathophysiological mechanisms (e.g., central sensitization, ectopic firing), but as yet this has not been implemented, primarily because the underlying knowledge of the mechanisms continues to evolve, and so we have retained the traditional classification here.

With respect to neuropathic pain, it is fair to say that there has been an overemphasis on the use of surgical nerve injury models since this only reflects a minority of clinical cases. However, these assays are attractive to many because the injury and timing can be controlled precisely, as is also true for assays of drug-induced neuropathic pain. Advances in the development of assays of more common disease-associated neuropathic pain (e.g., postherpetic neuralgia, painful diabetic neuropathy) would be welcome. The same case can be made for inflammation-based assays of pain, as the majority of studies are performed using chemicals to induce inflammation—such as complete Freund's adjuvant, carrageenan, zymosan, mono-iodoacetate, formalin, and mustard oil—which, although certainly capable of causing pain in humans (Gould, 2000) do not reflect situations or even possibly processes that would normally induce clinical inflammation. However, a surgical incision is a necessary component of surgery, and models such as laparotomy and hind paw incision act as excellent surrogates of such painful conditions.

III. Pain measures

Once a decision has been made on the subject to use (see below) and the assay to employ (e.g., genetic, surgical, chemical, or naturally occurring assay used to induce a pain state; see above), the critical decision remains: what to measure? The answer to this question has varied over the decades. Following early human studies of pain (Hardy et al., 1940), the first pain measures in common use in animals were withdrawals or other nocifensive reactions to heat or mechanical stimuli delivered to the tail or hind paws (D'Amour and Smith, 1941; Eddy and Leimbach, 1953), using psychophysical techniques that allowed the estimation of a pain threshold (Chaplan et al., 1994) (measuring pain tolerance in animals is obviously neither feasible nor necessary, and in humans, it is almost certainly more related to motivation than pain biology per se). This was followed by an era of irritant injections of algogens or inflammatory mediators into the abdominal cavity or hind paw (Dubuisson and Dennis, 1977; Taber et al., 1969), producing nocifensive and recuperative behaviors (e.g., shaking, licking, guarding) in the animal that could be summated as a measure of pain. The motivation for the shift was not only related to the fact that clinical pain is suprathreshold but also that the behaviors being measured lasted for longer: minutes to hours or even weeks, instead of seconds. That same impetus led to a third wave of assay development, featuring experimental nerve injuries similar to those producing causalgia (complex regional pain syndrome, type 2) (Bennett and Xie, 1988) in humans. However, although these injuries in rodents produce hypersensitivity to evoking mechanical and (sometimes) thermal stimuli lasting weeks to months, they are almost completely devoid of any other reliable nocifensive behaviors indicative of spontaneous pain, a symptom that is far more prevalent and bothersome clinically than hypersensitivity states (Backonja and Stacey, 2004; Maier et al., 2010). Thus, the pain field has been left in a bind: either use short-lasting assays with more face-valid measures (e.g., licking of the affected body part), or longer-lasting assays with less clinically relevant measures (e.g., reflexive withdrawal from a von Frey fiber).

A number of conceptually different measurement ideas have been forwarded, especially recently, as listed in Table 30.2. They include behaviors stimulated by pain,

TABLE 30.2 Nonreflexive measures of pain in animals.

Category	Measure	Key references[a]
Pain-stimulated behavior	Asymmetric limb-associated behaviors[b]	Mogil, Graham et al. (2010)
	Autotomy	Wall et al. (1979)
	Facial grimacing	McLennan et al. (2019), Mogil et al. (2020), Whittaker et al. (2021)
	Ultrasonic vocalization	Jourdan et al. (2002), Kurejova et al. (2010)
Pain-depressed behavior	Burrowing	Jirkof et al. (2010), Wodarski et al. (2016)
	Cage-lid hanging	Zhang et al. (2020)
	Nest building	Jirkof et al. (2013)
	Wheel running	Cobos et al. (2012), Sheahan et al. (2017)
Functional disability	Grip strength	Kehl et al. (2000)
	Locomotor activity	Urban et al. (2011)
	Weight bearing[c]	Clarke et al. (1997)
Conditioning/ Motivational	Classical conditioning[d]	Johansen et al. (2001), King et al. (2009), Sufka (1994)
	Operant conditioning[e]	LaBuda and Fuchs (2000), Mauderli et al. (2000), Negus (2019)

[a]*Cited reference(s) either first developed the measure, reviews its use, and/or reveals important facets of its use.*
[b]*Grooming, flinching, licking, lifting, scratching, shaking, turning.*
[c]*Dynamic weight bearing [gait], guarding, posture, static weight bearing.*
[d]*Conditioned place avoidance, conditioned place preference.*
[e]*Analgesic self-administration, intracranial self-stimulation, motivational conflicts, place escape/avoidance, responding for natural rewards.*

behaviors depressed by pain, measures of functional disability related to pain, and operant and classical conditioning procedures. Not listed in Table 30.2, but also the subject of renewed interest, are putative biomarkers of pain (in animals) and measures of comorbid states, including sleep, anxiety, and depression. Nonreflexive measures of pain are generally (and often considerably) more time-consuming and labor-intensive than reflexive measures, which is why the latter remains extraordinarily popular. The equipment required to measure nonreflexive measures is often considerably more expensive than that needed to measure reflexes.

Many of the newer concepts have other limitations as well. Classical conditioning techniques require extensive training and the addition of control groups to rule out motivation-related confounds and generally do not provide a real-time readout of pain levels. A recent multi-lab study of burrowing behavior revealed considerable interlaboratory variability, and the ubiquitous inflammatory mediator complete Freund's adjuvant (CFA) only produced statistically significant depression of burrowing for a single day (Wodarski et al., 2016), compared to several weeks of mechanical hypersensitivity. Similarly, facial grimacing to pain from spared nerve injury (SNI) lasts up to 3 weeks (Mogil et al., 2020), but the mechanical hypersensitivity from SNI lasts many months. Inflammatory mediators may only depress wheel running when delivered bilaterally (Cobos et al., 2012), preventing comparison to the contralateral side. Thus, it remains unclear what the optimal measure might be or even if the optimal measure has yet been identified (see Section 6). It is also possible, of course, that different measures might be optimal for each etiology.

IV. Organismic and environmental factors

As well as the complexities of what measure to use to determine the degree of pain, it is clearly apparent that there are robust effects of strain, sex, age, social factors, and the laboratory environment on pain even in inbred animals. The following are brief highlights of the main areas of influence:

A. Species

Rodents are overwhelmingly the subjects of preclinical pain research, with the mouse recently overtaking the rat as the modal species (Sadler et al., 2022) due to its size and ease of implementation of genetic modification. One new concept in the development of more "valid" assays of pain that is receiving increasing support is to take advantage of naturally occurring diseases or injuries in domesticated animals (see Klinck et al., 2017; Lascelles et al., 2018 for reviews). Examples include osteoarthritis in cats or cancer pain in dogs, in which considerable evidence is suggestive of similar pathophysiology to these painful states in humans (Guillot et al., 2015). Particularly intriguing is the idea of performing clinical trials on pets as a transitional, proof-of-concept step between rodent preclinical research and human clinical trials. Two such trials in companion dogs have provided evidence for the efficacy of resiniferatoxin for bone cancer pain (Brown et al., 2015) and grapiprant for osteoarthritis (Rausch-Derra et al., 2016). The challenge with this strategy relates to the measures taken. Perhaps the most common approach is to make use of subjective pain assessments by owners, caretakers, or veterinarians. For example, the Canine Brief Pain Inventory for the assessment of bone cancer pain in dogs was based directly on the human questionnaire (Brown et al., 2009). However, this type of pain assessment must be rigorously controlled, given how invested in the well-being of their pets the owners are. Quantitative sensory testing can also be adapted for many species, as, of course, can pain assessment via facial expression or gait/accelerometry. The paucity of high-quality pain research in species other than rodents has limited the emergence of any consensus on the usefulness of these measures. Whether or not switching from mice and rats to dogs and cats would facilitate preclinical pain research is also unknown, given the extremely limited evidence base on species differences in pain biology (Mogil, 2019b).

B. Strain

With the advent of modern molecular genetics as a research tool, it has become increasingly apparent that the precise genetic background of the rodent being tested for pain is critical to the results and conclusions that will be obtained from them. It is now clear, for example, that different mouse and rat strains differ robustly in their behavioral responses to every single pain assay they have been tested on (Mogil et al., 1999; Yoon et al., 1999). In addition to these ubiquitous quantitative differences, qualitative strain differences have been noted as well. For example, calcitonin gene-related peptide (CGRP) injected into the hind paw causes thermal hyperalgesia in some mouse strains but none at all (at any dosage) in others (Mogil et al., 2005). Despite these differences, 78% of papers using rats published between 2016 and 2020 in the flagship specialty journal, *PAIN*, used the Sprague-Dawley strain, and 60% of mouse papers used the C57BL/6 strain (Sadler et al., 2022). Apart from the highly restricted sampling of available genetic backgrounds these decisions imply, one might question the wisdom of so much experimentation being performed on the C57BL/6 strain, which is not only a phenotypic outlier when it comes to pain (Lariviere et al., 2001), but an inbred strain. Inbreeding, featuring loss of heterozygosity and inbreeding depression, is neither a natural nor a desirable situation. It is likely that the popularity of inbred strains derives from the expectation that they would feature less variability than outbred strains, but this has been shown empirically to be false (Chesler et al., 2002; Tuttle, Philip, et al., 2018).

C. Sex

Although the modal human chronic pain patient is a middle-aged woman, despite what was mentioned in the previous section regarding sex, the modal preclinical subject of a pain experiment is a male mouse. Although historically 80% of preclinical pain research was performed exclusively on male rodents, new policies from national funding agencies have caused a shift, such that by 2019 only 50% of studies published in *PAIN* were similarly male-biased (Mogil, 2020). These policies were wise and long overdue, and they have led to an explosion of documented sex differences in the operation of pain mechanisms that would have otherwise gone entirely unnoticed. Demonstrated sexually dimorphic pain biology includes spinal cord microglia (Sorge et al., 2015), transcriptomics (i.e., gene expression patterns) of sensory afferents (Mecklenburg et al., 2020; North et al., 2019), CGRP in the dura (Avona et al., 2019), prolactin and its receptor (Chen et al., 2020), dopamine in the periaqueductal gray/dorsal raphe and bed nucleus of the stria terminalis (Yu et al., 2021), human genetic associations (Freidin et al., 2021; Smith et al., 2019), and many more. Given the prevalence of sex-specificity in pain processing, it would seem to us to be ethically imperative to use both sexes in virtually all research going forward (Mogil, 2016).

D. Age and pain duration

In addition to concerns related to sex, another mismatch between clinical and preclinical realities is that the modal age of a preclinical research subject is from 8 to 11 weeks (Sadler et al., 2022). The decision to use young adult subjects is no doubt entirely driven by cost considerations, and as a result, there is a paucity of evidence to suggest that pain processing might differ in older animals, and the evidence that does exist is largely limited to acute, thermal pain (see Gagliese and Melzack, 2000). For example, only three studies that we are aware of have compared neuropathic mechanical allodynia in mice of different ages. Two studies observed no differences between young (2–4 months) and aging (12–24 months) animals (Millecamps et al., 2020; Ruiz-Medina et al., 2013). A recent study using mice of both sexes revealed a complete loss of allodynia in female mice 10 months after SNI, but unimpaired allodynia in mice given SNI surgery at 12 months of age (Muralidharan et al., 2020), suggestive of age-sex interactions and highlighting the fact that duration of injury is a factor that needs to be considered in addition to age per se. The interpretation of the "duration" of pain in animal models is complex, however. On the one hand, a comparison of the average life spans of humans versus rodents might suggest that typical durations of "chronic" pain experiments in the latter (7–28 days; Sadler et al., 2022) correspond to a year or more in humans. On the other hand, logic suggests that the pathophysiological processes thought to be responsible for chronic pain occur at similar rates in rodents and humans, and thus 1 month in the former might correspond to 1 month in the latter. If the latter interpretation of rodent versus human time is correct, then almost no rodent experiments of chronic pain (defined in humans as that lasting >3 months) have ever been performed.

E. Social environment

Almost entirely excluded from serious consideration by pain researchers has been the possibility that the social environment surrounding pain testing might affect results. Rodents are not tested in isolation, but rather lined up in cohorts to be tested in succession. Although individual animals are physically isolated from each other so that they can be independently manipulated, they are in olfactory, auditory, and often visual communication with each other during the testing process, and, of course, they live together in cages of 2–5 before and after that testing. It has been demonstrated that communication during testing can alter the pain sensitivity of mice with the same pain state (Chesler et al., 2002; Langford et al., 2006), that the proximity of a mouse not in pain can affect the pain behavior of one affected by pain (Langford et al., 2011), that (female) mice will respond to the pain of a conspecific with social approach (Langford et al., 2010), and that cohousing mice not in a pain state with mice in pain, or a 1-h social interaction between the two, will lead to pain hypersensitivity in the mice not previously in pain (Smith et al., 2016, 2021).

Since the modulatory factors described above have such fundamental impacts on the outcome of experiments, it is critical that the experimental methods and their resultant outcomes are reported in a transparent and detailed manner, such that others may replicate and build upon the work published. This is an area of experimental science that deals with the concept of validity and applies across all fields of science, though we will discuss it here in the context of experimental pain research.

V. External and internal validity

Experimental biology relies on the scientist assiduously paying attention to factors that, if not controlled, could lead to false conclusions. If the conclusions are wrongly interpreted as having relevance to the human condition, that is a problem of external validity. If the conclusions are erroneous due to factors affecting the experimental procedure itself, that is a problem of internal validity and primarily relates to experimental bias. Having a clear understanding and management of both forms of validity is therefore critical to the effective ethical use of animal models of human disorders. While the general concepts of validity are relevant to all in vivo modeling and experimentation, we are acutely aware that there has been a lot of attention placed on validity issues in the preclinical sphere. As mentioned earlier, this is primarily because of the failure of the drug industry to bring novel therapies to market either to treat acute pain (the development of nonopioids) or chronic pain. Putting aside the issues of poor target identification by industry or general lack of "druggability" of certain promising targets, this failure has been described as a failure of external validity ("the animal models do not model human pain accurately so there is a failure of translation from animals to patients") and/or internal validity ("the published results in the animal literature are biased and thus not to be trusted"). Whether in fact these points are correct has been the subject of great debate (e.g., Mao, 2002; Mogil, 2009; Yezierski and Hansson, 2018), but irrespective of where the blame truly lies, it is absolutely clear that validity must be addressed for animal models to be used effectively. Table 30.3 shows the definitions of external and internal validity and the issues associated with them as they relate to preclinical models of pain.

Options for improving the external validity of preclinical pain research have been described already in this manuscript in Sections 2, 3, and 4. One of the major drives to encourage scientists to improve internal validity in the field of experimental pain research has been to raise awareness of the perils of ignoring it. For example, in the U.S., the Society for Neuroscience has partnered with the National Institute of Neurological Disorders and Stroke (NINDS) and members of the scientific community to develop a multimodal training program aiming to inform and empower neuroscientists at all career stages to enhance the rigor and reproducibility of their research. In the U.K., the National Center for the 3Rs (NC3Rs) has promoted a set of reporting guidelines (**A**nimal **R**esearch: **R**eporting of **I**n Vivo **E**xperiments; (Kilkenny, Browne, Cuthill, Emerson, and Altman, 2010; Percie du Sert and Rice, 2014), used by many research journals, that aid transparency of

TABLE 30.3 The concept of validity as it applies to preclinical pain.

External validity	Definition	Defined by	Concern
Face	Symptomatic resemblance to the clinical condition	Reflexive withdrawal from painful stimulus (see Table 30.2 for nonreflex measures)	How does an animal show pain when it cannot verbalize it?
Predictive	Appropriate response to drugs which are clinically effective/ineffective giving a measure of specificity/sensitivity	Acute pain: e.g., morphine, Inflammatory pain: e.g., NSAIDs Neuropathic pain: e.g., gabapentinoids	If we want to detect novel mechanisms unrelated to current therapies, are models that respond to current drugs appropriate?
Construct	Theoretical rationale of the model with reference to clinical features		Can clinical pain be modeled in nonhuman species with sufficient confidence to translate to the clinic?
Internal validity	**Definition**	**Defined by**	**Concern**
Blinding	Operator and participants are unaware of treatment	For example, third party establishes pain model, third party labels drug vials	Sometimes this is not possible; e.g., how to blind someone to sex or a swollen foot?
Randomization[a]	A method based on chance alone by which study participants are assigned to a treatment group.	For example, treatments assigned using random number generator	Requires multiple scientists to run the experiment
Concealed allocation	Concealing the allocation sequence from those assigning participants to the intervention groups, until the moment of assignment	Third party assigns treatments to subjects	Requires multiple scientists to run the experiment
Adequate power	The likelihood that a significant effect will be found in a sample if such an effect exists in the population being studied	Power calculation using known variance	Needs prior knowledge of the variance within the experimental groups, which may not be apparent if experiment is completely novel
Sample size	The number of participants in a study		Cost can be prohibitive to have very large group sizes

[a]As long ago as 1947 it was recognized that randomization is critical to experimental rigor: "Randomization is necessary for trustworthiness, replication for efficiency and factorial design for comprehensiveness. Without these precautions, the experiment will at best give a poorer return than it need, for the labor and materials expended on it" (Fisher, 1947).

how the experiments were performed and executed. However, it should be noted that encouragement of such standards has not resulted in widespread adoption throughout the field (Leung et al., 2018), and much more needs to be done at the various levels, starting with university degree course materials, to improve standards. Specific to the field of pain research, the Analgesic, Anesthetic, and Addiction Clinical Trial Translations, Innovations, Opportunities, and Networks (ACTTION) initiative commissioned a 2-day meeting of leading pain research scientists from academia and industry, as well as journal editors and regulatory bodies, with the outcome being a set of reporting guidelines to aid transparency and reduce bias in the preclinical experimental pain literature (Andrews et al., 2016). Through such initiatives, not only should transparency in the reporting of such experiments increase (so that others can more easily repeat the published work), but awareness will also be raised of the need for increasingly high standards of experimental design.

VI. The future of preclinical pain research

Having put forward our reasons for the continued need for live animal research to delineate the mechanisms underlying pain signaling and processing, without ignoring the issues associated with the models and measures used in preclinical experimentation, we will finish by looking to the future, where we anticipate that there will be continued improvements in both *modeling* and *measuring* pain in species used in preclinical research.

Depending on the model being discussed, the level of refinement needed to more accurately model human clinical pain varies. Certain assays do indeed possess high face validity, modeling the painful condition as accurately as can be done in a different species (e.g., nerve trauma, ultraviolet light burn, and surgical incision), since that is how the pain is caused in the clinical situation. However, other assays, such as but certainly not limited to those of painful diabetic neuropathy and osteoarthritis, clearly need optimization if they are to serve as predictive models of pain in those diseases. The evolution of assays with greater construct validity will take time since improvements will be guided by information from the clinic and the laboratory and will always involve trade-offs with speed and simplicity.

On the other hand, changing how we measure pain in preclinical species is poised to make rapid advances thanks to the explosion in machine learning techniques for analyzing videos of the behavior of animals as apparently diverse as Hydra, flies, fish, rodents, and dogs (Bleuer-Elsner et al., 2019; Mathis et al., 2018; Mathis and Mathis, 2020; Robie et al., 2017; Shukla and Arac, 2020; Xu et al., 2020). We stated at the beginning of this chapter that there is almost universal support across the field of pain research that we cannot continue to exclusively measure pain in preclinical species as we have done in the past. Thus, the integration of computational techniques is timely and promises to facilitate pain measurements greatly. For example, facial grimacing can now be accurately scored using artificial intelligence (Tuttle, Molinaro, et al., 2018). The availability of advanced cameras that can capture images at up to 2000 frames per second (submillisecond timescale), promises to change how the humble reflex response to painful stimuli is perceived and measured. Such technological advances will assist fundamental studies of nociception and possibly analgesics for acute pain. For example, Browne and colleagues (2017) showed that optogenetic activation of cutaneous nociceptors activating only a single action potential leads to a primary response to injurious stimuli that is "not limited, fixed, or localized, but is dynamic and that it involves recruitment and gating of multiple circuits distributed throughout the central nervous system at a subsecond timescale to effectively both alert to the presence of danger and minimize the risk of harm." In another recent example, Jones et al. (2020) went even further by combining high-speed videography and automated paw tracking with the machine and deep learning approaches to define stereotyped subsecond paw trajectory patterns in response to four different mechanical stimuli: cotton swab, dynamic brush, light pinprick, and heavy pinprick. They found that there are specific categories of behavioral responses to these mechanical stimuli, and they were able to use the system to differentially phenotype several mouse strains. By word of caution, however, the system was not able to distinguish a response to CFA, suggesting further work is needed before general adoption.

Where we think the greatest advances in the measurement of pain will come is for models of chronic pain and the use of video analysis of behavior over longer periods, in the home-cage environment. This will be done automatically by computers and not human beings, with the additional benefit that once the algorithm has learned to detect a particular body pose or action, there will be no deviation, controlling for interobserver differences and errors when a human observer is distracted or becomes tired. Such methods have the potential to discover new relationships in how the body dynamics of animals fit together. For example, a technique called MoSeq (Wiltschko et al., 2015) using depth cameras to define 3-D body poses was able to effectively divide up the activity of mice in an open field into many smaller, identifiable components ("syllables"), showing it to be organized in a predictable fashion. We suggest that this type of analysis could then be used to understand how pain, for example, modifies this predictable organization. Computerized analysis will now make possible the capability to measure the home-cage activity of social groups of animals and to discover how they live with chronic pain, and whether interventions can normalize their behavior. It is highly plausible that in the absence of a human operator, laboratory species such as mice and rats will reveal a repertoire of behaviors that are otherwise concealed, as there is a popular notion that as prey species they may hide their pain in the presence of potential predators. Systems are being developed to measure behavior in real-time in the home cage (de Chaumont et al., 2019) that combine 3-D depth camera imaging with radio-frequency identification (RFID) to monitor the quality of the tracking. The combination of video tracking and RFID technology reduces the chances of the video analysis switching between mice in a group situation.

In conclusion, the next phase of algesiometry will likely be highly technology-based, involving the use of automation and unsupervised computational analysis of laboratory animal behavior. Basic pain experiments, using the accuracy of molecular genetics to define different populations of neurons that can then be stimulated selectively using opto- or chemo-genetics, or activity measured using fiber photometry for example, will facilitate understanding of nociceptive processes. Knowledge from such basic physiology will be applied to the study of chronic pain, finally enabling a reclassification of animal models of pain according to the underlying etiology, and ultimately leading to new therapies through more accurate targeting of specific pathologies.

References

Abboud, C., Duveau, A., Bouali-Benazzouz, R., Masse, K., Mattar, J., Brochoire, L., Landry, M., 2021. Animal models of pain: diversity and benefits. J. Neurosci. Methods 348, 108997.

Alvarado-Vazquez, P.A., Morado-Urbina, C.E., Castaneda-Corral, G., Acosta-Gonzalez, R.I., Kitaura, H., Kimura, K., Jimenez-Andrade, J.M., 2015. Intra-articular administration of an antibody against CSF-1 receptor reduces pain-related behaviors and inflammation in CFA-induced knee arthritis. Neurosci. Lett. 584, 39–44.

Andrews, N.A., Latremoliere, A., Basbaum, A.I., Mogil, J.S., Porreca, F., Rice, A.S., Whiteside, G., 2016. Ensuring transparency and minimization of methodologic bias in preclinical pain research: PPRECISE considerations. Pain 157, 901–909.

Avona, A., Burgos-Vega, C., Burton, M.D., Akopian, A.N., Price, T.J., Dussor, G., 2019. Dural calcitonin gene-related peptide produces female-specific responses in rodent migraine models. J. Neurosci. 39, 4323–4331.

Backonja, M.-M., Stacey, B., 2004. Neuropathic pain symptoms relation to overall pain rating. J. Pain 5, 491–497.

Bennett, G.J., Xie, Y.-K., 1988. A peripheral mononeuropathy in rat that produces disorders of pain sensation like those seen in man. Pain 33, 87–107.

Bleuer-Elsner, S., Zamansky, A., Fux, A., Kaplun, D., Romanov, S., Sinitca, A., van der Linden, D., 2019. Computational analysis of movement patterns of dogs with ADHD-like behavior. Animals 9, 9121140.

Boisvert, E.M., Engle, S.J., Hallowell, S.E., Liu, P., Wang, Z.W., Li, X.J., 2015. The specification and maturation of nociceptive neurons from human embryonic stem cells. Sci. Rep. 5, 16821.

Brennan, T.J., Vandermeulen, E.P., Gebhart, G.F., 1996. Characterization of a rat model of incisional pain. Pain 64 (3), 493–502.

Brown, D.C., Agnello, K., Iadarola, M.J., 2015. Intrathecal resiniferatoxin in a dog model: efficacy in bone cancer pain. Pain 156, 1018–1024.

Brown, D.C., Boston, R., Coyne, J.C., Farrar, J.T., 2009. A novel approach to the use of animals in studies of pain: validation of the canine brief pain inventory in canine bone cancer. Pain Med. 10, 133–142.

Browne, L.E., Latremoliere, A., Lehnert, B.P., Grantham, A., Ward, C., Alexandre, C., Woolf, C.J., 2017. Time-resolved fast mammalian behavior reveals the complexity of protective pain responses. Cell Rep. 20, 89–98.

Calvo, M., Zhu, N., Grist, J., Ma, Z., Loeb, J.A., Bennett, D.L., 2011. Following nerve injury neuregulin-1 drives microglial proliferation and neuropathic pain via the MEK/ERK pathway. Glia 59, 554–568.

Chambers, S.M., Qi, Y., Mica, Y., Lee, G., Zhang, X.J., Niu, L., Studer, L., 2012. Combined small-molecule inhibition accelerates developmental timing and converts human pluripotent stem cells into nociceptors. Nat. Biotech. 30, 715–720.

Chaplan, S.R., Bach, F.W., Pogrel, J.W., Chung, J.M., Yaksh, T.L., 1994. Quantitative assessment of tactile allodynia evoked by unilateral ligation of the fifth and sixth lumbar nerves in the rat. J. Neurosci. Methods 53, 55–63.

Chen, Y., Navratilova, E., Dodick, D.W., Porreca, F., 2020. An emerging role for prolactin in female-selective pain. Trends Neurosci. 43, 635–648.

Chesler, E.J., Wilson, S.G., Lariviere, W.R., Rodriguez-Zas, S.L., Mogil, J.S., 2002. Identification and ranking of genetic and laboratory environment factors influencing a behavioral trait, thermal nociception, via computational analysis of a large data archive. Neurosci. Biobehav. Rev. 26, 907–923.

Clark, A.J., Kaller, M.S., Galino, J., Willison, H.J., Rinaldi, S., Bennett, D.L.H., 2017. Co-cultures with stem cell-derived human sensory neurons reveal regulators of peripheral myelination. Brain 140, 898–913.

Clarke, K.A., Heitmeyer, S.A., Smith, A.G., Taiwo, Y.O., 1997. Gait analysis in a rat model of osteoarthrosis. Physiol. Behav. 62, 951–954.

Cobos, E.J., Ghasemlou, N., Araldi, D., Segal, D., Duong, K., Woolf, C.J., 2012. Inflammation-induced decrease in voluntary wheel running in mice: a nonreflexive test for evaluating inflammatory pain and analgesia. Pain 153, 876–884.

Coderre, T.J., Laferriere, A., 2020. The emergence of animal models of chronic pain and logistical and methodological issues concerning their use. J. Neural. Transm. 127, 393–406.

Coderre, T.J., Wall, P.D., 1987. Ankle joint urate arthritis (AJUA) in rats: an alternative animal model of arthritis to that produced by Freund's adjuvant. Pain 28, 379–393.

Coulombe, M.A., Lawrence, K.S., Moulin, D.E., Morley-Foster, P., Shokouhi, M., Nielson, W.R., Davis, K.D., 2017. Lower functional connectivity of the periaqueductal gray is related to negative affect and clinical manifestations of fibromyalgia. Front. Neuroanat. 11, 47.

Courteix, C., Eschalier, A., Lavarenne, J., 1993. Streptozotocin-induced diabetic rats: behavioural evidence for a model of chronic pain. Pain 53, 81–88.

Cox, J.J., Reimann, F., Nicholas, A.K., Thornton, G., Roberts, E., Springell, K., Woods, C.G., 2006. An *SCN9A* channelopathy causes congenital inability to experience pain. Nature 444, 894–898.

Crook, R.J., Dickson, K., Hanlon, R.T., Walters, E.T., 2014. Nociceptive sensitization reduces predation risk. Curr. Biol. 24, 1121–1125.

Cunha, A.M., Pereira-Mendes, J., Almeida, A., Guimaraes, M.R., Leite-Almeida, H., 2020. Chronic pain impact on rodents' behavioral repertoire. Neurosci. Biobehav. Rev. 119, 101–127.

D'Amour, F.E., Smith, D.L., 1941. A method for determining loss of pain sensation. J. Pharmacol. Exp. Therapeut. 72, 74–79.

Dalziel, R.G., Bingham, S., Sutton, D., Grant, D., Champion, J.M., Dennis, S.A., Mark, M.A., 2004. Allodynia in rats infected with varicella zoster virus–a small animal model for post-herpetic neuralgia. Brain Res. Rev. 46, 234–242.

de Chaumont, F., Ey, E., Torquet, N., Lagache, T., Dallongeville, S., Imbert, A., Olivo-Marin, J.C., 2019. Real-time analysis of the behaviour of groups of mice via a depth-sensing camera and machine learning. Nat. Biomed. Eng. 3, 930–942.

Decosterd, I., Woolf, C.J., 2000. Spared nerve injury: an animal model of persistent peripheral neuropathic pain. Pain 87, 149–158.

Deuis, J.R., Dvorakova, L.S., Vetter, I., 2017. Methods used to evaluate pain behaviors in rodents. Front. Mol. Neurosci. 10, 284.

Dougherty, P.M., Sluka, K.A., Sorkin, L.S., Westlund, K.N., Willis, W.D., 1992. Neural changes in acute arthritis in monkeys. I. Parallel enhancement of responses of spinothalamic tract neurons to mechanical stimulation and excitatory amino acids. Brain Res. Rev. 17, 1–13.

Dubuisson, D., Dennis, S.G., 1977. The formalin test: a quantitative study of the analgesic effects of morphine, meperidine, and brain stem stimulation in rats and cats. Pain 4, 161–174.

Eagles, D.A., Chow, C.Y., King, G.F., 2020. Fifteen years of $Na_V1.7$ channels as an analgesic target: why has excellent in vitro pharmacology not translated into in vivo analgesic efficacy? Br. J. Pharmacol. (in press).

Eddy, N.B., Leimbach, D., 1953. Synthetic analgesics II. Dithienylbutenyl- and dithienylbutylamines. J. Pharmacol. Exp. Therapeut. 107, 385–393.

Farmer, M.A., Taylor, A.M., Bailey, A.L., Tuttle, A.H., MacIntyre, L.C., Milagrosa, Z.E., Mogil, J.S., 2011. Repeated vulvovaginal fungal infections cause persistent pain in a mouse model of vulvodynia. Sci. Transl. Med. 3 (101), 101ra191.

Fattori, V., Franklin, N.S., Gonzalez-Cano, R., Peterse, D., Ghalali, A., Madrian, E., Rogers, M.S., 2020. Nonsurgical mouse model of endometriosis-associated pain that responds to clinically active drugs. Pain 161, 1321–1331.

Feng, Y., Cui, M., Willis, W.D., 2003. Gabapentin markedly reduces acetic acid-induced visceral nociception. Anesthesiology 98, 729–733.

Fisher, R.A., 1947. The design of experiments. Nature 160, 775.

Forstenpointner, J., Ruscheweyh, R., Attal, N., Baron, R., Bouhassira, D., Enax-Krumova, E.K., Vollert, J., 2021. No pain, still gain (of function): the relation between sensory profiles and the presence or absence of self-reported pain in a large multicenter cohort of patients with neuropathy. Pain 162, 718–727.

Freidin, M.B., Tsepilov, Y.A., Stanaway, I.B., Meng, W., Hayward, C., Smith, B.H., Williams, F.M.K., 2021. Sex- and age-specific genetic analysis of chronic back pain. Pain 162, 1176–1187.

Gagliese, L., Melzack, R., 2000. Age differences in nociception and pain behaviours in the rat. Neurosci. Biobehav. Rev. 24, 843–854.

Gasparotti, R., Padua, L., Briani, C., Lauria, G., 2017. New technologies for the assessment of neuropathies. Nat. Rev. Neurol. 13, 203–216.

Gaudio, E., Taddei, G., Vetuschi, A., Sferra, R., Frieri, G., Ricciardi, G., Caprilli, R., 1999. Dextran sulfate sodium (DSS) colitis in rats: clinical, structural, and ultrastructural aspects. Dig. Dis. Sci. 44, 1458–1475.

Gilchrist, H.D., Allard, B.L., Simone, D.A., 1996. Enhanced withdrawal responses to heat and mechanical stimuli following intraplantar injection of capsaicin in rats. Pain 67, 179–188.

Gold, M.S., Gebhart, G.F., 2010. Nociceptor sensitization in pain pathogenesis. Nat. Med. 16, 1248–1257.

Gonzalez-Cano, R., Montilla-Garcia, A., Perazzoli, G., Torres, J.M., Canizares, F.J., Fernandez-Segura, E., Cobos, E.J., 2020. Intracolonic mustard oil induces visceral pain in mice by TRPA1-dependent and -independent mechanisms: role of tissue injury and P2X receptors. Front. Pharmacol. 11, 613068.

Gould III., H.J., 2000. Complete Freund's adjuvant-induced hyperalgesia: a human perception. Pain 85, 301–303.

Guillot, M., Chartrand, G., Chav, R., Rousseau, J., Beaudoin, J.-F., Martel-Pelletier, J., Troncy, E., 2015. [^{18}F]-fluorodeoxyglucose positron emission tomography of the cat brain: a feasibility study to investigate osteoarthritis-associated pain. Vet. J. 204, 299–303.

Hardy, J.D., Wolff, H.G., Goodell, H., 1940. A new method for measuring pain threshold: observations on spatial summation of pain. J. Clin. Invest. 19, 649–657.

Hartman, K.G., Bortner Jr., J.D., Falk, G.W., Ginsberg, G.G., Jhala, N., Yu, J., Lynch, J.P., 2014. Modeling human gastrointestinal inflammatory diseases using microphysiological culture systems. Exp. Biol. Med. 239, 1108–1123.

Hayes, A.G., Arendt-Nielsen, L., Tate, S., 2014. Multiple mechanisms have been tested in pain — how can we improve the chances of success? Curr. Opin. Pharmacol. 14, 11–17.

He, Y., Li, Z., Alexander, P.G., Ocasio-Nieves, B.D., Yocum, L., Lin, H., Tuan, R.S., 2020. Pathogenesis of osteoarthritis: risk factors, regulatory pathways in chondrocytes, and experimental models. Biology 9, 9080194.

Hoke, A., Ray, M., 2014. Rodent models of chemotherapy-induced peripheral neuropathy. ILAR J. 54, 273–281.

Hucho, T., Levine, J.D., 2007. Signaling pathways in sensitization: toward a nociceptor cell biology. Neuron 55, 365–376.

Iadarola, M.J., Brady, L.S., Draisci, G., Dubner, R., 1988. Enhancement of dynorphin gene expression in spinal cord following experimental inflammation: stimulus specificity, behavioral parameters and opioid receptor binding. Pain 35, 313–326.

Ji, Y., Tang, B., Cao, D.-Y., Wang, G., Traub, R.J., 2012. Sex differences in spinal processing of transient and inflammatory colorectal stimuli in the rat. Pain 153, 1965–1973.

Jirkof, P., Cesarovic, N., Rettich, A., Nicholls, F., Seifert, B., Arras, M., 2010. Burrowing behavior as an indicator of post-laparotomy pain in mice. Front. Behav. Neurosci. 4, 165.

Jirkof, P., Fleischmann, T., Cesarovic, N., Rettich, A., Vogel, J., Arras, M., 2013. Assessment of postsurgical distress and pain in laboratory mice by nest complexity scoring. Lab. Anim. 47 (3), 153–161.

Johansen, J.P., Fields, H.L., Manning, B.H., 2001. The affective component of pain in rodents: direct evidence for a contribution of the anterior cingulate cortex. Proc. Natl. Acad. Sci. U. S. A. 98 (14), 8077–8082.

Jones, J.M., Foster, W., Twomey, C.R., Burdge, J., Ahmed, O.M., Pereira, T.D., Abdus-Saboor, I., 2020. A machine-vision approach for automated pain measurement at millisecond timescales. Elife 9, e57258.

Jourdan, D., Ardid, D., Eschalier, A., 2002. Analysis of ultrasonic vocalisation does not allow chronic pain to be evaluated in rats. Pain 95, 165–173.

Kehl, L.J., Trempe, T.M., Hargreaves, K.M., 2000. A new animal model for assessing mechanisms and management of muscle hyperalgesia. Pain 85, 333–343.

Khachigian, L.M., 2006. Collagen antibody-induced arthritis. Nat. Protoc. 1, 2512–2516.

Kilkenny, C., Browne, W.J., Cuthill, I.C., Emerson, M., Altman, D.G., 2010. Improving bioscience research reporting: the ARRIVE guidelines for reporting animal research. PLoS Biol. 8 (6), e1000412.

Kim, S.H., Chung, J.M., 1992. An experimental model for peripheral neuropathic produced by segmental spinal nerve ligation in the rat. Pain 50, 355–363.

King, T., Vera-Portocarrero, L., Gutierrez, T., Vanderah, T.W., Dussor, G., Lai, J., Porreca, F., 2009. Unmasking the tonic-aversive state in neuropathic pain. Nat. Neurosci. 12 (11), 1361–1363.

Klinck, M.P., Mogil, J.S., Moreau, M., Lascelles, B.D.X., Flecknell, P.A., Poitte, T., Troncy, E., 2017. Translational pain assessment: could natural animal models be the missing link? Pain 158 (9), 1633–1646.

Kurejova, M., Nattenmuller, U., Hildebrandt, U., Selvaraj, D., Stosser, S., Kuner, R., 2010. An improved behavioural assay demonstrates that ultrasound vocalizations constitute a reliable indicator of chronic cancer pain and neuropathic pain. Mol. Pain 6, 18.

LaBuda, C.J., Fuchs, P.N., 2000. A behavioral test paradigm to measure the aversive quality of inflammatory and neuropathic pain in rats. Exp. Neurol. 163, 490–494.

Langford, D.L., Crager, S.E., Shehzad, Z., Smith, S.B., Sotocinal, S.G., Levenstadt, J.S., Mogil, J.S., 2006. Social modulation of pain as evidence for empathy in mice. Science 312, 1967–1970.

Langford, D.L., Tuttle, A.H., Briscoe, C., Harvey-Lewis, C., Baran, I., Gleeson, P., Mogil, J.S., 2011. Varying perceived social threat modulates pain behavior in male mice. J. Pain 12 (1), 125–132.

Langford, D.L., Tuttle, A.H., Brown, K., Deschenes, S., Fischer, D.B., Mutso, A., Sternberg, W.F., 2010. Social approach to pain in laboratory mice. Soc. Neurosci. 5 (2), 163–170.

Langley, C.K., Aziz, Q., Bountra, C., Gordon, N., Hawkins, P., Jones, A., Tracey, I., 2008. Volunteer studies in pain research–opportunities and challenges to replace animal experiments: the report and recommendations of a Focus on Alternatives workshop. Neuroimage 42 (2), 467–473.

Lariviere, W.R., Chesler, E.J., Mogil, J.S., 2001. Transgenic studies of pain and analgesia: mutation or background phenotype? J. Pharmacol. Exp. Therapeut. 297 (2), 467–473.

Larson, A.A., Brown, D.R., El-Atrash, S., Walser, M.M., 1986. Pain threshold changes in adjuvant-induced inflammation: a possible model of chronic pain in the mouse. Pharmacol. Biochem. Behav. 24 (1), 49–53.

Lascelles, B.D.X., Brown, D.C., Maixner, W., Mogil, J.S., 2018. Spontaneous painful disease in companion animals can facilitate the development of chronic pain therapies for humans: osteoarthritis as a leading example. Osteoarthritis Cartilage 26, 175–183.

Latremoliere, A., Woolf, C.J., 2009. Central sensitization: a generator of pain hypersensitivity by central neural plasticity. J. Pain 10, 895–926.

Lee, B.H., Won, R., Baik, E.J., Lee, S.H., Moon, C.H., 2000. An animal model of neuropathic pain employing injury to the sciatic nerve branches. Neuroreport 11, 657–661.

Leung, V., Rousseau-Blass, F., Beauchamp, G., Pang, D.S.J., 2018. ARRIVE has not ARRIVEd: support for the ARRIVE (Animal Research: reporting of in vivo Experiments) guidelines does not improve the reporting quality of papers in animal welfare, analgesia or anesthesia. PLoS One 13, e1097882.

Lister, K.C., Maldonado-Bouchard, S., Markova, T., Aternali, A., Denecli, P., Donayre Pimentel, S., Mogil, J.S., 2020. Chronic pain produces hypervigilance to predator odor in mice. Curr. Biol. 30, R866–R867.

Liu, P., Okun, A., Ren, J., Guo, R.C., Ossipov, M.H., Xie, J., Porreca, F., 2011. Ongoing pain in the MIA model of osteoarthritis. Neurosci. Lett. 493, 72–75.

Mabuchi, T., Matsumura, S., Okuda-Ashitaka, E., Kitano, T., Kojima, H., Nagano, T., Ito, S., 2003. Attenuation of neuropathic pain by the nociceptin/orphanin FQ antagonist JTC-801 is mediated by inhibition of nitric oxide production. Eur. J. Neurosci. 17, 1384–1392.

Maier, C., Baron, R., Tolle, T.R., Binder, A., Birbaumer, N., Birklein, F., Treede, R.-D., 2010. Quantitative sensory testing in the German Research Network on Neuropathic Pain (DFNS): somatosensory abnormalities in 1236 patients with different neuropathic pain syndromes. Pain 150, 439–450.

Malmberg, A.B., Basbaum, A.I., 1998. Partial sciatic nerve injury in the mouse as a model of neuropathic pain: behavioral and neuroanatomical correlates. Pain 76, 215–222.

Mao, J., 2002. Translational pain research: bridging the gap between basic and clinical research. Pain 97, 183–187.

Mathis, A., Mamidanna, P., Cury, K.M., Abe, T., Murthy, V.N., Mathis, M.W., Bethge, M., 2018. DeepLabCut: markerless pose estimation of user-defined body parts with deep learning. Nat. Neurosci. 21, 1281–1289.

Mathis, M.W., Mathis, A., 2020. Deep learning tools for the measurement of animal behavior in neuroscience. Curr. Opin. Neurobiol. 60, 1–11.

Mauderli, A.P., Acosta-Rua, A., Vierck, C.J., 2000. An operant assay of thermal pain in conscious, unrestrained rats. J. Neurosci. Methods 97, 19–29.

McCoy, A.M., 2015. Animal models of osteoarthritis: comparisons and key considerations. Vet. Pathol. 52, 803–818.

McLennan, K.M., Miller, A.L., Dalla Costa, E., Stucke, D., Corke, M.J., Broom, D.M., Leach, M.C., 2019. Conceptual and methodological issues relating to pain assessment in mammals: the development and utilisation of pain facial expression scales. Appl. Anim. Behav. Sci. 217, 1–15.

McNamara, C.R., Mandel-Brehm, J., Bautista, D.M., Siemens, J., Deranian, K.L., Zhao, M., Fanger, C.M., 2007. TRPA1 mediates formalin-induced pain. Proc. Natl. Acad. Sci. U. S. A. 104 (33), 13525–13530.

Mecklenburg, J., Zou, Y., Wangzhou, A., Garcia, D., Lai, Z., Tumanov, A.V., Akopian, A.N., 2020. Transcriptomic sex differences in sensory neuronal populations of mice. Sci. Rep. 10, 15278.

Meents, J.E., Bressan, E., Sontag, S., Foerster, A., Hautvast, P., et al., 2019. The role of $Na_V1.7$ in human nociceptors: insights from human induced pluripotent stem cell-derived sensory neurons of erythromelalgia patients. Pain 160, 1327–1341.

Meller, S.T., Gebhart, G.F., 1997. Intraplantar zymosan as a reliable, quantifiable model of thermal and mechanical hyperalgesia in the rat. Eur. J. Pain 1, 43–52.

Millecamps, M., Shi, X.Q., Piltonen, M., Echeverry, S., Diatchenko, L., Zhang, J., Stone, L.S., 2020. The geriatric pain experience in mice: intact cutaneous thresholds but altered responses to tonic and chronic pain. Neurobiol. Aging (in press).

Mogil, J.S., 2009. Animal models of pain: progress and challenges. Nat. Rev. Neurosci. 10 (4), 283–294.

Mogil, J.S., 2016. Equality need not be painful. Nature 535, S7.

Mogil, J.S., 2019a. The measurement of pain in the laboratory rodent. In: Wood, J.N. (Ed.), The Oxford Handbook of the Neurobiology of Pain. Oxford Press, Oxford, U.K., pp. 28–60

Mogil, J.S., 2019b. The translatability of pain across species. Phil. Trans. R. Soc. B. 374, 20190286.

Mogil, J.S., 2020. Qualitative sex differences in pain processing: emerging evidence of a biased literature. Nat. Rev. Neurosci. 21, 353–365.

Mogil, J.S., Davis, K.D., Derbyshire, S.W., 2010. The necessity of animal models in pain research. Pain 151, 12–17.

Mogil, J.S., Graham, A.C., Ritchie, J., Hughes, S.F., Austin, J.-S., Schorscher-Petcu, A., Bennett, G.J., 2010. Hypolocomotion, asymmetrically directed behaviors (licking, lifting, flinching, and shaking) and dynamic weight bearing (gait) changes are not measures of neuropathic pain in mice. Mol. Pain 6 (1), 34.

Mogil, J.S., Meirmeister, F., Seifert, F., Strasburg, K., Zimmermann, K., Reinold, H., Reeh, P.W., 2005. Variable sensitivity to noxious heat is mediated by differential expression of the CGRP gene. Proc. Natl. Acad. Sci. U. S. A. 102, 12938–12943.

Mogil, J.S., Pang, D.S.J., Dutra, G.G.S., Chambers, C.T., 2020. The development and use of facial grimace scales for pain measurement in animals. Neurosci. Biobehav. Rev. 116, 480–493.

Mogil, J.S., Wilson, S.G., Bon, K., Lee, S.E., Chung, K., Raber, P., Devor, M., 1999. Heritability of nociception. I. Responses of eleven inbred mouse strains on twelve measures of nociception. Pain 80 (1-2), 67–82.

Moilanen, L.J., Hamalainen, M., Nummenmaa, E., Ilmarinen, P., Vuolteenaho, K., Nieminen, R.M., Moilanen, E., 2015. Monosodium iodoacetate-induced inflammation and joint pain are reduced in TRPA1 deficient mice–potential role of TRPA1 in osteoarthritis. Osteoarthr. Cartil. 23, 2017–2026.

Monach, P.A., Mathis, D., Benoist, C., 2008. The K/BxN arthritis model. Curr. Protoc. Neurosci. (Chapter 15), Unit 15 22.

Muralidharan, A., Sotocinal, S.G., Austin, J.-S., Mogil, J.S., 2020. The influence of aging and duration of nerve injury on the antiallodynic efficacy of analgesics in laboratory mice. Pain Rep. 5, e824.

Negus, S.S., 2019. Core outcome measures in preclinical assessment of candidate analgesics. Pharmacol. Rev. 71, 225–266.

North, R.Y., Li, Y., Ray, P., Rhines, L.D., Tatsui, C.E., Rao, G., Dougherty, P.M., 2019. Electrophysiological and transcriptomic correlates of neuropathic pain in human dorsal root ganglion neurons. Brain 142, 1215–1226.

O'Brien, P.D., Sakowski, S.A., Feldman, E.L., 2014. Mouse models of diabetic neuropathy. ILAR J. 54, 259–272.

Okayasu, I., Hatakeyama, S., Yamada, M., Ohkusa, T., Inagaki, Y., Nakaya, R., 1990. A novel method in the induction of reliable experimental acute and chronic ulcerative colitis in mice. Gastroenterology 98, 694–702.

Okuda, K., Nakahama, H., Miyakawa, H., Shima, K., 1984. Arthritis induced in cat by sodium urate: a possible animal model for tonic pain. Pain 18, 287–297.

Percie du Sert, N., Rice, A.S.C., 2014. Improving the translation of analgesic drugs to the clinic: animal models of neuropathic pain. Br. J. Pharmacol. 171, 2951–2963.

Pogatzki, E.M., Raja, S.N., 2003. A mouse model of incisional pain. Anesthesiology 99, 1023–1027.

Pollard, K.J., Bolon, B., Moore, M.J., 2021. Comparative analysis of chemotherapy-induced peripheral neuropathy in bioengineered sensory nerve tissue distinguishes mechanistic differences in early-stage vincristine-, cisplatin-, and paclitaxel-induced nerve damage. Toxicol. Sci. 180, 76–88.

Rausch-Derra, L., Huebner, M., Wofford, J., Rhodes, L., 2016. A prospecctive, randomized, masked, placebo-controlled multisite clinical study of grapiprant, an EP4 prostaglandin receptor antagonist (PRA), in dogs with osteoarthritis. J. Vet. Intern. Med. 30, 756–763.

Robie, A.A., Hirokawa, J., Edwards, A.W., Umayam, L.A., Lee, A., Philips, M.L., Branson, K., 2017. Mapping the neural substrates of behavior. Cell 170, 393–406.

Rocha, A.C., Fernandes, E.S., Quintao, N.L., Campos, M.M., Calixto, J.B., 2006. Relevance of tumour necrosis factor-a for the inflammatory and nociceptive responses evoked by carrageenan in the mouse paw. Br. J. Pharmacol. 148, 688–695.

Roughan, J.V., Flecknell, P.A., 2001. Behavioural effects of laparotomy and analgesic effects of ketoprofen and carprofen in rats. Pain 90, 65–74.

Ruiz-Medina, J., Baulies, A., Bura, S.A., Valverde, O., 2013. Paclitaxel-induced neuropathic pain is age dependent and devolves on glial response. Eur. J. Pain 17, 75–85.

Ruscheweyh, R., Forsthuber, L., Schoffnegger, D., Sandkuhler, J., 2007. Modification of classical neurochemical markers in identified primary afferent neurons with Ab-, Ad-, and C-fibers after chronic constriction injury in mice. J. Comp. Neurol. 502, 325–336.

Sadler, K.E., Langer, S.N., Menzel, A.D., Moehring, F., Erb, A.N., Brandow, A.M., Stucky, C.L., 2019. Gabapentin alleviates chronic spontaneous pain and acute hypoxia-related pain in a mouse model of sickle cell disease. Br. J. Haematol. 187, 246–260.

Sadler, K.E., Mogil, J.S., Stucky, C.L., 2022. Innovations and advances in modeling and measuring pain in animals. Nat. Rev. Neurosci. 23, 70–85.

Saito-Diaz, K., Street, J.R., Ulrichs, H., Zeitner, N., 2021. Derivation of peripheral nociceptive, mechanoreceptive, and proprioceptive sensory neurons from the same culture of human pluripotent stem cells. Stem Cell Rep. 16, 446–457.

Sanna, M.D., Manassero, G., Vercelli, A., Herdegen, T., Galeotti, N., 2020. The isoform-specific functions of the c-Jun N-terminal kinase (JNK) in a mouse model of antiretroviral-induced painful peripheral neuropathy. Eur. J. Pharmacol. 880, 173161.

Schaible, H.G., Schmidt, R.F., Willis, W.D., 1987. Enhancement of the responses of ascending tract cells in the cat spinal cord by acute inflammation of the knee joint. Exp. Brain Res. 66, 489–499.

Seltzer, Z., Dubner, R., Shir, Y., 1990. A novel behavioral model of causalgiform pain produced by partial sciatic nerve injury in rats. Pain 43, 205–218.

Sheahan, T.D., Siuda, E.R., Bruchas, M.R., Shepherd, A.J., Mohapatra, D.P., Gereau IV, R.W., Golden, J.P., 2017. Inflammation and nerve injury minimally affect mouse voluntary behaviors proposed as indicators of pain. Neurobiol. Pain 2, 1–12.

Shields, S.D., Eckert III, W.A., Basbaum, A.I., 2003. Spared nerve injury model of neuropathic pain in the mouse: a behavioral and anatomic analysis. J. Pain 4 (8), 465–470.

Shimada, S.G., Lamotte, R.H., 2008. Behavioral differentiation between itch and pain in mouse. Pain 139, 681–687.

Shukla, S., Arac, A., 2020. A step-by-step implementation of DeepBehavior, deep learning toolbox for automated behavior analysis. J. Vis. Exp. 156, 60763.

Silva, C.R., Melo, B.M.S., Silva, J.R., Lopes, A.H., Pereira, J.A., Cecilio, N.T., Cunha, T.M., 2020. S100A9 plays a pivotal role in a mouse model of herpetic neuralgia via TLR4/TNF pathway. Brain Behav. Immun. 88, 353–362.

Simone, D.A., Sorkin, L.S., Oh, U., Chung, J.M., Owens, C., LaMotte, R.H., Willis, W.D., 1991. Neurogenic hyperalgesia: central neural correlates in responses of spinothalamic tract neurons. J. Neurophysiol. 66, 228–246.

Sluka, K.A., Westlund, K.N., 1993. Behavioral and immunohistochemical changes in an experimental arthritis model in rats. Pain 55, 367–377.

Smith, M.L., Asada, N., Malenka, R.C., 2021. Anterior cingulate inputs to nucleus accumbens control the social transfer of pain and analgesia. Science 371, 153–159.

Smith, M.L., Hostetler, C.M., Heinricher, M.M., Ryabinin, A.E., 2016. Social transfer of pain in mice. Sci. Adv. 2, e1600855.

Smith, S.B., Parisien, M., Bair, E., Belfer, I., Chabot-Dore, A.-J., Gris, P., Diatchenko, L., 2019. Genome-wide association reveals contribution of MRAS to painful temporomandibular disorder in males. Pain 160, 579–591.

Smith, S.M., Dworkin, R.H., Turk, D.C., Baron, R., Polydefkis, M., et al., 2017. The potential role of sensory testing, skin biopsy, and functional brain imaging as biomarkers in chronic pain clinical trials: IMMPACT considerations. J. Pain 18, 757–777.

Sorge, R.E., Mapplebeck, J.C.S., Rosen, S., Beggs, S., Taves, S., Alexander, J.K., Mogil, J.S., 2015. Different immune cells mediate mechanical pain hypersensitivity in male and female mice. Nat. Neurosci. 18 (8), 1081–1083.

Staniland, A.A., Clark, A.K., Wodarski, R., Sasso, O., Maione, F., D'Acquisto, F., Malcangio, M., 2010. Reduced inflammatory and neuropathic pain and decreased spinal microglial response in fractalkine receptor (CX3CR1) knockout mice. J. Neurochem. 114, 1143–1157.

Staton, P.C., Wilson, A.W., Bountra, C., Chessell, I.P., Day, N.C., 2007. Changes in dorsal root ganglion CGRP expression in a chronic inflammatory model of the rat knee joint: differential modulation by rofecoxib and paracetamol. Eur. J. Pain 11, 283–289.

Stevenson, G.W., Bilsky, E.J., Negus, S.S., 2006. Targeting pain-suppressed behaviors in preclinical assays of pain and analgesia: effects of morphine on acetic acid-suppressed feeding in C57BL/6J mice. J. Pain 7 (6), 408–416.

Sufka, K.J., 1994. Conditioned place preference paradigm: a novel approach for analgesic drug assessment against chronic pain. Pain 58, 355–366.

Taber, R.I., Greenhouse, D.D., Rendell, J.K., Irwin, S., 1969. Agonist and antagonist interactions of opioids on acetic acid-induced abdominal stretching in mice. J. Pharmacol. Exp. Therapeut. 169 (1), 29–38.

Tappe-Theodor, A., King, T., Morgan, M.M., 2019. Pros and cons of clinically relevant methods to assess pain in rodents. Neurosci. Biobehav. Rev. 100, 335–343.

Tjolsen, A., Berge, O.-G., Hunskaar, S., Rosland, J.H., Hole, K., 1992. The formalin test: an evaluation of the method. Pain 51, 5–17.

Tracey, I., Woolf, C.J., Andrews, N.A., 2019. Composite pain biomarker signatures for objective assessment and effective treatment. Neuron 101, 783–800.

Tuttle, A.H., Molinaro, M.J., Jethwa, J.F., Sotocinal, S.G., Prieto, J.C., Styner, M.A., Zylka, M.J., 2018. A deep neural network to assess spontaneous pain from mouse facial expressions. Mol. Pain 14, 1–9.

Tuttle, A.H., Philip, V.M., Chesler, E.J., Mogil, J.S., 2018. Comparing phenotypic variation between inbred and outbred mice. Nat. Methods 15 (12), 994–996.

Urban, R., Scherrer, G., Goulding, E.H., Tecott, L.H., Basbaum, A.I., 2011. Behavioral indices of ongoing pain are largely unchanged in male mice with tissue or nerve injury-induced mechanical hypersensitivity. Pain 152, 990–1000.

Valek, L., Auburger, G., Tegeder, I., 2019. Sensory neuropathy and nociception in rodent models of Parkinson's disease. Dis. Model Mech. 12, 039396.

van der Wende, C., Margolin, S., 1956. Analgesic tests based upon experimentally induced acute abdominal pain in rats. Fed. Proc. 15, 494.

Vilceanu, D., Honore, P., Hogan, Q.H., Stucky, C.L., 2010. Spinal nerve ligation in mouse upregulates TRPV1 heat function in injured IB4-positive nociceptors. J. Pain 11, 588–599.

Vos, B.P., Strassman, A.M., Maciewicz, R.J., 1994. Behavioral evidence of trigeminal neuropathic pain following chronic constriction injury to the rat's infraorbital nerve. J. Neurosci. 14 (5), 2708–2723.

Wainger, B.J., Buttermore, E.D., Oliveira, J.T., Mellin, C., Lee, S., Saber, W.A., Woolf, C.J., 2015. Modeling pain in vitro using nociceptor neurons reprogrammed from fibroblasts. Nat. Neurosci. 18 (1), 17–23.

Wall, P.D., Devor, M., Inbal, R., Scadding, J.W., Schonfeld, D., Seltzer, Z., Tomkiewicz, M.M., 1979. Autotomy following peripheral nerve lesions: experimental anaesthesia dolorosa. Pain 7, 103–113.

Wallace, V.C.J., Blackbeard, J., Segerdahl, A.R., Hasnie, F., Pheby, T., McMahon, S.B., Rice, A.S.C., 2007. Characterization of rodent models of HIV-gp120 and anti-retroviral-associated neuropathic pain. Brain 130, 2688–2702.

Weng, Y., Batista-Schepman, P.A., Barabas, M.E., Harris, E.Q., Dinsmore, T.B., Kossyreva, E.A., Story, G.M., 2012. Prostaglandin metabolite induces inhibition of TRPA1 and channel-dependent nociception. Mol. Pain 8, 75.

Whittaker, A.L., Liu, Y., Barker, T.H., 2021. Methods used and application of the Mouse Grimace Scale in biomedical research 10 years on: a scoping review. Animals 11, 673.

Wilson, R., Ahmmed, A.A., Poll, A., Sakaue, M., Laude, A., Sieber-Blum, M., 2018. Human peptidergic nociceptive sensory neurons generated from human epidermal neural crest stem cells (hEPI-NCSC). PLoS One 13, e0199996.

Wiltschko, A.B., Johnson, M.J., Iurilli, G., peterson, R.E., Katon, J.M., Pashkovskik, S.L., Datta, S.R., 2015. Mapping sub-second structure in mouse behavior. Neuron 88, 1121–1135.

Wodarski, R., Delaney, A., Ultenius, C., Morland, C., Andrews, N., Baastrup, C., Rice, A.S.C., 2016. Cross-centre replication of suppressed burrowing behaviour as an ethologically relevant pain outcome measure in the rat: a prospective multicentre study. Pain 157, 2350–2365.

Wolfe, A.M., Kennedy, L.H., Na, J.J., Nemzek-Hamlin, J.A., 2015. Efficacy of tramadol as a sole analgesic for postoperative pain in male and female mice. J. Am. Assoc. Lab. Anim. Sci. 54, 411–419.

Woolf, C.J., Bennett, G.J., Doherty, M., Dubner, R., Kidd, B., Koltzenburg, M., Torebjork, E., 1998. Towards a mechanism-based classification of pain? Pain 77, 227–229.

Xu, W., Zhu, Z., Ge, F., Han, Z., Li, J., 2020. Analysis of behavior trajectory based on deep learning in ammonia environment for fish. Sensors 20, 20164425.

Yezierski, R.P., Hansson, P., 2018. Inflammatory and neuropathic pain from bench to bedside: what went wrong? J. Pain 19 (6), 571–588.

Yoon, Y.W., Lee, D.H., Lee, B.H., Chung, K., Chung, J.M., 1999. Different strains and substrains of rats show different levels of neuropathic pain behaviors. Exp. Brain Res. 129, 167–171.

Young, G.T., Gutteridge, A., Fox, H., Wilbrey, A.L., Cao, L., Cho, L.T., Stevens, E.B., 2014. Characterizing human stem cell-derived sensory neurons at the single-cell level reveals their ion channel expression and utility in pain research. Mol. Ther. 22, 1530–1543.

Yu, W., Pati, D., Pina, M.M., Schmidt, K.T., Boyt, K.M., Hunker, A.C., Kash, T.L., 2021. Periaqueductal gray/dorsal raphe dopamine neurons contribute to sex differences in pain-related behaviors. Neuron 109, 1365–11380.

Zhang, H., Lecker, I., Collymore, C., Dokova, A., Pham, M.C., Rosen, S.F., Bonin, R.P., 2021. Cage-lid hanging behavior as a translationally relevant measure of pain in mice. Pain 162, 1416–1425.

Index

'*Note:* Page numbers followed by "f" indicate figures, "t" indicate tables and "b" indicate boxes.'

B

C

F

G

H

J

K

L

M

N

Q

R